COMPUTED TOMOGRAPHY OF THE BODY

With Magnetic Resonance Imaging

COMPUTED TOMOGRAPHY OF THE BODY

With Magnetic Resonance Imaging

Second Edition

Albert A. Moss, M.D.
Professor and Chairman, Department of Radiology
University of Washington School of Medicine
Seattle, Washington

Gordon Gamsu, M.D.
Professor of Radiology and Medicine
University of California, San Francisco, School of Medicine
San Francisco, California

Harry K. Genant, M.D.
Professor of Radiology, Medicine, and Orthopaedic Surgery; Chief of the
Musculoskeletal Section; Director of the Osteoporosis Research Group
University of California, San Francisco, School of Medicine
San Francisco, California

Volume Three
Abdomen and Pelvis

W.B. SAUNDERS COMPANY
Harcourt Brace Jovanovich, Inc.
Philadelphia   London   Toronto   Montreal   Sydney   Tokyo

W. B. SAUNDERS COMPANY
Harcourt Brace Jovanovich, Inc.

The Curtis Center
Independence Square West
Philadelphia, Pennsylvania 19106

Library of Congress Cataloging-in-Publication Data

Moss, Albert A.

Computed tomography of the body with magnetic resonance
imaging / Albert A. Moss, Gordon Gamsu, Harry K. Genant.
— 2nd ed.

     p.   cm.

Rev. ed. of: Computed tomography of the body / Albert A.
Moss, Gordon Gamsu, Harry K. Genant.

Includes bibliographical references and index.

ISBN 0–7216–2415–4 (set)

1. Tomography.   2. Magnetic resonance imaging.
I. Gamsu, Gordon.   II. Genant, Harry K.
III. Moss, Albert A.   Computed tomography of the body.
IV. Title.

[DNLM: 1. Anatomy, Regional.   2. Magnetic
Resonance Imaging.   3. Tomography, X-Ray Computed.
WN 160 M913c]

RC78.7.T6M68   1992

DNLM/DLC   91–32837

Editor: Lisette Bralow
Designer: W.B. Saunders Staff
Production Manager: Peter Faber
Manuscript Editors: Lorraine Zawodny and Kendall Sterling
Illustration Coordinator: Walter Verbitski
Indexer: Nancy Newman
Cover Designer: Michelle Maloney

Computed Tomography of the Body With
Magnetic Resonance Imaging, 2/e.

ISBN Volume I 0–7216–4358–2
        Volume II 0–7216–4359–0
        Volume III 0–7216–4503–8
        Three Volume Set 0–7216–2415–4

Printed in the United States of America

Last digit is the print number: 9   8   7   6   5   4   3   2   1

CONTRIBUTORS FOR VOLUME THREE

RICHARD L. BARON, M.D.
Professor, Department of Radiology, University of Pittsburgh School of
Medicine; Director, Body CT/MRI; Co-Director, Abdominal Imaging,
Presbyterian-University Hospital; Pittsburgh, PA
> THE BILIARY TRACT
> THE LIVER

DOUGLAS P. BOYD, Ph.D.
Adjunct Professor of Radiology, University of California, San Francisco,
School of Medicine; Chairman of the Board, Imatron, Inc.; San Francisco, CA
> PRINCIPLES OF COMPUTED TOMOGRAPHY

DAVID K. BREWER, M.D.
Associate Professor of Radiology, Adjunct Assistant Professor of Pediatrics,
University of Washington School of Medicine; Children's Hospital and
Medical Center; Seattle, WA
> PEDIATRIC BODY IMAGING

WILLIAM H. BUSH, M.D.
Professor of Radiology, Chief, Uroradiology, Department of Radiology,
University of Washington School of Medicine, Seattle, WA
> THE KIDNEYS

PETER L. DAVIS, M.D.
Associate Professor, Department of Radiology, University of Pittsburgh
School of Medicine; Research Administrator, Pittsburgh NMR Institute;
Pittsburgh, PA
> PRINCIPLES OF MAGNETIC RESONANCE IMAGING

MICHAEL P. FEDERLE, M.D.
Professor and Chairman, Department of Radiology, University of Pittsburgh
School of Medicine; Attending Staff, Presbyterian-University Hospital;
Pittsburgh, PA
> THE PANCREAS
> THE SPLEEN

PATRICK C. FREENY, M.D.
Professor of Radiology and Director of Abdominal Imaging, University of
Washington School of Medicine, Seattle, WA
    THE LIVER

HENRY I. GOLDBERG, M.D.
Professor, Department of Radiology, University of California, San Francisco,
School of Medicine, San Francisco, CA
    THE PANCREAS

MITCHELL M. GOODSITT, Ph.D.
Assistant Professor of Radiology (Physics); Adjunct Assistant Professor of
Radiological Sciences; Adjunct Assistant Professor of Bioengineering;
University of Washington School of Medicine; Director, Diagnostic Physics,
Department of Radiology, University of Washington Medical Center,
Seattle, WA
    PRINCIPLES OF COMPUTED TOMOGRAPHY

R. BROOKE JEFFREY, JR., M.D.
Professor of Radiology, Stanford University School of Medicine; Chief of
Abdominal Imaging, Department of Diagnostic Radiology and Nuclear
Medicine, Stanford University Medical Center; Stanford, CA
    THE RETROPERITONEUM AND LYMPHOVASCULAR STRUCTURES
    THE PERITONEAL CAVITY AND MESENTERY

SHIRLEY M. McCARTHY, M.D., Ph.D.
Associate Professor, Diagnostic Radiology, Yale School of Medicine; Director,
Magnetic Resonance Imaging, Yale New Haven Hospital; New Haven, CT
    THE PELVIS

ALBERT A. MOSS, M.D.
Professor and Chairman, Department of Radiology, University of Washington
School of Medicine, Seattle, WA
    THE GASTROINTESTINAL TRACT
    THE LIVER
    THE KIDNEYS
    THE ADRENAL GLANDS
    THE PELVIS
    INTERVENTIONAL COMPUTED TOMOGRAPHY

DENNIS L. PARKER, Ph.D.
Associate Professor, Medical Informatics; Adjunct Associate Professor,
Department of Radiology; Adjunct Associate Professor, Department of
Bioengineering; University of Utah School of Medicine; Associate Professor,
LDS Hospital; Salt Lake City, UT
    PRINCIPLES OF COMPUTED TOMOGRAPHY

RANDALL M. PATTEN, M.D.
Assistant Professor of Radiology, University of Washington School of
Medicine, Seattle, WA; Medical Director, Rainier Medical Imaging Center,
Kirkland, WA
    THE RETROPERITONEUM AND LYMPHOVASCULAR STRUCTURES

LESLIE M. SCOUTT, M.D.
Assistant Professor, Yale University School of Medicine; Attending
Radiologist, Yale-New Haven Hospital; New Haven, CT
> THE PELVIS

WILLIAM P. SHUMAN, M.D.
Professor, University of Washington Medical School; Director, CT/MR,
University of Washington Medical Center; Seattle, WA
> THE ADRENAL GLANDS
> THE RETROPERITONEUM AND LYMPHOVASCULAR STRUCTURES

RUEDI F. THOENI, M.D.
Associate Professor of Radiology, Department of Radiology, University of
California, San Francisco School of Medicine; Chief, Section CT/GI, Medical
Center at the University of California, Long-Moffitt Hospital, San Francisco,
CA
> THE GASTROINTESTINAL TRACT

EDWARD WEINBERGER, M.D.
Assistant Professor of Radiology and Adjunct Assistant Professor of
Pediatrics, University of Washington School of Medicine; Children's Hospital
and Medical Center; University Hospital; Seattle, WA
> PEDIATRIC BODY IMAGING

PREFACE

The second edition of *Computed Tomography of the Body* has been extensively updated and is presented as a comprehensive, state-of-the-art text on computed tomography (CT) of the body that now includes an integration of magnetic resonance (MR) imaging in all sections of the book. Since the first edition, there have been great advances in CT and its application to patient care. Although the impact of CT has been enormous, magnetic resonance imaging is undergoing explosive growth and is having an ever-increasing impact on body imaging.

As in the first edition, this text is organized so that basic anatomy and CT and MR techniques are discussed for each region of the body. The features of disease entities in these two imaging modalities are described and illustrated, and the relationship of CT to MR and other imaging techniques is discussed in depth. Recommendations are offered as to the role of each modality in specific clinical situations. The book presents an integrated approach, reflecting our current standard of practice. Knowledge of CT and MR imaging will continue to expand, and recommendations, techniques, and patterns of use will undoubtedly change in the future.

In writing this book, now expanded to three volumes, there have been many people without whose support, guidance, insight, and help this work could not have been completed. We thank our colleagues who contributed their time and case material, and we acknowledge the illustration departments at the University of California, San Francisco, and the University of Washington, as well as the secretarial and editorial support of Jan Taylor, Isabel Rosenthal, and Denice Nakano.

ALBERT A. MOSS, M.D.
GORDON GAMSU, M.D.
HARRY K. GENANT, M.D.

INTRODUCTION TO VOLUME THREE

Owing to the rapid expansion of computed tomography and magnetic resonance imaging of the abdomen and pelvis, *Computed Tomography of the Body* has been expanded to three volumes, and magnetic resonance imaging has been completely integrated. Volume Three, Abdomen and Pelvis is designed as a comprehensive udpate and expansion of these topics in the first edition.

Since the first edition, high-resolution CT has become commonplace as has sub–3-second CT scanning. Magnetic resonance imaging has become a valuable procedure in the diagnosis of hepatic, adrenal, renal, prostate, and gynecologic abnormalities. Magnetic resonance imaging has been compared to computed tomography and where appropriate, recommendations are made as to the most rational use of each technology. Chapters on the physics of CT and MR imaging are included as are chapters on pediatric imagery and CT interventional procedures. The explosion of data on the use of CT and magnetic resonance imaging in the evaluation of liver and biliary tract abnormalities has necessitated expansion of the discussion of hepatobiliary tract disease into two new chapters, The Liver and The Biliary Tract.

I would like to thank the many who have helped to write this volume. In particular, I would like to thank my former colleagues at the University of California in San Francisco, my current colleagues at the University of Washington, and those from other institutions who have contributed their expertise. I would also like to thank the residents, fellows, and technicians at the University of Washington who have contributed so much to this volume. Finally, I would like to offer thanks to my secretary, Jan Taylor, for her secretarial and editorial support and to my former professors John Amberg, Richard Greenspan, Henry Goldberg, and Alexander R. Margulis.

ALBERT A. MOSS, M.D.

CONTENTS

CHAPTER 16

THE GASTROINTESTINAL TRACT

RUEDI F. THOENI ▪ ALBERT A. MOSS

Although barium radiography[1-3] and endoscopy[4] are safe and accurate initial diagnostic procedures for evaluating gastrointestinal abnormalities, neither assesses the extramucosal extent of disease. Angiography,[5] radionuclide scanning,[6] and ultrasonography[7, 8] have been employed as additional diagnostic and staging modalities, but because of the limitations of these techniques, surgical exploration has remained the only accepted method of accurately assessing the true extent of disease. Computed tomography (CT) displays the gastrointestinal tract in cross section and thus images both the inner and outer surfaces of the alimentary tube. In addition, by imaging both adjacent and distant organs, CT is capable of evaluating both local and distant spread of disease.[8-10] Thus CT can provide the radiotherapist, surgeon, internist, and oncologist with a clearer understanding of the true extent of a gastrointestinal abnormality. More recently, magnetic resonance imaging (MRI) and cine- or ultrafast CT have been added to the diagnostic armamentarium of the radiologist but have not been widely used for the gastrointestinal tract. One of the major advantages of MRI imaging lies in the fact that direct coronal and sagittal images can be obtained in addition to the transaxial sections. Ultrafast CT using magnetic deflection of an electron beam to replace mechanical motion demonstrates the walls of the gastrointestinal tract more clearly than conventional CT because of the rapid acquisition time and resulting absence of image distortion related to peristalsis. Such rapid image acquisition facilitates accurate detection of bowel wall abnormalities.

COMPUTED TOMOGRAPHY OF THE GASTROINTESTINAL TRACT

Esophagus

Anatomy

The esophagus connects the pharynx with the stomach and consists of extrathoracic, mediastinal, and abdominal segments. Throughout its length, the

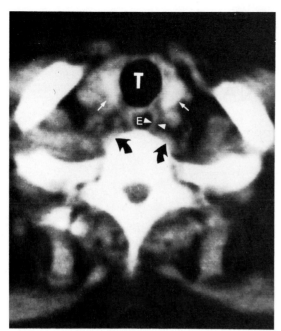

FIGURE 16–1 ■ Normal esophagus, cervical region. Cervical esophagus (E) at level of thyroid gland *(white arrows)* is positioned in the midline, just posterior to the trachea (T). The normal esophageal wall *(arrowheads)* is a thin, sharp structure outlined by air and mediastinal fat and measuring less than 3 mm in diameter. Longus colli muscles are indicated by black arrows.

esophagus is intimately related to a variety of vital vascular, pulmonary, cardiac, lymphatic, and neural structures. The esophagus is surrounded throughout most of its length by periesophageal fat that permits ready differentiation of the esophagus from adjacent structures.

The thickness of the normal esophageal wall as measured by CT in a well-distended esophagus is usually less than 3 mm (Fig. 16–1),[11, 12] and any

measurement of more than 5 mm should be considered abnormal.[11, 13] Air in the esophagus is present in 40 to 60 per cent of patients examined by CT[11, 14, 15] and should not be considered an abnormal finding. Air, when present in the normal esophagus, is centrally positioned, and an eccentric position of gas within the esophagus should raise the possibility of an esophageal abnormality.[11, 14]

UPPER ESOPHAGUS

The cervical esophagus is a midline structure intimately related to the posterior tracheal wall, indenting it in approximately 40 per cent of cases (see Fig. 16–1). A smooth, rounded esophageal impression on the trachea should not be interpreted as evidence of tracheal invasion by an esophageal mass. Lateral and dorsal to the esophagus on either side are the long muscles (longus colli) of the neck. The thyroid gland is seen as a high-density structure lying anterior and lateral to the trachea and esophagus. Air is present within the cervical esophagus more frequently than in any other part of the esophagus.

MIDDLE ESOPHAGUS

At the level just below the sternal notch, the trachea deviates slightly to the right of the esophagus, with the esophagus remaining midline or shifting slightly to the left (Fig. 16–2).[11] The esophagus is closely applied to the thoracic spine, and no normal structure is found posterior to the esophagus at this level. A retrotracheal space of up to 4 mm can be present between the trachea and esophagus,[11] and a portion of lung can extend retrotracheally. The subclavian artery, common carotid artery, brachiocephalic artery, and brachiocephalic veins are also clearly identified at this level.

At the level of the aortic arch, the esophagus is closely related to the left posterolateral portion of the trachea (Fig. 16–3). The azygos vein is located to the

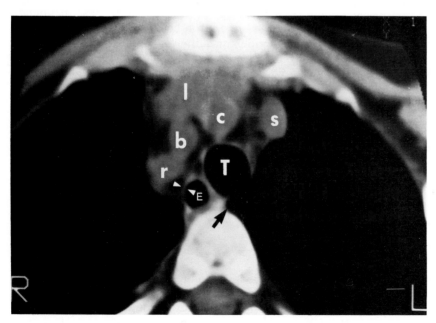

FIGURE 16–2 ■ Normal esophagus, level of sternal notch. In this patient the trachea (T) is slightly to the left of the esophagus (E). The retrotracheal extension of lung *(arrow)* is a normal finding. The left subclavian artery (s), common carotid artery (c), brachiocephalic artery (b), right (r) and left (l) brachiocephalic veins, and thin wall of the normal esophagus *(arrowheads)* are clearly identified.

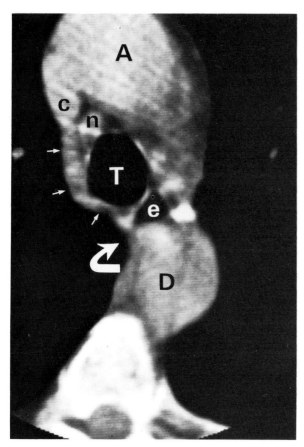

FIGURE 16–3 ■ Normal esophagus, level of aortic arch. The esophagus (e) is slightly to the right of the trachea (T), and the ascending (A) and descending (D) aorta, arch of the azygos vein *(straight arrows)* entering the superior vena cava (c) and azygoesophageal recess *(curved arrow)* are identified at this level. n = Normal-sized pretracheal lymph node.

right, posterior and lateral to the esophagus, and the arch of the azygos can be identified at this level (see Fig. 16–3). The lung is in direct contact with the right side of the esophagus, forming the azygoesophageal recess.[14] Just below the carina, the esophagus is closely related to the left main stem bronchus, separated only by a small amount of mediastinal fat (Fig. 16–4).[11, 14] At this level, a lung recess is present in 10 per cent to 20 per cent of patients between the esophagus and the left pulmonary artery.[14]

LOWER ESOPHAGUS

Below the left main stem bronchus, the esophagus comes in contact with the pericardium surrounding the posterior wall of the left atrium and is positioned near the left pulmonary vein as it enters into the left atrium. At this level the azygos vein is visible as a midline structure (Fig. 16–5). Below the level of the left atrium, the esophagus moves slightly to the left of midline just anterior to the descending aorta (Fig. 16–6), with only mediastinal fat separating the esophagus from the pericardium.

Just after the esophagus passes through the diaphragm, it turns left and courses in a horizontal

plane to enter the gastric fundus (Fig. 16–7). On CT scans, the region of the gastroesophageal junction appears as a thickening along the medial cephalic aspect of the stomach in approximately one third of patients.[11, 16, 17] The apparent mass is produced as a result of the transverse plane's of axial CT sections passing through the horizontally directed normal esophagogastric junction (see Fig. 16–7).

Knowledge of the anatomy of the esophagogastric region usually permits a distinction of a true mass from a normal gastroesophageal junction. The gastrohepatic ligament courses between the lesser curvature of the stomach and liver, and the distal esophagus is enveloped by the cranialmost aspect of the ligament (Fig. 16–8).[16] The gastrohepatic ligament fuses with the fissure of the ligamentum venosum to pass anterior to the caudate lobe. Thus the cleft seen on transverse CT images separating the caudate lobe from the lateral segment of the left lobe points directly to the region of the esophagogastric junction (see Fig. 16–7).[16]

When a soft tissue mass is noted high along the lesser curvature of the stomach, its relation to the fissure plane anterior to the caudate lobe should be studied. If the mass and fissure plane are present on

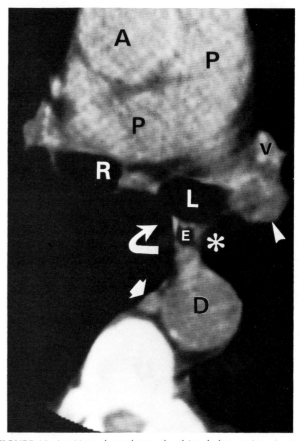

FIGURE 16–4 ■ Normal esophagus, level just below carina. A scan at this level demonstrates the relationships of the right (R) and left (L) main stem bronchi, esophagus (E), descending aorta (D), azygos vein *(straight arrow)*, pulmonary artery (P), ascending aorta (A), and azygoesophageal recess *(curved arrow)*. The left lung recess *(asterisk)* is shown abutting on the left main stem bronchus, esophagus, and left pulmonary artery *(arrowhead)*. V = Left pulmonary vein.

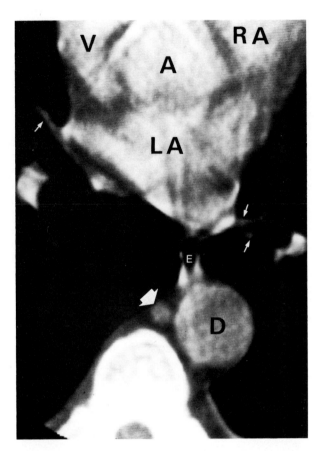

FIGURE 16–5 ■ Normal esophagus, level of left atrium. The esophagus (E) is in contact with pericardium surrounding the left atrium (LA). Pulmonary veins *(small arrows)*, right ventricle (V), right atrium (RA), ascending aorta (A), descending aorta (D), and azygos vein *(large arrow)* are also seen. At this level the esophagus is separated from lung by only the thickness of the esophageal wall and pleura.

FIGURE 16–6 ■ Normal esophagus, level of left ventricle. The esophagus (E) is just to the left of midline, closely related to the left ventricle (LV) and separated from the descending aorta (D) by the posterior junction line *(arrow)*. RV = Right ventricle; V = inferior vena cava.

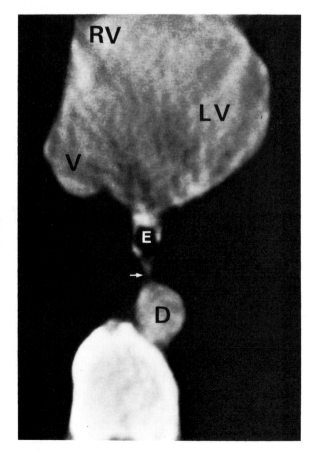

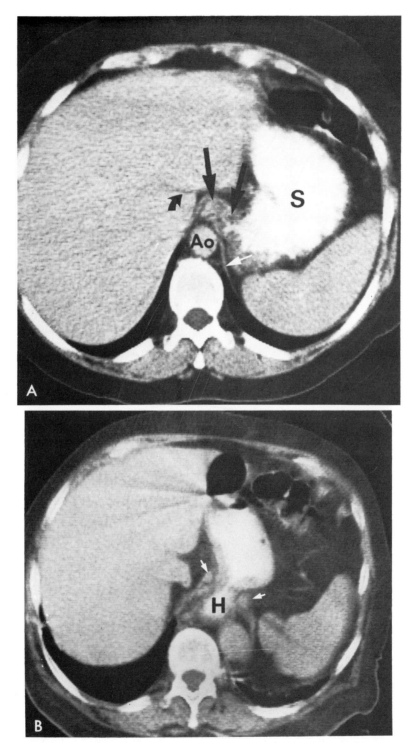

FIGURE 16–7 ■ Normal esophagus, level of gastroesophageal junction. *A,* The normal esophagus *(straight arrows)* courses in a horizontal plane to enter the fundus of the stomach (S). The cleft above the caudate lobe *(curved arrow)* points to gastroesophageal junction. Left diaphragmatic crus *(small arrow)* is closely applied to the abdominal aorta (Ao). *B,* Hiatus hernia (H) producing a mass in region of gastroesophageal junction. Note that the crura of the diaphragm *(arrows)* at the level of the esophageal hiatus are widely separated instead of tightly surrounding the descending aorta and esophagus. *(A from Marks WM, Callen PW, Moss AA: AJR 136:359, 1981. © 1981, American Roentgen Ray Society. Reprinted by permission.)*

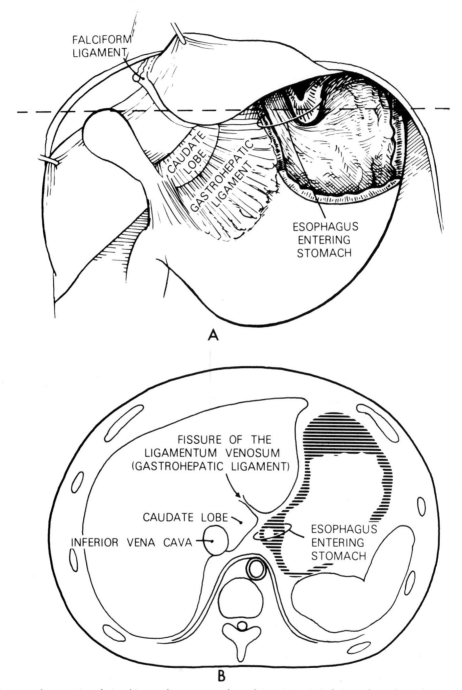

FIGURE 16–8 ■ Diagram of anatomic relationships at the gastroesophageal junction. *A*, Relation of esophageal entrance into stomach and gastrohepatic ligament (lesser omentum). *B*, Illustration of CT scan at level of esophageal entrance into stomach *(dashed line* in *A)* demonstrating the location of the gastroesophageal junction to be opposite the fissure of ligamentum venosum (gastrohepatic ligament). (From Marks WM, Callen PW, Moss AA: AJR 136:359, 1981. © 1981, American Roentgen Ray Society. Reprinted by permission.)

the same or adjoining sections, a pseudotumor should be suspected.

Techniques of Examination

Patients are routinely fasted, except for water by mouth, from midnight until the CT examination in the morning. CT scans 1 cm in thickness are taken contiguously at 1-cm intervals from the sternal notch to the umbilicus, with the patient in the supine position. The examination is extended to the umbilicus to detect abdominal lymphadenopathy, commonly found in esophageal carcinoma. CT scans of the neck are obtained if barium esophagography or endoscopy suggests a cervical esophageal lesion. Scans are obtained using the shortest available scan time with the scanner gantry at 0° angulation. CT sections thinner than 1 cm are routinely employed through areas of esophageal abnormality to better define the relationship of the esophagus to adjacent structures. In certain instances, placement of a nasogastric tube or decubitus positioning is employed to evaluate the esophagogastric junction more accurately.

An intravenous bolus of 150 to 180 mL of 60 per cent methylglucamine diatrizoate or a nonionic contrast material (iopamidol or iohexol) is administered during the scanning procedure to define the mediastinal vascular structures. Patients are not routinely given oral contrast medium to drink, but in some patients additional CT scans are obtained during or immediately following a swallow of a 1 per cent to 2 per cent solution of diatrizoate meglumine (Gastrografin) or barium sulfate in order to identify the esophageal lumen or distend the esophagus.[18, 19]

CT scans of the cervical esophagus are reconstructed using the infant or cranial reconstruction file, and the rest of the esophagus is displayed on the appropriate adult whole-body reconstruction file. The CT images of the esophagus and adjacent mediastinal structures can be magnified 1.5 to 2.5 times prior to filming to ensure optimal display of the esophagus and paraesophageal tissues.

Pathology

MALIGNANT ESOPHAGEAL TUMORS

Malignant esophageal tumors outnumber benign tumors by more than 4 to 1.[20] The majority of malignant esophageal tumors are squamous cell carcinomas, although there are scattered examples of primary esophageal adenocarcinoma, carcinosarcoma, lymphoma, sarcoma, and melanoma.[21–24] Carcinoma of the esophagus is rarely diagnosed prior to extraesophageal spread to the mediastinum, abdomen, or liver.[21–23, 25] As a result of the usually advanced state of the disease at the time of diagnosis, the overall 5-year survival rate has remained between 4 and 10 per cent,[21, 23, 26–36] despite more aggressive surgical and radiation therapy regimens. With the esophagus lacking a serosa, esophageal carcinoma can spread rapidly by way of lymphatic channels to regional lymph

TABLE 16–1 ■ CT Staging of Esophageal Carcinoma

Stage I	Intraluminal polypoid mass or localized thickening of esophageal wall (3 to 5 mm); no mediastinal extension or metastases.
Stage II	Thickened esophageal wall (> 5 mm) without invasion of adjacent organs or distant metastases.
Stage III	Thickened esophageal wall with direct extension into surrounding tissue; local or regional mediastinal adenopathy may or may not be present; no distant metastases.
Stage IV	Any tumor stage with distant metastatic disease.

nodes and directly to contiguous structures such as the trachea, bronchi, and pericardium.[21, 22, 28, 29, 37]

An accurate diagnosis of esophageal carcinoma is made in more than 90 per cent of patients by esophagography or endoscopy. Chest radiography, mediastinal tomography, azygous venography, mediastinoscopy, and bronchoscopy have been used to assess the extent of disease,[37–42] although they have not proved accurate in staging carcinoma of the esophagus.[21, 22, 37, 43] Because CT accurately displays the anatomy and relationships between the esophagus and mediastinal structures,[11–15, 44–46] it has become the imaging procedure of choice to assess the degree of the spread of carcinoma into extraesophageal tissues and to determine the effect of therapy.[12, 13, 44]

CT Staging ■ Based on the CT findings, esophageal carcinoma can be classified into one of four stages (Table 16–1):

1. *Stage I:* esophageal carcinoma produces an intraluminal mass or localized esophageal wall thickening measuring 3 to 5 mm without mediastinal extension or distant metastasis. (The normal esophageal wall measures <3 mm in thickness.)

2. *Stage II:* esophageal malignancy thickens the esophageal wall to greater than 5 mm, but there is no evidence of metastatic disease or mediastinal tumor extension (Fig. 16–9).

3. *Stage III:* carcinoma thickens the esophageal wall to more than 5 mm and extends directly into the surrounding tissue (Fig. 16–10). Local or regional mediastinal lymphadenopathy may be present, but distant metastases are not seen.

4. *Stage IV:* there is evidence of distant metastatic spread with esophageal carcinoma (Fig. 16–11).

Differentiating among an esophageal squamous cell carcinoma and less frequent adenocarcinoma, melanoma, sarcoma, or mesenchymoma[47] on the basis of CT findings alone is usually not possible. Squamous cell carcinoma and esophageal adenocarcinoma are solid lesions without calcification that have a CT number close to or identical with that of adjacent soft tissues. All other esophageal malignancies except liposarcomas (Fig. 16–12), which can have a CT attenuation value close to that of periesophageal fat, also appear similar to squamous cell carcinoma of the esophagus. The administration of intravenous contrast material has not aided in differentiating

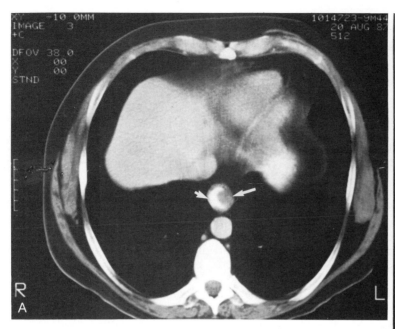

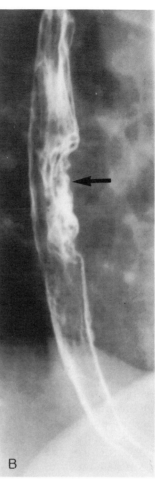

FIGURE 16–9 ■ Stage II esophageal carcinoma. *A*, CT scan showing focal thickening of the left lateral esophageal wall *(large arrow)*, which causes the esophageal lumen *(small arrow)* to have an eccentric position. Fat planes surrounding the esophagus are preserved. *B*, Esophagogram of focal nonobstructing mass *(arrow)* in distal third of esophagus.

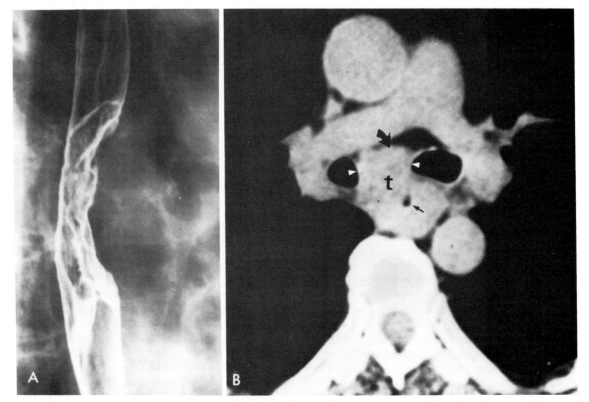

FIGURE 16–10 ■ Stage III esophageal carcinoma. *A*, Esophagogram of large infiltrating carcinoma of the midesophagus. *B*, CT scan of a tumor mass (t) causing thickening of the esophageal wall and narrowing of the esophageal lumen *(straight arrow)* and invading the subcarinal space *(curved arrow)*. Tumor obliterates the fat plane *(arrowheads)* between the esophagus and bronchial wall of the right and left main stem bronchi. (From Moss AA, Schnyder P, Thoeni RF, Margulis AR: AJR 136:1051, 1981. © 1981, American Roentgen Ray Society. Reprinted by permission.)

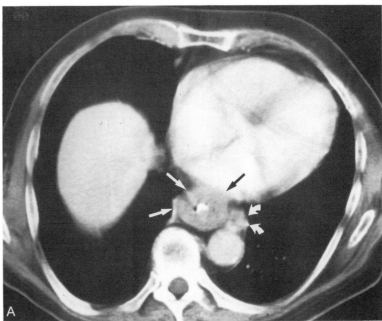

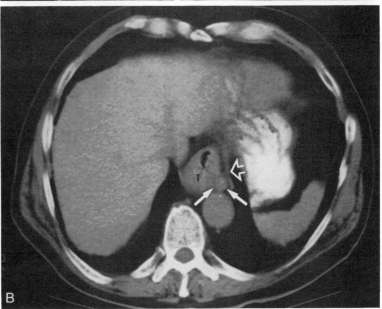

FIGURE 16–11 ■ Stage IV esophageal carcinoma. *A,* Diffusely thickened esophageal wall *(straight arrows)* without invasion of mediastinum but with a positive node *(curved arrows)* between the distal esophagus and the aorta. *B,* Node *(solid arrows)* next to crus *(open arrow)* in abdomen. T = Tumor.

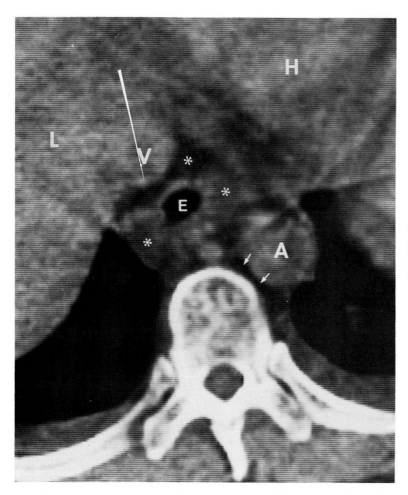

FIGURE 16–12 ■ Liposarcoma of the esophagus. Air is seen in the esophageal lumen (E), surrounded by a mass lesion (asterisks) that has a density only slightly greater than that of periaortic fat (arrows). A = Aorta; H = heart; L = liver; V = inferior vena cava.

among the various forms of primary esophageal malignancy.

CT Findings ■ Accurate determination of extraesophageal tumor extension can be difficult and demands excellent technique and careful evaluation of the periesophageal tissues. One of the most useful CT findings in determining extraesophageal spread of esophageal carcinoma is the loss of tissue fat planes between an esophageal mass and contiguous mediastinal structures (Fig. 16–10). When direct extension of esophageal carcinoma has occurred, normal fat planes are invariably lost; however, in patients with sparse mediastinal fat, it can be difficult to determine whether esophageal carcinoma has invaded or is just contiguous with an adjacent mediastinal structure. Administration of intravenous contrast material may be helpful in determining whether actual obliteration of the periesophageal fat plane has occurred (Fig. 16–13).

An interpretation of direct tumor extension requires demonstration by CT of loss of the periesophageal fat and the presence of a definite mass extending into an adjacent structure. Identification of a polypoid mass extending from the esophagus into the trachea or bronchi (Fig. 16–14), compression or displacement of the airways by tumor, and demonstration of an esophagobronchial fistula (Fig. 16–15)

prior to therapy are all accurate indicators of extraesophageal tumor spread.[12, 44] However, because the cartilage rings are incomplete posteriorly in the trachea and main stem bronchi, concavity of the tracheobronchial walls may be caused by a normal esophagus and may lead to false-positive results. Tumor invasion of the aorta is diagnosed based on the degree of contact between tumor and aortic circumference: contact along an arc of 90° or more strongly suggests invasion, whereas contact of 0° to 45° indicates absence of aortic tumor invasion. Contact between 45° and 90° may be considered indeterminate. Using these criteria, one study showed that invasion of aorta by esophageal tumor was correctly diagnosed in 80 per cent,[48] and in another report, the accuracy was increased if any contact of less than 90° was considered to represent absence of invasion.[49] CT identification of hepatic, pulmonary, local (Fig. 16–16) or abdominal lymphatic (see Fig. 16–11), or bony metastases is also proof of extraesophageal disease.

In staging esophageal carcinoma, care must be taken in evaluating mediastinal adenopathy. Mediastinal lymphadenopathy (nodes larger than 1 cm in diameter), especially in nodal groups close to an esophageal carcinoma, usually is secondary to metastatic spread of esophageal carcinoma. However,

FIGURE 16–13 ■ Value of intravenous contrast medium administration. *A,* Scan performed prior to rapid infusion of contrast material. There is circumferential thickening of the esophageal wall *(arrows)* and apparent obliteration of the fat plane between the tumor and the left atrium. Pulmonary veins are indicated by *arrowheads. B,* Scan during rapid contrast infusion. A normal fat plane *(arrows)* is now apparent between the thickened esophageal wall, the left atrium (LA), and the descending aorta (D). Pulmonary veins are indicated by *arrowheads.*

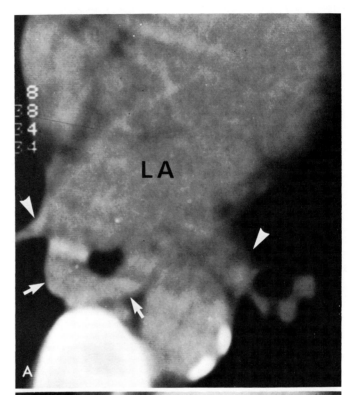

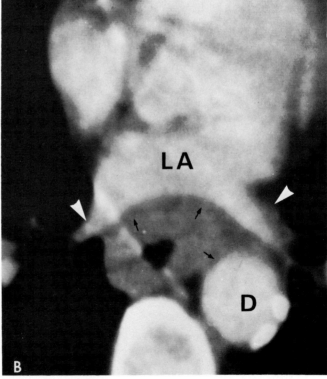

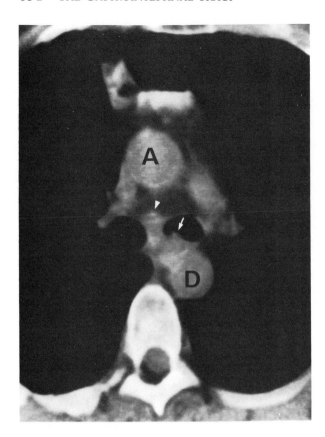

FIGURE 16–14 ■ Extraesophageal spread of esophageal carcinoma. CT scan at level of tracheal bifurcation demonstrates a polypoid mass *(arrow)* extending into the left main stem bronchus. Tumor also involves the subcarinal space *(arrowhead)* and has obliterated the fat plane surrounding the descending aorta (D). A = Ascending aorta. (From Moss AA, Schnyder P, Thoeni RF, Margulis AR: AJR 136:1051, 1981. © 1981, American Roentgen Ray Society. Reprinted by permission.)

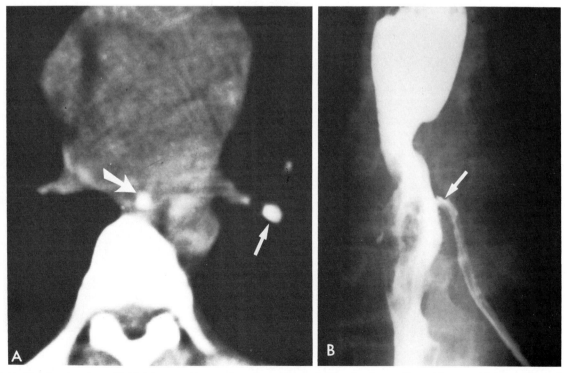

FIGURE 16–15 ■ Esophagobronchial fistula caused by esophageal carcinoma. *A,* CT scan after swallow of 2 per cent barium sulfate. Esophageal lumen *(large arrow)* and left bronchial tree *(small arrow)* are opacified by barium. *B,* Esophagogram of esophagobronchial fistula *(arrow).* (From Moss AA, Schnyder P, Thoeni RF, Margulis AR: AJR 136:1051, 1981. © 1981, American Roentgen Ray Society. Reprinted by permission.)

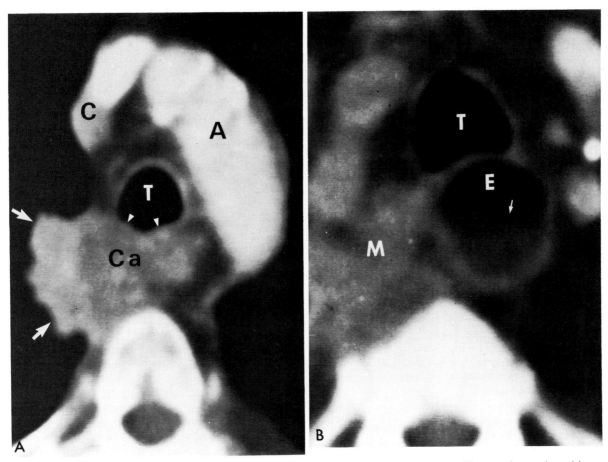

FIGURE 16–16 ■ Esophageal obstruction by esophageal carcinoma. *A*, A large esophageal cancer (Ca) obliterates the esophageal lumen and extends into the right paraesophageal soft tissues *(arrows)*. The tumor invades the trachea (T), causing the posterior wall to have an irregular appearance *(arrowheads)*. A = Aortic arch; C = superior vena cava. *B*, Scan 2 cm cephalad from *A* demonstrates a dilated esophagus (E) with an air-fluid-food level *(arrow)*. The spread of esophageal cancer has produced a mass (M) in the right paraesophageal soft tissues. T = Trachea.

reactive hyperplasia or lymphadenopathy resulting from prior inflammatory disease can produce CT findings that cannot be distinguished from metastatic disease. If clinically indicated, histologic sampling by means of mediastinoscopy or CT-directed biopsy can be performed to determine whether the enlarged lymph nodes are caused by benign or malignant disease. Frequently, pathologic positive nodes are smaller than 1 cm and cannot be distinguished from normal nodes. As metastasis to small local periesophageal nodes does not contraindicate surgical resection, this limitation of CT usually does not change the decision for performing surgery. However, the presence of positive nodes carries a decreased postoperative survival.

A variety of CT findings are encountered in patients with esophageal carcinoma. Most commonly found are focal esophageal wall thickening, which produces an eccentrically positioned esophageal lumen (see Fig. 16–9) and large esophageal masses that obliterate the esophageal lumen (see Fig. 16–16). Subtle eccentricities of the esophageal lumen may be indicators of early esophageal carcinomas (see Fig. 16–9), although detection may be impossible without a prior endoscopic or radiologic examination. A di-

lated esophagus above an obstructing carcinoma is evidence that an advanced malignancy is present (see Fig. 16–16). The length of esophageal carcinoma as judged by CT closely correlates with tumor lengths measured by esophagography,[12] and CT measurement of tumor thickness permits accurate esophageal tumor volumes to be calculated.

Computed tomography can detect direct extension of esophageal carcinoma into a variety of mediastinal structures (trachea, bronchi, pericardium) and identifies metastatic disease to the liver, adrenal gland, lung, and cervical, retrocrural, celiac, retroperitoneal, and mediastinal lymph nodes (Table 16–2).[12, 48, 49] Extraesophageal spread of carcinoma was found in 87 per cent of patients studied by Moss and coworkers.[12] Most frequently involved by direct extension were the trachea, bronchi, and aorta, whereas spread to abdominal lymph nodes was the most frequent site of distant metastases. Because positive nodes in the celiac and left gastric chains usually are larger than 1 cm when invaded by tumor, CT enables better detection of these nodes than of those in the mediastinal area. Invasion of the crura of the hemidiaphragms and of the pleura by esophageal tumor is not always correctly identified but does not signif-

TABLE 16–2 ■ Extraesophageal Extent of Esophageal Carcinoma in 52 Patients

DIRECT INVASION		METASTATIC DISEASE	
Location	No.	Location	No.
Trachea	24	Liver	3
Carina	12	Adrenals	1
Bronchi		Lung	1
Right main	6	Pleura	2
Left main	14	Lymph nodes	
Fistula	2	Right paratracheal	5
Left atrium	8	Left paratracheal	3
Aorta	17	Pulmonary aortic window	4
Pulmonary vessels		Pretracheal space	3
Artery	3	Cervical	1
Veins	2	Retrocrural	1
Azygos vein	3	Celiac	7
Vertebra	1	Paraaortic, paracaval	3
		Jugular	2
		Superior mediastinum	1

Source: Adapted from Moss AA, Schnyder P, Thoeni RF, Margulis AR: AJR 136:1051, 1981.

icantly influence surgical management. The gastric wall needs to be carefully analyzed for the presence of localized wall thickening caused by metastases from esophageal tumor. The incidence of esophageal metastases to the stomach ranges from 2.4 per cent to 15 per cent[50] and occurs by way of spread through the submucosal lymphatics.

CT Accuracy ■ Preoperative tumor staging that can reliably differentiate patients with potentially curable cancer from those with advanced tumors is necessary because of the higher operative mortality rate for attempted curative resections (about 20 per cent)[51] compared with that for palliative surgical procedures (about 10 per cent). Palliative surgical procedures that leave the esophageal tumor in place but bypass the obstruction include colonic interposition, retrosternal esophagogastrostomy, and placement of Beck tubes or stents. Patients are not considered for curative resection of an esophageal cancer if the pulmonary, cardiovascular, or nutritional status precludes major surgery; if tumor invasion of the aorta or tracheobronchial tree prevents tumor dissection; or if metastases to distant sites are detected. Local adenopathy does not prevent curative surgery. Surgery may be used alone or may be combined with radiation therapy or chemotherapy.[52]

Based on results to date, many investigators advocate that CT be routinely employed prior to surgery or radiation therapy in patients with esophageal carcinoma.[12, 43, 48, 49, 52–54] While the reported accuracy of CT staging for esophageal carcinomas ranges between 84 per cent and 100 per cent,[12, 45, 48–51, 53] the CT staging results are better for tumors in the esophagus proper (94 per cent accuracy) than for those in the gastroesophageal junction (42 per cent accuracy).[53] Recently Quint et al.[55] reported that CT had a low accuracy rate for staging esophageal tumors. However, visual inspection of the tumor site during surgery was prevented in their study, because only transhiatal and cervical incisions using blunt mediastinal dissection without thoracotomies were performed. Furthermore, indeterminate results for aortic

invasion were considered positive, and their analysis included patients who had received radiation therapy and it considered all tumor types together (adenocarcinomas, squamous cell carcinomas, and sarcomas). It is well established that radiation fibrosis obliterates tissue planes, and therefore a lack of tissue planes in these patients cannot be used as a sign of direct tumor invasion. Furthermore, adenocarcinomas, the most common type of malignant esophageal tumor found in Quint et al.'s series (48 per cent), behave differently than do squamous cell carcinomas of the esophagus.

Following therapy, CT can be used to evaluate the effectiveness of radiation therapy and can be employed to predict survival of patients with esophageal carcinoma. One study[51] found that regardless of therapy, patients with CT evidence of mediastinal invasion, liver metastases, or abdominal adenopathy had a statistically shortened survival. Also, patients who underwent attempted curative surgery had a longer mean survival rate than those who underwent palliative or no surgery. An association between tumor width greater than 3 cm (shown by CT) and extraesophageal spread and overall survival has been demonstrated.[56]

CT Evaluation After Esophagogastrectomy ■ CT is useful in patients who have undergone esophagogastrectomies for esophageal cancer to establish the presence or absence of recurrence or of early or late complications[57, 58] (Figs. 16–17 and 16–18). Early complications consist of anastomotic leak, gastric necrosis, and gastric outlet obstruction; late complications are reflux esophagitis and benign stricture.

In patients with extensive esophageal resection and high anastomosis, the esophagogastric junction is located in the right paravertebral region, and in patients with resection of distal esophagus and low anastomosis, the stomach is brought through the left side of the diaphragm and projects into the left paravertebral area. Frequently, in the normal patient with esophagogastrectomy and high anastomosis, the esophagus above the anastomosis is dilated, and

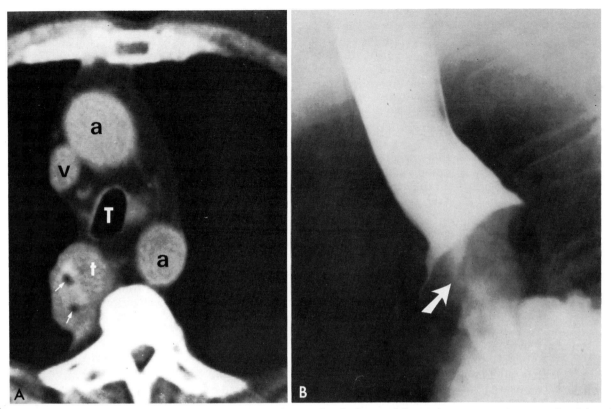

FIGURE 16–17 ■ Recurrent esophageal carcinoma. *A*, CT scan showing that the lumen of the esophagus *(arrows)* is narrowed and there is a solid tumor mass (t) that does not fill with contrast material. a = Aorta; T = trachea; v = superior vena cava. *B*, Esophagogram. A tumor mass *(arrow)* is present at the esophageal-enteric anastomosis.

the stomach is located anterolaterally to the right side of the vertebral column (see Fig. 16–15A). The retrotracheal and retrocardiac areas contain increased amounts of fat because omentum has been brought up with the stomach. On some CT sections of these patients, the crus appears displaced laterally because of surgical division of the right crus. Therefore displacement of the right crus does not constitute recurrence of tumor.

Good filling of the intradiaphragmatic portion of the stomach is essential to rule out local recurrence of neoplasm. Although recurrence of tumor can be

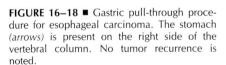

FIGURE 16–18 ■ Gastric pull-through procedure for esophageal carcinoma. The stomach *(arrows)* is present on the right side of the vertebral column. No tumor recurrence is noted.

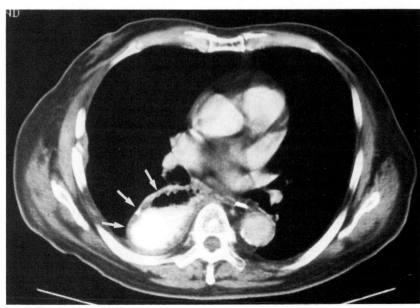

variable in appearance, it usually is extramucosal and presents as esophageal or anastomotic wall thickening (see Fig. 16–16).

Although mucosal abnormalities in patients after esophagogastrectomy are better evaluated by barium esophagography, CT is superior for detecting extramucosal tumor or distant metastases. Because many recurrent lesions originate outside the interposed stomach, CT is more useful than barium studies in detecting early recurrence.[59]

CT is also helpful in patients with suspected tracheobronchial fistula or perforation caused by bougienage. In these patients, fluid collections in the left lung base (or rarely in the lesser sac), mediastinitis, and thickening of esophageal wall are demonstrated.[60, 61] Although esophagography usually visualizes fistulae well, CT is superior in assessing the presence or absence of fluid collections resulting from an esophageal leak.

BENIGN ESOPHAGEAL TUMORS

Benign esophageal tumors are relatively rare lesions found in less than 1 per cent of autopsies performed at the Mayo Clinic.[62] The esophageal leiomyoma accounts for 45 per cent to 73 per cent of all benign esophageal tumors.[58, 59] Most frequently, esophageal leiomyomas occur in the lower third of the esophagus (60 per cent) and are detected in early or middle adult life.[63] Most leiomyomas are solitary tumors, but occasionally multiple tumors are present.[39] Leiomyomas usually cause no symptoms, but when lesions become large, they can produce dysphagia. Another rare benign esophageal tumor is the giant fibrovascular polyp, which presents as an intraluminal pedunculated mass, often containing low-attenuation elements.[64]

Diagnosis by esophagography is usually straightforward; an intramural lesion producing a smooth, crescent-shaped defect in the barium column is found. CT typically reveals an esophageal mass, which may contain calcium (Fig. 16–19). Preservation of adjacent fat planes and calcifications distinguish a benign leiomyoma from a malignant squamous cell carcinoma.

ESOPHAGEAL VARICES

Esophageal varices can be suggested by CT in patients with superior vena cava obstruction or liver cirrhosis. In these patients, CT demonstrates thickening of the esophageal wall; evidence of oval, grape-like masses resulting from enlarged veins located in the distal esophagus, periesophageal region (Fig. 16–20), gastrohepatic ligament, or gastric wall.[65] Dynamic CT studies facilitate the diagnosis by enhancing the varicoid vessels within the esophageal wall.[66, 67] For detecting esophageal varices, CT has a sensitivity similar to that of barium studies, but periesophageal varices and portal hypertension are better shown by CT. In the absence of a bolus injection of contrast material, small varices may be missed on CT scans.

Endoscopic esophageal sclerotherapy has gained widespread acceptance for the management of bleeding esophageal varices. CT is often used in these patients to assess complications such as esophageal perforation, wall necrosis, hemorrhage, esophagopleural fistula, abscess, and pleural effusions. In the normal postsclerotherapy patient, CT shows thickening of the esophageal wall with areas of low attenuation that give the esophagus a laminated appearance. Following sclerotherapy there may be obliteration of mediastinal fat planes, thickening of

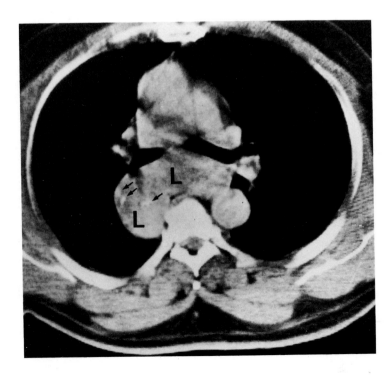

FIGURE 16–19 ■ Leiomyoma of the esophagus. A large esophageal leiomyoma (L) extending primarily to the right has a sharp, rounded, well-defined outer margin and multiple foci of calcification (arrows).

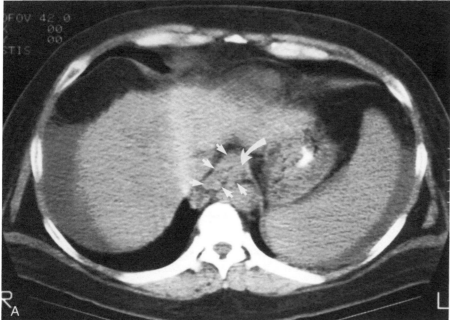

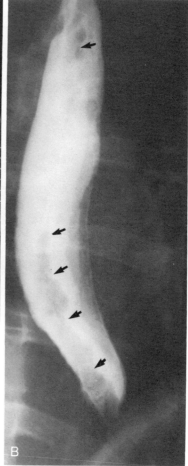

FIGURE 16–20 ■ Esophageal varices. *A,* Several nodular soft tissue densities *(straight arrows)* surround the distal esophagus *(curved arrow).* The liver surface is slightly nodular because of cirrhosis, and mild ascites is present in the perihepatic and perisplenic areas. *B,* The esophagogram in the same patient demonstrates the varices as beaded, thickened folds *(arrows).*

diaphragmatic crura, pleural effusions, and subsegmental atelectases.[67] Understanding of the normal CT findings in patients who have undergone esophageal sclerotherapy permits determination of the presence or absence of complications.

CONGENITAL ABNORMALITIES

Esophageal duplication cysts account for 10 per cent to 15 per cent of all duplications in the alimentary tract. Sixty per cent of all esophageal duplication cysts occur in the lower esophagus and are paraesophageal or intramural in location. They protrude into the posterior mediastinum and usually are symptomatic early in life but can remain asymptomatic until adulthood. Alimentary tract duplication cysts result from developmental errors and are lined with epithelium and a double layer of smooth muscles. On CT scans they appear as homogeneous, low-attenuation masses with smooth borders.[68, 69] The differential diagnosis includes abscess, old hematoma, neurofibroma, lipoma, leiomyoma, or other foregut duplications. Usually CT can establish the cystic nature of the mass and its relationship to other adjacent structures.

Stomach

Anatomy

The stomach joins the esophagus to the duodenum and is usually divided into fundal, body, and antral segments. The normal gastric wall as measured by CT in a well-distended stomach usually ranges from 2 to 5 mm thick, and any measurement greater than 1 cm is considered abnormal.[70–72] Rugal thickness varies greatly, but the normal gastric wall when measured at the depth of a rugal fold is usually less than 5 mm thick.

GASTRIC FUNDUS

As the esophagus becomes an intraabdominal organ and joins the stomach, it may produce either a focal thickening involving the cranial aspect of the medial gastric wall or an apparent mass projecting into the gastric lumen (Figs. 16–7 and 16–21).[16, 17] Marks and colleagues[16] found one of these features in 38 per cent of patients retrospectively reviewed and in 33 per cent of those studied in a prospective manner. The configuration seen on CT scans relates to the transverse anatomic plane section through the

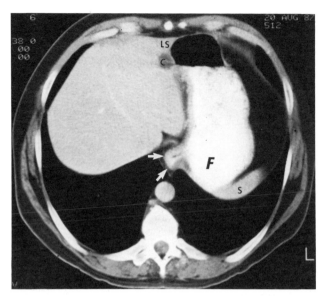

FIGURE 16–21 ■ Normal stomach, level of fundus. The normal gastric fundus (F) is related to the spleen (S) and lateral segment of the left lobe of the liver (LS). The gastroesophageal junction (arrows) is well seen, but if it is not filled with contrast material, it can simulate a mass. C = Liver cyst.

normal esophagogastric junction and cardia and should not be interpreted as a mass lesion. Variations in anatomic configuration and gastric distention most likely are responsible for the different CT profiles of this anatomic region.

The stomach at the level of the gastroesophageal junction is also related intimately to the spleen, the lateral segment of the left lobe of the liver, and the diaphragmatic crus (see Fig. 16–21). Frequently, an air-fluid level is present in the fundus that can produce streak artifacts, making evaluation of the lateral segment of the left hepatic lobe difficult. When this occurs, scanning in the lateral decubitus position helps to eliminate the problem. This artifact also can be reduced if, after respiration, the beginning of a scan is delayed to allow fluid motion to cease.[73]

BODY OF THE STOMACH

The body of the stomach is related to the spleen, lateral segment of the left hepatic lobe, jejunum, tail of the pancreas, and in some patients, the splenic flexure of the colon (Fig. 16–22). The lesser and greater curvatures of the stomach are depicted in cross section, and frequently either the celiac or superior mesenteric artery can be identified.

ANTRUM

The gastric antrum is an anteriorly positioned horizontal structure crossing the midline of the body. It is contiguous with the first portion of the duodenum and frequently receives an impression from the left lobe of the liver or gallbladder (Fig. 16–23). The body of the pancreas lies immediately dorsal to the antrum, and the head of the pancreas lies just medial to the duodenum. The superior mesenteric artery is seen in cross section as it arises from the

aorta, and the splenic vein is identified dorsal to the pancreas. The antrum and duodenal sweep surround the head of the pancreas, and in some patients the antrum often can still be identified at the level where the third portion of the duodenum crosses the spine dorsal to the superior mesenteric artery and vein. In some patients, because of the horizontal course of the distal antrum and duodenum, thickening of the antral and duodenal walls is simulated and should not be confused with abnormality. If necessary, scanning in the decubitus position can help to solve this problem.

Techniques of Examination

To ensure that the stomach is empty of solid food prior to the CT examination, patients are allowed water but no food from midnight until the CT scan in the morning or for 8 hours before the examination. Thirty minutes before the CT examination, 450 to 500 mL of a 0.5 per cent to 2 per cent solution of diatrizoate meglumine (Gastrografin) is given orally. This contrast material rapidly passes into the proximal small bowel; thus 200 to 300 mL of the same solution or a 1 per cent barium sulfate mixture is administered just prior to the patient's being placed on the CT scan table. The barium sulfate mixture may coat the stomach and duodenum better than diatrizoate meglumine and tends to move more slowly out of the stomach. Alternatively, water[74] or oily solutions can be used; these permit excellent demonstration of mucosa and wall thickness. The use of large volumes of dilute contrast media ensures that the stomach will be fully distended during the CT scan. Foaming agents and hypotonic agents are

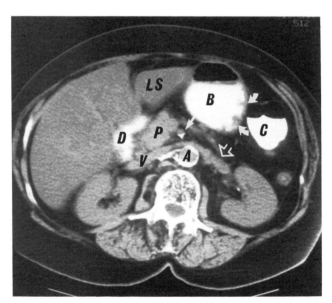

FIGURE 16–22 ■ Normal stomach, level of body. CT scan is through the body of the stomach (B) at a level just below the spleen. The lateral segment of the left lobe of the liver (LS), head of the pancreas (P), and spenic flexure of the colon (C) are adjacent structures. A = Aorta; D = duodenum; V = inferior vena cava; solid arrow = superior mesenteric artery; open arrow = renal vein. The rugae (curved arrows) are well seen.

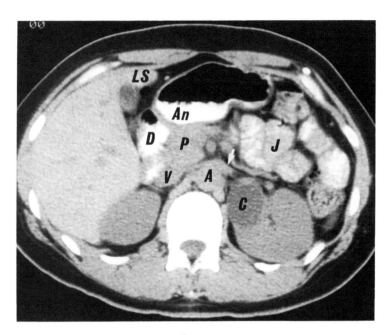

FIGURE 16–23 ■ Normal stomach (level of antrum) and proximal duodenum. The gastric antrum (An) crosses the midline of the body and appears contiguous with the proximal duodenum (D). Important adjacent or nearby structures are the lateral segment of the left hepatic lobe (LS), left renal cyst (C), and left renal vein *(arrow)*. A = Aorta; J = jejunum; P = pancreas; V = inferior vena cava.

not routinely administered but should be employed in instances of rapid gastric emptying and in all cases of staging of gastric neoplasms. If the jejunum and ileum in the lower abdomen need to be well visualized, metoclopramide (Reglan) is given with the first dose of diatrizoate meglumine.

The scanner gantry is positioned at 0°, and CT scans of sections 1 cm thick are taken at 1-cm intervals from the xiphoid to the umbilicus with the patient supine. Prone or lateral decubitus scans are performed if better delineation and distention of the fundus, antrum, and duodenal sweep are required. Intravenous contrast material is routinely administered, and a rapid intravenous bolus of 150 to 180 mL of 60 per cent methylglucamine diatrizoate or nonionic contrast material followed by a dynamic scan sequence has been of value in determining the vascularity of mass lesions, in distinguishing between lymph nodes and vascular structures, and in demonstrating associated lower esophageal and upper abdominal varices.

Whenever a mass lesion is demonstrated, it is useful to confirm that the mass is not a pseudotumor by giving additional contrast material, effervescent agents, or glucagon (1 mg) and rescanning the patient in the prone, decubitus, or left posterior oblique position. These maneuvers help distinguish true masses from pseudotumors, because the additional contrast and change in position combine to distend the stomach, particularly in the antral and gastroesophageal regions. Pseudotumors, but not true pathologic lesions, are usually obliterated by such positional changes. Passage of a nasogastric tube also can be of help in evaluating the gastroesophageal junction (Fig. 16–24). Incomplete distention can be seen in the dependent portion of the stomach, with a sharp transition to normal gastric wall thickness at or slightly above the gastric air-fluid level (the "gastric air-fluid sign").[75]

All CT scans are analyzed for gastric wall thickness, contour of the inner and outer gastric margins, ulcerations, extension of a mass into adjacent organs, local adenopathy, and distant metastases. Vascular anatomy and change in the CT density of a mass are best evaluated after intravenous contrast administration.

The criteria employed to determine direct tumor extension include loss of the fat plane between a gastric mass and the pancreas, liver, spleen, mesocolon, or duodenum; a mass extending anterior and posterior to the pancreas; thickening of the esophageal wall; and obliteration of the periportal fat in the liver hilum. Ascites and metastases to the liver, adrenal glands, mesentery, lymph nodes, kidney, or peritoneal cavity are shown by CT as features of extensive spread of gastric tumors.

Pathology

MALIGNANT GASTRIC TUMORS

Adenocarcinoma ■ Gastric adenocarcinoma is the most common form of primary gastric malignancy, with more than 23,000 new cases encountered yearly in the United States.[76] Preoperative evaluation of gastric adenocarcinoma has been largely dependent on radiography and endoscopy of the upper gastrointestinal tract, despite the limitations of these techniques in detecting local, regional, or distant spread.[77, 78] Arteriography,[5] radionuclide imaging,[6] and ultrasonography[8] have been used to detect tumor spread, but each has serious limitations as a staging technique. In contrast, CT has been shown capable of accurately detecting and staging gastric adenocarcinoma.[8, 70–72, 79–84]

Based on the CT findings, gastric adenocarcinoma can be classified into one of four stages (Table 16–3):

1. A *stage I* gastric adenocarcinoma produces an intraluminal mass without gastric wall thickening or evidence of spread to distant or adjacent organs.

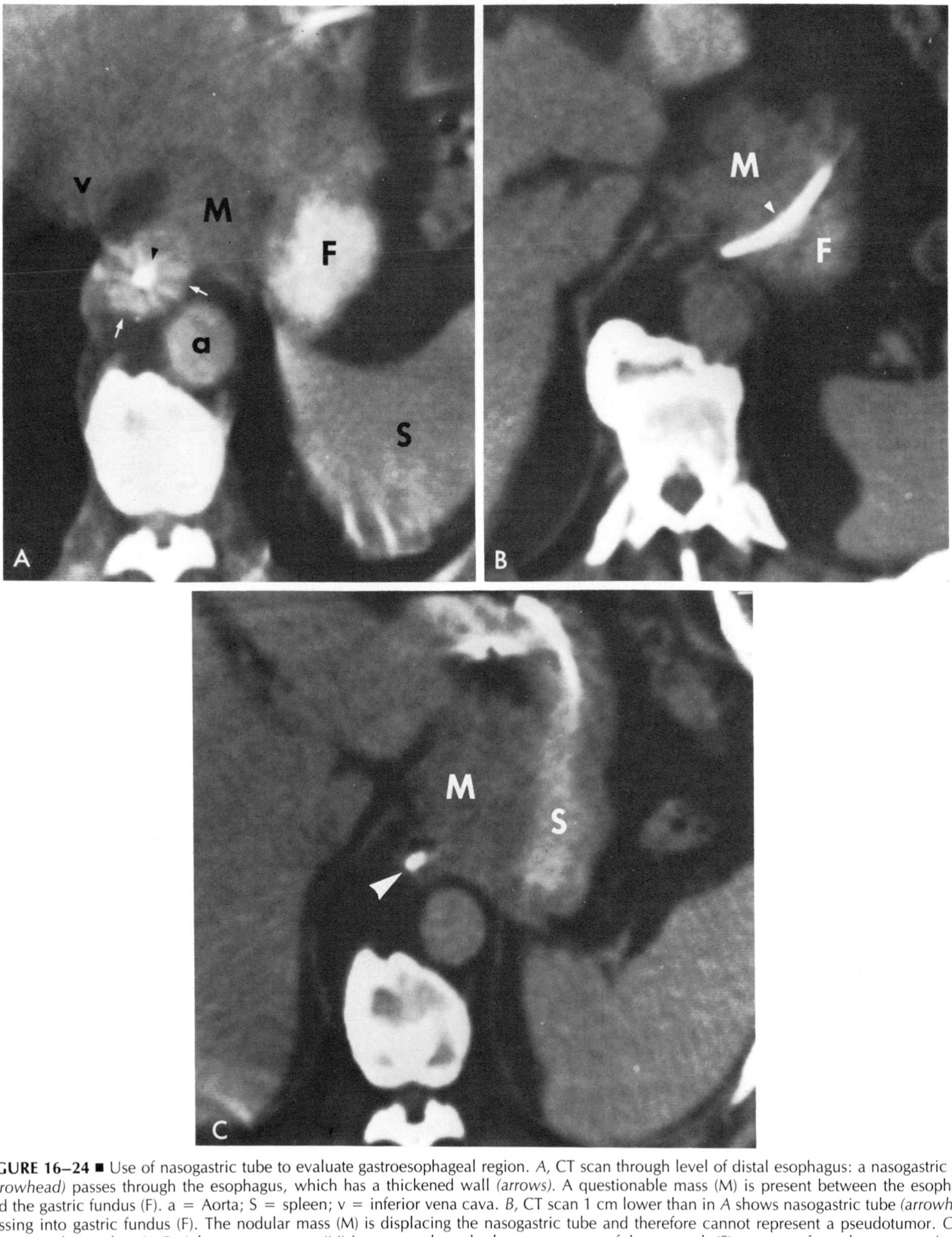

FIGURE 16–24 ■ Use of nasogastric tube to evaluate gastroesophageal region. *A,* CT scan through level of distal esophagus: a nasogastric tube *(arrowhead)* passes through the esophagus, which has a thickened wall *(arrows).* A questionable mass (M) is present between the esophagus and the gastric fundus (F). a = Aorta; S = spleen; v = inferior vena cava. *B,* CT scan 1 cm lower than in *A* shows nasogastric tube *(arrowhead)* passing into gastric fundus (F). The nodular mass (M) is displacing the nasogastric tube and therefore cannot represent a pseudotumor. *C,* CT scan 1 cm lower than in *B.* A large tumor mass (M) is present along the lesser curvature of the stomach (S), separate from the nasogastric tube *(arrowhead)* in the distal esophagus. Diagnosis: gastric adenocarcinoma spreading up the esophagus.

TABLE 16–3 ■ CT Staging of Gastric Adenocarcinoma

Stage I	Intraluminal gastric mass without gastric wall thickening; no evidence of local or distant spread of disease.
Stage II	Thickened gastric wall (> 1 cm) without invasion of adjacent organs or distant metastases.
Stage III	Thickened gastric wall with direct extension into adjacent organs; no distant metastases.
Stage IV	Any tumor stage with distant metastatic disease.

2. *Stage II* gastric cancers show gastric wall thickening to greater than 1 cm but have not spread beyond the stomach (Figs. 16–25 and 16–26). (Normal gastric wall thickness is ≤5 mm.)

3. Thickening of the gastric wall with direct extension of tumor into adjacent organs but without evidence of distant metastatic disease is classified as *stage III* (Fig. 16–27).

4. Distant spread of tumor is evident in *stage IV* disease (Figs. 16–28 through 16–30).

The most frequently demonstrated CT abnormality is focal gastric wall thickening (see Figs. 16–25 through 16–29), but diffuse gastric wall thickening can also be encountered. Diffuse low attenuation in the thickened gastric wall may be produced by mucinous adenocarcinoma.[80] Other abnormalities frequently demonstrated by CT are irregular outer and inner gastric margins (see Fig. 16–27), ulcerated masses (see Fig. 16–28), and gastric outlet obstruction. Direct invasion of gastric adenocarcinoma into the pancreas, esophagus (see Fig. 16–28), spleen, liver (see Fig. 16–30), and transverse mesocolon and metastatic involvement of the liver (see Fig. 16–30), adrenal glands, lymph nodes (see Fig. 16–29), kidneys, ovaries, and peritoneal cavity (see Fig. 16–29A) can also be demonstrated by CT.

In the early reports of CT use, correlation of CT staging with surgical, laparoscopic, or autopsy findings showed a high accuracy of CT staging of gastric adenocarcinoma.[79] Preoperative CT studies have correctly predicted patients who had locally confined gastric adenocarcinoma and those whose gastric adenocarcinoma had spread to adjacent or distant structures. However, three more recent series have clearly indicated that CT staging in gastric cancer is limited. In one study of 49 patients, an overall accuracy of 72 per cent for CT staging when compared with surgery was achieved.[85, 86, 87] The authors of that study observed that CT assessment of regional lymph node metastases and invasion of adjacent organs was unreliable. In another study,[86] 37 patients were examined in whom both preoperative CT and laparotomy staging were available. CT understaged 19 of 31 patients (61 per cent) as stage I, whereas clinically they had stage III disease. This was principally because of missed metastases in the liver, regional lymph nodes, and omentum. Additionally, CT overstaged three of six patients who were considered unresectable by CT when in fact the tumors were operable. The most comprehensive study, performed by Sussman and co-workers,[87] compared preoperative CT and operative staging in 75 patients. Thirty-one per cent were understaged, and 16 per cent were overstaged by CT. Regional lymph node metastases were diagnosed with a sensitivity of 67 per cent and

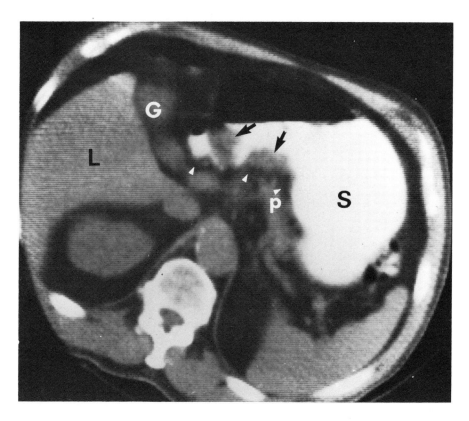

FIGURE 16–25 ■ Stage II gastric adenocarcinoma. There is a slight focal thickening of the lesser gastric curvature *(arrows)*. The fat plane *(arrowheads)* surrounding the stomach (S) is preserved. The liver (L), gall bladder (G), and pancreas (p) are uninvolved.

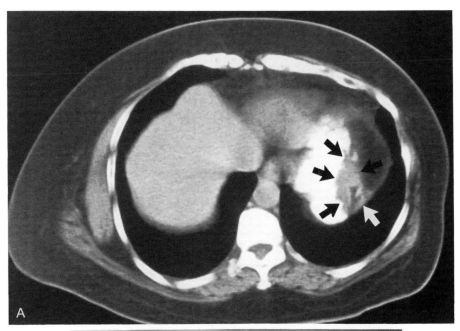

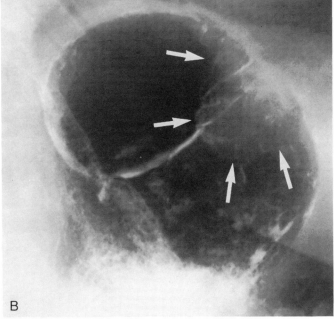

FIGURE 16–26 ■ Stage II gastric carcinoma. *A,* An irregular mass is seen in the fundus *(black arrows)* without extension into surrounding tissue. The white arrow indicates the tip of the spleen. *B,* Upper gastrointestinal scan shows a large, irregular soft tissue mass *(arrows)* in the fundus of the stomach.

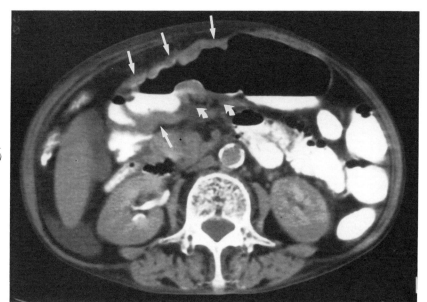

FIGURE 16–27 ■ Stage III gastric adenocarcinoma. An irregular mass in the antrum *(straight arrows)* extends into the lesser sac *(curved arrows).*

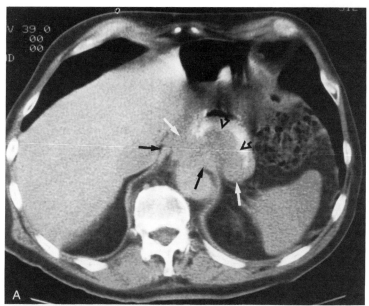

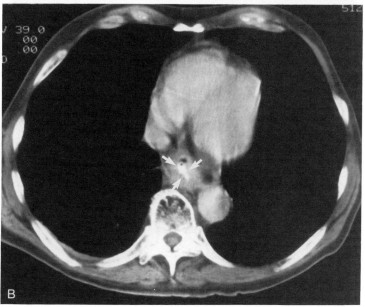

FIGURE 16–28 ■ Stage IV gastric adenocarcinoma. *A,* Scan reveals a mass *(white arrows)* along the posterior wall of the gastric fundus. The stomach has an irregular margin because of multiple ulcerations *(open arrows).* The mass extends to the crura *(black arrows). B,* Scan through the lower esophagus demonstrates a thickened esophageal wall caused by gastric tumor extension, which is causing the irregular contour of the lumen of the esophagus *(arrows).*

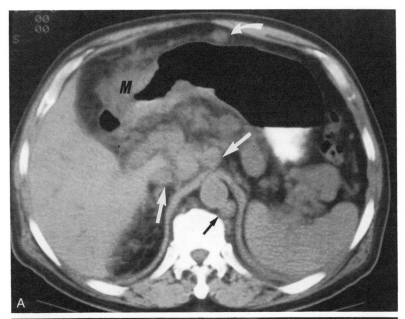

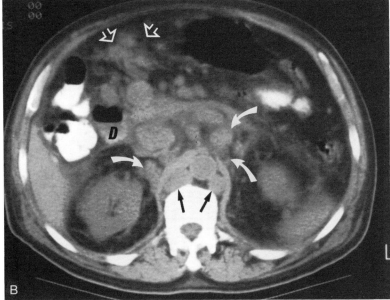

FIGURE 16–29 ■ Stage IV gastric adenocarcinoma. *A,* Irregular thickening (M) of the antrum with direct extension of tumor into perigastric fat is noted. Peritoneal implant *(curved arrow)* and retrocrural *(black arrow)* and pericaval nodes *(white straight arrows)* are seen. *B,* Retrocrural *(black solid arrows)* and retroperitoneal *(white curved arrows)* adenopathy and mesenteric tumor infiltration *(open arrows)* are present. D = Duodenum.

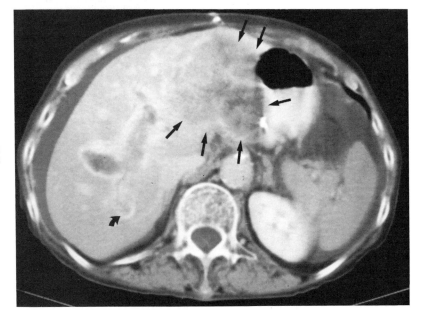

FIGURE 16–30 ■ Stage IV gastric adenocarcinoma. Direct invasion of gastric carcinoma into the left lobe of the liver *(straight arrows)* and liver metastasis *(curved arrow)* are identified.

specificity of 61 per cent. Whereas the inability of CT to detect metastases in normal-sized lymph nodes was the major contributor to the limited sensitivity, pancreatic invasion and peritoneal carcinomatosis were also frequently missed.

Based on these results, radiologists and clinicians must assume a more realistic posture when CT is used for staging gastric adenocarcinoma. Patients who have gross hepatic and intraperitoneal metastases detected and percutaneously biopsied under CT guidance can be spared all except palliative surgery. However, patients with limited abnormalities apparent on CT scans and who are deemed to be operative candidates require laparotomy for accurate staging of their tumors, although advanced disease will be discovered in many of these patients. In debilitated patients who are poor surgical risks, CT may be helpful in expeditiously detecting and histologically confirming distant metastases. In addition to preoperatively staging gastric adenocarcinoma, CT has also been shown to be valuable in planning radiation fields, assessing tumor response to therapy, and detecting tumor recurrence (Fig. 16–31).

CT After Gastrectomy ■ The primary methods used to evaluate patients for local recurrence of gastric cancer after gastrectomy are endoscopy and upper gastrointestinal (UGI) studies as tumor recurrence usually occurs at the anastomotic site or gastric stump. In addition to local disease CT is excellent in demonstrating recurrent disease in the left upper quadrant and anterior abdominal wall, as well as metastases to regional nodes or to liver. CT features that suggest tumor recurrence include soft tissue masses in the area of the gastric stump (see Fig. 16–31) and obliteration of fascial planes between the area of anastomosis and pancreatic bed.[88] In these

patients it is important that the gastric remnant be well distended by using intravenous glucagon and sufficient oral contrast or air. Local adenopathy and evidence of distant metastases are further CT indications of recurrence. Care must be taken not to confuse tumor recurrence with postoperative fibrosis, hematoma, or unopacified bowel loops of small bowel. A baseline CT examination 2 months after gastrectomy helps to avoid such diagnostic errors.

Lymphoma ■ Gastric lymphomas represent 1 per cent to 5 per cent of the malignant tumors of the stomach, and the stomach is the most common site of involvement in the gastrointestinal tract.[89] Lymphomas either occur as part of a generalized lymphomatous process or, in 10 per cent of instances, arise as an isolated primary gastric malignancy.[90, 91] The lymphomatous process usually extends submucosally, producing thickening of the gastric wall and rugal folds without mucosal abnormalities until ulceration occurs. As a result of the submucosal pattern of spread, barium sulfate studies of the upper gastrointestinal tract often reveal only thickened gastric folds; endoscopy and mucosal biopsy are frequently nondiagnostic and even if positive are unable to determine the extent of spread.[92–94] By directly imaging the entire gastric wall and adjacent structures, CT has proved capable of diagnosing and determining the extent of spread of gastric lymphoma with a high degree of accuracy.[95, 96]

In our personal experience and in that of other investigators, gastric wall thickening greater than 1 cm has been seen in virtually all patients with gastric lymphoma[71, 79, 81, 89, 95] (mean gastric wall thickness, 4 cm; range, 1.1 to 7.7 cm) (Fig. 16–32). Most commonly, gastric lymphoma results in thickening of the wall of the entire stomach (50 per cent of cases) or

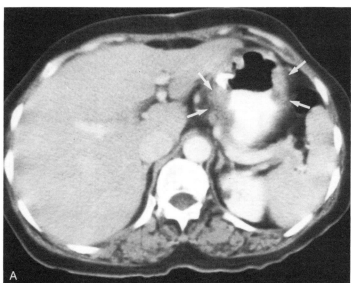
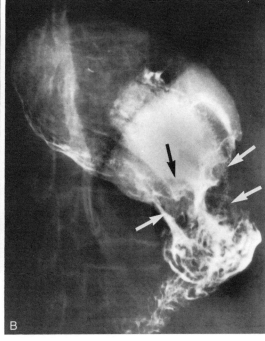

FIGURE 16–31 ■ Recurrent gastric carcinoma with lymphoma in a patient with a Billroth II gastrojejunostomy. *A,* CT scan shows irregular thickening of lesser and greater curvature *(arrows). B,* Upper gastrointestinal scan shows nodular masses *(black and white arrows)* at and above gastrojejunostomy site.

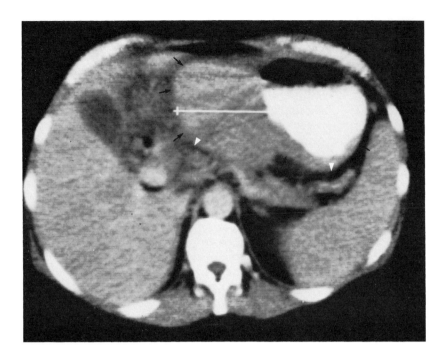

FIGURE 16–32 ■ Gastric lymphoma producing thickening of the gastric wall (measured distance 7.7 cm). The outer margin of the thickened gastric wall (arrows) is smooth, and the perigastric fat plane (arrowheads) is preserved. (From Buy J-N, Moss AA: AJR 138:859, 1982. © 1982, American Roentgen Ray Society. Reprinted by permission.)

thickening of the antrum and body or fundus and body of the stomach. The abnormally thickened portion of the gastric wall typically involves greater than half the circumference of the stomach (Fig. 16–33). Focal lymphomatous lesions of the stomach presenting as submucosal ulcerated masses ("bull's-eye" lesions) may be missed by CT.[89]

The CT attenuation value of the gastric wall measured at the site of maximum width of the lymphoma varies from patient to patient within a range of 34 to 74 Hounsfield units (H). However, there are areas within lymphomatous tissue that have lower CT attenuation values than the major portion of the gastric mass. Most commonly, these hypodense re-

gions are located just below the inner surface of the lymphoma and give the tumor an inhomogeneous appearance (Figs. 16–33 and 16–34). Whether these areas of low attenuation represent true tissue inhomogeneity of the lymphomatous tissue or necrosis, hemorrhage, submucosal edema, or artifact has not been proved. However, pathologic studies commonly reveal areas of necrosis and hemorrhage within gastric lymphoma with a distribution similar to that of the hypodense lesions detected by CT.[97, 98] CT can visualize perforation or fistulization of a gastric lymphoma by demonstrating fluid collections in the lesser sac or subphrenic space. Frequently such a perforation is silent. Perforation may occur

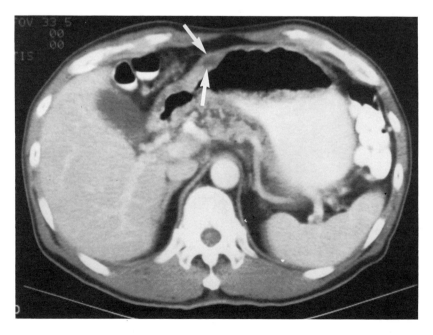

FIGURE 16–33 ■ Stage III lymphoma of stomach. Thickening of gastric wall in area of antrum and body with one area of low density (arrows) is seen. Outer margins are smooth, and inner margins are slightly irregular.

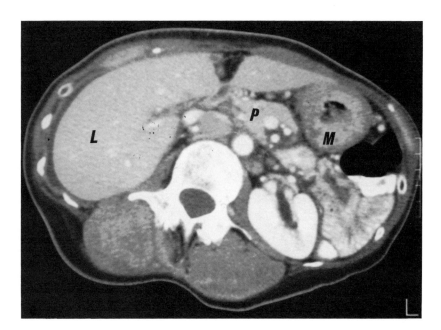

FIGURE 16–34 ■ Gastric lymphoma. Diffuse thickening of the gastric wall (M) with marked inhomogeneity is identified. The outer margins are smooth. L = Liver; P = pancreatic head.

because of the lack of desmoplastic response, rapid growth of tumor, or as a response to therapy.[99] Perforations are not uncommon, being seen in 9 per cent to 47 per cent of patients.[97]

The outer gastric margin is smooth or lobulated in approximately two thirds of patients with gastric lymphoma, and the fat plane between the outer wall of the stomach and adjacent abdominal organs is preserved in a similar percentage of patients (Figs. 16–33, 16–34, and 16–35). The inner gastric wall is frequently irregular in contour (see Fig. 16–33). In one third of patients, at least a portion of the outer gastric margin is ill defined, and the perigastric fat plane is lost. Although preservation of the perigastric fat plane is strong evidence for lack of extension of lymphoma into adjacent organs, obliteration of the fat plane is found to be secondary to direct invasion

in only 70 per cent to 75 per cent of instances.[93] Most frequently, gastric lymphoma invades the pancreas, but extension to the spleen (Fig. 16–36), transverse mesocolon, and pleura is also found.

Although perigastric lymphadenopathy is most frequent, lymph node enlargement both above and below the renal hilum is also common. Lymphadenopathy in patients with gastric lymphoma usually indicates disseminated disease but can also be secondary to reactive hyperplasia; thus care must be exercised in equating lymph node enlargement with lymphomatous involvement, even in patients with known gastric lymphoma.

As in patients with gastric adenocarcinoma, CT scanning is useful in following the effects of radiation or chemotherapy on gastric lymphomas and in assessing complications. In successful treatment, dis-

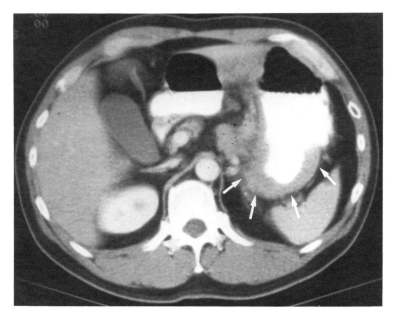

FIGURE 16–35 ■ Gastric lymphoma. There is thickening of the body of the stomach with preservation of the perigastric fat plane (arrows).

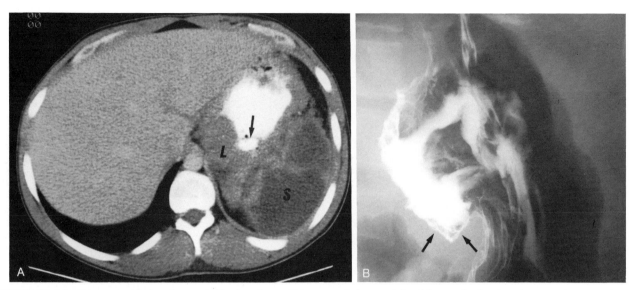

FIGURE 16–36 ■ Primary gastric lymphoma. *A,* The lymphoma (L) has extended to partially obliterate the fat plane between the stomach and spleen (S). Surgery confirmed direct lymphomatous extension into spleen. An ulcer within the mass *(arrow)* is also seen. *B,* Upper gastrointestinal scan shows a large ulcerating mass in fundus *(arrows).*

appearance of the gastric mass is documented; recurrent disease may be detected by CT prior to recurrence of symptoms (Fig. 16–37).

The individual CT features of gastric carcinoma and gastric lymphoma overlap, but the pattern of gastric involvement, the incidence of particular CT findings, and the location of extragastric metastases vary enough to permit a differentiation to be made in some patients (Table 16–4), particularly if findings from barium studies are also used. Occasionally it is difficult to distinguish gastric lymphoma from severe peptic gastritis or other benign inflammatory

gastric changes. CT features highly suggestive of a diagnosis of gastric lymphoma include the following:

1. Gastric wall thickening that diffusely involves the entire circumference of the gastric lumen or encompasses an entire region of the stomach and has an outer contour that is smooth or slightly lobulated.

2. Preservation of the fat plane between the stomach and adjacent organs.

3. Lymphadenopathy above and below the renal pedicle and/or massive periaortic lymph node enlargement.

4. Gastric wall thickening greater than 3 cm.

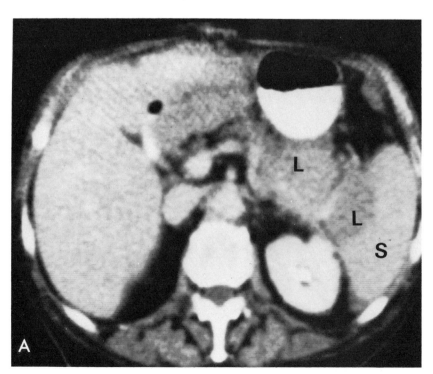

FIGURE 16–37 ■ Histiocytic lymphoma. *A,* Before treatment. There is marked thickening of the gastric wall by lymphoma (L), which has invaded the spleen (S) and pancreas.

FIGURE 16–37 *Continued* ■ *B,* Two months after chemotherapy. Gastric wall is of normal thickness; restoration of fat planes *(arrows)* between stomach and spleen (S) and between stomach and pancreatic vein (p) can be seen. *C,* CT scan 1 year after chemotherapy, while patient was asymptomatic. Note thickening of the gastric fundus *(small arrows)* and evidence of an extragastric mass *(large arrow).* After another course of therapy, the mass and gastric thickening again resolved. (Courtesy of J. Kaiser, MD. From Buy J-N, Moss AA: AJR 138:859, 1982. © 1982, American Roentgen Ray Society. Reprinted by permission.)

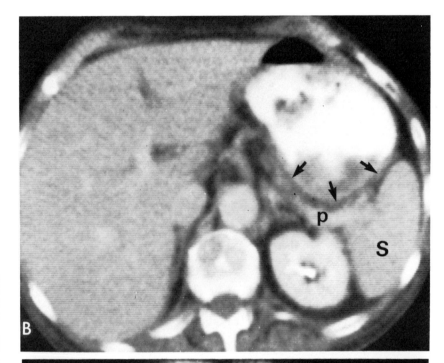

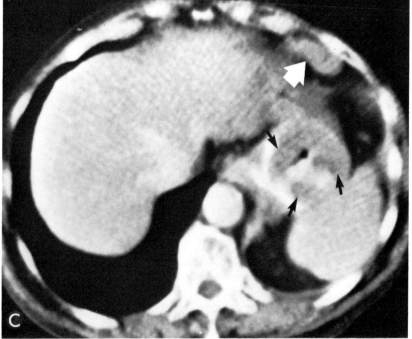

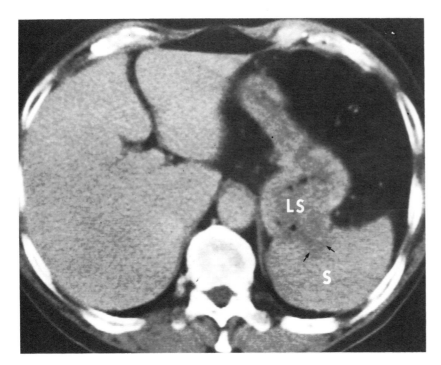

FIGURE 16–38 ■ Leiomyosarcoma of the stomach. The tumor (LS) appears as a large, pedunculated, extraluminal tumor that has obliterated the perigastric fat plane *(arrows)* and invaded the spleen (S).

Leiomyosarcoma ■ Leiomyosarcomas are malignant tumors arising from smooth muscle of the gastrointestinal tract. While 60 per cent arise in the stomach, gastric leiomyosarcomas make up only 0.5 per cent of gastric neoplasms.[100] Leiomyosarcomas are often large (50 per cent are greater than 10 cm across) and irregular in shape. Growth tends to be extraluminal, with often only a small mural or luminal component (Fig. 16–38).[100] Because of a predilection for exophytic growth, these gastric lesions are difficult to detect until they are very large. Central tumor necrosis is common, and calcification does occur. Leiomyosarcomas have a nonhomogeneous CT appearance both before and after contrast enhancement.[101] Metastases to the liver are common and, when present, typically show areas of necrosis within the metastatic deposits. Spread to local nodes and adrenal glands also may be present.

Metastatic Tumors ■ The stomach may be secondarily involved with neoplasms from the ovary, breast, thyroid, lung, or skin (melanoma) (Fig. 16–39), but in most instances blood-borne metastases are too small to be detected by routine CT scans. Direct gastric invasion from colonic, retroperitoneal (Fig. 16–40), or pancreatic neoplasms is more often detected by CT, but it is difficult to distinguish direct invasion from a primary gastric malignancy.

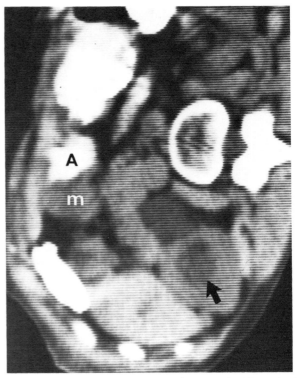

FIGURE 16–39 ■ Ovarian metastasis to the stomach. CT scan in the right lateral decubitus position demonstrates a solid mass (m) affecting the gastric antrum (A). Note hydronephrosis *(arrow)* of the right kidney due to obstruction by pelvic tumor.

TABLE 16–4 ■ Features of Gastric Lymphoma and Adenocarcinoma as Shown by Computed Tomography

CT FINDINGS	LYMPHOMA	CARCINOMA
Wall thickness		
Mean	4.0 cm	1.8 cm
Range	1.1–7.7 cm	1.1–3.2 cm
Contour	Regular: 42%	Regular: 27%
	Irregular: 58%	Irregular: 73%
Extent	Diffuse: 83%	Focal: 91%
Direct spread to adjacent organs	42%	73%
Lymphadenopathy above, below renal hilum	42%	0%

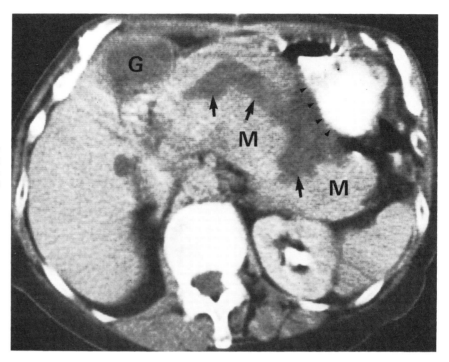

FIGURE 16–40 ■ Retroperitoneal paraganglioma. Paraganglioma produces a large mass (M) that directly invades the stomach *(arrowheads)*. The low-density central portion of the tumor *(arrows)* was necrotic at surgery. G = Gallbladder.

BENIGN GASTRIC TUMORS

Benign gastric tumors are usually asymptomatic but occasionally cause obstruction, bleeding, and epigastric pain.

Adenomatous Polyp ■ Hyperplastic polyps are the most common benign growth, but adenomatous polyps (Fig. 16–41) are the most frequent benign neoplastic gastric tumors,[102] followed by, in order of decreasing occurrence, tumors of smooth muscle, neurogenic and fibrous tissue, lipomas, vascular tumors, glomus tumors, hemangiopericytomas, and granular cell myoblastomas.[103, 104]

Leiomyoma ■ A leiomyoma may be present in any portion of the stomach but is most common in the antrum and body of the stomach.[105] It may be intramural, submucosal, or subserosal in location, but usually it is a submucosal lesion that appears on examination of the upper gastrointestinal tract as a round or egg-shaped mass with smooth borders (Fig. 16–42A)[72] with an intact or ulcerated mucosa.

Leiomyomas usually appear on CT scans as solid mass lesions of uniform density producing a focal thickening of the gastric wall (see Fig. 16–42B).[101] The outer border of the leiomyoma is smooth, and the

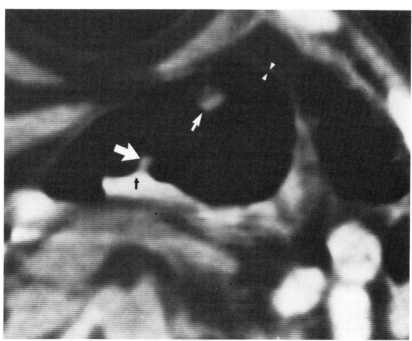

FIGURE 16–41 ■ Adenomatous polyp and polypoid carcinoma. A pedunculated adenomatous polyp *(small arrow)* produces no thickening of the adjacent gastric wall *(arrowheads)*. The polypoid mass *(large arrow)* with adjacent thickening (t) of the gastric wall proved to be gastric adenocarcinoma. (From Moss AA, Schnyder PP, Candardjis G, Margulis AR: J Clin Gastroenterol 2:401, 1980. Reprinted by permission.)

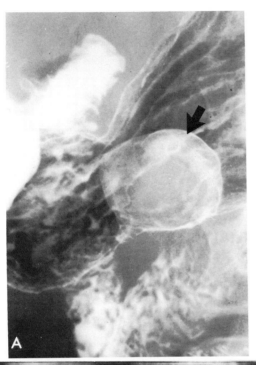

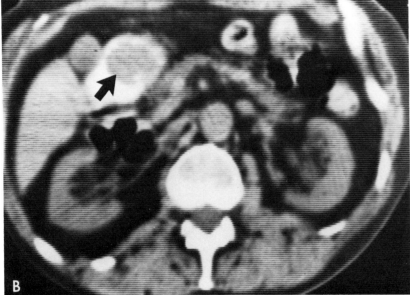

FIGURE 16–42 ■ Gastric leiomyoma. *A*, upper gastrointestinal tract examination demonstrates a submucosal leiomyoma (*arrow*) to have sharp margins and an intact mucosa. *B*, CT scan showing rounded, solid mass (*arrow*) without extragastric extension.

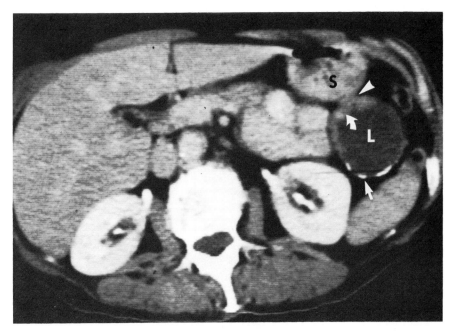

FIGURE 16–43 ■ Pedunculated leiomyoma. Leiomyoma (L) has a partially calcified rim *(arrow)* and a narrow zone of attachment *(arrowhead)* to the greater curvature of the stomach (S). The center of the leiomyoma has a low CT number because of necrosis of the tumor, whereas a portion near the attachment *(curved arrow)* has a higher CT density. The perigastric fat plane is preserved.

fat plane between the tumor and adjacent organs is preserved;[101] however, the inner margin of the leiomyoma may be irregular as a result of ulceration. Calcification is frequently identified (Fig. 16–43), as leiomyomas are one of the most commonly calcified benign gastric tumors. Leiomyomas can demonstrate a dramatic and diffuse increase in attenuation value following a bolus injection of contrast material. However, CT differentiation of a benign leiomyoma from other solid benign gastric tumors, such as neurogenic or fibrous tumors, and from focal gastric malignancies is not usually possible.

Lipoma ■ Lipomas are rare gastric tumors that occur predominantly in the gastric antrum. They are sub-mucosal, produce oval or spherical masses, and may become quite large before causing symptoms.

On CT scans, a gastric lipoma appears as a well-circumscribed antral mass having a CT attenuation value equivalent to that of fat (Fig. 16–44).[68, 106] A comparison of supine and decubitus scans may reveal a change in shape of the soft lipomatous tumor, but the CT finding of gastric mass having a CT density equivalent to fat is pathognomonic for a gastric lipoma and may obviate the need for fiberoptic endoscopy, biopsy, or surgical exploration.

Teratoma ■ Teratomas in the gastrointestinal tract are rare and occur mainly in the pediatric age group. While they are usually derived from all three germ

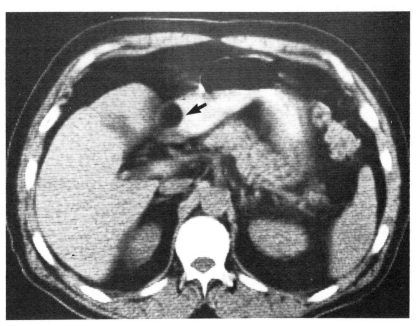

FIGURE 16–44 ■ Gastric lipoma. A rounded antral mass *(arrow)* is present and has a measured CT number of −104 H, equivalent to the CT density of retroperitoneal and perigastric fatty tissue.

layers, the presence of only two germ layers is still adequate for a diagnosis of teratoma to be made. Histologically, gastrointestinal teratomas are similar to gonadal teratomas. They frequently contain skin appendages, cartilage, bone, teeth, adipose tissue, and, less often, glial elements and glandular structures. All reported gastric teratomas have been benign.[107]

The appearance of gastrointestinal teratoma on CT scans is that of a well-marginated mass with one or more cystic components of variable size, frequently containing areas of fat and calcification. Based on these CT criteria, a correct preoperative diagnosis can often be made.[108]

INFLAMMATORY LESIONS

Peptic ulceration can result in thickening of the gastric wall, a condition that is difficult to distinguish from malignancy (Fig. 16–45) unless a CT scan reveals a return of the gastric wall to normal.[71, 72] CT demonstrates gastric ulcers as collections of contrast medium protruding into the gastric wall or as an irregularity of the gastric wall. Following intravenous contrast administration, the inflammatory tissue around the ulcer can show marked contrast enhancement.[109]

Pancreatitis is a very common cause of gastric wall thickening, but distinction from carcinoma invading the pancreas is usually possible by clinical means.

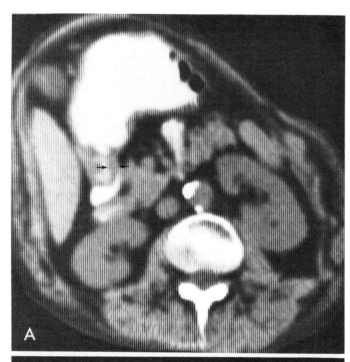

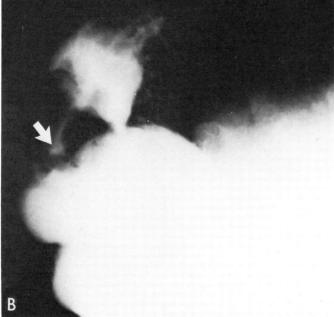

FIGURE 16–45 ■ Peptic ulcer simulating gastric malignancy. *A,* CT scan in right lateral decubitus position. The antrum is circumferentially thickened *(arrows). B,* Upper gastrointestinal series reveals antral narrowing and a small antral ulcer *(arrow).* Follow-up endoscopy documented complete healing of benign gastric ulcer. (From Moss AA, Schnyder P, Candardjis G, Margulis AR: J Clin Gastroenterol 2:401, 1980. Reprinted by permission.)

Occasionally an intramural mass caused by a pseudocyst can be identified.[110]

Eosinophilic granuloma, pseudolymphoma, tuberculosis, syphilis, Crohn's disease, and radiation can produce thickening of the gastric wall simulating gastric malignancy. In immunocompromised patients such as in patients with acquired immunodeficiency syndrome (AIDS), CT may be the most sensitive modality for detecting changes caused by invasive, enteric pathogens such as cytomegalovirus and cryptosporidiosis.[111]

Emphysematous gastritis is a rare infectious gastritis with a grave prognosis. On CT scans it produces a thickening of the gastric wall that contains air bubbles. Associated findings are large amounts of secretions, debris, and gas within the gastric lumen.[112]

Ménétrier's disease is a condition characterized by hyperrugosity, mucosal hypertrophy, and hyposecretion of acid with or without protein loss into the stomach. The rugae are most prominent along the greater curvature, and the antrum is usually spared (Fig. 16–46A).[71] The CT findings of Ménétrier's disease are not completely defined, but a normal gastric

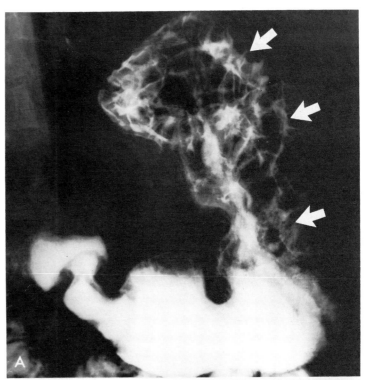

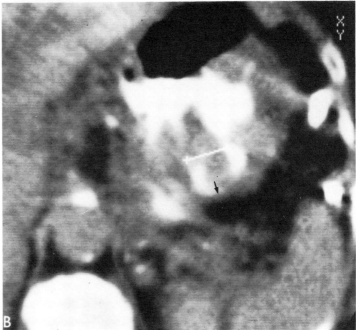

FIGURE 16–46 ■ Ménétrier's disease. *A,* Upper gastrointestinal series reveals thickened folds in fundus and body of stomach *(arrows)* that are particularly prominent along the greater gastric curvature in this view. *B,* CT scan demonstrates elongation and thickening of the rugal folds (measured distance 1.9 cm). Gastric wall measured between folds *(arrow)* is of normal thickness.

wall with elongated and thickening gastric rugae has been described (see Fig. 16–46B).[79]

The *Zollinger-Ellison syndrome* consists of elevated gastric acid secretion and severe upper gastrointestinal ulceration resulting from overproduction of gastrin by a nonbeta islet cell tumor of the pancreas. CT is most frequently employed to detect pancreatic tumors, to screen for metastatic disease, or to evaluate patients having features of multiple endocrine adenomatosis. In patients with the Zollinger-Ellison syndrome, CT has demonstrated the stomach wall to be of normal thickness but has revealed thickening of the rugal folds in some patients (Fig. 16–47).

The use of CT to distinguish thick rugal folds from true thickening of the gastric wall is helpful in differentiating benign from malignant gastric disease. Thickened gastric folds are present in many benign diseases, and the determination that the underlying gastric wall is normal may permit an accurate distinction between benign and malignant gastric disease to be made without surgery.

GASTRIC VARICES

Gastric varices may be seen in any part of the stomach but are seen most frequently in the fundus. Varices may develop in portal hypertension as a result of intrahepatic (cirrhosis) or extrahepatic obstruction, such as in portal or splenic vein occlusion. Intra- or extrahepatic portal vein obstruction leads to gastric and esophageal varices fed mainly by the left gastric (coronary) vein. If the splenic vein is occluded, gastric varices develop by way of short gastric and gastroepiploic veins that drain into the coronary and portal veins, generally without development of esophageal varices. The CT diagnosis of gastric varices is based on the following features:[113]

1. Well-defined clusters of round or tubular soft tissue densities within the posterior and posteromedial wall of the proximal stomach that enhance during contrast administration and are inseparable from the gastric wall.

2. Tubular structures running along the circumference of the gastric fundus, mostly on the posteromedial gastric wall (Fig. 16–48).

3. Other evidence of intra-abdominal collateral venous channels indicating portal hypertension.

In patients with portal hypertension, CT demonstrates umbilical and retroperitoneal varices better than angiography.[114] Angiography is superior for detection of peripancreatic varices and cavernous transformation. Both methods in combination offer more information than either alone in identifying coronary or gastroesophageal, retrogastric, and perisplenic-mesenteric varices. This information is helpful in patient management before and after shunt procedures.

CONGENITAL ABNORMALITIES

Gastric duplication is a rare congenital abnormality of the stomach that is usually located posteriorly on the greater gastric curvature, lined by gastric mucosa, and does not communicate with the lumen of the stomach.[115] Pathologically, the smooth muscle wall of the duplication cyst is contiguous with the gastric wall. The CT findings have ranged from an 11-cm, rounded left upper quadrant cystic mass with marginal calcification[115] to a noncalcified lesion in a child that simulated a renal or suprarenal cyst (Fig. 16–49). Although CT probably is capable of detecting most gastric duplications, distinction from a pancreatic, omental, splenic, or mesenteric cyst adjacent to the stomach is usually not possible.

Gastric diverticula may be acquired or congenital. The congenital form is thought to be caused by herniation of the posterior wall of the gastric fundus through an area of dorsal mesentery before its fusion with the left posterior body wall. After fusion of dorsal mesentery and posterior body wall, the gastric

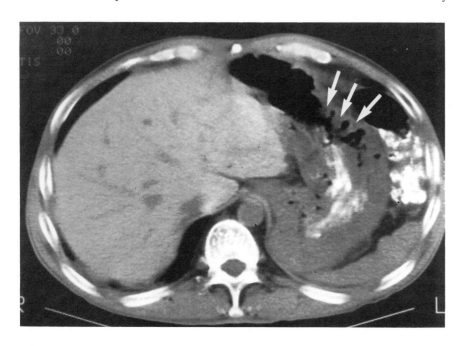

FIGURE 16–47 ■ Zollinger-Ellison syndrome. Thickening of the gastric wall, particularly in the area of the rugae (*arrows*), is noted.

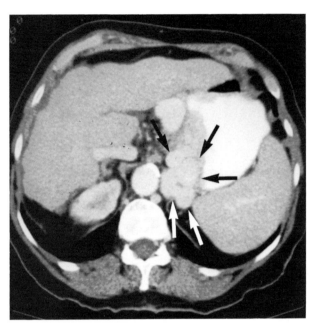

FIGURE 16–48 ■ Gastric varices. Large enhancing varicoid structures are seen in the gastrohepatic ligament *(arrows)*, gastric wall, and posterior to stomach. The liver shows a nodular surface compatible with cirrhosis.

diverticulum becomes trapped within the retroperitoneum. In this position, it lies adjacent to Gerota's fascia and the left adrenal gland and can be confused with an adrenal mass.[116, 117] The differential diagnosis includes adrenal, pancreatic, and renal cyst, duplication cyst, and diverticulum of bowel. In contradistinction to necrotic neoplasms or abscesses, which have thick, shaggy walls with or without gas bubbles, a gastric diverticulum is demonstrated by CT as a thin-walled, cystic-appearing mass having a low-attenuation coefficient.

Small Intestine

Computed tomography has been employed only rarely in the evaluation of small bowel disease, because conventional radiographic procedures, particularly enteroclysis, combine a high degree of diagnostic accuracy with safety and low cost. However, CT has been valuable in recognizing abnormalities of the wall of the small bowel and adjacent mesentery when determining the extent and nature of abnormalities such as Crohn's disease and in detecting and characterizing primary and secondary tumors affecting the small intestine.[118]

Anatomy

The wall of a normal contrast-filled loop of small bowel measures less than 3 mm in thickness. Normally there is no appreciable separation between small bowel loops except by intra-abdominal fat, and the folds of the jejunum and ileum measure no more than 2 to 3 mm in thickness and are feathery in appearance (Fig. 16–50). The small bowel is suspended by a mesentery in which fatty tissue and blood vessels are routinely demonstrated.

MESENTERY AND SMALL BOWEL

The small bowel and its mesentery can be seen on sections at the level of the renal hilum and the aortic bifurcation. The superior mesenteric artery is visualized at the level of the third portion of the duodenum, and to its right is the superior mesenteric vein (see Figs. 16–11 through 16–23). At or near this level, the origin of the inferior mesenteric artery may be seen on the left anterolateral surface of the aorta. The transverse duodenum courses between the aorta and the superior mesenteric artery. If sufficient intraperitoneal fat is present, jejunal and ileal mesenteric

FIGURE 16–49 ■ Gastric duplication cyst. Patient is a 3-year-old child. An oval mass (d) having a CT number of 6 H proved to be a gastric duplication cyst. The duplication simulated an adrenal or upper pole renal mass but was attached along the greater gastric curvature *(arrowheads)*.

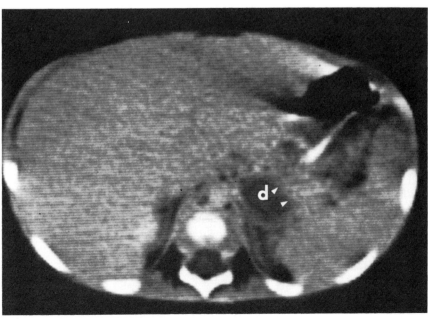

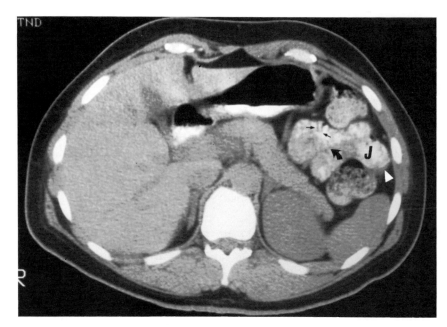

FIGURE 16–50 ■ Normal small bowel. CT scan through the jejunum (J) demonstrates a barely perceptible jejunal wall *(arrowhead),* only slight separation of bowel loops *(curved arrow),* and folds *(small arrows)* that measure less than 3 mm in thickness.

vessels can be identified and appear as round, oval, or short tubular structures.

A multitude of small lymph nodes may be seen surrounding the aorta and the inferior vena cava on high-resolution CT scans. The cecum and the ileocecal valve are demonstrated on lower sections.

Techniques of Examination

In large part the success of a CT examination of the small bowel depends on the degree to which the small bowel is filled with contrast material. To ensure optimal filling, patients are given 400 to 600 mL of a 1 per cent to 2 per cent solution of contrast medium to drink 45 minutes prior to the examination, a second cup with the same amount at 30 minutes, and an additional 250 mL 5 to 10 minutes prior to the CT scan. Administration of the contrast material in distinct phases helps ensure that the proximal and distal portions of the small intestine will be filled with contrast when the CT scans are obtained. Dilute diatrizoate meglumine (Gastrografin) can be employed, but a dilute mixture of barium sulfate (E-Z-CAT) has also proved satisfactory.[119]

If a lesion is suspected in the terminal ileum, pelvis, or right colon, additional time is allowed before the CT scan is obtained to ensure that the region in question contains sufficient contrast material (Fig. 16–51). Preferably, contrast medium is given several hours prior to the CT scan and then again beginning 30 to 45 minutes before the study.[120, 121] Rectal contrast material is given as an enema just prior to the small bowel CT study if the pelvis is also to be examined.[122]

Another method is to use drugs to propel the contrast material into the distal small bowel. Using this approach, the small bowel may be first stimulated by a cholecystokinin-like drug,[123] and immediately before obtaining the CT scan, the gut is paralyzed with glucagon. Metoclopramide (Reglan) is another agent that accelerates the transit time of the contrast material through the small bowel.[124] Reglan is given orally as a 10-mg tablet with the first cup of contrast material at 45 minutes, followed by the same amount of contrast medium at 30 minutes. The increased peristalsis ensuing from the drug subsides by the time the CT examination is performed approximately 30 to 45 minutes later, and glucagon is not needed. However, because of the rapid emptying from the stomach and proximal small bowel, a large cup of oral contrast material must be administered 5 to 10 minutes before the examination to ensure filling of stomach, duodenum, and proximal small bowel loops.

Pathology

TUMORS

Tumors of the small bowel are uncommon, accounting for no more than 6 per cent of gastrointestinal tract neoplasms; about one third are located in the duodenum. Common benign tumors of the small bowel are leiomyomas, adenomatous polyps, and lipomas. Common malignant small bowel neoplasms include adenocarcinomas, leiomyosarcomas (Fig. 16–52), lymphomas, malignant neurogenic tumors such as neurofibrosarcomas, carcinoids, and metastases.[118, 125–128]

Benign tumors appear as intraluminal filling defects without evidence of invasion unless malignant degeneration has occurred. Leiomyomas may be large and either are of homogeneous density or show central areas of low density resulting from necrosis with or without calcifications. Lipomas and lipohyperplasia appear as smooth masses that have characteristic densities.[128–131] Malignant tumors produce

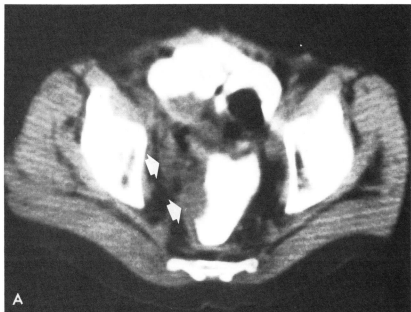

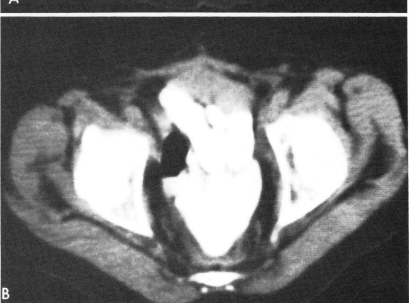

FIGURE 16–51 ■ Technique of delayed CT scans to evaluate a possible pelvic mass. *A,* Initial CT scan. There is a soft tissue density in the pelvis *(arrows)* that could not definitely be identified as bowel. *B,* CT scan 2 hours later. Contrast medium has now filled the area of the suspected mass, proving the mass was really an intestinal "pseudotumor" resulting from unopacified bowel.

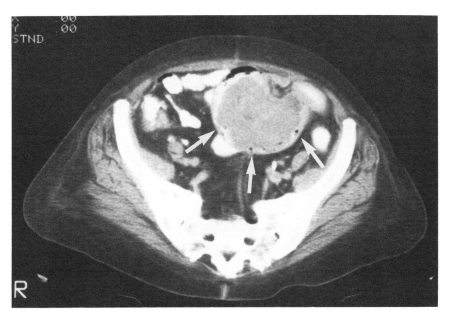

FIGURE 16–52 ■ Leiomyosarcoma of the jejunum. An inhomogeneous mass *(arrows)* associated with an exophytic component is seen that markedly expands the lumen of the jejunum.

thickening of the bowel wall or mesentery (Figs. 16–52, 16–53, and 16–54). In the duodenum, CT frequently is able to determine that a mass arises from the duodenum rather than from pancreas or kidney. At times the CT features may be sufficiently characteristic to enable a specific diagnosis to be suggested. Large, annular, aneurysmally dilated, ulcerated masses associated with bulky adenopathy are typical for lymphoma. Dilated small bowel caused by an annular solid mass with ulceration is seen in adenocarcinoma; a mesenteric mass associated with desmoplastic changes with or without hepatic metastases or lymphadenopathy is typical for carcinoid; a large, locally spreading, bulky inhomogenous and occasionally calcified mass, for leiomyosarcoma; and a well-circumscribed, homogeneous, fat-density mass, for lipoma.[132] Associated features of carcinoid consist of a mass of soft tissue density in the mesenteric fat (see Fig. 16–54) having spiculated margins, retraction of bowel loops toward the mesenteric

mass, and frequently liver metastases. CT scans in patients with small bowel lymphomas may reveal intussusceptions.[133, 134]

Metastatic disease to the small bowel from tumors of the lung, breast, colon,[135] pancreas, kidney, uterus, and skin can produce soft tissue nodules adjacent to or impinging on the bowel lumen, scirrhous lesions, intramural deposits, or polypoid intraluminal masses. Most commonly, the greatest portion of metastatic deposit is located in the mesentery adjacent to the wall of the small bowel (Fig. 16–55), and metastatic lesions often become very large and ulcerate before symptoms are produced. Occasionally, when the greater omentum is diffusely infiltrated, an omental cake may be recognized as an extensive soft tissue mass separating colon or small bowel from the anterior abdominal wall.[136] Serosal implants in the small bowel wall may be missed by CT because of their small size. Although CT is not advocated as a screening method for detecting meta-

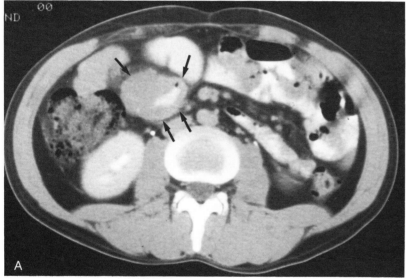

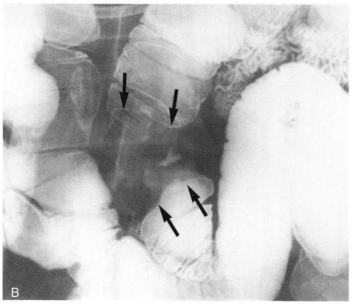

FIGURE 16–53 ■ Lymphoma of the jejunum. A, Marked thickening of a jejunal loop (arrows) with an eccentric component is seen. B, Enteroclysis demonstrates the large mass (arrows).

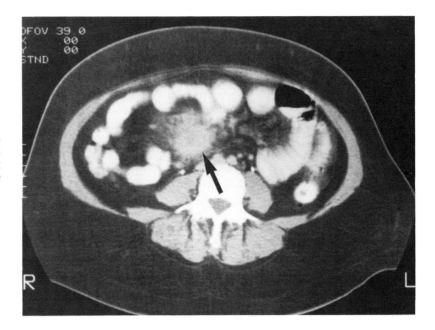

FIGURE 16–54 ■ Carcinoid tumor. The tumor produces a mass *(arrow)* in the mesentery, which has poorly defined margins owing to a fibrotic reaction in the mesenteric fat stimulated by the tumor.

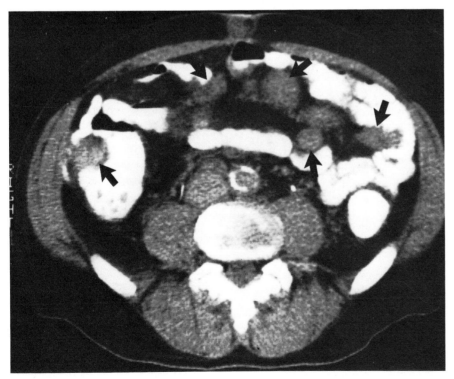

FIGURE 16–55 ■ Metastatic melanoma to the small bowel. The tumor *(arrows)* forms soft tissue masses located in the mesentery adjacent to the wall of the small intestine.

static disease to the small intestine, it provides unique information about extent and location of lesions detected or suggested by other diagnostic techniques.

PSEUDOTUMORS

Unopacified small bowel may appear as a mass lesion anywhere within the abdomen. These small bowel "pseudotumors" are commonly located in the pelvis, in the upper abdomen, or adjacent to the aorta and inferior vena cava, where they appear as enlarged lymph nodes.[122] An unopacified duodenal diverticulum may simulate a pancreatic mass,[137] and a malrotation of the small bowel may suggest a pancreatic tumor, pelvic mass, or intraabdominal neoplasm.[138, 139] Unopacified small bowel can simulate a variety of tumor masses; thus whenever there is doubt as to the nature of an abdominal mass, the area should be rescanned following administration of additional oral contrast medium (see Fig. 16–51).

CROHN'S DISEASE

The diagnosis of Crohn's disease is best made by barium examinations of the small bowel, such as by small bowel follow-through or enteroclysis. However, although conventional barium studies demonstrate the mucosal abnormalities of Crohn's disease very accurately, they only indirectly evaluate the adjacent mesentery and extraluminal extent of disease. In contrast, CT provides information concerning the presence or absence of an extraluminal abscess, degree of mesenteric involvement, the relationship of fistulous tracts to adjacent structures, and the extent of perirectal disease.[118, 140–142]

The most common abnormality detected by CT is thickening of the bowel wall.[143] If the thickened bowel wall is imaged in a transaxial plane, it appears as a thickened sphere with a small dot of contrast material in the center (see Fig. 16–56A,B). When imaged longitudinally, longer segments of thickened bowel wall may be seen (Figs. 16–56C and 16–57).

In patients with Crohn's disease who are suspected of having a frank abdominal abscess, CT is useful to determine whether the separation of bowel loops on barium studies is the result of an abscess or mesenteric and bowel wall thickening. A frank abscess produces a circumscribed mass of fluid density that may contain gas (see Fig. 16–56). Although mesenteric abscesses occur in Crohn's disease, more frequently CT demonstrates fibrofatty proliferation of the mesentery, which is responsible for the mass palpated and identified on barium studies (Fig. 16–58). Fibrofatty proliferation causes the mesenteric fat to increase in density from its normal -100 to -120 H to -40 to -90 H but does not produce CT evidence of a focal mass containing fluid or air.[118, 140, 141]

In one third of patients with Crohn's disease, separation of bowel loops is caused by an ill-defined solid inflammatory mass within the mesentery. Less frequently, a solid mesenteric mass contains contrast material, indicating the existence of a fistulous communication from the bowel to the mesenteric mass

(Fig. 16–59). The full extent of fistulae frequently are best detected by CT, particularly in the perirectal and ischiorectal portions of the fossa.[144] Some enterovesical fistulae may be demonstrated only by CT.

It is clear that CT will continue to play a secondary role in the evaluation of patients with Crohn's disease. However, in patients with active disease, fever, and an abdominal mass, CT is an accurate method for distinguishing among the various causes of the abdominal mass and, by so doing, preventing abdominal surgery except in patients with frank intraabdominal abscesses. Other abnormalities that may not have been suspected initially on clinical grounds can be detected by CT: vascular necrosis of femoral head, sacral osteomyelitis, hydronephrosis, and venous thrombosis.[144, 145]

THICKENED FOLDS

Thickening of the folds of the small bowel to more than 2 mm is a nonspecific abnormality that may be caused by hypoproteinemia, radiation enteritis, inflammatory bowel disease (see Fig. 16–56), Whipple's disease,[146] infectious enteritis,[147] ischemic disease (Fig. 16–60), or an adjacent inflammatory process. The underlying bowel wall may be of normal thickness in patients with ascites and mild hypoproteinemia, but it is frequently thickened in patients with Crohn's disease or infectious enteritis, an adjacent inflammatory mass, or radiation damage.

Patients with overwhelming secretory diarrhea after bone marrow transplantation associated with acute graft-versus-host disease frequently show diffuse wall thickening in small bowel, colon, or mesentery with or without target lesions in the bowel caused by submucosal edema or hemorrhage.[148] In patients who are immunocompromised (e.g., those with AIDS), opportunistic infections of the gastrointestinal tract may be demonstrated on CT scans.[149] CT findings in such infections, which include cryptosporidiosis, cytomegalovirus infection, and tuberculosis, consist of thickening of the mucosal folds and bowel walls of small intestines and colon and additionally, in tuberculosis adenopathy, hepatosplenomegaly, ascites, masses in liver and spleen, and mesenteric thickening ("dirty mesentery"). Frequently, in patients with infections by *Mycobacterium tuberculosis* or *M. avium–intracellulare* (Fig. 16–61), peripancreatic and mesenteric adenopathy is prominent and is often associated with low-attenuation centers.[150]

In patients with documented hypoalbuminemia resulting from cirrhosis, nephrosis, or intestinal lymphangiectasia or in patients with superior mesenteric vein thrombosis, diffuse mesenteric edema may be suggested by CT based on the findings of an increase in density of mesenteric fat, poor definition of segmental mesenteric veins, relative sparing of retroperitoneal fat, and association with subcutaneous edema.[151] In these cases, the root of the mesentery must be carefully evaluated to exclude a focal tumor mass that obstructs mesentery vessels and creates secondary edema. Occasionally, diffuse malignant

Text continued on page 689

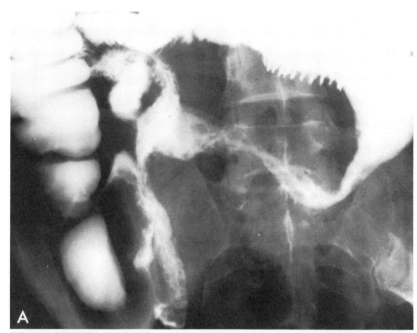

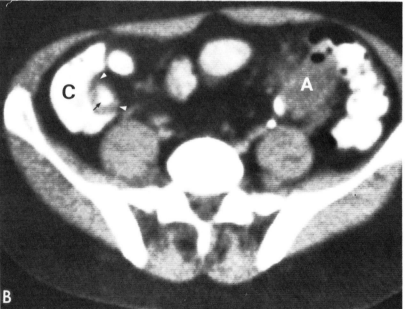

FIGURE 16–56 ■ Crohn's disease; clinical suspicion of abscess. *A,* Small bowel follow-through study. Note narrowing of the terminal ileum with separation of bowel loops. There is mucosal ulceration typical of Crohn's disease. *B,* CT scan. The lumen of the terminal ileum *(arrow)* is imaged in cross section just as it enters the colon (C), and it appears as a dot of contrast material surrounded by the thickened wall of the terminal ileum *(arrowheads).* There is a gas-containing abscess (A) in the mesentery.

Illustration continued on following page

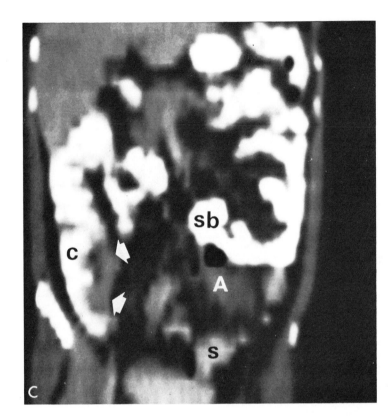

FIGURE 16–56 *Continued* ■ *C,* Coronal reformation of CT scan. The longitudinal extent of the thickened terminal ileum *(arrows)* is better appreciated. The close relationship of the abscess (A) to the small bowel (sb) is also demonstrated. c = Right colon; s = sigmoid colon. (*B* from Goldberg HI, Bore RM, Margulis AR, Moss AA, Baker EL: AJR 140:277, 1983. © 1983, American Roentgen Ray Society. Reprinted by permission.)

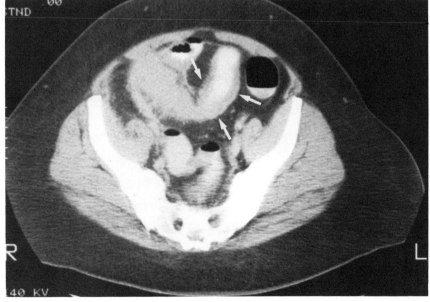

FIGURE 16–57 ■ Crohn's disease of terminal ileum. Thickened ileal walls *(arrows)* are well demonstrated.

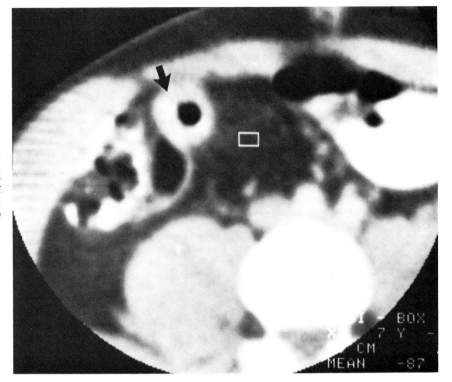

FIGURE 16–58 ■ Crohn's disease with mesenteric fibrofatty proliferation. There is a thickened terminal ileum *(arrow)*, and the mesenteric fat *(box)* has a CT number of −87 H, whereas remaining retroperitoneal fat measures −120 H. There is no evidence of a focal mesenteric mass.

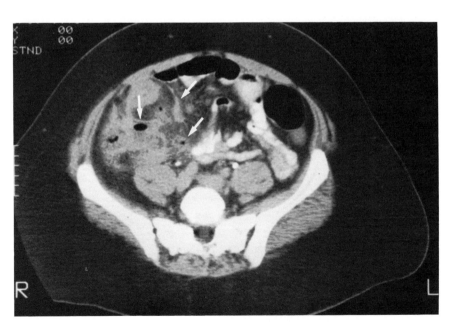

FIGURE 16–59 ■ Crohn's disease. Multiple fistulae *(arrows)* and inflammatory reaction in the mesentery are present in the ileocecal region.

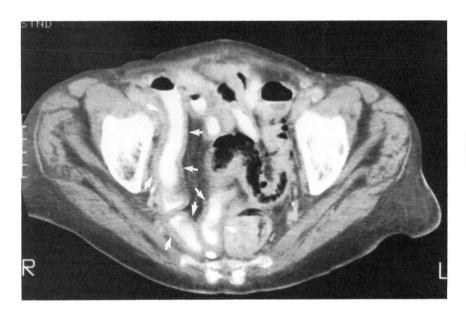

FIGURE 16–60 ■ Ischemia of the ileum. Several loops of ileum in the right pelvis show thickened walls *(arrows)* as a result of ischemic disease involving the ileocolic branch of the superior mesenteric artery.

FIGURE 16–61 ■ Infection with *Mycobacterium avium–intracellulare* in a patient with AIDS. Multiple masses in the mesentery caused by adenopathy compress *(arrows)* the proximal jejunum.

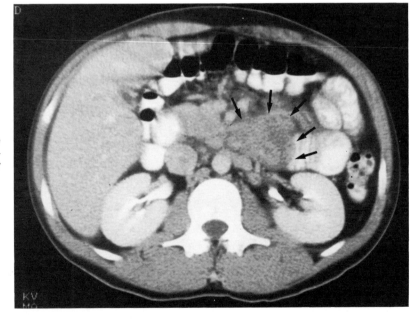

infiltration may create thickening of the mesenteric leaves, which can be distinguished from mesenteric edema by the absence of increased density throughout the mesentery and by the lack of change in prone and decubitus scans. Mesenteric edema frequently is associated with bowel wall thickening.

DIVERTICULAR DISEASE

When duodenal or small bowel diverticula fill with air or contrast material, the CT diagnosis is apparent. However, diverticula may not fill with contrast material or air when the patient is supine, and unfilled diverticula or those that are filled with food or bowel fluid may simulate neoplastic or inflammatory masses.[137, 152] In these cases, additional scans with the patient in the decubitus or prone position usually opacify the diverticulum adequately. Small bowel diverticulitis is a rare entity that frequently is confused clinically with Crohn's disease, appendicitis with abscess, perforated cecal mass, or perforated right-sided diverticulum. Although CT is not diagnostic of ileodiverticulitis, if the abnormality is located in the right lower quadrant, it may suggest an abscess based on the presence of a soft tissue mass and edema of the surrounding mesentery with or without gas in the mass.[153]

OBSTRUCTION

Small bowel obstruction produces dilated loops of small intestine that have thin walls (Fig. 16–62). The obstructed small bowel may be fluid-filled or contain air-fluid levels. Orally administered contrast medium often layers in the most dependent portions of the dilated small intestine (see Fig. 16–62). An obstructed afferent loop can be demonstrated as a U-shaped cystic mass located caudal to the superior mesenteric artery and in direct contiguity with the biliary system.[154–156] CT cholangiography or radionuclide hepatobiliary scanning permits differentiation from a pancreatic pseudocyst by proving contiguity of the afferent loop with the biliary system.

Intussusception of a bypassed jejunoileal segment occurs in 4 per cent of patients following jejunoileal bypass for morbid obesity.[157] As conventional radiographic studies do not visualize the bypassed segment of small bowel, the diagnosis is often missed. CT can identify the intussuscepted bypassed segment of small bowel as a rounded, oval abdominal mass with a "targetlike" appearance.[157–161] The mass has a well-defined, enhancing rim and a low-density center that does not fill with oral contrast.

The mechanism and CT appearance of intussusception have been described.[134] Three concentric circles are formed as the small bowel invaginates. The central portion is the entering layer of the intussusceptum. Just peripheral to this is the entrapped mesentery. Beyond the mesentery is the intussusceptum and intussuscipiens. Features demonstrated by CT include a soft tissue mass containing an eccentric crescent of mesenteric fat, contrast material peripheral to the intussusceptum, and evidence of a leading lesion that is responsible for the intussusceptum.[134]

Closed loop obstruction is a form of mechanical obstruction in which a loop of bowel is occluded at two points along its course. The occluded segments are adjacent to each other, and the cause usually is adhesive bands. CT findings of closed loop obstruction are characteristic and may be more diagnostic than plain films in a patient with sudden onset of severe and constant abdominal pain and a history of surgery. The CT criteria of closed loop obstruction include fluid-filled proximal small bowel loops, abrupt point of transition with collapsed distal intestinal loops, and a grossly distended fluid-filled U-shaped loop with two adjacent limbs showing a zone of abrupt transition of both limbs. If the closed loop is oriented horizontally, it can be recognized on a few CT sections, but if it is oriented vertically, mul-

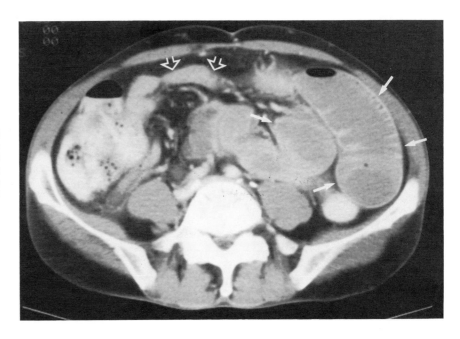

FIGURE 16–62 ■ Obstruction of the distal jejunum caused by an adhesive band. Dilated loops of the jejunum (*solid arrows*) are well demonstrated, but the actual point of obstruction could not be visualized. The ileum (*open arrows*) beyond the obstruction is not distended.

tiple distended fluid-filled rings of decreasing size are seen on multiple sections down to the site of occlusion.[162, 163]

Occasionally a pseudotumor in the small bowel is created by loops of bowel that have altered motility, such as in patients after Whipple's or Billroth II procedures. In these patients, afferent, or Roux-en-Y, loops are isolated from the normal flow of contrast material through the small bowel. In these cases, a CT-guided percutaneous loopogram can help to evaluate suspected pathologic abnormalities in these isolated gastrointestinal loops such as obstruction resulting from strictures or recurrent tumor.[164]

A gallstone ileus may be suggested on CT scans if the three signs of Rigler's triad are demonstrated: multiple dilated loops of bowel filled with gas or fluid; an ectopic, calcified gallstone in the lower abdomen; and a small amount of air in the gallbladder or biliary tree.[165] CT is better able to diagnose air in the gallbladder or biliary tree and faintly or moderately calcified gallstones than plain film radiography.

TRAUMA

Blunt abdominal trauma can injure the small bowel, resulting in bleeding that produces a mass with intraluminal, intramural, and/or mesenteric components.[166–169] The duodenum is the most frequently injured segment of small bowel, with obstruction secondary to a duodenal hematoma being the most common sequela. More severe injury can result in rupture of the duodenum into either the peritoneal cavity or retroperitoneal space.[170]

The duodenal bulb and a small segment of duodenum near the ligament of Treitz lie intraperitoneally, and perforation of these portions of the duodenum usually produces a pneumoperitoneum detectable by conventional radiologic studies. Retroperitoneal rupture of the duodenum is often not apparent on abdominal radiographs,[171, 172] but is evident on CT studies.[170, 173]

Gas and fluid liberated from retroperitoneal duodenal rupture are most frequently confined to the right anterior pararenal space (Fig. 16–63). Trauma can result in rupture of the fascial planes and permits gas to be found either intraperitoneally or in other retroperitoneal spaces. Right perirenal gas usually occurs from a rent in the anterior renal fascia that allows gas to escape from the anterior pararenal space into the perirenal space. The anterior and posterior pararenal spaces join below the apex of the cone of renal fascia at about the level of the iliac crest; below the apex, gas can escape the anterior pararenal space and proceed up to the flank into the properitoneal fat. Because of its greater contrast resolution and tomographic nature, CT can detect small amounts of retroperitoneal gas that are not seen on plain film examinations.

CT is recommended in patients with blunt abdominal trauma who do not require immediate surgery and in patients with suspected iatrogenic trauma resulting from endoscopic duodenal biopsy or sphincterotomy. In this subset of patients, the increased sensitivity of CT to retroperitoneal abnormalities permits the most accurate nonsurgical assessment of the duodenum and surrounding organs.[167] In blunt abdominal trauma, detection of a pneumoperitoneum alone is not diagnostic but is useful for suggesting possible bowel perforation.[168, 169] A dense collection near a bowel loop, the so-called "sentinel clot sign," indicates the source of bleeding.

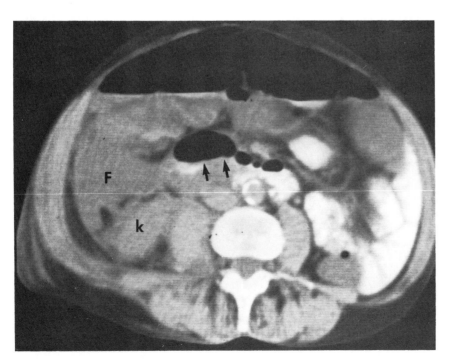

FIGURE 16–63 ■ Duodenal perforation secondary to endoscopic sphincterotomy. CT scan is through the lower pole of the right kidney (k). Fluid (F) and gas *(arrows)* are present in anterior perirenal space. Note the dilated transverse colon with long air-fluid level in the anterior abdomen. At surgery 800 mL of fluid was drained.

ISCHEMIA AND HEMATOMA

Because of the increased general aging of the population, ischemic changes are seen more frequently and intestinal infarction is a common cause of hospital admission among older people. Although these patients usually present with severe abdominal pain, often clinical findings alone are not specific enough for an accurate diagnosis. This fact leads to increased reliance on radiographic evaluation. Plain films and barium or diatrizoate sodium studies of the gastrointestinal tract may not be sufficient. CT demonstrates features that are similar to those seen on plain films: thickening of bowel wall, sometimes resulting in "thumb-printing"; irregular bowel wall; distended fluid-filled bowel loops; portal venous and/or mesenteric venous gas; and intramural air.[174, 175] In addition, CT may detect mesenteric arterial occlusion or extraluminal gas not apparent on the plain films. However, intramural gas is not diagnostic of bowel infarction and may be seen in pneumatosis intestinalis resulting from benign or idiopathic non–life-threatening conditions such as scleroderma. Because CT is used increasingly for evaluation of abdominal pain, CT scans of the elderly patient must be closely analyzed for signs of bowel infarction.

Intramural hematomas in the small bowel may be seen in patients following blunt abdominal trauma (incidence: 50 per cent), in patients under anticoagulation treatment (incidence: 10 per cent), in alcoholic pancreatitis or pancreatic disease (incidence: 10 per cent), and in collagenosis. Intramural bleeding of the small bowel appears as thickening of the bowel wall and valvulae conniventes, similar to the "stack of coins" appearance on small bowel follow-through; as a solid mass of high density; or as a partially cystic mass, frequently with fluid layers if the hematoma is caused by anticoagulation. The density of the bowel wall in an intramural bleed is frequently high (52 to 80 H).[176] If a mass is present in the small bowel without increased density, tumors such as lymphoma or melanoma and inflammatory conditions such as Crohn's disease must be ruled out.

CONGENITAL ABNORMALITIES

Duplication cysts can occur anywhere in the alimentary tract but are most common in the small bowel and esophagus.[177, 178] They are tubular structures lined by epithelium and fibromuscular layers, usually adherent to a segment of small bowel and, rarely, directly communicating with the small intestine. Other congenital anomalies such as deformities in the cervical or thoracic spine or other bowel abnormalities may be associated with duplication cysts. They may be discovered because of pain, a palpable mass, partial or complete bowel obstruction, or occasionally gastrointestinal bleeding. Plain films usually are not diagnostic. Ectopic gastric mucosa is common in duplication cysts of abdomen and chest, and sodium pertechnetate technetium 99m scintigraphy can be used for localization and verification of a duplication cyst. CT may help in demonstrating a cystic nonenhancing mass contiguous to a segment of normal small bowel, but if small bowel obstruction is present, the correct diagnosis is usually difficult to make because of multiple dilated loops of small bowel. For confirmation of a suspected duplication cyst, a CT-guided aspiration biopsy and injection of contrast material into the duplication cyst can be performed.[179]

Colon

Anatomy

The wall of the normal colon (Fig. 16–64) measures 3 mm or less in thickness.[180, 181] Walls measuring between 4 and 6 mm in thickness are considered suspicious; if they are more than 6 mm in thickness, they are considered definitely abnormal, unless it can be determined that the colonic wall was scanned obliquely or that the colon was partially collapsed. The luminal margin is usually smooth, being well outlined on the mucosal side by contrast or air. The outer colonic margin is sharply outlined by surrounding pericolonic fat (see Fig. 16–64). Inflammation adjacent to the colonic wall obliterates the sharpness of the outer colonic margin by increasing the density of the pericolonic fat.

CT scans after resection of a rectal or rectosigmoid tumor and reanastomosis demonstrate a shorter rectosigmoid area and can reveal a slight thickening or irregularity at the anastomotic site (Fig. 16–65). Therefore it is important to obtain a baseline CT scan following surgery to avoid interpreting slight anastomotic irregularity as evidence of recurrence of tumor on later examinations. In patients having total abdominoperineal resections, the bladder extends far posteriorly (Fig. 16–66), and the pelvic fat may be normal or contain linear, streaky densities representing scar tissue (see Fig. 16–66B). The linear nature of scar tissue usually permits scar tissue to be distinguished from recurrent tumor, which generally appears as a globular soft tissue mass.[182, 183] However, scar tissue can be asymmetric, have a rounded shape, and simulate a tumor mass (Fig. 16–67).

PELVIC INLET TO SYMPHYSIS

The midportion of the pelvis is filled with small bowel loops. Laterally the cecum or ascending colon is demonstrated on the right, and the descending colon is on the left (Fig. 16–68). On lower sections, the symmetric piriform muscles extend from the sacrum through the greater sciatic foramen. Immediately anterior to these muscles, the internal iliac arteries and veins are seen. The obturator arteries and veins and the ureters are visible bilaterally, in close proximity to the obturator internus muscles at the lower portion of the ilium and ischium. Occasionally the inferior epigastric vessels can be seen posterior to the rectus abdominis muscle, and the superficial epigastric vessels can be seen in the subcutaneous soft tissue. The sigmoid colon appears as a curved structure that passes posteriorly to the

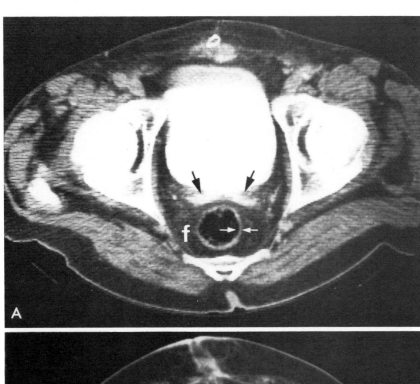

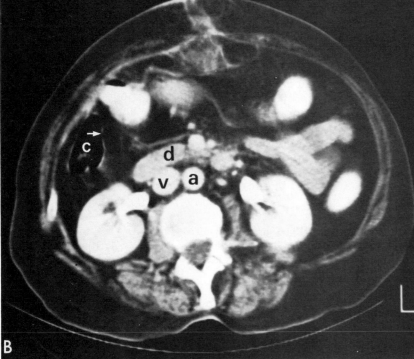

FIGURE 16–64 ■ Normal colon. *A,* Rectosigmoid colon; the wall of the colon *(white arrows)* is less than 1 cm thick. The outer colonic margin is surrounded by pericolonic fat (f), and a clear tissue plane is seen between the colon and seminal vesicles *(black arrows). B,* The ascending colon (c) has a thin wall *(arrow)* and is filled with air. A bolus injection of contrast material demonstrates normal anatomy of the inferior vena cava (v) and aorta (a). d = Duodenum.

FIGURE 16–65 ■ A normal rectosigmoid anastomosis 14 months following resection for carcinoma. The colonic wall is thin *(straight arrows)*, with only a slight posterior irregularity *(curved arrow)* due to to a plication defect at the surgical anastomosis. (From Moss AA, Thoeni RF, Schnyder P, Margulis AR: J Comput Assist Tomogr 5:870, 1981. Reprinted by permission.)

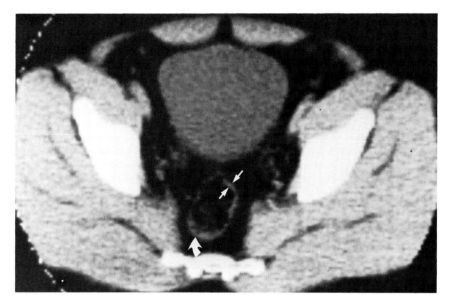

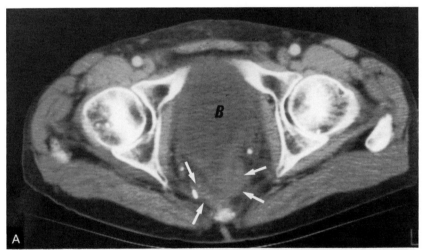

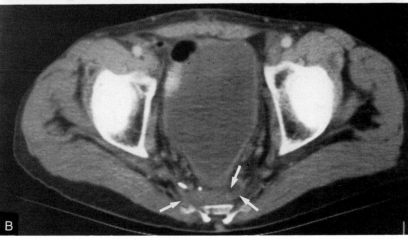

FIGURE 16–66 ■ *A,* Pelvis in a male patient following abdominal-perineal resection. The bladder (B) extends posteriorly, and the seminal vesicles *(arrows)* are displaced dorsally. No scar tissue is present. *B,* Symmetric streaky linear densities *(arrows)* are seen in the presacral space in a patient following an abdominal-perineal resection. No recurrent tumor was found on subsequent studies.

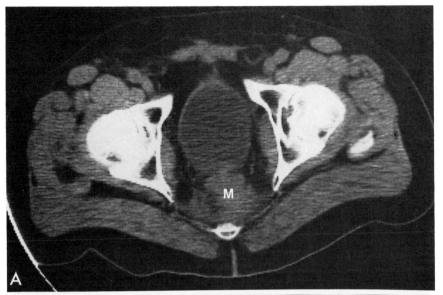

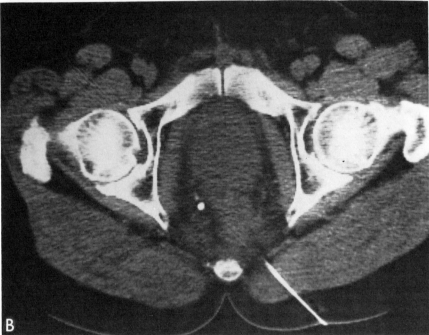

FIGURE 16–67 ■ Scar tissue simulating recurrent tumor. *A*, Globular soft tissue mass (M) is present in the presacral space of a patient 9 months following total abdominal-perineal resection for a primary rectosigmoid carcinoma. *B*, A CT-guided biopsy of the mass revealed extensive scar tissue but no evidence of recurrent tumor. Biopsy findings were confirmed at surgery.

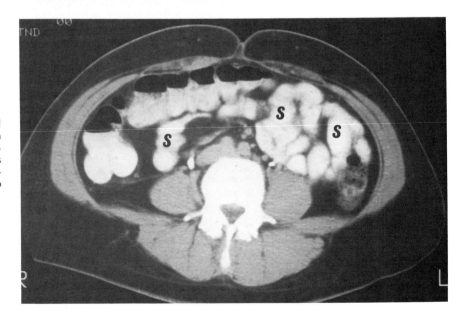

FIGURE 16–68 ■ Oral contrast material given the night before or together with metoclopramide hydrochloride (Reglan) 45 minutes before the examination ensures good filling of proximal and transverse segments of the colon. Contrast (S) is also present in the small bowel.

694

midline to become the rectum in the retroperitoneum.

SYMPHYSIS TO ANAL CANAL

The bladder dome is frequently indented superiorly by small bowel loops, and portions of the sigmoid colon and multiple small bowel loops are seen above the bladder. The rectal ampulla is identified as a round to oval, air-filled structure. Between rectum and bladder, the seminal vesicles are seen as oval or tubular structures. The rectum is surrounded by the perirectal adipose tissue. Lateral and superior to the anal canal, the superior rectal and sacral vessels are demonstrated.

Techniques of Examination

CT scans of patients with suspected colonic tumors are obtained from the dome of the liver to the anal verge. The entire abdomen is scanned, because even though most patients have colonic adenocarcinoma limited to only one area of the colon, a significant number (25 per cent) prove to have disease elsewhere in the abdomen.[180, 184] The entire abdomen and pelvis are also examined after surgery, because liver and lymph node metastases can be detected while the site of the primary tumor remains normal.[185]

Dynamic CT scans are obtained at 1-cm intervals from the tip of the liver through the entire liver toward the dome during injection of a bolus of 150 mL of intravenous contrast material, to allow for optimal differentiation between normal liver parenchyma and possible pathologic changes such as metastases. Following this bolus, dynamic CT scans of the pelvis and remaining abdomen are obtained, starting at the symphysis. Routine scanning is done with the patient supine, but decubitus or prone scans are occasionally performed.

Approximately 45 minutes prior to the examination, patients drink 400 to 600 mL of a 1 per cent to 2 per cent solution of diatrizoate meglumine. They can then be given 10 mg of oral metoclopramide to hasten transit of the oral contrast material through the small bowel so that the distal small bowel and the right colon are opacified. Such an approach is useful for outpatients and for emergency studies in inpatients. Alternatively, 400 to 600 mL of a 1 per cent to 2 per cent solution of diatrizoate meglumine can be given the evening before or 2 to 3 hours prior to the CT study to ensure good filling of the distal small and proximal large bowel (see Fig. 16–68). The more proximal small bowel is opacified by giving a second cup of 500 mL of diatrizoate meglumine approximately 30 minutes before the examination. Immediately prior to the CT study, another 250 mL of a 1 per cent to 2 per cent diatrizoate meglumine or a barium sulfate solution is given to fill the stomach and duodenum. Also, 200 to 500 mL of a 1 per cent diatrizoate sodium solution or air is given as an enema in order to distend the distal colon and rectum and avoid interpreting a normal but collapsed colon as being thickened by tumor or inflammation.

If a rectal enema is contraindicated, 30 mL of undiluted diatrizoate meglumine can be given the night before the examination; this permits complete opacification of the entire colon, with particularly good opacification in the rectosigmoid area.[186] Intravenous contrast material is not routinely given, but fluids are given to ensure that the bladder is adequately distended. The bladder is distended with unopacified urine rather than with intravenous contrast material, because the density of contrast material can obscure slight thickening of the wall of the bladder. A vaginal tampon may be inserted to better identify the vagina and cervix in female patients.

An injection of 1 mg of glucagon permits maximum distention of the rectum and rectosigmoid colon, ensuring accurate delineation, measurement, and staging of small tumors prior to endocavitary radiation.[187] In these patients, a rapid bolus of iodinated contrast material permits better delineation of tumor and bowel wall thickening. Tumors of the transverse colon, colonic flexures, and incompletely distended areas of the large bowel are also better examined following an intravenous injection of glucagon and administration of 500 to 700 mL of air per rectum. The use of glucagon may aid in differentiating an intrinsic colonic tumor from other pathologic conditions, particularly those that are extracolonic in origin, without confusing them with fecal material.[188]

Pathology

CARCINOMA OF THE COLON

More than 100,000 new cases of carcinoma of the colon are identified each year in the United States.[189] Endoscopic and double-contrast radiographic examinations are the primary modalities used to evaluate patients who are suspected of having colonic tumors. Although both of these techniques afford high accuracy, neither permits an assessment of the depths of tumor infiltration or detection of the spread of tumor to distant sites. CT cross sections of the abdomen and pelvis permit precise measurements of the thickness of the colonic wall, determination of the relationship of abdominal and pelvic organs, and detection of the presence of metastases to lymph nodes, adrenal glands, liver, bony structures, or adjacent musculature. The rectum and rectosigmoid are easily evaluated by CT because of the fixed position of these organs in the pelvis; the ascending and descending segments of the colon also can be readily assessed because of their fixed retroperitoneal positions. Tumors in the flexures and transverse colon are less readily examined by CT, because colonic peristalsis and diaphragmatic excursions make these parts of the colon more difficult to evaluate.

Although CT offers many advantages for obtaining information about the extent of tumor in and beyond the colonic wall,[190] CT is not the primary modality for evaluating patients with suspected tumors of the colon. Early and subtle changes of the mucosal surface and lesions less than 6 mm in diameter are usually not detected by CT because of retained fecal material and incomplete distention of parts of the large bowel. However, an aggressive diagnostic approach that includes pretherapy staging of advanced colonic malignancies can enable the most appropriate treatment regimen to be planned. Pretherapy staging is useful in patients in whom resection of the tumor is not immediately feasible but may become possible after irradiation, in patients with suspected advanced disease in whom a decision for or against extensive abdominal surgery needs to be made, and in patients who may benefit from local endocavitary irradiation.[180, 187]

Following surgery, evaluation of the surgical site is important, as local recurrence of colonic carcinoma after surgery is not uncommon.[191] In a study of 280 patients with complete resection of primary adenocarcinoma of the colon, Cass and associates[192] showed that 105 patients (37 per cent) had recurrence of the tumor within the first 2 years after surgery. Among these 105 patients, 60 per cent had local recurrence alone, 14 per cent had concomitant local recurrence and distant metastases, and 26 per cent had isolated distant metastases. In 92 per cent of the patients with local recurrences, the recurrent tumor was contiguous to the operative area of the incision. In postsurgical patients CT has proved to be most valuable in assessing the success of therapy, in determining the presence or absence of recurrence, and in designing radiation ports for patients having recurrent tumors that are unresectable.[181, 182, 185, 190, 191]

Because of the high frequency of tumor recurrence in the first 24 months after surgery, a series of follow-up CT examinations has been recommended to detect early tumor recurrence. In addition, a CT scan should be obtained whenever a patient is found to have a rising carcinoembryonic antigen (CEA) titer.

The staging of colonic tumors has been most frequently based on Dukes' classification[193] or a modification thereof.[194] However, because CT is unable to determine whether a tumor is localized to the mucosa or extends to the muscularis, CT staging is based on an analysis of thickness of the colon wall and the presence or absence of tumor spread to adjacent and distant organs.[195] The size of a recurrent or primary colon tumor can be measured and the tumor placed into one of the following four stages depending on the CT findings[195] (Table 16–5):

TABLE 16–5 ■ CT Staging of Primary and Recurrent Colonic Tumors

Stage I	Intraluminal polypoid mass without thickening of colonic wall.
Stage II	Thickened colonic wall (>6 mm) or pelvic mass without invasion of adjacent organs or extension to pelvic sidewalls.
Stage IIIA	Thickened colonic wall or pelvic mass with invasion of adjacent muscles and/or organs.
Stage IIIB	Thickened colonic wall or pelvic mass extending to pelvic sidewalls and/or abdominal wall.
Stage IV	Metastatic disease with or without local abnormality.

1. An intramural mass without thickening of the wall of the colon is classified as a *stage I* tumor (Fig. 16–69).

2. A *stage II* carcinoma produces thickening of the colonic wall to greater than 6 mm without invasion of adjacent organs (Fig. 16–70).

3. Tumors invading adjacent pelvic muscles or organs but not extending to the pelvic sidewalls are considered *stage IIIA* (Figs. 16–71 and 16–72). If a rectal or sigmoid carcinoma reaches the pelvic sidewalls, it is considered *stage IIIB* (Fig. 16–73). Adenopathy may or may not be present.

4. *Stage IV* colonic carcinoma has spread to distant sites within the body (Fig. 16–74).

Extracolonic tumor spread is suggested by loss of tissue fat planes between the large bowel and surrounding muscles (levator ani, obturator internus, piriform, coccygeal, and gluteus maximus). However, invasion is definite only when a tumor mass extends directly into an adjacent muscle, obliterating the fat plane and enlarging the individual muscle (see Fig. 16–73). Spread to contiguous organs in the pelvis can be simulated by the absence of tissue planes between the viscera and the tumor mass without actual invasion. Therefore invasion should be cautiously diagnosed and considered definite only if a major portion of the viscera is enveloped or if an obvious mass involves an adjacent organ (Figs. 16–73, 16–75, 16–76, and 16–77). Distinction between tumor infiltration of adjacent muscle and simple absence of fat separating normal structures is particularly difficult in the area of lower rectum and anal verge.

Primary and recurrent colonic cancer can invade the seminal vesicles, sciatic nerves, prostate, bladder, uterus, and ovaries and can produce hydronephrosis by obstructing the ureters. Occasionally tumors of the prostate, uterus, or ovaries that invade or are contiguous with the rectum or sigmoid colon can be indistinguishable from an invasive colonic neoplasm. Tumor necrosis is suggested by areas of low attenuation within the mass, and tumor calcifications indicate a mucinous adenocarcinoma.

Colonic tumors can destroy adjacent bone. Destruction most frequently involves the sacrum and coccyx, but large tumors can involve the ilium. When advanced, invasion of bone is easily diagnosed by identifying destruction of bone and evidence of a soft tissue mass adjacent to and within bone. However, minor invasion of bone can be diagnosed only if cortical destruction is seen.

Liver metastases are usually recognized as areas of low attenuation before contrast enhancement, although foci or calcification can be seen within metastatic mucinous adenocarcinomas (Fig. 16–78). Following a bolus injection of contrast material, the CT density of hepatic colonic metastasis can change rapidly. The metastatic deposits often show early rim enhancement or become uniformly hyperdense, go through an isodense phase, and finally again become

Text continued on page 702

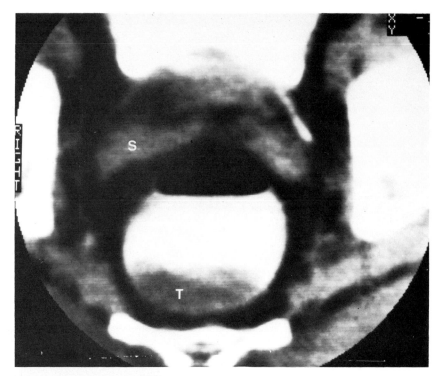

FIGURE 16–69 ■ Stage I rectal carcinoma. An intraluminal tumor mass (T) without thickening of the bowel wall is present in a patient with a primary adenocarcinoma of the rectum. S = Seminal vesicles.

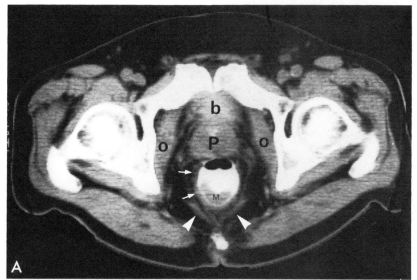

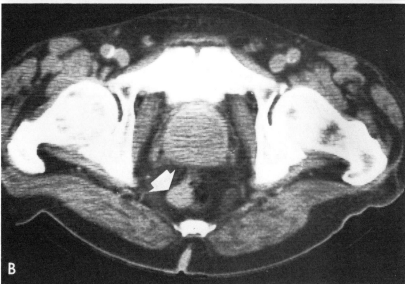

FIGURE 16–70 ■ Stage II rectal carcinoma. *A,* Thickening of the posterolateral rectal wall *(arrows)* and an intraluminal mass (M) are present in a patient with primary adenocarcinoma of the rectum. The perirectal fat planes are preserved. The levator muscle *(arrowheads)* is not invaded. The prostate (P) is slightly enlarged. b = Bladder; O = internal obturator muscle. *B,* Recurrent rectal carcinoma detected 3 months after resection. A polypoid mass 2 × 2 cm in dimensions *(arrow)* is demonstrated along the right posterolateral wall of the rectum. The thickness of the uninvolved rectal wall is normal. There is no invasion of adjacent organs or pelvic sidewalls.

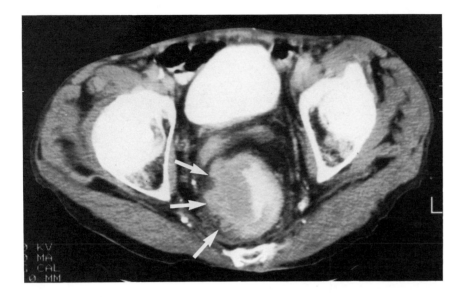

FIGURE 16–71 ■ Stage IIIA rectal carcinoma. An irregular mass is noted to primarily occupy the right lateral wall with extension beyond the outer margins *(arrows)*.

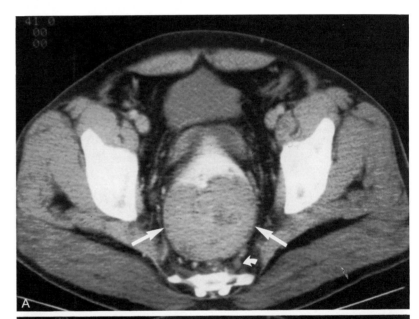

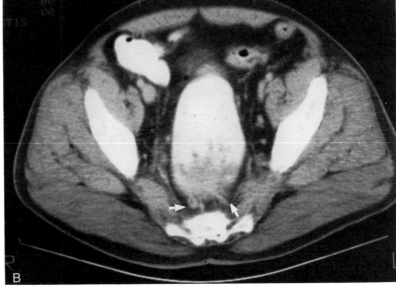

FIGURE 16–72 ■ Stage IIIA colonic carcinoma. *A,* A large mass in the rectum *(straight arrows)* is noted. In addition, a small (5-mm) node *(curved arrow)* is present posteriorly. *B,* On a higher section, the tumor mass is noted to extend beyond the rectal wall *(arrows)* but not to the pelvic sidewall.

698

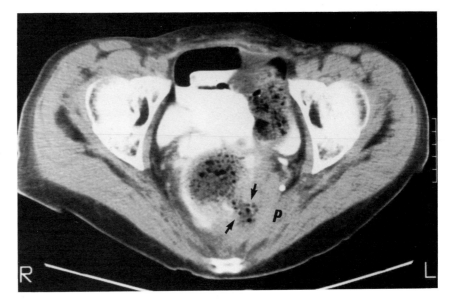

FIGURE 16–73 ■ Stage IIIB rectal carcinoma. Extension of tumor beyond the left lateral rectal wall with perforation *(arrows)* and invasion of the piriformis muscle (P), which appears thickened, is well demonstrated.

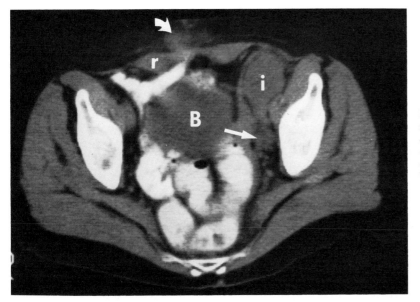

FIGURE 16–74 ■ Stage IV colonic carcinoma. Metastatic spread of recurrent rectal carcinoma *(curved arrow)* has occurred to the subcutaneous tissue, abdominal rectus muscle (r), obturator *(straight arrow)*, and external iliac lymph nodes (i). Liver metastasis was seen on scans at a more cephalic level. B = Bladder.

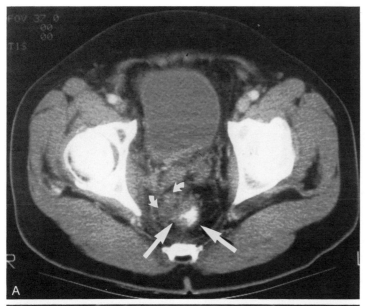

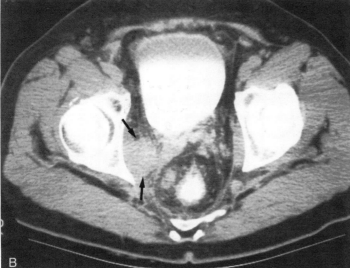

FIGURE 16–75 ■ Local recurrence of stage IIIB rectal tumor following AP resection and reanastomosis. *A,* Thickening of rectal wall caused by tumor recurrence *(straight arrows)* and adenopathy *(curved arrows)* are noted. *B,* The right obturator vein *(arrows)* is enlarged because of tumor invasion.

FIGURE 16–76 ■ Stage II recurrent rectal tumor. The tumor, mostly with extrinsic mass *(arrows),* is seen elevating the bladder floor. Patient had undergone a hysterectomy previously.

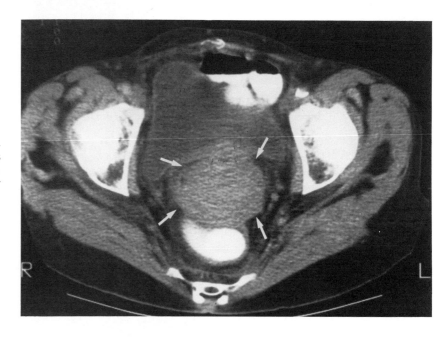

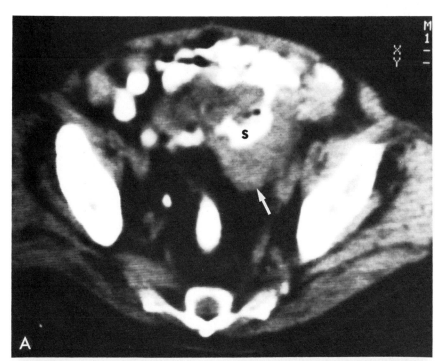

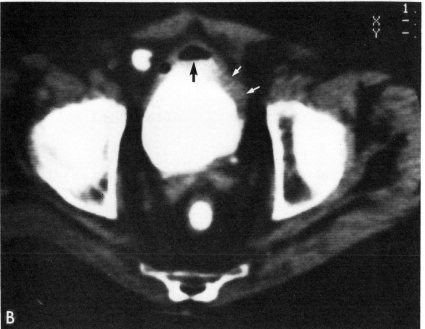

FIGURE 16–77 ■ Sigmoid carcinoma producing colovesical fistula. *A,* A large carcinoma *(arrow)* of the sigmoid colon (s) extends beyond the bowel wall. *B,* The bladder wall is thickened *(white arrows)* by tumor, and an air-fluid level is present *(black arrow)* in the bladder. Surgery confirmed a colovesical fistula.

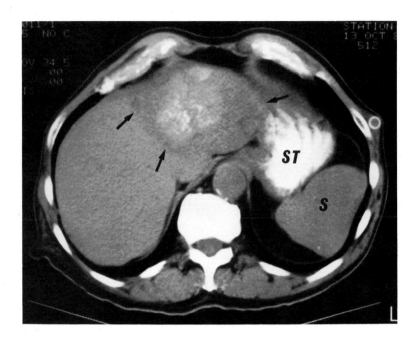

FIGURE 16–78 ■ Metastases from colon carcinoma. A large low-density lesion with multiple small calcifications is noted in the left lobe of the liver *(arrows).* S = Spleen; ST = stomach with partially collapsed gastroesophageal junction.

low-density lesions. Optimal bolus technique is necessary to avoid false-negative results with metastases that have become isointense with normal liver parenchyma. When hepatic metastasis is detected that is confined to one hepatic lobe or segment, an aggressive approach appears warranted, because an improved 5-year survival rate has been demonstrated after removal of metastatic foci.[196] Selective catheterization and intraarterial chemotherapy of the liver are also used. Adrenal metastasis occurs in up to 14 per cent of patients with colon carcinoma, producing enlarged, often inhomogeneous, adrenal glands. Generally rectal or rectosigmoid carcinoma metastasizes to lymph nodes along the external iliac arteries and to the inguinal and paraaortic chains (see Fig. 16–74). Occasionally metastasis to portal hepatic nodes occurs.

Lymph nodes measuring larger than 1.5 cm in diameter in the abdomen and 1 cm in the pelvis are considered abnormal, but although asymmetry and size can be used to determine lymph node abnormality, the pathologic nature of the enlargement cannot be absolutely determined by CT.[197] Benign as well as malignant disease can produce lymphadenopathy, and only lymphangiography or guided biopsy can give a definite diagnosis. Many metastatic foci are found in normal-sized lymph nodes (<1 cm) that cannot be considered abnormal by CT criteria.

Although interpretation of CT scans in patients with colonic tumors is usually not difficult, there are potential pitfalls in accurate interpretation.[198] CT scans obtained during or soon after surgery or irradiation can demonstrate edema or hemorrhage of the pelvic structures that simulates recurrent neoplasm. Chronic radiation changes in the pelvis[182, 183, 198] may be difficult or impossible to distinguish from colonic tumors without CT-guided biopsies (Fig. 16–79). Benign bony defects can simulate metastatic foci, and

nonopacified bowel loops can be mistaken for a tumor mass. Perforation of a colonic cancer can result in an inflammatory mass or abscess, which makes diagnosis of the underlying cancer difficult (Fig. 16–80).[199]

Little information is available about the detection and staging of tumors in the cecum and ascending, transverse, and descending segments of the colon.[200–202] Most tumors in these areas are easily demonstrated (Figs. 16–81 and 16–82), but no investigation has analyzed these lesions in detail.

CT Accuracy ■ Computed tomography has been reported to have a wide range of accuracy rates (47.5 per cent to 100 per cent) in detecting and staging primary and recurrent rectal and rectosigmoid tumors.[180, 181, 185, 190, 191, 200–207] Reports that appeared early after CT became available showed a very high accuracy, which was largely because of the more advanced cases in these series. For primary colon cancer, CT is more accurate in showing extensive invasion of surrounding tissue and distant metastases, such as those in liver and adrenals, than in demonstrating local adenopathy or minimal tumor extension. CT frequently understages patients with microinvasion of pericolonic or perirectal fat or small tumor foci in normal-sized nodes. In one study, the sensitivity and specificity of local extension of tumor were 61.2 per cent and 80.6 per cent, respectively, whereas sensitivity and specificity for detection of lymph node metastases were 25.9 per cent and 96 per cent, respectively.[203]

At present CT remains the best modality for the detection and staging of recurrent rectal or rectosigmoid carcinomas, because almost all recurrent tumors in patients with sphincter-saving resection of rectal and rectosigomoid carcinomas develop extraluminally, infiltrating the suture lines secondarily, with tumor extension beyond the bowel confines in

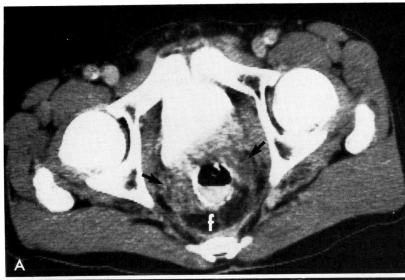

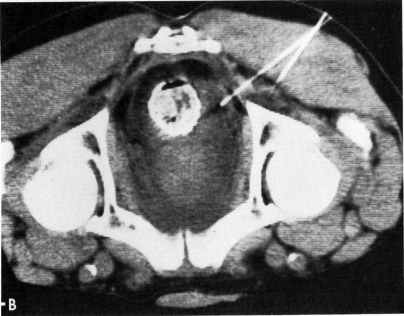

FIGURE 16–79 ■ Radiation change simulating recurrent tumor. *A,* There is an increased density in the anterior perirectal soft tissue *(arrows)* that cannot be distinguished from recurrent tumor. f = Posterior perirectal fat. *B,* CT-guided biopsy of perirectal tissues. Final diagnosis: fibrofatty proliferation as a result of radiation damage.

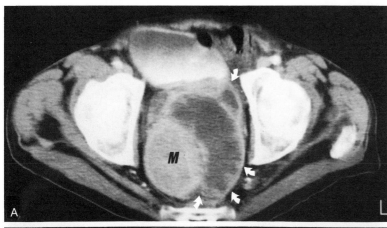

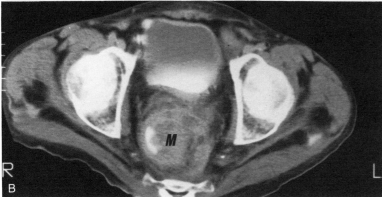

FIGURE 16–80 ■ Stage IIIA rectal carcinoma with perforation. *A,* A large rectal tumor (M) with perirectal abscess *(curved arrows)* is present. *B,* A large tumor mass (M) remains after abscess drainage and radiation. Soft tissue strands in left lateral and posterior perirectal space may represent tumor, scar, or radiation change.

FIGURE 16–81 ■ Carcinoma of cecum. An apple core lesion is well demonstrated *(arrows).*

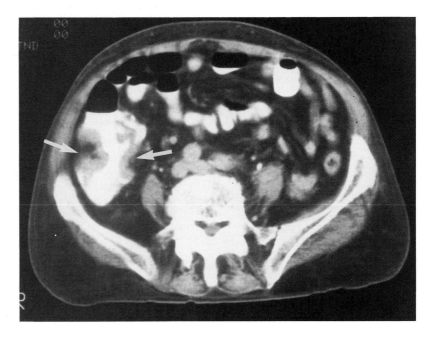

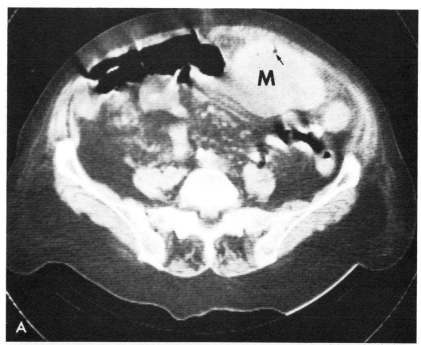

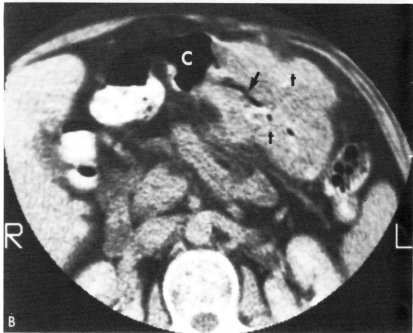

FIGURE 16–82 ■ Carcinoma of the transverse colon. *A,* CT scan reveals a large soft tissue mass (M) that contains a focus of gas *(arrow).* At surgery a perforated carcinoma of the transverse colon was found. *B,* A large tumor mass (t) thickens the wall and narrows the lumen *(arrow)* of the distal portion of the transverse colon. The wall of the proximal transverse colon (C) is normal.

one fourth of all cases.[204] For accurately staging these patients, CT is superior to endoscopy and barium examinations, both of which permit the diagnosis of recurrence and show mucosal detail to better advantage than CT. However, without careful distention of colon using rectal contrast material and glucagon, some of the local recurrences may be missed by CT.[205] Although colonoscopy and barium enemas provide information on local disease, CT is able to accurately show recurrence remote from the anastomotic side. In patients with complete anteroposterior resections, CT is the only modality for evaluating recurrent tumor. Therefore barium enema and CT are complementary methods for evaluating patients with suspected recurrent colonic tumor. Definition of full extent of disease, particularly to distant sites, is necessary if repeat resection is contemplated. Several studies have demonstrated that liver function tests and CEA levels are unreliable indicators of recurrent disease,[203, 204] unless a sudden rise in the CEA level is observed and other causes of CEA level rises can be excluded.

Role of CT in Patient Management ■ CT may aid in the differential diagnosis of focal masses by changing the diagnosis or by increasing diagnostic confidence. However, CT is more valuable than any other modality in demonstrating the extent of disease, particularly in the late stages, and by doing so, altering patient management.[208]

Because of the inherent limitations of CT in recognizing microinfiltration of tumor into pericolonic tissue and small metastatic foci in normal-sized nodes, CT should not be used for routine staging of primary colonic tumors. However, CT is helpful in differentiating between patients with initially inoperable tumors who would benefit from preoperative radiation and subsequent attempted curative surgery and those patients in whom only palliative surgery can be performed. It is also helpful for recognizing

patients who could undergo endocavitary radiation to save the rectum.

Because local recurrence of cancer occurs in 50 per cent of patients within the first year and in 80 per cent within the second year, it is recommended that patients undergo a baseline study 2 to 3 months after initial surgery, when postsurgical acute changes such as edema and hemorrhage have cleared, and follow-up examinations every 6 months during the first 2 years and then at yearly intervals (Fig. 16–83). These follow-up examinations should be compared with the baseline study to avoid unnecessary biopsies. A study is considered positive if a mass or nodes are detected that were not seen on the baseline study or that have enlarged since the original study. Any new mass or nodes should be biopsied using a transgluteal percutaneous approach in the case of rectosigmoid tumor masses.[207] Although CT should not be used as the primary modality for examining patients with suspected colonic tumors, CT represents the best method, short of performing surgery, for reliably assessing the presence or absence of recurrent colonic tumors, particularly in patients with abdominal-perineal resections. This is particularly important in men, in whom a recurrent mass cannot be easily palpated following complete anteroposterior resection of a rectal tumor. In women recurrent masses frequently can be examined through a vaginal approach.

As CT is used more frequently to follow patients with resected colonic tumors, it is probable that small tumor recurrences will be detected. However, it remains to be seen whether the detection and staging of these recurrent tumors by CT will ultimately improve the overall 5-year survival rate of these patients.

Metastatic Tumors ■ Pelvic and abdominal masses caused by tumors of the uterus, ovary, prostate, bladder, pancreas, kidney, stomach, retroperito-

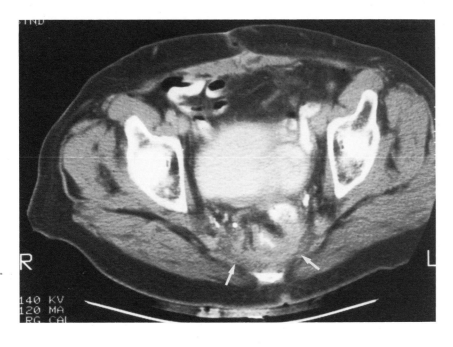

FIGURE 16–83 ■ Marked increase in perirectal tissue (arrows) as a result of postsurgical changes 11 months after surgery.

neum, or mesentery can displace, invade, or constrict the colon.[209, 210] In most instances CT is able to demonstrate the organ in which the tumor arises, but in some patients it is impossible to distinguish direct invasion of the colon by an adjacent neoplasm from a colonic tumor invading a nearby organ unless a needle biopsy is performed. It is important to remember that in 3 per cent to 8 per cent of women operated on for colorectal carcinoma, ovarian metastases are found.[210] Such metachronous ovarian metastases after resection of colon cancer are particularly common in premenopausal women in the fifth decade. Therefore if a primary or recurrent colonic tumor is suspected, the ovaries must be carefully evaluated on CT examinations. Also, if a malignancy in the ovary is suspected clinically, the stomach and colon should be carefully examined on the CT scans, as well as on gastrointestinal barium studies, to rule out Krukenberg's tumors.

BENIGN TUMORS

Benign lesions of the colon such as hyperplastic polyps or adenomatous polyps usually are not examined by CT. These are demonstrated by barium examinations or endoscopy and are seen during CT examinations only incidentally. CT may detect benign tumors when they become very large. One published report suggested that villous adenomas have a characteristic CT appearance based on their high mucus content.[211] Villous adenomas are seen as solid mass lesions containing a homogeneous water density (<10 H) component that occupies more than half of the lesion. The water density mass is eccentrically positioned an the luminal side of the villous adenoma.[211] No air-fluid level is seen, and the lesion should not have a round cystic configuration. When using CT to evaluate a suspected villous adenoma, oral or rectal contrast material should not be used.

Occasionally, anorectal giant condyloma acuminatum (Buschke-Löwenstein tumor) can be detected on CT scans as an infiltrating mass with a cauliflower-like appearance on the surface and infiltration of the subcutaneous tissue and perirectal fascial planes.[212] In some cases, rectal wall thickening and narrowing of the lumen are also seen. CT is useful in accurately demonstrating the exact location and extent of the lesion. The inherently invasive lesion may show malignant degeneration histologically. CT is used in these cases to preoperatively stage the lesions and determine the type of surgical approach and extent of resection needed. Although the morphology of the lesion is accurately appreciated, CT does not discriminate among different histologic types of soft tissue infiltration. Therefore inflammatory and fibrotic induration associated with the condyloma and benign or malignant tumor infiltration have generally similar CT characteristics.

INFLAMMATORY DISEASES

Computed tomography can detect abnormalities of the colon produced by granulomatous or ulcerative colitis[213, 214] (Figs. 16–84 and 16–85), amebiasis (Fig. 16–86), pseudomembranous colitis,[215] ischemia[174, 216] (Figs. 16–87 and 16–88), and appendicitis. Abdominal or pelvic abscesses and fistulae[217, 218] with or without abscess formation and colonic perforation,[199] can be detected and related to adjacent structures (see Fig. 16–86). In patients with Crohn's disease, the degree of thickening of the bowel (see Fig. 16–84) and mesentery can be assessed, fistulous tracts around a stoma detected (Fig. 16–89), and abscesses identified that cannot be demonstrated by conventional studies. Barium studies have been and remain the most effective radiographic technique for establishing the diagnosis of inflammatory bowel disease, and CT is reserved for cases in which displacement of bowel loops seen on barium studies must be elucidated first or if complications such as extent of fistulae or abscesses must be assessed. Appendiceal abscesses appear as well-demarcated fluid collections in the right lower abdominal quadrant or pelvis.

Pneumatosis coli is diagnosed by demonstrating gas within a colon wall of normal thickness (Fig. 16–90). When pneumatosis coli is caused by ischemia, gas may also be seen in the portal venous system (Fig. 16–91). A thick colon wall is also seen in patients with an edematous colon related to cirrhosis, hypoproteinemia, ascites, ischemia, or a local inflammatory process such as pancreatitis.

Neutropenic colitis, also called *typhlitis* or *necrotizing enteropathy*, is an infectious condition associated with severe neutropenia. It is a complication of acute leukemia, aplastic anemia, or cyclic neutropenia. The cecum is most commonly involved, but other portions of the colon or the terminal ileum also may be affected. In patients with typhlitis, CT shows thickening of the cecal wall or other bowel areas with attenuation similar to that of normal bowel wall or with areas of low density as a result of edema, hemorrhage, necrosis, or even pneumatosis.[219, 220] The thickening of the cecal wall is caused by mucosal ulcerations resulting from ischemia, which may be related to distention of the bowel alone and may be increased by intramural hemorrhage and the effects of steroids, antimetabolites, and folic acid antagonists. The damaged mucosa is then penetrated by bacteria, viruses, and fungi, which grow profusely in the absence of neutrophils. All these changes lead to the wall thickening observed on CT scans. Frequently the remaining bowel loops are distended because of a paralytic ileus. Decrease of wall thickening on follow-up examinations indicates recovery from neutropenic colitis. CT is useful in patients with leukemia and nonspecific symptoms of abdominal pain, nausea, and vomiting (which could be considered side effects of chemotherapy), because in these instances, recognition on CT scans of thickened cecal wall permits timely and effective medical and surgical management.

CT is helpful in patients with perirectal inflammatory disease and suspected perirectal abscesses.[221] Such abscesses also can be seen in patients following corrective surgery for Hirschsprung's disease[222] or after total colectomy and ileoanal anastomosis with

Text continued on page 713

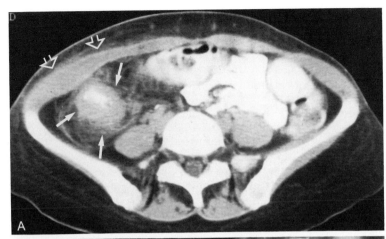

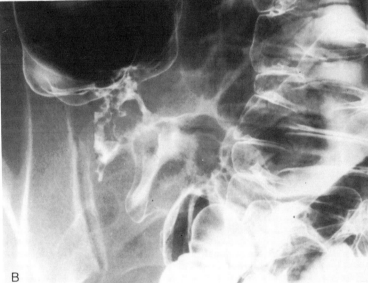

FIGURE 16–84 ■ Crohn's disease of ileocecal area and abdominal wall abscess. A, Thickening of cecal wall with pericolonic inflammation (solid arrows) and thickened anterior abdominal wall (open arrows) is identified. B, A double-contrast barium enema shows dilated terminal ileum and several fistulae.

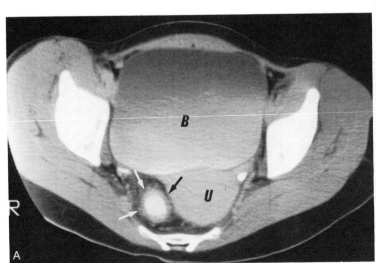

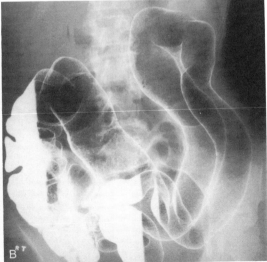

FIGURE 16–85 ■ Ulcerative colitis. A, A thickened rectal wall (arrows) with only minor perirectal inflammation is seen. U = Uterus; B = bladder. B, Double-contrast barium enema in the same patient shows acute ulcerative colitis with a granular mucosal pattern.

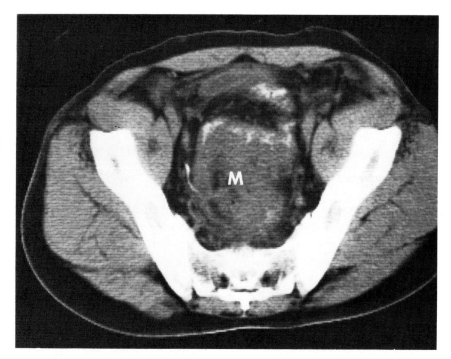

FIGURE 16–86 ■ Amebiasis producing a large soft tissue mass (M) in the presacral space. The wall of the colon appears irregular and cannot be separated from the mass. Differentiation from a primary adenocarcinoma or a paracolic abscess caused by diverticulitis is not possible. Final diagnosis: paracolonic abscess resulting from amebiasis.

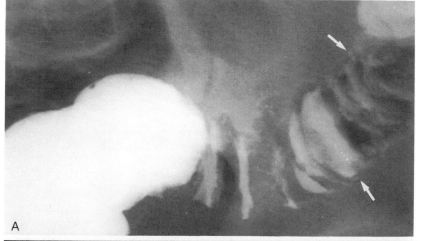

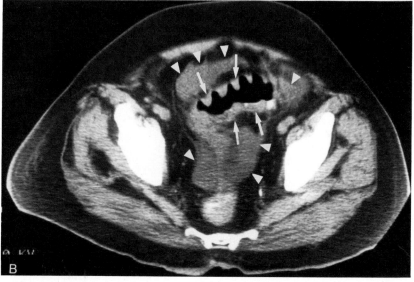

FIGURE 16–87 ■ Ischemic colitis. *A,* The diatrizoate sodium (Hypaque) enema shows marked thickening of haustra in sigmoid colon and mucosal ulcerations *(arrows). B,* CT scan shows thickening of the colonic wall and haustra *(arrows)* and ascites *(arrowheads)* in a patient with renal cell carcinoma who was being treated with chemotherapy and phenylephrine hydrochloride (e.g., Neo-Synephrine).

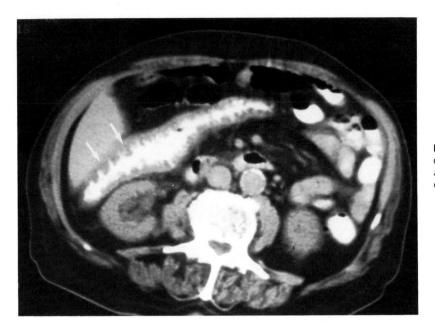

FIGURE 16–88 ■ Ischemic colitis. The CT scan demonstrates markedly thickened hepatic flexure and transverse colon, with diatrizoate meglumine outlining typical thumbprinting *(arrows)*.

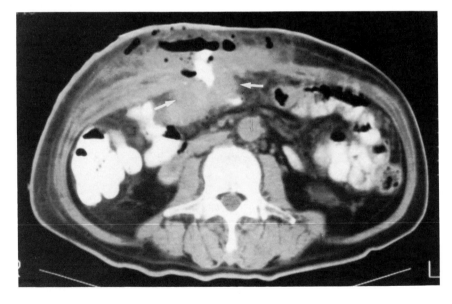

FIGURE 16–89 ■ Multiple bubbles and soft tissue strands are seen in the subcutaneous tissue of a patient with Crohn's disease and fistulae. Also, the colonic wall *(arrows)* is thickened at the stoma site.

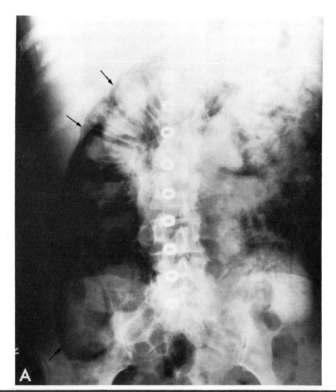

FIGURE 16–90 ■ Pneumatosis coli of the ascending colon. *A,* Plain abdominal radiograph reveals gas *(arrows)* in the wall of the ascending colon. The colonic wall is of normal thickness. *B,* CT scan photographed at wide window width demonstrates gas (g) in the wall of the right colon (C), which is filled with contrast material. A small amount of air *(arrow)* is present in the retroperitoneal tissue.

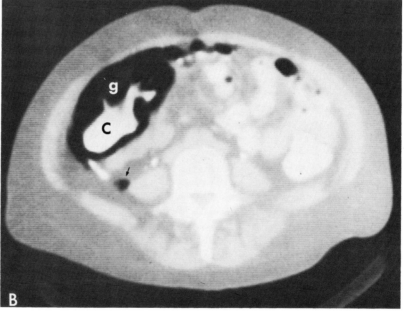

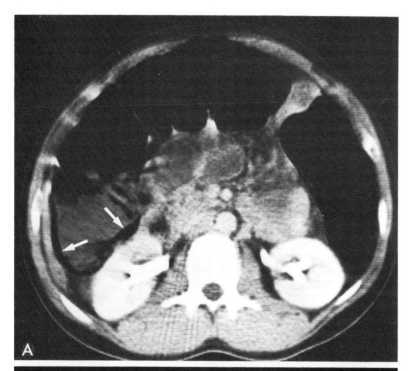

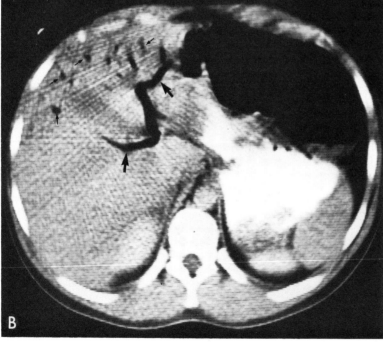

FIGURE 16–91 ■ Pneumatosis coli and portal vein gas as the result of ischemic bowel disease. *A,* CT scan reveals gas *(arrows)* in the wall of the ascending colon and cecum. *B,* CT scan through the liver demonstrates gas in the portal vein *(large arrows),* as well as in the periphery of the liver *(small arrows).* (From Hoddick W, Jeffrey RB, Federle MP: J Comput Assist Tomogr 6:633, 1982. Reprinted by permission.)

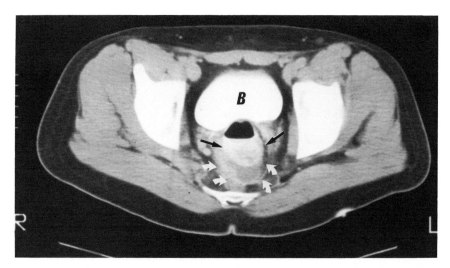

FIGURE 16–92 ■ Ileoanal anastomosis with ileal pouch. Posterior to the ileal pouch *(black arrows)* a low-density mass with an enhancing rim *(white curved arrows)* represents a postsurgical abscess. B = Bladder.

creation of a rectal pouch. In patients with perirectal inflammation, clinical examination without anesthesia may be quite difficult; CT provides a noninvasive means to assess the perirectal space reliably (Fig. 16–92) and can differentiate patients who need percutaneous drainage or surgery from those who can be managed conservatively. In particular, CT can distinguish between supralevator and infralevator abscess. It is important to differentiate between a simple perianal or ischiorectal abscess and one that is a caudal extension of a large supralevator abscess. Failure to recognize such extension of a supralevator abscess leads to recurrence of abscesses and inadequate surgical drainage.

DIVERTICULAR DISEASE

Diverticula in the sigmoid colon frequently are well demonstrated because of the horizontal or oblique course of the colon in that area. They appear as small, flask-shaped outpouchings of the colonic wall filled with contrast material or air, with an appearance similar to that on barium enema examinations. Muscular hypertrophy can also be appreciated on CT scans as slight thickening of the colonic wall and accordion-like appearance of the sigmoid colon.

An unusual complication of diverticular disease is giant sigmoid diverticulum, which is a pulsion diverticulum with superimposed infection. The infectious changes narrow the neck of the diverticulum, with a resultant ball valve mechanism that increases the size of the diverticulum. Torsion and perforation are complications associated with the giant diverticulum and occur in about 10 per cent of these cases. Patients who become symptomatic should undergo surgical resection of the diverticulum. The diagnosis usually is made on plain films and barium enema examinations, but CT enables diagnostic exclusion of an abscess or perforation associated with this diverticulum. The CT appearance of a giant sigmoid diverticulum is that of a large cystic structure with thin, smooth walls, usually containing contrast material,[223] whereas an abscess has shaggy, thickened walls and frequently peridiverticular streaking as a result of inflammation. The differential diagnosis of a giant sigmoid diverticulum includes abscess, sigmoid volvulus, colonic duplication, and emphysematous cystitis.

Diverticulitis results from obstruction of the neck of the diverticulum; subsequent bacterial proliferation and mucus production lead to distention of the diverticulum and peridiverticular inflammation. Usually the inflammation is confined by the serosa. In general, microperforations are quickly sealed off, but continued infection can lead to peritonitis or fistulae. Also, the inflammatory process can dissect intramurally, producing a sinus tract in the colonic wall that can lead to inflammation of other diverticula nearby. Although barium enema examinations have long been used to depict diverticulitis, they can only reveal changes that affect the colonic lumen. Frequently pericolonic changes cannot be accurately assessed, and in early cases of diverticulitis, the barium enema may not reveal any changes other than diverticula. Colonoscopy or barium enema examinations are often deferred in patients with acute symptoms until the inflammation has subsided under conservative therapy, and in toxic patients, barium enemas and colonoscopy are contraindicated.

CT should be performed routinely in any patient with signs and symptoms of diverticulitis if the diagnosis is clinically in doubt (Fig. 16–93). It is the initial method of examination in toxic patients. CT can be used to demonstrate the full extent of the inflammation, which is largely pericolonic in location, and to assess for complications such as perforation, abscess, and fistulae. In one study,[224] CT depicted the extent and complications of diverticulitis more accurately than did conventional radiographic examination of the colon. In our experience, CT is the most accurate method to establish the presence of diverticulitis. Contrary to our experience, one study[225] stated that the barium enema examination should remain the initial method, because it is more often correct than CT.

The CT signs of early diverticulitis include colonic diverticula; pericolonic inflammation evidenced as

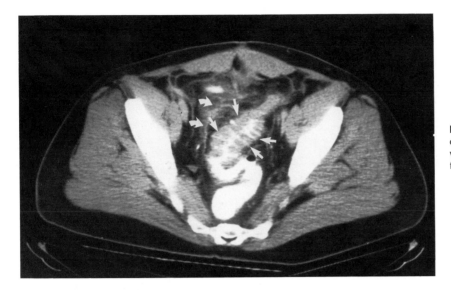

FIGURE 16–93 ■ Early diverticulitis. Thickened colonic wall *(straight arrows)* and pericolonic wispy strands *(curved arrows)* caused by inflammation are present.

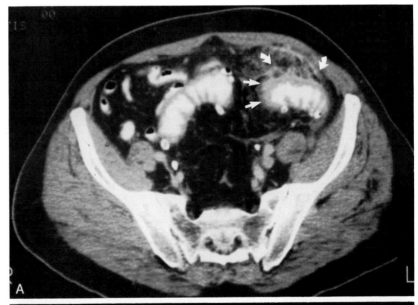

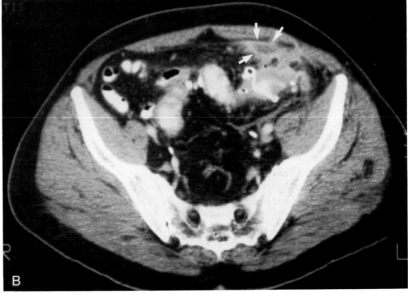

FIGURE 16–94 ■ Diverticulitis. *A,* Thickening of rectosigmoid wall *(straight arrows)* and perirectal stranding *(curved arrows)* are noted. *B,* On a higher section, a small abscess cavity *(arrows)* is present anteriorly, close to the rectus abdominis.

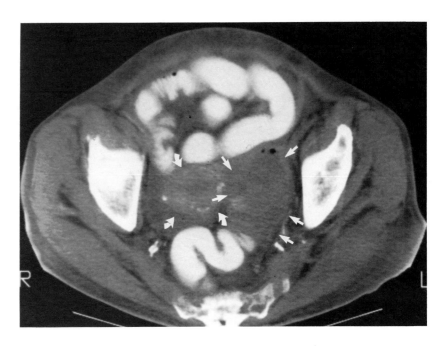

FIGURE 16–95 ■ Diverticulitis and pericolonic abscess. A soft tissue mass *(straight arrows)* containing an air bubble is seen immediately adjacent to the sigmoid colon. In the right adnexal area, a calcified fibroid *(curved arrows)* is also seen.

wispy, streaky densities in the pericolonic fat; and slight thickening of the colonic wall, defined as more than 4 mm on scans perpendicular to or through the long axis of a slightly distended colon lumen (see Fig. 16–93). More advanced cases of diverticulitis show soft tissue masses of variable sizes, with or without low-density centers, representing the full gamut from simple phlegmon to full-blown abscess formation (Fig. 16–94). If diverticulitis is located in the cecum, it cannot be distinguished from appendicitis unless an intramural abscess or diverticulum is present in the cecum.[226] Frequently gas is present within the abscess cavity (Fig. 16–95). In severe cases of diverticulitis, peritonitis (evidenced as diffuse, hazy densities, linear strands, and pockets of fluid in the pelvis or peritoneal cavity), sinus tracts (appearing as linear fluid collections within thickened colonic wall), and free air and fistulae (usually inferred by air in bladder, vagina, or abdominal wall) may be seen. Occasionally, ureteral obstruction resulting from diverticulitis is demonstrated based on dilated ureter and intrarenal collecting system.

OBSTRUCTION

CT is rarely used for evaluating patients with suspected colonic obstruction. Plain films and barium studies of the large bowel usually are diagnostic. In cases of suspected colonic malignancy, sigmoidoscopy and colonoscopy also are employed. CT is used only in selected instances, but because of the increased frequency with which CT is employed for the investigation of abdominal disorders of unknown origin, colonic obstruction may be first seen on CT.

The CT sign of colonic volvulus is the so-called *whorl*,[227] a term that was first used for volvulus of the small bowel.[138] The whorl is composed of the afferent and efferent limbs leading to the volvulus. The central portion of the whorl is composed of tightly twisted bowel and mesentery with fat of low density. The distal loop typically shows the "beak sign," similar to the one observed on barium enema examinations. Rarely, retained foreign bodies following surgery can assume the appearance of the whorl sign,[228] but usually metallic markers and air in the foreign body or signs of inflammation such as bowel wall thickening are diagnostic of retained surgical sponges or laparotomy pads.

Another type of colonic obstruction that might be first seen on CT scans is ileocolonic or colocolonic intussusception.[229, 230] CT features of intussusception include a target mass with enveloped, eccentrically located areas of low density, frequently associated with a linear structure representing the intussusceptum leading into the area of fat density.[229] This latter area represents the invaginated fat. Other CT features are low- and high-density stripes producing a layered or stratified pattern within the intussusception, which occurs when the invagination increases in length. These layers are caused by the differential attenuation characteristics of mesenteric fat, air in bowel lumen of intussuscipiens and intussusceptum, and soft tissue representing the layers of the bowel wall. In advanced stages, edema ensues, with intra- and extraluminal exudation and obscured fascial planes. The final stage is the gangrenous state, in which all planes, including the outer plane toward the pericolonic fat, are completely obliterated, and intramural air may be seen.

Massive cecal distention can occur in colonic obstruction caused by volvulus, cancer, stricture, or idiopathic pseudo-obstruction (Ogilvie's syndrome). Such massive cecal distention may result in perforation or necrosis of the right colon, with frequent fatal outcome as a result of fecal peritonitis. Conservative standard treatment in these patients includes fluid and electrolyte replacement and nasogastric suction. If distention progresses under conservative treatment, decompression is necessary when the cecal

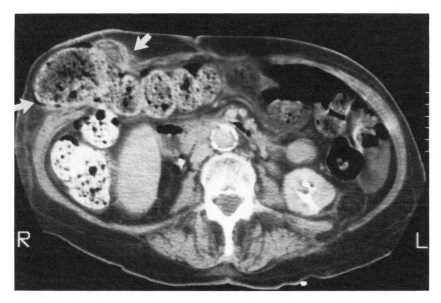

FIGURE 16–96 ■ Spigelian hernia. Herniation of the right colon *(arrows)* through the anterior abdominal wall, next to the linea semilunaris of the aponeurosis of the transversalis muscle, can be seen.

diameter reaches 12 cm. Decompression can be achieved by colonoscopy in 85 per cent of patients, but in the remaining cases, surgery or percutaneous cecostomy must be performed. CT can be used for guidance of needle and trocar and for placement of catheters.[231, 232] A posterior approach through the retroperitoneum avoids spillage of feces into the peritoneum. However, an anterior approach also can be taken.[231] Using an anterior approach, the catheter can be safely removed after 10 days when a fistulous tract between the cecum and abdominal wall is well established. The fistulous tract will heal spontaneously once the catheter is removed, if no mechanical obstruction is present in the colon.

Occasionally hernias produce intermittent obstruction. Internal hernias, spigelian hernias (Fig. 16–96), inguinal hernias, and femoral hernias (Fig. 16–97) are abnormalities that can be easily detected by CT.

CONGENITAL ABNORMALITIES

Normal anatomic variants of the colon include the retrorenal colon and anterior or posterior hepatodia-

phragmatic interposition of the colon. Retrorenal position of colon of varying degrees is found in 1 per cent to 1.9 per cent of patients in the supine position and in 10 per cent of patients in the prone position.[233, 234] Retrorenal colon is more frequently seen in older patients. This anomaly is caused by a more posterior fusion of the anterior and posterior renal fascia and the lateroconal fascia. Therefore the location of the ascending and descending segments of the colon, both of which are located in the anterior pararenal space, is determined by the presence of the lateroconal fascia and the level at which the lateroconal fascia fuses with the anterior abdominal wall. Knowledge of the location of ascending and descending colon is important if percutaneous procedures such as nephrostomies are planned.

Anterior or posterior hepatodiaphragmatic interposition of the colon may lead to misinterpretations on conventional radiographs, radionuclide scans, or sonograms.[235] Occasionally the ascending colon and hepatic flexure retain a long mesocolon from embryonic development and become very mobile. Exten-

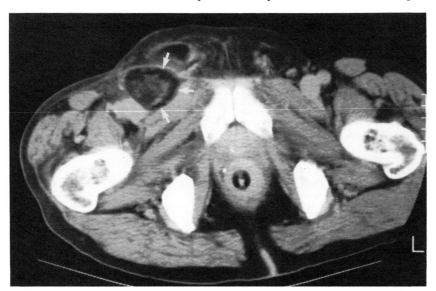

FIGURE 16–97 ■ Femoral hernia. Mesenteric fat *(arrows)* herniating into the femoral foramen is noted.

sion of the right colon anteriorly to the diaphragm is referred to as *Chilaiditi's syndrome.* Only rarely does the patient present with symptoms such as abdominal pain and vomiting. Posterior interposition is seen much more rarely and may be present without any other abnormality or may be associated with right renal agenesis, ectopia, or nephrectomy. CT can easily assess the anatomic relationships in the right upper abdomen and clarify the presence of anterior or posterior interposition.

Colonic duplication cysts similar to duplication cysts in other areas of the gastrointestinal tract appear as cystic structures adherent to segments of the colon. They are tubular or spherical if sectioned through their long axis or perpendicular to it. They are mostly diagnosed in infancy or childhood but occasionally are seen in adulthood. A rare complication is malignancy within a duplication cyst that presents as a discrete soft tissue density nodule within the cystic wall.[236] The differential diagnosis includes other cystic structures such as renal, mesenteric, splenic, or adrenal cyst, pancreatic pseudocyst, abscess, and loculated ascites.

In congenital anomalies of the anorectal area CT can be helpful[237] by depicting the anatomy of the anal sphincter muscles in relation to intestine and amount of muscle present. The external and internal sphincters and the levator ani are the three muscle compartments. On axial CT sections, the anal sphincter is seen as a ring-shaped soft tissue mass composed of external and internal sphincter muscles that cannot be differentiated from one another. The puborectal muscle is seen as a band surrounding the soft tissue ring and extending anteriorly to the pubic bones. The levator ani is composed of the pubococcygeus, levator prostatae (in males) or pubovaginalis (in females), puborectalis, and ileococcygeus muscles. The puborectalis muscle is the most important muscle for control of bowel function after surgical repair, and CT can help the assess the success of surgery after pull-through procedures by demonstrating the relationship between levator sling and pulled-through intestine and the size of the levator sling.

MAGNETIC RESONANCE IMAGING OF THE GASTROINTESTINAL TRACT

At the present time, only a few articles have addressed the use of magnetic resonance imaging (MRI) in the evaluation of the gastrointestinal tract.[238–247] It is uncertain whether MRI will be similar to CT for staging of gastrointestinal tumors, but it is already clear that direct coronal and sagittal images add additional information in selected instances. For instance, on coronal images, magnetic resonance (MR) detects the presence or absence of tumor invasion into the crus of the diaphragm in patients with esophageal or gastric tumor, and on the sagittal plane, MRI may visualize the presence or absence of tumor extension into the bladder neck or prostate in patients with rectal tumors. Gastrointestinal pathologic changes other than neoplasms have not yet been sufficiently investigated to reach any conclusions. In its present status, MR images of the gastrointestinal tract are of inferior quality to CT scans, with the exception of images of the rectosigmoid area.

Anatomy

Transaxial anatomy is similar to that already described in the CT section of this chapter (Figs. 16–98 through 16–103).

Coronal Plane

MIDPORTION OF THE LUMBAR SPINE

At the midportion of the lumbar spine (Fig. 16–104) all of the vertebral bodies of the normal lumbar spine and some of the vertebral bodies of the lower thoracic spine can be seen. In patients with exaggerated lordosis, not all the vertebral bodies will be in the plane of section. On T1-weighted images, the normal disk appears as a central signal of intermediate intensity surrounded by a low-intensity signal rim related to the annulus fibrosus and the end plates of the vertebral bodies. The psoas muscles are seen as low-intensity structures that assume a cephalocaudal and slightly anterior course.

On more anterior sections, the lower portion of the iliopsoas muscle is easily identified. The liver and spleen appear in the right and left upper quadrants as medium-intensity areas, of higher intensity than the psoas muscles. At this level, the right

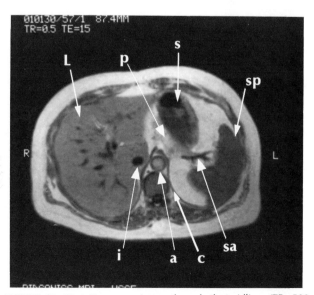

FIGURE 16–98 ■ Transverse image through the midliver (TR, 500 msec; TE, 50 msec). a = Aorta; c = crus of diaphragm; i = inferior vena cava; L = liver; p = pancreas; s = stomach; sa = splenic artery; sp = spleen.

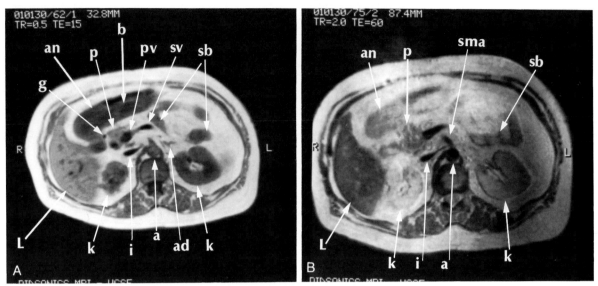

FIGURE 16–99 ■ Transverse images through the antrum. *A,* TR, 500 msec; TE, 15 msec. *B,* TR, 2000 msec; TE, 60 msec. a = Aorta; ad = adrenal; an = antrum; b = body of stomach; g = gastroduodenal artery; i = inferior vena cava; k = kidney; L = liver; p = pancreas; pv = portal vein; sb = small bowel loops; sma = superior mesenteric artery; sv = splenic vein.

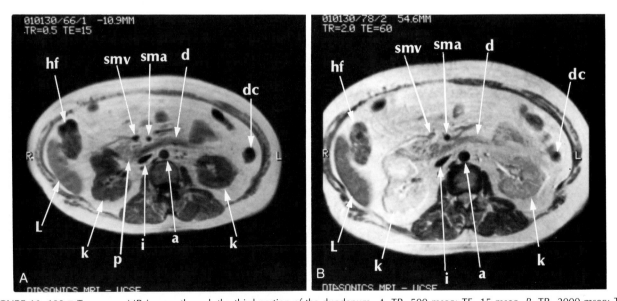

FIGURE 16–100 ■ Transverse MR images through the third portion of the duodenum. *A,* TR, 500 msec; TE, 15 msec. *B,* TR, 2000 msec; TE, 60 msec. a = Aorta; d = duodenum; dc = descending colon; hf = hepatic failure; i = inferior vena cava; k = kidney (right kidney with mass); L = liver tip; p = pancreas; sma = superior mesenteric artery; smv = superior mesenteric vein.

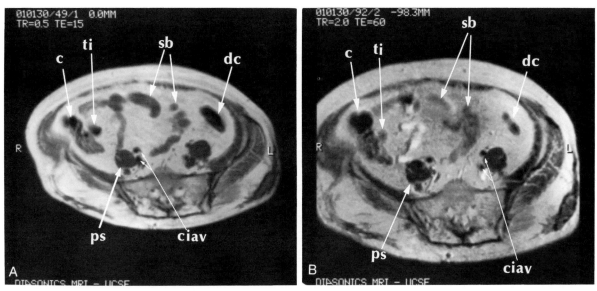

FIGURE 16–101 ■ Transverse images through the cecum. *A,* TR, 500 msec; TE, 15 msec. *B,* TR, 2000 msec; TE, 60 msec. c = Cecum; ciav = common iliac artery and vein; dc = descending colon; ps = psoas; sb = small bowel loops; ti = terminal ileum.

hepatic vein is frequently visualized coursing obliquely from the lower lateral portion of the liver toward the inferior vena cava. The branches of the hepatic artery are usually not seen. The posterior margins of the inferior vena cava and portions of the aorta are both visualized as structures void of signal.

The splenic hilus can usually be seen at this level, with the adrenal gland medial to it. The kidneys are clearly outlined bilaterally because of the high contrast between them and the perirenal fat. Gerota's fascia frequently is seen as a line of very low intensity. Depending on the axis of the kidneys, the renal hilus may be seen at this level or slightly anterior to it. On T1-weighted images, the higher-intensity cor-

tex can be differentiated from the lower-intensity medulla. Occasionally the tail of the pancreas is seen superior to the kidneys and next to the splenic hilus. The muscle layers of lateral portions of the abdominal walls have low intensity and are bordered on either side by high-intensity fat. Because they contain urine, the renal hilus, renal pelvis, and proximal ureters are seen as low-intensity structures 1 to 2 cm anterior to the midportion of the vertebral bodies. The ureters are often seen to turn medially and caudally to follow a slightly curved course over the psoas muscles. At this level, the middle hepatic vein runs obliquely cephalad into the inferior vena cava. The left hepatic vein is infrequently visualized.

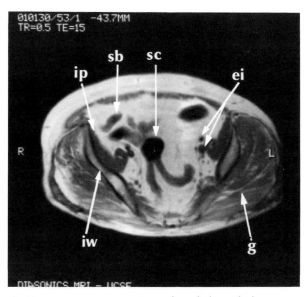

FIGURE 16–102 ■ Transverse image through the midpelvis. TR, 500 msec; TE, 50 msec. ei = External iliac artery and vein; g = gluteus muscles; ip = iliopsoas muscle; iw = iliac wing; sb = small bowel loops; sc = sigmoid colon.

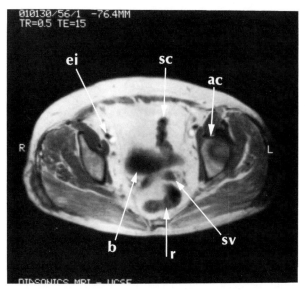

FIGURE 16–103 ■ Transverse image through the acetabular roof. TR, 500 msec; TE, 15 msec. ac = Acetabulum; b = top of bladder; ei = external iliac artery and vein; r = rectum; sc = sigmoid colon; sv = seminal vesicles.

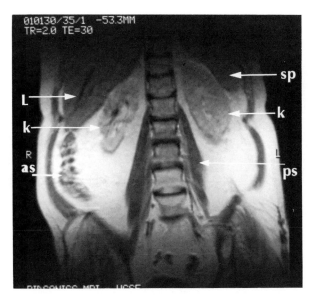

FIGURE 16–104 ■ Coronal image through the midportion of the lumbar spine. TR, 2000 msec; TE, 60 msec. as = Ascending colon; k = kidney; L = liver; ps = psoas muscle; sp = spleen.

Portions of the stomach may be noted next to the proximal abdominal aorta and the spleen and superior to the splenic artery and vein. Immediately below these vessels, the body of the pancreas may be identified. The renal arteries are well outlined bilaterally as signal-void structures coursing obliquely toward the aorta. The confluence of the splenic vein and the superior mesenteric veins is directly visualized, and some small bowel loops and portions of the ascending colon are also clearly outlined.

INFERIOR VENA CAVA

The inferior vena cava (Fig. 16–105) is outlined as a signal-void structure with the proximal portal vein

originating near it and coursing toward the right and cephalad. The right portal vein is usually observed heading to the right for a short distance before dividing into the anterosuperior and posteroinferior branches. The left portal vein and its branches are occasionally seen, usually slightly anterior to the level of the right portal vein. The renal veins may be seen bilaterally, with the left renal vein coursing anterior to the abdominal aorta. The distal abdominal aorta and its bilateral bifurcation into the common iliac arteries are well demonstrated. At this level the splenic artery and vein frequently are seen as round to oval signal-void areas. The ascending and descending segments of the colon are shown in each flank as low-intensity signal or signal-void areas because of the air within their lumens. The celiac axis, with the main hepatic artery and proximal splenic artery, may also be seen at this level. Although the pancreas can be demonstrated, it cannot always be separated from small bowel loops.

GALLBLADDER FOSSA

The gallbladder (Fig. 16–106) is visualized at this level as a low- or high-intensity area on the undersurface of the liver with its neck extending toward the porta hepatis. The branches of the right and left portal veins are seen as round to oval structures within the liver parenchyma, but branches of the left proximal portal vein may be seen as tubular low-signal-intensity areas.

The ascending and descending colon are seen at this level, but the transverse colon is visualized 1 to 2 cm anteriorly. Multiple small bowel loops are also demonstrated, but they can be separated from one another only when sufficient mesenteric fat is present. Portions of the sigmoid colon may be identified in the lower abdomen, depending on the gaseous

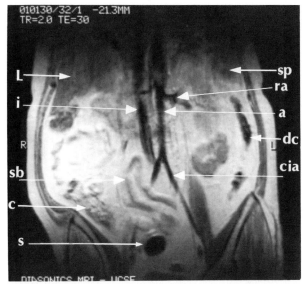

FIGURE 16–105 ■ Coronal image at the level of the inferior vena cava. TR, 2000 msec; TE, 30 msec. a = Aorta; c = cecum; cia = common iliac artery; dc = descending colon; i = inferior vena cava; L = liver; ra = renal artery; sb = small bowel loops; sc = sigmoid colon; sp = spleen.

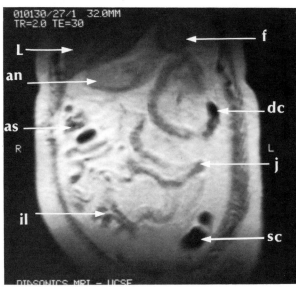

FIGURE 16–106 ■ Coronal image at the level of the gastric fundus. TR, 2000 msec; TE, 30 msec. an = Antrum of stomach; as = ascending colon; dc = descending colon; f = fundus of stomach; j = jejunum; il = ileum; L = liver; sc = sigmoid colon.

distention of the large bowel and the redundancy of the sigmoid colon.

Sagittal Plane

RIGHT PARASAGITTAL PLANE

At the right parasagittal level (Fig. 16–107) the inferior vena cava is seen throughout its abdominal and intrahepatic course as a signal-free channel located posteriorly and entering the right atrium. The right coronary ligament suspends the liver from the diaphragm posteriorly and divides the peritoneal cavity around the right lobe of the liver into subphrenic and subhepatic spaces. In a normal individual, the right posterior subhepatic space (Morison's pouch) is a potential space, and it has the same high signal intensity as that of fat.

The liver occupies the entire anterior upper abdomen in this plane. The right hepatic vein is visualized to the right of the midline, coursing obliquely cephalad. On the right, the branches of the right hepatic vein often are seen as round, signal-free structures. The middle hepatic vein is seen as a channel in or just to the right of midline. Occasionally it is in the same section as the inferior vena cava and is joined by the left hepatic vein before entering the inferior vena cava. The main portal vein is a signal-free channel located anteriorly to the inferior vena cava as it enters the liver. The right portal vein and its branches are seen as signal-free structures bisecting the anterior and posterior segments of the right lobe of the liver. The common hepatic artery is identified only rarely in the sagittal plane, and the intrahepatic arteries and biliary tree are not seen.

The duodenum, small bowel loops, and transverse colon may be observed inferior to the liver. The head of the pancreas is located immediately anterior to the inferior vena cava and above the horizontal portion of the duodenum but is difficult to clearly identify.

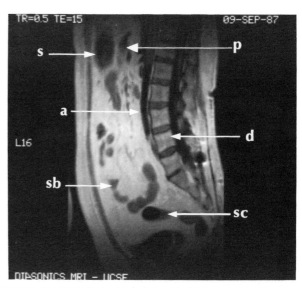

FIGURE 16–108 ■ Midsagittal plane. TR, 500 msec; TE, 15 msec. a = Aorta; d = dorsal spine; p = pancreas; s = stomach; sb = small bowel loops; sc = sigmoid colon.

MIDSAGITTAL PLANE

In the midsagittal plane (Fig. 16–108), the aorta, unless very tortuous, is well outlined as a signal-free, tubular structure. Posterior to it, the lumbar vertebrae and the spinal cord are visible. The left lobe of the liver is visualized as a tear-shaped organ with its tip located anteriorly and caudally. The body of the pancreas and the stomach are seen immediately anterior to the aorta, and portions of the crura of the hemidiaphragms are also located anterior to the aorta. The transverse colon and small bowel loops are seen inferiorly.

LEFT PARASAGITTAL PLANE

In the left parasagittal plane (Fig. 16–109) the left kidney is demonstrated along its longitudinal axis.

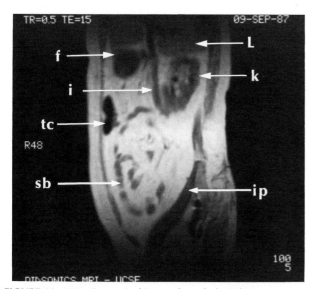

FIGURE 16–107 ■ Parasagittal image through the inferior vena cava. TR, 500 msec; TE, 50 msec. f = Fundus of stomach; i = inferior vena cava; ip = iliopsoas; k = medial portion of kidney; L = liver; sb = small bowel loops; tc = transverse colon.

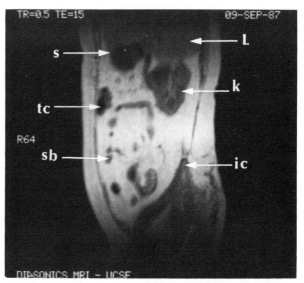

FIGURE 16–109 ■ Parasagittal image through the kidney. TR, 500 msec; TE, 15 msec. ic = Top of iliac crest; k = kidney; L = liver; s = stomach; sb = small bowel loops; tc = transverse colon.

The left adrenal gland may be seen slightly anterior to the superior pole. More anteriorly, the left lobe of the liver can be identified. The left portal vein is easily seen. The ascending colon and small bowel loops may be identified inferior to the liver. Posteriorly, the quadratus lumborum muscle can be noted.

Techniques of Examination

At present, for the examination of the gastrointestinal tract, we use in the midfield (0.35 to 0.6 T) spin-echo sequences (SE) with short repetition time (TR) (TR, 125 to 250 ms; echo time [TE], 15 ms; number of excitations [NEX], 8) and/or gradient-echo sequences (TR, 250 ms; TE, 20 ms; 70° angle) and long TR (TR, 2000 ms; TE, 30/60 ms). For the high field (1.5 T), we use inversion recovery (IR: TR, 2000 ms; TE, 20 ms; inversion time [TI], 650 ms; NEX, 2) or SE (TR, 300 ms; TE, 15 ms; NEX, 4), for T1-weighted sequences and SE sequences (TR, 2000 to 2500 ms; TE, 20/70 ms) for T2 weighting. Images with short TR and first echo are considered T1 weighted, and images with long TR and second or later echoes are considered T2 weighted. Echo sequences and imaging results vary with different field strengths and areas imaged, and the choice of best imaging sequence for any given area or suspected pathology is still under investigation. Also, results depend on the field strength used (low [0.1 T], medium [0.35 to 0.6 T],[248] and high [1 to 2T]). The contrast between bowel wall and perigastrointestinal fat is shown best on T1-weighted images because of the short T1 of fat and the longer T1 of the bowel wall. On T1-weighted images, the low-intensity signal of the bowel wall is equal to or slightly greater than the intensity of skeletal muscle. On T2-weighted images, tissue contrast is decreased, and the margins of the bowel wall are sometimes not clearly visualized because of motion. These MR characteristics are important factors in staging gastrointestinal tumors. However, T2-weighted images can be helpful in the upper abdomen to distinguish the stomach, duodenum, and small bowel from the pancreas.[204]

MR imaging of the gastrointestinal tract is degraded by both respiratory motion and peristalsis. Artifacts from peristalsis can be decreased by administration of glucagon (1 mg intramuscularly) just prior to the examination. In the colon, bowel preparation is necessary to avoid misinterpreting stool for an abnormally thickened bowel wall (Fig. 16–110). Effervescent agents also help outline the bowel wall, because air creates a signal void that can be used as a natural contrast material.

Oral administration of paramagnetic substances is being studied to determine whether it can improve MRI of the gastrointestinal tract, because as with CT, identification of gut without the use of bowel-labeling agents is difficult with MR. Positive or negative oral contrast enhancement can be employed.[244–246] Ferric ammonium citrate, which is the major ingredient in Geritol, is paramagnetic and produces a high MR signal intensity because of shortening of T1 relaxation times. Water is diamagnetic and produces a low MR signal intensity if T1-weighted sequences are used. Because fat is depicted as a very high signal intensity, positive agents such as dilute iron solutions or other paramagnetic agents such as gadolinium administered with mannitol[247] may become isointense with fat. Proper selection of radiofrequencies or gradient pulse sequences (proper TR and TE sequences) may overcome this problem. Negative contrast enhancement with air or water may be a better gastrointestinal labeling method for MR imaging.

Ferric ammonium citrate can aid in differentiating the esophagus, stomach, duodenum, and small bowel from adjacent tumor, vessels, and viscera and helps to delineate pancreas, liver, and kidney from gastrointestinal tract in areas where these organs abut the bowel.[246] However, distinction between bowel and fat is better made with water. The stomach is reliably seen by MRI with ferric ammonium citrate

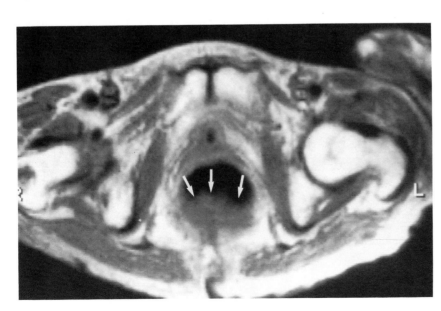

FIGURE 16–110 ■ Feces in rectum, transverse image. TR, 2000 msec; TE, 60 msec. Feces (*arrows*) mimic the appearance of a tumor in the posterior rectal wall.

or with water, but iron solutions identify the duodenum more consistently. The jejunum and ileum are difficult to depict well by MRI with or without iron solutions or water, which probably is related to peristalsis of gut and resulting image distortion. Better overall resolution and thus improvement in identification of the small bowel and colon by oral agents could be achieved with the use of shorter acquisition times, shorter pulse repetition times, and respiratory gating coupled with glucagon injection to minimize degradation of anatomic detail induced by peristalsis in the gut. Iron oxide particles have also been used for labeling the gastrointestinal tract, and a preliminary report indicated the usefulness of this form of iron as a negative contrast agent[238] (Fig. 16–111).

Intravenous paramagnetic substances such as gadolinium-diethylenetriamine pentaacetic acid (Gd-DTPA) have been employed to enhance detection of liver metastases, but no final results are available as yet.[249] The clinical usefulness of intravenous paramagnetic agents depends on the way contrast changes between different pathologic processes and normal tissue. High levels of contrast enhancement may lead to a loss of definition of a lesion, and spin-echo sequences that are useful before injection of the paramagnetic contrast material may not be adequate after injection of such paramagnetic substances. In the liver, Gd-DTPA decreases the T1 of normal liver to a moderated degree but usually decreases the T1 of tumors to a greater degree. Therefore with spin-echo sequences, the net result may be a decrease in the contrast between the tumor and normal tissue. However, if fast imaging sequences are used, contrast between lesion and liver or pancreas parenchyma is increased, and lesions can become more conspicuous. The enhancement pattern in these cases is similar to the one seen with iodinated intravenous contrast material for CT.

At the present time, the use of oral and intravenous paramagnetic and diamagnetic substances is still in its research phase. To achieve the high resolution seen with CT of the gastrointestinal tract, many more trials need to be made with different scanning sequences and administration of different contrast media.

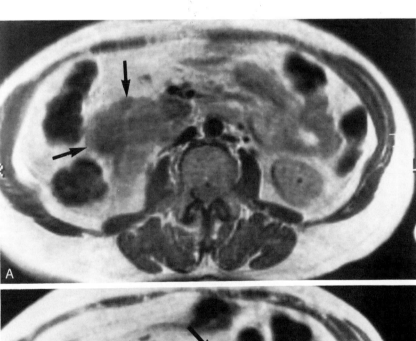

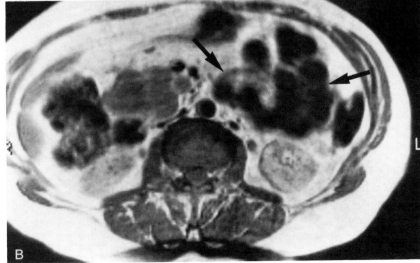

FIGURE 16–111 ■ MR scans of pancreatic carcinoma with and without oral contrast material. *A,* Proton density image (TR, 2000 msec; TE, 30 msec; NEX, 4 at 0.35 T) shows a mass in the head of the pancreas *(arrows).* Separation of mass from bowel is difficult. *B,* Proton density image after oral administration of a solution of iron oxide particles outlines the pancreas to great advantage. Also the jejunal loops *(arrows)* are well seen.

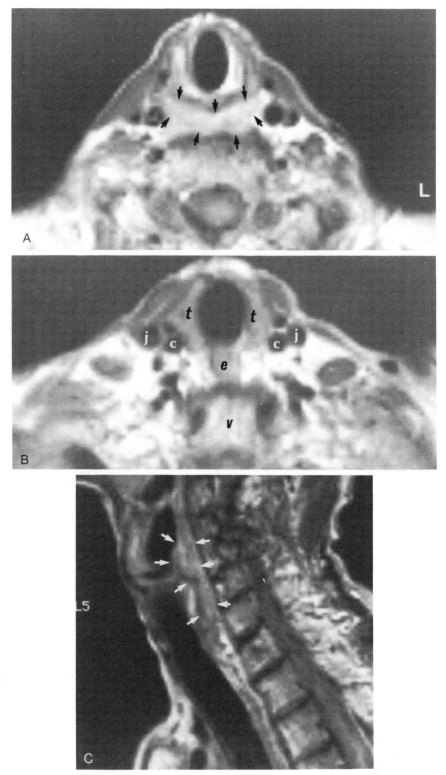

FIGURE 16–112 ■ MR scans showing esophageal carcinoma invading the larynx. *A,* Transverse image. TR, 2000 msec; TE, 30 msec. A mass *(arrows)* in the area of the esophagus is seen, which on higher sections invades the left piriform sinus and the left neurovascular bundle. This mass was of intermediate signal intensity on T1-weighted images and increased in intensity relative to fat on T2-weighted images. *B,* Transverse image. TR, 2000 msec; TE, 30 msec. At this level the esophagus (e) is normal. c = Common carotid artery; j = jugular vein; t = thyroid gland; v = vertebral body. *C,* Sagittal image. TR, 2000 msec; TE, 40 msec. Invasion of the larynx by the esophageal mass *(arrows)* can be seen.

Pathology

The normal esophagus is well visualized by MR[239] except for the area immediately posterior to the left atrium, where the esophagus is flattened. However, the current MR techniques do not permit accurate staging of esophageal tumors (Fig. 16–112).[239] If cardiac and respiratory gating are used, the extent of mediastinal disease in patients with esophageal carcinoma may be more precisely determined. As calculated relaxation times (T1 and T2) show a wide variety for both normal and abnormal esophagi, they cannot be used to establish a histologic diagnosis or in staging of esophageal tumors. Esophageal varices can be accurately depicted by MR without the use of contrast material based on the lack of signal in the varicoid venous structures of the distal esophagus.

Thickening of the gastric wall can be easily shown by MR on axial, coronal, and sagittal images, but its appearance is nonspecific. Diffuse involvement of the stomach favors lymphoma, inflammatory processes, or systemic conditions involving the stomach. The ability of MR relaxation characteristics to provide insight into the pathologic nature of the tissue causing gastric wall thickening occasionally can add specificity to the findings of MR imaging. In one case report, gastric wall thickening was noted to have very short T2 signal characteristics, a finding that suggests the presence of fibrous tissue, which has lower signal intensity than what would be expected from muscle or mucosal tumors.[240]

Because of the fixed position in the pelvis and as with CT, detection and staging of rectosigmoid tumors by MRI can be done more accurately than can detection and staging in the other areas of the colon. For correct depiction of the intraluminal component of tumors, particularly for smaller tumors, colonic preparation (to avoid confusion with feces), air insufflation, and prone positioning are necessary. On T1-weighted images (SE: TR, 500 ms; TE, 15 ms for midfield; and TR, 700 ms; TE, 20 ms for high field), rectosigmoid tumors appear as wall thickening with signal intensity similar to or slightly higher than skeletal muscle (long T1) (Figs. 16–113 and 16–114). Because perirectal fat has high signal intensity (short T1), air has no signal intensity, and tumor has moderate signal intensity (long T1), tumors are well shown because of the high contrast among these different areas. For the same reasons, extension of tumor beyond the colonic wall is well seen on T1-weighted images. On T2-weighted images (SE: TR, 2000 ms; TE, 30/60 ms for midfield; and TR, 2000 to 2500 ms; TE, 20/70 ms for high field), the signal intensity of tumor increases relative to that of muscle; however, the contrast between tumor and the perirectal fat decreases, because both tissues have long T2 relaxation times. Therefore T2-weighted images are not as useful as T1-weighted sequences, particularly for determination of extracolonic tumor extension. However, if uterine or pelvic sidewall invasion is suspected, T2-weighted sequences are useful because of the differences in signal intensities of tumor with its long T2 and muscle with its short T2. In general, perirectal tumor invasion is better seen by MR than by CT because of the higher contrast between tumor and fat.[241]

Both CT and MR are unable to distinguish between tumors localized to mucosa (stage I) and those that infiltrate the entire colonic wall (stage II). Also, microinvasion cannot be detected by MR or CT, and tumor foci in normal-sized nodes go unrecognized.[250] Like CT, MR bases the diagnosis of lymph node abnormality on the size of the nodes. In one series,[241] in five out of six cases in which lymph nodes were seen, the nodes were normal in size but contained tumor, and in one case with enlarged nodes (>15 mm in diameter), reactive hyperplasia was present. Using a medium magnetic field (0.35 T), lymph nodes are well seen on T1-weighted images but are difficult to detect on T2-weighted images because of their high signal intensity similar to that of fat. Using a high magnetic field, nodes can also be detected with T2-weighted images, because with high field strength the signal intensity of fat decreases and that of lymph nodes increases, resulting in better image contrast. Liver and adrenal metastases are as well demonstrated by MR as by CT. Final comparison of the two modalities is not available yet, but it appears that some liver lesions, particularly in the left lobe, are better seen on MR images, especially if gating is used.

Invasion of adjacent organs is best demonstrated on transverse or coronal MR images, and MR is superior to CT in demonstrating invasion of the levator ani. Lateral extension of tumor is difficult to detect on sagittal MR images. Extension into prostate, seminal vesicles, vagina, and cervix can be shown, but extension into bladder may be missed if the bladder is not well distended.

Overall, when CT and MR are compared, both stage rectosigmoid tumors equally well, but perirectal disease is better delineated by MR.[251] In the detection of lymph node abnormalities, MR and CT demonstrate lymphadenopathy equally well, but both fail to distinguish among benign hyperactive hyperplasia, metastatic adenopathy, and lymphoma.[252] For normal-sized nodes (<10 mm), CT is better than MR because of its superior spatial resolution.[253] CT offers shorter examination times and better delineation of the gastrointestinal tract because of the well-established use of oral contrast materials. Following surgery, MR may be helpful in patients with large surgical clips for whom CT results are inadequate because of artifacts (see Fig. 16–114).

For recurrent colorectal tumors, MR was initially considered to be very accurate[254–256] and superior to CT. It was suggested that based on signal intensity of a pelvic mass, MRI could replace CT-guided biopsy for assessing presence or absence of recurrent tumors. However, recent studies have shown that while MRI determines extent quite well, no correlation was found between tumor histology and signal intensity. de Lange and co-workers found that high signal intensity on T2-weighted sequences may in-

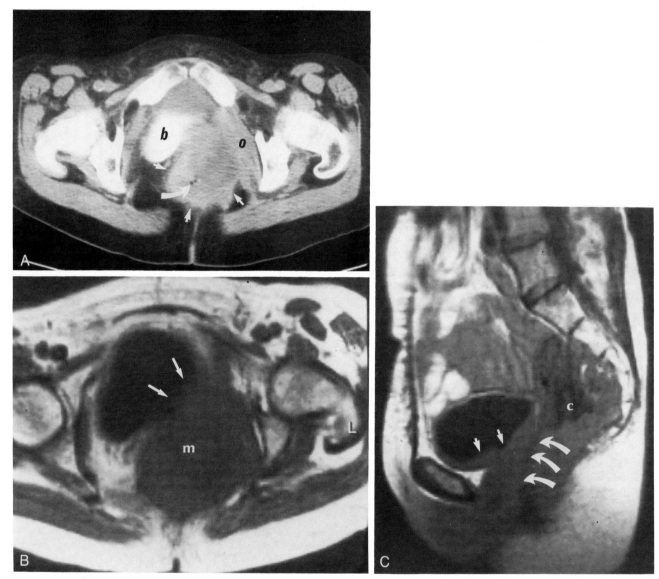

FIGURE 16–113 ■ Rectal carcinoma, stage IIIB. *A,* CT scan shows a large mass *(straight arrows)* with a low-density center involving the obturator muscle (o), but involvement of the bladder (b) by tumor is uncertain. Air density *(curved arrow)* represents the top of a large necrotic tumor cavity in the perineum. *B,* MR scan, transverse plane. TR, 500 msec; TE, 30 msec. A large mass (m) with clear invasion of bladder *(arrows)* and posterior vagina is demonstrated. *C,* MR scan, sagittal plane. TR, 500 msec; TE, 30 msec. This MR scan shows infiltration of the bladder *(straight arrows)* and posterior vagina *(curved arrows),* but the cervix (c) is clearly spared.

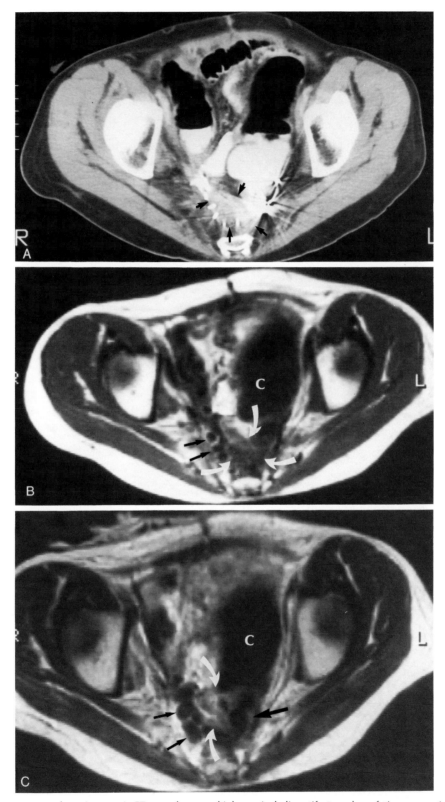

FIGURE 16–114 ■ Recurrent rectal carcinoma. *A,* CT scan shows multiple surgical clip artifacts and a soft tissue mass *(arrows)* in the presacral area. *B,* MR scan, transverse image. TR, 500 msec; TE, 15 msec. At the level corresponding to the CT scan, signal dropout *(black straight arrows)* from the surgical clips is identified, but there are no streak artifacts. The mass *(white curved arrows)* is seen, and the colon (c) anterior to it is dilated. *C,* MR scan, transverse image. TR, 2000 msec; TE, 60 msec. Again, signal dropout *(black straight arrows)* from the surgical clips is noted. On this T2-weighted image, the mass *(white curved arrows)* increased in signal intensity relative to fat when compared with T1-weighted images. Although no streak artifacts disturb the image, a biopsy of a mass seen on such MR images still must be performed under CT guidance.

dicate viable tumor, tumor necrosis, edematous tissue, or benign inflammation.[257] Low signal intensity on T1-weighted spin-echo images may indicate tumor-induced desmoplastic reaction or benign fibrosis without neoplasia.[257] Also, areas of early fibrosis (within 1 year of surgery) contain enough granulation tissue, vascular changes, and edema to elevate the MR signal so that fibrosis cannot be diagnosed unequivocally. The MRI diagnosis of fibrosis is based on low signal intensity in the area of a suspected scar on T1- and T2-weighted sequences (Fig. 16–115). Therefore at the present time, the role of MRI for recurrent rectal carcinoma is uncertain. MRI is very sensitive in detecting a tumor mass, but because of its desmoplastic nature, small tumor sheaths mixed with fibrotic material may not be correctly diagnosed based on the intermediate-to-low signal intensity.

MRI also can be used for evaluating congenital anorectal malformations.[242] Depending on the position of the most distal rectal segment in relationship to the levator sling, a low, intermediate, or high anal atresia or imperforated anus can be distinguished. Other extraintestinal abnormalities associated with anorectal malformations may be present and are more common with supralevator location of the segment of atresia. MRI can easily depict these extraintestinal abnormalities and visualize anorectal malformations as a result of the good tissue contrast among perirectal fat, rectal sphincter muscles, levator sling, and air in the rectal pouch.

Diverticulitis has been demonstrated by MRI as wall thickening with indistinct margins on T1 and increased signal intensity on T2 caused by edema (Fig. 16–116).

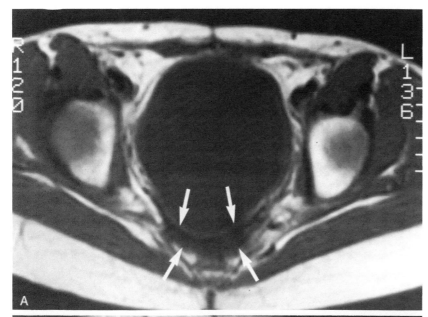
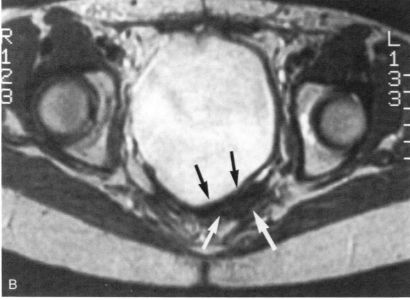

FIGURE 16–115 ■ Scar tissue versus recurrent rectal carcinoma. *A,* A T1-weighted image (TR, 250 msec; TE, 15 msec; NEX, 8) shows an area of low signal intensity *(arrows)* anterior to the sacrum. *B,* On T2-weighted scans (TR, 2000 msec; TE, 60 msec; NEX, 2), the same area *(arrows)* remains low in signal intensity, indicative of scar tissue.

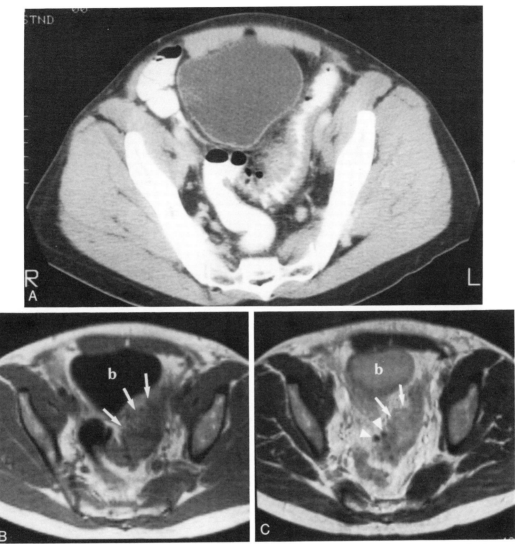

FIGURE 16–116 ■ Diverticulitis without abscess. *A*, CT scan shows wall thickening and increased soft tissue strands in fat due to inflammation. *B*, Transverse image. TR, 500 msec; TE, 15 msec. Thickened wall and irregular margins *(arrows)* are seen in the sigmoid colon. b = Bladder. *C*, Transverse image. TR, 2000 msec; TE, 60 msec. The sigmoid wall shows increased signal intensity *(arrows)*, suggesting edema in this patient with known diverticulitis. A well-defined abscess is not seen. *Arrowheads* indicate the diverticula.

References

1. Laufer I, Mullens JE, Hamilton J: The diagnostic accuracy of barium studies of the stomach and duodenum: correlation with endoscopy. Radiology 115:569, 1975.
2. Herlinger G, Glanville JN, Kreel L: An evaluation of the double-contrast barium meal (DCBM) against endoscopy. Clin Radiol 28:307, 1977.
3. Moss AA, Beneventano TC, Gohel V, Larger I, Margulis AR: The current status of upper gastrointestinal radiography. Invest Radiology 15:92, 1980.
4. Moule EB, Cochrane KM, Sokhi GS: A comparative study of the diagnostic value of upper gastrointestinal endoscopy and radiography. Gut 16:411, 1975.
5. Efsen F, Fisherman K: Angiography in gastric tumors. Acta Radiol (Diagn) 15:193, 1974.
6. Marsden DS, Alexander CH, Yeung PK: The use of ⁹⁹ᵐTc to detect gastric malignancy. Am J Gastroenterol 59:410, 1973.
7. Walls WJ: The evaluation of malignant gastric neoplasms by ultrasound B scanning. Radiology 118:159, 1976.
8. Komaiko MS: Gastric neoplasm: ultrasound and CT evaluation. Gastrointest Radiol 4:131, 1979.
9. Kressel HY, Callen PW, Montagne JP, Korobkin M, Goldberg HI, et al: Computed tomographic evaluation of disorders affecting the alimentary tract. Radiology 129:451, 1978.
10. Parienty RA, Smolarski N, Pradel J, Ducellier R, Lubrano JM: Computed tomography of the gastrointestinal tract: lesion recognition and pitfalls. J Comput Assist Tomogr 3:615, 1979.
11. Halber MD, Daffner RH, Thompson WM: CT of the esophagus: 1. Normal appearance. AJR 133:1047, 1979.
12. Moss AA, Schnyder P, Thoeni RF, Margulis AR: Esophageal carcinoma: pre-therapy staging by computed tomography. AJR 136:1051, 1981.
13. Moss AA, Schnyder P, Margulis AR: Computed tomographic evaluation of esophageal and gastric tumors. In Goldberg HE (ed): Interventional Radiology and Diagnostic Imaging Modalities. San Francisco, University of California Press, 1982, pp 215–225.
14. Goldwin RL, Heitzman ER, Proto AV: Computed tomography of the mediastinum: normal anatomy and indications for the use of CT. Radiology 124:235, 1977.
15. Jost RG, Sagel SS, Stanley RJ, Levitt RG: Computed tomography of the thorax. Radiology 126:125, 1978.
16. Marks WM, Callen PW, Moss AA: Gastroesophageal region: source of confusion on CT. AJR 136:359, 1981.
17. Kaye MD, Young SW, Hayward R, Castellino RA: Gastric pseudotumor on CT scanning. AJR 135:1980.

18. Nyman U, Dinnetz G, Andersson I: On oral contrast medium for use in computed tomography of the abdomen. Acta Radiol (Diagn) 25:121, 1984.

19. Cayea PD, Seltzer SE: A new barium paste for computed tomography of the esophagus. J Comput Assist Tomogr 9(1):214, 1985.

20. Plachta A: Benign tumors of the esophagus: review of literature and report of 99 cases. Am J Gastroenterol 38:639, 1962.

21. Drucker MH, Mansour KA, Hatcher CR Jr, Symbas PN: Esophageal carcinoma: an aggressive approach. Ann Thorac Surg 28:133, 1979.

22. Guerney JM, Knudsen DF: Abdominal exploration in evaluation of patients with carcinoma of the thoracic esophagus. J Thorac Cardiovasc Surg 59:62, 1970.

23. Beatty JD, DeBoer G, Rider ND: Carcinoma of the esophagus: pretreatment assessment, correlation of radiation treatment parameters with survival, and identification and management of radiation treatment failure. Cancer 43:2254, 1979.

24. Halvorsen RA, Foster WL, Williford ME, Roberts L Jr, Postlethwait RW, Thompson WM: Pseudosarcoma of the esophagus: barium swallow and CT findings. J Can Assoc Radiol 34:278, 1983.

25. Cukingnan RA, Casey JS: Carcinoma of the esphagus. Ann Thorac Surg 26:274, 1978.

26. Van Andel JG, Dees J, Dijkhuis CM: Carcinoma of the esophagus: results of treatment. Ann Surg 190:684, 1979.

27. Nakayama K, Hirota K: Experience of about 3000 cases with cancer of the esophagus and the cardia. Aust NZ J Surg 31:222, 1962.

28. Cederqvist C, Nielsen J, Berthelsen A, Hansen HS: Cancer of the esophagus: I: 1002 cases survey and survival. Acta Chir Scand 144:227, 1978.

29. Cederqvist C, Nielsen J, Berthelsen A, Hansen HS: Cancer of the esophagus: II: therapy and outcome. Acta Chir Scand 144:233, 1978.

30. Schuchmann GF, Heydorn WH, Hall RV: Treatment of esophageal carcinoma: a retrospective review. J Thorac Cardiovasc Surg 79:67, 1980.

31. Earlam R, Cunha-Melo JR: Esophageal squamous cell carcinoma: I. A critical review of surgery. Br J Surg 67:381, 1980.

32. Earlam R, Cunha-Melo JR: Esophageal squamous cell carcinoma: II. A critical review of radiotherapy. Br J Surg 67:457, 1980.

33. Giuli R, Gignoux M: Treatment of carcinoma of the esophagus. Ann Surg 192:44, 1980.

34. Heck HA, Rosse NP: Esophageal and gastroesophageal junction carcinoma: an evolved philosophy of management. Cancer 46:1873, 1980.

35. Postlethwait PW: Surgery of the Esophagus. New York, Appleton-Century-Crofts, 1979, pp 341–414.

36. Rosenberg JC, Schwade JG, Vaitkevicius VK: Cancer of the esophagus. In DeVita JR, Hellman S, Rosenberg SA (eds): Cancer Principles and Practice of Oncology. Philadelphia, JB Lippincott, 1982, pp 499–533.

37. Mori S, Kasai M, Watanabe T, Shibuya I: Preoperative assessment of resectability for carcinoma of the thoracic esophagus. Ann Surg 190:100, 1979.

38. Daffner RH, Postlethwait RW, Putman CE: Retrotracheal abnormalities in esophageal carcinoma. Prognostic implications. AJR 130:719, 1978.

39. Akiyama H, Kogure T, Itai Y: The esophageal axis and its relationship to resectability of carcinoma of the esophagus. Ann Surg 176:30, 1972.

40. Segarra MS, Cardus JC: The value of azygography in carcinoma of the esophagus. Surg Gynecol Obstet 141:248, 1973.

41. Saito J: Submucosal esophagography: a new method for demonstrating the depth of invasion of esophageal cancer. Jpn J Surg 9:37, 1979.

42. Yamada A: Radiologic assessment of resectability and prognosis in esophageal carcinoma. Gastrointest Radiol 4:213, 1979.

43. Murray GF, Wilcox BR, Stareck PJK: The assessment of operability of esophageal carcinoma. Ann Thorac Surg 23:393, 1977.

44. Daffner RH, Halber MD, Postlethwait RW, Korobkin M, Thompson WM: CT of the esophagus: II. Carcinoma. AJR 133:1051, 1979.

45. Heitzman ER, Goldwin RL, Proto AV: Radiologic analysis of the mediastinum utilizing computed tomography. Radiol Clin North Am 15:309, 1977.

46. Crowe JK, Brown LR, Muhm JR: Computed tomography of the mediastinum. Radiology 128:75, 1978.

47. Onomura K, Ohno M, Uchino A, Nakata H, Haratake J: CT of malignant mesenchymoma of the esophagus. Gastrointest Radiol 14:202–204, 1989.

48. Picus D, Balfe DM, Koehler RE, Roper CL, Owen JW: Computed tomography in the staging of esophageal carcinoma. Radiology 146:433, 1983.

49. Becker CD, Barbier P, Porcellini B: CT evaluation of patients undergoing transhiatal esophagectomy for cancer. J Comput Assist Tomogr 10:607, 1986.

50. Glick SN, Teplick SK, Levine MS, Caroline DF: Gastric cardia metastasis in esophageal carcinoma. Radiology 160:627, 1986.

51. Halvorsen RA Jr, Magruder-Habib K, Foster WL, Roberts L Jr, Postlethwait RW, Thompson WM: Esophageal cancer staging by CT: long-term follow-up study. Radiology 161:147, 1986.

52. Rosenberg JC, Franklin R, Steiger Z: Squamous cell carcinoma of the thoracic esophagus: an interdisciplinary approach. Curr Probl Cancer 5:1, 1981.

53. Thompson WM, Halvorsen RA, Foster WL, Williford ME, Postlethwait RW, Korobkin M: Computed tomography for staging esophageal and gastroesophageal cancer: reevaluation. AJR 141:951, 1983.

54. Terrier F, Schapria C, Fuchs WA: CT assessment of operability in carcinoma of the esophagogastric junction. Eur J Radiol 4:114, 1984.

55. Quint LE, Glazer GM, Orringer MB, Gross BH: Esophageal carcinoma: CT findings. Radiology 155:171, 1985.

56. Lefor AT, Merino MM, Steinberg SM, et al: Computerized tomographic prediction of extraluminal spread and prognostic implications of lesion width in esophageal cancer. Abstract. Radiology 171:290, 1989.

57. Heiken JP, Balfe DM, Roper CL: CT evaluation after esophagogastrectomy. AJR 143:555, 1984.

58. Gross BH, Agha FP, Glazer GM, Orringer MB: Gastric interposition following transhiatal esophagectomy: CT evaluation. Radiology 155:177, 1985.

59. Becker CD, Barbier PA, Terrier F, Porcellini B: Patterns of recurrence of esophageal carcinoma after transhiatal esophagectomy and gastric interposition. AJR 148:273, 1987.

60. Allen KS, Barry N, Siskind, Burrell MI: Perforation of distal esophagus with lesser sac extension: CT demonstration. J Comput Assist Tomogr 10:612, 1986.

61. Vaid YN, Shin MS: Computed tomography evaluation of tracheoesophageal fistula. J Comput Tomogr 10:281, 1986.

62. Moersch HJ, Harrington SW: Benign tumors of the esophagus. Ann Otol 53:800, 1944.

63. Godard JE, McCranie D: Multiple leiomyomas of the esophagus. AJR 117:259, 1973.

64. Whitman GJ, Borkowski GP: Giant fibrovascular polyp of the esophagus: CT and MR findings. AJR 152:518–520, 1989.

65. Balthazar EJ, Naidich DP, Megibow AJ, LeFleur RS: CT evaluation of esophageal varices. AJR 148:131, 1987.

66. Hirose J, Takashima T, Suzuki M, Matsui O: "Downhill" esophageal varices demonstrated by dynamic computed tomography. J Comput Assist Tomogr 8:1007, 1984.

67. Mauro MA, Jacques PF, Swantkowski TM, Staab EV, Bozymski EM: CT after uncomplicated esophageal sclerotherapy. AJR 147:57, 1986.

68. Kuhlman JE, Fishman EK, Wang KP, Siegelman SS: Esophageal duplication cyst: CT and transesophageal needle aspiration. AJR 145:531, 1985.

69. Weiss L, Fagelman D, Warhit JM: CT demonstration of an esophageal duplication cyst. J Comput Assist Tomogr 7:716, 1983.

70. Moss AA, Schnyder P, Marks W, Margulis AR: Gastric adenocarcinoma: a comparison of the accuracy and economics of staging by computed tomography and surgery. Gastroenterology 80:45, 1981.

71. Balfe DM, Koehler RE, Karstaedt MB, Stanley RJ, Sagel SS: Computed tomography of gastric neoplasms. Radiology 140:431, 1981.

72. Moss AA, Schnyder P, Candardjis G, Margulis AR: Computed tomography of benign and malignant gastric abnormalities. J Clin Gastroenterol 2:401, 1980.

73. Scott RL, Payne S, Pinstein ML: Fluid-level motion artifact in computed tomography. J Assoc Can Radiol 34:294, 1983.

74. Baert AL, Roex L, Marchal G, Hermans P, Dewilde D, Wilms G: Computed tomography of the stomach with water as an oral contrast agent: technique and preliminary results. J Comput Assist Tomogr 13:633–636, 1989.

75. Hammerman AM, Mirowitz SA, Susman N: Gastric air-fluid sign: aid in CT assessment of gastric wall thickening. Gastrointest Radiol 14:109–112, 1989.

76. Silverberg E: Cancer statistics 1980. CA 30:23, 1980.

77. Friedland GW: Stomach. In Steckel RJ, Kugan AR (eds): Diagnosis and Staging of Cancer: A Radiologic Approach. Philadelphia, WB Saunders, 1976, pp 129–155.

78. Frik W: Neoplastic diseases of the stomach. In Margulis AR, Burhenne HJ (eds): Alimentary Tract, 2nd ed, Vol I. St Louis, CV Mosby, 1973, pp 662–709.

79. Lee KR, Levine E, Moffat RE, Bigongiari LR, Hermreck AS: Computed tomographic staging of malignant gastric neoplasms. Radiology 133:151, 1979.

80. Miyake H, Maeda H, Kurauchi S, Watanabe H, Kawaguchi M, Tsuji K: Thickened gastric walls showing diffuse low attenuation on CT. J Comput Assist Tomogr 13:253–255, 1989.

81. Yeh H-C, Rabinowitz JG: Ultrasonography and computed tomography of gastric wall lesions. Radiology 141:147, 1981.

82. Phatak MG, Dobben GD, Asselmeir GH: CT demonstration of scirrhous carcinoma of the stomach: a case report. Comput Radiol 6:31, 1982.

83. Freeny PC, Marks WM: Adenocarcinoma of the gastroesophageal junction. Barium and CT examination. AJR 138:1077, 1982.

84. Scatarige JC, DiSantis DJ: CT of the stomach and duodenum. Radiol Clin North Am 27:687–706, 1989.

85. Kleinhaus U, Militianu D: Computed tomography in the preoperative evaluation of gastric carcinoma. Gastrointest Radiol 13:97–101, 1984.

86. Cook AO, Levine BA, Sirinek KR, Gaskill HV: Evaluation of gastric adenocarcinoma: abdominal computed tomography does not replace celiotomy. Arch Surg 121:603–606, 1986.

87. Sussman DK, Halvorsen RA, Illescas FF, et al: Gastric adenocarcinoma: CT versus surgical staging. Radiology 167:335–340, 1988.

88. Mullin D, Shirkhoda A: Computed tomography after gastrectomy in primary gastric carcinoma. J Comput Assist Tomogr 9:30, 1985.

89. Megibow AJ, Balthazar EJ, Naidich DP, Bosniak MA: Computed tomography of gastrointestinal lymphoma. AJR 141:541, 1983.

90. Rosenberg SA, Diamond HD, Jaslowitz B, Craver LF: Lymphosarcoma: a review of 1296 cases. Medicine 40:31, 1961.

91. Brady LW, Asbell O: Malignant lymphoma of the gastrointestinal tract. Radiology 137:291, 1980.

92. Sherrick DW, Hudson JR, Dockerty MB: The roentgenologic diagnosis of primary gastric lymphoma. Radiology 86:925, 1965.

93. Nelson RS, Lanza FL: The endoscopic diagnosis of gastric lymphoma: gross characteristics and histology. Gastrointest Endosc 21:66, 1976.

94. Katz S, Klein MS, Winawer SJ, Sherlock P: Disseminated lymphoma involving the stomach: correlation of endoscopy with directed cytology and biopsy. Am J Digest Dis 18:370, 1973.

95. Buy J-N, Moss AA: Computed tomography of gastric lymphoma. AJR 138:859, 1982.

96. Krudy AG, Dunnick NR, Magrath IT, Shawker TH, Doppman JL, Speigel R: CT of American Burkitt lymphoma. AJR 136:747, 1981.

97. Hertzer NR, Hoerr SO: An interpretive review of lymphoma of the stomach. Surg Gynecol Obstet 143:113, 1976.

98. Ellis HA, Lannigan R: Primary lymphoid neoplasms of the stomach. Gut 4:145, 1963.

99. Megibow AJ: Gastrointestinal lymphoma: the role of CT on diagnosis and management. Semin US CT MR 7(1):43, 1986.

100. Clark RA, Alexander ES: Computed tomography of gastrointestinal leiomyosarcoma. Gastrointest Radiol 7:127, 1982.

101. Megibow AJ, Balthazar EJ, Hulnick DH, Naidich DP, Bosniak MA: CT evaluation of gastrointestinal leiomyomas and leiomyosarcomas. AJR 144:727, 1985.

102. Kriss N: Some unusual features of gastric adenomas. Am J Digest Dis 15:103, 1970.

103. Kleyn KA, Mandell GH, Sakawa S, Kobernick SD: Glomus tumor of the stomach. Arch Surg 97:111, 1968.

104. Stout AP: Tumors of the Stomach. Washington, DC, Armed Forces Institute of Pathology, 1953.

105. Palmer ED: Benign intramural tumors of the stomach: a review with special reference to gross pathology. Medicine 30:81, 1951.

106. Heiken JP, Forde KA, Gold RP: Computed tomography as a definitive method for diagnosing gastrointestinal lipomas. Radiology 142:409, 1982.

107. Moruichi A, Nakayama I, Muta H, Taira Y, Takahara O, Yokoyama S: Gastric teratoma of children: a case report with review of the literature. Acta Pathol Jpn 27:749, 1977.

108. Bowen B, Ros PR, McCarthy MJ, Olmstead WW, Hjermstad BM: Gastrointestinal teratomas: CT and US appearance with pathologic correlation. Radiology 162:431, 1987.

109. Coin CG, Coin JT, Howiler WE, Phillips CA, Tart JA: Computed tomography in peptic ulcer: a preliminary report. Comput Tomogr 5:225, 1981.

110. Milici LP, Markowitz SK: Gastric intramural pseudocyst: computed tomographic diagnosis. Gastrointest Radiol 14:113–114, 1989.

111. Soulen MC, Elliot FK, Scatarige JC, Hutchins D, Zerhouni EA: Cryptosporidiosis of the gastric antrum: detection using CT. Radiology 159:705, 1986.

112. de Lange EE, Slutsky VS, Swanson S, Shaffer HA Jr: Computed tomography of emphysematous gastritis. J Comput Assist Tomogr 10:139, 1986.

113. McCain AH, Bernardino ME, Sones PJ, Berkman WA, Casarella WJ: Varices from portal hypertension: correlation of CT and angiography. Radiology 154:63, 1985.

114. Balthazar EJ, Megibow A, Naidich D, LeFleur RS: Computed tomographic recognition of gastric varices. AJR 142:1121, 1984.

115. Omojola MF, Hood IC, Stevenson GW: Calcified gastric duplication. Gastrointest Radiol 5:235, 1980.

116. Schwartz AN, Goiney RC, Graney DO: Gastric diverticulum simulating and adrenal mass: CT appearance and embryogenesis. AJR 146:553, 1986.

117. Silverman PM: Gastric diverticulum mimicking adrenal mass: CT demonstration. J Comput Assist Tomogr 10:709, 1986.

118. Goldberg HI: Computed tomographic evaluation of the gastrointestinal tract in diseases other than primary adenocarcinoma. In Goldberg HI (ed): Interventional Radiology and Diagnostic Imaging Modality. San Francisco, University of California Press, 1982, pp 236–250.

119. Megibow AJ, Bosniak MA: Dilute barium as a contrast agent for abdominal CT. AJR 134:1273, 1980.

120. Kreel L: Computerized tomography using the EMI general purpose scanner. Br J Radiol 50:2, 1977.

121. Ruijs SHJ: A simple procedure for patient preparation in abdominal CT. AJR 133:551, 1979.

122. Marks WM, Goldberg HI, Moss AA, Koehler FR, Federle MP: Intestinal pseudotumors: a problem in abdominal computed tomography solved by direct techniques. Gastrointest Radiol 5:155, 1980.

123. Demas BE, McCarthy SM, Moss AA, Wall SD, Goldberg HI: Utility of ceruletide in promoting opacification for abdominal and pelvic computed tomography. Gastrointest Radiol 11:197, 1986.

124. Thoeni RF, Filson RG: Abdominal and pelvic CT: use of oral metoclopramide to enhance bowel opacification. Radiology 169:391, 1988.

125. Seigel RS, Kuhns LR, Borlaza GS: Computed tomography

and angiography in ileal carcinoid tumor and retractile mesenteritis. Radiology 134:437, 1980.

126. Pagani JJ, Bernardino ME: CT-radiographic correlation of ulcerating small bowel lymphomas. AJR 136:998, 1981.

127. Schaefer PS, Friedman AC: Nodular lymphoid hyperplasia of the small intestine with Burkitt's lymphoma and dysgammaglobulinemia. Gastrointest Radiol 6:325, 1981.

128. Farah MC, Jafri SZH, Schwab RE, Mezwa DG, Francis IR, et al: Duodenal neoplasms: role of CT. Radiology 162:839, 1987.

129. Megibow AJ, Redmond PE, Bosniak MA, Horowitz L: Diagnosis of gastrointestinal lipomas by CT. AJR 133:743, 1979.

130. Cohen WN, Seidelman FE, Bryan PJ: Computed tomography of localized adipose deposits presenting as tumor masses. AJR 128:1007, 1977.

131. Ormson MJ, Stephens DH, Carlson HC: CT recognition of intestinal lipomatosis. AJR 144:313, 1985.

132. Dudiak KM, Johnson CD, Stephens DH: Primary tumors of the small intestine: CT evaluation. AJR 152:995–998, 1989.

133. Parienty RA, Lepreux JF, Gruson B: Sonographic and CT features of ileocolic intussusception. AJR 136:608, 1981.

134. Donovan AT, Goldman SM: Computed tomography of ileocecal intussusception. Mechanism and appearance. J Comput Assist Tomogr 6:603, 1982.

135. Diamond RT, Greenberg HM, Boult IF: Direct metastatic spread of right colon adenocarcinoma to duodenum—barium and computed tomographic findings. Gastrointest Radiol 6:339, 1981.

136. Rubesin SE, Levine MS: Omental cakes: colonic involvement by omental metastases. Radiology 154:593, 1985.

137. Ginaldi S, Zornosa J: Large duodenal diverticulum simulating a pancreatic mass by computed tomography. Comput Tomogr 4:169, 1980.

138. Fisher JF: Computed tomographic diagnosis of volvulus in intestinal malrotation. Radiology 140:145, 1981.

139. Hoyt TS: Malrotation of small bowel simulating a neoplastic mass in the right upper quadrant. Comput Radiol 6:27, 1982.

140. Goldberg HI, Gore RM, Margulis AR, Moss AA, Baker EL: Computed tomography in the evaluation of Crohn's disease. AJR 140:277, 1983.

141. Carey LS: Regional enteritis: the rubbery mesentery. J Can Assoc Radiol 31:269, 1980.

142. Yeh CH, Rabinowitz JG: Granulomatous enterocolitis: findings by ultrasonography and computed tomography. Radiology 149:253, 1983.

143. Schnor MJ, Winer SN: The "string sign" in computerized tomography. Gastrointest Radiol 7:43, 1982.

144. Fishman EK, Wolf EJ, Jones B, Bayless TM, Siegelman SS: CT evaluation of Crohn's disease: effect on patient management. AJR 148:537, 1987.

145. Megibow AJ, Bosniak MA, Ambos MA, Redmond PE: Crohn's disease causing hydronephrosis. J Comput Assist Tomogr 5:909, 1981.

146. Le DKB, Rennie CS: Abdominal computed tomography in Whipple's disease. J Comput Assist Tomogr 6:193, 1982.

147. Greyson-Fleg RT, Jones B, Fishman EK, Siegelman SS: Computed tomography findings in gastrointestinal involvement by opportunistic organisms in acquired immune deficiency syndrome. J Comput Tomogr 10:175, 1986.

148. Jones B, Fishman EK, Kramer SS, Siegelman SS, Saral R, et al: Computed tomography of gastrointestinal inflammation after bone marrow transplantation. AJR 146:691, 1986.

149. Frager DH, Frager JD, Brandt LJ, Wolf EL, Rand LG, et al: Gastrointestinal complications of AIDS: radiologic features. Radiology 158:597, 1986.

150. Hulnick DH, Megibow AJ, Naidich DP, Hilton S, Cho KC, Balthazar EJ: Abdominal tuberculosis: CT evaluation. Radiology 157:199, 1985.

151. Silverman PM, Baker ME, Cooper C, Kelvin FM: CT appearance of diffuse mesenteric edema. J Comput Assist Tomogr 10:67, 1986.

152. Downey EF Jr, Pyatt RS Jr, Vincent M, Evans DR, Daye S: Upper gastrointestinal diverticula. J Comput Assist Tomogr 6:193, 1982.

153. Greenstein S, Jones B, Fishman EK, Cameron JL, Siegelman SS: Small-bowel diverticulitis: CT findings. AJR 147:271, 1986.

154. Kuwabara Y, Nishitani H, Numaguchi Y, Kamoi I, Matsuura K, Saito S: Afferent loop syndrome. J Comput Assist Tomogr 4:687, 1980.

155. Robbins AH: CT appearance of afferent loop obstruction. AJR 138:1085, 1982.

156. Cho KC, Hoffman-Tretin JC, Alterman DD: Closed-loop obstruction of the small bowel: CT and sonographic appearance. J Comput Assist Tomogr 13:256–258, 1989.

157. Parienty RA, Lepreux JF, Gruson B: Sonographic and CT features of ileocolic intussusception. AJR 136:608, 1981.

158. Lo G, Fisch AE, Brodey PA: CT of the intussuscepted excluded loop after intestinal bypass. AJR 137:157, 1981.

159. Billimoria PE, Fabian TM, Schulz EE: Computed tomography of intussusception in the bypassed jejunoileal segment. J Comput Assist Tomogr 6:86, 1982.

160. Cholankeril JV, Ketyer S, Kessler MA, Kogan E: Computerized tomography and ultrasonography in intussusception of the small bowel. Comput Tomogr 6:167, 1982.

161. Merine D, Fishman EK, Jones B, Siegelman SS: Enteroenteric intussusception: CT findings in nine patients. AJR 148:1129, 1987.

162. Balthazar EJ, Bauman JS, Megibow AJ: CT diagnosis of closed loop obstruction. J Comput Assist Tomogr 9:953, 1985.

163. Leyman P, Ponette E, Marchal G, Vercruyssen J, Timmermans G, Ceulemans R, Baert AL: Computed tomography of acute jejunogastric intussusception. J Comput Assist Tomogr 13:531–533, 1989.

164. Hoddick WK, Demas B, Moss AA: CT-guided percutaneous bowel loopogram. AJR 143:1098, 1984.

165. Grumbach K, Levine MS, Wexler JA: Gallstone ileus diagnosed by computed tomography. J Comput Assist Tomogr 10:146, 1986.

166. Federle MP, Goldberg HI, Kaiser JA, Moss AA, Jeffrey RB, Mall JC: Evaluation of abdominal trauma by computed tomography. Radiology 138:637, 1981.

167. Mohamed G, Reyes HM, Fantus R, Ramilo J, Radhakrishna J: Computed tomography in the assessment of pediatric abdominal trauma. Arch Surg 121:703, 1986.

168. Bulas DI, Taylor GA, Eichelberger MR: Value of CT in detecting bowel perforation in children after blunt abdominal trauma. AJR 153:561–564, 1989.

169. Rizzo MJ, Federle MP, Griffiths BG: Bowel and mesenteric injury following blunt abdominal trauma: evaluation with CT. Radiology 173:143–148, 1989.

170. Glazer GM, Buy J-N, Moss AA, Goldberg HI, Federle AP: CT detection of duodenal perforation. AJR 137:333, 1981.

171. Toxopeus MD, Lucas CE, Krabbenhoft KL: Roentgenographic diagnosis in blunt retroperitoneal duodenal rupture. Radiology 115:281, 1972.

172. Kelly G, Norton L, Moore G, Eiseman B: The continuing challenge of duodenal injuries. J Trauma 18:160, 1978.

173. Karnaze GC, Sheedy PF II, Stephens DH, McLeod RA: Computed tomography in duodenal rupture due to blunt abdominal trauma. J Comput Assist Tomogr 5:267, 1981.

174. Federle MP, Chun G, Jeffrey RB, Rayor R: Computed tomographic findings in bowel infarction. AJR 142:91, 1984.

175. Pérez C, Llauger J, Puig J, Palmer J: Computed tomographic findings in bowel ischemia. Gastrointest Radiol 14:241–245, 1989.

176. Plojoux O, Hauser H, Wettstein P: Computed tomography of intramural hematoma of the small intestine. Radiology 144:559, 1982.

177. Anderson MC, Silberman WW, Shields TW: Duplications of the alimentary tract in the adult. Arch Surg 85:94, 1962.

178. Bower RJ, Sieber WK, Kieswetter WB: Alimentary tract duplications in children. Ann Surg 188:669, 1978.

179. Kelly RB, Mahoney PD, Johnson JF: CT demonstration of an unusual enteric duplication cyst. J Comput Assist Tomogr 10:506, 1986.

180. Thoeni RF, Moss AA, Schnyder P, Margulis AR: Staging of primary rectal and rectosigmoid tumors by computed tomography. Radiology 141:135, 1981.

181. Moss AA, Thoeni RF, Schnyder P, Margulis AR: The value of computed tomography in detecting recurrent rectal carcinomas. J Comput Assist Tomogr 5:870, 1981.

182. Lee JKT, Stanley RJ, Sagel SS, Levit RG, McClennan BL: CT appearance of the pelvis after abdomino-perineal resection for rectal carcinoma. Radiology 14:737, 1981.

183. Doubleday LC, Bernardino ME: CT findings in the perirectal area following radiation therapy. J Comput Assist Tomogr 4:634, 1980.

184. Mayers GB, Zornoza J: Computed tomography of colon carcinoma. AJR 135:43, 1980.

185. Ellert J, Dreel L: The value of CT in malignant colonic tumors. CT 4:225, 1980.

186. Mitchell DG, Bjorgvinsson E, terMeulen D, Lane P, Greberman M, Friedman AC: Gastrografin versus dilute barium for colonic CT examination: a blind, randomized study. J Comput Assist Tomogr 9:451–453, 1985.

187. Hamlin DF, Burgener FA, Sischy B: New techniques to stage early rectal carcinoma by computed tomography. Radiology 141:539, 1981.

188. Solomon A, Michowitz M, Papo J, Yust I: Computed tomographic air enema technique to demonstrate colonic neoplasms. Gastrointest Radiol 11:194, 1986.

189. Silverberg E: Cancer statistics 1977. CA 27:26, 1977.

190. Husband JE, Hodson NJ, Parsons CA: The use of computed tomography in recurrent rectal tumors. Radiology 134:677, 1980.

191. Grabbe E, Winkler R: Radiologische Diagnostik nach abdomino-perinealer Rektumamputation. ROEFO 131:127, 1979.

192. Cass AW, Million RR, Pfaff WW: Patterns of recurrence following surgery alone for adenocarcinoma of the colon and rectum. Cancer 37:2861, 1976.

193. Dukes CE: The classification of cancer of the rectum. J Pathol Bacteriol 35:232, 1932.

194. Astler VB, Coller FA: The prognostic significance of direct extension of carcinoma of the colon and rectum. Am Surg 139:846, 1954.

195. Moss AA, Margulis AR, Schnyder P, Thoeni RF: A uniform, CT-based staging system for malignant neoplasms of the alimentary tube. Editorial. AJR 136:1251, 1981.

196. Wilson SM, Adson MA: The surgical treatment of hepatic metastases from colorectal cancers. Arch Surg 111:330, 1976.

197. Lee KT, Stanley RJ, Sagel SS, McClennan BL: Accuracy of CT in detecting intra-abdominal and pelvic lymph node metastases from pelvic cancers. AJR 131:675, 1978.

198. Zaunbauer W, Haertel M, Fuchs WA: Computed tomography in carcinoma of the rectum. Gastrointest Radiol 6:79, 1981.

199. Colley DP, Farrell JA, Clark RA: Perforated colon carcinoma presenting as a suprarenal mass. Comput Tomogr 5:55, 1981.

200. Grabbe E, Buurman R, Winkler R, Buechler E, Shreiber HW: Computer-tomographische Befunde nach Rektumamputation. ROEFO 131:135, 1979.

201. Thoeni RF: Computed tomography of rectosigmoid tumors. In Goldberg HI (ed): Interventional Radiology and Diagnostic Imaging Modalities. San Francisco, University of California Press, 1982, pp 227–236.

202. Keeney G, Jafir SZH, Mezwa DG: Computed tomographic evaluation and staging of cecal carcinoma. Gastrointest Radiol 14:65–69, 1989.

203. Freeny PC, Marks WM, Ryan JA, Bolen JW: Colorectal carcinoma evaluation with CT: preoperative staging and detection of postoperative recurrence. Radiology 158:347, 1986.

204. Grabbe E, Winkler R: Local recurrence after sphincter-saving resection for rectal and rectosigmoid carcinoma. Value of various diagnostic methods. Radiology 155:305–310, 1985.

205. Chen YM, Ott DJ, Wolfman NT, Gelfand DW, Karsteadt N, Bechtold RE: Recurrent colorectal carcinoma: evaluation with barium enema examination and CT. Radiology 163:307, 1987.

206. McCarthy SM, Barnes D, Deveney K, Moss AA, Goldberg HI: Detection of recurrent rectosigmoid carcinoma: prospective evaluation of CT and clinical factors. AJR 144:577, 1985.

207. Butch RJ, Wittenberg J, Mueller PR, Simeone JF, Meyer JE, Ferrucci JT Jr: Presacral masses after abdominoperineal resection for colorectal carcinoma: the need for needle biopsy. AJR 144:309, 1985.

208. Coscina WF, Arger PH, Levine MS, Herlinger H, Cohen S, et al: Gastrointestinal tract focal mass lesions: role of CT and barium evaluations. Radiology 158:581, 1986.

209. Walsh JW, Amendola MA, Hall D, Tisnado J, Goplerud DR: Recurrent carcinoma of the cervix: CT diagnosis. AJR 136:117, 1981.

210. Cho KC, Gold BM: Computed tomography of Krukenberg tumors. AJR 145:285, 1985.

211. Coscina WF, Arger PH, Herlinger H, Levine MS, Coleman BG, Mintz MC: CT diagnosis of villous adenoma. J Comput Assist Tomogr 10:764, 1986.

212. Balthazar EJ, Streiter M, Megibow AJ: Anorectal giant condyloma acuminatum (Buschke-Loewenstein tumor): CT and radiographic manifestations. Radiology 150:651, 1984.

213. Gore RM, Goldberg HI: Computed tomographic evaluation of the gastrointestinal tract in diseases other than primary adenocarcinoma. Radiol Clin North Am 20:781, 1982.

214. Gore RM, Marn CS, Kirby DF, Vogelzang RL, Neiman HL: CT findings in ulcerative, granulomatous, and indeterminate colitis. AJR 143:279, 1984.

215. Goodman PC, Federle MP: Pseudomembranous colitis. J Comput Assist Tomogr 4:403, 1980.

216. Hoddick W, Jeffrey RB, Federle MP: CT differentiation of portal venous air from biliary air. J Comput Assist Tomogr 6:633, 1982.

217. Frick MP, Feinberg SB, Stenlund RR, Gedgaudas E: Evaluation of abdominal fistulas with computed body tomography (CT). Comput Radiol 6:17, 1982.

218. Alexander ES, Weinberg S, Clark RA, Belkin RD: Fistulas and sinus tracts: radiologic evaluation, management and outcome. Gastrointest Radiol 7:135, 1982.

219. Adams GW, Rauch RF, Kelvin FM, Silverman PM, Korobkin M: CT detection of typhlitis. J Comput Assist Tomogr 9:363, 1985.

220. Frick MP, Maile CW, Crass JR, Goldberg ME, Delaney JP: Computed tomography of neutropenic colitis. AJR 143:763, 1984.

221. Guillaumin E, Jeffrey RB, Shea WJ, Asling CW, Goldberg HI: Perirectal inflammatory disease: CT findings. Radiology 161:153, 1986.

222. Donaldson JS, Gilsanz V: CT findings in rectal cuff abscess following surgery for Hirschsprung disease. J Comput Assist Tomogr 10:151–153, 1986.

223. Siskind BN, Burrell MI, Richter JO, Radin DR: CT appearance of giant sigmoid diverticulum. J Comput Assist Tomogr 10:543–544, 1986.

224. Hulnick DH, Megibow AJ, Balthazar EJ, Naidich DP, Bosniak MA: Computed tomography in the evaluation of diverticulitis. Radiology 152:491, 1984.

225. Johnson CD, Baker ME, Silverman P, Thompson WM: Diagnosis of acute colonic diverticulitis: comparison of barium enema and CT. AJR 148:541, 1987.

226. Balthazar EJ, Megibow AJ, Gordon RB, Hulnick D: Cecal diverticulitis: evaluation with CT. Radiology 162:79, 1987.

227. Shaff MI, Himmelfarb E, Sacks GA, Burks DD, Kulkarni MV: The whirl sign: a CT finding in volvulus of the large bowel. J Comput Assist Tomogr 9:410, 1985.

228. Sheward SE, Williams AG Jr, Mettler FA Jr, Lacey SR: CT appearance of a surgically retained towel (gossypiboma). J Comput Assist Tomogr 10:343, 1986.

229. Iko BO, Teal JS, Siram SM, Chinwuba CE, Roux VJ, Scott VF: Computed tomography of adult colonic intussusception: clinical and experimental studies. AJR 143:769, 1984.

230. Styles RA, Larsen CR: CT appearance of adult intussusception. J Comput Assist Tomogr 7:331, 1983.

231. Casola G, Withers C, vanSonnenberg E, Herba MJ, Saba RM, Brown RA: Percutaneous cecostomy for decompression of the massively distended cecum. Radiology 158:793, 1986.

232. Crass JR, Simmons RL, Frick MP, Maile CW: Percutaneous decompression of the colon using CT guidance in Ogilvie syndrome. AJR 144:475, 1985.

233. Sherman JL, Hopper KD, Greene AJ, Johns TT: The retrorenal colon on computed tomography: a normal variant. J Comput Assist Tomogr 9:339, 1985.

234. Hopper KD, Sherman JL, Luethke JM, Ghaed N: The retro-

renal colon in the supine and prone patient. Radiology 162:443, 1987.

235. Auh YH, Pardes JG, Chung BK, Rubenstein WA, Kazam E: Posterior hepatodiaphragmatic interposition of the colon: ultrasonographic and computed tomographic appearance. J Ultrasound Med 4:113, 1985.

236. Rice CA, Anderson TM, Sepahdari S: Computed tomography and ultrasonography of carcinoma in duplication cysts. J Comput Assist Tomogr 10:233, 1986.

237. Kohda E, Fujioka M, Ikawa H, Yokoyama J: Congenital anorectal anomaly: CT evaluation. Radiology 157:349, 1985.

238. Hahn PF, Stark DD, Lewis JM, Saini S, Elizondo G, et al: First clinical trial of a new superparamagnetic iron oxide for use as an oral gastrointestinal contrast agent in MR imaging. Radiology 175:695–700, 1990.

239. Quint LE, Glazer GM, Orringer MB: Esophageal imaging by MR and CT: study of normal anatomy and neoplasms. Radiology 156:727, 1985.

240. Winkler ML, Hricak H, Higgins CB: MR imaging of diffusely infiltrating gastric carcinoma. J Comput Assist Tomogr 11:337, 1987.

241. Butch RJ, Stark DD, Wittenberg J, Tepper JE, Saini S, et al: Staging rectal cancer by MR and CT. AJR 146:1155, 1986.

242. Pomeranz SJ, Altman N, Sheldon JJ, Tobias JA, Soila KP, et al: Magnetic resonance of congenital anorectal malformations. Magn Reson Imaging 4:69, 1986.

243. Tscholakoff D, Hricak H, Thoeni R, Winkler ML, Margulis AR: MR imaging in the diagnosis of pancreatic disease. AJR 148:703, 1987.

244. Wesbey GE, Brasch RC, Engelstad BL, Moss AA, Crooks LE, Brito AC: Nuclear magnetic resonance contrast enhancement study of the gastrointestinal tract of rats and a human volunteer using nontoxic oral iron solutions. Radiology 149:175, 1983.

245. Wesbey GE, Engelstad BL, Brasch RC: Paramagnetic pharmaceuticals for magnetic resonance imaging. Physiol Chem Phys Med NMR 16:145, 1984.

246. Wesbey GE, Brasch RC, Goldberg HI, Engelstad BL, Moss AA: Dilute oral iron solutions as gastrointestinal contrast agents for magnetic resonance imaging; initial clinical experience. Magn Reson Imaging 3:57, 1985.

247. Kaminsky S, Laniado M, Kornmesser W, Claussen CD, Felix R: Use of Gd-DTPA as a positive contrast agent in abdominal MR imaging. Radiology 169(P):221, 1988.

248. Crooks L, Arakawa M, Hoenninger J, Watts J, McRee R, et al: Nuclear magnetic resonance whole-body imager operating at 3.5 kgauss. Radiology 143:169–174, 1982.

249. Carr DH, Brown J, Bydder GM, Steiner RE, Weinmann HJ, et al: Gadolinium-DTPA as a contrast agent in MRI: initial clinical experience in 20 patients. AJR 143:215, 1984.

250. Moss AA: Imaging of colorectal carcinoma. Radiology 170:308–310, 1989.

251. Krestin GP, Steinbrich W, Friedmann G: Recurrent rectal cancer: diagnosis with MR imaging versus CT. Radiology 168:307–311, 1988.

252. Lee JKT, Heiken JP, Ling D, Glazer HS, Balfe DM, et al: Magnetic resonance imaging of abdominal and pelvic lymphadenopathy. Radiology 153:181, 1984.

253. Dooms GC, Hricak H, Crooks LE, Higgins CB: Magnetic resonance imaging of the lymph nodes: comparison with CT. Radiology 153:719, 1984.

254. Blum L, Kressel HY, de Roos A, Gefter WB: MR imaging differentiation of fibrosis versus recurrent colorectal carcinoma in the pelvis: quantitative assessment. Radiology 169(P):167, 1988.

255. Glazer HS, Lee JKT, Levitt RG, Heiken JP, Ling D, et al: Radiation fibrosis: differentiation from recurrent tumor by MR imaging (work in progress). Radiology 156:721–726, 1985.

256. Ebner F, Kressel HY, Mintz MC, Carlson JA, Cohen EK, et al: Tumor recurrence versus fibrosis in the female pelvis: differentiation with MR imaging at 1.5 T. Radiology 166:333–340, 1988.

257. de Lange EE, Fechner RE, Wanebo HJ: Suspected recurrent rectosigmoid carcinoma after abdominoperineal resection: MR imaging and histopathologic findings. Radiology 170:323–328, 1989.

CHAPTER 17

THE LIVER

RICHARD L. BARON ▪ *PATRICK C. FREENY* ▪ *ALBERT A. MOSS*

Computed tomography (CT) and magnetic resonance imaging (MRI) have been applied to the liver since their introduction to body imaging. In each instance, the liver has become the organ most often studied in the truncal body with both modalities, predominantly because the liver is a common site of metastatic disease. CT and MR techniques to evaluate the liver have advanced during the past decade and undoubtedly will continue to evolve. We now have a better definition of when and how to utilize these examinations, although as we learn more and MR images improve in quality, choosing which method to use may occasionally be difficult. This chapter will review liver anatomy and disease processes that can be evaluated with CT and MR imaging.

Anatomy

Computed Tomography

GROSS MORPHOLOGY

The liver is the largest organ in the body, lying in the right upper quadrant of the abdomen. Cross-sectional CT images readily display most border-forming perihepatic structures, including the anterior abdominal wall, posterior diaphragm, right kidney, right colon, stomach, inferior vena cava, and right adrenal gland. The liver is covered by peritoneum, except for the fossa for the inferior vena cava, the fossa for the gallbladder, and the bare area of the liver, where the posterior surface of the liver comes

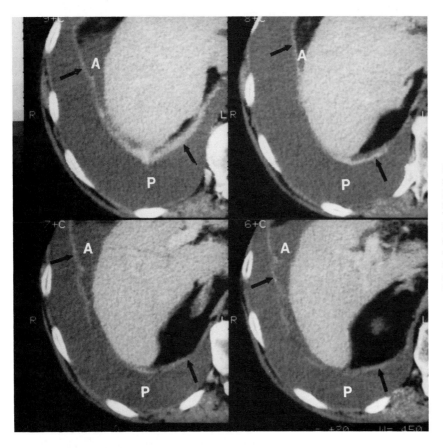

FIGURE 17–1 ■ Bare area of the liver. CT scans at four levels in a patient with a right pleural effusion and ascites. The pleural effusion (P) extends medially to the vertebral body. The peritoneal ascites (A) is seen abutting the liver surface laterally but does not extend medially where the liver surface comes in direct contact with the diaphragm without peritoneal surfaces. The diaphragm *(arrows)* is well delineated from the pleural and peritoneal fluid and intraabdominal fat.

in direct contact with the diaphragm. This lack of a peritoneal surface against the diaphragm can be used to aid in differentiating the origins of fluid collections (Fig. 17–1). Pleural fluid collections are seen throughout the entire posterior aspect of the posterior perihepatic space, whereas peritoneal fluid stops medially at the bare area of the liver.[1]

The shape of the liver is complex; superiorly it is dome shaped, conforming to the undersurface of the diaphragm. This surface is usually smooth, although accessory fissures containing fat and slips of the diaphragm can cause peripheral indentation and scalloping of the liver margin or liver and simulate a peripheral lesion (Fig. 17–2).[2] Inferiorly, the undersurface of the liver is concave and slopes downward to a sharp border. The complex hepatic shape accounts for the varied appearance of the liver on CT scans obtained at different levels (Fig. 17–3). Sections obtained near the diaphragm reveal that the liver occupies nearly the entire right half of the abdomen.

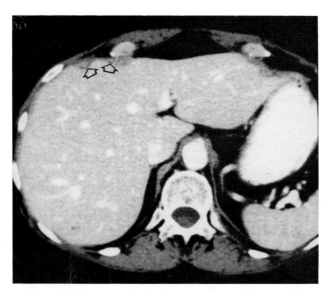

FIGURE 17–2 ■ Slips of the diaphragm can be seen indenting the anterior margin of the liver. These diaphragmatic slips appear as lower attenuation regions when compared with the contrast-enhanced liver parenchyma and can simulate a peripheral parenchymal liver lesion. A thin rim of fat *(open arrows)* may be seen insinuating against the liver parenchyma and confirms the extrahepatic nature of these structures.

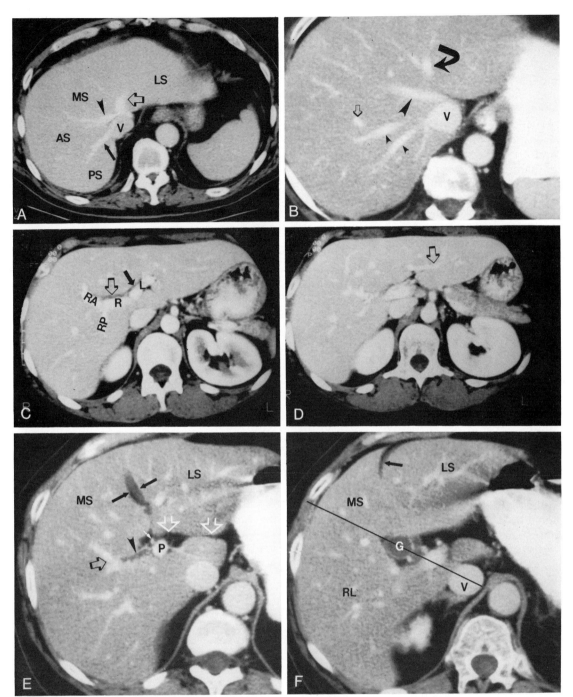

FIGURE 17–3 ■ Normal liver anatomy. *A,* The hepatic veins delineate the segmental anatomy in the superior aspects of the liver. The left hepatic vein *(open arrow)* bisects the left lobe into the lateral segment (LS) and the medial segment (MS). The middle hepatic vein *(arrowhead)* bisects the right and left hepatic lobes. The right hepatic vein *(solid arrow)* bisects the right lobe into the anterior segment (AS) and the posterior segment (PS). The hepatic veins converge and often share common trunks as they empty into the inferior vena cava (V). *B,* Scan from another patient slightly caudal to the level in *A* shows the left hepatic vein *(curved arrow)* and middle hepatic vein *(large arrowhead)* as single large veins. Two major branches of the right hepatic vein *(small arrowheads)* are seen. A right portal vein branch *(open arrow)* is imaged in cross section. V = Inferior vena cava. *C,* Scan from the patient in *B* at a lower level shows the right (R) and left (L) branches of the portal vein. The right portal vein further bifurcates into the right anterior (RA) and right posterior (RP) portal vein branches. These latter portal vein branches run through the central portion of the anterior and posterior right lobe segments, respectively, unlike the hepatic veins, which run in the margins of the segments. The left *(solid arrow)* and right *(open arrow)* hepatic ducts are identified just proximal to their confluence into the common hepatic duct. *D,* At a slightly lower level than *C,* the left portal vein *(open arrow)* can be seen in its linear course through the lateral segment of the left lobe. There is not a well-defined left intersegmental fissure in this patient to demarcate the segments of the left lobe. *E,* Scan from the same patient as in *B* at the level of the porta hepatis and main portal vein (P) shows a prominent fissure for the ligamentum teres *(solid black arrows),* separating the lateral segment (LS) from the medial segment (MS). The fissure for the ligamentum venosum *(open white arrows)* separates the caudate lobe from the lateral segment of the left lobe. Frequently the right lobe landmarks are not as well delineated on CT at this level, although the right anterior portal vein branches *(open black arrow)* courses through the interior of the right anterior segment. Arrowhead = Right common hepatic duct; solid white arrow = hepatic artery. *F,* Scan at a slightly lower level than *E* shows the anterior extension of the fissure for the ligamentum teres *(arrow),* delineating the lateral (LS) and medial (MS) segments of the left lobe. A line drawn through the plane of the inferior vena cava (V) and gallbladder (G) and its fossa demarcates the interlobar fissure, which is often incomplete, as in this patient. The right lobe (RL) segmental landmarks are incomplete at this level, and it is difficult to differentiate the anterior and posterior segments.

More caudally located images reveal that the volume of the liver gradually decreases, the right lobe becoming indented by the kidney and assuming a more anterior and lateral position. The gallbladder lies on the visceral surface of the liver in a fossa between the right hepatic lobe and medial segment of the left hepatic lobe. Caudally the gallbladder is located more laterally and anteriorly and at times may reach the anterior abdominal wall or press on the duodenal sweep, colon, or gastric antrum.

The liver is composed of a large right hepatic lobe, a smaller left hepatic lobe, and an anatomically distinct caudate lobe. A total of four intrahepatic fissures define the margins of the intrahepatic lobes and the principal lobar segments.

The left intersegmental fissure (see Fig. 17–3E, F) contains fat and the ligamentum teres and produces a vertical cleft in the anterior surface of the left hepatic lobe. This fissure separates the medial and lateral segments of the left hepatic lobe. The fissure of the ligamentum venosum (see Fig. 17–3E) courses obliquely from the posterior aspect of the left intersegmental fissure deeply into the liver anterior to the caudate lobe and contains the two layers of the lesser omentum. It separates the posteriorly positioned caudate lobe from the posterior aspect of the medial and lateral segments of the left hepatic lobe. At its lower end, it curves laterally in front of the papillary process of the caudate lobe to reach the left extremity of the porta hepatis.

The sagittally oriented interlobar fissure (see Fig. 17–3F), separating the right and left hepatic lobes, is approximated by a plane extending from the superior recess of the gallbladder through the fossa of the inferior vena cava. This fissure is an incomplete structure, occasionally present inferiorly above the gallbladder as a fat-filled cleft containing the main portal vein and smaller accompanying portal triad structures. Superiorly, the same vertical plane runs through the plane of the middle hepatic vein, the superior landmark delineating the right and left hepatic lobes.[3]

The right intersegmental fissure is ill defined and is best seen by examining hepatic casts; it cannot be visualized directly by computed tomography, because it produces no detectable surface alterations. An approximation of its location may be made by drawing a line that bisects the liver parenchyma between the anterior and posterior branches of the right portal vein and extends superiorly to run in the plane of the right hepatic vein.

Variations in size and configuration of the normal liver are common. The lateral segment of the left lobe may appear bulbous or extend anteriorly across the midline to varying degrees, reaching the posterior left side of the upper abdomen in some patients (Fig. 17–4). Following surgical resection of the right lobe of the liver, the left lateral segment may enlarge to such an extent that the total liver mass returns almost to normal. Congenital absence of either the right or the left lobe of the liver is a rare anomalous variant

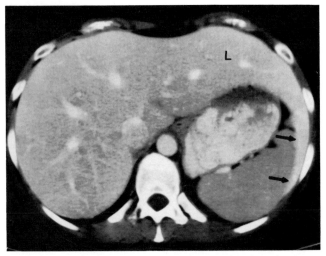

FIGURE 17–4 ■ Normal variation in the shape of the lateral segment of left hepatic lobe. Prominent lateral segment of the left lobe (L) of the liver can be seen crossing the left abdomen with an extension lateral and posterior to the spleen (arrows).

without clinical significance, usually with hypertrophy of the contralateral lobe and the caudate lobe (Fig. 17–5).[4-7] It is important to recognize this variant so as not to mistake the lack of lobar tissue as atrophy from cirrhosis or chronic biliary obstruction, which may have a similar appearance,[8] although in the latter condition, crowded bile ducts and vessels in the atrophied lobe may be a clue to the diagnosis.[8, 9] Another normal structure, occasionally mistaken for an abnormal mass, is the inferior process of the caudate lobe, the papillary process (Fig. 17–6). On transverse images below its attachment to the caudate lobe, it may appear separate from the liver and simulate an abnormal, extrinsic mass.[10, 11]

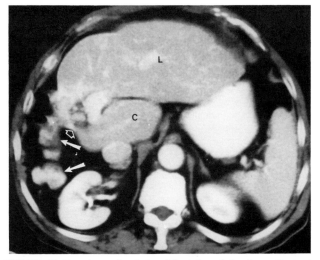

FIGURE 17–5 ■ Agenesis of the right lobe of the liver. Contrast-enhanced scan shows absence of the right lobe of the liver, with the right colon (solid arrows) and fat in the posterior right upper abdomen. Enlargement of the left (L) and caudate (C) lobes is seen; these are connected by a thin slip of liver parenchyma (open arrow).

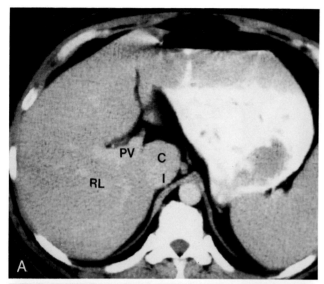

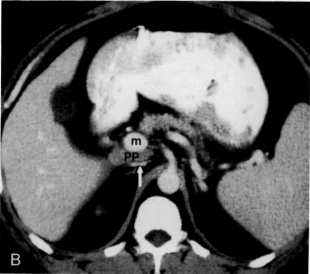

FIGURE 17–6 ■ Papillary process of the caudate lobe. *A*, Caudate lobe (C) can be seen between the portal vein (PV) and inferior vena cava (I), contiguous with the right lobe of the liver (RL). *B*, Scan at an inferior level to *A* shows the papillary process (PP) as separate from the right lobe, lying between the superior mesenteric vein (m) and the inferior vena cava *(arrow)*. This can simulate an abnormal mass at this one level, without visualizing the connection of the papillary process to the liver.

An appreciation of the landmarks of the segmental anatomy of the liver is important as an aid for planning surgical resection of malignant liver lesions.[12, 13] Surgical approaches are limited by the fact that there are no functional intersegmental anastomoses for the vascular and biliary channels, thus requiring procedures more extensive than a wedge resection to be performed along intersegmental/interlobar planes.[12]

SEGMENTAL AND VASCULAR ANATOMY

Intrahepatic vascular structures are well delineated as enhancing structures following intravenous contrast administration. They also are generally seen on non–contrast-enhanced images as slightly hypo-

dense to liver parenchyma. When fatty infiltration of the liver is present, the vessels often have higher attenuation than liver parenchyma, even on non–contrast-enhanced scans. Conversely, in severely anemic patients, the vascular structures can be easily seen as significantly lower in attenuation than the liver parenchyma.

The hepatic veins comprise the efferent vascular system of the liver. The three major hepatic vein trunks—the right, middle, and left—are routinely displayed on CT as they drain into the inferior vena cava at the posterior superior margin of the liver (see Fig. 17–3A). The hepatic veins are all intersegmental or interlobar in position and provide CT and MR landmarks for distinguishing the segments of the liver. The right hepatic vein runs in a coronal plane at the superior aspect of the right intersegmental fissure, which separates the anterior and posterior segments of the right lobe, and enters the right lateral margin of the inferior vena cava. The middle hepatic vein is located at the top of the interlobar fissure separating the right and left hepatic lobes and enters the left anterior aspect of the inferior vena cava. The left hepatic vein courses in the left intersegmental fissure separating the medial and lateral segments of the left lobe and enters the anterior left portion of the inferior vena cava either alone or after joining with the middle hepatic vein.[13, 14] Smaller accessory veins may also enter directly into the inferior vena cava. The caudate lobe drains separately via multiple short hepatic veins emptying directly into the inferior vena cava from the posterior margin of the caudate lobe.[14–17]

The main portal vein extends in a relatively straight course from its retropancreatic origin at the confluence of the superior mesenteric vein and splenic vein, through the hepatoduodenal ligament (free edge of the lesser omentum) at the anterior margin of the inferior vena cava, and into the porta hepatis, where it bifurcates into the right and left portal vein (see Fig. 17–3C).[18] The main hepatic artery and the common hepatic and bile ducts also course within the hepatoduodenal ligament and lie anterior to the main portal vein.

At its origin the initial portion of the left portal vein, or pars transversa, extends anteriorly, leftward, and cranially over the anterior surface of the caudate lobe, giving off small caudate lobe branches. At the left intersegmental fissure, the left portal vein turns sharply cranially and ascends as the second portion, or umbilical segment, of the left portal vein within the left intersegmental fissure (see Fig. 17–3C). The umbilical segment gives horizontal branches to the medial and lateral segments of the left hepatic lobe. The undivided right portal vein courses rightward and cranially, giving several small caudal lobe branches. Within the substance of the right hepatic lobe, the right portal vein divides into anterior and posterior branches (see Fig. 17–3C) that supply the corresponding segments of the right hepatic lobe. Unlike the hepatic venous trunks, which course

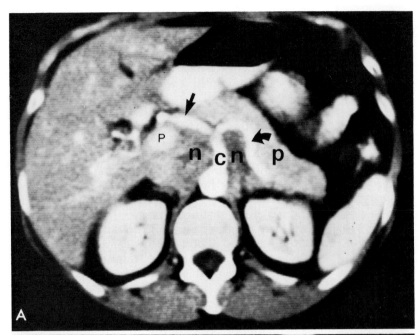

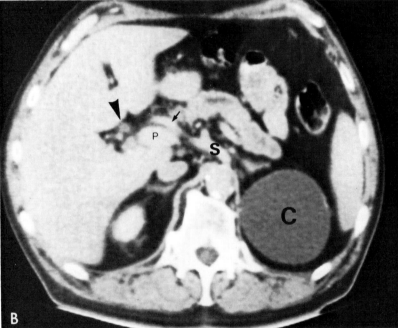

FIGURE 17–7 ■ Hepatic arterial anatomy. *A,* Celiac axis (C) gives off proper hepatic *(straight arrow)* and splenic arteries *(curved arrow)*. The hepatic artery lies ventral to the portal vein (P). n = Enlarged celiac nodes as a result of lymphoma. *B,* Replaced right hepatic artery *(arrow)* arising from the superior mesenteric artery (S). A dilated pancreatic duct is present. Arrowhead = Common hepatic duct; C = renal cyst; P = portal vein.

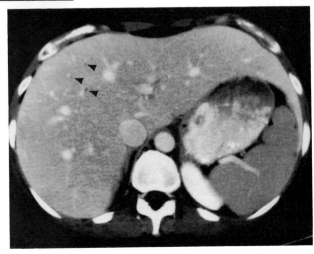

FIGURE 17–8 ■ Normal intrahepatic bile ducts. Intrahepatic bile ducts can be seen on CT as small (≤2 mm) foci of low attenuation *(arrowheads)* coursing adjacent to peripheral portal venous branches.

between segments, the portal vein branches run *within* segments. The angulation of the venous branches relative to the axial plane appears to determine the likelihood of visualization of these vessels on transverse CT images. Horizontally oriented vessels (right portal vein) and vertically oriented vessels (right hepatic vein, inferior vena cava, and the umbilical segment of the left portal vein) are more readily identified on axial CT sections than are obliquely directed vessels (middle hepatic vein and pars transversa of the left portal vein).

The proper hepatic artery usually arises from the celiac axis (Fig. 17–7), continues as the common hepatic artery after giving rise to the gastroduodenal artery, and branches into the right and left arteries in the porta hepatis. Within the hepatoduodenal ligament, the artery lies anterior to the portal vein and medial to the common hepatic duct. Unlike the proximal portal veins, the initial hepatic arterial trunks display considerable variability in their origins and proximal course. In up to 45 per cent of cases, anomalous origins of the common, left, and other hepatic arteries are present with replacement either to the superior mesenteric (see Fig. 17–7B) or left gastric arteries.[14] Smaller, intrahepatic arteries are identified only infrequently as they course in the portal triad. As with the portal venous system, every distal hepatic artery supplies a definite hepatic segment and courses within the segment parenchyma.

The intrahepatic peripheral bile ducts course in the portal triad with the portal veins and hepatic arteries. With older CT equipment, the normal peripheral intrahepatic bile ducts were not visible, but the high resolution available with current scanners allows visualization of intrahepatic bile ducts on CT in up to 40 per cent of patients. Therefore the mere presence of small intrahepatic ducts on CT does not indicate biliary obstruction.[19] These small intrahepatic bile ducts typically measure 1 to 3 mm in diameter and are seen adjacent to contrast enhancing portal venous radicles (Fig. 17–8). The course of these structures is toward the liver hilus, where the right and left hepatic ducts are usually visualized. These two main bile ducts exit from the liver and join in the right side of the porta hepatis to form the common hepatic duct.

HEPATIC PARENCHYMA

The CT attenuation measurements of normal adult livers vary between 38 and 80 Hounsfield units (H) on non–contrast-enhanced images.[20–22] However, the range in the individual patient is much narrower, causing the normal liver to appear relatively homogeneous. The broad range of reported hepatic CT numbers is largely the result of attenuation values being obtained on different CT scanners, using different scanning energies and methods of calibration. In addition, varying amounts of liver glycogen in fasting and recently fed patients may affect hepatic CT attenuation values,[23] and CT numbers vary with variations in fat content.

The non–contrast-enhanced liver parenchyma has a higher density than that of the pancreas, kidneys, or spleen. The average liver-spleen difference is 7 to 8 H, with high normal hepatic CT numbers always associated with high normal splenic attenuation values; the converse is also true.[21] The relatively higher attenuation value of liver parenchyma compared with other organs is a result of the high concentration of glycogen within the liver.[24]

Usually the hepatic parenchyma has a greater attenuation than that of blood, and the portal and hepatic venous systems are seen as lower attenuation branching structures within the liver on non–contrast-enhanced CT scans. Delineation of the status of the intrahepatic biliary tree is difficult without the use of intravenous contrast to enhance the liver parenchyma and portal vascular structures, allowing for accurate evaluation of the bile ducts, which remain near water density.

Magnetic Resonance Imaging

The liver parenchyma appears homogeneous on both T1- and T2-weighted images. The liver shows moderate signal intensity on T1-weighted images (Fig. 17–9), similar to the pancreas but brighter than the kidneys or spleen. The T1 and T2 relaxation times of the spleen are similar to those of many neoplastic lesions, so the spleen can be a helpful marker to determine whether adequate T1 weighting has been achieved to evaluate for liver metastases (see Fig. 17–63). If adequate contrast between the liver and spleen are present, then adequate T1 weighting is present to detect liver neoplasms.[25] On T2-weighted images the liver appears darker (Fig. 17–10) and has a signal intensity similar to that of muscle and significantly less than that of the kidneys and spleen.

The intrahepatic venous structures are well delineated on MR spin-echo images. The axial plane has been found to be significantly superior to other planes for depiction of the vascular structures and anatomic landmarks of the liver.[26] With routine spin-echo imaging, both the hepatic and portal veins appear as signal-void structures (see Fig. 17–9), although occasionally slow-flowing blood may have increased signal on T2-weighted images. Use of flow compensation techniques also increases the signal intensity of these structures (see Fig. 17–10). These venous structures are identified in nearly all patients, whereas the hepatic artery and branches are identified less often.[26] Intrahepatic bile ducts are difficult to identify in normal patients, although the branches just proximal to and within the porta hepatis can be identified as high signal intensity tubular structures on T2-weighted images, in contrast to the flow-void appearance of vascular structures.[27]

Examination Techniques

The imaging modality and specific techniques used should be tailored to the individual patient situation.

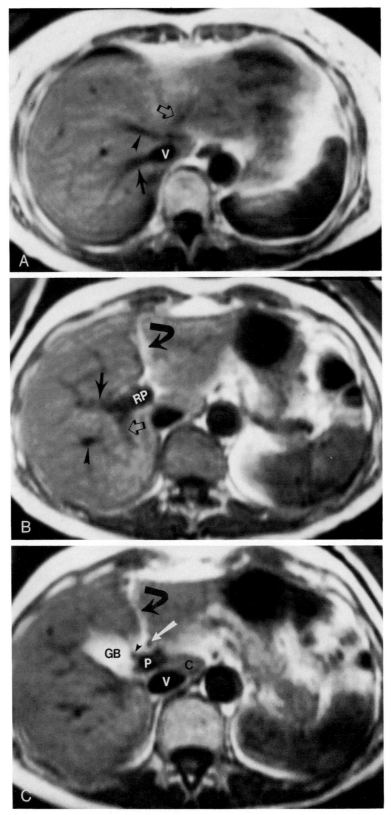

FIGURE 17–9 ■ Normal liver anatomy on T1-weighted spin-echo images (1.5 T). *A,* Cephalic section shows the right *(solid arrow),* middle *(arrowhead),* and left *(open arrow)* hepatic veins as they join the inferior vena cava (V). These veins course in the anatomic boundaries of the hepatic segments. The liver parenchyma is of medium signal intensity, less than that of the high-intensity fat. *B,* Scan at the level of the right portal vein (RP) demonstrates the right anterior *(solid straight arrow)* and posterior *(open arrow)* branches. The right portal vein *(arrowhead)* is imaged in cross section. Fat in the left intersegmental fissure is evident by high signal intensity *(curved arrow). C,* Scan at the level of the gallbladder fossa shows the gallbladder (GB) as it abuts the liver. An imaginary line from the inferior vena cava (V) through the gallbladder fossa demarcates the right and left hepatic lobes. The high signal intensity from the fat in the left intersegmental fissure *(curved arrow)* separates the medial and lateral segments of the left lobe. Arrowhead = Common hepatic duct; C = caudate lobe; P = portal vein; white arrow = hepatic artery.

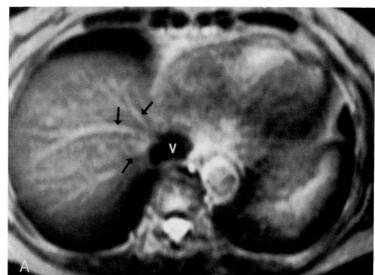

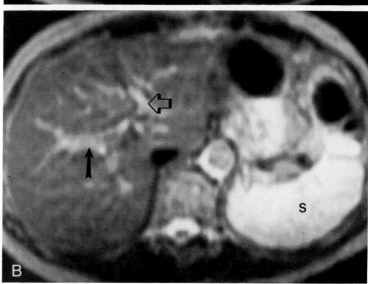

FIGURE 17–10 ■ Normal liver anatomy on T2-weighted spin-echo images using flow compensation techniques, thereby increasing the signal intensity in the portal and hepatic veins. *A,* Cephalic scan shows the liver parenchyma with lower signal intensity than on T1-weighted images. The hepatic veins *(arrows)* are of high signal intensity. V = Inferior vena cava. *B,* A more caudal scan shows the right *(solid arrow)* and left *(open arrow)* portal vein branches. Note the larger difference in signal intensity between liver and splenic (S) parenchyma.

Unlike techniques used with CT scanning, techniques employed with MR to optimize lesion detection and characterization may differ among units of differing manufacturers and field strength. In comparative studies, although the techniques reported to optimize lesion detection may be different, there has been no significant difference found in the abilities of low versus high field strength technology in detecting hepatic lesions.[28, 29]

There are four levels of evaluating the liver in abdominal scanning, and the appropriate CT/MR techniques vary depending on the clinical indication. First, an abdominal survey without specific liver indications may be required. This is the case, for example, when evaluating a patient for abdominal pain, trauma, fever of unknown origin, or source of unknown primary neoplasm. In this instance, liver evaluation should be optimized, but not at the expense of other organ evaluation. Second, liver screening may be the primary source of interest, such as a search for liver metastases in a patient with a known malignancy, but in whom the entire abdomen must also be evaluated. Third, the liver may be the sole area of interest, such as in patients referred for surgical resection of a known solitary hepatic neoplastic lesion. Exclusion of other liver lesions would preclude this therapeutic approach. Fourth, a patient with a known solitary lesion within the liver may be referred for characterization of the lesion. Although knowledge of whether other liver lesions are present may aid in establishing a diagnosis, characteristics of the lesion in question are the primary concern, and imaging techniques should be optimized for this specific evaluation, which may affect evaluation of the remainder of the liver.

CT Techniques

Detection of hepatic abnormalities by computed tomography is dependent on differentiating normal from pathologically altered hepatic tissue. Abnormalities in hepatic contour may permit detection of hepatic disease, but most abnormalities are identified on CT by visualizing regions of altered hepatic density. Generally, a difference of at least 10 H between the abnormal and normal regions of liver must be present for accurate detection of liver lesions.[30] Although many of these abnormalities can be detected on non–contrast-enhanced CT, attempts to increase the differences in CT attenuation between normal liver and hepatic abnormalities have focused on the administration of various intravenous contrast media,[31–35] on the timing of contrast administration,[30, 36–39] and on varying CT technical factors.[40–46]

NON–CONTRAST-ENHANCED CT

Non–contrast-enhanced CT is usually utilized in patients with a history of prior contrast reactions, with renal impairment, or in conjunction with a contrast-enhanced CT examination. Noncontrast scans are helpful in detecting metastases from hypervascular tumors (carcinoid, pancreatic islet cell tumors, renal cell carcinomas, breast carcinoma, sarcomas)[47, 48] and in visualizing calcifications or hemorrhage that may aid in characterizing lesions, but generally they do not provide additional information to that obtained with a properly performed dynamic, bolus contrast CT. In addition, because nonenhanced vessels appear as low-attenuation masses compared with liver parenchyma, contrast images must also be obtained to accurately differentiate vessels from small metastases.

INCREMENTAL-BOLUS DYNAMIC CT

Numerous studies have confirmed that optimal detection of the majority of types of malignant liver lesions requires a rapid, sustained infusion of contrast, generally administered over a period no longer than 2 minutes. It is essential to image the liver during the bolus phase of vascular and parenchymal enhancement and prior to the equilibrium phase when the intravascular and interstitial concentrations of contrast equilibrate. Hypovascular lesions, often with fibrosis or necrosis, thus appear hypodense compared with the enhanced liver parenchyma. With more delayed imaging—either following a rapid bolus or during a slower, drip infusion—it is possible for a liver tumor to increase its enhancement at a time when the liver is less than optimally enhanced. At this time, the lesion may be isodense with liver parenchyma and not visualized. Several reports, in fact, have shown that non–contrast-enhanced CT scans have a higher sensitivity for liver neoplasms than scans obtained during the equilibrium phase of contrast kinetics.[30, 37] Clinically this is relevant in situations where the liver is scanned late during an examination, such as at the end of a chest examination. This should be avoided, and in such circumstances, scanning and contrast administration should begin inferiorly through the liver and continued cephalad through the chest (Fig. 17–11).[30] Hypervascular tumors may markedly increase their enhancement very early during dynamic incremental-bolus

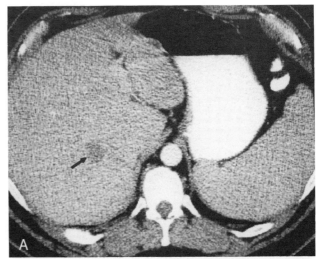

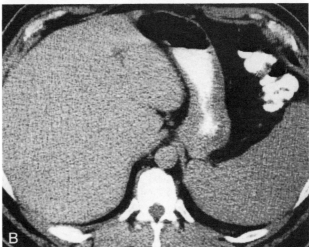

FIGURE 17–11 ■ Liver metastasis (lung primary) seen only on initial dynamic CT images. *A*, Scan initiated inferiorly shows a hypodense mass in the right lobe of the liver *(arrow)*, subsequently shown by biopsy to be a metastasis. Note the lack of peripheral enhancement typical of hemangiomas. *B*, Scan at the same level as *A* obtained 10 minutes later shows the lesion to have achieved the same attenuation as normal liver parenchyma.

scanning and thus become isodense with liver parenchyma, despite rapid contrast administration and scanning (Fig. 17–12).[47, 48] For this reason, non–contrast-enhanced scans have been recommended in conjunction with contrast-enhanced scanning when searching for metastases from a vascular primary tumor, such as islet cell carcinoma, leiomyosarcoma, pheochromocytoma, and renal cell carcinoma.

Incremental-bolus dynamic CT of the liver is best done using a 60 per cent contrast agent, with either a two-phase bolus administration (with 50 to 90 mL administered at 1.5 to 2.5 mL/sec, followed by 90 to 130 mL at 1 mL/sec) or as a one-rate rapid infusion of 100 to 180 mL at 1 to 1.5 mL/sec.[30, 37, 39] A delay of 45 sec following injection is recommended to allow for adequate liver parenchymal enhancement and for visualization of hepatic veins for anatomic location of visualized masses.[49] Use of a power injector to achieve a precise and sustained contrast injection

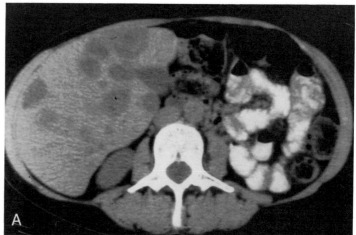

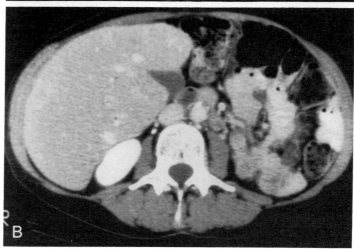

FIGURE 17–12 ■ Metastases from a leiomyosarcoma seen only on non–contrast-enhanced CT scan. *A,* Non–contrast-enhanced CT scan demonstrates numerous metastases as hypodense masses compared with adjacent liver parenchyma. *B,* Scan at the same level as *A* during incremental dynamic bolus contrast administration. Despite the rapid administration of contrast and rapid scan time, with excellent enhancement of the hepatic vascular structures, the metastases have enhanced to the same degree as liver parenchyma and are no longer discernible.

greatly improves enhancement of the liver parenchyma.[30, 50, 51]

A variant of this technique, single-level bolus dynamic CT, utilizes a bolus of contrast administered with rapid scanning at the same level to visualize the contrast enhancement characteristics of a single lesion, such as a hemangioma. Following this evaluation, a smaller bolus of contrast can be administered and sequential images obtained over the following seconds and minutes.

ANGIOGRAPHY-ASSISTED CT

The most sensitive technique for detecting liver lesions uses contrast administered through an indwelling angiographic catheter placed in either the hepatic artery (CT-angiography) or the superior mesenteric artery (CT-portography).[41, 45, 46, 52] CT-angiography (CT-A) detects the vascular enhancement found in the periphery of even markedly hypovascular malignant lesions but is used most often in evaluating suspected hypervascular tumors (Fig. 17–13).[30] CT-portography (CT-P) rapidly delivers contrast to normal hepatic parenchyma via the portal vein, and when rapid scanning is utilized before significant contrast reaches the hepatic arterial circulation, neoplastic lesions (supplied by the hepatic artery) appear as nonenhanced defects contrasted with the enhanced liver parenchyma (Fig. 17–14). Although CT-P has been shown to be more sensitive to small neoplastic lesions than CT-A, it also shows nonneoplastic changes as defects similar in appearance to areas of fibrotic scarring. Benign neoplasms and small cysts do not enhance with contrast supplied by the portal vein. Thus small lesions that cannot undergo percutaneous biopsy should not deter the surgeon from an otherwise indicated surgical approach. In these situations we utilize intraoperative ultrasound prior to liver resection to evaluate these lesions. CT-A, although slightly less sensitive than CT-P, is more specific.

Because of the invasive nature of these examinations, they are generally performed only when documentation of the presence of liver lesions will dramatically alter patient therapy. Usually these are patients referred for surgical resection of presumed solitary neoplastic lesions in whom it is essential to maximize the evaluation of the remainder of the liver to exclude other neoplastic lesions. When performing CT-A, a 30 per cent contrast material is generally utilized, usually as intermittent boluses of 15 mL during clusters of two to three dynamic scans, repeated sequentially until the entire liver has been

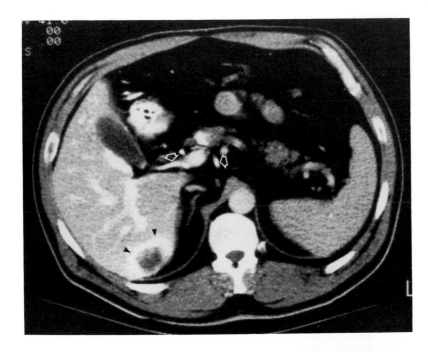

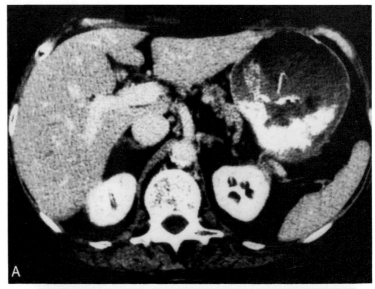

FIGURE 17–13 ■ Liver metastasis (colon primary) appearance at CT angiography. Contrast has been administered using an indwelling hepatic artery catheter with marked enhancement seen in the hepatic artery *(open arrows)*. Marked peripheral enhancement of the metastasis *(arrowheads)* is seen surrounding a lower attenuation center.

FIGURE 17–14 ■ CT portography detects metastatic lesions (colon primary) not detected with dynamic incremental bolus technique. *A,* Dynamic scans fail to identify any liver lesions at this level. *B,* CT portography at the same level as *A* detects numerous space-occupying lesions *(arrowheads)* proven to be metastases. Note the marked enhancement of the portal vein with absence of inferior vena cava enhancement *(arrow)*, which is typical of the portography technique.

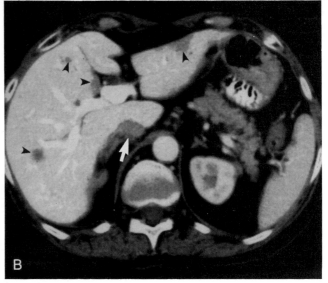

evaluated.[30, 46] The CT-P technique uses 60 per cent contrast agents infused at 1 to 1.5 mL/sec and combined with dynamic imaging through the liver, with scans obtained following a 20-sec delay after initiation of the bolus and scanning the entire liver performed within 2 to 2.5 min.

DELAYED HIGH-DOSE CONTRAST CT (DELAYED CT)

Delayed CT has been shown to be a sensitive technique for the detection of liver neoplasms.[40, 44] The scan technique requires the use of 60 g of iodine administered intravenously 4 to 6 hours prior to CT scanning. Iodine is retained within normal liver parenchyma prior to excreting one to two per cent of the iodine load into the biliary tract. This results in an increase in normal liver attenuation of approximately 20 H over noncontrast images.[53] In contrast, focal hepatic lesions do not retain iodine over the prolonged period to scanning and thus appear as lower attenuation defects (Fig. 17–15). Because the liver vessels also appear as hypodense defects on delayed CT, this examination is usually performed in conjunction with incremental-bolus dynamic CT or angiography-assisted CT, which provides a "road map" of the normal vessels. In these instances, delayed CT can be used to clarify confusing or uncertain findings on the contrast examinations.

IODOLIPID CT

A decade of investigations with intravenous use of iodolipids (iodinated, emulsified fat globules such as EOE-13) has shown that selective and persistent enhancement of the liver parenchyma can be obtained on CT, resulting in high sensitivity in detecting space-occupying lesions. Although iodolipids may possess desirable features, they require a 20- to

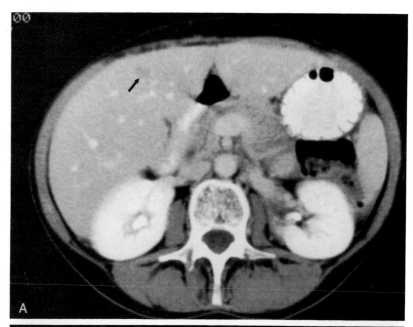

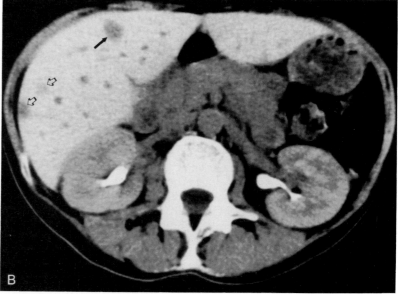

FIGURE 17–15 ■ Metastases (colon primary) seen best on delayed high-dose contrast CT. *A,* Dynamic scan made with incremental bolus administration shows a solitary lesion in the medial segment of the left lobe *(arrow). B,* Delayed scan shows better delineation of lesion seen in *A (solid arrow),* as well as two additional lesions in the right lobe *(open arrows).* Intrahepatic vessels also appear as hypodense regions *(arrowheads)* and can be confused with small lesions.

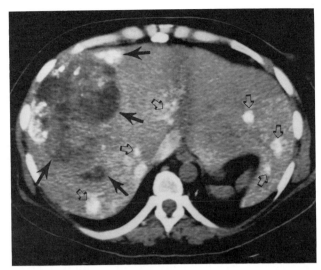

FIGURE 17–16 ■ CT using iodized oil (Lipiodol) with delayed scanning. CT without intravenous contrast obtained 14 days following intraarterial (hepatic artery) injection of iodized oil shows a large hepatocellular carcinoma in the right lobe of the liver (solid arrows), predominately hypodense with liver parenchyma but with foci of retained iodized oil. In addition, numerous scattered other foci of hepatocellular carcinoma, not detected on conventional CT examinations, also retain iodized oil (open arrows).

60-minute period of infusion, are more toxic than urographic type contrast agents, provide no information about hepatic and tumor vascularity, and are difficult to manufacture. They have not achieved commercial availability, and it does not appear that they will in the near future.

Intraarterial injection of iodolipids into the hepatic artery followed by CT scanning 5 to 7 days later has been shown to be highly sensitive in the detection of small hepatocellular carcinoma nodules.[54–57] High-attenuation iodized oil (Lipiodol) is rapidly cleared from normal liver parenchyma via the reticuloendothelial system but is retained within liver neoplasms for prolonged periods of time and allows for the detection of very small nodules on the delayed scans (Fig. 17–16).

Magnetic Resonance Imaging Techniques

Unlike CT, MR offers the capabilities of multiplanar imaging. Axial images, however, optimally display intrahepatic mass lesions and the anatomic structures of the liver. When the relationship of the liver or abdominal masses to the right kidney, adrenal gland, or hemidiaphragm are of concern, sagittal or coronal views are helpful. Axial spin-echo imaging is usually performed with 8 to 10-mm-thick sections obtained with a 3 to 5-mm interslice gap. The interslice gap is required with T2-weighted spin-echo imaging to avoid cross talk, which will shorten the effective TR and increase T1 weighting.[58] Generally T1-weighted images give the best anatomic definition using a repetition time (TR) of ≤300 ms and an echo delay time (TE) of <20 ms. Because of the short TR and acquisition time, multiple acquisitions (generally 4 to

12) can be used to decrease motion artifact. Using midfield strength units (0.5 to 0.6 T), some authors have reported that T1-weighted spin-echo sequences are superior to T2-weighted images in the detection of liver lesions, with a greater signal-to-noise, as well as contrast-to-noise, ratio.[29, 59] Steinberg et al., however, found that at 0.5 T T1-weighted inversion recovery sequences were most sensitive, detecting 98 of 106 lesions, with T2-weighted spin-echo sequences almost as sensitive, detecting 96 of 106

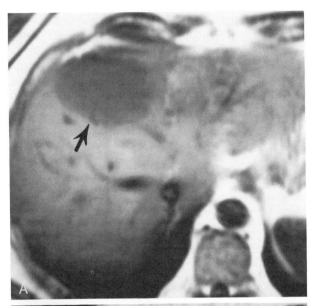

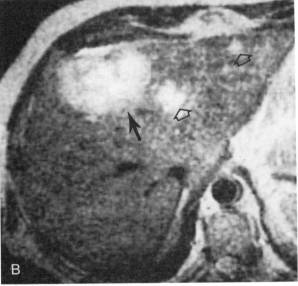

FIGURE 17–17 ■ Metastases (colon primary) seen better on T2-weighted images at 1.5 T. A, T1-weighted image show a single large liver metastasis as a homogeneous low-intensity lesion (arrow) when compared with surrounding parenchyma. Small vessels seen in cross section can have a similar appearance. B, T2-weighted image at the same level as A shows the lesion (solid arrow) as a heterogeneous region of moderately high signal intensity. Two similar but smaller lesions are seen (open arrows) that were not identified on T1-weighted images. Despite the increased image noise present, the lesions are better seen because of increased contrast between the metastases and normal liver parenchyma.

lesions.[28] T1-weighted spin-echo images detected only 86 of 106 lesions.

At 1.0 and 1.5 T, as a result of reduced T1 differences between normal liver and liver tumors, T1-weighted spin sequences are less effective in detecting lesions than T2-weighted sequences (Fig. 17–17).[28, 29, 60] However, when T1 weighting is obtained by using inversion recovery sequences at 1.5 T, contrast can be obtained between normal tissue and tumors, resulting in lesion detection rates equal to those of T2-weighted spin-echo sequences.[28, 29]

Use of short T1 inversion recovery (STIR) sequences has been reported to maximize contrast-to-noise ratios and subjective liver lesion visibility at all field strengths (Fig. 17–18).[61–64] The STIR images suppress the fat signal, and the additive T1 and T2 contrast results in high tumor-liver contrast. In addition, suppression of the abdominal wall fat reduces the ghost artifact displayed over the liver from abdominal wall motion. Phase-contrast pulse sequences also reduce the signal from fat.[65–67] This can also give increased tumor-liver contrast when utilizing T2-weighted sequences for lesion detection,[68, 69] but is not helpful with T1-weighted sequences.

Gradient-echo techniques permit multislice images to be obtained with a single breathhold,[70, 71] and current scan times down to 1 sec are commercially available with these sequences. The obvious advantage with these techniques is that they decrease motion artifacts and motion-related signal losses. These techniques are under investigation, and their efficacy at this time in detecting liver disease has not been significantly evaluated against other spin-echo and inversion recovery techniques. These techniques are often used in conjunction with gadolinium contrast injections. The rapid scan times allow for evaluation of contrast enhancement characteristics over time, similar to CT contrast techniques. Because they are capable of demonstrating blood flow as increased signal intensity, gradient-echo techniques are also used to delineate vascular structures and to document vascular patency or tumor involvement.

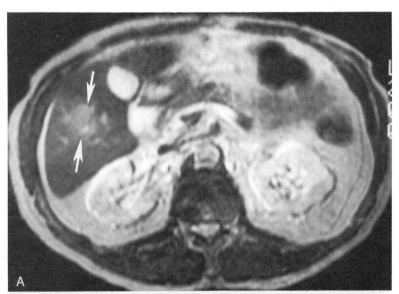
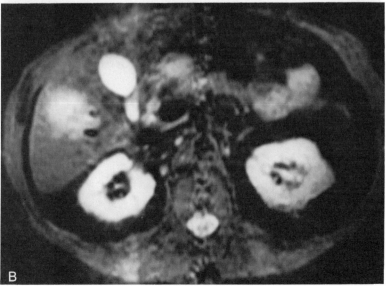

FIGURE 17–18 ■ Increased conspicuousness of liver metastasis (colon primary) with STIR imaging. *A,* T2-weighted spin-echo image shows an ill-defined region of slightly increased signal intensity within the right lobe of the liver. Flow compensation techniques increased the signal intensity of the hepatic vessels. *B,* STIR image at the same level more clearly delineates the abnormality and allows for a confident diagnosis.

At all field strengths, T2-weighted sequences are generally superior for characterization of liver masses.[72–74] As discussed later in this chapter, benign cysts and hemangiomas characteristically demonstrate homogenous marked enhancement (termed a *light bulb sign*), whereas metastatic lesions are usually more heterogeneous, appearing as (1) an amorphous pattern of mild to moderate increased signal intensity, (2) a peripheral rim of increased signal intensity (halo), or (3) a central region of high signal intensity surrounded by an outer margin of lesser intensity than the center, but greater than normal liver (simulating a target).[72] Malignant lesions tend to have irregular or indistinct margins, whereas benign lesions tend to have sharply marginated borders. These findings are guidelines, and there is some overlap between benign and malignant lesions.[72]

As with elsewhere in the body, certain techniques are helpful in decreasing artifacts and increasing the diagnostic quality of MR images. Respiratory compensation techniques should be used to decrease both blurring of images from liver motion during respiration and ghost artifacts from abdominal wall motion. Presaturation techniques, which decrease signal from blood vessels, also decrease the ghost artifact in the phase-encoded direction that is displayed over the liver parenchyma from the aorta. If these flow-related ghost artifacts obscure portions of the liver parenchyma, repeat images swapping the phase- and frequency-encoding directions should be obtained to ensure that all regions of the liver are adequately visualized. Unfortunately this is usually only of concern with T2-weighted images, which require longer imaging times. Flow compensation techniques, which decrease motion-related signal artifacts, can also enhance the clarity of liver parenchyma with T2-weighted images, but caution must be used with this technique, as it causes vessels to become bright. Because pathologic lesions of the liver have increased signal intensity on T2-weighted images, small lesions may be mistaken for vessels with flow compensation techniques or small vessels may be mistaken for a lesion (Fig. 17–19). In uncertain situations, clarification should be obtained with gradient-echo sequences that are flow sensitive.

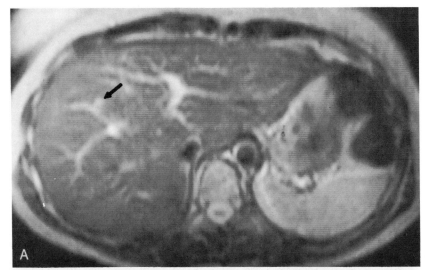

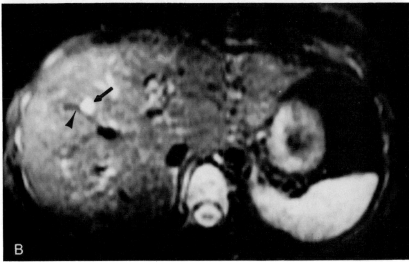

FIGURE 17–19 ■ Flow compensation techniques obscuring a liver metastasis (colon primary). *A,* The metastasis *(arrow)* is of high signal intensity on this T2-weighted image. The lesion abuts a vessel (which is of similar signal intensity as a result of flow compensation techniques) and simulates a branching vessel. *B,* STIR image at the same level shows the lesion *(arrow)* with very high signal intensity but the adjacent vessel *(arrowhead)* with a signal void.

CONTRAST MRI TECHNIQUES

Gadolinium ■ Gadolinium DPTA (Gd-DTPA) is a paramagnetic contrast agent that reduces T1 and T2 relaxation times, producing signal enhancement as a result of T1 shortening.[75] Similar to iodinated contrast agents used for CT, Gd-DTPA rapidly distributes into the extravascular space. Thus by using fast scan techniques (gradient-echo or fast T1-weighted spin-echo sequences), scans obtained immediately after contrast administration may show liver lesions as hypointense to the enhanced surrounding liver parenchyma, with an improvement in lesion-liver signal intensity differences.[76, 77] However, preliminary studies have not shown this agent to significantly increase the detection rate of liver lesions when compared with noncontrast techniques.[76] Preliminary studies show that this agent may be helpful in characterizing hepatic hemangiomas.[78, 79]

Iron Oxide (Ferrite Particles) ■ Small crystalline ferrite particles have been used in clinical trials as a liver contrast agent.[8, 80] These small particles are cleared by the reticuloendothelial system and are not taken up by liver neoplasms. The marked T2 shortening caused by the ferrite particles causes dramatic signal loss in normal liver parenchyma, whereas liver tumors are not affected by the contrast and are more clearly visible as regions of higher signal intensity. Stark et al.[80] reported a reduction in the threshold of lesion size for MR visualization to 3 mm and a significant increase in the detection rate of tumors at 0.6 T. At 1.5 T, however, Marchal et al.,[80a] while finding an increase in lesion-to-liver contrast, did not find an increased lesion detection rate in the 15 patients studied. Further studies are needed to delineate the future role of these contrast agents.

Diffuse Diseases

Fatty Infiltration of the Liver

Fatty infiltration of the liver is the result of excessive deposition of triglycerides, which occurs in association with a variety of disorders, including obesity, malnutrition, chemotherapy, hyperalimentation, alcohol abuse, diabetes, steroid administration, Cushing's syndrome, and radiation hepatitis.[23, 81–83] Fatty infiltration appears to be a nonspecific response of the liver cells to certain metabolic insults[82] and, although indicative of significant hepatic abnormality, is reversible.

COMPUTED TOMOGRAPHY

Although the attenuation of normal liver on CT can vary, there is a constant relationship between the attenuation values of the nonenhanced liver and the spleen, with the liver averaging 8 H greater than the spleen and not measuring less than the spleen.[21] Thus fatty infiltration results in the liver having an attenuation less than the spleen on noncontrast CT (Figs. 17–20 and 17–21). Although these relationships generally also are seen following contrast administration, the spleen may demonstrate more contrast enhancement immediately following a bolus injection, making this an unreliable time to evaluate for fatty infiltration.[84] Measurement of absolute liver attenuation values is not helpful in diagnosing this disorder. Although some lesions of fatty infiltration demonstrate attenuation values similar to those of fat,[85] the majority of lesions are in the 0 to 30 H range, resulting in significant overlap with primary and metastatic neoplasms as well.[83] Diffuse fatty infiltration may obscure dilated biliary ducts[86] or low-attenuation lesions within the liver (see Fig. 17–21).[87]

Fatty infiltration may have a focal or diffuse distribution within the liver. When diffuse and severe, the portal and hepatic veins appear as high-attenuation structures surrounded by a background of lower attenuation hepatic parenchyma (see Fig. 17–20). When focal, the involved parenchymal region of lower attenuation more commonly has a lobar distribution or has linear margins that suggest the diagnosis (Fig. 17–22). Vessels traversing through the area of infiltration may aid in identifying this as a

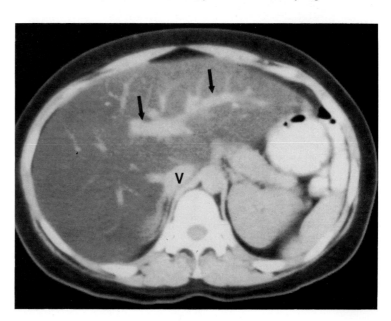

FIGURE 17–20 ■ Diffuse fatty infiltration of the liver. Noncontrast CT scan demonstrates the liver parenchyma to be homogeneously decreased in attenuation, providing a greater than usual contrast with portal vessels *(arrows)*. The inferior vena cava (V) and portal vein branches are of higher attenuation than the liver parenchyma, thus simulating a contrast-enhanced scan.

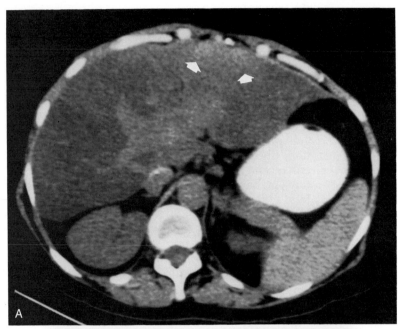

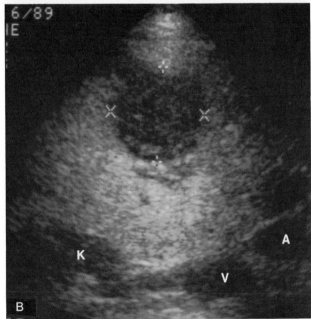

FIGURE 17–21 ■ Hepatic abscess in patient with fatty infiltration. *A,* Noncontrast CT scan shows diffuse low-attenuation liver parenchyma from fatty infiltration, with a residual focus of higher attenuation liver parenchyma *(arrows)* that simulates a space-occupying lesion within the liver. A large pyogenic abscess is present in the right lobe of the liver but is not visualized because it is of the same attenuation as the fatty infiltrated liver parenchyma. *B,* Transverse ultrasound approximating the plane of section in *A* shows the hypoechoic abscess (delineated by electronic cursors) in contrast to the echogenic liver parenchyma. A = Aorta; K = right kidney; V = inferior vena cava.

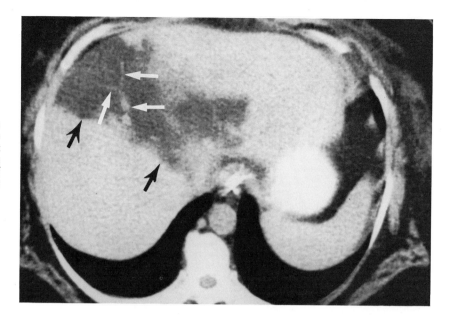

FIGURE 17–22 ■ Focal fat infiltration with linear distribution. In this case the fat deposition is lobar in distribution, involving the left lobe. The straight line margin *(black arrows)* is typical of fatty infiltration. Note the lack of displacement of vessels *(white arrows)* within the lesion.

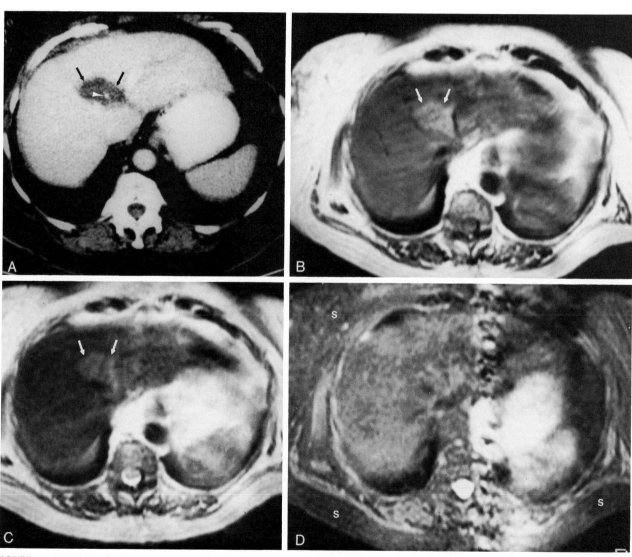

FIGURE 17–23 ■ CT and MR appearances of focal fatty infiltration. *A,* Contrast-enhanced CT scan shows a focal low-attenuation area *(arrows)* within the liver parenchyma, not displacing vascular structures *(arrowhead). B,* T1-weighted spin-echo MR image shows the lesion as increased intensity *(arrows)* when compared with normal liver. *C,* T2-weighted MR image also shows increased intensity in the lesion *(arrows)* when compared with normal liver parenchyma. *D,* MR image at same level as *A* through *C,* using the STIR sequence to suppress fat, shows suppression of the signal in the region of abnormality seen on prior sequences. The signal from subcutaneous fat (s) has also been suppressed.

753

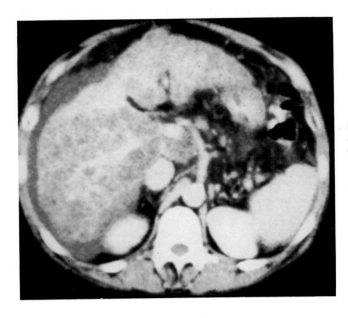

FIGURE 17–24 ■ Diffuse, irregular fatty infiltration in a patient with alcohol-induced cirrhosis. Contrast-enhanced CT scan shows heterogeneous, irregular, low-attenuation infiltration of the liver, a pattern not dissimilar to that of infiltrating neoplastic lesions. One month later, a follow-up CT scan was normal. Such rapid changes are typical of fatty infiltration.

region of fatty infiltration (Figs. 17–22 and 17–23), although rarely hepatocellular carcinoma with fat may not displace vessels, but surround them, and can simulate fatty infiltration. Occasionally small nodules of infiltration or diffuse infiltration occurring in a patchy, rounded, or heterogeneous fashion can simulate metastatic disease (Figs. 17–23 through 17–25)[88] and may require biopsy for documentation.[89, 90] The medial segment of the liver adjacent to the falciform ligament has been reported as particularly susceptible to focal fatty infiltration (see Fig. 17–25).[90, 91] Occasionally small islands of normal hepatic parenchyma can persist within an otherwise diffusely infiltrated fatty liver (see Fig. 17–21). In such cases, it can be difficult to distinguish among normal liver parenchyma, regenerating nodules, hemangiomas, or metastases.[81]

A further aid to the diagnosis of focal fatty infiltration can be a rapid change in appearance over time.

Focal areas of infiltration may resolve over a period as short as 6 days.[92]

MAGNETIC RESONANCE IMAGING

Although fatty infiltration in some cases may demonstrate increased MR signal intensity compared with adjacent liver parenchyma on both T1- and T2-weighted spin-echo images (see Fig. 17–23B, C),[93] in general MR has proved insensitive in detecting fatty infiltration.[94, 95] Stark et al. showed that even with massive increases in hepatic triglyceride content, the signal intensity of the liver increased only minimally.[94]

Although spin-echo imaging is insensitive, phase-contrast and proton spectroscopic imaging[67, 68, 96] are sensitive methods of detecting fatty infiltration. These techniques are particularly useful in differentiating focal metastatic lesions from fatty infiltration, as metastatic lesions appear bright when using these

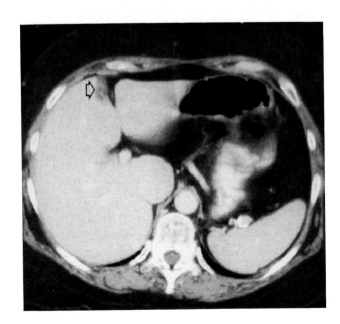

FIGURE 17–25 ■ Focal fat. Contrast-enhanced CT scan shows a low-attenuation region (open arrow) adjacent to the fissure for the ligamentum teres. Biopsy revealed fat accumulation. Note the small central vessel within the fat.

sequences, in contrast to regions of focal fatty infiltration, which are of low signal intensity. At high field strength (1.5 T), we have found STIR imaging to be similarly useful in differentiating metastatic lesions from local fat. STIR images demonstrate metastatic foci as high-signal-intensity masses, whereas regions of fatty infiltration do not demonstrate high signal, appearing isointense or hypointense with liver parenchyma (see Fig. 17–23D).

Cirrhosis

COMPUTED TOMOGRAPHY

Cirrhosis resulting from a variety of causes can produce changes in the liver that are detectable by CT scanning. Occasionally the attenuation of liver parenchyma may be mildly increased and may reflect the mild increase in hepatocyte iron found in up to 50 per cent of patients with cirrhosis.[97] However, the basic pathologic process characterizing cirrhosis—that of extensive collagen deposition with replacement of hepatocytes and distortion of the normal hepatic lobular architecture—does not alter the mean CT number beyond the range of normal.[20] Therefore measurement of CT attenuation is of little value in identifying the presence of cirrhosis.

Although no hepatic CT abnormalities may be detectable in some patients with proven cirrhosis, frequently there are changes in liver contour or size or homogeneity of liver parenchyma.[98–100] A small liver with a nodular contour results from focal atrophy, fibrosis, and/or regenerating nodules (Fig. 17–26). Enlargement of the caudate lobe and lateral segment of the left lobe with associated shrinkage of the right lobe of the liver has been noted.[98, 99] The ratio of the transverse caudate lobe width (measured from the medial aspect of the caudate lobe to the lateral aspect of the main portal vein) to the transverse right hepatic lobe width (measured from the lateral aspect of the main portal vein to the right

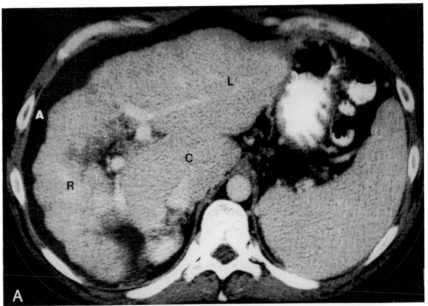

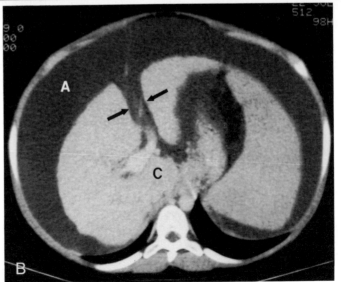

FIGURE 17–26 ■ Liver cirrhosis. *A,* CT scan shows typical findings of cirrhosis: nodular liver margins resulting from regenerating nodules, atrophy of the right lobe (R), and hypertrophy of the caudate lobe (C) and lateral segment (L) of the left lobe. Ascites (A) is also present. *B,* Scan from another patient shows widening of the left intersegmental fissure *(arrows)* from the fibrosis and atrophy associated with cirrhosis. Enlargement of the caudate lobe (C), a nodular contour of the liver, and ascites (A) are also present.

lateral liver margin) increased from a mean of 0.37 in a normal population to 0.83 in patients with cirrhosis.[98] No normal liver had a value above 0.55, and only one cirrhotic liver had a ratio less than 0.6.[98] The increase in caudate lobe–to–right lobe ratio in cirrhotic livers results both from actual caudate lobe enlargement and greater fibrotic scarring and shrinkage of the right hepatic lobe. The shrinkage of the right lobe and medial segment of the left lobe results in a prominence of the intersegmental fissures and porta hepatis (see Fig. 17–26).[98, 100]

Other CT findings in cirrhosis include ascites, regenerating nodules, hepatocellular carcinoma (HCC), and portal hypertension. Regenerating nodules are usually of the same density as normal liver parenchyma but can be detected by an irregular, lobular liver contour (see Fig. 17–26). Rarely, they may present with increased attenuation compared with normal, nonenhanced liver parenchyma (Figs. 17–27 and 17–28).[101, 102] Regenerating nodules, when large, may simulate a mass lesion. Fibrosis and irregular fatty infiltration often may be seen on noncontrast CT as areas of low attenuation that are isodense with liver parenchyma on contrast images. Caution must be used, however, in assuming all such lesions to be benign, as a small percentage of hepatomas may be seen only on noncontrast images and become isodense with liver after contrast. Portal hypertension may be evident by splenomegaly and enlarged collateral vessels. Collateral vessels produce numerous round, serpiginous structures in the porta hepatis, perigastric, esophageal, paraumbilical, and splenic regions that increase in CT attenuation after intravenous contrast administration (Figs. 17–29 and 17–30). Ascites, often found in patients with cirrhosis, can easily be seen on CT.

Findings of HCC, a known complication of cirrhosis, should be searched for in all patients with cirrhosis. Unlike regenerating nodules, HCC has a large spectrum of CT appearances but is most often hypodense with contrast-enhanced liver parenchyma.

MAGNETIC RESONANCE IMAGING

The morphologic changes in the liver associated with cirrhosis are delineated on MR images in a similar pattern to that seen on CT. These include a nodular liver contour, hypertrophied caudate lobe and lateral segment of the left lobe, widening of the hepatic fissures, splenomegaly, and ascites. Collateral vessels can be demonstrated on MR as a signal void on spin-echo sequences or with high-intensity signal on flow-sensitive sequences (see Fig. 17–30B).[103] The patency of portal venous structures or portosystemic shunts[104] can also be documented using these techniques.

Regenerating nodules can be seen on MR as small foci of low signal intensity on T2-weighted and proton density images and, less commonly, (also as low-signal-intensity foci) on T1-weighted images (see Fig. 17–28).[101] These lesions have been reported to be more prominent at high field strength (1.5 T).[101]

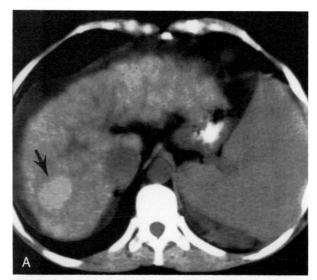

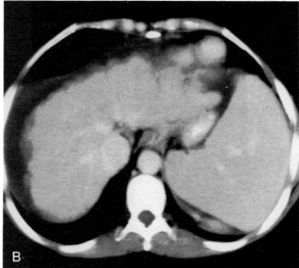

FIGURE 17–27 ■ Large regenerating nodule in liver cirrhosis. *A,* Noncontrast CT scan shows a large regenerating nodule *(arrow)* as higher attenuation than remaining liver parenchyma. *B,* Contrast CT scan shows enhancement of the nodule to the same degree as remaining parenchyma, obscuring the nodule. Numerous smaller isodense nodules are noted along the liver margin, resulting in a nodular surface contour.

Adenomatous hyperplastic nodules (or macroregenerative nodules), thought to be a premalignant condition, have a different MR appearance, with high signal intensity on T1-weighted images and low signal intensity on T2-weighted images.[105] Although up to a third of hepatomas have high signal intensity on T1-weighted sequences, they do not typically present as low-signal-intensity lesions on T2-weighted images,[105] a feature that differentiates them from adenomatous hyperplastic nodules.

Hemochromatosis

Excessive total body iron stores can result from a primary process (idiopathic hemochromatosis) or develop as a secondary disorder in patients with con-

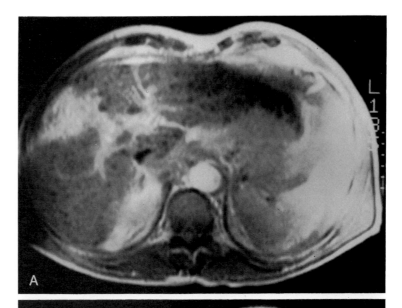

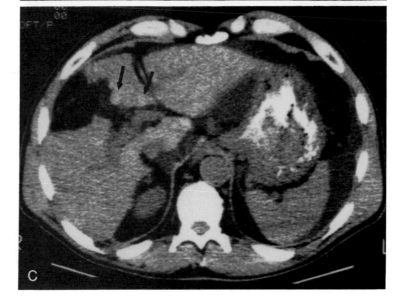

FIGURE 17–28 ■ Regenerating liver nodules in a patient with cirrhosis. A, Proton density MR image shows numerous low-intensity nodules throughout the liver. B, T2-weighted image at a different level also shows low-intensity nodules throughout, although they are less discernible because of the lower intensity of liver parenchyma. C, Noncontrast CT scan at the same level as A shows the largest nodules as foci of slightly higher attenuation (arrows) than liver parenchyma. Smaller nodules of increased attenuation can also be seen scattered throughout both lobes.

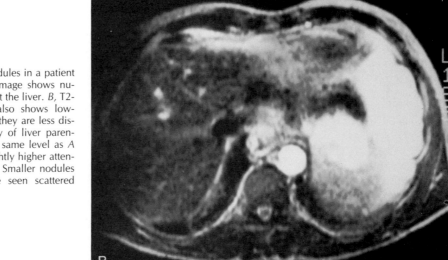

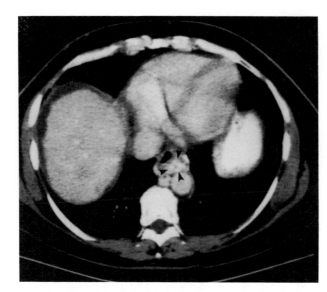

FIGURE 17–29 ■ Esophageal varices. Contrast CT scan shows numerous small enhancing varices *(arrowheads)* within the thickened esophageal wall.

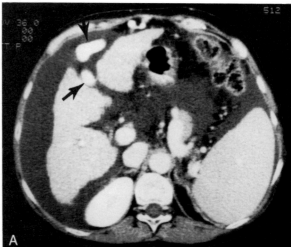

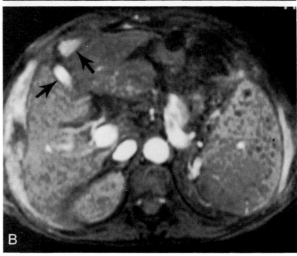

FIGURE 17–30 ■ Venous collaterals with portal hypertension. *A,* Distended paraumbilical vein collateral seen on contrast CT scan as an enhancing tubular structure *(arrows)* within the left intersegmental fissure and in the region of the falciform ligament. *B,* Gradient-recalled acquisition in the steady state (GRASS) MR image in the same patient at the same level as *A* shows the collateral vessels *(arrows)* with high signal intensity, indicative of flow.

genital or acquired anemia who receive repeated blood transfusions. Patients with idiopathic hemochromatosis have increased iron absorption as a result of a defect in intestinal mucosal cells, leading to excess iron deposition within hepatic parenchyma, as well as other organs (pancreas, heart, spleen, lymph nodes, kidney, endocrine glands, and skin).[106] These patients typically present with cirrhosis (or complications of cirrhosis), diabetes mellitus, and hyperpigmentation.[107] Secondary hemochromatosis is most frequently seen in patients having thalassemia, sickle cell anemia, and sideroblastic anemia[107–110] and is secondary to increased iron deposition within the reticuloendothelial cells of the spleen, liver, and bone marrow. Such iron deposition does not usually result in underlying organ dysfunction.[111]

COMPUTED TOMOGRAPHY

The diagnosis of primary or secondary hemochromatosis is readily made by CT when images reveal a diffuse and homogeneous increase in attenuation of the hepatic parenchyma (Fig. 17–31). The primary disorder may demonstrate increased liver attenuation with normal splenic attenuation. The secondary form, caused by increased iron stores in the reticuloendothelial system, may demonstrate an increase in both liver and splenic attenuation. Rarely, this disorder can appear as a focal process.[112] At scanning energies of 120 kV(p), the average CT attenuation values of the liver in patients with hemochromatosis range between 75 and 132 H.[23, 107, 109, 113, 114] As a result of the diffuse increase in hepatic CT attenuation, the portal and hepatic venous structures appear as low-attenuation, tubular branching structures against the background of the hyperdense liver. An associated increase in iron may increase attenuation values in the spleen, pancreas, lymph nodes, pituitary, heart, adrenals, bowel wall, parathyroid, and thyroid glands. The liver findings can be similar to those in other diffuse diseases with elevated attenuation val-

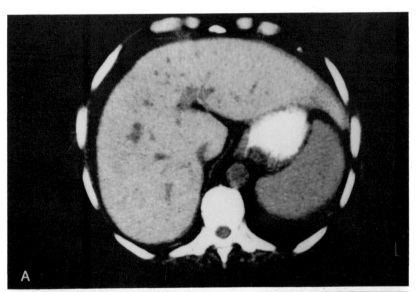
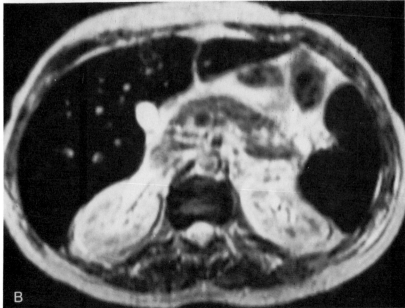

FIGURE 17–31 ■ Hemochromatosis. *A*, Noncontrast CT scan shows a marked diffuse increase in liver attenuation when compared with the attenuation of other soft tissue structures. The portal and venous structures appear as low attenuation against the abnormally high attenuation of liver parenchyma. *B*, T2-weighted image. The liver and spleen are homogeneously displayed as very low signal intensity organs.

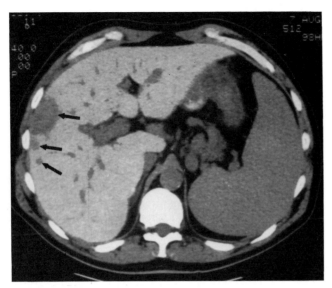

FIGURE 17–32 ■ Hepatocellular carcinoma in a patient with hemochromatosis. Noncontrast CT scan shows the liver to be of higher attenuation than other organs. Multifocal hepatoma (arrows) appears as soft tissue attenuation masses, hypodense when compared with abnormal liver parenchyma.

ues (e.g., amiodarone toxicity, glycogen storage disease, or the heterozygote carrier state for Wilson's disease).[115] Interruption of the diffuse increase in parenchymal attenuation with focal areas of soft tissue attenuation can be seen with malignant involvement of the liver, either by metastases or by HCC (a known complication of hemochromatosis) (Fig. 17–32).

By using dual-energy scanning techniques, computed tomography is capable of quantitating the amount of iron present within the liver.[116, 117] Experimental work has shown a constant change in CT

attenuation value for each gram of iron present within the liver.[116, 117] Dual-energy scanning for liver densitometry is applicable not only in detecting hemochromatosis, but also in following the progress of therapy. The hepatic CT attenuation has been found to be more specific for iron overload than a serum ferritin measurement.[118]

MAGNETIC RESONANCE IMAGING

Hemochromatosis causes excessive hemosiderin deposition, which shortens T2 but has a lesser effect on T1. The shortening of T2 results in a marked decrease in hepatic signal intensity throughout the liver (see Fig. 17–31B),[119, 120] approaching that of background noise. When involved, the spleen, pancreas, and heart may also show decreased signal intensity. Although more sensitive than CT to the presence of iron, MR does not appear to be able to quantitate iron content.[121]

Glycogen Storage Disease

Glycogen storage diseases are genetic disorders of carbohydrate metabolism categorized into six groups on the basis of the specific enzyme defect.[122] In all forms of glycogen storage disease there is excessive storage of glycogen, and in types I, II, III, IV, and VI the liver is involved.[122] Although the diseases are present at birth, except for type IV, they may not be detected until late childhood, when hepatomegaly is discovered. Patients with glycogen storage disease may demonstrate an increase[116, 123] (Fig. 17–33) or a decrease[123, 124] in liver CT attenuation values. Livers having CT attenuation values greater than normal are more common. The excessive amount of glycogen packed into the liver produces an increased hepatic attenuation value, which is related to the single

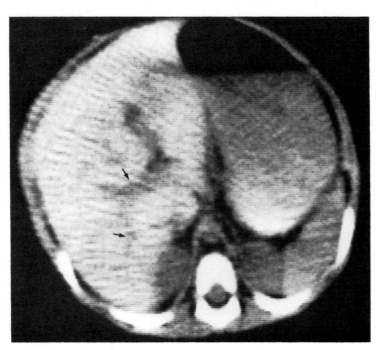

FIGURE 17–33 ■ Type II glycogen storage disease. A diffuse increase in hepatic attenuation is present on noncontrast CT scan (liver = 66 H) with hepatomegaly. Portal vessels (arrows) appear as low-attenuation structures compared with high-attenuation liver. The kidneys and spleen are normal.

power of the physical density of the glycogen. Attenuation values of 55 to 90 can be seen, which overlaps the range seen in hemochromatosis. Separation of the two entities is usually not difficult clinically, but when necessary, dual-energy CT can be employed to determine whether the high liver attenuation is caused by iron or glycogen.[116] Unlike the great increase in hepatic CT attenuation observed in hemochromatosis when the liver is scanned at 80 kV(p) compared with 120 kV(p), the glycogen-laden liver has a much smaller attenuation change. Dual-energy CT can be employed to quantitate the amount of glycogen present in the liver without biopsy.

Low-attenuation changes may be seen in these diseases as a result of the fatty infiltration that occurs in longstanding glycogen storage disease.[123, 124] The areas of fatty infiltration may be nonhomogeneous, with foci of normal hepatic attenuation scattered throughout the liver. These areas of normal attenuation may be difficult to distinguish from tumor foci. Additional abnormalities that may be identified by CT in glycogen storage disease are renomegaly with increased cortical density (type I), splenomegaly (types I, III, and VI), renal calculi (type I), and liver cell adenoma or hepatoma (type I).[124]

Radiation Changes

Hepatocellular damage induced by radiation therapy can result in a focal hypodense area of the liver with a geographic distribution corresponding to the region of the radiation ports with a sharp, straight border (Fig. 17–34).[125, 126] Clinically, the acute form of radiation damage has its onset 2 to 6 weeks after therapy and is generally not seen in patients receiving less than 3500 rad (35 Gy) to the liver.[127] The CT changes of radiation may be seen several weeks after

initiation of therapy. The changes resolve on CT by 3 to 5 months, and follow-up scans are either normal or demonstrate atrophy of the affected liver.[125, 126] Histologically, acute hepatic injury is characterized by panlobular congestion, hemorrhagic foci, variable amounts of fatty change, lipofuscin-laden macrophages, and marked venous occlusion. The MR findings of decreased signal intensity on T1-weighted images and increased signal intensity on T2-weighted images, as well as on proton spectroscopic images, confirm that the imaging appearance of radiation change is caused by an increased water content.[126] Unger et al. hypothesized that vascular congestion may play a role in the CT appearance. They reported one patient in whom CT-portography demonstrated a decrease attenuation in the affected liver during the dynamic phase, but a reversal of the appearance, with increased density noted in the region of the radiation port, on the later equilibrium phase images.[126] Increased attenuation in the affected portions of the liver can also be seen following routine intravenous administration of contrast (Fig. 17–35).

Other Diffuse Disorders

Other disorders that can diffusely increase liver CT attenuation include prior thorotrast administration (Fig. 17–36), amiodarone toxicity,[128, 129] and accumulations of gold from preparations injected for the treatment of rheumatoid arthritis.[130] Cisplatin therapy has been reported to homogeneously increase liver attenuation if the liver is imaged immediately following therapy, but attenuation returns to normal 1 month following therapy.[131] Although the heterozygous carrier state for Wilson's disease has been reported to increase liver CT attenuation values,[115] patients with Wilson's disease have not demon-

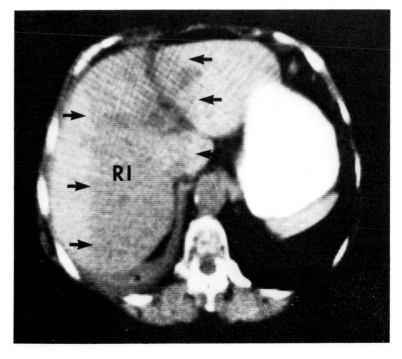

FIGURE 17–34 ■ Radiation injury (RI) following therapy for gallbladder carcinoma produces a zone of low attenuation within the liver, with straight margins (arrows) corresponding to the radiation port. (From Jeffrey RB Jr, Moss AA, Quivey JM, Federle MP, Wara WM: AJR 135:495, 1980. © American Roentgen Ray Society. Used with permission.)

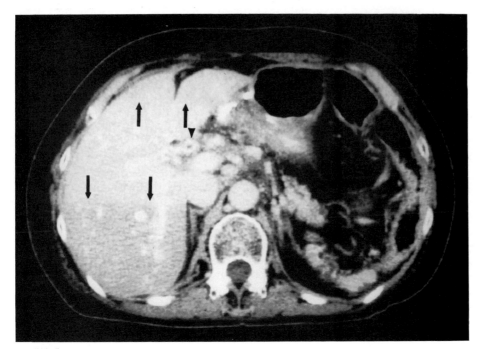

FIGURE 17–35 ■ Radiation changes to the liver. Contrast-enhanced CT scan shows a sharp linear zone of transition *(arrow)* between areas of increased and decreased attenuation in the liver. In this instance, a lateral radiation port was utilized to radiate the porta hepatis and pancreas, and the areas affected within the liver are of increased attenuation. Tumor and radiation changes in the porta hepatis are evident by infiltration of fat and the thickened, enhancing wall of the common hepatic duct *(arrowhead).*

strated an increase in liver attenuation beyond the range of normal.[132, 133] The liver in such patients may demonstrate a heterogeneous, nodular appearance on CT, but this is not a diagnostic appearance and can also be seen in other diseases such as cirrhosis.[133]

Hepatic Cysts

Hepatic cysts are common and are found either as isolated lesions or in association with congenital cystic disease of the liver. Pathologically thought to be congenital, they usually reach a detectable size in the fifth to seventh decade. They usually do not cause symptoms but can rarely present with clinical signs when torsion, rupture into the peritoneum, or intracystic hemorrhage has occurred.[134]

Computed Tomography

Hepatic cysts vary in size from a few millimeters to several centimeters in diameter. When of larger size, they appear on CT as homogeneous, sharply delineated, round or oval low-attenuation lesions with imperceptible or thin, smooth walls and an absence of internal structures (Figs. 17–37 and 17–

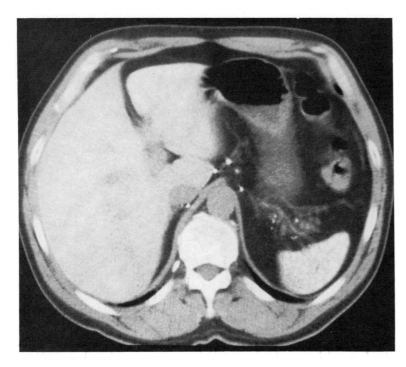

FIGURE 17–36 ■ Thorotrast deposition in liver and spleen. Noncontrast CT scan shows a heterogeneously diffuse increase in attenuation of the liver and spleen. Portal venous structures appear as radiating areas of lower attenuation within liver parenchyma.

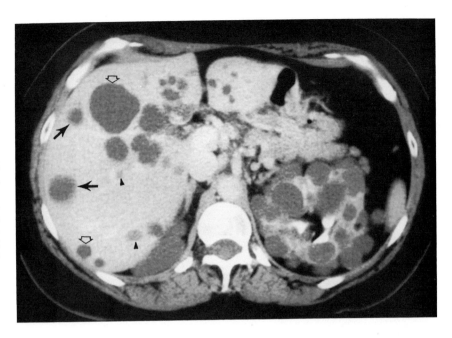

FIGURE 17–37 ■ Polycystic disease of the liver and kidneys. Multiple cysts of varying size are seen throughout the liver and renal parenchyma. Scan obtained through the center of the cysts *(open arrows)* shows classic features of simple cysts: homogeneous, near-water attenuation and a sharp zone of transition with normal parenchyma. Cysts scanned through their curving margin *(solid arrows)* show a hazy transition with liver parenchyma because of volume averaging. Smaller lesions not scanned through the center may result in volume averaging throughout *(arrowheads)*, raising the attenuation value centrally as well. These lesions cannot be differentiated from a solid lesion such as a metastasis.

38).[135] The attenuation value of cysts range from 0 to 15 H, although unfortunately, some necrotic metastases, abscesses, and chronic hematomas may also have attenuation coefficients in this range.[136–138] These abnormalities usually do not meet all of the criteria for a cyst and may demonstrate a thick or irregular wall, increased attenuation following contrast, or internal heterogeneity (Fig. 17–39). Cysts should not demonstrate an increase in attenuation following intravenous contrast administration, as is most often seen in hypodense liver metastases. Intrahepatic extension of pancreatic pseudocysts may simulate a simple hepatic cyst. Bilomas can also have a similar

appearance, although these usually occur in the perihepatic space adjacent to the liver.[135, 139]

Small cysts often demonstrate attenuation values greater than water density as a result of volume averaging with adjacent hepatic parenchyma (see Fig. 17–38), again resulting in an overlap between the CT appearance of cysts and that of other lesions such as metastases (although the utilization of thin collimation sections (1.5 mm) can overcome this in many cases).

Cystic neoplasms may rarely have attenuation values identical to simple hepatic cysts[136] and not demonstrate mural abnormalities suggestive of neoplastic

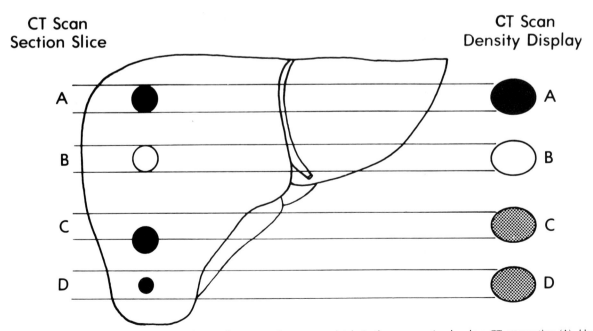

FIGURE 17–38 ■ Diagram illustrating partial volume effect. Hepatic cyst completely in the scan section has low CT attenuation (A). Hepatic solid mass completely in the scan section has high CT attenuation (B). A large hepatic cyst only partially within the CT section has intermediate CT attenuation (C). A hepatic cyst smaller than the CT slice thickness also has intermediate CT attenuation (D).

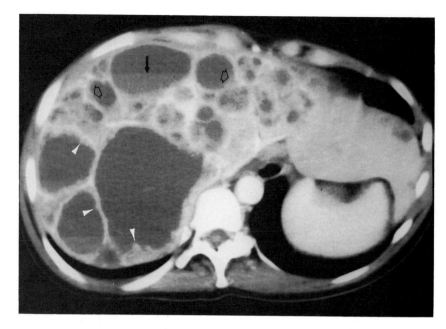

FIGURE 17–39 ■ Carcinoid tumor with cystic liver metastases. These cystic lesions do not meet CT criteria for simple cysts. Although many are of predominantly low, near-water attenuation, mural nodularity *(arrowheads)*, wall thickening *(open arrows)* and the fluid-fluid level *(solid arrow)* seen in this example are not seen in simple cysts.

change. In these cases, ultrasonography may permit differentiation by demonstrating internal septations and irregularities of the inner margin of the wall of cystic tumors, characteristics not seen in non-neoplastic hepatic cysts.[140] In rare instances, a percutaneous aspiration or biopsy may be needed to differentiate a simple cyst from a necrotic or cystic metastasis.

Magnetic Resonance Imaging

Because of their morphology (well-marginated and homogeneous) and the very long T1 and T2 relaxation times, simple cysts have a relatively characteristic MR appearance (Fig. 17–40). They appear as sharply circumscribed, homogeneous areas of low signal intensity on T1-weighted images and of very high intensity on T2-weighted images (the latter referred to as similar to a light bulb).[72] Unfortunately the MR appearance of cysts is not pathognomonic, as up to nine per cent of patients with metastatic lesions can demonstrate the high, homogeneous intensity on T2 images similar to the light bulb sign.[72] These tend to be metastases from vascular primary tumors.

Hemorrhage into a cyst increases the signal intensity of cysts on T1-weighted images as a result of the T1 shortening caused by methemoglobin.[141]

Liver Neoplasms

Benign Neoplasms

CAVERNOUS HEMANGIOMA

Hemangiomas are the most common benign hepatic neoplasms, with an autopsy incidence of about four per cent.[142, 143] They are usually unifocal, but multiple lesions are not infrequent. The tumors are classified into two types: capillary hemangiomas, which are small lesions, usually less than 2 cm in diameter; and cavernous hemangiomas, which are large lesions, ranging in size from 3 to 5 cm to almost complete replacement of one or more hepatic lobes. In both types, the histology is similar. The lesions are composed of multiple small or large vascular spaces lined with endothelial cells containing varying amounts of fibrous tissue. Calcifications (phleboliths) can occur within the vascular spaces but are rare.

Nonspecific symptoms such as fever, abdominal pain, a palpable abdominal mass, and anemia occur in about 30 to 50 per cent of patients with hemangiomas. Symptoms are usually caused by large tumors (greater than 5 cm in diameter) that exert pressure on adjacent structures or stretch the liver capsule. Tumors located near the porta hepatis produce symptoms most often. In addition, because hemangiomas are quite common, they are not infrequently identified in patients who have symptoms from a known primary or metastatic malignant tumor.

Fifty to 70 per cent of patients with hemangiomas are asymptomatic, and the lesions are discovered incidentally, usually by sonography or CT performed for some other reason. Asymptomatic hemangiomas rarely require treatment.[143] Thus it is important to be able to differentiate hemangioma from other benign (e.g., liver cell adenoma) or malignant hepatic neoplasms that do require therapy.

Computed Tomography ■ The CT features of hemangiomas are quite varied. On non–contrast-enhanced scans, they appear as well-marginated, low-attenuation lesions when compared with normal surrounding hepatic parenchyma (Figs. 17–41*B* and 17–42*A*). However, if they arise in a liver with diffuse fatty infiltration, they may be of greater attenuation than the liver parenchyma (see Fig. 17–41*A*). Calci-

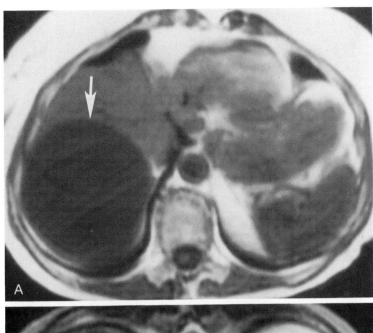

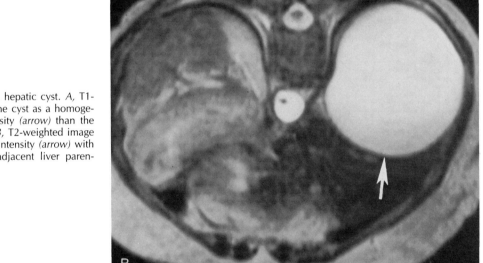

FIGURE 17–40 ■ MR imaging of a hepatic cyst. *A*, T1-weighted spin-echo image shows the cyst as a homogeneous lesion of lower signal intensity *(arrow)* than the surrounding hepatic parenchyma. *B*, T2-weighted image shows homogeneous bright signal intensity *(arrow)* with a sharp zone of transition from adjacent liver parenchyma.

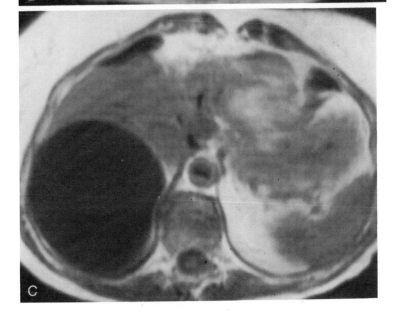

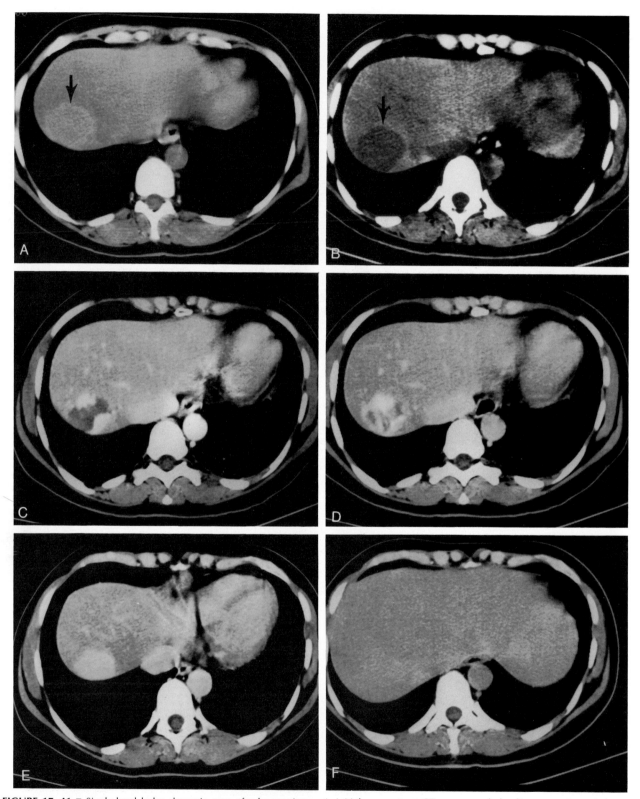

FIGURE 17–41 ■ Single-level bolus dynamic scan of a hemangioma. *A,* Initial noncontrast CT scan revealed a liver mass *(arrow)* that was hyperdense when compared with liver parenchyma because of diffuse fatty infiltration of the liver. *B,* Noncontrast scan 4 months later with clearing of the fatty infiltration shows the lesion *(arrow)* to be hypodense to normal liver. *C,* Scan at 83 seconds following a bolus of 150 mL of 60 per cent contrast material shows intense, nodular, peripheral enhancement. The degree of enhancement is similar to that of the liver vessels. *D,* Delayed scan at 5 minutes shows further central enhancement, with the degree of enhancement paralleling that of the vessels. *E,* Scan at 10 minutes shows complete enhancement of the lesion, maintaining similar lesion and vessel enhancement intensity. *F,* Scan at 30 minutes reveals the lesion and the vessels to be isodense when compared with liver parenchyma.

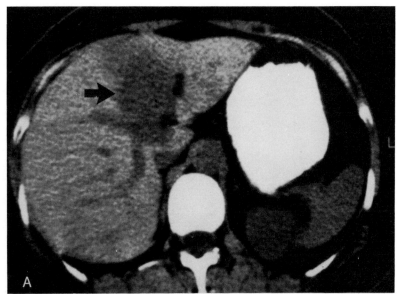

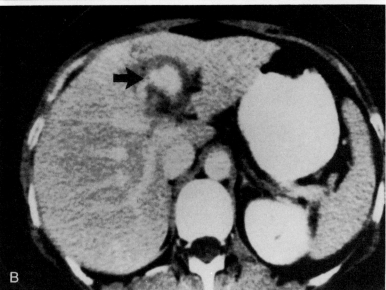

FIGURE 17–42 ■ Single-level bolus dynamic scans of an atypical hemangioma. *A,* Scan without contrast shows a low-attenuation mass in the left lobe *(arrow)*. *B,* Scan at 87 seconds following a bolus of 150 mL of 60 per cent contrast material shows intense central contrast enhancement. Note the similarity to Figures 17–60 and 17–68.

fications are rare but can easily be detected by CT if present.

Hemangiomas display several different patterns of enhancement following intravenous infusion of iodinated contrast. If a single-level bolus dynamic technique is used (2 sec scan time, with 16 images collected in 92 sec) during rapid bolus injection of 75 to 150 mL of 60 per cent contrast, 97 per cent of hemangiomas will show some type of contrast enhancement during the initial vascular phase. The most common pattern is peripheral contrast enhancement. It occurs in 74 per cent of cases and is characterized by focal, discontinuous, nodular areas of relatively intense enhancement around the lesion (see Fig. 17–41). The pattern of enhancement also may be central (12 per cent), mixed (simultaneously peripheral and central) (nine per cent), or diffuse (homogeneous enhancement of the entire lesion) (two per cent) (see Fig. 17–42*B*). However, single-level bolus dynamic scans are performed only to evaluate lesions that are already known to be present, usually by sonography or by a previous incremental dynamic CT.

Many hemangiomas are detected during routine incremental-bolus dynamic CT scans of the liver or abdomen. Thus evaluation of the patterns of enhancement is not as precise as with single-level scans. However, if typical dense, peripheral enhancement of a centrally hypodense lesion is seen, delayed scans often enable an accurate diagnosis to be made (Fig. 17–43). Usually the degree of enhancement seen in these lesions parallels the degree of enhancement in the hepatic vasculature (Figs. 17–41 through 17–44).

Delayed scans, following either single-level or incremental scans of the liver, should be collected from 2 to 60 min following the contrast bolus if a lesion is suspected of being a hemangioma. Delayed images will show some degree of isodense contrast fill-in

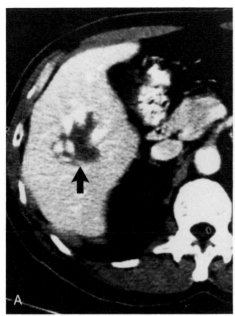

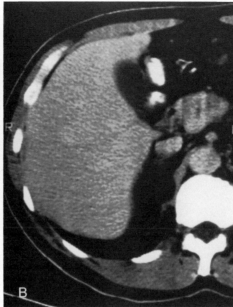

FIGURE 17–43 ■ Incremental bolus dynamic scan of a hemangioma. *A,* Scan during bolus infusion of 150 mL of 60 per cent contrast shows lesion with decreased attenuation centrally and intense peripheral contrast enhancement. *B,* Delayed scan 15 minutes after contrast infusion shows complete isodense fill-in of the lesion.

FIGURE 17–44 ■ Incremental bolus dynamic scan of an atypical hemangioma. *A,* Scan during bolus infusion of contrast shows a heterogeneous contrast-enhancing lesion in the left lobe *(arrow),* predominantly hypodense to normal liver parenchyma. *B,* Delayed scan 20 minutes after contrast infusion shows almost complete isodense fill-in with only a small central hypodense zone *(arrowhead).*

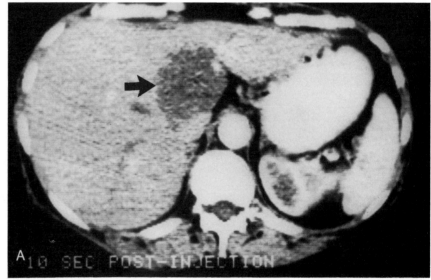

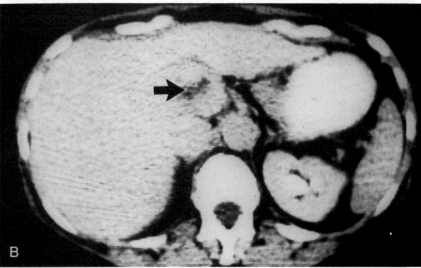

within 93 per cent of hemangiomas (Figs. 17–41 and 17–43). Only seven per cent of hemangiomas fail to show any significant fill-in. The most characteristic pattern is gradual, centripetal fill-in from the periphery, with the hemangioma becoming completely isodense with the surrounding hepatic parenchyma within 5 to 60 min after contrast. This occurs in about 72 per cent of cases. Not infrequently, many of the lesions appear homogeneously hyperdense for 5 to 15 min prior to becoming isodense (see Fig. 17–41E).

Hemangiomas show central zones of diminished attenuation on delayed scans in 21 per cent of cases. These zones may be round, oval, or angular (clefts) (see Fig. 17–44). The lack of fill-in in these cases probably is the result of fibrosis or thrombosis of vascular spaces near the central portion of the tumor. If fibrosis or thrombosis are more widespread, the lesions may have a very inhomogeneous appearance.

The time required for isodense fill-in is independent from the size of the lesion. However, large tumors (10 to 20 cm) generally require more time to fill-in than smaller lesions. Most lesions achieve maximum fill-in by 30 min.

There has been considerable controversy regarding the criteria required to make a specific CT diagnosis of hemangioma. This has generally revolved around the degree of delayed isodense fill-in. It is generally accepted that a CT diagnosis of hemangioma can be made *only* if the lesion shows peripheral contrast enhancement, usually nodular, discontinuous, and equal in intensity to adjacent enhancing blood vessels during the bolus infusion of contrast. It is also accepted that they should slowly fill in centripetally, eventually becoming isodense with adjacent liver. The controversy involves whether it is necessary for hemangiomas to become completely isodense or only partially isodense with a remaining hypodense central zone cleft.

The accuracy of CT obviously increases as the criteria become more strict. Some investigators believe that an accurate diagnosis can be made if a low-density lesion demonstrates intense peripheral contrast enhancement and subsequently shows only partial centripetal isodense fill-in, whereas others have added additional criteria, such as a delay of at least 3 min following contrast before partial or complete isodense fill-in occurs or requiring complete isodense fill-in.[144–146] We believe that three strict criteria generally must be present to make an accurate CT diagnosis of hemangioma: a low-density lesion prior to contrast, intense peripheral enhancement, and complete isodense fill-in.[145] However, these criteria are seen in only 55 per cent of hemangiomas and thus have been judged by some to be too strict.[145] However, in a comparison study of malignant hepatic tumors, only 1 in 63 (1.6 per cent) malignant lesions met these criteria, whereas 25 (39.6 per cent) met the criteria of hemangioma if only partial isodense fill-in was required.[145]

If less strict criteria are used, there are several features of the patterns of enhancement that can be helpful in differential diagnosis. First, the intensity of peripheral enhancement in hemangiomas is usually equal to that of adjacent contrast-enhancing blood vessels, whereas in hepatocellular carcinoma and most metastases it is usually less. Second, the rapidity of fill-in that occurs in some malignant lesions tends to be more rapid than in hemangiomas.

Atypical CT features are seen in 45 per cent of hemangiomas. These include lesions with increased attenuation prior to contrast administration, lack of peripheral contrast enhancement, central or mixed enhancement of the lesion, and incomplete or inhomogeneous isodense fill-in delayed scans (see Figs. 17–42 and 17–44).[147, 148] These atypical patterns were seen in 52 of 63 malignant tumors (83 per cent) and thus should not be used for CT diagnosis of hemangioma (Fig. 17–45).[147]

Magnetic Resonance Imaging ■ Reports indicate that many hemangiomas have typical or diagnostic MR patterns. Stark, using a 0.6-T scanner, demonstrated that T2-weighted sequences (spin-echo; TR, 2000; TE, 120) produced the most useful images.[149] Using several spin-echo T1- and T2-weighted and inversion recovery sequences, MR correctly differentiated hemangioma from malignant tumor with a 90 per cent sensitivity and a 92 per cent specificity (overall accuracy, 90 per cent).[149] Birnbaum et al.[150] showed MR sensitivity to exceed labeled RBC-SPECT imaging in detecting and characterizing hemangiomas.

Four MR features of hemangiomas can be evaluated: signal intensity, morphology, T2 values, and tumor-liver signal intensity ratio. In addition, evaluation of patterns of contrast enhancement using Gd-DTPA also may be of value.[78, 151]

It has been shown that most hemangiomas have higher signal intensities than most metastases, particularly when long TE (90- to 120-ms) intervals are used. However, Li et al. and Wittenberg and co-workers have shown that there is an overlap of signal intensity of hemangiomas and metastases.[72, 152] Wittenberg et al. showed that morphology was important for diagnosis. Hemangiomas typically demonstrate a homogeneously increased signal (light bulb sign) (Fig. 17–46), whereas metastases show amorphous (45 per cent), doughnut (28 per cent), target (27 per cent), or halo (13 per cent) appearances.[72] However, some overlap was still present, with nine per cent of metastases showing the light bulb sign (usually vascular tumors such as islet cell carcinoma, carcinoid, and sarcoma) and six per cent of hemangiomas showing the doughnut sign. Ros and colleagues[153] recently showed that 80 per cent of hemangiomas in their series had a heterogeneous appearance on T2-weighted images, although different scanners and sequences were used: 0.3 T, 0.35 T, and 0.5 T with spin-echo sequences; TR, 1600 to 2154 ms; TE, 70 to 120 ms (Fig. 17–47). The giant cavernous hemangiomas typically demonstrate internal heterogeneity on both T1- and T2-weighted images, presumably because of the spectrum of histopathologic changes such as hemorrhage, thrombosis, and fibrosis.[154]

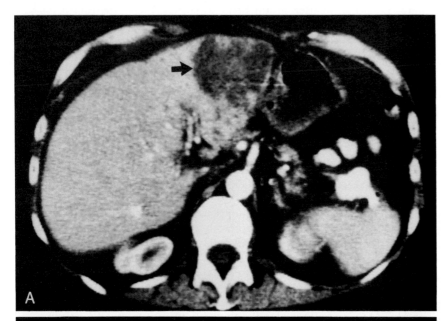

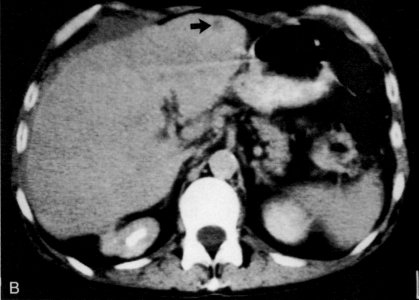

FIGURE 17–45 ■ Incremental bolus dynamic scan of a metastasis. *A,* Scan during bolus infusion of contrast shows inhomogeneous contrast enhancement of lesion in left lobe. *B,* Delayed scan 20 minutes after contrast infusion shows lesion to be isodense except for a small, round zone of decreased attenuation *(arrow).*

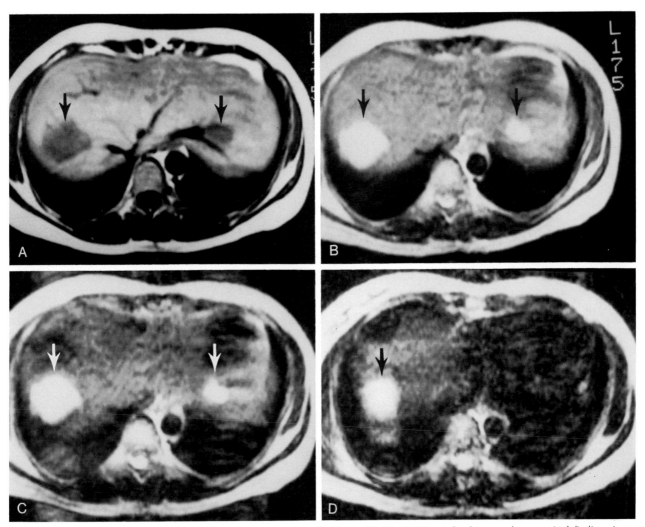

FIGURE 17–46 ■ MR appearance of hemangioma (same patient as in Figure 17–41). *A*, T1-weighted image shows typical findings in two hemangiomas *(arrows)*, which appear hypointense with normal liver parenchyma. *B,* Proton density image (TR/TE = 2300/30) shows both lesions *(arrows)* to be of homogeneous high signal intensity. A progressive increase in T2 weighting (*C* = TR, 2300; TE, 90; *D* = TR, 2300; TE, 120) shows retention of homogeneous high signal intensity throughout the lesions *(arrows)* compared with decreasing intensity in the liver parenchyma. *D* was obtained at a level slightly higher than that of *A* through *C* and did not visualize the left lobe lesion.

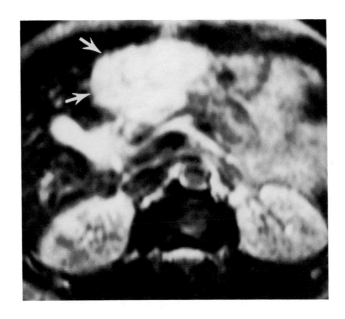

FIGURE 17–47 ■ Hemangioma with heterogeneous MR appearance. T2-weighted image shows a large mass in the left lobe (*arrows*). Although the mass is predominantly of high signal intensity, irregular linear regions of lower signal intensity are seen throughout.

A report by Ohtomo and Itai using single breath-holding fast, low-angle shot (FLASH) images (gradient-echo imaging: 2 T; TR, 20 ms; TE, 12 ms; flip angle 90°) showed high accuracy in distinguishing hemangioma from hepatocellular carcinoma by using T2 values and tumor-to-liver signal intensity ratios.[155] Hemangiomas had high T2 values (88 ms vs. 48 ms for hepatocellular carcinoma) and low tumor-to-liver signal intensity ratios (0.86 vs. 1.46 for hepatocellular carcinoma). Using a cutoff of >80 ms for T2 and >0.9 for the tumor-to-liver signal intensity ratio for hemangioma, 92 per cent of lesions were identified correctly.

Ohtomo and colleagues have used a bolus of gadolinium during MR (1.5 T; T1-weighted sequence: 100/15 or 100/20) to aid in differentiation of hemangioma from malignant hepatic tumors.[151] Hemangiomas showed contrast enhancement patterns similar to dynamic CT: lesions of decreased signal on precontrast scans, peripheral contrast enhancement during the bolus, and increased signal (prolonged contrast enhancement) on delayed images (Figs. 17–48 and 17–49). Hepatocellular carcinoma showed lack of fill-in and absence of prolonged, increased signal on delayed images. Shuman et al.[78] reported that 100 per cent of small hemangiomas demonstrated a lesion-to-liver intensity ratio of >1.3 at 12-minute images (T1-weighted) following Gd-DTPA administration. This delayed increase in signal intensity is unusual with malignant lesions.[76, 79, 156] As in CT, the giant hemangiomas and many small hemangiomas may not achieve homogeneous enhancement throughout (Fig. 17–50). However, MR appears to be more sensitive to gadolinium retention than CT is to iodinated contrast, and persisting high-signal-intensity regions within masses on delayed 12- to 15-minute images appear to be relatively specific for hemangioma. More extensive evaluation of the specificity of these findings is necessary.

Approach to Diagnosis ■ Patients can be divided into two groups, depending on the modality that detects the lesion. Group I consists of patients who have liver lesions detected incidentally during sonography. If the lesion is well marginated and hyperechoic and the patient has normal liver function tests and no known primary tumor, we recommend only a follow-up sonogram in 3 to 6 months to assess lesion stability. Gibney and co-workers recently showed that 82 per cent of hemangiomas rescanned from 1 to 6 years after the initial study were unchanged in size and appearance.[157] However, 18 per cent did show change: three disappeared, seven were less echogenic, one was smaller, and one was enlarged.

Patients with an atypical sonographic pattern (hypoechoic or mixed) or those with abnormal liver function tests or a known primary tumor, should have a technetium Tc 99m erythrocyte (RBC) scan.[158, 159] If the radionuclide scan is negative, MR should be performed.

Group II consists of patients who have lesions detected by incremental dynamic CT. If the lesion shows intense peripheral contrast enhancement during the bolus phase, delayed images should be obtained. If the lesion shows typical isodense fill-in on delayed images, a diagnosis of hemangioma can be made (see Fig. 17–43). If the lesion has atypical CT features, a technetium Tc 99m RBC scan should be performed.

Technetium Tc 99m RBC scans are inexpensive, highly accurate, and easy to interpret compared with MR. However, MR has a specific role. In both groups I and II, we recommend MR instead of a technetium Tc 99m RBC scan if the lesions are small (<1.5 to 2 cm) or if they are located near the porta hepatis, locations that are difficult for SPECT RBC imaging.[150]

The role of fine-needle aspiration biopsy recently has been evaluated in several reports. Solbiati and colleagues sampled 33 hemangiomas, obtaining only blood in 73 per cent and endothelial cells in 27 per

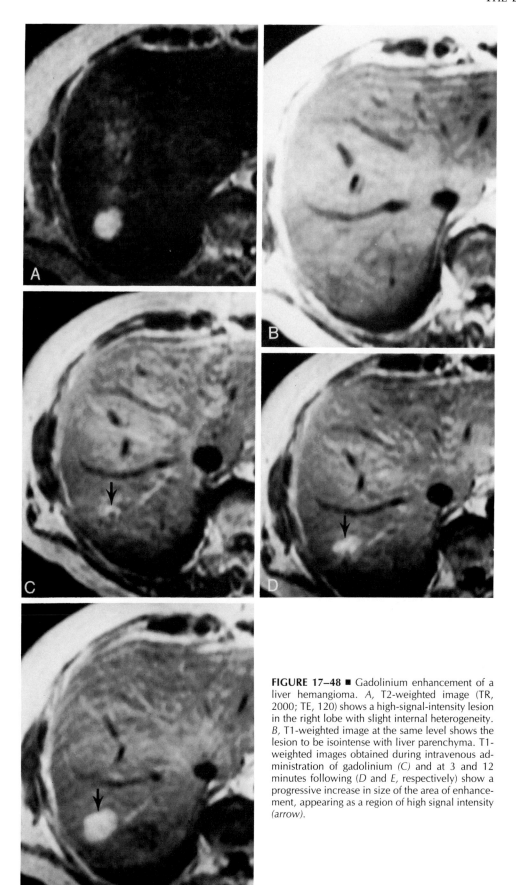

FIGURE 17–48 ■ Gadolinium enhancement of a liver hemangioma. *A,* T2-weighted image (TR, 2000; TE, 120) shows a high-signal-intensity lesion in the right lobe with slight internal heterogeneity. *B,* T1-weighted image at the same level shows the lesion to be isointense with liver parenchyma. T1-weighted images obtained during intravenous administration of gadolinium *(C)* and at 3 and 12 minutes following *(D* and *E,* respectively) show a progressive increase in size of the area of enhancement, appearing as a region of high signal intensity *(arrow).*

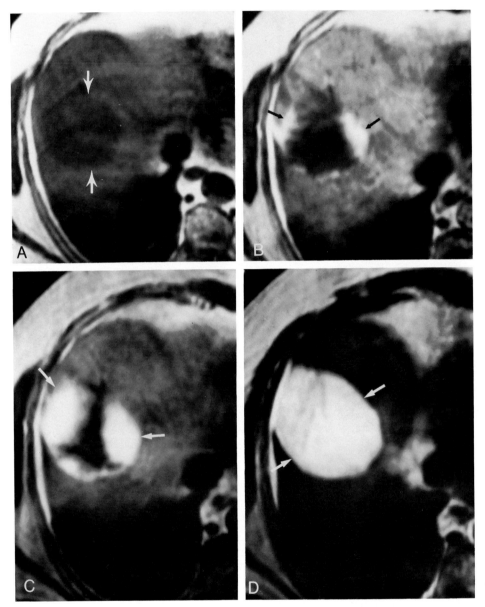

FIGURE 17–49 ■ Large hemangioma with characteristic MR enhancement features. *A*, T1-weighted image before contrast enhancement shows a hypointense mass in the right lobe *(arrows)*. Serial T1-weighted images during administration of gadolinium *(B)* and at 6 *(C)* and 15 minutes *(D)* following administration show progressive peripheral enhancement leading to a homogeneous high signal intensity *(arrows)*.

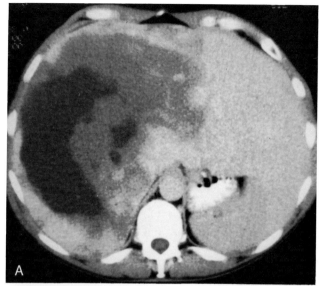

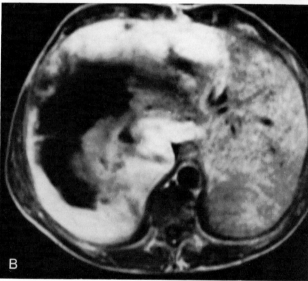

FIGURE 17–50 ■ Giant cavernous hemangiomas. *A,* Contrast-enhanced CT shows a large hemangioma in the right lobe with varying degrees of peripheral enhancement and central lower attenuation. Delayed images failed to show complete central enhancement. *B,* T1-weighted MR image 12 minutes after gadolinium DTPA administration shows only peripheral enhancement with low central signal intensity similar to that on CT.

cent.[160] The latter finding was considered diagnostic of hemangioma. No complications occurred (all biopsies were performed with sonographic guidance using 23-gauge needles with angulation adjusted so that normal liver parenchyma was interposed between the liver capsule and the lesion). Cronan and Spamer used 20-gauge Franseen cutting needles and obtained tissue cores that histologically showed hemangioma.[161, 162] Again, no complications or bleeding occurred. These reports suggest that if a cutting needle is used, a specific diagnosis may be reached quickly with fine-needle biopsy, obviating additional imaging such as technetium Tc 99m RBC scans, MR, CT, and angiography.

HEPATIC ADENOMA

Liver cell adenomas are benign, well-encapsulated, true hepatic neoplasms composed entirely of hepatocytes.[163, 164] The hepatocytes and capsule may be vacuolated by fat globules,[164] but fibrous septations and bile ducts are not found. Liver cell adenomas are usually solitary tumors occurring predominantly in women taking oral contraceptives.[165] Clinically, liver cell adenomas are usually asymptomatic until growth of the tumor produces an abdominal mass or tumoral hemorrhage results in abdominal pain; if the hemorrhage is massive, shock and even death may result. Liver cell adenomas can regress or completely disappear following withdrawal of oral contraceptives or hormonal therapy.[166, 167] However, hemorrhage and growth of liver cell adenomas may occur despite stoppage of oral contraceptives,[168] and therefore surgical resection remains the therapy of choice for symptomatic liver cell adenomas.

Liver cell adenomas usually appear on non–contrast-enhanced CT as a discrete mass hypodense to the normal liver parenchyma (Fig. 17–51*A*), but isodense adenomas, detectable only by contour abnormalities, have been described.[169] Although the CT attenuation of liver cell adenomas does not permit differentiation from other solid hepatic masses, the capsule may contain an excess of lipid-laden hepatocytes, permitting a low-attenuation peripheral ring to be identified.[164] Foci of high attenuation (75 to 90 H) representing areas of hemorrhage may be seen within these lesions on noncontrast CT (Fig. 17–52).[169, 170] Areas of old hemorrhage or necrosis may result in areas of marked hypodensity, particularly after contrast administration.[169]

Following the rapid administration of intravenous contrast, these lesions typically demonstrate significant enhancement during the arterial phase (see Fig. 17–51) that can rapidly diminish on more delayed images, resulting in an isodense or even hypodense appearance during the portal phase.[169] A minority of cases demonstrate hypodense enhancement when compared with the adjacent normal liver parenchyma.[169]

The MR appearance of these tumors is nonspecific and simulates other benign and malignant neoplasms. They appear isointense with liver parenchyma on T1-weighted images and with higher signal intensity than liver on T2-weighted sequences (see Fig. 17–52).[74, 171, 172] A peripheral low-signal-intensity rim, similar to that reported with hepatocellular carcinoma, can be seen in liver cell adenomas.[74] As with CT, when foci of hemorrhage are present, corresponding changes are identified on MR images as well (see Fig. 17–52) and may be the clue to the diagnosis.

FOCAL NODULAR HYPERPLASIA

Focal nodular hyperplasia is a rare, benign liver lesion composed of Kupffer cells, hepatocytes, and bile ducts.[173] It is usually well circumscribed but not encapsulated and is subdivided into nodules by a

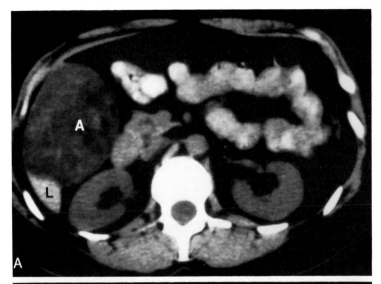

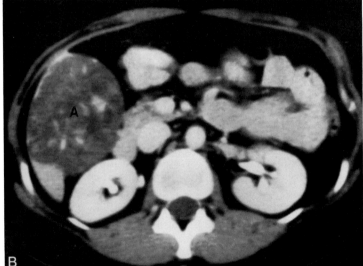

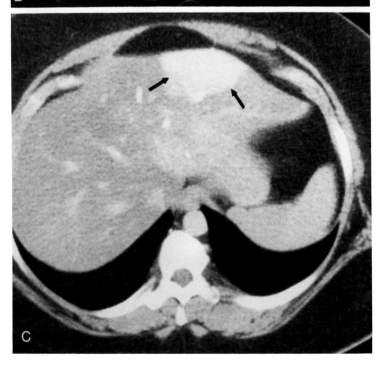

FIGURE 17–51 ■ Hepatic adenoma. *A*, Noncontrast CT scan shows the adenoma (A) as a sharply defined lesion of lower attenuation than adjacent liver parenchyma (L). *B*, Contrast CT scan shows a mild diffuse increase in attenuation throughout the adenoma (A), with a heterogeneous pattern and regions of more marked enhancement. *C*, Early contrast-enhanced image from a different patient with a hepatic adenoma shows marked, diffuse enhancement of the lesion *(arrows)*.

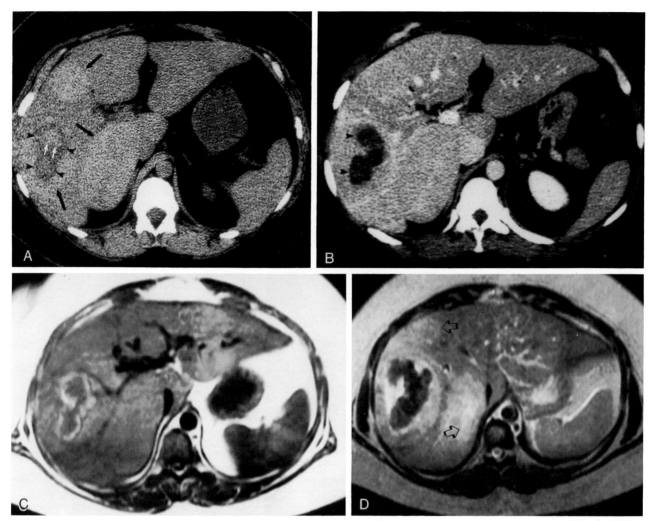

FIGURE 17–52 ■ Hepatic adenomas with hemorrhage. *A,* Noncontrast CT scan in a patient with mild fatty infiltration of the liver shows three liver lesions *(black arrows)* of higher attenuation than liver parenchyma. Subacute hemorrhage within one lesion has resulted in central low attenuation *(arrowheads)* with foci of higher attenuation *(white arrows)*. *B,* Contrast administration results in the lesions becoming isodense with liver parenchyma, except for the central lower attenuation in the region of hemorrhage *(arrowheads)*. *C,* T1-weighted MR image (1.5 T) shows two of the lesions as isointense with normal liver parenchyma. The lesion with hemorrhage is identifiable because of the focus of hemorrhage. The hemorrhage shows central hypointensity with a surrounding hyperintense rim resulting from methemoglobin accumulation, which shortens T1. The peripheral dark rim present is caused by hemosiderin deposition. *D,* T2-weighted MR image at a slightly different level shows a slight increase in signal intensity in the nonhemorrhagic lesions *(open arrows)*. The hemorrhagic lesion shows a heterogeneous signal intensity pattern. Centrally the lesion is dark because of T2 shortening caused by deoxyhemoglobin, and the progressive increase in signal intensity peripherally parallels methemoglobin formation, as on the T1-weighted images.

central fibrous core or scar and radiating septa containing arterial and venous channels and proliferating bile ducts.[174, 175] It occurs in all age groups and is predominantly found in women, although 10 to 20 per cent of cases occur in men.[169, 175] The lesion arises in an otherwise normal liver, is multiple in 20 per cent of cases, and typically is 4 to 7 cm in diameter. Hemorrhage, necrosis, or malignant degeneration is very rare, and the vast majority of patients remain entirely asymptomatic. As a result of the benign nature of focal nodular hyperplasia, no therapy is recommended unless torsion, infarction, or lesion size forces surgical resection.

Diagnosis may be possible by correlating the findings of the radionuclide colloid scintigram and hepatic angiography. Radionuclide colloid scintigrams often appear normal, as the Kupffer cells in the area of focal nodular hyperplasia concentrate colloid.[175] However, hyperconcentration of colloid may be seen, and in 30 to 35 per cent of patients the region of hyperplasia may be photopenic.[170, 174, 175] Angiographically, the lesions are hypervascular, with fine radiating septations identifiable in the parenchymal stain.[175, 176] The combination of a normal radionuclide scan and a hypervascular mass or masses usually allows focal nodular hyperplasia to be distinguished from liver cell adenoma and other malignant lesions. A biopsy may have to be performed when the radionuclide scan is photopenic or the angiographic features are atypical. Ultrasound findings are nonspecific, with hyperechoic, hypoechoic, and mixed echogenic patterns seen.[169, 170]

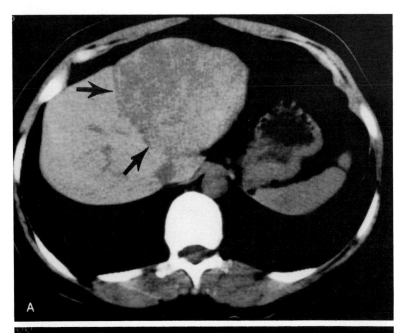

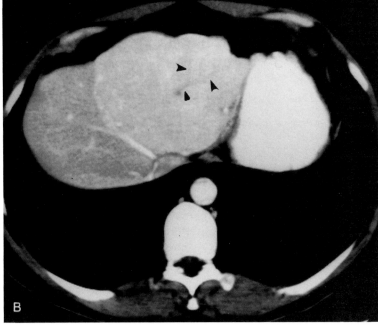

FIGURE 17–53 ■ Focal nodular hyperplasia. *A,* Non-contrast CT scan shows a hypodense mass *(arrows)* in the left lobe. *B,* Early contrast CT scan demonstrates marked diffuse enhancement within the lesion, with a linear, branching lower attenuation region *(arrowheads)* that proved to be a central fibrous scar.

Computed Tomography ■ The lesions may be single or multiple and usually appear as discrete, slightly hypodense lesions on non–contrast-enhanced images (Fig. 17–53), although a minority may appear isodense.[169, 170] Although these lesions have been noted to be isodense or mildly hypodense following intravenous contrast administration (Fig. 17–54),[170, 177] when dynamic, rapid scan techniques are utilized, the early arterial phase usually demonstrates significant enhancement (see Fig. 17–53).[169] The central fibrous core, or scar, is visible on CT images in 14 to 44 per cent of patients[169, 170] as a central, stellate region of lower attenuation, visible on the noncontrast or contrast-enhanced images (see Fig. 17–53). Unfortunately, these central scars can also be seen in other lesions, such as fibrolamellar hepatoma,[178] and is therefore not always a helpful identifying feature. Central necrosis or hemorrhage is unusual in focal nodular hyperplasia and can be a helpful feature in differentiating it from hepatic adenoma.

Magnetic Resonance Imaging ■ Focal nodular hyperplasia has been reported to have a characteristic appearance on MR images.[179] Although the lesions usually are isointense with normal liver parenchyma on T1-weighted images and isointense or minimally hyperintense on T2-weighted images,[179, 180] lesions with areas of marked hyperintensity on T2-weighted images have been reported at 1.5 T.[181] The margins of the lesions are most often ill defined or indiscernible. In one series,[179] 50 per cent of lesions demonstrated a central scar with characteristic findings. The central scar was hypointense on T1-weighted images but hyperintense on T2-weighted images, presumably because of the presence of bile duct and vascular channels within the scar.[179, 180] These findings are in contradistinction to the central scars seen on MR in patients with fibrolamellar hepatomas that were of low signal intensity on both sequences.[179]

RARE MISCELLANEOUS TUMORS

Rare primary benign hepatic tumors may arise from mesodermal derivatives or lymphangiomatous elements. Lipomas and angiomyolipoma in the liver have been reported with a homogeneous, low-attenuation appearance (< -20 H) in the majority of cases, although fine septations or small vessels may be seen within these lesions (Fig. 17–55).[182–184] They may occur as an isolated lesion but are found in many patients with underlying renal angiomyolipoma and tuberous sclerosis.[183] With hepatic angiomyolipomas, as in the kidney, a spectrum of CT attenuation values can be seen, depending on the amount of fat present within the lesion. Frequently ten per cent or less of these lesions are composed of fat.[185] Because of this, Roberts et al.[183] hypothesized that these lesions may be more prevalent than thought, but the lack of fat attenuation present obscures the diagnosis. Myelolipoma, a benign tumor containing a combination of mature fat cells and normal myeloid and erythroid precursors, may occur in the liver with regions of low attenuation (< -30 H) and soft tissue attenuation.[186] Caution must be used in diagnosing a benign fatty lesion if significant soft tissue regions are present within a liver mass, as hepatomas may contain regions of low attenuation with fat accumulation.[182]

Because of the short T1 and long T2 of fat, fatty tumors appear as high-intensity masses on both T1- and T2-weighted images.[182] Thus the T1-weighted sequence is essential to differentiate fatty tumors from hemangiomas, cysts, or other neoplasms. Although hepatomas may contain fat and also have increased signal intensity on T1-weighted images, these cases usually demonstrate heterogeneous signal intensity, rather than the homogeneous appearance typical of benign fatty masses.[182]

Mesenchymal hamartoma of the liver (also known as lymphangioma, hamartoma, and cystic hamar-

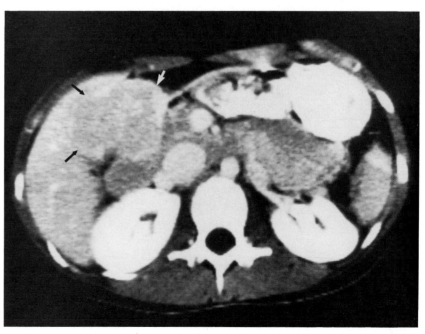

FIGURE 17–54 ■ Focal nodular hyperplasia. Contrast-enhanced CT scan shows the lesion *(arrows)* to be predominantly isodense with normal liver.

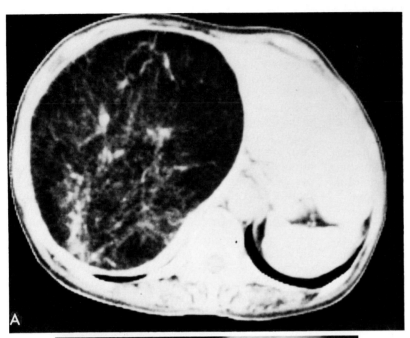

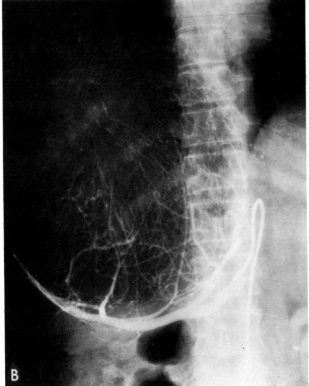

FIGURE 17–55 ■ Benign hepatic tumor composed almost entirely of fat. *A,* CT scan shows the lesion to be sharply marginated from the normal liver and containing multiple linear densities, which enhanced after contrast administration. *B,* Hepatic angiogram shows displacement of the hepatic artery and a number of small, thin vessels entering the center of the tumor from the periphery.

toma) is an uncommon lesion occurring in children younger than 2 years of age. It is thought to be a developmental anomaly rather than a neoplasm, with large liver masses up to 20 cm in size representing an admixture of bile ducts and mesenchymal tissue.[187] The appearance can range from a solid-appearing mass with cystic areas to a predominantly cystic mass with septations.[187, 188] These lesions can simulate dilated intrahepatic biliary ducts.[189]

Hemangioendothelioma, a tumor of vascular origin presenting in the infantile period, is a benign lesion that may present with potential life-threatening complications of hepatic rupture, consumptive coagulopathy, or congestive heart failure.[190] It may involve the liver focally or diffusely.[191] The typical noncontrast CT appearance is that of a hypodense mass that may contain small calcifications. Contrast enhancement is usually present, either peripherally or centrally, and (similarly to cavernous hemangiomas) tends to progress over time to become isodense with normal liver parenchyma by the equilibrium contrast phase.[190, 191]

Biliary cystadenoma and its malignant counterpart, biliary cystadenocarcinoma, although of bile duct origin, almost always occur as large masses within the liver parenchyma, ranging up to 27 cm in diameter.[192, 193] The masses appear as predominantly cystic masses of low attenuation (<30 H) and are usually multilocular with numerous septations (Fig. 17–56). Calcifications can occur in the wall and septations in both benign and malignant cases.[192, 193] Although the cystadenocarcinoma is more likely to show thick, irregular septations or mural nodules,[192, 193] there is an overlap in these appearances, and thus CT cannot reliably differentiate these lesions. Percutaneous biopsy does not help in many instances, as regions of benign appearance can be seen in the cystadenocarcinoma.[192] Because cystadenoma is considered a premalignant lesion, both of these lesions require surgical treatment. Only rarely do they have a unilocular appearance that could be mistaken for a simple cyst.[193]

Primary Malignant Tumors

HEPATOCELLULAR CARCINOMA

Hepatocellular carcinoma (HCC) is the most common primary malignant tumor of the liver, representing more than 80 per cent of all primary hepatic malignancies. Although relatively common in equatorial Africa and Asia, it is rare in the United States. When seen in the United States, these tumors are usually found in patients with preexisting liver disease such as cirrhosis or hemochromatosis (see Fig. 17–32), or in patients with positive hepatitis B surface antigen levels.

Pathologically, HCC is characterized by a tendency toward intravascular growth into the hepatic veins and portal system. The usual angiographic appearance of a hepatocellular carcinoma is that of a hypervascular mass being supplied by an enlarged hepatic artery, with prominent tumor neovascularization, arteriovenous shunting, capillary staining, arterial encasement, and portal vein occlusion.[194–197] Although hypervascularity is the most frequent finding, hypovascular HCC and HCC with a mixed hypovascular-hypervascular pattern occur,[194, 195] particularly in smaller lesions.[196, 197] Avascular areas result from vascular obstruction, tumor necrosis, or hemorrhage. Invasion of portal veins results in a high incidence of portal vein thrombosis. The initial presentation of these patients may be a result of spontaneous hemorrhage (intrahepatic, subcapsular, or intraperitoneal).[198, 199]

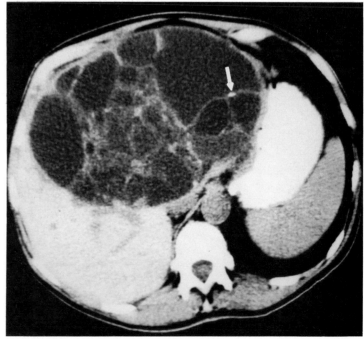

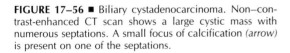

FIGURE 17–56 ■ Biliary cystadenocarcinoma. Non–contrast-enhanced CT scan shows a large cystic mass with numerous septations. A small focus of calcification *(arrow)* is present on one of the septations.

Fibrolamellar hepatocellular carcinoma is a histologic subtype seen in younger patients (15 to 35 years of age) and has a better patient prognosis than hepatocellular carcinoma.[200, 201] It occurs in noncirrhotic livers and often does not result in an increased serum alpha-fetoprotein level,[202] although mild increases[201, 203] and, rarely, marked elevation[178] may be seen.

Computed Tomography ■ The CT appearance of HCC is varied, reflecting differences in extent, differentiation, vascularity, necrosis, and venous occlusion. There are three predominant patterns of appearance of HCC on CT. Most frequently HCC appears as either solitary or multiple discrete hepatic mass lesions (Figs. 17–57 and 17–58). In approximately five per cent of cases it appears as diffuse, ill-defined infiltration of the liver parenchyma (Fig. 17–59).[204] On non–contrast-enhanced images, HCC most often appears hypodense with normal liver parenchyma, but up to 12 per cent may be isodense.[204–206] In these latter instances, contour abnormalities of the liver may suggest the diagnosis. In many instances, although the bulk of the lesion may appear isodense, a hypodense rim can be seen on the noncontrast images.[206] Calcification has been reported in 2 to 25 per cent of cases (Fig. 17–60),[204–206] and high-attenuation foci may also be seen within these lesions following hemorrhage. Rarely, fatty metamorphosis

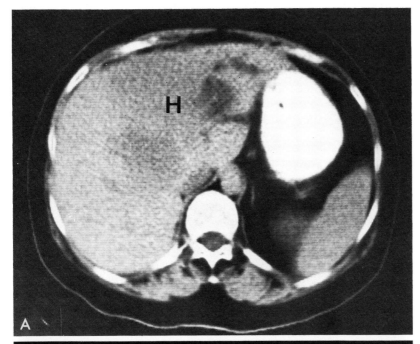

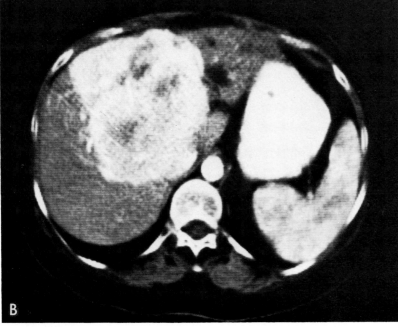

FIGURE 17–57 ■ Single-level dynamic scan of hepatocellular carcinoma. *A,* Precontrast scan shows the lesion (H) as an ill-defined, low-attenuation mass. *B,* Scan during peak arterial contrast. The hepatocellular carcinoma dramatically enhances throughout. *C,* Scan 30 seconds after contrast administration shows the tumor to have a hyperdense rim; it is predominantly hypodense with respect to normal liver.

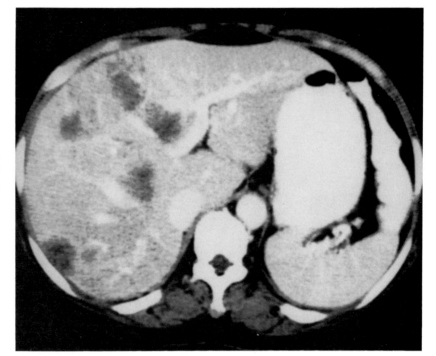

FIGURE 17–58 ■ Multifocal hepatocellular carcinoma. Contrast CT scan reveals numerous masses that are hypodense to normal liver parenchyma. This is a nonspecific appearance and cannot be differentiated from metastatic disease.

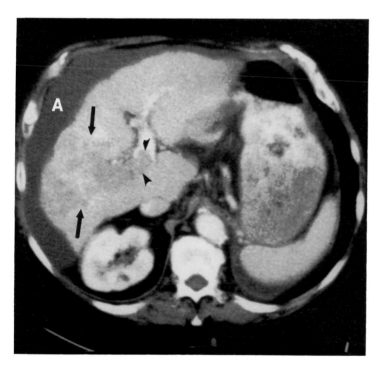

FIGURE 17–59 ■ Hepatocellular carcinoma with diffuse infiltration. Rather than appearing as a well-defined, solitary lesion, this hepatocellular carcinoma presents on contrast CT scan as a large area of diffuse tumoral infiltration throughout the right lobe of the liver *(arrows)*. Portal vein tumor thrombus *(arrowheads)* is also present. A = Ascites.

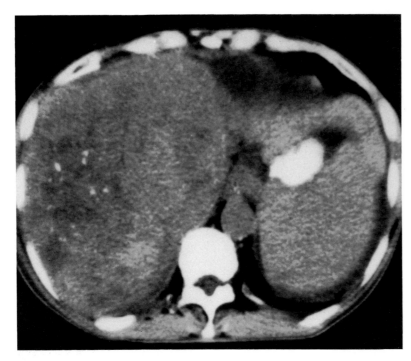

FIGURE 17–60 ■ Hepatocellular carcinoma. Noncontrast CT scan shows a large right lobe tumor appearing predominantly hypodense to normal liver parenchyma but with scattered foci of high-attenuation calcification.

can be detected on CT, with lesions exhibiting regions of low attenuation (< -10 H) (Fig. 17–61).[91]

The CT appearance of hepatomas following intravenous contrast varies depending on the vascularity of the tumor and the time sequence used for scanning (see Fig. 17–57). Most often these lesions show diffuse inhomogeneous enhancement,[204, 206] with significant areas of decreased enhancement indicating areas of necrosis or old hemorrhage. Scanning during the early, arterial phase may demonstrate marked diffuse enhancement (see Fig. 17–57), but this is always transient, rapidly changing to either a heterogeneous or isodense appearance. Utilizing current dynamic scan techniques, only rarely (usually in the infiltrating, diffuse type of lesion) does the tumor appear isodense with adjacent liver parenchyma on contrast-enhanced images.[207] The capsule seen on noncontrast images as decreased density can exhibit prolonged enhancement following contrast administration; this was seen in 50 per cent of cases in Japan (see Fig. 17–57).[208]

There is a high incidence of vascular complications in the liver in patients with HCC. Arterioportal shunting is evident angiographically, and similar findings can be demonstrated on CT, with early and prolonged enhancement of the portal vein.[208] Central portal vein thrombosis can be identified in 11 to 40 per cent of cases (see Figs. 17–59 and 17–61)[204, 209, 210] and peripheral involvement in 16 per cent.[210] This may lead to an increased attenuation in contralateral lobes following contrast administration, with portal blood flow increasing to the nonaffected lobe.

Fibrolamellar hepatocellular carcinoma usually presents on CT as a large solitary mass or, less commonly, as multiple lesions.[178, 202] Similar to usual HCC, these lesions are hypodense on noncontrast scans and demonstrate heterogeneous enhancement

with contrast in varying degrees (Fig. 17–62). There is an increased incidence of calcification in these tumors (in up to 55 per cent of cases),[178] which are usually punctate and central. In addition, a central low-attenuation scar can be seen on both noncontrast and contrast scans in up to 45 per cent of patients.[178] Although suggestive, these findings are not diagnostic and overlap the spectrum of usual HCC and other benign lesions. Ultimately, a biopsy is required for accurate diagnosis.

As has been found for metastatic disease with colon cancer, CT portography has been found to be the most accurate method of detecting the full extent of HCC. Matsui et al.[43] found that for lesions >3 cm in diameter, CT portography detected 95 per cent of lesions, compared with 58 per cent for noncontrast and contrast-enhanced CT combined, 63 per cent for ultrasound, and 83 per cent for angiography. Several Japanese investigators have found that iodized oil is retained within hepatocellular carcinoma for prolonged periods of time. CT scans obtained approximately 1 week after intraarterial injection of iodized oil have resulted in high detection rates of primary and satellite lesions of HCC (see Fig. 17–16).[54–56] Merine et al.[57] reported that CT portography was more sensitive than CT enhanced with iodized oil in detecting main lesions of hepatocellular carcinoma (94 per cent vs. 82 per cent), but the iodized oil CT was more sensitive in detecting the small, satellite metastatic lesions (50 per cent vs. 38 per cent).

Magnetic Resonance Imaging ■ The capability of MRI to detect HCC varies directly with lesion size and is comparable to incremental bolus dynamic CT.[211, 212] Ebara et al.[212] detected 100 per cent of lesions 3 cm or greater in diameter, but only 33 per cent of lesions less than 2 cm in diameter. At middle field strength, unlike metastatic disease, hepatomas are

FIGURE 17–61 ■ Hepatocellular carcinoma containing fat. *A,* Noncontrast CT scan shows a heterogeneous right lobe mass with foci of low attenuation *(arrows)* measuring −15 H. *B,* Contrast CT scan at a different level shows the heterogeneous mass with foci of low attenuation *(white arrows)* that measure >0 H with contrast enhancement. Tumor thrombus is seen in the right portal vein *(black arrow).*

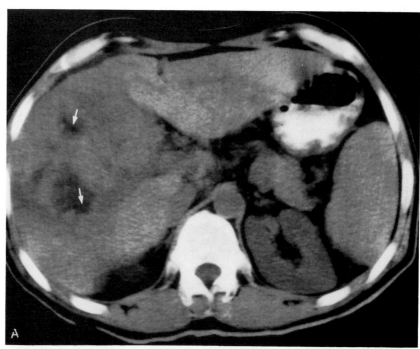

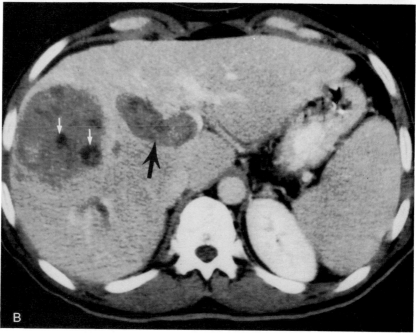

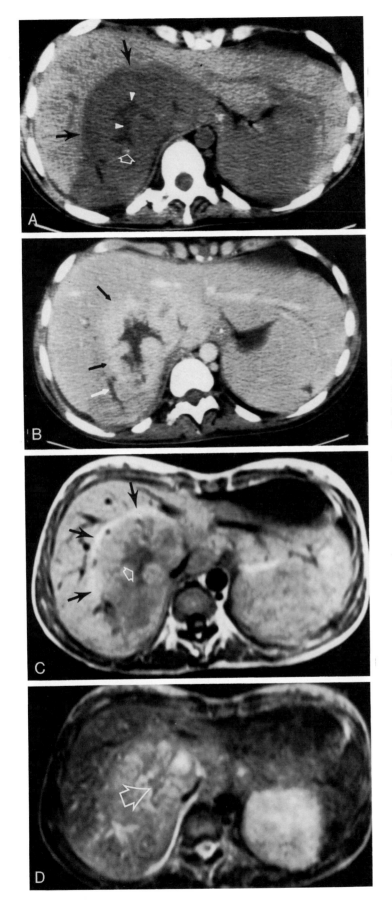

FIGURE 17–62 ■ Fibrolamellar hepatocellular carcinoma. *A,* Noncontrast CT scan shows the lesion as a hypodense mass *(solid arrows)* with a central stellate lower attenuation region *(arrowheads)* and calcification *(open arrow)*. *B,* Contrast-enhanced CT scan shows the lesion to peripherally enhance *(black arrows)* more than liver parenchyma, with the central low-attenuation scar more prominent than on noncontrast images. Focal peripheral bile duct dilatation caused by obstructed bile ducts is seen *(white arrow)*. *C,* T1-weighted MR image (0.5 T) shows a hyperintense rim to the mass *(solid arrows)*, which is otherwise isointense or slightly hypointense to the liver. The central scar is of low signal intensity *(open arrow)*. *D,* T2-weighted image shows the lesion as predominantly slightly hyperintense to liver, with smaller central low signal intensity in the region of the central scar *(open arrow)*.

best detected with T2-weighted pulse sequences.[73, 74] Although the lesions are almost always hyperintense with liver parenchyma on T2-weighted sequences, two per cent of cases may be isointense.[211–213] The signal intensity seen on T1-weighted images demonstrates more variety, including hypointense, isointense and hyperintense with normal liver parenchyma (Figs. 17–63 through 17–65).[74, 105, 156, 211] The increased T1 signal intensity often relates to the fat content present in many hepatomas (Fig. 17–64),[74, 214] although it may be seen in tumors without fat content as well.[105] This finding may be helpful in suggesting the diagnosis of HCC, but caution must be used, as other masses with fat or hemorrhage, as well as complicated cysts with hemorrhage or proteinaceous contents, can have a similar appearance. Many of these latter lesions are of homogeneous high signal intensity on T2-weighted images; however, they are unlike HCC lesions, which are usually heterogeneous and with a signal intensity less than that of cysts. A dark surrounding rim thought to represent the pseudocapsule identified pathologically has been identi-

fied in up to 45 per cent of HCC lesions on inversion recovery and spin-echo T1-weighted images (Fig. 17–65)[74, 212] and can be a differentiating feature of HCC (although it can also be seen in benign lesions such as adenomas).[74] At 1.5 T, these pseudocapsules are also identified on T2-weighted images with an inner dark band (thought to represent the fibrous tumor capsule) and an outer bright band (thought to represent compressed vessels or new bile duct formation).[211] The encapsulated lesions tend to have slower growth and a better prognosis than nonencapsulated types.[211, 215]

Like CT, MR is capable of demonstrating the tumor thrombi that occur frequently with HCC (Fig. 17–66). The sensitivity of spin-echo MR techniques in detecting the vascular involvement is equal to that of CT,[211] although the use of flow-sensitive techniques such as gradient refocused images would be expected to increase the sensitivity of MR.

The use of gadolinium contrast has been advocated to differentiate HCC from hemangiomas using fast scan techniques.[79, 156] HCC typically demonstrates

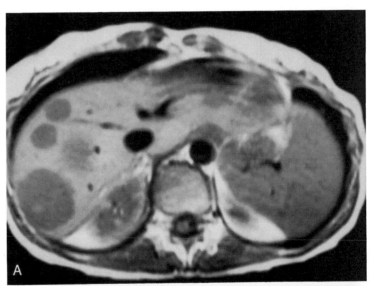
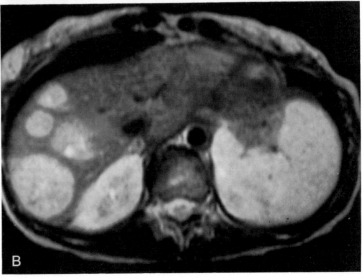

FIGURE 17–63 ■ Multifocal hepatocellular carcinoma. *A*, T1-weighted image shows the lesions as well-defined foci of lower signal intensity than adjacent liver parenchyma. *B*, T2-weighted scan shows the lesions as well-defined foci of higher signal intensity when compared with liver parenchyma, approximating the intensity of the spleen.

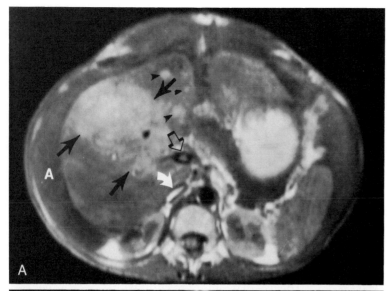

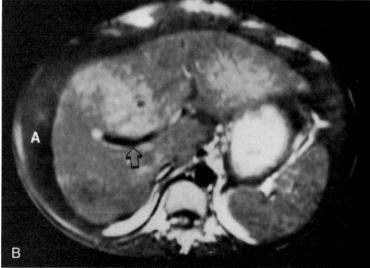

FIGURE 17–64 ■ Hepatocellular carcinoma in a patient with cirrhosis. *A,* T1-weighted image shows a large right lobe lesion *(black solid arrows)* and several smaller satellite nodules *(arrowheads).* The lesions are of high signal intensity because of high fat content. Increased signal is seen within the lumens of the portal vein *(open arrow)* and inferior vena cava *(curved arrow)* because of slow flow and not thrombosis. *B,* T1-weighted scan cephalic to *A* shows the portal vein *(open arrow)* as a signal void without thrombosis.

FIGURE 17–65 ■ Hepatocellular carcinoma. T1-weighted MR image shows a low-signal-intensity rim *(arrows)* surrounding the mass in the right lobe.

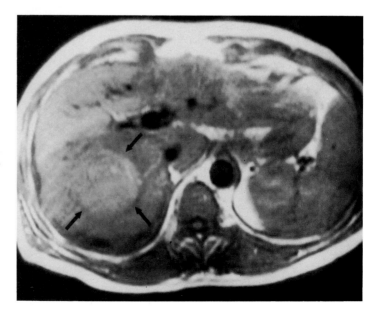

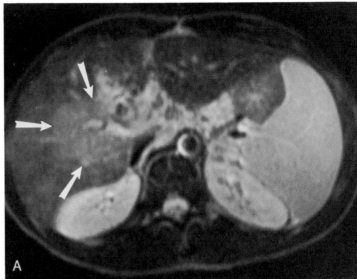

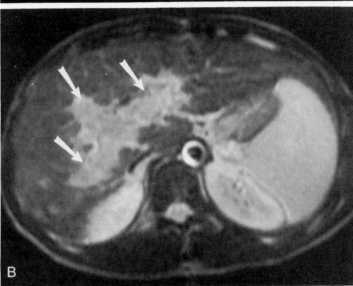

FIGURE 17–66 ■ Hepatocellular carcinoma with portal vein thrombosis. *A,* T2-weighted image shows the carcinoma *(arrows)* invading the porta hepatis. *B,* A more cephalic image shows diffuse enlargement of the portal vein *(arrows)* with tumor thrombus of moderately increased signal intensity.

enhancement early (peak enhancement within 10 seconds after injection), achieves only mild or moderate peak contrast enhancement, and does not exhibit prolonged enhancement at 10 to 12 minutes (Fig. 17–67).[79, 156] This is in contrast to hemangiomas, which typically demonstrate marked peak enhancement occurring more than 2 minutes after injection, with marked delayed enhancement at 10 to 12 minutes.[78, 79] As with CT contrast, the pseudocapsule demonstrates enhancement on MR in 55 per cent of cases.[156]

Limited reports of the MR appearance of fibrolamellar hepatocellular carcinoma have been published.[179, 216] Similarly to usual HCC, the lesions are of lower signal intensity than normal liver on T1-weighted images and of increased signal intensity of varying degrees on T2-weighted images (see Fig. 17–62). When present, the central branching scan is of low signal intensity on both T1- and T2-weighted images. The central scan of focal nodular hyperplasia may be of increased signal intensity on T2-weighted images, a discriminating feature.[180, 181] In addition, focal nodular hyperplasia is usually isointense with normal liver on T1-weighted sequences.

CHOLANGIOCARCINOMA

Although most often occurring in the extrahepatic biliary tree, cholangiocarcinoma can arise from the intrahepatic bile ducts and present as a parenchymal liver mass. Similar to hepatomas, they can occur as focal masses or as diffuse or multifocal masses and can have a varied CT appearance, in part because of varied histology. When the tumors are small and surround an intrahepatic bile duct, only the proximal ductal obstruction, lobar or segmental in distribution, will be identified on CT.[217] When larger, these lesions have a nonspecific appearance and are generally of lower attenuation than liver parenchyma on noncontrast and contrast-enhanced images. Although usually less vascular than hepatomas, vascular lesions can occasionally be identified on angiography and CT, and these lesions may have some features similar

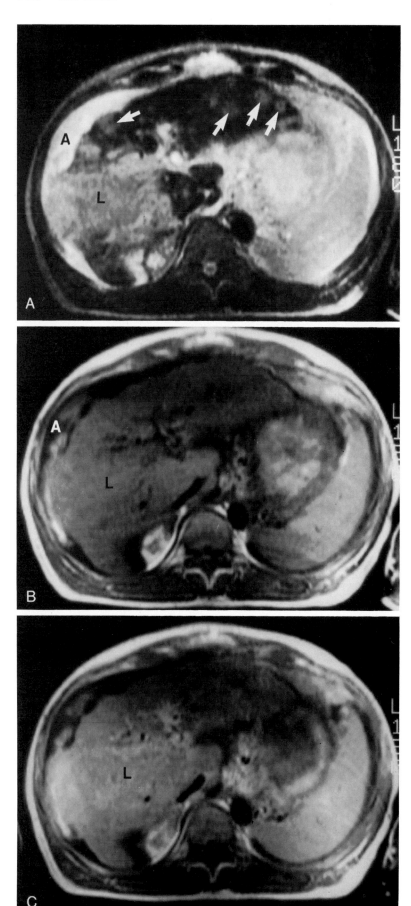

FIGURE 17–67 ■ MR contrast enhancement of hepatocellular carcinoma. *A,* T2-weighted noncontrast image shows a large right lobe lesion of moderately increased signal intensity (L). Numerous smaller nodules *(arrows)* of increased signal intensity are seen throughout the liver. A = Ascites. *B,* T1-weighted precontrast image shows the carcinoma (L) as a region of increased signal intensity compared with liver parenchyma. The numerous small nodules are not seen. A = Ascites. *C,* T1-weighted image following intravenous gadolinium contrast administration shows the lesion (L) as having slightly increased signal intensity compared with liver parenchyma, but less conspicuous than in *A.* The other nodules are not well seen, as they are isointense with the enhanced liver parenchyma.

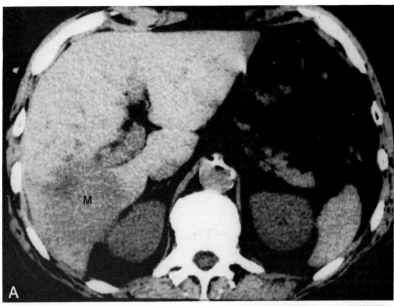

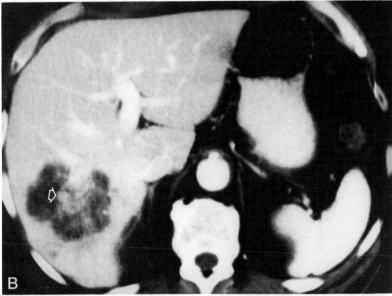

FIGURE 17–68 ■ Intrahepatic cholangiocarcinoma. *A,* Noncontrast CT scan shows the mass (M) as hypodense compared with adjacent liver parenchyma. *B,* Early contrast-enhanced image shows central enhancement *(open arrow)* within the mass. *C,* Delayed scan 20 minutes after *B* shows further enhancement persisting throughout nearly the entire lesion. The lesion has not become homogeneously enhanced, however, sparing a thin peripheral rim of low attenuation *(arrowheads);* therefore it does not meet the criteria for a diagnosis of hemangioma. Note the similarity of appearance to Figure 17–42.

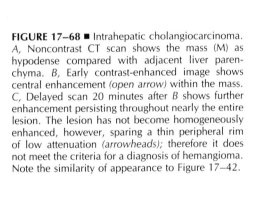

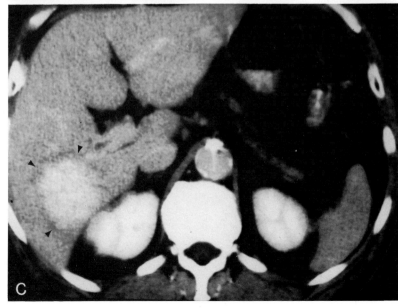

to atypical hemangiomas on CT with significant delayed enhancement (Fig. 17–68). Intrahepatic cholangiocarcinoma can present as a cystic mass with papillary projections[217] and simulate other complex cystic lesions, including cystadenoma or adenocarcinoma, echinococcal cyst, cystic hamartomas, old hematoma, and abscess.

LYMPHOMA

Primary lymphoma of the liver is rare, although the incidence may be increased in organ transplant recipients.[218, 219] Secondary involvement, however, occurs frequently. Autopsy series have shown that the liver is a secondary site of involvement in 60 per cent of patients with Hodgkin's lymphoma and in 50 per cent of those with non-Hodgkin's lymphoma.[220, 221] Diffuse infiltration is more frequent in Hodgkin's disease, whereas diffuse and nodular hepatic involvement are equally frequent in non-Hodgkin's lymphoma.[222] The CT appearances of lymphomatous involvement are not characteristic and cannot be differentiated from other space-occupying lesions or infiltrative disorders. When seen, the most common CT appearance of hepatic lymphoma is heterogeneous-appearing liver parenchyma with ill-defined regions of decreased contrast enhancement.[218] Generally, however, the small, diffusely infiltrating lesions are not detected with CT. Less commonly, they appear as focal, hypodense lesions in the liver, best seen following intravenous contrast administration. The B-cell lymphomas seen in organ transplant recipients have a propensity for central necrosis and can appear as low-attenuation liver lesions (Fig. 17–69).[223] Initial studies[218] showed CT to have a low sensitivity for detecting hepatic lymphoma (57 per cent). Another study using optimal techniques reported greater than 80 per cent sensitivity in detecting hepatic involvement.[224] Although hepatomegaly is frequently seen with lymphomatous involvement in the liver, CT demonstration of hepatomegaly alone should not be interpreted as evidence of lymphomatous involvement, as lymphoma is histologically absent in 43 per cent of patients with non-Hodgkin's lymphoma and hepatomegaly.[221]

MRI has been shown to have a poor sensitivity for lymphomatous involvement of the liver.[225, 226] Rarely, lesions are seen within the liver of increased signal intensity[225] compared with adjacent liver parenchyma. Unfortunately, because of the diffuse, microscopic involvement in this disease process, no difference is generally discerned in MRI parameters between normal livers and livers with malignant lymphoma,[226, 227] unless it is associated with fibrosis, necrosis, or edema. Preliminary animal studies show that ferrite-enhanced MR images also fail to detect the diffuse lymphomatous liver involvement.[227]

HEPATOBLASTOMA

Hepatoblastomas are encountered during the first 5 years of life and usually are asymptomatic except for a palpable abdominal mass. The CT features of this mass are similar to those of hepatoma, except that up to 50 per cent of these lesions may demonstrate amorphous calcifications.[228, 229] The lesions are often large, appearing hypodense or isodense on noncontrast CT and hypodense to normal liver parenchyma on contrast-enhanced images.[228, 229] CT has been shown to be helpful in assessing the extent of tumor when planning surgical resection,[228, 230] as well as evaluating the response to nonoperative therapy.

RARE MISCELLANEOUS TUMORS

Angiosarcoma (also known as hemangioendothelial sarcoma, hemangiosarcoma, or Kupffer cell sarcoma) originates in the vascular endothelium and

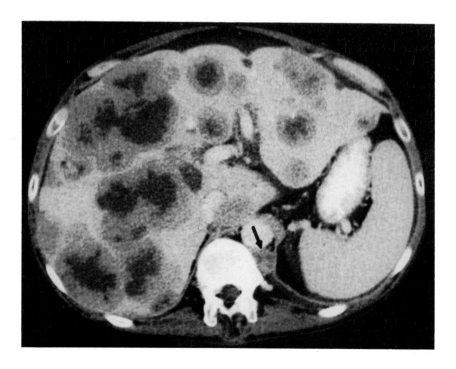

FIGURE 17–69 ■ Non-Hodgkin's lymphoma. Contrast-enhanced CT scan shows multifocal involvement by numerous low-attenuation lesions. Centrally, lower attenuation resulting from necrosis is present. Retrocrural adenopathy is also present (arrow). This appearance of the liver is unusual for lymphoma but is often seen in immunosuppressed patients following organ transplantation (posttransplant lymphoproliferative disorder).

may arise in a number of organs.[231] It has been reported to have been induced by therapeutic radiation, chemotherapy, exposure to vinyl chloride, arsenic, and thorotrast.[232–234] The lesion may present as a solitary nodule, but most often is multinodular or infiltrating extensively through the liver. On noncontrast CT the lesions appear as hypodense masses without other characterizing features, although if thorotrast exposure has been present, the increased attenuation of the liver may be a clue to the diagnosis.[235] Because of a propensity to hemorrhage, regions of the tumor may appear of high attenuation if fresh and of lower attenuation if older.[236] As a result of its vascular nature, there is extensive contrast enhancement in a heterogeneous fashion.[237]

Undifferentiated embryonal sarcoma is the malignant counterpart to the mesenchymal hamartoma. It occurs predominantly in young children and adults ranging from 3 to 27 years of age.[238] The CT spectrum, like that in the mesenchymal hamartoma, ranges from a predominantly solid tumor with small cystic changes to a predominantly cystic mass (near-water attenuation) with septations of varying thickness.[238]

Secondary Malignant Tumors (Metastases)

Metastases are the most common malignant tumors of the liver. Metastases have varied appearances, none of which are diagnostic; when such a lesion is detected on CT or MR, the diagnosis is usually made based on the clinical presentation of the patient in conjunction with the imaging findings in the liver and elsewhere. Many physicians are under the mistaken impression that biochemical liver function tests, rather than imaging tests such as CT or MR, can be used as a preliminary screen for metastatic disease. One recent study showed that one third of all patients with proven liver metastases had normal liver function tests.[239] The spectrum of imaging appearances of metastases can overlap that of primary malignant lesions, as well as benign lesions such as hemangiomas, abscess, and benign neoplasms. Definitive diagnosis requires a biopsy, which can usually be easily performed under ultrasound or CT guidance.

Computed Tomography ■ The accuracy of CT in detecting metastases varies with the techniques utilized and underlying primary disease. Dynamic incremental bolus contrast-enhanced scanning is accepted as the optimal routine CT technique for evaluating the liver.[30, 37, 38, 42, 240] Sensitivities for detecting patients with liver metastases using this technique have been reported to be between 72.5 and 100 per cent.[25, 241–246] Carefully performed studies with surgical correlation have shown that optimally performed screening CT detects 80 to 90 per cent of patients with liver metastatic disease, a figure comparable to the reported MR sensitivity.[245, 246] Accuracy in detecting the specific lesion number, however, is far less for both CT and MR. This information is essential prior to consideration of surgical resection of isolated lesions. Studies in patients following liver resection have

afforded an excellent opportunity to compare preoperative imaging tests with complete pathologic evaluation, thereby rendering a true evaluation of CT and MR accuracies.[41, 45] Dynamic incremental bolus CT detected only 38 per cent of lesions in one series,[41] failing to detect all lesions less than 1 cm in size and most lesions less than 2 cm. In contrast, MRI (combining a variety of pulse sequences) detected 52 per cent of lesions. In similar studies with pathologic confirmation,[41, 45] delayed high-dose CT has been shown to detect 52 to 73 per cent of lesions when used in conjunction with dynamic contrast-enhanced or angiography-assisted CT, and angiography-assisted CT had sensitivities of 82 to 87 per cent. Extensive research into lipid-soluble contrast agents has shown ethiodized oil emulsions (most recently EOE-13) to be more sensitive than dynamic contrast-enhanced liver CT in detecting metastatic lesions,[247–249] equalling the sensitivity of delay high-dose CT and angiography-assisted CT.[44] However, because of contrast reactions and production difficulties, this agent remains experimental.[32, 44]

The CT appearance of metastatic lesions generally correlates with the degree of tumor vascularity. On non–contrast-enhanced CT, most lesions appear as either hypodense or isodense with adjacent parenchyma, unless fresh hemorrhage or calcification is present, which can increase the attenuation (Fig. 17–70). Calcifications are seen most often with metastases from mucinous colon carcinomas and can also be seen with ovarian, breast, lung, renal, and thyroid primaries.[250–253] The patterns of calcification can vary, and no features exist to differentiate among histologic types of lesions, (e.g., hepatoma and benign liver tumors such as adenoma and focal nodular hyperplasia).[250]

The margins of the lesions vary from sharp and well defined to ill defined and infiltrating. Many metastases show peripheral enhancement around a hypodense lesion (Fig. 17–71), which can be confused with an hemangioma. The presence of a fatty liver can obscure metastases on either noncontrast or contrast-enhanced images.

Most metastatic lesions are hypovascular and thus appear hypodense to adjacent enhanced liver parenchyma. Central low attenuation may be marked, either because of central necrosis or as a result of cystic changes in lesions, and can simulate a cyst[136, 137, 140] in some instances (see Fig. 17–39). Large tumors and sarcomas have a propensity to undergo necrosis,[254] and cystic primaries such as ovarian or pancreatic cystic malignancies typically develop cystic metastases in the liver. Even in these situations, however, typical characteristics (such as a thick or nodular wall, internal heterogeneity, or attenuation values greater than water) are present and lead to the diagnosis of a potentially malignant liver lesion (see Fig. 17–39). Ultrasound can be helpful in confirming the nature of such questionable liver lesions.[140]

In tumors with increased vascularity, some metastases may not be well demonstrated with contrast

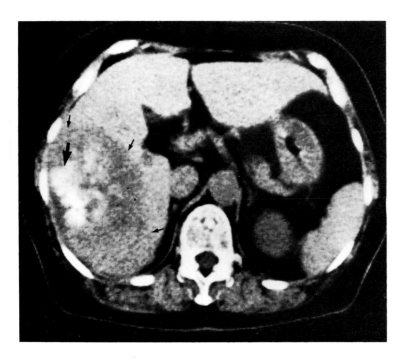

FIGURE 17–70 ■ Mucinous colon carcinoma metastatic to the liver. Noncontrast CT scan shows the calcified portion of the metastasis *(large arrow)* surrounded by a larger noncalcified zone of tumor *(small arrows)*.

CT, as they rapidly become isodense with normal liver (Figs. 17–12 and 17–72). Bressler et al.[47] reported that 37 per cent of liver metastases were not identified on dynamic contrast-enhanced images but were seen on noncontrast images in patients with vascular primary tumors, including renal cell carcinoma, pheochromocytoma, and islet cell tumors. Other vascular tumors we have seen with this propensity include breast carcinoma (see Fig. 17–72), melanoma, and sarcoma (see Fig. 17–12). Depending on the rate of contrast administration and time of scanning, vascular lesions may appear to be of greater attenuation than liver parenchyma, approximating the attenuation of hepatic vessels and similar in appearance to hemangiomas (Fig. 17–73). Vascular metastases, however, become homogeneously enhanced only during the early phase of contrast administration, whereas hemangiomas generally require at least 3 minutes[144] to completely fill in.

The presence of diffuse fatty infiltration can give the appearance of a homogeneously enhancing lesion in the liver that would otherwise be isodense or even hypodense to liver parenchyma (Fig. 17–74). Realizing the presence of fatty infiltration is the key to the proper diagnosis.

Occasionally the location of liver lesions can aid in diagnosing or characterizing liver metastases. Metastases distributed via peritoneal spread (most often seen with ovarian carcinoma) typically are found in a peripheral distribution or initially may be seen as

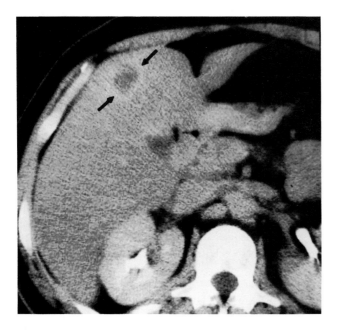

FIGURE 17–71 ■ Metastasis (colon primary). Contrast-enhanced CT scan shows the lesion as predominantly hypodense to liver parenchyma, with a thin hyperdense enhancing margin *(arrows)*.

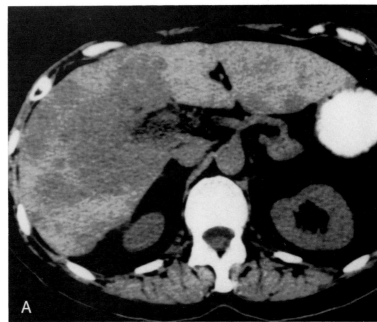
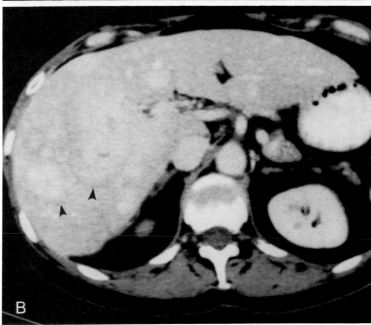

FIGURE 17–72 ■ Metastases (breast primary). *A,* Non-contrast CT scan shows numerous low-attenuation metastases throughout the liver. *B,* Contrast CT scan shows many of the lesions enhancing to a greater degree than liver parenchyma. Some are homogeneously increased in attenuation, and others are surrounded by a thin rim of low attenuation *(arrowheads).* Many lesions well seen in *A* are isodense with liver parenchyma following contrast and are not seen in *B.*

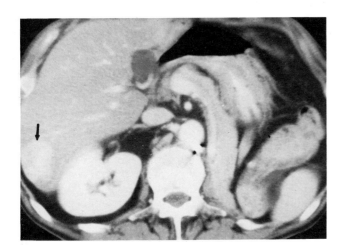

FIGURE 17–73 ■ Metastasis (kidney primary). The metastasis shows intense diffuse enhancement greater than that of adjacent liver parenchyma *(arrow)* during this early dynamic image.

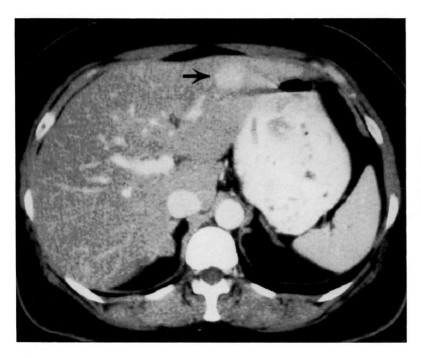

FIGURE 17–74 ■ Metastasis *(arrow)* has the appearance of a hypervascular lesion as it enhances throughout to a greater degree than adjacent liver parenchyma. The liver parenchyma, however, is diffusely low in attenuation because of fatty infiltration. The enhancing lesion is less dense than the spleen and, if not for the fatty liver, would be isodense or hypodense with liver parenchyma.

liver surface irregularity as a result of metastases studding the liver surface (Fig. 17–75).

Magnetic Resonance Imaging ■ Compared with incremental-bolus dynamic CT, MR has been found to be as accurate or more accurate in detecting liver metastases.[41, 45, 96, 245–247] As discussed fully in the techniques section, optimizing detection of metastatic lesions varies with the field strength and pulse sequences utilized. Techniques for screening for liver metastases, therefore, must be tailored to the equipment being used.

Because of the longer T1 and T2 relaxation times compared with normal liver parenchyma, most metastatic lesions appear darker than liver on T1-weighted images and brighter than liver on T2-weighted images. Whereas T1-weighted images have been reported in some instances to have a higher detection rate of metastases, there is no controversy over the necessity of T2-weighted images to characterize liver lesions. Unlike benign liver cysts and most hemangiomas (which are homogeneous, well circumscribed, and extremely bright on T2-weighted images), most metastatic lesions exhibit a heterogeneous appearance and are of lesser signal intensity (Figs. 17–17, 17–18, and 17–75 through 17–77). However, nine per cent of metastases can have a homogeneous bright appearance similar to that of benign cysts and hemangiomas; these are generally the vascular lesions such as islet cell tumors, carcinoid, and sarcomas.[72] On T2-weighted images metastatic lesions more typically appear as one of three patterns: amorphous, target, or halo (Figs. 17–17, 17–18, and 17–75 through 17–77).[72] The target pattern (see Fig. 17–76) is one of central high intensity (often because of necrosis with liquefaction) surrounded by areas of lesser signal intensity than centrally, but still greater than that of normal liver. The halo appearance is a

mass with the highest signal intensity seen peripherally (see Fig. 17–77), which may be because of surrounding edema. The amorphous pattern represents a heterogeneous mass of variable increased signal intensity, usually with indistinct margins.

Inflammatory Masses

Pyogenic Abscess

COMPUTED TOMOGRAPHY

Patients with a pyogenic liver abscess usually present with fever and abdominal pain, occasionally hepatomegaly, and rarely jaundice. CT is highly sensitive in diagnosing pyogenic liver abscesses, with two large series reporting 95 to 98 per cent sensitivity.[255, 256] Hepatic abscesses are readily detected on CT as low-density masses with attenuation values hypodense with either nonenhanced or enhanced liver parenchyma (Figs. 17–78 and 17–79). Attenuation values for these lesions range from near-water density (2 H) to 36 H,[255] thus overlapping the appearances of cysts and hypodense neoplasms. This variance reflects the varying contents within abscesses, ranging from thin fluid to thick, viscous material. The presence of gas collections (see Fig. 17–78) is most helpful in suggesting the diagnosis, but this finding is only present in approximately 20 per cent of cases.[255, 256] Usually gas is seen as small air bubbles but may appear as an air-fluid level. Large air-fluid levels suggest communication with the gastrointestinal tract.[257] The central appearance of abscesses may be unilocular (see Fig. 17–78) or multilocular (see Fig. 17–79). The multilocular components are often in free communication and thus should not deter percutaneous drainage. Bernardino

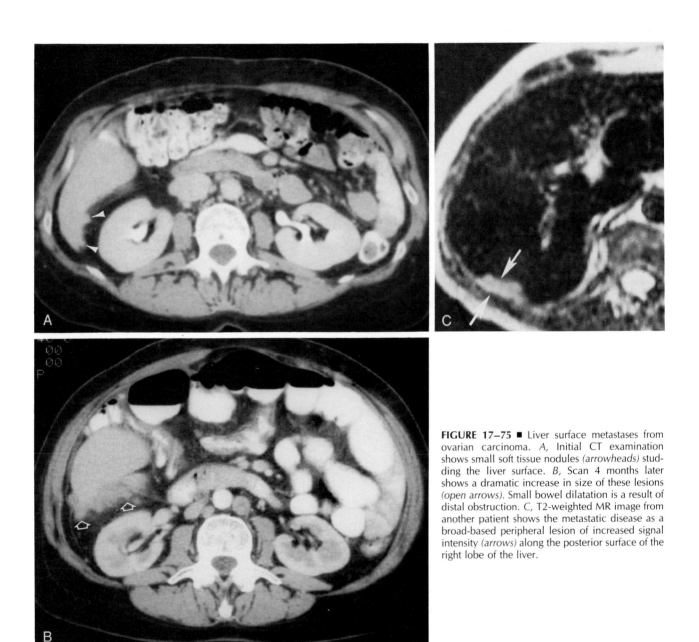

FIGURE 17–75 ■ Liver surface metastases from ovarian carcinoma. *A,* Initial CT examination shows small soft tissue nodules *(arrowheads)* studding the liver surface. *B,* Scan 4 months later shows a dramatic increase in size of these lesions *(open arrows).* Small bowel dilatation is a result of distal obstruction. *C,* T2-weighted MR image from another patient shows the metastatic disease as a broad-based peripheral lesion of increased signal intensity *(arrows)* along the posterior surface of the right lobe of the liver.

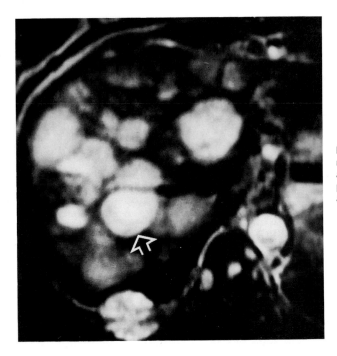

FIGURE 17–76 ■ Metastases (melanoma primary). STIR image shows numerous metastatic foci in the liver and abdominal wall as areas of amorphous increased signal intensity. In one lesion, a typical target pattern is seen *(arrow)*, with a central region of very high signal intensity and lesser peripheral signal intensity.

FIGURE 17–77 ■ Hepatocellular carcinoma with a halo appearance on MRI. A large right lobe tumor *(open arrow)* has a heterogeneous signal intensity pattern, predominantly slightly greater than that of normal liver. A surrounding zone of higher signal intensity *(solid arrows)* is present because of edema.

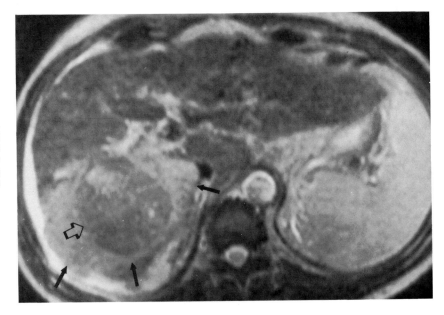

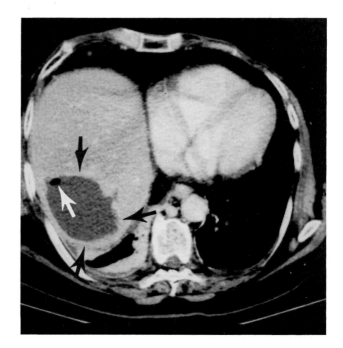

FIGURE 17–78 ■ Pyogenic liver abscess. Contrast CT scan shows the abscess as a low-attenuation (near water) collection with an enhancing rim *(black arrows)*. Air *(white arrow)* within the collection is characteristic of infected collections.

et al.[258] reported successful percutaneous drainage in 11 of 13 multiloculated hepatic abscesses. Similarly, Jaques et al.[257] reported no correlation between CT appearance of abdominal abscesses and eventual outcome at percutaneous drainage. Of abdominal abscesses in this series, the hepatic abscesses had the highest cure rate, with success occurring in multilocular- and unilocular-appearing collections in 86 per cent of cases.

Although the peripheral margin of abscesses may demonstrate an increase in attenuation following intravenous contrast administration (see Fig. 17–78), central portions do not.[255, 256] This peripheral rim of enhancement may be greater than that of adjacent normal parenchyma, creating a ringed appearance on contrast-enhanced CT seen in 6 to 22 per cent of cases.[255, 256]

With the exception of the presence of central gas collections, the varied appearances of abscesses are not diagnostic, and the abscesses require aspiration for diagnosis. If the diagnosis is confirmed, CT-guided percutaneous drainage is therapeutic in 86 to 92 per cent of cases.[257, 258]

MAGNETIC RESONANCE IMAGING

There have been few MR investigations into the appearance of pyogenic liver abscesses. Hepatic pyogenic abscesses have an MR appearance similar to that of cysts, although the central signal intensity may vary with varying central contents.[172]

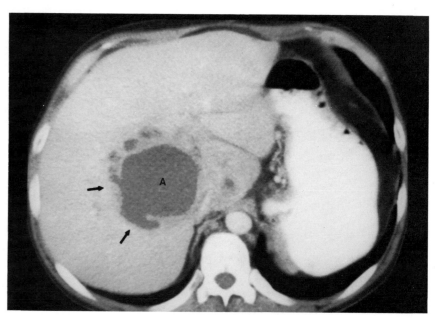

FIGURE 17–79 ■ Pyogenic liver abscess. The abscess (A) appears as a near-water-attenuation mass with a cluster of smaller adjacent lesions around the periphery. This cluster of lesions is typical of early pyogenic abscesses. A faint hyperemic rim *(arrow)* is seen.

Fungal Abscess

Fungal infections of the liver occur in immunocompromised patients, usually with underlying hematologic malignancies.[259–261] The most common agent is *Candida*, followed by *Aspergillus*.[259, 260] The typical CT appearance is that of numerous small, round, low-density lesions scattered throughout the liver and splenic parenchyma (Fig. 17–80). Faint peripheral contrast enhancement may be seen in some lesions,[259, 261] although the majority of lesions do not show enhancement. Rarely, small central densities can be identified within the lesions thought to represent hyphae.[261] To optimize detection sensitivity, both non- and postcontrast images are required, as not all lesions are best seen with any one technique.[261] Although no large series have studied the sensitivity of ultrasound and CT in detecting these lesions, small series have shown that both examinations can fail to diagnose biopsy-proven disease, and when strong clinical suspicion of disease exists, laparoscopy or laparotomy should be performed so that a histologic diagnosis may be made.[261]

The CT appearance of these lesions is not specific and can be simulated by metastatic disease and bacterial abscesses. Most often, hepatic biopsy is required for confirmation of the diagnosis prior to initiation of antifungal therapy.

CT can be used to evaluate patient response to therapy. Successful treatment usually results in a decrease in number and size of the visualized lesions, with eventual clearing of the CT abnormality.[259, 260] The persistence of the liver lesions, however, does not preclude successful sterilization, as granulomas and focal areas of necrosis can be seen in the healing phase without persisting infection.[259]

Hydatid Disease

Hydatid disease is caused by the larval stage of either *Echinococcus granulosus* or *Echinococcus alveolaris*. Infection by *E. granulosus* is more common and is prevalent in Australia, New Zealand, southern Europe, North Africa, South America, and the Near and Middle East. *E. alveolaris* infection is found in central Europe, Russia, Alaska, Japan, and the United States. In both forms, the liver is the most frequently involved organ.[262]

E. granulosus produces well-defined cysts that may appear on CT as uni- or multilocular with thin or thick walls (Figs. 17–81 and 17–82).[87, 262, 263] Calcifications may occur either peripherally or centrally within septations (see Fig. 17–82). The wall of the cysts, even when not calcified, may demonstrate marked contrast enhancement and appear of higher attenuation.[87, 264] Daughter cysts can be seen within the interior of the larger cyst as smaller cysts with septations (see Fig. 17–82), usually oriented in the periphery of the lesion. The daughter cysts usually are of lower attenuation than the mother cyst,[263] which may be helpful in recognizing the origin of these lesions. Daughter cysts can also be discharged from the germinal layer of the cyst wall and float freely within the lumen of the mother cyst. In this case, altering the patient position during scanning may show a change in position of internal vesicles in these cases, confirming the diagnosis of hydatid disease.[265] Infected cysts may demonstrate ill-defined margins, air within the lesions, or an increased central density,[87, 262] although these same findings can be seen in noninfected, ruptured cysts.

Following surgical treatment of these lesions, it can be difficult to differentiate recurrent disease from

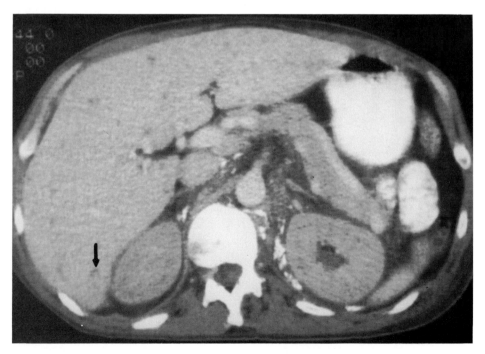

FIGURE 17–80 ■ Hepatic candidiasis. Contrast-enhanced CT scan shows the typical appearance of disseminated hepatic fungal infection as scattered, low-attenuation, rounded lesions. Central high-attenuation densities can be seen in some lesions (*arrow*). Retroperitoneal calcifications in regions of prior lymphoma following radiation therapy are also seen.

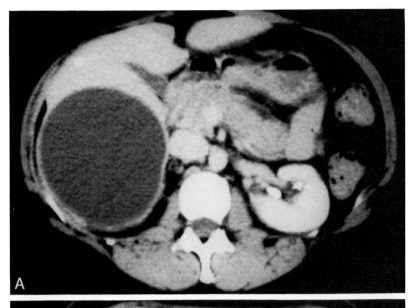

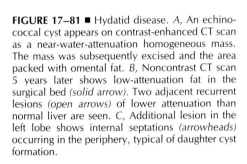

FIGURE 17–81 ■ Hydatid disease. *A,* An echino-coccal cyst appears on contrast-enhanced CT scan as a near-water-attenuation homogeneous mass. The mass was subsequently excised and the area packed with omental fat. *B,* Noncontrast CT scan 5 years later shows low-attenuation fat in the surgical bed *(solid arrow).* Two adjacent recurrent lesions *(open arrows)* of lower attenuation than normal liver are seen. *C,* Additional lesion in the left lobe shows internal septations *(arrowheads)* occurring in the periphery, typical of daughter cyst formation.

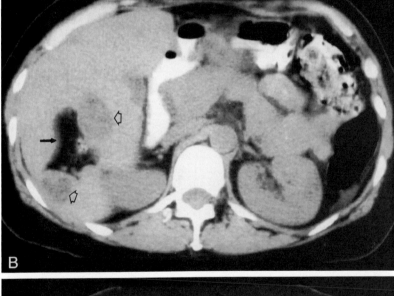

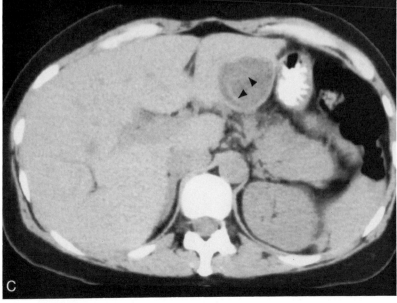

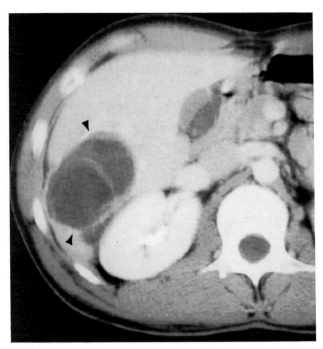

FIGURE 17–82 ■ Echinococcal cyst. The mass is predominantly of water attenuation and demonstrates internal septation and peripheral calcification (arrowheads).

appearance, with a signal intensity similar to that of other cysts; the lesions have low signal intensity on T1-weighted images and higher intensity on T2-weighted images. Unlike simple hepatic cysts, however, these lesions demonstrate a low-intensity rim on both T1- and T2-weighted images. This rim may be the result of the short T2 of the fibrous capsule (pericyst) typical of these lesions.[264, 267] Although this rim is seen in the majority of liver echinococcal cysts, low-intensity rims on both T1- and T2-weighted sequences can also be found in malignant hepatomas and other benign lesions such as adenoma.[73, 211]

The imaging appearance of hydatid disease due to *E. alveolaris* is different from that caused by *E. granulosus. E. alveolaris* produces geographic, infiltrating lesions without sharp margins or dense rims.[268, 269] The lesions have the appearance and attenuation values (14 to 40 H) of low-density, solid mass lesions rather than cysts, but they do not demonstrate contrast enhancement.[269] Calcification is amorphous or nodular, rather than ringlike, and the infection frequently extends directly to the abdominal wall, diaphragm, or porta hepatis. The CT appearance of hepatic *E. alveolaris* infection is not pathognomonic, as it closely resembles infiltrating malignant lesions.

Amebic Abscess

Amebic abscess, caused by the parasite *Entamoeba histolytica,* is endemic in tropical and subtropical climates and is present in the southern areas of the United States. The CT appearance of these lesions is variable and nonspecific.[270] Generally, well-defined round or oval low-attenuation lesions are seen. The central attenuation is usually slightly greater than water (10 to 20 H),[270] often accompanied by a peripheral rim of slightly higher attenuation on noncontrast

pseudocysts filling the removed space.[266] Because omentum may be packed in these areas surgically, the postoperative CT appearance may demonstrate masses with low attenuation similar to that of fat (see Fig. 17–81B)[266] The MR scan in such cases shows lesions of high signal intensity on T1-weighted images.[264]

The MR appearance of echinococcal cysts has been reported.[264, 267] The cyst component is nonspecific in

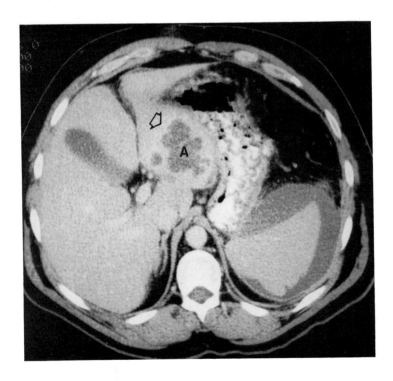

FIGURE 17–83 ■ Amebic liver abscess. Abscess (A) appears as a low-attenuation mass with a hyperemic rim (open arrow). The mass is multilocular with nodular margins.

examinations that can demonstrate marked contrast enhancement (Fig. 17–83). The lesion may appear unilocular or multilocular and may demonstrate nodularity of the margins.[270] Extrahepatic abnormalities may be present in complicated cases, including pleural effusions, perihepatic fluid collections, gastric or colonic involvement, and retroperitoneal extension.[270] Air seen centrally may be caused by pyogenic infection or hepatobronchial or hepatocolic fistula.[270]

MR appearances of amebic abscesses have been described.[271, 272] Although a variety of MRI patterns have been reported, no pattern of intensity or morphology is seen that could be considered specific for amebic abscess.[271, 272] Most abscesses appeared on MR as sharply defined round or oval lesions of low intensity on T1-weighted images and high intensity on T2-weighted images (Fig. 17–84). The T2-weighted images particularly demonstrate diffuse central heterogeneity.[271] One to three zones of varying signal intensity are often seen peripherally on both T1- and T2-weighted images, but they do not appear to demonstrate consistent intensity patterns.[271, 272]

Because of the large size of amebic lesions and the ease of visibility with CT, MR, and ultrasound, all three modalities are virtually 100 per cent sensitive in detecting such lesions in the liver.[271] Therefore ultrasound will probably remain the imaging method of choice in suspected amebic abscess.

Schistosomiasis

Schistosomiasis japonica is endemic to regions of the Far East, particularly China, Taiwan, and the Philippines. The adult worms of this parasite reside in the portal tributaries, and the eggs produced are carried through the portal vein to the liver. The pathologic changes take place mainly in the liver capsule and in the portal space, and the CT appearance reflects these changes. The CT appearance is

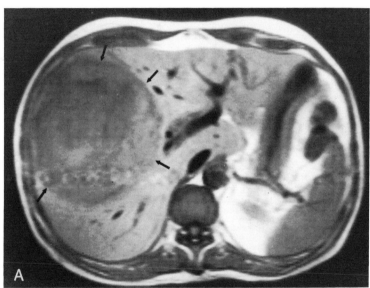

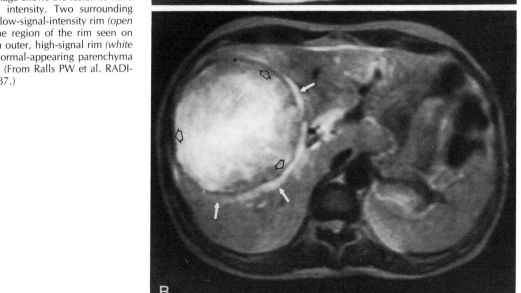

FIGURE 17–84 ■ MR imaging of an amebic liver abscess. *A,* T1-weighted image shows a large heterogeneous right lobe lesion hypointense to liver parenchyma. A peripheral rim of low signal intensity defines the margin of the lesion *(arrows). B,* T2-weighted image shows the lesion to have predominantly high signal intensity. Two surrounding rims are present: an inner, low-signal-intensity rim *(open arrow)* corresponding to the region of the rim seen on T2-weighted images and an outer, high-signal rim *(white arrows)* corresponding to normal-appearing parenchyma on the T1-weighted image. (From Ralls PW et al. RADIOLOGY 165:801–804, 1987.)

characterized by capsular calcification, as well as branching liver parenchymal calcifications along fibrous scars, creating a lattice appearance of calcification.[273, 274] Parenchymal fibrosis and shrinkage result in an increase in periportal fat, seen on CT as increased low-attenuation regions in the periportal regions.[273] Hepatocellular carcinoma is a known complication of this disease, and findings of such should be searched for on CT in all infected patients.[273]

Less commonly, schistosomiasis mansoni can produce significant liver infection.[273] The periportal fibrosis seen in this infection results in periportal low-attenuation regions on non–contrast-enhanced scans. Contrast-enhanced images can show either enhancement to the same degree as normal liver parenchyma or marked enhancement, which can simulate neoplastic disease.[275]

Other Infections

The CT findings in hepatic fascioliasis have been described[276, 277] as low-attenuation nodular and tortuous, sometimes branching, lesions, best seen on dynamic contrast-enhanced images. Their appearance is nonspecific and is similar to that of necrotic neoplasms or more common abscesses.[278] The MR appearance is also nonspecific, with poorly defined nodular areas of increased signal intensity on T2-weighted images.[277]

Vascular Diseases

Portal Vein Thrombosis

Thrombosis of the portal vein may be caused by neoplasm, infection, cirrhosis, trauma, hypercoagulable states, or hepatic venous obstruction.[210, 256, 279] In the acute phase, the vein is usually enlarged and appears on CT with an attenuation value equal to that of unopacified blood on noncontrast images; it does not undergo central enhancement with contrast (Fig. 17–85). Rarely, the thrombus may be of higher attenuation typical of freshly clotted blood.[256] The vessel wall may be thickened and demonstrate marked enhancement from a dilated vaso vasorum.[256] In cases of partial thrombosis, the thrombus appears as a filling defect surrounded by contrast in the open portions of the vessel.[280] There may be a segmental or focal decrease in hepatic enhancement to the segment or segments of the liver that are supplied by the occluded portal vein branches. Chronic portal vein thrombosis may show recanalization of portions of the thrombus or enlarged collateral venous channels adjacent to a shrunken, thrombosed portal vein, often termed *cavernous transformation of the portal vein* (Fig. 17–86).[256, 281] The course of the thrombus may be seen extending into the splenic or superior mesenteric vein.

MR has been shown to be an excellent tool in evaluating flow within vessels and particularly within the portal vein.[282–285] With spin-echo imaging, the presence of intraluminal signal within the portal vein, excluding such artifacts as entry slice phenomena and even-echo rephasing, is suggestive of portal vein thrombosis (Fig. 17–87), although slow flow within veins in patients with portal hypertension can cause intraluminal signal (see Fig. 17–64).[286] Levy and Newhouse[282] found no false-positive cases of portal vein thrombus when they used the following strict criteria: the thrombus signal (1) involved the entire width of the portal vein lumen; (2) was isointense or slightly hypointense to liver parenchyma with T1 weighting; and (3) exceeded the intensity of hepatic parenchyma on T2-weighted images that showed a flow void in the hepatic veins. Fresh thrombi may also appear as high-intensity signal on T1-weighted images.[285] In addition, the diagnosis of thrombosis can be suggested when extensive periportal collateral vessels are identified.[282, 286]

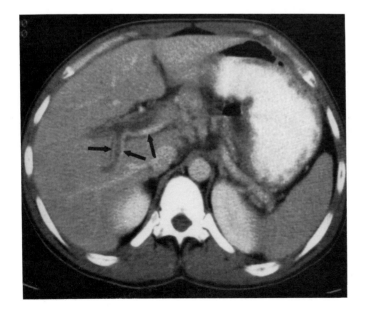

FIGURE 17–85 ■ Portal vein thrombosis in a patient with chronic pancreatitis. Contrast CT scan shows the central portal vein as low attenuation with peripheral tracking of contrast (arrows), creating a "train track" appearance.

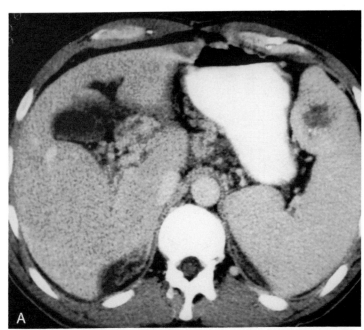

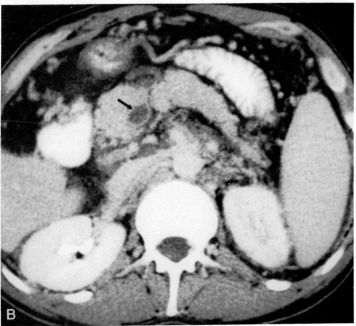

FIGURE 17–86 ■ Chronic portal vein thrombosis with collateral veins. *A*, Contrast-enhanced CT scan fails to identify a single large portal vein but demonstrates numerous small contrast-enhancing collateral vessels in the porta hepatis. *B*, Chronic thrombus extends retrograde back into the superior mesenteric vein *(arrow)*, which does not enhance and instead appears as a low-attenuation structure.

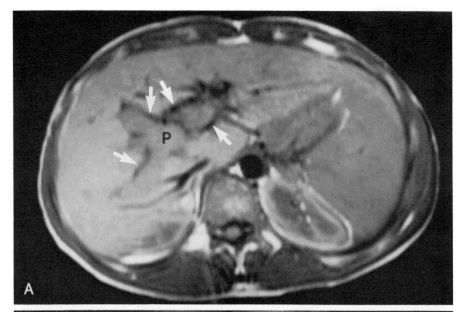

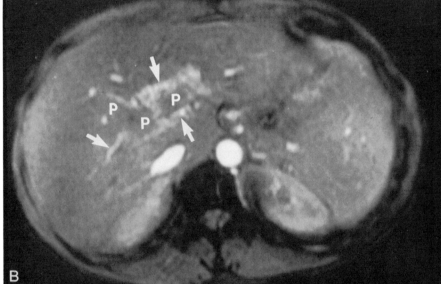

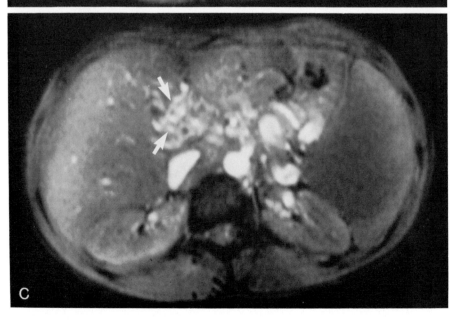

FIGURE 17–87 ■ Portal vein thrombosis in a patient with hepatocellular carcinoma (same patient as in Figure 17–66). *A,* T1-weighted spin-echo image shows increased signal diffusely within the portal vein branches (P), with signal void seen in numerous adjacent collaterals *(arrows).* *B* and *C,* GRASS MR images show absence of flow in the portal vein (P) and numerous collateral vessels appearing as small high-intensity foci *(arrows).*

Quantitative measurements of portal blood flow are possible using MR and correlate well with findings at Doppler ultrasound.[283, 284] In patients in whom Doppler ultrasound cannot be performed, MR measurements may offer a useful noninvasive alternative.

Hepatic Venous Occlusion Disease (Budd-Chiari Syndrome)

The Budd-Chiari syndrome is a rare clinical entity of obstruction of hepatic venous outflow and is associated with hypercoagulopathy states, oral contraceptives, pregnancy, invading tumors, and congenital webs.[287] The level of occlusion may occur at the intrahepatic venules, the hepatic veins, or the inferior vena cava.

COMPUTED TOMOGRAPHY

Hepatomegaly and ascites are seen in nearly all patients,[279, 288] with enlargement of the caudate lobe being a particular feature in chronic cases. Mathieu et al.[288] reported diffuse hepatomegaly in the acute phase and described lobar atrophic changes with contralateral hypertrophy in some patients with chronic disease.

Regional attenuation differences throughout the liver characterize this abnormality.[279, 288] Noncontrast CT typically demonstrates peripheral low attenuation of the liver, with higher attenuation seen in the caudate lobe and central portions of the left lobe. Early dynamic contrast-enhanced images demonstrate patchy enhancement centrally with less enhancement noted peripherally (Fig. 17–88). Later equilibrium images may show a reversal of this pattern, with a delayed increase in attenuation peripherally, or they may show persistence of the patchy central enhancement, with progression toward the periphery.

The hepatic veins are usually not visualized, although in some cases thrombus may be seen within these veins, which appear as radiating, linear low-density structures (Fig. 17–89), occasionally with peripheral enhancement.[279, 288] Thrombus can also be seen in the inferior vena cava. In the acute stage, the thrombi may be of higher attenuation and clearly visible on noncontrast CT images.[289] Associated thrombi may be found in the portal circulation, and hepatic venous occlusion should be considered as a cause of portal thrombosis.[279]

Other associated findings include narrowing of the inferior vena cava and dilated collateral veins (azygous, hemiazygous, or subcutaneous).[290]

MAGNETIC RESONANCE IMAGING

Morphologic changes of the liver and associated vessels similar to those seen on CT are demonstrated at MR and include diffuse hepatomegaly and ascites, reduction in caliber or absence of visualization of the hepatic veins (Fig. 17–90), and marked narrowing of the intrahepatic inferior vena cava (Fig. 17–91).[291] With its excellent vascular depiction, MR may demonstrate intrahepatic collateral veins, which appear as comma-shaped signal voids on spin-echo images,[291] and vascular webs in the inferior vena cava.

Liver Infarction

Because of the dual blood supply to the liver, hepatic infarctions caused by hepatic artery occlusion are rare. Hepatic arterial occlusion may be caused by atherosclerosis, embolism, thrombosis, vasculitis, or hypotension/shock. Rarely, hepatic arterial thrombosis occurs following pregnancy or oral contraceptive use.[292, 293]

The CT appearance of infarcts may take on several appearances. Like infarcts in the spleen and kidney, the lesions have been reported as peripheral, wedge-shaped, low-attenuation lesions on contrast-enhanced images.[293] Rarely, the infarct may involve an entire lobe, resulting in diffuse low attenuation

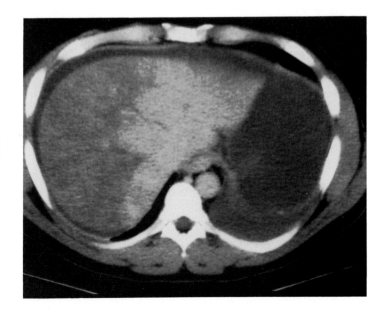

FIGURE 17–88 ■ Budd-Chiari syndrome. In the typical early dynamic contrast-enhanced image, the greatest enhancement is seen centrally, with lesser, patchy enhancement peripherally.

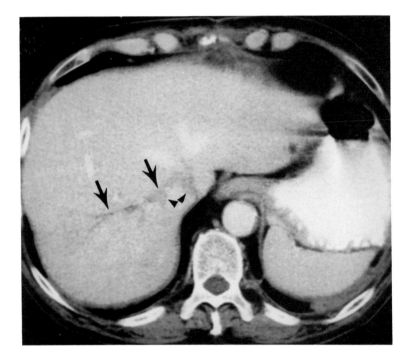

FIGURE 17–89 ■ Hepatic vein thrombosis in a patient with extensive renal cell carcinoma. Tumoral extension into the inferior vena cava *(arrowheads)* has occluded the drainage of the right hepatic vein, with subsequent thrombosis *(arrows)*. The thrombosed vein appears as a linear, branching, low-attenuation structure on the contrast-enhanced CT scan. The middle and left hepatic veins enhance normally. The affected right posterior hepatic segment shows a mottled contrast enhancement pattern.

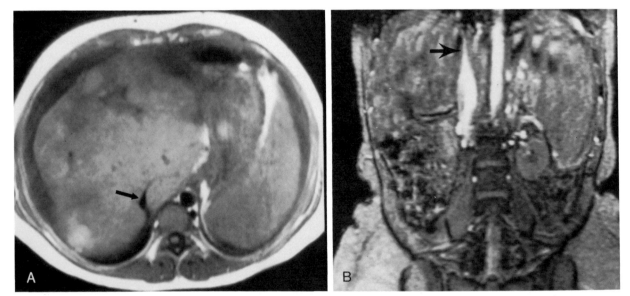

FIGURE 17–90 ■ Budd-Chiari syndrome. *A,* T1-weighted MR image shows narrowing of the inferior vena cava *(arrow)*. No hepatic veins were identified at any level. *B,* Coronal GRASS image demonstrates the marked narrowing of the intrahepatic inferior vena cava *(arrow)*.

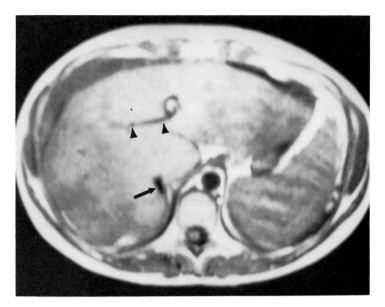

FIGURE 17–91 ■ Budd-Chiari syndrome. *A,* T1-weighted MR image shows narrowing of the inferior vena cava *(arrow).* A collateral intrahepatic vein is seen *(arrowheads).*

throughout the lobe (Fig. 17–92). In contrast, Lev-Toaff et al. reported the majority of liver infarcts to be round and central in location (see Fig. 17–92).[294] Liver infarct appearances evolve over time, initially being poorly marginated and then becoming more discrete, with sharp margins and having lower attenuation.[294] Subsequent necrosis may result in air collections centrally without infection present (see Fig. 17–92).[294] Chronic findings include atrophy of the involved liver segment with residual hypodense areas and cystic changes (Fig. 17–93).[292, 294, 295] The cystic areas have been shown to be caused by bile

duct cyst formation from the necrosis of bile duct epithelium and subsequent bile extravasation.[295]

Passive Hepatic Congestion

Passive hepatic congestion is a constellation of clinical and pathologic findings resulting from congestive heart failure or constrictive pericarditis.[234, 296] Elevated central venous pressure is transmitted back to the hepatic venous system, resulting in centrilobular congestion with subsequent hepatic enlargement and dysfunction. Patients present with hepatomegaly

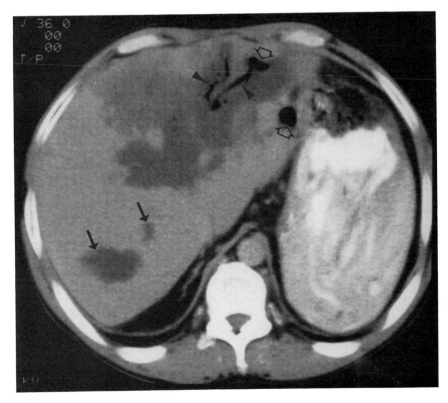

FIGURE 17–92 ■ Hepatic artery thrombosis and liver infarct 1 year following liver transplantation. Diffuse low-attenuation changes are seen throughout the left lobe of the liver as a result of parenchymal infarction. Despite the presence of parenchymal air collections *(open arrows)* that communicate with the biliary tree *(arrowheads),* no infection was present. In the right lobe of the liver, regions of infarction appear as central, round areas of decreased attenuation *(solid arrows).*

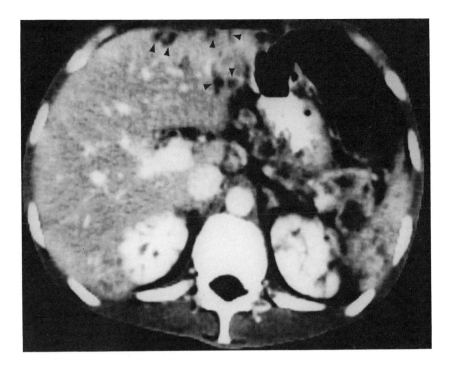

FIGURE 17–93 ■ Liver infarcts secondary to vasculitis (polyarteritis nodosa). Numerous areas of focal infarction are seen in the periphery of the left lobe, appearing as irregular-shaped foci of low attenuation without contrast enhancement *(arrowheads)*. In this patient with chronic changes, these are cystic lesions representing bile lake formation. Other areas of infarction and chronic changes are seen in the spleen, kidneys, and pancreas.

and liver tenderness. This elevation of venous pressure can result on CT in a patchy, inhomogeneous pattern of liver parenchymal contrast enhancement during early scans, which with delay images become isodense throughout (Fig. 17–94).[297, 298] Circumferential low-attenuation edema surrounding portal vessels can be seen in some cases.[299] Other accompanying CT findings include prominent size of the inferior vena cava and hepatic veins, often with retrograde hepatic venous opacification prior to the parenchymal enhancement seen during early dynamic images.[297, 298] The prominence of the inferior vena cava and hepatic veins in this condition can help differentiate these patients from those with hepatic venous occlusive disease (Budd-Chiari syndrome), which has a similar patchy parenchymal enhancement pattern but with nonvisualized hepatic veins and an attenuated inferior vena cava size.

Trauma

Traumatic injuries to the liver can occur as the result of blunt or penetrating abdominal trauma and as complications of surgery, percutaneous cholangiography, biopsy, or biliary drainage procedures. Injuries include capsular tears, parenchymal lacerations or contusions, intrahepatic and subcapsular hematomas, parenchymal avulsions, parenchymal infarction, bile pseudocyst, pseudoaneurysm, arteriovenous and arterioportal fistula, and intraperitoneal hemorrhage. Mortality in patients with major liver trauma ranges from 7 to 26 per cent,[300, 301] but is less if only isolated liver abnormalities are present.[302, 303] Prior to the availability of CT, surgical intervention was the treatment of choice for liver

trauma, determined by the patient's clinical status and by peritoneal lavage detecting evidence of hemorrhage. More recently, CT has become widely accepted as a useful method of diagnosing significant hepatobiliary trauma and provides an excellent tool for following and guiding the management of these patients,[304–309] decreasing the incidence of angiography and nontherapeutic, exploratory laparotomy in hemodynamically stable patients.[304, 306, 307] The necessity for surgery does not appear to correlate with the severity of findings on CT, but instead depends on the hemodynamic status of the patient. Mirvis et al.[307] reported that none of the grade 4 liver injury patients in their series who were hemodynamically stable required surgery. Nonoperative, conservative management of these patients requires constant patient monitoring and serial CT examinations demonstrating clearing or significant reduction in size of liver lesions and associated hemoperitoneum.[304, 306, 307]

Computed Tomography

Lacerations of the liver appear as linear or branching, poorly demarcated lesions that may be isolated or contiguous with areas of contusion or hematoma and often extend to the periphery of the liver (Figs. 17–95 and 17–96). These lesions usually are of lower attenuation than adjacent parenchyma, although acute blood clot can be of higher attenuation (see Fig. 17–96). Blunt trauma may produce a stellate or radiating laceration pattern.[307] These lesions show a typical evolutionary pattern, with sharper demarcation of the margins and decreased attenuation at 1 week and demonstrating a decreasing width and margins at 2 to 3 weeks, then becoming indistinct.[306]

Hematomas can appear as single or multifocal

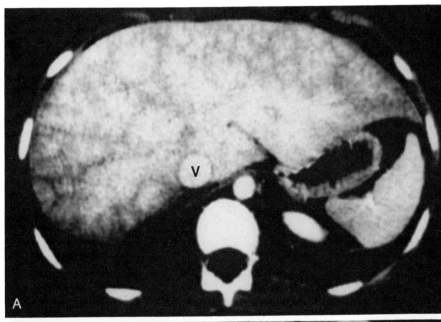

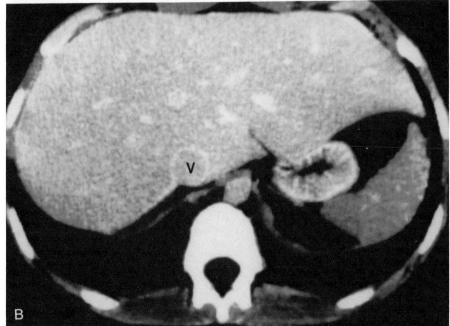

FIGURE 17–94 ■ Vascular hepatic congestion. *A,* Early dynamic contrast-enhanced image shows a mottled enhancement pattern within the hepatic parenchyma, with greatest enhancement seen centrally and less peripherally. *B,* Scan at the same level 20 minutes later shows a homogeneous parenchymal enhancement pattern. Note the large size of the inferior vena cava (V), a helpful feature in differentiating this appearance from that seen in hepatic venous occlusive disease.

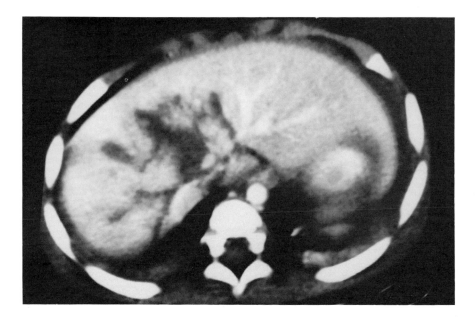

FIGURE 17–95 ■ Acute stellate liver fracture following a motor vehicle accident. Contrast-enhanced CT scan shows typical radiating low-attenuation collections of fluid and blood within areas of liver laceration.

FIGURE 17–96 ■ Liver laceration and subcapsular hematoma following penetrating trauma. *A,* Liver laceration is seen as an expanding linear collection of high-attenuation blood *(solid arrows)* with an adjacent subcapsular collection *(open arrows)* comprised of high-attenuation blood and lower attenuation fluid. *B,* A more cephalic scan shows the more typical elliptical configuration *(arrows)* of the subcapsular hematoma.

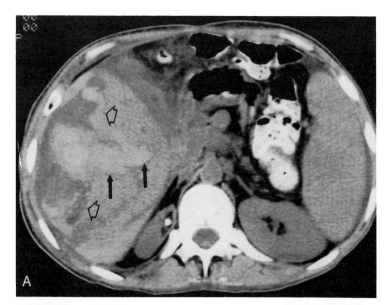

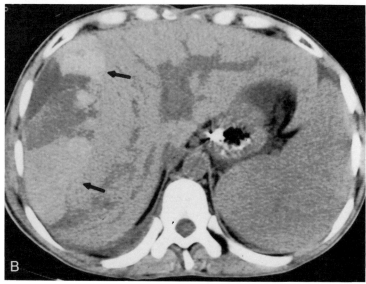

lesions within the liver parenchyma or in a subcapsular location. Subcapsular hematomas usually appear as crescent-shaped or lenticular, well-marginated collections located just beneath the hepatic capsule (see Fig. 17–96). The density of the collection depends on the age of the hematoma, being of higher attenuation than non–contrast-enhanced liver early when clotted blood is present and decreasing in attenuation over time to low attenuation.[310] Most hematomas appear hypodense when compared with contrast-enhanced liver parenchyma, although freshly clotted blood usually remains hyperdense with enhanced liver parenchyma.[311] The value of non–contrast-enhanced images in detecting subtle hematomas remains somewhat controversial. Mirvis and Whitley[311] and Federle[312] suggest that the detection yield is not significantly increased with noncontrast images, whereas Kelly et al.[313] increased their sensitivity and accuracy in detecting visceral injuries by adding noncontrast images.

Parenchymal hematomas also show typical changes over time.[306, 307, 310] Initially they appear with central high attenuation because of clotted blood surrounded by regions of lower attenuation from liquid blood, edema, and contused and necrotic liver. As the central clot lyses, the attenuation decreases until it becomes similar to other fluid collections such as bilomas (Fig. 17–97). Hepatic contusions appear as ill-defined areas of lower attenuation than surrounding parenchyma because of a combination of edematous liver, hemorrhage, necrosis, and extravasated bile.[311] Areas of fragmentation of the liver or infarcted portions of the liver appear as irregular or wedge-shaped areas that do not enhance with contrast administration.

Periportal lymphedema can be seen in liver trauma caused by obstruction of lymphatics and appears as circumferential hypodensity around portal vessels

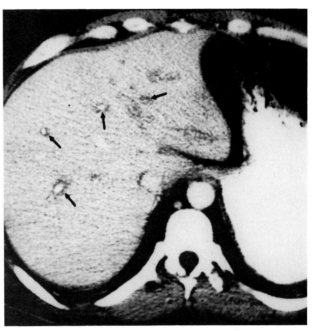

FIGURE 17–98 ■ Periportal edema following blunt trauma. Contrast-enhanced CT scan shows periportal edema *(arrows)* as circumferential low-attenuation collections surrounding the portal venous radicals. Following trauma this can be caused by lymphedema or by blood tracking along the portal vessels.

(Fig. 17–98).[299] This same appearance can be seen secondary to blood tracking along the portal vessels.

Bile pseudocysts, or bilomas, represent a loculated collection of bile, usually occurring within or immediately adjacent to the liver. Most often occurring following penetrating injuries or surgery, they may be seen with blunt trauma as well and may take days to weeks to become clinically evident.[314] They appear as low-attenuation collections, with an appearance similar to that of hematoma, abscess, or extrapancreatic pseudocyst.[311, 315] Confirmation requires aspiration or demonstration of biliary communication by cholangiography or cholescintigraphy. Although they may have nonspecific attenuation values on CT, the sonographic appearance usually is anechoic with enhanced through-sound transmission, an uncommon finding in hematomas or abscesses. The MR appearance is similar to that of other cysts, with a sharply defined, low-intensity mass on T1-weighted images and a very high-intensity mass on T2-weighted images (Fig. 17–99).

Traumatic liver lesions can become infected and develop into an abscess. There are no characteristic CT features that allow the differentiation of abscess from evolving liver hematoma.[305] Although the presence of air within such lesions may suggest abscess,[305] hepatic parenchymal gas has been reported without abscess following blunt trauma.[316]

Hepatic artery pseudoaneurysm[317] and arterioportal fistulae[318–320] are potential sequelae of hepatic vascular injury. The CT diagnosis of a traumatic pseudoaneurysm may be made by identifying a mass that markedly enhances after a bolus injection of contrast

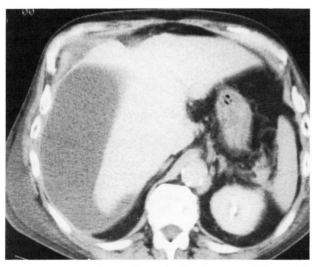

FIGURE 17–97 ■ Evolving subcapsular liver hematoma. Three weeks following blunt trauma, a contrast-enhanced CT scan shows the subcapsular collection as a low-attenuation fluid collection.

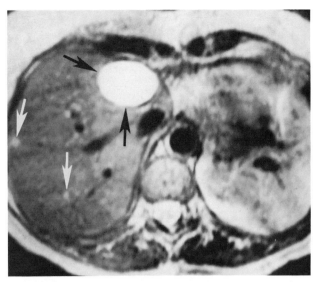

FIGURE 17–99 ■ Postsurgical biloma. T2-weighted MR image shows a homogeneously hyperintense lesion typical of fluid collections *(black arrows)*. A focus of recurrent metastatic disease *(white arrows)* is seen as less intense than the biloma.

material.[317] Arterioportal fistulae can occur in association with hematoma,[208] as well as with penetrating trauma to the liver, most often iatrogenic (i.e., following liver biopsy or transhepatic catheterization).[319] A dynamic scan sequence following a bolus injection of contrast best demonstrates arterial communications with the hepatic venous or portal system. In these cases, postcontrast images show a triangular, hyperdense, enhancing segment of the hepatic parenchyma, extending to the liver surface as a result of an increase in arterial flow from the fistula. This hyperdensity persists for only 45 sec during the early dynamic phase and returns to isodensity when the remaining hepatic parenchyma receives its normal portal contribution.[319]

Magnetic Resonance Imaging

There has been little reported experience with MR imaging in liver trauma. In an acutely traumatized patient, there is not adequate time for MR imaging with the current requirements for spin-echo sequences, compared with the fast CT scanning now available. Monitoring the acutely ill patient is awkward at best in most MR imaging suites. The follow-up of liver traumatic lesions is usually also performed with CT, which allows comparison with a prior CT performed during the immediate posttraumatic period.

The MR appearances of lacerations and hematomas within liver parenchyma vary depending on the time course of the hematoma and the field strength of the MR scanner. Most knowledge concerning the MR appearances of hematomas has been from reports studying intracranial hemorrhage.[321] The timing and MR appearances of changes in liver and abdominal hematomas are less predictable than those of intracranial hematomas.[172] With low and middle field strengths, the appearance in the acute phase of a hemorrhage is usually that of low signal intensity on T1-weighted images and high signal intensity on T2-weighted images because of the long T1 and T2 of fresh blood. At high field strength, however, there is often central hypointensity on T2-weighted images because of preferential T2 shortening of deoxyhemoglobin.[321] In the subacute phase, typically beginning around 72 hours, the methemoglobin present shortens the T1 of blood, resulting in hyperintensity on T1-weighted images as well.[321, 322] This is initially seen at the periphery of hematomas and increases centrally over time (see Fig. 17–52). In the chronic hematoma, a peripheral low signal rim may be seen[321, 322] as a result of formation of hemosiderin. In the liver, this progression may be altered by various body responses, including resorption of the hematoma and fluid or bile collections in the hematoma.

References

1. Rubinstein WA, Auh YH, Whalen JP, Kazam E: The perihepatic spaces: computed tomographic and ultrasound imaging. Radiology 149:231–239, 1983.
2. Auh YH, Rubinstein WA, Zirinsky K, et al: Accessory fissures of the liver: CT and sonographic appearance. AJR 143:565–572, 1984.
3. Sexton CC, Zeman RK: Correlation of computed tomography, sonography and gross anatomy of the liver. AJR 141:711–718, 1983.
4. Demirci A, Diren HB, Selcuk MB: Computed tomography in agenesis of the right lobe of the liver. Acta Radiol 31:105–106, 1990.
5. Belton RL, VanZandt TF: Congenital absence of the left lobe of the liver: a radiologic diagnosis. Radiology 147:184, 1983.
6. Radin DR, Colletti PM, Ralls PW, Boswell WDJ, Halls JM: Agenesis of the right lobe of the liver. Radiology 164:639–642, 1987.
7. Yamamoto S, Kojoh K, Saito I, et al: Computed tomography of congenital absence of the left lobe of the liver. J Comput Assist Tomogr 12:206–208, 1988.
8. Demaerel P, Marchal G, Van Steenbergen W, Fevery J, Van Damme B, Baert AL: CT demonstration of right hepatic lobe atrophy. J Comput Assist Tomogr 13:351–353, 1989.
9. Czerniak A, Soreide O, Gibson RN, et al: Liver atrophy complicating benign bile duct strictures. Surgical and interventional radiologic approaches. Am J Surg 152:294–300, 1986.
10. Auh YH, Rosen A, Rubenstein WA, Engel IA, Whalen JP, Kazam E: CT of the papillary process of the caudate lobe of the liver. AJR 142:535–538, 1984.
11. Dodds WJ, Erickson SJ, Taylor WJ, Lawson TL, Stewart ET: Caudate lobe of the liver: anatomy, embryology, and pathology. AJR 154:87–93, 1990.
12. Pagani JJ: Intrahepatic vascular territories shown by computed tomography. Radiology 147:173–178, 1983.
13. Mukai JK, Stack CM, Turner DA, et al: Imaging of surgically relevant hepatic vascular and segmental anatomy. Part 2. Extent and resectability of hepatic neoplasms. AJR 149:293–297, 1987.
14. Michels NA: Normal anatomy of the liver and its variant blood supply and collateral circulation. Am J Surg 112:337–347, 1966.
15. Healey JEJ, Schroy PC: Anatomy of the biliary ducts within the human liver. Arch Surg 66:599–616, 1953.
16. Marks WM, Filly RA, Callen PW: Ultrasonic anatomy of the liver: a review with new applications. J Clin Ultrasound 7:137–146, 1979.

17. Starzl RE, Bell RH, Beart RW, Putman CW: Hepatic trisegmentectomy and other liver resections. Surg Gynecol Obstet 141:429–437, 1975.
18. Weinstein JB, Heiken JP, Lee JKT, et al: High resolution CT of the porta hepatis and hepatoduodenal ligament. RadioGraphics 6:55–74, 1986.
19. Liddell RM, Baron RL, Ekstrom JE, Varnell RM, Shuman WP: CT depiction of intrahepatic bile ducts. Radiology 176:633–635, 1990.
20. Ritchings RJT, Pullman BR, Lucas SB, et al: An analysis of the spatial distribution of attenuation values in computed tomographic scans of liver and spleen. J Comput Assist Tomogr 3:36–39, 1979.
21. Piekarski J, Goldberg HI, Royal SA, Axel L, Moss AA: Difference between liver and spleen CT numbers in the normal adult: its usefulness in predicting the presence of diffuse liver disease. Radiology 137:727–729, 1980.
22. Stephens DH, Sheedy PFI, Hattery RR, MacCarty RL: Computed tomography of the liver. AJR 128:579–590, 1977.
23. Goldberg HI: Recognition of hepatocellular disorders by computed tomography. In Moss AA, Goldberg HI, Norman D (eds): Interventional Radiologic Techniques: Computed Tomography and Ultrasonography. New York, Academic Press, 1981.
24. Dwyer A, Doppman JL, Adams AJ, Girton ME, Chernick SS, Cornblath M: Influence of glycogen on liver density: computed tomography from a metabolic perspective. J Comput Assist Tomogr 7:70–73, 1983.
25. Ferrucci JT, Freeny PC, Stark DD, et al: Advances in hepatobiliary radiology. Radiology 168:319–338, 1988.
26. Fisher MR, Wall SD, Hricak H, McCarthy S, Kerlan RK: Hepatic vascular anatomy on magnetic resonance imaging. AJR 144:739–746, 1985.
27. Spritzer CE, Kressel HY, Mitchell D, Axel L: MR imaging of normal extrahepatic bile ducts. J Comput Assist Tomogr 11:248–252, 1987.
28. Steinberg HV, Alarcon JJ, Bernardino ME: Focal hepatic lesions: comparative MR imaging at 0.5 and 1.5 T. Radiology 174:153–156, 1990.
29. Reinig JW, Dwyer AJ, Miller DL, Frank JA, Adams GW, Chang AE: Liver metastases: detection with MR imaging at 0.5 and 1.5T. Radiology 170:149–153, 1989.
30. Foley WD: Dynamic hepatic CT. Radiology 170:617–622, 1989.
31. Seltzer SE, Hamilton C, VanDeripe D. Experimental evaluation of iosefamate meglumine and its derivatives as hepatobiliary CT contrast agents. AJR 145:67–72, 1985.
32. Miller DL, Vermess M, Doppman JL, et al: CT of the liver and spleen with EOE-13: review of 225 examinations. AJR 143:235–243, 1984.
33. Nelson RJ, Chezmar JL, Peterson JE, Bernardino ME: Contrast-enhanced CT of the liver and spleen: comparison of ionic and nonionic contrast agents. AJR 153:973–976, 1989.
34. Young SW, Enzmann DR, Long DM, Muller HH: Perfluoroctylbromide contrast enhancement of malignant neoplasms: preliminary observations. AJR 137:141–146, 1981.
35. Berland LL, Lawson TL, Foley WD, Melrose BL, Chintapalli KN, Taylor AJ: Comparison of pre- and post-contrast CT in hepatic masses. AJR 138:853–858, 1982.
36. Araki T, Itai Y, Furui S, Tasaka A: Dynamic CT densitometry of hepatic tumors. AJR 135:1037–1043, 1980.
37. Paushter DM, Zeman RK, Scheibler ML, Choyke PL, Jaffe MH, Clark LR: CT evaluation of suspected hepatic metastases: comparison of techniques for IV contrast enhancement. AJR 152:267–271, 1989.
38. Burgener FA, Hamlin DJ: Contrast enhancement of hepatic tumors in CT: comparison between bolus and infusion techniques. AJR 140:291–295, 1983.
39. Berland LL, Lee JY: Comparison of contrast media injection rates and volumes for hepatic dynamic incremented computed tomography. Invest Radiol 23:918–922, 1988.
40. Bernardino ME, Erwin BC, Steinberg HV, Baumgartner BR, Torres WE, Gedgaudas-McClees RK: Delayed hepatic CT scanning: increased confidence and improved detection of hepatic metastases. Radiology 159:71–74, 1986.
41. Heiken JP, Weyman PJ, Lee JKT, et al: Detection of focal
42. Moss AA, Dean PB, Axel L, Goldberg HI, Glazer GM, Friedman MA: Dynamic CT of hepatic masses with intravenous and intraarterial contrast material. AJR 138:847–852, 1982.
43. Matsui O, Takashima T, Kadoya M, et al: Dynamic computed tomography during arterial portography: the most sensitive examination for small hepatocellular carcinomas. J Comput Assist Tomogr 9:19–24, 1985.
44. Miller DL, Simmons JT, Chang R, et al: Hepatic metastasis detection: comparison of three CT contrast enhancement methods. Radiology 165:785–790, 1987.
45. Nelson RC, Chezmar JL, Sugarbaker PH, Bernardino ME: Hepatic tumors: comparison of CT during arterial portography, delayed CT, and MR imaging for preoperative evaluation. Radiology 172:27–34, 1989.
46. Freeny PC, Marks WM: Computed tomographic arteriography of the liver. Radiology 148:193–197, 1983.
47. Bressler EL, Alpern MB, Glazer GM, Francis IR, Ensminger WD: Hypervascular hepatic metastases: CT evaluation. Radiology 162:49–51, 1987.
48. DuBrow RA, David CL, Lorigan JG, Libshitz HI, Shirkhoda A: Hepatic metastasis detection in breast cancer: role of pre- and postcontrast CT. Radiology 169(P):347, 1988.
49. Foley WD. Dynamic hepatic CT scanning. AJR 152:272–274, 1989.
50. McCarthy S, Moss AA: Use of flow-rate injector for contrast-enhanced computed tomography. Radiology 151:800, 1984.
51. Shuman WP, Adam JL, Schoenecker SA, et al: Use of a power injector during dynamic computed tomography. J Comput Assist Tomogr 10:1000–1002, 1986.
52. Matsui O, Takashima T, Kadoya M, et al: Liver metastases from colorectal cancers: detection with CT during arterial portography. Radiology 165:65–70, 1987.
53. Phillips VM, Erwin BC, Bernardino ME: Delayed iodine scanning of the liver: promising CT technique. J Comput Assist Tomogr 9:415–416, 1985.
54. Yumoto Y, Jinno K, Tokuyama K, et al: Hepatocellular carcinoma detected by iodized oil. Radiology 154:19–24, 1985.
55. Nakakuma K, Tashiro S, Hiraoka T, Ogata K, Ootsuka K: Hepatocellular carcinoma and metastatic cancer detected by iodized oil. Radiology 154:15–17, 1985.
56. Ohishi H, Uchida H, Yoshimura H: Hepatocellular carcinoma detected by iodized oil: use of anticancer agents. Radiology 154:25–29, 1985.
57. Merine D, Takayasu K, Wakao F: Detection of hepatocellular carcinoma: comparison of CT during arterial portography with CT after intraarterial injection of iodized oil. Radiology 175:707–710, 1990.
58. Kneeland JB, Shimakawa A, Wehrli FW: Effect of intersection spacing on MR image contrast and study time. Radiology 158:819–822, 1986.
59. Stark DD, Wittenberg J, Edelman RR, et al: Detection of hepatic metastases: analysis of pulse sequence performance in MR imaging. Radiology 159:365–370, 1986.
60. Foley WD, Kneeland JB, Cates JD, et al: Contrast optimization for the detection of focal hepatic lesions by MR imaging at 1.5T. AJR 149:1155–1160, 1987.
61. Dwyer AJ, Frank JA, Sank VJ, Reinig JW, Hickey AM, Doppman JL: Short-T1 inversion-recovery pulse sequence: analysis and initial experience in cancer imaging. Radiology 168:827–836, 1988.
62. Paling MR, Abbitt PL, Mugler JP, Brookeman JR: Liver metastases: optimization of MR imaging pulse sequences at 1.0 T. Radiology 167:695–699, 1988.
63. Dousset M, Weissleder R, Hendrick RE: Short T1 inversion-recovery imaging of the liver: pulse-sequence optimization and comparison with spin-echo imaging. Radiology 171:327–333, 1989.
64. Shuman WP, Baron RL, Peters MJ, Tazioli PK: Comparison of STIR and spin-echo MR imaging at 1.5T in 90 lesions of the chest, liver, and pelvis. AJR 152:853–859, 1989.
65. Lee JKT, Heiken JP, Dixon WT: Detection of hepatic metas-

tases by proton spectroscopic imaging. Radiology 156:429–433, 1985.

66. Stark DD, Wittenberg J, Middleton MS, Ferrucci JT Jr: Liver metastases: detection by phase-contrast MR imaging. Radiology 158:327–332, 1986.

67. Dixon WT: Simple proton spectroscopic imaging. Radiology 153:189–194, 1984.

68. Schertz LD, Lee JKT, Heiken JP, Molina PL, Totty WG: Proton spectroscopic imaging (Dixon method) of the liver: clinical utility. Radiology 173:401–405, 1989.

69. Rummeny E, Saini S, Stark DD, Weissleder R, Compton CC, Ferrucci JT: Detection of hepatic metastases with MR imaging: spin-echo vs phase-contrast pulse sequences at 0.6T. AJR 153:1207–1211, 1989.

70. Winkler ML, Thoeni RF, Luh N, Kaufman L, Margulis AR: Hepatic neoplasia: breath-hold MR imaging. Radiology 170:801–806, 1989.

71. Edelman RJ, Hahn PF, Buxton R, et al: Rapid MR imaging with suspended respiration: clinical application in the liver. Radiology 161:125–131, 1986.

72. Wittenberg J, Stark DD, Forman BH, et al: Differentiation of hepatic metastases from hepatic hemangiomas and cysts by using MR imaging. AJR 151:79–84, 1988.

73. Rummeny E, Saini S, Wittenberg J, et al: MR imaging of liver neoplasms. AJR 152:493–499, 1989.

74. Rummeny E, Weissleder R, Stark DD, et al: Primary liver tumors: diagnosis by MR imaging. AJR 152:63–72, 1989.

75. Runge VM, Clanton JA, Herzer WA, et al: Intravascular contrast agents suitable for MRI. Radiology 153:171–176, 1984.

76. Edelman RR, Siegel JB, Singer A, Dupuis K, Longmaid HE: Dynamic MR imaging of the liver with Gd-DTPA: initial clinical results. AJR 153:1213–1219, 1989.

77. Hamm B, Wolf K-J, Felix R: Conventional and rapid MR imaging of the liver with Gd-DTPA. Radiology 164:313–320, 1987.

78. Shuman WP, Baron RL, Patten RM, Ekstrom JE: Dynamic gadolinium-enhanced MR imaging of small liver hemangiomas. Radiology 173(P):270–271, 1989.

79. Mano I, Yoshida H, Nakabayashi K, Yashiro N, Iio M: Fast spin echo imaging with suspended respiration: gadolinium enhanced MR imaging of liver tumors. J Comput Assist Tomogr 11:73–80, 1987.

80. Stark DD, Weissleder R, Elizondo G, et al: Superparamagnetic iron oxide: clinical application as a contrast agent for MR imaging of the liver. Radiology 168:297–301, 1988.

80a. Marchal G, VanHeckep E, Demaerel P, Decro P, Kennis C, et al. Detection of liver metastases with superparamagnetic iron oxide in 15 patients: Results of MR imaging at 1.5 T. AJR 152:771–775, 1989.

81. Lewis E, Bernardino ME, Barnes PA, Parvey HR, Soo C, Chuang VP: The fatty liver: pitfalls in the CT and angiographic evaluation of metastatic disease. J Comput Assist Tomogr 7:235–241, 1983.

82. Leevy CM: Fatty liver: a study of 270 patients with biopsy proven fatty liver and a review of the literature. Medicine 41:249–276, 1962.

83. Halvorsen RA, Korobkin M, Ram RC, Thompson WM: CT appearance of focal fatty infiltration of the liver. AJR 139:277–281, 1982.

84. Berland LL, Van Dyke JA: Decreased splenic enhancement on CT in traumatized hypotensive patients. Radiology 156:469–471, 1985.

85. Scott WW, Sanders RC, Siegelman SS: Irregular fatty infiltration of the liver: diagnostic dilemmas. AJR 135:67–71, 1980.

86. Quint LE, Glazer GM: CT evaluation of the bile ducts in patients with fatty liver. Radiology 153:755–756, 1984.

87. Choliz JD, Olaverri FJL, Casa TF, Zubieta SO: Computed tomography in hepatic echinococcosis. AJR 139:699–702, 1982.

88. Baker ME, Silverman PM: Nodular focal fatty infiltration of the liver: CT appearance. AJR 145:79–80, 1985.

89. Yates CK, Streight RA: Focal fatty infiltration of the liver simulating metastatic disease. Radiology 159:83–84, 1986.

90. Kawashima A, Suehiro SM, Russell WJ: Focal fatty infiltration of the liver mimicking a tumor: sonographic and CT features. J Comput Assist Tomogr 10:329–331, 1986.

91. Yoshikawa J, Matsui O, Takashima T, et al: Fatty metamorphosis in hepatocellular carcinoma: radiologic features in 10 cases. AJR 151:717–720, 1988.

92. Bashist B, Hecht HL, Harley WD: Computed tomographic demonstration of rapid changes in fatty infiltration of the liver. Radiology 142:691–692, 1982.

93. Wenker JC, Baker MK, Ellis JH, Glant MD: Focal fatty infiltration of the liver: demonstration by magnetic resonance imaging. AJR 143:573–574, 1984.

94. Stark DD, Bass NM, Moss AA, et al: Nuclear magnetic resonance imaging of experimentally induced liver disease. Radiology 148:743–751, 1983.

95. Stark DD, Goldberg HI, Moss AA, Bass NM: Chronic liver disease: evaluation by magnetic resonance. Radiology 150:149–151, 1984.

96. Heiken JP, Lee JKT, Glazer HS, Ling D: Hepatic metastases studied with MR and CT. Radiology 156:423–427, 1985.

97. Williams R, Williams HS, Scheuer PJ, et al: Iron absorption and siderosis in chronic liver disease. Q J Med 36:151–165, 1967.

98. Harbin WP, Robert NJ, Ferrucci JT: Diagnosis of cirrhosis based on regional changes in hepatic morphology. Radiology 135:273–283, 1980.

99. Torres WE, Whitmire LF, Gedgaudas-McClees K, Bernardino ME: Computed tomography of hepatic morphologic changes in cirrhosis of the liver. J Comput Assist Tomogr 10:47–50, 1986.

100. Waller RM, Oliver TW, McCain AH, Sones PJ, Bernardino ME: Computed tomography and sonography of hepatic cirrhosis and portal hypertension. RadioGraphics 4:677–715, 1984.

101. Itai Y, Ohnishi S, Ohtomo K, et al: Regenerating nodules of liver cirrhosis: MR imaging. Radiology 165:419–423, 1987.

102. Ishikawa N, Nakagawa S, Hirata K, et al: Long-term follow-up of hepatitis using computed tomography. 13:645–649, 1989.

103. Ohtomo K, Itai Y, Makita K, et al: Portosystemic collaterals on MR imaging. J Comput Assist Tomogr 10:751–755, 1986.

104. Bernardino ME, Steinberg HV, Pearson TC, Gedgaudas-McClees RK, Torres WE, Henderson JM: Shunts for portal hypertension: MR and angiography for determination of patency. Radiology 158:57–61, 1986.

105. Matsui O, Kadoya M, Kameyama T, et al: Adenomatous hyperplastic nodules in the cirrhotic liver: differentiation from hepatocellular carcinoma with MR imaging. Radiology 173:123–126, 1989.

106. Jensen PS: Hemochromatosis: a disease often silent but not invisible. AJR 126:343–351, 1976.

107. Mills SR, Doppman JL, Nienhus AW: Computed tomography in the diagnosis of disorders of excessive iron storage of the liver. J Comput Assist Tomogr 1:101–104, 1977.

108. Long JA, Doppman JL, Nienhus AW, Mills ST: Computed tomographic analysis of beta-thalassemic syndromes with hemochromatosis: pathologic findings with clinical and laboratory correlations. J Comput Assist Tomogr 4:159–165, 1980.

109. Mitnick JS, Bosniak MA, Megibow AJ, et al: CT in B-thalassemia: iron deposition in the liver, spleen and lymph nodes. AJR 136:1191–1194, 1981.

110. Houang MTW, Arozena X, Skalicka A, Huehns ER, Shaw DG: Correlation between computed tomographic values and liver iron content in thalassemia major with iron overload. Lancet 1:1322–1323, 1979.

111. Powell LW, Bassett ML, Halliday JW: Hemochromatosis: 1980 update. Gastroenterology 78:374–381, 1980.

112. Murphy FB, Bernardino ME: MR imaging of focal hemochromatosis. J Comput Assist Tomogr 10:1044–1046, 1986.

113. Scherer U, Santos M, Lissner J: CT studies of the liver in vitro: a report on 82 cases with pathological correlation. J Comput Assist Tomogr 3:589–595, 1979.

114. Chapman RWG, Williams G, Bydder G: Computed tomography for determining liver iron content in primary hemochromatosis. Br Med J 280:440–442, 1980.

115. Mayer DP, Kressel HY, Soloway RS: Asymptomatic carrier state in Wilson's disease. J Comput Assist Tomogr 7:146–147, 1983.

116. Royal SA, Beiderman BA, Goldberg HI, Koerper MM, Thaler MM: Detection and estimation of iron, glycogen and fat in liver of children with hepatomegaly using computed tomography (CT). Pediatr Res 13:408, 1979.

117. Goldberg HI, Cann CE, Moss AA, Ohto M, Brito A, Federle M: Noninvasive quantitation of liver iron in dogs with hemochromatosis using dual energy CT scanning. Invest Radiol 17:375–380, 1982.

118. Howard JM, Ghent CN, Carey LS, Flanagan PR, Valberg LS: Diagnostic efficacy of hepatic computed tomography in the detection of body iron overload. Gastroenterology 84:209–215, 1983.

119. Brasch RC, Wesbey GE, Gooding CA, Koerper MA: MRI of transfusional hemosiderosis complicating thalassemia major. Radiology 150:767–771, 1984.

120. Stark DD, Moseley ME, Bacon BR, et al: MRI and spectroscopy of hepatic iron overload. Radiology 154:137–142, 1985.

121. Brown DW, Henkelman RM, Poon PY, Fisher MM: Nuclear magnetic resonance study of iron overload in liver tissue. Magn Reson Imaging 3:275–282, 1985.

122. Miller JH, Stanley P, Gates GF: Radiography of glycogen storage diseases. AJR 132:379–387, 1979.

123. Doppman JL, Cornblath M, Dwyer AJ, Adams AJ, Girton ME, Sidbury J: Computed tomography of the liver and kidneys in glycogen storage disease. J Comput Assist Tomogr 6:67–71, 1982.

124. Biondetti PR, Fiore D, Muzzio PC: Computed tomography of the liver in Von Gierke's disease. J Comput Assist Tomogr 4:685–686, 1980.

125. Jeffrey RB, Moss AA, Quivey JM, Federle MP, Wara WM: CT of radiation-induced hepatic injury. AJR 135:445–448, 1980.

126. Unger EC, Lee JKT, Weyman PW: CT and MR imaging of radiation hepatitis. J Comput Assist Tomogr 11:264–268, 1987.

127. Ingold J, Reed GB, Kaplan HS, Bagshaw MA: Radiation hepatitis. AJR 93:200–208, 1965.

128. Markos J, Veronese ME, Nicholson MR, McLean S, Shevland JE: Value of hepatic computerized tomographic scanning during amiodarone therapy. Am J Cardiol 56:89–92, 1985.

129. Goldman IS, Winkler ML, Raper SE, et al: Increased hepatic density and phospholipidosis due to aminodarone. AJR 144:541–546, 1985.

130. DeMaria M, DeSimone G, Laconi A, Mercadante G, Pavone P, Rossi P: Gold storage in the liver: appearance on CT scans. Radiology 159:355–356, 1986.

131. Aihara T, Fujioka M, Yamamoto K: Increased CT density of the liver due to cis-diaminedichloro platinum (II). Pediatr Radiol 17:75–76, 1987.

132. Lawler GA, Pennock JM, Steiner RE, Jenkins WJ, Sherlock S, Young IR: Nuclear magnetic resonance (NMR) imaging in Wilson's disease. J Comput Assist Tomogr 7:1–8, 1983.

133. Dixon AK, Walsh JM: Computed tomography of the liver in Wilson disease. J Comput Assist Tomogr 8:46–49, 1984.

134. San Felippo PM, Beahrs OH, Weiland LH: Cystic disease of the liver. Ann Surg 179:922–925, 1974.

135. Murphy BJ, Casillas J, Ros PR, Morillo G, Albores-Saavedra J, Rolfes DB: The CT appearance of cystic masses of the liver. RadioGraphics 9:307–322, 1989.

136. Barnes PA, Thomas JL, Bernardino ME: Pitfalls in the diagnosis of hepatic cysts by computed tomography. Radiology 141:129–133, 1981.

137. Wooten WB, Bernardino ME, Goldstein HM: Computed tomography of necrotic hepatic metastases. AJR 131:839–842, 1978.

138. Callen PW: Computed tomographic evaluation of abdominal and pelvic abscesses. Radiology 131:171–175, 1979.

139. Mueller PR, Ferrucci JT Jr, Simeone JF, et al: Detection and drainage of bilomas: special considerations. AJR 140:715–720, 1983.

140. Federle MP, Filly RA, Moss AA: Cystic hepatic neoplasms: complementary roles of CT and sonography. AJR 136:345–348, 1981.

141. Wilcox DM, Weinreb JC, Lesh P: MR imaging of a hemorrhagic hepatic cyst in a patient with polycystic liver disease. J Comput Assist Tomogr 9:183–185, 1985.

142. Edmondson H: Tumors of the liver and intrahepatic bile ducts. In Atlas of Tumor Pathology. Washington, DC, Armed Forces Institute of Pathology, 1958.

143. Trastek VF, van Heerden JA, Sheedy PF, et al: Cavernous hemangiomas of the liver: resect or observe. Am J Surg 145:49–53, 1983.

144. Ashida C, Fishman EK, Zerhouni EA, et al: Computed tomography of hepatic cavernous hemangioma. J Comput Assist Tomogr 11:455–460, 1987.

145. Freeny PC, Marks WM: Hepatic hemangioma: dynamic bolus CT. AJR 147:711–719, 1986.

146. Johnson CM, Sheedy PFI, Stanson AW, et al: Computed tomography and angiography of cavernous hemangiomas of the liver. Radiology 138:115–121, 1981.

147. Freeny PC, Marks WM: Patterns of contrast enhancement of benign and malignant hepatic neoplasms during bolus dynamic and delayed CT. Radiology 160:613, 1986.

148. Mikulis DJ, Costello P, Clouse ME: Hepatic hemangioma: atypical appearance. AJR 145:77–78, 1985.

149. Stark DD, Felder RC, Wittenberg J, et al: Magnetic resonance imaging of cavernous hemangioma of the liver: tissue-specific characterization. AJR 145:213–222, 1985.

150. Birnbaum BA, Weinreb JC, Megibow AJ, et al: Definitive diagnosis of hepatic hemangiomas: MR imaging versus Tc-99m-labeled red blood cell SPECT. Radiology 176:95–101, 1990.

151. Ohtomo K, Itai Y, Yoshikawa K, et al: Hepatic tumors: dynamic MR imaging. Radiology 163:27–31, 1987.

152. Li KC, Glazer GM, Quint LE, et al: Distinction of hepatic cavernous hemangioma from hepatic metastases with MR imaging. Radiology 169:409–415, 1988.

153. Ros PR, Lubbers PR, Olmstead WW, Morillo G: Hemangioma of the liver: heterogeneous appearance on T-2 weighted images. AJR 149:1167–1170, 1987.

154. Choi BI, Han MC, Park JH, Kim SH, Han MH, Kim C-W: Giant cavernous hemangioma of the liver: CT and MR imaging in 10 cases. AJR 152:1221–1226, 1989.

155. Ohtomo K, Itai Y, Yoshida H, et al: MR differentiation of hepatocellular carcinoma from cavernous hemangioma: complementary roles of FLASH and T2 values. AJR 152:505–507, 1989.

156. Yoshida H, Itai Y, Ohtomo K, Kokubo T, Minami M, Yashiro N: Small hepatocellular carcinoma and cavernous hemangioma: differentiation with dynamic FLASH MR imaging with Gd-DTPA. Radiology 171:339–342, 1989.

157. Gibney RG, Hendin AP, Cooperberg PL: Sonographically detected hepatic hemangiomas: absence of change over time. AJR 149:953–957, 1987.

158. Kudo M, Ikekubo K, Yamamoto K, et al: Distinction between hemangioma of the liver and hepatocellular carcinoma: value of labeled RBC-SPECT scanning. AJR 152:977–983, 1989.

159. Tumeh SS, Benson C, Nagel JS, et al: Cavernous hemangioma of the liver: detection with single-photon emission computed tomography. Radiology 164:353–356, 1987.

160. Solbiati L, Livraghi T, De Pra L, et al: Fine-needle biopsy of hepatic hemangioma with sonographic guidance. AJR 144:471–474, 1985.

161. Cronan JJ, Esparza AR, Dorfman GS, et al: Cavernous hemangioma of the liver: role of percutaneous biopsy. Radiology 166:135–138, 1988.

162. Spamer C, Brambs C, Koch H, et al: Benign circumscribed lesions of the liver diagnosed by ultrasonically guided fine needle biopsy. JCU 14:83–88, 1986.

163. Casarella WJ, Knowles DM, Wolff M, Johnson PM: Focal nodular hyperplasia and liver cell adenoma: radiologic and pathologic differentiation. AJR 131:393–402, 1978.

164. Angres G, Carter JB, Velasco JM: Unusual ring in liver cell adenoma. AJR 135:172–174, 1980.

165. Rooks JB, Ory HW, Ishak KG, et al: Epidemiology of hepa-

tocellular adenoma: the role of oral contraceptive use. JAMA 242:644–648, 1979.

166. Brum JK, Bookstein J, Holtz F, Klein EW: Possible association between benign hepatomas and oral contraceptives. Lancet 2:926, 1973.

167. Andersen P, Packer JT: Hepatic adenoma: Observations after estrogen withdrawal. Arch Surg 111:898–900, 1976.

168. Mariani A, Livingstone AS, Pereiras RV Jr: Progressive enlargement of an hepatic adenoma. Gastroenterology 77:1319–1325, 1979.

169. Mathieu D, Bruneton JN, Drouillard J, Pointreau CC, Vasile N: Hepatic adenomas and focal nodular hyperplasia: dynamic CT study. Radiology 160:53–58, 1986.

170. Welch TJ, Sheedy PF, Johnson CM, et al: Focal nodular hyperplasia and hepatic adenoma: comparison of angiography, CT, US, and scintigraphy. Radiology 156:593–595, 1985.

171. Moss AA, Goldberg HI, Stark DB, et al: Hepatic tumors: magnetic resonance and CT appearance. Radiology 150:141–147, 1984.

172. Mattrey R, Trambert M, Edelman RR: MR imaging of the upper abdomen and adrenal glands. In Edelman RR, Hesselink JR (eds): Clinical Magnetic Resonance Imaging. Philadelphia, WB Saunders, 1990.

173. Ishak K, Rabin L: Benign tumors of the liver. Med Clin North Am 59:995–1013, 1975.

174. Freeny PC: Radiologic diagnosis of focal hepatic masses: an integrated approach. In Moss AA, Goldberg HI, Norman D (eds): Interventional Radiologic Techniques: Computed Tomography and Ultrasonography. New York, Academic Press, 1981.

175. Rogers JV, Mack LA, Freeny PC, Johnson ML, Sones PJ: Hepatic focal nodular hyperplasia: angiography, CT, sonography, and scintigraphy. AJR 137:983–990, 1981.

176. McMullen CT, Montgomery JL: Arteriographic findings of focal nodular hyperplasia of the liver and review of the literature. AJR 117:380–387, 1973.

177. Ros PR: Computed tomography—pathologic correlation in hepatic tumors. In Ferrucci JT, Mathieu DG (eds): Advances in Hepatobiliary Radiology. St Louis, CV Mosby, 1990.

178. Brandt DJ, Johnson CD, Stephens DH, Weiland LH: Imaging of fibrolamellar hepatocellular carcinoma. AJR 151:295–299, 1988.

179. Mattison GR, Glazer GM, Quint LE, Francis IR, Bree RL, Ensminger WD: MR imaging of hepatic focal nodular hyperplasia: characterization and distinction from primary malignant hepatic tumors. AJR 148:711–715, 1987.

180. Butch RJ, Stark DD, Malt RA: MR imaging of hepatic focal nodular hyperplasia. J Comput Assist Tomogr 10:874–877, 1986.

181. Schiebler ML, Kressel HY, Saul SH, Yeager BA, Axel L, Gefter WB: MR imaging of focal nodular hyperplasia of the liver. J Comput Assist Tomogr 11:651–654, 1987.

182. Itai Y, Ohtomo K, Kokubo T, et al: CT and MR imaging of fatty tumors of the liver. J Comput Assist Tomogr 11:253–257, 1987.

183. Roberts JL, Fishman EK, Hartman DS, Sanders R, Goodman Z, Siegelman SS: Lipomatous tumors of the liver: evaluation with CT and US. Radiology 158:613–617, 1986.

184. Bruneton JN, Kerboul P, Drouillard J, Menu Y, Normand R, Santini N: Hepatic lipomas: ultrasound and computed tomographic findings. Gastrointest Radiol 12:299–303, 1987.

185. Goodman ZD, Ishak KG: Angiomyolipomas of the liver. Am J Surg Pathol 8:745–750, 1984.

186. Kaurich JD, Coombs RJ, Zeiss J: Myelolipoma of the liver: CT features. J Comput Assist Tomogr 12:660–661, 1988.

187. Ros PR, Goodman ZD, Ishak KG, et al: Mesenchymal hamartoma of the liver: radiologic-pathologic correlation. Radiology 158:619–624, 1986.

188. Giyanani VL, Meyers PC, Wolfson JJ: Mesenchymal hamartoma of the liver: computed tomography and ultrasonography. J Comput Assist Tomogr 10:51–54, 1986.

189. Arenson AM, Rosen IE, McKee JD, Hamilton PA: Ultrasonography and CT of multiple bile duct hamartomas simulating dilated intrahepatic ducts. J Can Assoc Radiol 39:26–28, 1988.

190. Lucaya J, Enriquez G, Amat L, Gonzalez-Rivero MA: Computed tomography of infantile hepatic hemangioendothelioma. AJR 144:821–826, 1985.

191. Dachman AH, Lichtenstein JE, Friedman AC, et al: Infantile hemangioendothelioma of the liver: a radiologic-pathologic-clinical correlation. AJR 140:1091–1096, 1983.

192. Korobkin M, Stephens DH, Lee JKT, et al: Biliary cystadenoma and cystadenocarcinoma: CT and sonographic findings. AJR 153:507–511, 1989.

193. Choi BI, Lim JH, Han MC, et al: Biliary cystadenoma and cystadenocarcinoma: CT and sonographic findings. Radiology 171:57–61, 1989.

194. Inamoto K, Sugiki K, Yamasaki H, Nakao N, Miura T: Computed tomography and angiography of hepatocellular carcinoma. J Comput Assist Tomogr 4:832–839, 1980.

195. Inamoto K, Sugiki K, Yamasaki H, Miura T: CT of hepatoma: effects of portal vein obstruction. AJR 136:349–353, 1981.

196. Sumida M, Ohto M, Ebara M, Kimura K, Okuda K, Hirooka N: Accuracy of angiography in the diagnosis of small hepatocellular carcinoma. AJR 147:531–536, 1986.

197. Takayasu K, Shima Y, Muramatsu Y, et al: Angiography of small hepatocellular carcinomas: analysis of 105 resected tumors. AJR 147:525–529, 1986.

198. Merine D, Fishman EK, Zerhouni EA: Spontaneous hepatic hemorrhage, clinical and CT findings. J Comput Assist Tomogr 12:397–400, 1988.

199. Clarkston W, Inciardi M, Kirkpatrick S, McEwen G, Ediger S, Schubert T: Acute hemoperitoneum from rupture of a hepatocellular carcinoma. J Clin Gastroenterol 10:221–225, 1988.

200. Chuong JJH, Livstone EM, Barwick KW: The histopathologic and clinical indicators of prognosis in hepatoma. J Clin Gastroenterol 4:547–552, 1982.

201. Craig JR, Peters RL, Edmondson HA, Omata M: Fibrolamellar carcinoma of the liver: a tumor of adolescents and young adults with distinctive clinicopathologic features. Cancer 46:372–379, 1980.

202. Friedman AC, Lichtenstein JE, Goodman Z, Fishman EK, Siegelman SS, Dachman AH: Fibrolamellar hepatocellular carcinoma. 157:583–587, 1985.

203. Lack EE, Neave C, Vawter GF: Hepatocellular carcinoma: review of 32 cases in childhood and adolescence. Cancer 52:1510–1515, 1983.

204. Teefey SA, Stephens DH, James EM, et al: Computed tomography and ultrasonography of hepatoma. Clin Radiol 37:339–345, 1986.

205. Kunstlinger F, Federle MP, Moss AA, Marks W: Computed tomography of hepatocellular carcinoma. AJR 134:431–437, 1980.

206. Itai Y, Araki T, Furui S, Tasaka A: Differential diagnosis of hepatic masses on computed tomography, with particular reference to hepatocellular carcinoma. J Comput Assist Tomogr 5:834–842, 1981.

207. Hosoki T, Toyonaga Y, Araki Y, Mori S: Dynamic computed tomography of isodense hepatocellular carcinoma. J Comput Assist Tomogr 8:263–268, 1984.

208. Itai Y, Furui S, Ohtomo K, et al: Dynamic CT features of arterioportal shunts in hepatocellular carcinoma. AJR 146:723–727, 1986.

209. LaBerge JM, Laing FC, Federle MP, Jeffrey RB Jr, Lim RC Jr: Hepatocellular carcinoma: assessment of resectability by computed tomography and ultrasound. Radiology 152:485–490, 1984.

210. Mathieu D, Grenier P, Larde D, Vasile N: Portal vein involvement in hepatocellular carcinoma: dynamic CT features. Radiology 152:127–132, 1984.

211. Itoh K, Nishimura K, Togashi K, et al: Hepatocellular carcinoma: MR imaging. Radiology 164:21–25, 1987.

212. Ebara M, Ohto M, Watanabe Y, et al: Diagnosis of small hepatocellular carcinoma: correlation of MR imaging and tumor histologic studies. Radiology 159:371–377, 1986.

213. Itai Y, Ohtomo K, Furui S, et al: MR imaging of hepatocellular carcinoma. J Comput Assist Tomogr 10:963–968, 1986.

214. Matsui O, Kadoya M, Takashima T, Kameyama T, Yoshikawa J, Tamura S: Intrahepatic periportal abnormal intensity on

MR images: an indication of various hepatobiliary diseases. Radiology 171:335–338, 1989.

215. Okuda K, Obata H, Jinnouchi S, et al: Angiographic assessment of gross anatomy of hepatocellular carcinoma: comparison of celiac angiograms and liver pathology in 100 cases. Radiology 123:21–29, 1977.

216. Titelbaum DS, Hiroto H, Schiebler ML, Kressel HY, Burke DR, Saul SH: Fibrolamellar hepatocellular carcinoma: MR appearance. 12:588–591, 1988.

217. Itai Y, Araki T, Furui S, Yashiro N, Ohtomo K, Iio M: Computed tomography of primary intrahepatic biliary malignancy. Radiology 147:485–490, 1983.

218. Zornoza J, Ginaldi S: Computed tomography in hepatic lymphoma. Radiology 138:405–410, 1981.

219. Honda H, Franken EAJ, Barloon TJ, Smith JL: Hepatic lymphoma in cyclosporine-treated transplant recipients: sonographic and CT findings. AJR 152:501–503, 1989.

220. Levitan R, Diamond HD, Craver LF: The liver in Hodgkin's disease. Gut 2:60–71, 1971.

221. Rosenberg SA, Diamond HD, Jaslowitz B, et al: Lymphosarcoma: a review of 1,269 cases. Medicine 40:31–84, 1961.

222. Scheuer PJ: Liver Biopsy Interpretation. Baltimore, Williams & Wilkins, 1973.

223. Tubman DE, Frick MP, Hanto DW: Lymphoma after organ transplantation: radiologic manifestations in the central nervous system, thorax, and abdomen. Radiology 149:625–631, 1983.

224. Mathieu D, Bruneton J-N, Vasile N, Dao T-H, Normand F, Balu-Maestro C: Value of CT for the diagnosis of hepatic involvement by lymphoma. Radiology 165(P):200, 1987.

225. Weinreb J, Brateman L, Maravilla K: Magnetic resonance imaging of hepatic lymphoma. AJR 143:1211–1214, 1984.

226. Nyman R, Rhen S, Ericsson A, et al: An attempt to characterize malignant lymphoma in spleen, liver and lymph nodes with magnetic resonance imaging. Acta Radiol 28:527–533, 1987.

227. Weissleder R, Stark DD, Compton CC, Wittenberg J, Ferrucci JT: Ferrite-enhanced MR imaging of hepatic lymphoma: an experimental study in rats. AJR 149:1161–1165, 1987.

228. Amendola MA, Blane CE, Amendola BE, Glazer GM: CT findings in hepatoblastoma. J Comput Assist Tomogr 8:1105–1109, 1984.

229. Dachman AH, Pakter RL, Ros PR, Fishman EK, Goodman ZD, Lichtenstein JE: Hepatoblastoma: radiologic-pathologic correlation in 50 cases. Radiology 164:15–19, 1987.

230. Korobkin M, Kirks DR, Sullivan DC, Mills SR, Bowie JD: Computed tomography of primary liver tumors in children. Radiology 139:431–435, 1981.

231. Coldwell DM, Baron RL, Charnsangavej C: Angiosarcoma: diagnosis and clinical course. Acta Radiol 30:627–631, 1989.

232. Lockner GY, Doroshow JH, Zwelling LA, Chabner BA: The clinical features of hepatic angiosarcoma. A report of four cases and a review of the English literature. Medicine 58:48–64, 1979.

233. Schonland MM, Millward-Sadler GH, Wright DH, Wright R: Hepatic tumors. In Wright R, Alberti KGMM, Karran S, Millward-Sadler GH (eds): Liver and Biliary Disease. Philadelphia, WB Saunders, 1979.

234. Sherlock S: Diseases of the Liver and Biliary System. Oxford, England, Blackwell Scientific Publications, 1989.

235. Silverman PM, Ram PC, Korobkin M: CT appearance of abdominal thorotrast deposition and thorotrast-induced angiosarcoma of the liver. J Comput Assist Tomogr 7:655–658, 1983.

236. Mahoney B, Jeffrey RB, Federle MP: Spontaneous rupture of hepatic and splenic angiosarcoma demonstrated by CT. AJR 138:965–966, 1982.

237. Vasile N, Larde D, Zafrani ES, Berard H, Mathieu D: Hepatic angiosarcoma. J Comput Assist Tomogr 7:899–901, 1983.

238. Ros PR, Olmsted WW, Dachman AH, Goodman ZD, Ishak KG, Hartman DS: Undifferentiated (embryonal) sarcoma of the liver: radiologic-pathologic correlation. Radiology 161:141–145, 1986.

239. Ottmar MD, Gonda RLJ, Leithauser KJ, Gutierrez OH: Liver function tests in patients with computed tomography demonstrated hepatic metastases. Gastrointest Radiol 14:55–58, 1989.

240. Foley WD, Berland LL, Lawson TL, Smith DF, Thorsen MK: Contrast enhancement technique for dynamic hepatic computed tomographic scanning. Radiology 147:797–803, 1983.

241. Freeny PC, Marks WM, Ryan JA, Bolen JW: Colorectal carcinoma evaluation with CT: preoperative staging and detection of postoperative recurrence. Radiology 158:347–353, 1986.

242. Brendel A, Leccia F, Drouillard J, et al: Single photon emission computed tomography (SPECT), planar scintigraphy, and transmission computed tomography: a comparison of accuracy in diagnosing focal hepatic disease. Radiology 153:527–532, 1984.

243. Knopf DR, Torres WE, Fajman WJ, et al: Liver lesions: comparative accuracy of scintigraphy and computed tomography. AJR 138:623–627, 1982.

244. Alderson PO, Adams DF, McNeil BJ, et al: Computed tomography, ultrasound and scintigraphy of the liver in patients with colon or breast carcinoma: a prospective comparison. Radiology 149:225–230, 1983.

245. Stark DD, Wittenberg J, Butch RJ, Ferrucci JT: Hepatic metastases: randomized, controlled comparison of detection with MR imaging and CT. Radiology 165:399–406, 1987.

246. Chezmar JL, Rumancik WM, Megibow AJ, Hulnick DH, Nelson RC, Bernardino ME: Liver and abdominal screening in patients with cancer: CT versus MR imaging. Radiology 168:43–47, 1988.

247. Reinig JW, Dwyer AJ, Miller DL, et al: Liver metastasis detection: comparative sensitivities of MR imaging and CT scanning. Radiology 162:43–47, 1987.

248. Sugarbaker PH, Vermess M, Doppman JL, Miller DL, Simon R: Improved detection of focal lesions with computerized tomographic examination of the liver using ethiodized oil emulsion (EOE-13) liver contrast. Cancer 54:1489–1495, 1984.

249. Miller DL, Rosenbaum RC, Sugarbaker PH, et al: Detection of hepatic metastases: comparison of EOE-13 CT and ^{99m}Tc-MAA scintigraphy. AJR 141:931–935, 1983.

250. Scatarige JC, Fishman EK, Saksouk FA, Siegelman SS: Computed tomography of calcified liver masses. J Comput Assist Tomogr 7:83–89, 1983.

251. Bernardino M: Computed tomography of calcified liver metastases. J Comput Assist Tomogr 3:527–530, 1979.

252. Federle MP, Jeffrey RBJ, Minagi H: Calcified liver metastases from renal cell carcinoma. J Comput Assist Tomogr 5:771–772, 1981.

253. McDonnell CH, Fishman EK, Zerhouni EA: CT demonstration of calcified liver metastases in medullary thyroid carcinoma. J Comput Assist Tomogr 10:976–978, 1986.

254. McLeod AJ, Zornosa J, Shirkhoda A: Leiomosarcoma: computed tomographic findings. Radiology 152:133–136, 1984.

255. Halvorsen RA, Korobkin M, Foster WL, Silverman PM, Thompson WM: The variable CT appearance of hepatic abscesses. AJR 142:941–946, 1984.

256. Mathieu D, Vasile N, Grenier P: Portal thrombosis: dynamic CT features and course. Radiology 154:737–741, 1985.

257. Jaques P, Mauro M, Safrit H, Yankaskas B, Piggott G: CT features of intraabdominal abscesses: prediction of successful percutaneous drainage. AJR 146:1041–1045, 1986.

258. Bernardino ME, Berkman WA, Plemmons M, Sones PJ, Barton RB, Casarella WJ: Percutaneous drainage of multiseptated hepatic abscess. J Comput Assist Tomogr 8:38–41, 1984.

259. Shirkhoda A, Lopez-Berestein G, Holbert JM, Lunga MA: Hepatosplenic fungal infection: CT and pathologic evaluation after treatment with liposomal amphotericin B. Radiology 159:349–353, 1986.

260. Berlow ME, Sprit BA, Weil L: CT follow-up of hepatic and splenic fungal microabscesses. J Comput Assist Tomogr 8:42–45, 1984.

261. Pastakia B, Shawker TH, Thaler M, O'Leary T, Pizzo PA: Hepatosplenic candidiasis: wheels within wheels. Radiology 166:417–421, 1988.

262. Beggs I: The radiology of hydatid disease. AJR 145:639–648, 1985.

263. Kalovidouris A, Pissiotis C, Pontifex G, Gouliamos A, Pentea

S, Papavassiliou C: CT characterization of multivesicular hydatid cysts. J Comput Assist Tomogr 10:428–431, 1986.

264. Hoff FL, Aisen AM, Walden ME, Glazer GM: MR imaging of hydatid disease of the liver. Gastrointest Radiol 12:39–42, 1987.

265. Parizel P, Van Gijesegem D, Vereycken H, De Schepper A: CT demonstration of mobile echinococcal daughter cysts. J Comput Assist Tomogr 8:179–180, 1984.

266. Kalovidouris A, Gouliamos A, Demou L, Vassilopoulos P, Vlachos L, Papavassiliou K: Postsurgical evaluation of hydatid disease with CT: diagnostic pitfalls. J Comput Assist Tomogr 8:1114–1119, 1984.

267. Marani SAD, Canossi GC, Nicoli FA, Albertis GP, Monni SJ, Casolo P: Hydatid disease: MR imaging study. Radiology 175:701–706, 1990.

268. Scherer U, Weinzieri M, Sturm R, Schildberg F, Zrenner M, Lissner J: Computed tomography in hydatid disease of the liver: a report of 13 cases. J Comput Assist Tomogr 2:612, 1978.

269. Didier D, Weiler S, Rohmer P, et al: Hepatic alveolar echinococcosis: correlative US and CT study. Radiology 154:179–186, 1985.

270. Radin DR, Ralls PW, Colletti PM, Halls JM: CT of amebic liver abscess. AJR 150:1297–1301, 1988.

271. Ralls PW, Henley DS, Colletti PM, et al: Amebic liver abscess: MR imaging. Radiology 165:801–804, 1987.

272. Elizondo G, Weissleder R, Stark DD, et al: Amebic liver abscess: diagnosis and treatment evaluation with MR imaging. Radiology 165:795–800, 1987.

273. Araki T, Hayakawa K, Okada J, Hayashi S, Uchiyama G, Yamada K: Hepatic schistosomiasis japonica identified by CT. Radiology 157:757–760, 1985.

274. Hamada M, Ohta M, Yasuda Y, et al: Hepatic calcification in schistosomiasis japonica. J Comput Assist Tomogr 6:76–78, 1982.

275. Fataar S, Bassiony H, Satyanath S, et al: CT of hepatic schistosomiasis mansoni. AJR 145:63–66, 1985.

276. Serrano MAP, Vega A, Ortega E, Gonzalez A: Computed tomography of hepatic fascioliasis. J Comput Assist Tomogr 11:269–272, 1987.

277. Van Beers B, Pringot J, Geubel A, Trigaux J-P, Bigaignon G, Dooms G: Hepatobiliary fascioliasis: noninvasive imaging findings. Radiology 174:809–810, 1990.

278. Takeyama N, Okumura N, Sakai Y, et al: Computed tomography findings of hepatic lesions in human fascioliasis: report of two cases. Am J Gastroenterol 81:1078–1081, 1986.

279. Vogelzang RL, Anschuetz SL, Gore RM: Budd-Chiari syndrome: CT observations. Radiology 163:329–333, 1987.

280. Miller VE, Berland LL: Pulsed Doppler duplex sonography and CT of portal vein thrombosis. AJR 145:73–76, 1985.

281. Reinig JW, Sanchez FW, Vujic I: Hemodynamics of portal blood flow shown by CT portography. Radiology 154:473–476, 1985.

282. Levy HM, Newhouse JH: MR imaging of portal vein thrombosis. AJR 151:283–286, 1988.

283. Tamada T, Moriyasu F, Ono S, et al: Portal blood flow: measurement with MR imaging. Radiology 173:639–644, 1989.

284. Edelman RR, Zhao B, Liu C, et al: MR angiography and dynamic flow evaluation of the portal venous system. AJR 153:755–760, 1989.

285. Zirinsky K, Markisz JA, Auh YH, et al: MR imaging of portal venous thrombosis: correlation with CT and sonography. AJR 150:283–288, 1988.

286. Williams DK, Cho KJ, Aisen AM, Eckhauser FE: Portal hypertension evaluated by MR imaging. Radiology 157:703–706, 1985.

287. Stanley P: Budd-Chiari syndrome. Radiology 170:625–627, 1989.

288. Mathieu D, Vasile N, Menu Y, Van Beers B, Lorphelin JM, Pringot J: Budd-Chiari syndrome: dynamic CT. Radiology 165:409–413, 1987.

289. Mori H, Maeda H, Fukuda T, et al: Acute thrombosis of the inferior vena cava and hepatic veins in patients with Budd-Chiari syndrome: CT demonstration. AJR 153:987–991, 1989.

290. Baert AL, Fevery J, Marchal G, Guddeeris P, Wilms G, et al: Early diagnosis of Budd-Chiari syndrome by computed tomography and ultrasonography: report of five cases. Gastroenterology 84:587–595, 1983.

291. Stark DD, Hahn PF, Trey C, Clouse ME, Ferrucci JTJ: MRI of the Budd-Chiari syndrome. AJR 146:1141–1148, 1986.

292. Peterson IM, Neumann CH: Focal hepatic infarction with bile lake formation. AJR 142:1155–1156, 1984.

293. Adler DD, Glazer GM, Silver TM: Computed tomography of liver infarction. AJR 142:315–318, 1984.

294. Lev-Toaff AS, Friedman AC, Cohen LM, Radecki PD, Caroline DF: Hepatic infarcts: new observations by CT and sonography. AJR 149:87–90, 1987.

295. Doppman JL, Dunnick NR, Girton M, Fauci AS, Popovsky M: Bile duct cysts secondary to liver infarction. Radiology 130:1–5, 1979.

296. White TJ, Leevy CM, Brusca AM, Guassi AM: The liver in congestive heart failure. Am Heart J 49:250–257, 1955.

297. Holley HC, Koslin DB, Berland LL, Stanley RJ: Inhomogeneous enhancement of liver parenchyma secondary to passive congestion: contrast-enhanced CT. Radiology 170:795–800, 1989.

298. Moulton JS, Miller BL, Dodd GDI, Vu DN: Passive hepatic congestion in heart failure: CT abnormalities. AJR 151:939–942, 1988.

299. Koslin DB, Stanley RJ, Berland LL, et al: Hepatic perivascular lymphedema: CT appearance. AJR 150:111–113, 1988.

300. Toombs BD, Sandler CM: Acute abdominal trauma. In Toombs BD, Sandler CM (eds): Computed Tomography in Trauma. Philadelphia, WB Saunders, 1987.

301. Moore FA, Moore EE, Seagraves AS: Nonresectional management of major hepatic trauma. Am J Surg 150:725–729, 1985.

302. Trunkey DD, Shires GT, McClelland R: Management of liver trauma in 811 consecutive patients. Ann Surg 179:722–728, 1974.

303. Defore WW, Mattox KL, Jordan GL, et al: Management of 1,590 consecutive cases of liver trauma. Arch Surg 111:493–496, 1976.

304. Moon KL, Federle MP: Computed tomography in hepatic trauma. AJR 141:309–314, 1983.

305. Haney PJ, Whitley NO, Brotman S, Cunat JS, Whitley J: Liver injury and complications in the postoperative trauma patient: CT evaluation. AJR 139:271–275, 1982.

306. Foley WD, Cates JD, Kellman GM, et al: Treatment of blunt hepatic injuries: role of CT. Radiology 164:635–638, 1987.

307. Mirvis SE, Whitley NO, Vainwright JR, Gens DR: Blunt hepatic trauma in adults: CT-based classification and correlation with prognosis and treatment. Radiology 171:27–32, 1989.

308. Federle MP, Jeffrey RB: Hemoperitoneum studied by computed tomography. Radiology 148:187–192, 1983.

309. Federle MP: Computed tomography of blunt abdominal trauma. Radiol Clin North Am 21:461–476, 1983.

310. Savolaine ER, Grecos GP, Howard J, White P: Evolution of CT findings in hepatic hematoma. J Comput Assist Tomogr 9:1090–1096, 1985.

311. Mirvis SE, Whitley NO: Computed tomography in hepatobiliary trauma. In Ferrucci JT, Mathieu DG (eds): Advances in Hepatobiliary Radiology. St Louis, CV Mosby, 1990.

312. Federle MP: CT of upper abdominal trauma. Semin Roentgenol 19:269–280, 1984.

313. Kelly J, Raptopoulos V, Davidoff A, Waite R, Norton P: The value of non–contrast-enhanced CT in blunt abdominal trauma. AJR 152:41–46, 1989.

314. Esensten M, Ralls PW, Colletti P, Halls J: Posttraumatic intrahepatic biloma: sonographic diagnosis. AJR 140:303–305, 1983.

315. Vazquez JL, Thorsen MK, Dodds WJ, et al: Evaluation and treatment of intraabdominal bilomas. AJR 144:933–938, 1985.

316. Panicek DM, Paquet DJ, Clark KG, Urrutia EJ, Brinsko RE: Hepatic parenchymal gas after blunt trauma. Radiology 159:343–344, 1986.

317. Foley WD, Berland LL, Lawson TL, Maddison FE: Computed tomography in the demonstration of hepatic pseudoaneu-

rysm with hemobilia. J Comput Assist Tomogr 4:863–865, 1980.

318. Hoiem L, Kvam G: Arterio-portal fistula diagnosed by computerized tomography. Eur J Radiol 1:57–59, 1981.

319. Mathieu D, Larde D, Vasile N: CT features of iatrogenic hepatic arterioportal fistulae. J Comput Assist Tomogr 7:810–814, 1983.

320. Axel L, Moss AA, Berninger W: Dynamic computed tomog-

raphy demonstration of hepatic arteriovenous fistula. J Comput Assist Tomogr 5:95–98, 1981.

321. Gomori J, Grossman RI, Goldberg HI, et al: Intracranial hematomas: imaging by high-field MR. Radiology 157:87–93, 1985.

322. Unger EC, Glazer HS, Lee JKT, Ling D: MRI of extracranial hematomas: preliminary observations. AJR 146:403–407, 1986.

CHAPTER 18

THE BILIARY TRACT

RICHARD L. BARON

Indications

Although nonobstructive abnormalities of the biliary tract can be identified, computed tomography (CT) of the biliary tree most often involves three basic questions: (1) Is biliary obstruction present? (2) If obstruction is present, what is the etiology? and (3) What is the stage (extent) of the disease process present? CT is highly accurate in indicating the presence or absence of biliary obstruction, correctly differentiating obstructed from nonobstructed bile ducts in 93 per cent of patients in one large series.[1] In addition, CT can predict the level and etiology of biliary obstruction in the majority of cases.[1, 2] In a manner similar to that of ultrasound, false-negative and false-positive diagnoses can occur, owing to obstruction without dilatation and dilatation without obstruction. In addition, the presence of diffuse fatty changes in the liver can obscure dilated intrahepatic bile ducts.[3] Relative disadvantages for routine use of CT in evaluating the biliary tract include the need for intravenous contrast, cost relative to other types of examinations, and ease of performing other examinations such as portable ultrasound. Although ultrasonography is the screening examination of choice in most evaluations of the biliary tract, certain patient populations can be more efficiently screened with CT. In patients in whom there is a strong clinical suggestion that an underlying malignancy is causing biliary obstruction (elderly patients with markedly abnormal liver function tests and a strong clinical suggestion of malignant disease), CT will more efficiently assist diagnosis and staging of the extent of potential disease.[1] Many patients are not optimal candidates for ultrasonographic evaluation, particularly obese patients or those with prominent bowel loops that obscure distal bile ducts. For planning therapeutic procedures, presentation of the entire abdomen in cross section on a CT scan is easy to comprehend and affords a reproducible method for follow-up evaluation. For this same reason, CT is often helpful in evaluating confusing findings seen in ultrasonography or cholangiography.

There have been few investigations into the efficacy of MR in evaluating the biliary tract.[4-7] Magnetic resonance (MR) can show the abnormal biliary tree and extrahepatic bile ducts in many situations[8] and can image gallstones in vitro and in vivo with great sensitivity.[9-11] However, the value of magnetic resonance imaging (MRI) of biliary tract disease in clinical situations remains mostly unproved.

Special Techniques

Although CT techniques used for the biliary tract are similar to those used for evaluating the liver, there are certain techniques that can optimize biliary tract delineation. The hallmark of the CT appearance in diagnosis of biliary obstruction has been the presence of dilated intrahepatic and extrahepatic biliary ducts. Intrahepatic duct dilatation can usually be demonstrated on noncontrast CT as low-attenuation branching structures, but minimal dilatation requires the use of intravenous contrast material to increase liver attenuation and to avoid mistaking portal venous structures for dilated biliary ducts. Although with older equipment, normal intrahepatic bile ducts generally were not visible, with the high resolution now available in the current generation of CT scanners, normal intrahepatic bile ducts can be visualized on dynamic contrast–enhanced images in 40 per cent of patients (Fig. 18–1). Merely the presence of small intrahepatic ducts does not indicate obstruction.[12] These normal intrahepatic ducts do not exceed 3 mm in diameter, are usually between 1.5 and 2 mm, and are seen as small, scattered structures that are not confluent. Whereas these features can help differentiate normal ducts from those that are obstructed, certain disease processes remain problematic. Sclerosing cholangitis and obstructive diseases that are superimposed on cirrhosis may not show confluent intrahepatic dilatation.[13–15] In addition, early in the course of biliary obstruction, the intrahepatic ducts do not dilate (animal studies suggest that it takes more than 4 days after complete occlusion for intrahepatic dilatation to occur).[16] Extrahepatic bile duct dilatation usually occurs earlier in the course of obstruction. Normal extrahepatic bile ducts are seen on CT in 67 to 80 per cent of normal patients[17] and usually are 8 mm or less in diameter.[18] Using the short axis of the duct for measurements avoids artificially increasing the diameter owing to the oblique course of the duct.[18, 19] As with use of ultrasonography, because of dilatation without obstruction and obstruction without dilatation, these findings are guidelines, not absolutes. Although biliary contrast agents have been reported to be helpful in conjunction with CT of the biliary tract,[20, 21] they have not generally been found useful. Rarely, when the question of localizing confusing low-attenuation structures within the porta hepatis or pancreas is indicated, such opacification can be of assistance. Similarly, CT examinations following cholangiographic instillation of contrast material can be helpful in delineating ductal structures from other low-attenuation masses or collections. Conversely, CT images in such situations may also clarify confusing cholangiographic appearances.

By obtaining sequential images through the liver, porta hepatis, and pancreas, the longitudinal course of the extrahepatic bile ducts can be translated on sequential axial images into sequential near–water-attenuation circles.[2, 22] Normally, these show gradual tapering as the duct approaches the ampulla of Vater. The disease processes that affect the cholangiographic appearance of the bile ducts produce similar changes on the cross-sectional images, and it is the ability to understand these changes that allows accurate diagnoses with use of CT scans. For example, abrupt termination of the duct is a characteristic cholangiographic sign of malignancy, and this can similarly be demonstrated on CT images (Figs. 18–2 and 18–3).[2, 23] In contrast, patients with a nonobstructed duct or a benign stricture usually demonstrate a gradual tapering of the distal duct at both cholangiography and axial CT sections (Figs. 18–2

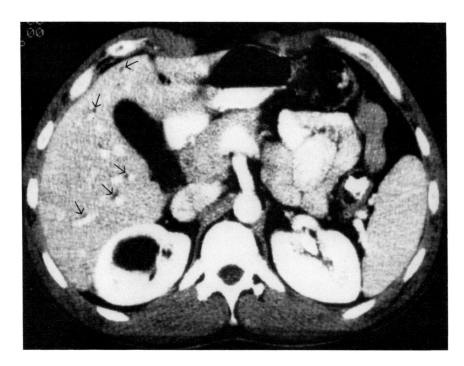

FIGURE 18–1 ■ Normal intrahepatic bile ducts. Contrast-enhanced CT scan shows normal bile ducts as small, low-attenuation structures (*arrows*) adjacent to portal venous radicles. (From Rohrman CA Jr, Baron RL: Radiol Clin North Am 27:93–104, 1989.)

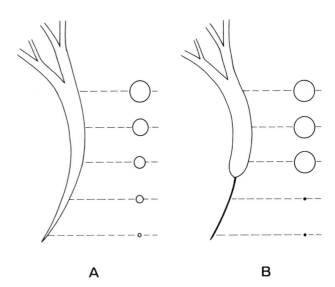

FIGURE 18–2 ■ Line drawings demonstrating correlation of cholangiography and serial transaxial images of the common bile duct (CBD) in normal patients or patients with mild dilatation from a benign stricture (A) and those with pancreatic carcinoma (B). With benign strictures (A), the most common cholangiographic pattern of gradual tapering correlates on axial images to circles of gradually decreasing diameter. Pancreatic carcinoma (B) more typically causes abrupt termination of the CBD, resulting in a sudden loss of visualization of the duct circles on axial images. (From Rohrman CA Jr, Baron RL: Radiol Clin North Am 27:93–104, 1989.)

A   B

and 18–4). Evaluation of the duct wall just proximal to the level of biliary obstruction may show specific features of thickening of the duct wall that can provide clues to the underlying cause of obstruction.[17] Utilizing these criteria for scanning to diagnose malignancy requires obtaining scans at close intervals through the transition zone of duct visualization so as not to miss a region of gradual tapering or subtle evidence of ductal calculi. We usually obtain scans at 3- to 5-mm intervals, with 3- to 5-mm collimation through the transition zone, using a small field of view. These techniques increase the detection rates of subtle, small pancreatic neoplasms that do not enlarge the pancreatic head, and they increase the ability to demonstrate the finding of a duct stone missed on the initial scans.

Other technical factors can greatly affect CT images of the biliary tract and must be optimized for each patient and each clinical situation. When evaluating for biliary tract stone disease, maximal kVp should be utilized, since this will optimize visualization of cholesterol gallstones[24] that demonstrate maximal attenuation using high kVp technique. Use of reconstructed small-field-of-view images also increases resolution of duct detail and should be used rather than magnification images. When conditions strongly suggest that a stone is present in the common bile duct (CBD), oral contrast should be withheld so as not to obscure a stone impacted at the ampulla of Vater. In these cases, an effervescent agent may be used to distend the duodenum.

Anatomy

CT

The intrahepatic peripheral bile ducts course in the portal triad with the portal veins and hepatic arteries. Normal peripheral intrahepatic bile ducts are visible, with the high resolution available with the current generation of scanners, as small intrahepatic lucen-

cies measuring 1 to 3 mm in diameter and are seen adjacent to contrast-enhancing portal venous radicles (see Fig. 18–2). Normal bile ducts, when visualized, are seen as random, scattered structures, and the course of normal intrahepatic bile ducts cannot be ascertained on CT until the right and left hepatic ducts are seen near the liver hilus. These two main bile ducts exit from the liver and join in the right side of the porta hepatis to form the common hepatic duct (Fig. 18–5). In contrast, the obstructed biliary tree will usually demonstrate either a more confluent appearance of the ducts or more generalized, ordered visualization of minimally dilated ducts (see Fig. 18–3).

The common hepatic duct is a thin-walled structure 3 to 6 mm in diameter, located anterolateral to the portal vein in the porta hepatis, best appreciated after intravenous contrast administration. In 66 per cent of patients, the common hepatic duct is visualized as a separate, distinct structure[17] lying anterior to the portal vein and lateral to the hepatic artery (see Fig. 18–3B). With central low attenuation of bile, the wall is usually thin, less than 1.5 mm thick.[17] Occasionally, the cystic duct can be seen paralleling the common hepatic duct as they course within the hepatoduodenal ligament.[25]

The CBD often has a slightly larger diameter than the common hepatic duct, generally up to 8 mm, although it occasionally is larger in normal patients.[18] The CBD initially courses in the free edge of the lesser omentum (hepatoduodenal ligament) then lies behind the first duodenum, sloping away from the portal vein. The final course of this duct lies either within the pancreatic parenchyma (Fig. 18–5C to E) or within a groove on the posterior surface, where it joins the main pancreatic duct in the ampulla of Vater.[26] Because of its vertical course, the CBD is more often seen on CT than the hepatic duct and is visualized on CT in 82 per cent of patients, being best appreciated on contrast-enhanced images as a low-attenuation structure against the contrast-en-

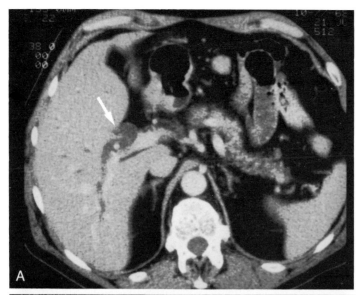

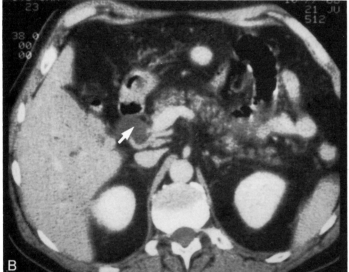

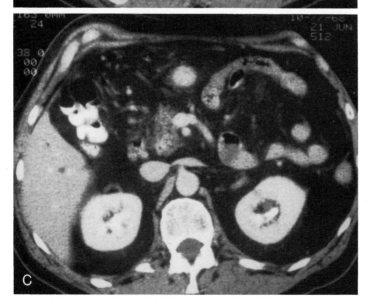

FIGURE 18–3 ■ Pancreatic carcinoma. *A,* Scattered intrahepatic bile ducts that in some ways resemble normal ducts are seen (as in Fig. 18–1), but the confluent intrahepatic duct dilatation shown *(arrows)* is indicative of the obstructive abnormality. In addition, the diffuse nature of the ductal dilatation, in contrast to random visualization, is abnormal. *B,* Scan 2 cm lower than *A* shows dilatation of the suprapancreatic common bile duct *(arrow). C,* Scan 1 cm lower than *B* reveals abrupt loss of visualization of the duct. Despite normal appearance of the pancreatic head, this is highly suggestive of pancreatic carcinoma. At surgery a 1.5 cm pancreatic carcinoma was found.

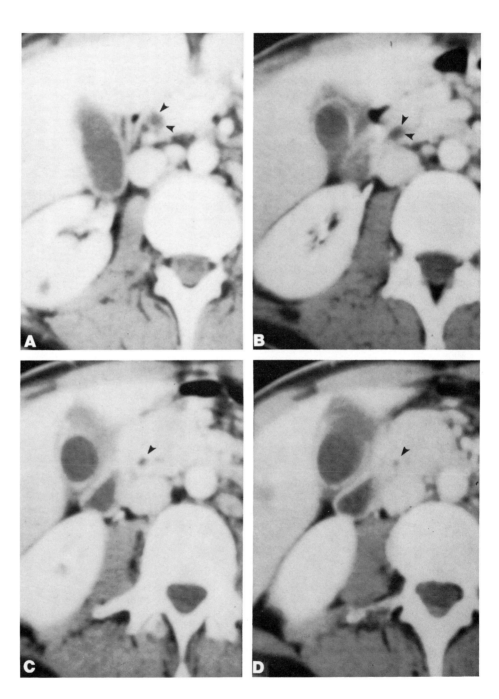

FIGURE 18–4 ■ Benign stricture of the common bile duct secondary to chronic pancreatitis. *A* to *D,* Serial CT images demonstrate biliary ductal dilatation, greatest proximally. There is progressive gradual narrowing of the distal common bile duct *(arrowheads)* as it traverses the pancreatic head, which is focally enlarged from chronic pancreatitis. (From Rohrmann CA Jr, Baron RL: Radiol Clin North Am 27:93–104, 1989.)

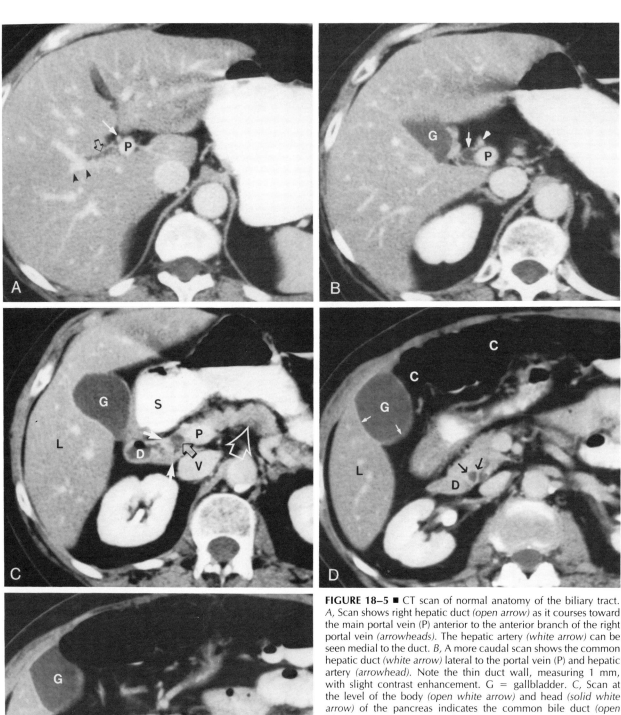

FIGURE 18–5 ■ CT scan of normal anatomy of the biliary tract. *A,* Scan shows right hepatic duct *(open arrow)* as it courses toward the main portal vein (P) anterior to the anterior branch of the right portal vein *(arrowheads).* The hepatic artery *(white arrow)* can be seen medial to the duct. *B,* A more caudal scan shows the common hepatic duct *(white arrow)* lateral to the portal vein (P) and hepatic artery *(arrowhead).* Note the thin duct wall, measuring 1 mm, with slight contrast enhancement. G = gallbladder. *C,* Scan at the level of the body *(open white arrow)* and head *(solid white arrow)* of the pancreas indicates the common bile duct *(open black arrow)* as a structure having an attenuation value close to that of water, surrounded by the parenchyma of the pancreas. The duodenum (D), lateral to this, also contains fluid and can simulate the bile duct at times. The relationships of the gallbladder (G) to the liver (L) and antrum of the stomach (S) are well demonstrated on CT.

D, A scan more caudal to *C,* through the head of the pancreas, shows the common bile duct, which has a thin, enhancing duct wall *(black arrows).* The adjacent duodenum (D) lies posterior to the head of the pancreas and duct. The gallbladder (G) wall shows similar normal contrast enhancement *(white arrows)* as it abuts the liver (L) and transverse colon (C). *E,* Scan just proximal to the ampulla shows an oblique course of the common bile duct *(black arrows)* as it passes posterior to and lateral to the duodenum. The enhancing wall helps identify this structure as duct. G = gallbladder.

hanced pancreatic parenchyma. The duct wall is often identified in this region, measuring 1.5 mm or less in thickness. Contrast enhancement of the duct wall is a normal finding and should not be construed as indicative of pathology.[17]

The gallbladder is well seen when it is distended as an oval sac of near-water density lying in a fossa along the inferior hepatic surface (see Fig. 18–5B to E). The wall of the gallbladder is thin (1 to 2 mm) when seen in profile and may enhance after intravenous contrast administration. If the gallbladder (G) is folded on itself, the normal wall may appear in cross section and simulate a rimmed gallstone (Fig. 18–6). The relationship of the gallbladder to the liver, anterior abdominal wall, duodenum, colon, right kidney, and stomach are readily displayed by axial CT images. Occasionally, the cystic duct can be identified as a separate structure coursing between the gallbladder and the common hepatic duct.

MRI

Nondilated peripheral intrahepatic bile ducts are not visualized on MR images, although the distal left and right hepatic ducts can occasionally be seen just proximal to the porta hepatis. When dilated, the intrahepatic ducts appear as branching structures of low signal intensity on T1-weighted images and high signal intensity on T2-weighted images (Fig. 18–7).[6] The normal extrahepatic bile ducts are best depicted on T2-weighted axial images and can be seen in 50 per cent of normal patients. The ducts are seen in cross section and follow the signal intensity patterns of near-water fluid collections, being dark on T1-weighted sequences and very bright on T2-weighted images (Figs. 18–8 and 18–9). Despite the usual better

anatomic definition on T1-weighted spin-echo images, the extrahepatic bile ducts are seen less often owing to poorer contrast resolution.[8] No studies have been published to establish the normal size of the common hepatic duct or CBD as seen on MR, although the size should not differ significantly from that seen on CT or ultrasonography, and a maximal cross-sectional diameter in most patients is less than 8 mm. Coursing through the hepatoduodenal ligament, the common hepatic duct can be seen in cross section anterolateral to the portal vein and medial to the hepatic artery. More distally, it is often identified as it courses either through or dorsal to the pancreatic head, just proximal to the ampulla. The duct appears darker than pancreatic parenchyma on T1-weighted images and is significantly brighter on T2-weighted images.[8]

As on CT scans, the gallbladder is easily identified on MR images, usually along the inferior surface of the liver. The MR signal intensity of the liver varies with the fasting state of the patient.[27] Fresh, nonconcentrated bile shows signal intensities similar to other fluid collections, appearing hypointense or isointense with liver on T1-weighted images and hyperintense on T2-weighted images (Figs. 18–8 and 18–9).[11, 27] However, concentrated gallbladder bile seen in fasting patients appears hyperintense compared with liver on T1-weighted images. Demas and colleagues,[28] using proton MR spectroscopy, showed that the increase in signal intensity in concentrated bile is caused by water proton T1 and T2 shortening and not by a contribution from lipid signal. Often a fluid-fluid level can be seen, with the concentrated bile in the dependent portion of the gallbladder appearing hyperintense and fresh bile, above it, appearing hypointense (see Fig. 18–8B).

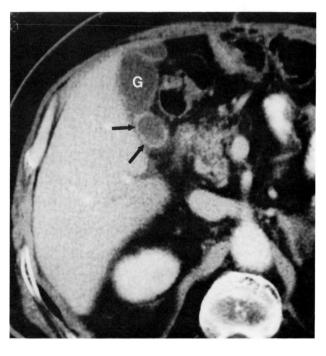

FIGURE 18–6 ■ Gallbladder fold simulating a gallstone. The gallbladder (G) is folded on itself, and the cross-section appearance of the proximal gallbladder wall (arrows) simulates a rimmed gallstone.

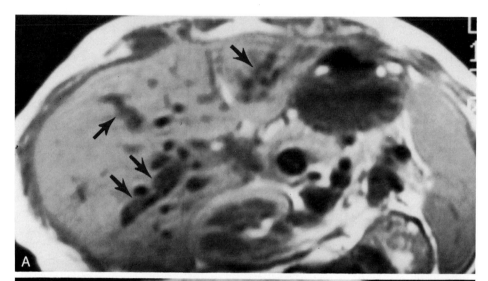

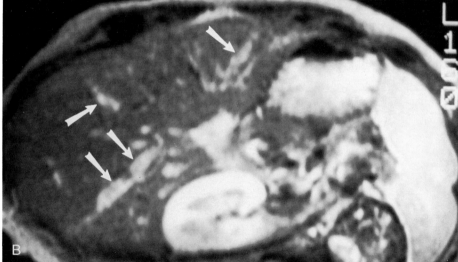

FIGURE 18–7 ■ MR appearance of dilated intrahepatic bile ducts due to cholangiocarcinoma. *A*, T1-weighted MR image shows intrahepatic vascular structures as radiating areas of signal void. The dilated bile ducts appear as regions of low signal intensity *(arrows)*, but the intensity is higher than that of adjacent portal venous radicles. *B*, T2-weighted image at the same level shows the ducts *(arrows)* as high signal intensity. The use of flow compensation techniques also displays vessels with high signal intensity, which can make it difficult to detect dilated bile ducts.

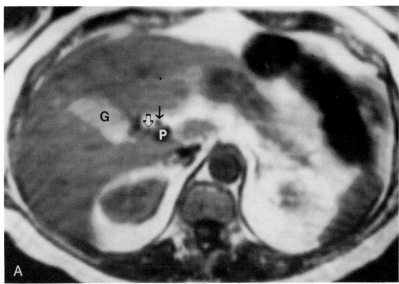

FIGURE 18–8 ■ T1-weighted MRI of normal anatomy of the biliary tract. *A,* Scan at the level of the porta hepatis shows concentrated bile in the gallbladder (G) with high signal intensity. Anterior to the portal vein (P) are the common hepatic duct *(open arrow)* and hepatic artery *(solid arrow),* both of low signal intensity. *B,* In another patient, a more caudal scan, at the level of the body of the pancreas (Pa), shows the low-intensity common bile duct *(open arrow)* posterior to and lateral to the portal vein (P) in the suprapancreatic region. The gallbladder (G) demonstrates a fluid-fluid level *(solid arrows)* with fresh bile layering superiorly with low signal intensity and concentrated bile of high signal intensity in the dependent portion. V = inferior vena cava. *C,* Scan at the level of the head of the pancreas shows the distal common bile duct *(open arrow)* as low intensity, surrounded by the higher-intensity pancreatic parenchyma. G = gallbladder; P = portal vein; V = inferior vena cava.

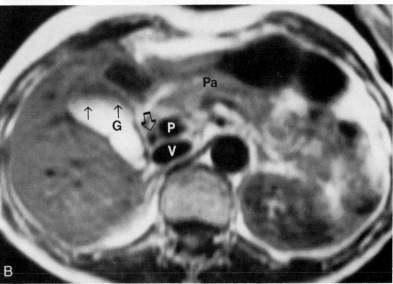

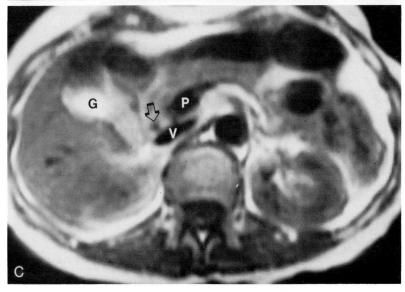

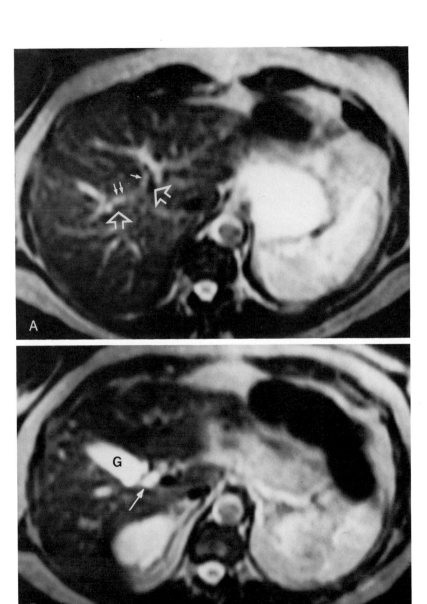

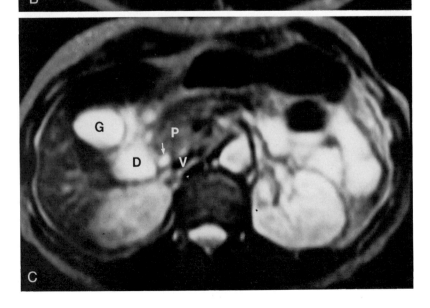

FIGURE 18–9 ■ T2-weighted MRI of normal anatomy of the biliary tract. (Flow compensation technique increases signal intensity of vessels flowing in the direction of the plane of section). *A,* Scan at the level of the confluence of the right *(double arrows)* and left *(single arrow)* hepatic ducts, anterior to portal venous branches *(open arrows). B,* Scan at the level of the porta hepatis shows high signal intensity within the gallbladder (G) and the common hepatic duct *(arrow). C,* Scan at the level of the head of the pancreas (P) shows the distal common bile duct *(arrow)* with high signal intensity. G = gallbladder; D = duodenum; V = inferior vena cava.

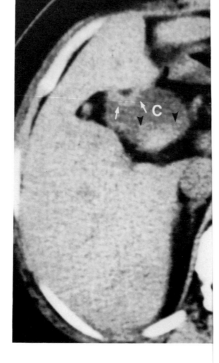

FIGURE 18–12 ■ Cholangiocarcinoma in a choledochal cyst. The cyst (C) contains material of high attenuation *(arrowheads)* layering in the dependent portion as a result of prior administration of an oral cholecystographic agent. Focal wall thickening *(arrows)* is due to cholangiocarcinoma. (From Montana MA, Rohrmann CA Jr: Cholangiocarcinoma in a choledochal cyst: preoperative diagnosis. AJR 147:516–517, 1986. © by Williams and Wilkins.)

Congenital Abnormalities

Gallbladder

Congenital anomalies of the gallbladder are rare. The most common presentation is that of a positional variant. The gallbladder can be seen in the left abdomen, suprahepaticly, intrahepaticly (Fig. 18–10), retrorenally, and in other rare locations.[29] Duplication of the gallbladder and cystic duct occurs rarely, but usually in close proximity.[30]

Bile Ducts

Cystic diseases of the biliary tree include choledochal cysts, choledochoceles, CBD diverticula, and Caroli's disease.

CHOLEDOCHAL CYSTS

True choledochal cysts represent focal dilatation of the extrahepatic bile duct. The dilatation may be mild (and may simulate a duct dilated as a result of obstruction), or it may exceed diameters seen with ducts dilated owing to obstruction (up to 15 cm in diameter).[31] The dilatation may occur only in the extrahepatic ducts or may also be accompanied by central intrahepatic dilatation. The CT scan appearance is that of a large, near–water density mass in the porta hepatis contiguous with the proximal and distal ductal system (Fig. 18–11). The clue to the diagnosis is a marked disparity between the extrahepatic and intrahepatic duct dilatation, making biliary obstruction and subsequent duct dilatation less likely. Other cystic lesions in the region of the porta hepatis (hepatic and pancreatic cystic lesions, fluid collections, and enteric duplication cysts) may be confused with these lesions. In these instances, administration of a biliary contrast agent may demonstrate accumulation of contrast in choledochal cysts and confirm the diagnosis (Fig. 18–12).[32]

MR imaging demonstrates anatomic changes similar to those seen on CT. The MR signal intensity within the choledochal cyst corresponds to that of fluid with low signal intensity on T1-weighted images and high intensity on T2-weighted images.[33]

Secondary complications of stone disease and biliary tract carcinoma should be sought on scans in all patients with this disorder. In one series, CT detected 8 gallbladder and bile duct carcinomas in 35 cases being followed.[34] The malignancies appeared as either a soft tissue attenuation mass lesion or irregular thickening of the bile duct or cyst wall (see Fig. 18–12).[34]

CHOLEDOCHOCELES

Choledochoceles (also referred to as type III choledochal cysts) represent focal dilatation of the distal CBD, which protrudes into the wall and lumen of the duodenum. Analogous to ureteroceles, they have a characteristic appearance at cholangiography. These are difficult to diagnose on CT scans or ultrasonography studies unless they are large and appear as well-circumscribed, near–water density masses in the wall or lumen of the duodenum (Fig. 18–13).[35, 36] Even then, they are often indistinguishable from other pancreatic-duodenal cystic lesions. Administration of a biliary contrast agent may be helpful in suggesting the correct diagnosis. Choledocholithiasis may be seen in association with choledochocele and may be demonstrated on CT images as small foci of higher attenuation (soft tissue or high attenuation) within the choledochocele.

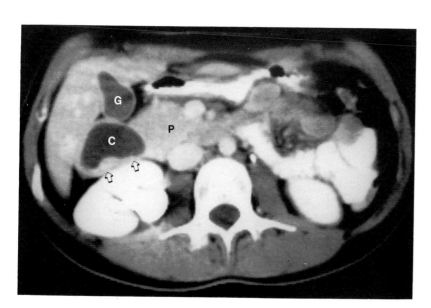

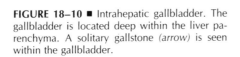

FIGURE 18–13 ■ Choledochocele (C) appears as a ho... water attenuation lying adjace... pancreas (P) and spreading ... *(open arrows)* at the level of th...

FIGURE 18–10 ■ Intrahepatic gallbladder. The gallbladder is located deep within the liver parenchyma. A solitary gallstone *(arrow)* is seen within the gallbladder.

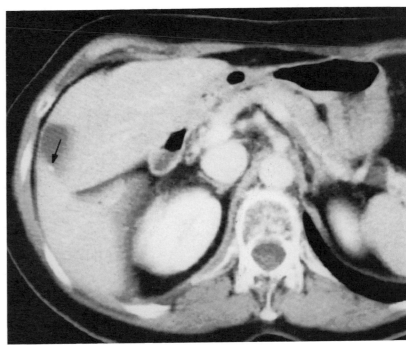

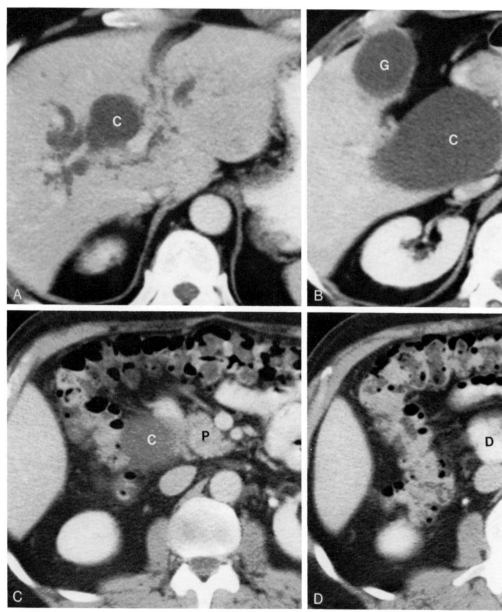

FIGURE 18–11 ■ Choledochal cyst. *A,* Contrast-enhanced CT scan shows the contiguity of the dilated intrahepa[...] proximal portion of the choledochal cyst (C). The cyst appears as a large mass having an attenuation value close to t[...] position of the extrahepatic bile duct. No significant soft tissue attenuation components are seen. *B,* Scan inferior to [...] of the cyst (C) as it approaches the pancreas (P). G = gallbladder.

C, Scan at the level of the head of the pancreas (P) shows a smaller diameter of the cyst (C) as a result of taperin[...] ampulla. *D,* Scan 1 cm inferior to C shows a normal head of pancreas (P) and duodenum (D), without residual c[...] level of the ampulla.

CAROLI'S DISEASE

Caroli's disease is a rare congenital abnormality characterized by segmental dilatation of the intrahepatic bile ducts. It is almost always associated with cystic lesions of the kidney.[37, 38] CT demonstrates multiple low-attenuation cystic lesions throughout the liver in these patients (Fig. 18–14). Although these often simulate polycystic liver disease, CT scans can often demonstrate the branching nature of these lesions and the contiguity with dilated intrahepatic bile ducts that accompany this condition. As with other cystic lesions of the biliary tree, administration of a biliary contrast agent prior to CT scanning may demonstrate contiguity of these lesions with the biliary tree and confirm the diagnosis.[39] The abnormal, dilated bile ducts may surround the accompanying portal vein radicles. On CT this can create the appearance of a central dot within the center of low attenuation or cystic-appearing masses, proposed as pathognomonic of Caroli's disease.[40] Associated intrahepatic stone disease is often present and visualized on CT images as well.

Gallbladder Disease

Adenomyomatosis

Adenomyomatosis refers to abnormalities of the gallbladder characterized by hyperplastic changes, which may involve overgrowth of the mucosa, thickening of the muscle wall, or development of intramural diverticula or sinus tracts (Rokitansky-Aschoff sinuses).[41] The abnormality may be diffuse, segmental, or localized. When it is segmental, it usually occurs in the fundus of the gallbladder.[42] Although it can be diagnosed more readily with oral cholecystography or ultrasonography,[42, 43] nonspecific gallbladder wall thickening can be seen on CT (Fig. 18–15). Visualization on CT scans of the Rokitansky-Aschoff sinuses has been reported only when scans

were performed in conjunction with an oral cholecystogram.[44]

Neoplasms

Gallbladder Carcinoma

Gallbladder carcinoma is an uncommon malignancy, representing 1 to 3 per cent of malignancies at autopsy.[45] It occurs primarily in the sixth and seventh decades of life and is four to five times more common in women.[46, 47] Gallstones and chronic cholecystitis are found in 65 to 95 per cent of patients with carcinoma of the gallbladder.[48, 49] Patients with calcification of the gallbladder wall (porcelain gallbladder) also have an increased incidence of carcinoma of the gallbladder (Fig. 18–16).[50, 51] Approximately 90 per cent of carcinomas of the gallbladder are adenocarcinomas, although, rarely, squamous cell carcinoma, adenosquamous carcinoma, anaplastic carcinoma, or sarcomas can be found.[52]

CT

The most common finding on CT scans in gallbladder carcinoma is that of a mass replacing the gallbladder lumen (Fig. 18–17), less common appearances being eccentric thickening of the gallbladder wall (Fig. 18–18) and the presence of a focal mass protruding into the gallbladder lumen (Fig. 18–19).[47, 53–55] In rare cases, thickening of the gallbladder wall may be smooth and symmetric, simulating cholecystitis.[53] Often the mass or gallbladder wall shows marked contrast enhancement, but this can also be seen with cholecystitis and in normal patients and thus is not a differentiating feature. Intraluminal papillary carcinomas have been shown to have a better prognosis than the other patterns.[56]

CT depiction of tumoral extension and metastases may aid in making the diagnosis of gallbladder carcinoma, as well as staging the extent of disease (see

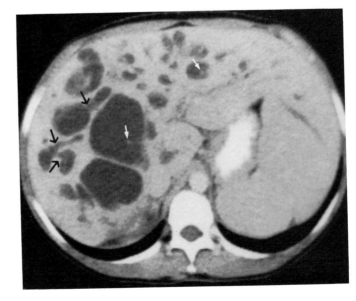

FIGURE 18–14 ■ Caroli's disease. Contrast-enhanced CT scan shows numerous cystic lesions throughout the liver, many of which can be seen in communication with dilated bile ducts *(black arrows)*. Some of these cysts contain a central dot *(white arrows)* thought to represent portal vein radicles.

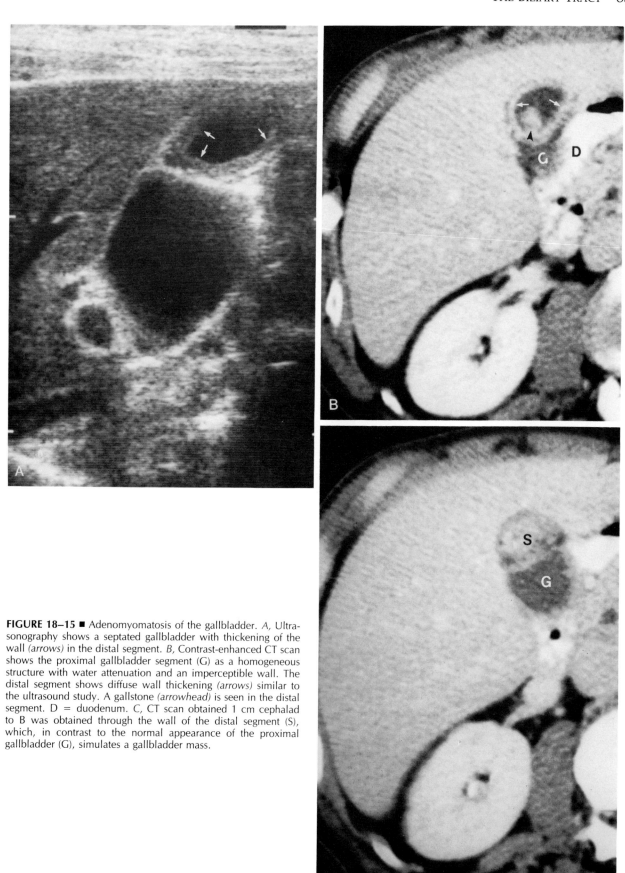

FIGURE 18–15 ■ Adenomyomatosis of the gallbladder. *A,* Ultrasonography shows a septated gallbladder with thickening of the wall *(arrows)* in the distal segment. *B,* Contrast-enhanced CT scan shows the proximal gallbladder segment (G) as a homogeneous structure with water attenuation and an imperceptible wall. The distal segment shows diffuse wall thickening *(arrows)* similar to the ultrasound study. A gallstone *(arrowhead)* is seen in the distal segment. D = duodenum. *C,* CT scan obtained 1 cm cephalad to B was obtained through the wall of the distal segment (S), which, in contrast to the normal appearance of the proximal gallbladder (G), simulates a gallbladder mass.

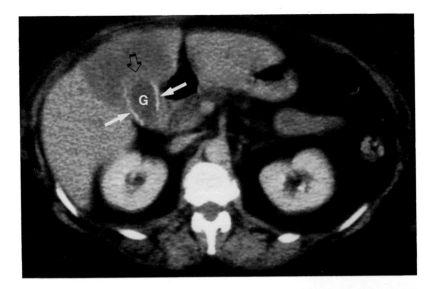

FIGURE 18–16 ■ Gallbladder carcinoma with porcelain gallbladder. The gallbladder (G) wall displays diffuse high attenuation *(solid arrows)*. In the fundus, the calcification is disrupted *(open arrow)* owing to gallbladder carcinoma, which has invaded the liver.

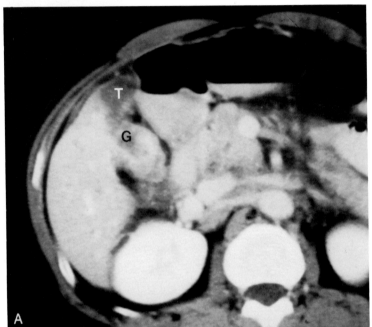

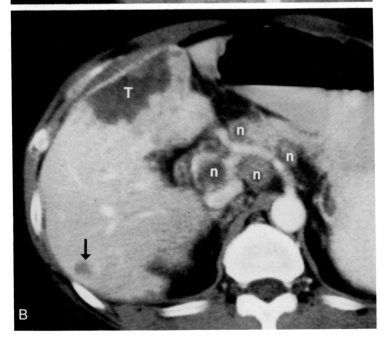

FIGURE 18–17 ■ Gallbladder carcinoma. *A,* Contrast-enhanced CT scan shows a heterogeneous mass replacing the gallbladder lumen (G). Adjacent tumor invasion (T) of the liver is of low attenuation compared with the adjacent liver parenchyma. *B,* Scan, more cephalad, shows the extent of direct tumor invasion (T) into the liver and a remote liver metastasis *(arrow).* Lymph node metastases (n) are seen throughout the porta hepatis.

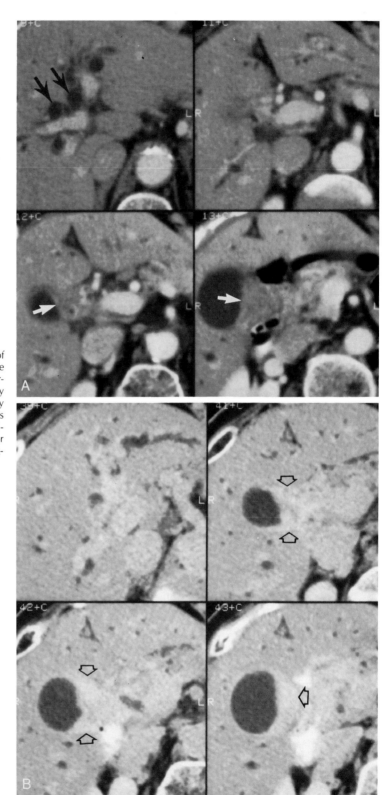

FIGURE 18–18 ■ Gallbladder carcinoma. *A,* A series of four contrast-enhanced images shows eccentric soft tissue attenuation thickening of the gallbladder wall *(white arrows)* and infiltration of the adjacent porta hepatis. Biliary obstruction from the tumor extension is characterized by dilated bile ducts seen only to the level of the porta hepatis *(black arrows)*. *B,* Series of four images delayed an additional 25 minutes shows delayed enhancement of the tumor *(open arrows)*, a feature often seen with biliary tract malignancies.

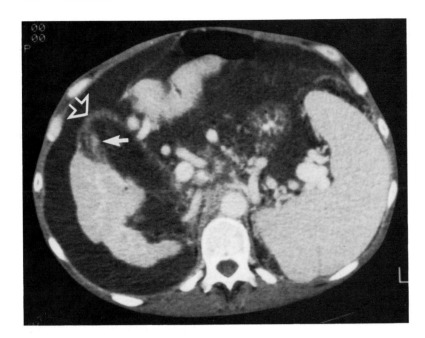

FIGURE 18–19 ■ Early gallbladder carcinoma in a patient with cirrhosis. Contrast-enhanced CT scan shows eccentric thickening of the gallbladder wall in the fundus *(open arrow)* with a small protruding intraluminal mass *(solid arrow)*.

Fig. 18–17).[55, 57] Direct tumoral extension into the liver is a frequent finding on CT; this has been reported to be uncommon with complicated cholecystitis and can thus be a differentiating feature.[58] Caution in using this criterion is recommended, however, since inflammatory gallbladder disease can occasionally extend into the liver parenchyma. Another differentiating feature can be tumoral extension to porta hepatis nodes, causing biliary obstruction at the porta hepatis (see Fig. 18–16). Lymph node drainage for these tumors extends through the hepatoduodenal ligament to the celiac and peripancreatic region and can result in a peripancreatic mass simulating pancreatic carcinoma. CT can also depict direct tumoral invasion into adjacent duodenum or colon, and peritoneal carcinomatosis can be seen in advanced cases.[57] CT has proved extremely accurate in detecting the extent of metastatic involvement, except for spread to peritoneal surfaces.[57] In some instances, the gallbladder carcinoma may be difficult to visualize, particularly when numerous gallstones are present, and when local adjacent liver invasion is present, it can simulate inflammatory gallbladder disease (see Fig. 18–21C).

MRI

The morphologic appearances of gallbladder carcinoma are similar on MRI and CT. The limited reports of MRI in gallbladder carcinoma have shown that MR can detect the tumor and depict the tumoral extent with high reliability.[7, 59] In all cases, the tumor appeared hypointense with adjacent liver parenchyma on T1-weighted images, and hyperintense on T2-weighted images. Gallstones are more frequently visualized on MRI than on CT and appear as low signal intensity structures, often trapped within the mass.[7] Although no direct comparison with CT has been made, anecdotal studies indicate that MR better

delineates direct liver invasion[7, 59] and tumoral extension to vascular structures in the hepatoduodenal ligament.[7]

Metastatic Disease

Rarely, the gallbladder can be involved with metastatic involvement. In one series, two thirds of these lesions were from melanoma,[60] and this has been our experience as well. Blood-borne metastases usually appear as focal thickening of the gallbladder wall or as focal protruding luminal masses (Fig. 18–20). Direct extension into the gallbladder can also occur from adjacent tumors, most often gastric and pancreatic tumors, although metastatic lesions in the porta hepatis can also extend into the gallbladder.

Cholecystolithiasis

CT

CT detects 74 to 79 per cent of gallstones,[61, 62] whereas the remainder are isodense with bile and are not visualized. Because of low detection sensitivity, cost, and use of ionizing radiation, CT is not a screening tool for cholecystolithiasis. However, because of its ability to characterize gallstones, in the future CT may play a role in predicting chemical composition of gallstones and in selecting patients for the variety of gallstone treatment options currently available.[61–64] In addition, CT is being used with increasing frequency in patients with underlying biliary tract pathology and can be critical in detecting and documenting stone disease of the gallbladder or CBD in these patients.

Gallstones can be categorized by their CT attenuation values and imaging patterns (Fig. 18–21). Homogeneously dense stones (>90 H), constitute 20 to 38 per cent of stones[61, 62] and are readily detected.

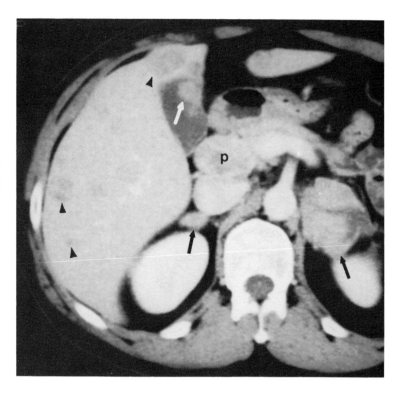

FIGURE 18–20 ■ Melanoma metastases to the gallbladder and liver. Metastasis appears as focal attenuation—a soft tissue mass *(white arrow)* protruding into the gallbladder lumen. Metastases to the liver *(arrowheads)*, a peripancreatic lymph node (p), and both adrenal glands *(black arrows)* are also seen.

Stones with a homogeneous attenuation slightly greater than bile (30 to 89 H) are termed faint or soft tissue density stones;[61, 62] these make up 21 to 26 per cent of stones. Rimmed stones, 17 to 32 per cent of stones, are those with a peripheral rim of higher CT attenuation surrounding a homogeneous lower-density center. More complex variations of lower and higher densities on CT scans can be seen in laminated stones (up to 14 per cent of stones). Stones isodense with bile and not visualized constitute 21 to 26 per cent of stones. Rarely, a stone will appear as homogeneously lower in density than bile. These stones are felt to represent calculi high in cholesterol content.[62] Rarely, gas located centrally within a gallbladder can be depicted on a CT scan.[65]

A gallbladder folded on itself may simulate a gallstone, giving the appearance of a rimmed stone within the gallbladder (see Fig. 18–6). Marked, eccentric, low-attenuation thickening of the gallbladder wall may simulate a fluid-filled gallbladder, with the higher attenuation mucosa appearing as a rimmed gallstone (Fig. 18–22). Ultrasonography can clarify both these situations and should be used when any uncertainty exists.

Although some investigators using CT have found a close correlation between gallstone attenuation value and chemical composition,[63, 66, 67] others have not.[61, 68] Several reports have shown a better correlation between gallstone attenuation and cholesterol than between attenuation and calcium content.[61, 68] It is the ability of CT to react to changes in cholesterol content that may be the determining factor in the appearance of gallstones on a CT scan. Cholesterol is one of the few compounds in the human body

that demonstrate maximal attenuation on CT scanning at high kV(p). Similarly, the majority of gallstones, composed predominantly of cholesterol, demonstrate maximal attenuation using the highest CT kVp source (140 kVp).[24] Thus, unlike plain film radiography, CT detection of gallstones is optimized using high kVp technique. When biliary tract stone detection is of concern, use of the highest kVp technique will increase CT visualization.

Some investigators use CT to select gallstones with high cholesterol content in order to predict successful gallstone dissolution with MTBE.[64, 69] Other sites use CT prior to gallstone lithotripsy as a means of predicting successful shock wave treatment.[70, 71] Although Ell and associates[71] found that with stones of attenuation ≤ 50 H, better stone fragmentation and eventual stone clearance following in vivo lithotripsy resulted, Franke and colleagues[72] found no difference in fragment clearance rates following lithotripsy. Whether CT will become an accepted tool for predicting outcome of these treatments awaits further investigation.

MRI

Early MR investigations utilizing low field strength scanners (0.2 to 0.35 tesla T) reported that the majority of gallstones were visualized as a signal void, with a small minority of gallstones demonstrating central foci of faint signal intensity.[9, 73] More recently, investigations at higher field strengths have reported a higher incidence of visualizing MR signals within gallstones (up to 73 per cent) and have shown a variety of gallstone patterns (Fig. 18–23).[10, 11] Unfortunately, MR images do not appear able to differen-

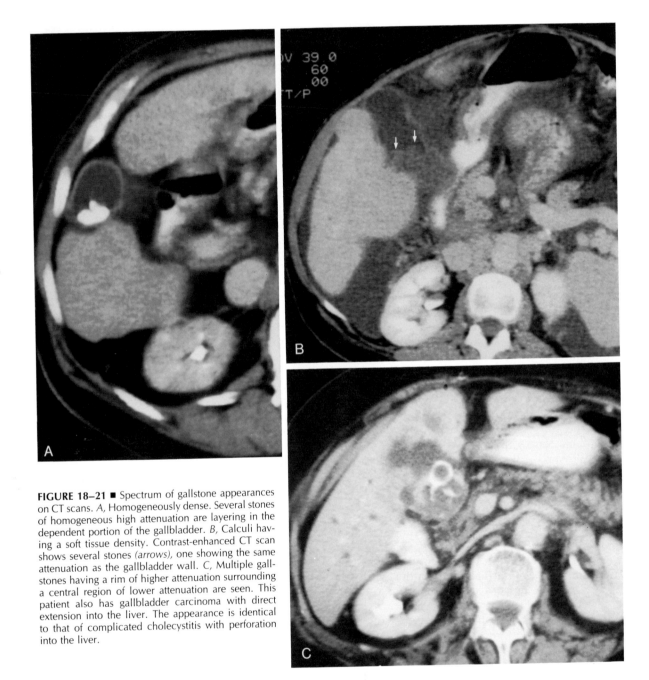

FIGURE 18–21 ■ Spectrum of gallstone appearances on CT scans. *A,* Homogeneously dense. Several stones of homogeneous high attenuation are layering in the dependent portion of the gallbladder. *B,* Calculi having a soft tissue density. Contrast-enhanced CT scan shows several stones *(arrows),* one showing the same attenuation as the gallbladder wall. *C,* Multiple gallstones having a rim of higher attenuation surrounding a central region of lower attenuation are seen. This patient also has gallbladder carcinoma with direct extension into the liver. The appearance is identical to that of complicated cholecystitis with perforation into the liver.

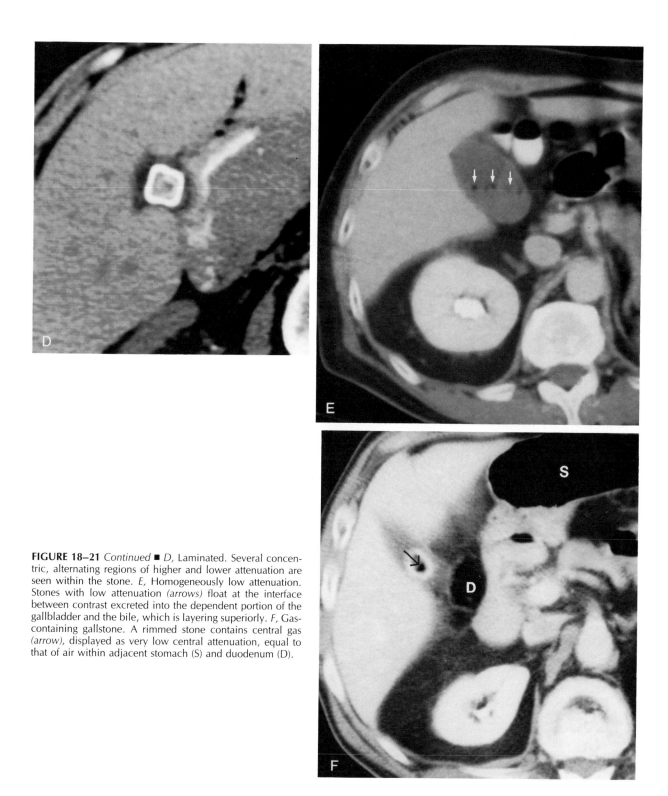

FIGURE 18–21 *Continued* ■ *D,* Laminated. Several concentric, alternating regions of higher and lower attenuation are seen within the stone. *E,* Homogeneously low attenuation. Stones with low attenuation *(arrows)* float at the interface between contrast excreted into the dependent portion of the gallbladder and the bile, which is layering superiorly. *F,* Gas-containing gallstone. A rimmed stone contains central gas *(arrow),* displayed as very low central attenuation, equal to that of air within adjacent stomach (S) and duodenum (D).

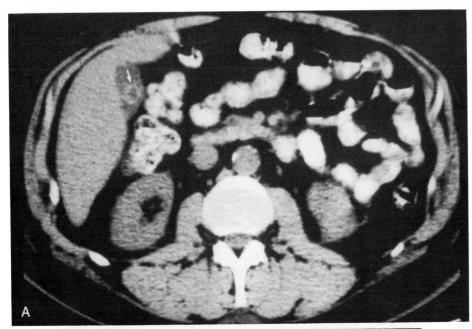

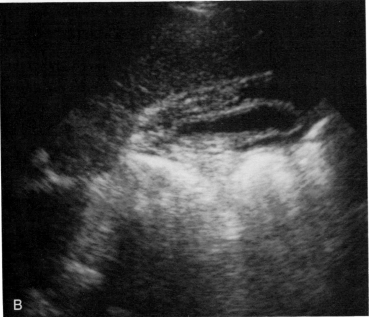

FIGURE 18–22 ■ Thickened gallbladder wall with gallbladder mucosa simulating a gallstone. A, The marked, eccentric low-attenuation thickening of the gallbladder wall in this patient with cirrhosis simulates a fluid-filled gallbladder, with the higher-attenuation mucosa *(arrow)* simulating a rimmed gallstone. The fact that the rimmed structure does not fall to the dependent portion of the gallbladder provides a clue to the correct diagnosis. B, Ultrasound examination confirms the marked and eccentric thickening of the gallbladder wall, with a striated wall pattern and large areas of sonolucency.

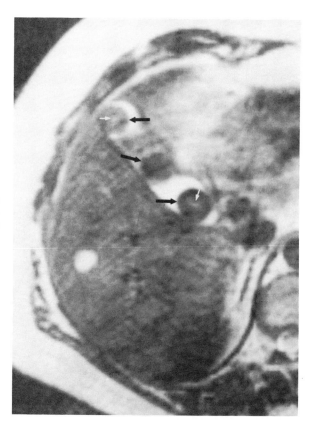

FIGURE 18–23 ■ MR imaging of gallstones. T1-weighted image shows three gallstones *(black arrows)* as low-intensity structures in contrast to the surrounding high-intensity bile. Central high signal intensity regions *(white arrows)* can be seen on T1-weighted images in many gallstones.

tiate among gallstone types. Gallstone MR signal is due to water with a shortened T1 relaxation time within gallstones and does not predict cholesterol content.[10]

Cholecystitis

CT

Although CT is not a screening tool for cholecystitis, sick patients with confusing presentations may undergo CT scanning as the initial diagnostic examination. It is important, therefore, to recognize the CT findings of acute or complicated cholecystitis. Indeed, in one series[74] of complicated cholecystitis, gallbladder disease was clinically suspected at presentation in only 7 of 23 patients.

The most common CT findings in cholecystitis are gallbladder wall thickening (> 3 mm) and cholelithiasis (Fig. 18–24).[75] These findings are not specific, however, and are often found with gallbladder carcinoma and hyperplastic cholecystosis. Other CT findings more suggestive of the diagnosis include an increased density of the bile (>20 H),[75, 76] loss of clear definition of the gallbladder wall (Fig. 18–25),[75] and gallbladder lumen dilatation. Although some authors have suggested that marked contrast enhancement of the gallbladder wall (Fig. 18–26) is indicative of cholecystitis,[77] this can also be seen in normal subjects and in other diseases.[78]

CT can detect changes suggestive of complicated cholecystitis, often as zones of low density within a thickened gallbladder wall or pericholecystic fluid collections (Fig. 18–25). A low attenuation halo around the gallbladder may be indicative of edema or minimal fluid collection and is a useful clue in differentiating complicated cholecystitis from carcinoma on CT.[58] Air within the gallbladder wall or lumen is indicative of emphysematous cholecystitis and is virtually pathognomonic of complicated cholecystitis (Fig. 18–26).[79] Still, many patients with gangrenous cholecystitis have a normal gallbladder appearance on CT. Air can also be seen in the gallbladder and bile ducts following catheterization procedures such as endoscopic retrograde cholangiopancreatography (ERCP), following surgical procedures such as sphincterotomy or bile duct anastomoses to bowel, and with fistulization from the gallbladder or bile ducts to bowel, whether posttraumatic, iatrogenic, from peptic ulcer disease, or with gallstone ileus (Fig. 18–27).

Benign gallbladder wall thickening on CT often is of low attenuation, and because of higher attenuation of the gallbladder mucosa, it may simulate fluid in the gallbladder bed (Fig. 18–28). Benign causes of wall thickening such as hepatitis and hypoalbuminemia may thus simulate cholecystitis with perforation.

Xanthogranulomatous cholecystitis is a rare inflammatory disease characterized histologically by foamy histiocytes, foreign body giant cells, and chronic inflammatory cells. The CT appearance of irregular gallbladder wall thickening, occasionally with calcification, and pericholecystic extension can simulate gallbladder carcinoma.[80–82]

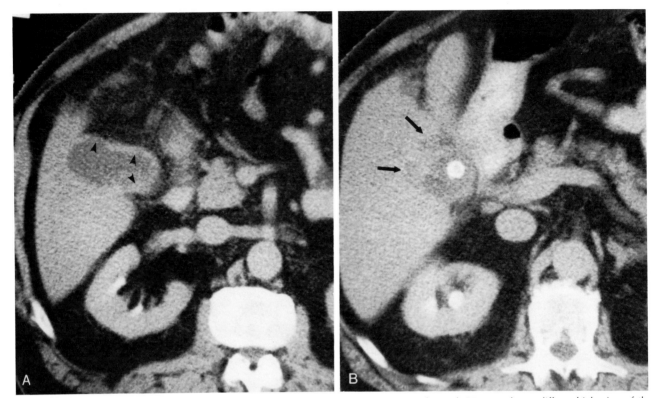

FIGURE 18–24 ■ Gangrenous cholecystitis with perforation into the liver. *A,* Contrast-enhanced CT scan shows diffuse thickening of the gallbladder wall *(arrowheads).* The bile is of higher attenuation here than normal bile and measured 30 H. *B,* CT scan slightly more cephalad from same patient shows a high-density gallstone within the gallbladder. The stone does not fall to the dependent portion of the gallbladder, however, confirming the presence of inflammatory debris within the gallbladder. The gallbladder wall is indistinct and blends gradually with the increased attenuation of the bile and gallbladder contents. Adjacent inflammatory changes from perforation into the liver appear as foci of low attenuation *(arrows).*

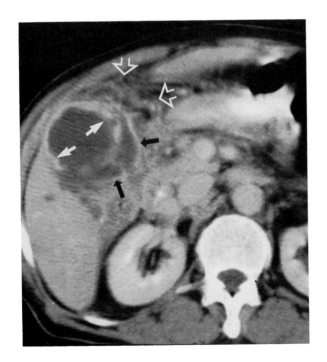

FIGURE 18–25 ■ Gangrenous cholecystitis with perforation. Contrast-enhanced CT scan shows marked enhancement of the thickened gallbladder wall *(white arrows).* A septated pericholecystic fluid collection is present *(black arrows).* Diffuse haziness is present in the pericholecystic fat *(open arrows).*

FIGURE 18–26 ■ Emphysematous cholecystitis. In this condition, air can be seen within the gallbladder lumen *(arrow),* within the gallbladder wall *(white arrowhead),* or within both, as here. Additional findings, associated with complicated cholecystitis, seen in this patient include inflammatory infiltration of the pericholecystic fat (increasing the attenuation value of surrounding fat, *open arrow),* and associated pericholecystic fluid collection *(black arrowheads).*

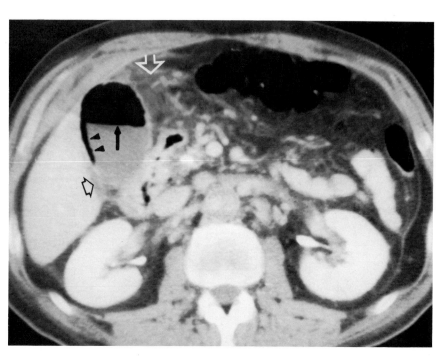

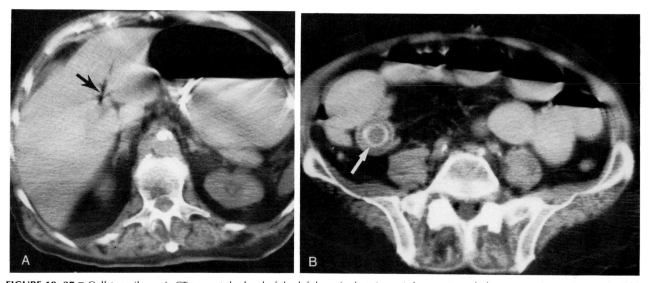

FIGURE 18–27 ■ Gallstone ileus. *A,* CT scan at the level of the left hepatic duct *(arrow)* shows extremely low attenuation owing to air within the duct. *B,* Scan at the level of the distal ileum shows a rimmed gallstone *(arrow)* in the distal ileum, causing a small bowel obstruction, with dilated proximal small bowel loops.

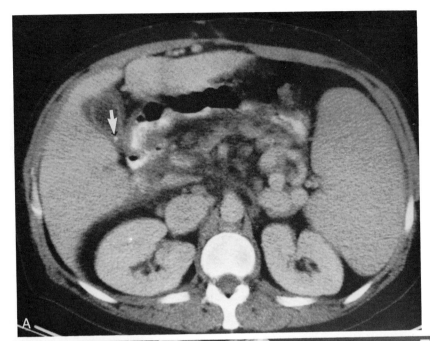

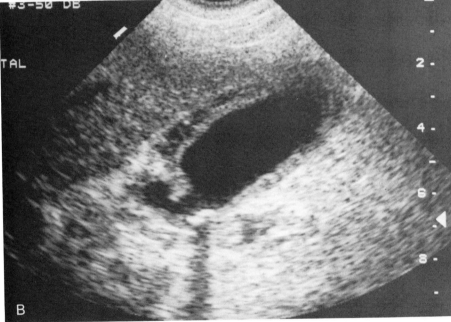

FIGURE 18–28 ■ Gallbladder wall thickening simulating pericholecystic fluid. A, Contrast-enhanced CT scan shows low attenuation indicating symmetric thickening of the gallbladder wall surrounding the higher-attenuation mucosa. This simulates a pericholecystic fluid collection, which is worrisome, for it suggests cholecystitis and perforation in this patient with gallstones (arrow). B, Ultrasound examination delineates the wall thickening rather than the pericholecystic fluid. Patient had no symptoms of cholecystitis, and wall thickening was due to chronic liver disease.

MRI

A normal, functioning gallbladder is able to concentrate bile within the gallbladder. This results in a changing pattern of MR signal intensity in the gallbladder between fasting and nonfasting states.[28] McCarthy and co-workers[11] found that the inflamed gallbladder, presumably unable to concentrate bile, showed an abnormal signal intensity on spin-echo images obtained with a repetition time TR of 500 and interpulse delay time TE of 56. All normal patients demonstrated fasting gallbladder bile hyperintense with the liver at these parameters, compared with only 5 of 18 patients with cholecystitis. No normal patients demonstrated hypointense or isointense

bile, compared with 13 of 18 patients with cholecystitis. These authors proposed that MRI may provide functional information about the gallbladder that could be an aid in the diagnosis of cholecystitis. In contrast, Loflin and associates[83] reported no significant difference in the in vitro T1 and T2 values of gallbladder bile obtained from normal gallbladders and those with documented cholecystitis.

MRI can also display, similarly to CT, the morphologic features of complicated cholecystitis. Thickening of the gallbladder walls and pericholecystic fluid can be identified on MRI. High–signal intensity foci within the gallbladder wall on T2-weighted images, presumably due to intramural fluid and edema,[84] have been reported.

Traumatic Lesions

Gallbladder trauma or bleeding into the biliary tract from liver trauma can be identified by high attenuation of the bile contents.[85, 86] Such changes may cause the bile to diffusely increase in attenuation or as the blood retracts into a clot, may pool in the dependent portions of the gallbladder.[86] Based on studies in monkeys, it has been found that this effect can persist for days following the cessation of bleeding.[86] Occasionally, similar findings can be seen in the bile ducts.

Caution should be used in making the diagnosis of hemobilia when visualizing high-density contents within the gallbladder, since other processes can cause an increase in attenuation of bile, including contrast material, milk of calcium bile, and gallstones.

Bile Duct Diseases

Neoplasms

PRIMARY NEOPLASMS

The most common primary malignancy of the bile ducts is cholangiocarcinoma, which has been associated with ulcerative colitis, sclerosing cholangitis, liver fluke disease, gallstones, and choledochal cysts.[87, 88] The tumor usually arises in the larger bile ducts, and reported series have shown varying incidence of sites of origin as follows: 8 to 31 per cent in intrahepatic ducts; 37 to 50 per cent in proximal extrahepatic ducts; and 4 to 36 per cent in the distal extrahepatic ducts.[47, 87, 89, 90] A small percentage of cases can arise from the cystic duct.[47] Three morphologic patterns of tumor are seen: most commonly, an infiltrating stenotic mass; less commonly, a bulky, exophytic mass; and uncommonly, a polypoid, intramural tumor.[87, 91]

CT ■ The CT appearance of these lesions depends on the location and morphology of the tumor. Intrahepatic lesions (Fig. 18–29) demonstrate nonspecific appearances, usually as low attenuation masses with minimal contrast-enhancement or none on early images,[47] but they may show delayed enhancement (see Fig. 17–68). These lesions cannot be differentiated on CT from other liver lesions, including hepatoma or metastatic disease.

The key to the diagnosis of extrahepatic or confluence lesions with the aid of CT is the presence of dilated biliary ducts to the level of the tumor. A tumor mass at the level of biliary obstruction can be seen (Fig. 18–30), but the tumors may be small and may not be identifiable. In such cases, the recognition of an abrupt termination of dilated ducts without a visible mass allows one to suspect the correct diagnosis, although benign stricture or a cholesterol gallstone can simulate this appearance. Because stone disease usually produces a distal obstruction, when the level of obstruction is between the level of confluence of hepatic ducts and the pancreatic portion of the CBD, there should be a strong suspicion of cholangiocarcinoma. The primary mass can be detected in approximately 70 per cent of patients by CT scanning.[91]

When the cholangiocarcinoma is proximal and infiltrates adjacent liver, the tumor may envelop the porta hepatis and extend into the liver parenchyma, making differentiation from a primary or secondary liver neoplasm difficult (Fig. 18–31; see also Fig. 18–29). Such lesions may appear to be of lower attenuation than liver parenchyma (see Fig. 18–29) or may appear to be an infiltrating enhancing mass (see Fig. 18–31). When the extent of involvement of liver

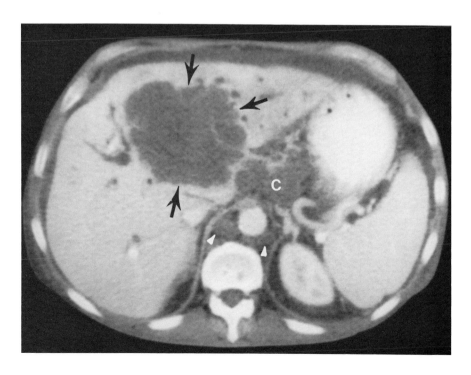

FIGURE 18–29 ■ Cholangiocarcinoma. An infiltrating large mass showing low attenuation *(arrows)*, originating in the proximal common hepatic duct, has extensively invaded the adjacent liver parenchyma. Metastases of low attenuation are seen to celiac (c) and retrocrural *(white arrowheads)* lymph nodes. Proximal biliary obstruction is evident by dilated intrahepatic ducts.

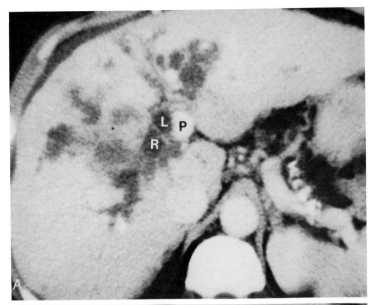

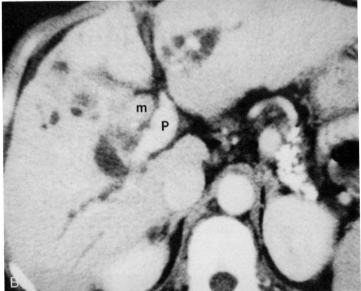

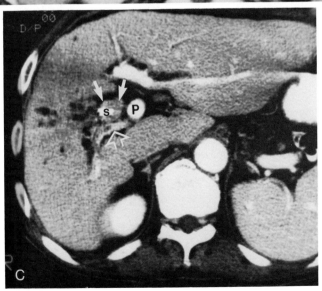

FIGURE 18–30 ■ Cholangiocarcinoma at the confluence of the hepatic ducts. *A*, Contrast-enhanced CT scan shows marked bile duct dilatation at the level at which the left (L) and right (R) hepatic ducts converge. P = portal vein. *B*, Scan 1 cm caudad shows no visualization of a dilated common hepatic duct, indicating an abrupt termination and a proximal level of obstruction. Anterior to the portal vein (P), in the expected location of the duct, is an enhancing mass (M), representing replacement of the duct by a cholangiocarcinoma. *C*, Another patient with a proximal cholangiocarcinoma of the common hepatic duct. There is a soft tissue mass *(solid arrows)* lateral to the main portal (P) and anterior to the right portal vein *(open arrow)*, replacing the common hepatic duct, similar to that in the patient in *B*. The high-attenuation biliary stent(s) through the central lumen of the duct and tumor allows for easy recognition of this structure as the common hepatic duct, with walls markedly thickened circumferentially by the cholangiocarcinoma.

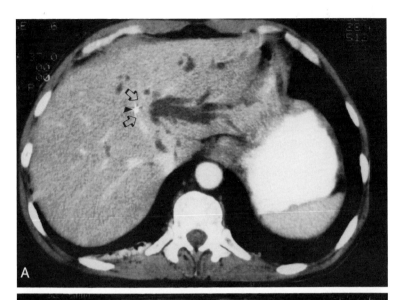

FIGURE 18–31 ■ Cholangiocarcinoma. *A* and *B,* Incremental, dynamic, contrast-enhanced CT shows the cholangiocarcinoma as an enhancing mass *(open arrows)* infiltrating the porta hepatis, with dilated intrahepatic biliary ducts despite an indwelling stent *(arrowhead).* Portions of the tumor enhance to lesser degrees *(solid arrows). C,* CT-angioportogram at same level as *B* shows the full extent of the tumor found at surgery that is infiltrating the left *(solid arrows)* and caudate *(open arrow)* lobes, which appeared isointense with the liver in *B.*

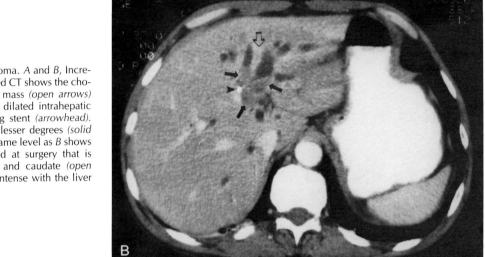

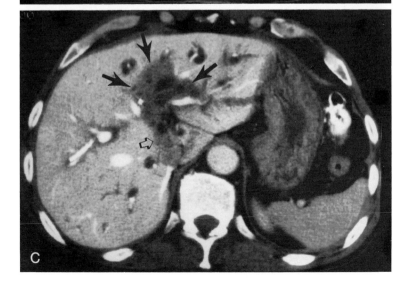

parenchyma is uncertain, CT-angioportography evaluation will delineate more completely the extent of tumor (see Fig. 18–31). When the tumors are small or are visualized more distally in the extrahepatic system, they usually have a soft tissue attenuation. Large tumors may have regions of necrosis and have a low CT density. Often, just proximal to the high-grade duct obstruction, CT will show eccentric thickening of the CBD wall, suggesting the diagnosis of cholangiocarcinoma (Figs. 18–32 and 18–33).[17] The rare papillary form of cholangiocarcinoma, as depicted on cholangiography, is more difficult to detect on a CT scan unless it achieves a large size. When seen, the lesion can simulate a common bile duct calculus.

MRI ■ Cholangiocarcinoma can be a difficult diag-

nosis on CT or MR when the primary lesion is small. Dooms and colleagues[4] reported MR findings in nine patients, but it should be noted that five of these patients had received prior irradiation, which may have affected the imaging appearance of the lesions. In seven of nine instances, MR imaging was able to display the tumors as either hypodense or isointense with liver on T1-weighted images, and hyperintense to liver on T2-weighted sequences (Fig. 18–34). The four patients with a scirrhous subtype showed only slightly higher signal intensity than liver on T2-weighted images, presumably owing to the higher fibrous content shortening the T2 of these lesions. Encasement of vascular structures in the porta hepatis and liver invasion was better delineated on MRI than CT. As with many other areas of the abdomen,

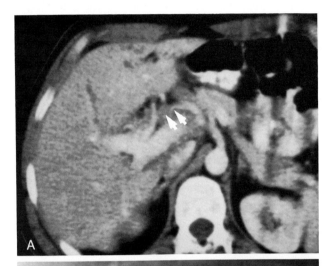

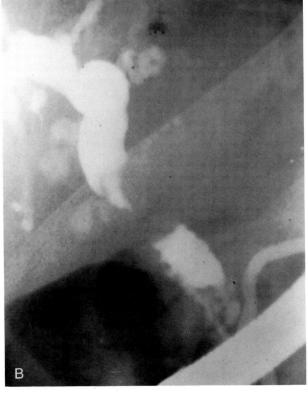

FIGURE 18–32 ■ Cholangiocarcinoma. *A,* CT scan at the level of the porta hepatis shows eccentric thickening of the common hepatic duct wall posteromedially *(arrowheads)* and posteriorly, separating the lumen with water attenuation from the portal vein. *B,* Cholangiogram shows marked circumferential narrowing. (*B,* from Teefey SA, et al: RADIOLOGY 169:635–639, 1983.)

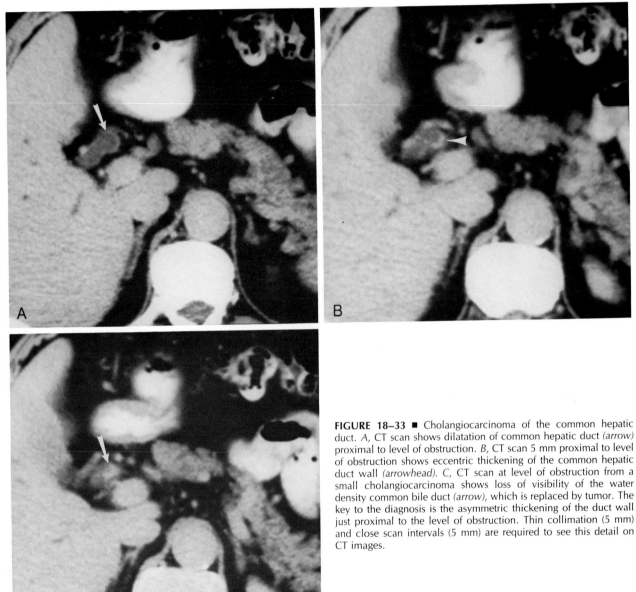

FIGURE 18–33 ■ Cholangiocarcinoma of the common hepatic duct. *A,* CT scan shows dilatation of common hepatic duct *(arrow)* proximal to level of obstruction. *B,* CT scan 5 mm proximal to level of obstruction shows eccentric thickening of the common hepatic duct wall *(arrowhead). C,* CT scan at level of obstruction from a small cholangiocarcinoma shows loss of visibility of the water density common bile duct *(arrow),* which is replaced by tumor. The key to the diagnosis is the asymmetric thickening of the duct wall just proximal to the level of obstruction. Thin collimation (5 mm) and close scan intervals (5 mm) are required to see this detail on CT images.

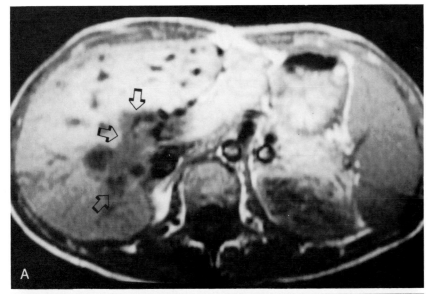

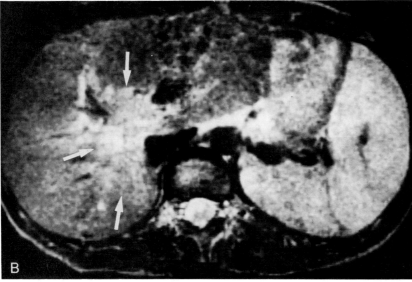

FIGURE 18–34 ■ MR appearance of infiltrating cholangiocarcinoma. *A*, T1-weighted image shows the tumor *(arrows)* as hypointense compared with the liver parenchyma and infiltrating the porta hepatis. *B*, T2-weighted image slightly cephalad shows the tumor *(arrows)* is of higher intensity than liver parenchyma and is infiltrating around vascular structures in the porta hepatis.

the exact role of MRI in evaluating cholangiocarcinoma remains uncertain at this time.

METASTATIC DISEASE

Metastasis to the porta hepatis can involve the extrahepatic bile ducts. This can be in the form of direct invasion into the porta hepatis from gallbladder (see Fig. 18–16) or pancreatic carcinoma, or it can occur as metastases to lymph nodes in the porta hepatis from lymphoma or other carcinomas. The CT appearance of bile duct metastases is similar to that of other masses obstructing the bile duct. Metastases usually produce abrupt termination of the bile duct due to a surrounding mass of soft tissue attenuation density.

Inflammation

ASCENDING CHOLANGITIS

Ascending cholangitis (or acute cholangitis) is usually seen in patients with underlying biliary tract obstruction. It can be caused by a variety of organisms, most commonly by *Escherichia coli* infection. Most patients demonstrate dilated intrahepatic and extrahepatic biliary ducts, although with an acute or partial obstruction, this may not be present. Suppurative material within the bile ducts may result in an increase in attenuation of bile on CT that is similar to changes seen in infected gallbladder bile.

Thickening of the bile duct wall can be seen and is usually diffuse and concentric, often demonstrating marked contrast enhancement (Fig. 18–35).[17] Gas can be seen as low density within the biliary tree in the case of infection with gas-forming organisms, and gas within the portal vein in association with acute cholangitis has been reported.[92] Acute suppurative cholangitis can progress to frank liver abscesses demonstrated on CT as low attenuation areas in the liver in contiguity with the biliary tree.

SCLEROSING CHOLANGITIS

Sclerosing cholangitis can occur as a primary form (either idiopathic or in association with ulcerative

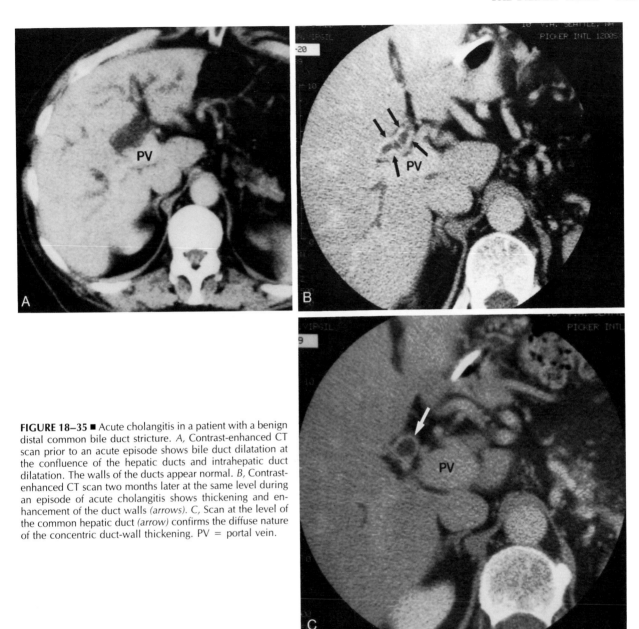

FIGURE 18–35 ■ Acute cholangitis in a patient with a benign distal common bile duct stricture. *A,* Contrast-enhanced CT scan prior to an acute episode shows bile duct dilatation at the confluence of the hepatic ducts and intrahepatic duct dilatation. The walls of the ducts appear normal. *B,* Contrast-enhanced CT scan two months later at the same level during an episode of acute cholangitis shows thickening and enhancement of the duct walls *(arrows). C,* Scan at the level of the common hepatic duct *(arrow)* confirms the diffuse nature of the concentric duct-wall thickening. PV = portal vein.

colitis, Crohn's disease, or retroperitoneal fibrosis) or secondary to prior biliary infection, stone disease, or surgery.

Cholangiography demonstrates characteristic findings in the intrahepatic and extrahepatic biliary tree, including multifocal strictures, pruning of duct branches, duct wall nodularity, and duct diverticula. The CT findings reflect these changes. Intrahepatic stenoses are suggested on CT scans by the presence of scattered, dilated peripheral ducts with no apparent connection to the central ducts (Fig. 18–36).[13–15] Rarely, CT may demonstrate intrahepatic duct strictures as regions of duct narrowing between two dilated portions of the biliary tree (Fig. 18–37). Irregular intrahepatic duct dilatation results in a beaded appearance on both CT (Fig. 18–38) and cholangiography. Although some authors[13, 15] think these findings are suggestive of primary sclerosing cholangitis, to date there have been no studies evaluating the specificity of this finding. Similarly, CT may demonstrate pruning of the intrahepatic ducts by demonstrating a long segment of a dilated intrahepatic duct without the expected side branches (see Fig. 18–37),[14] but the specificity of this finding has yet to be determined.

Findings of sclerosing cholangitis in the extrahepatic ducts can be demonstrated on CT. The cholangiographic findings of mural irregularity and diverticula are evident on CT as bile duct wall thickening (>2 mm), nodularity, and wall enhancement (Figs. 18–39 and 18–40).[14] The wall thickening may be focal or diffuse, and eccentric or concentric. However, the thickening is usually < 5 mm and does not reach the proportions seen with some cholangiocarcinomas.[17]

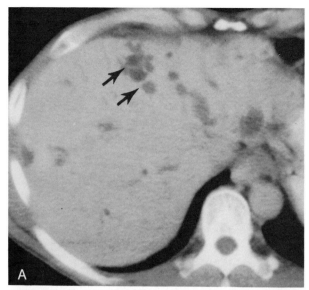

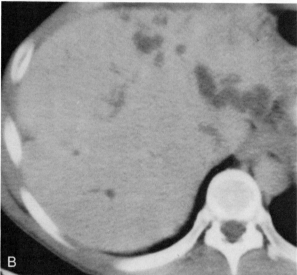

FIGURE 18–36 ■ Sclerosing cholangitis. *A* and *B,* Sequential CT images of the liver show dilated peripheral biliary ducts, some of which have a beaded appearance *(arrows)*. The dilated peripheral ducts are not contiguous from one section to the next, indicating interval stenoses. These scattered, "skip," dilatations are typical of sclerosing cholangitis.

FIGURE 18–37 ■ Sclerosing cholangitis. Contrast-enhanced CT scan shows dilatation of the peripheral intrahepatic ducts *(open arrow)* in the left lobe and the distal left hepatic duct *(solid arrow),* with a long segmental stricture between visualized as a narrowed segment *(arrowheads).* Pruning is demonstrated by the lack of visualized side branches expected on the long duct. (From Teefey SA et al: RADIOLOGY 169:635–639, 1988.)

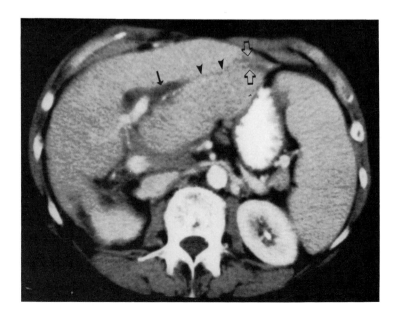

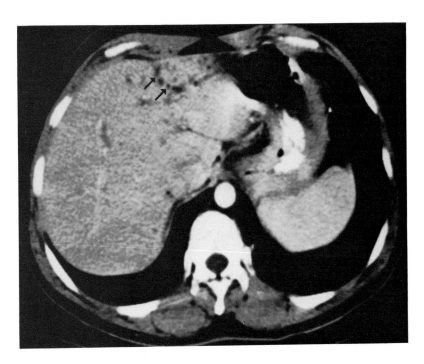

FIGURE 18–38 ■ Sclerosing cholangitis. Scattered regions of intrahepatic bile duct dilatation are present. A "beaded" appearance of the left lobe ducts *(arrows)* is due to multiple, closely attenuating regions of saccular dilatation and strictures. (From Teefey SA et al: RADIOLOGY 169:635–639, 1988.)

Rarely, strictures of the extrahepatic ducts can be directly visualized on CT (see Fig. 18–40). Small field-of-view, thin collimation images may optimize visualization of these findings.

Complications from primary sclerosing cholangitis (PSC) should be sought on CT images in these patients; complications include findings of cirrhosis and portal hypertension. Cholangiocarcinoma is a known complication of PSC[93] and may be both difficult to detect and to differentiate from findings of sclerosing cholangitis at cholangiography. CT may be able to provide the diagnosis because of its ability to visualize beyond the duct lumen; it may visualize the primary tumor or detect metastatic disease.[14]

RECURRENT PYOGENIC CHOLANGITIS

Recurrent pyogenic cholangitis is also known as oriental cholangiohepatitis, intrahepatic pigment stone disease, and the biliary obstruction syndrome of the Chinese.[94–96]

The disease is endemic to areas of eastern Asia (Japan, China, Korea, and Hong Kong), usually in patients of low socioeconomic status. As its name implies, patients usually present with recurrent cholangitis manifested by abdominal pain, jaundice, and sepsis. The recurrent nature of the disease leads to multiple areas of progressive biliary strictures. Marked ductal dilatation and stone disease of the biliary tract results. The disease often progresses, resulting in cirrhosis. Although the etiology remains uncertain, infection with parasites *(Clonorchis sinensis, Ascaris, Entamoeba coli)* and bacteria *(E. coli)* has been postulated as the cause of biliary strictures and stone formation.[94]

The characteristic CT findings are the marked intrahepatic and extrahepatic bile duct dilatation (often to 3 or 4 cm in diameter) with associated biliary calculi and debris (Figs. 18–41 and 18–42).[94] The stones are composed mostly of bile pigment, with varying degrees of calcification, and thus the stones appear on CT with densities ranging from isodense with bile to extremely dense. Owing to the soft, mud-like consistency of many of the stones, CT is often better able to depict them than ultrasonography.[94] Thickening of the bile duct wall can be identified. Usually, it is mild, ranging from 2 to 3 mm in an eccentric and diffuse distribution (Fig. 18–42).[17] Pneumobilia from infection with a gas-forming organism can be seen in a small number of cases.

Stone Disease

Common bile duct (CBD) stones are found in 15 per cent of patients undergoing cholecystectomy and develop in 2 to 4 per cent of patients following the operation.[97] Thus, stone disease is a common cause of biliary obstruction, accounting for 20 to 42 per cent of cases of biliary obstruction.[98] Documenting stone disease in the CBD in these patients can be a challenging imaging task and requires meticulous techniques to achieve high detection rates. When the specific imaging question is to document whether or not CBD stones are present, the examination of choice is a cholangiogram, which has an accuracy approaching 100 per cent. Most often, however, patients present with evidence of biliary obstruction, and the imaging studies center on determining whether or not the patient has biliary tract obstruction and if so at what level and what the cause is. In these cases, both ultrasonography and CT scans can be used as screening tools. Generally, ultrasonography is the initial examination of choice because of

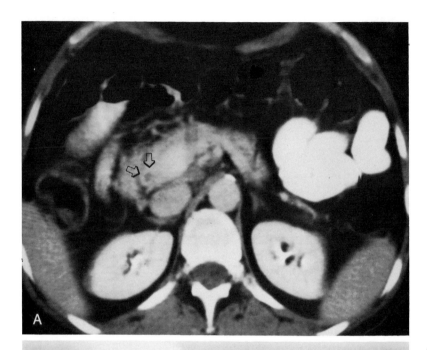

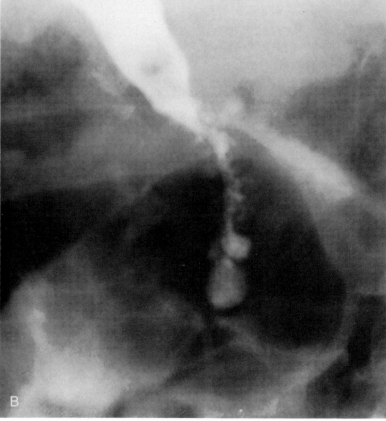

FIGURE 18–39 ■ Sclerosing cholangitis. *A*, CT shows concentric wall thickening and mural enhancement of the intrapancreatic common bile duct *(arrows)*. *B*, Cholangiogram shows distal duct wall irregularity, diverticula, and nodularity, which contribute to the observation of wall thickening on the CT image. (*B*, from Teefey SA et al: RADIOLOGY 169:635–639, 1988.)

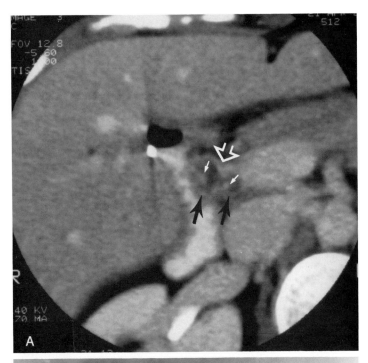

FIGURE 18–40 ■ Sclerosing cholangitis: mural nodules. *A,* Small field-of-view (target) image shows an oblique course of the suprapancreatic common bile duct *(black arrows).* Note the stricture of the duct *(open white arrow)* and multiple, enhancing nodules *(solid white arrows). B,* Cholangiogram confirms beaded common bile duct due to multiple mural nodules. *(A,* from Teefey SA et al: RADIOLOGY 169:635–639, 1988.)

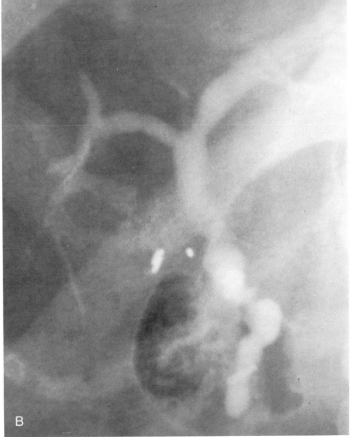

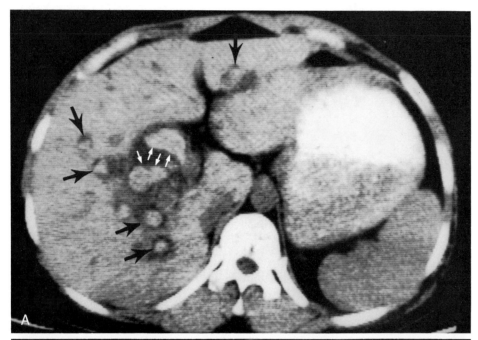

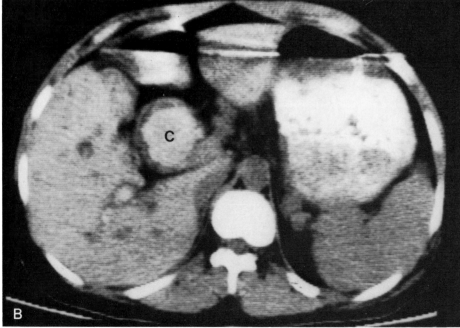

FIGURE 18–41 ■ Recurrent pyogenic cholangitis. *A,* CT scan without use of contrast agent shows dilatation of intrahepatic ducts filled with high-attenuation calculi *(black arrows).* Large calculi *(white arrows)* are seen emanating from the right and left hepatic ducts into the common hepatic duct. *B,* Scan several centimeters caudad shows a giant high-attenuation calculus (C) in the common hepatic duct.

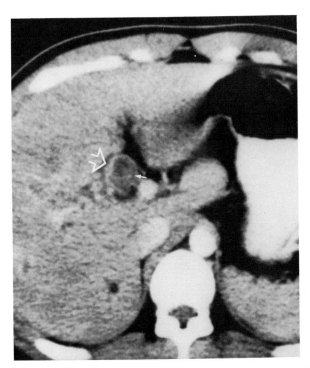

FIGURE 18–42 ■ Recurrent pyogenic cholangitis. Contrast-enhanced CT scan shows marked dilatation of the common hepatic duct. A large calculus within the duct is of slightly greater attenuation than bile, with a thin rim of bile *(white arrow)* seen between the calculus and duct wall. Eccentric thickening of the duct wall is present *(open arrow)*.

the easy availability, lower cost, and the lack of ionizing radiation or requirement for intravenous contrast agents. The reported sensitivity of CT for detection of stones in the CBD varies from 45 to 90 per cent.[1, 2, 23, 99–101] The higher figures generally reflect series with selected patient populations, often patients with known dilated ducts detected at sonography. Ultrasound literature has revealed that 24 to 36 per cent of patients with CBD stones do not have dilated biliary ducts.[102–104] These cases are more difficult to detect on both ultrasonography and CT, and inclusion of such patients would lessen the CT results reported in series without such patients.

The CT appearance of stones in the CBD depends on the chemical composition of each stone and demonstrates the same range of appearances as gallbladder calculi. A densely calcified CBD stone can be seen on CT images as a high-density structure within the water attenuation lumen of the CBD (Fig. 18–43). Even if they are impacted, without the surrounding bile visible, such calcified stones can be detected by appreciating that the calcification lies in the expected course of the CBD predicted from the prior serial images. Unfortunately, only approximately 20 per cent of CBD stones are of homogeneous high attenuation on CT images.[100] Approximately 50 per cent of these stones are of soft tissue density and can be recognized by visualizing the faint density stone in the CBD lumen surrounded by a rim of

FIGURE 18–43 ■ Common bile duct stone. Sequential CT images demonstrate the stone *(arrowheads)* as homogeneous high attenuation surrounded by the soft tissue attenuation of the pancreas, just medial to and abutting the duodenum *(solid arrows)*. Although no bile showing water attenuation is seen around the stone, the calcific density lies in the expected course of the duct as visualized on the more cephalad section *(open arrow)*. Oral contrast was not administered; if it had been, the high attenuation of the contrast agent might have obscured the stone. (From Baron RL: RADIOLOGY 162:419–424, 1987.)

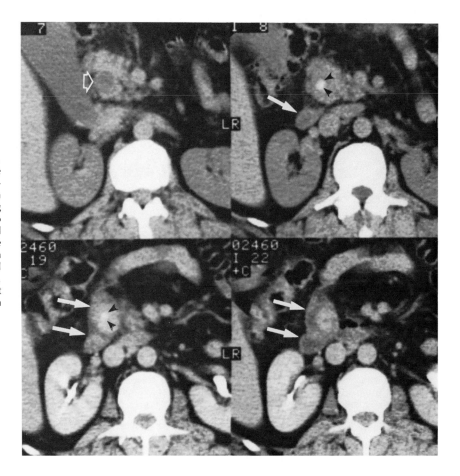

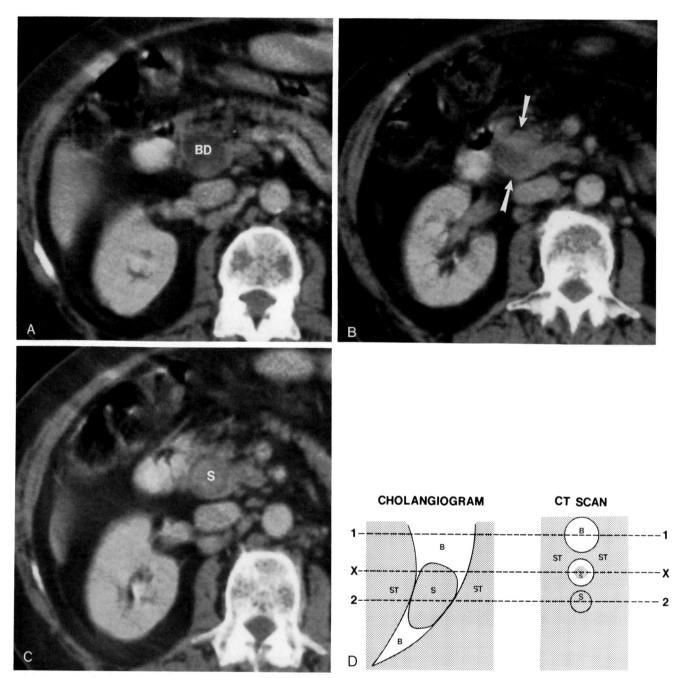

FIGURE 18–44 ■ Common bile duct stone. *A,* Scan at the level of the head of the pancreas shows a markedly dilated duct with water attenuation (BD) proximal to the stone. *B,* Scan 1 cm lower shows abrupt termination of the duct without evidence of a stone or mass in the pancreas *(arrows)* at the level where the stone is impacted in the duct. No bile is visible, as the stone with soft tissue attenuation abuts the wall of the duct and the soft tissues of the pancreas. *C,* An additional scan between the levels of A and B, through the convex margin of the stone (S), reveals a surrounding rim of bile with water attenuation around the stone.

D, Line drawing of a cholangiogram *(left)* and corresponding axial CT scan sections in a patient with an impacted common bile duct stone. CT scan at level 1 (similar to A) would show the soft tissues (ST) of the pancreas around the circle of bile with water attenuation, representing the common bile duct proximal to the stone (S). A scan at level 2 (similar to B) through the site of impaction of a stone (S) with soft tissue attenuation would not cut through the bile with water attenuation and would demonstrate only soft tissue densities, obscuring the outline of the stone. A scan centered several millimeters proximally at level X (similar to C), between levels 1 and 2, would section through the convex margin of the impacted stone and would demonstrate a rim of surrounding bile. If only scans at level 1 and 2 were obtained, abrupt termination of the duct without visualization of an intraluminal stone would result in a nondiagnostic CT examination and would in fact be suggestive of malignancy. (From Baron RL: RADIOLOGY 162:419–424, 1987.)

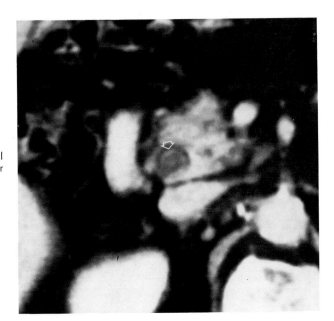

FIGURE 18–45 ■ Common bile duct stone. The stone is seen with central low attenuation and a peripheral rim *(open arrows)* of slightly higher attenuation. Bile can be seen surrounding the stone.

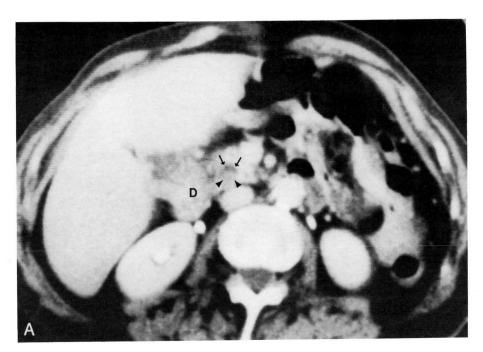

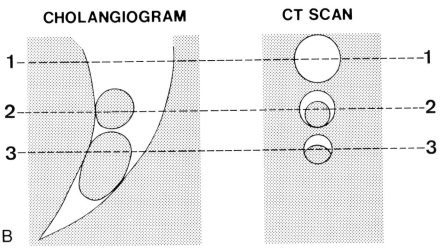

CHOLANGIOGRAM   CT SCAN

FIGURE 18–46 ■ Common bile duct stone: crescent sign. *A,* CT scan shows the stone with soft tissue attenuation *(arrowheads)* in the dependent portion of the common bile duct, medial to the duodenum (D). The bile with water attenuation is draped over the stone in the shape of a crescent *(arrows). B,* Line drawing of a cholangiogram *(left)* and corresponding axial CT sections *(right)* demonstrating the etiology of the crescent sign. A scan at level 1 would demonstrate soft tissues of the pancreas around the bile with water attenuation of the duct in a patient lying in a supine position. The water attenuation bile changes its shape from the ring at level 1 to a crescent at levels 2 and 3 and represents a characteristic appearance. The stone at level 2 is in a dependent position within the duct, and the bile as it drapes over the stone has a crescent shape. Oblique sectioning through an impacted stone (level 3) scans through one margin of the stone as it abuts the wall of the common bile duct and surrounding pancreas creates a similar appearance.

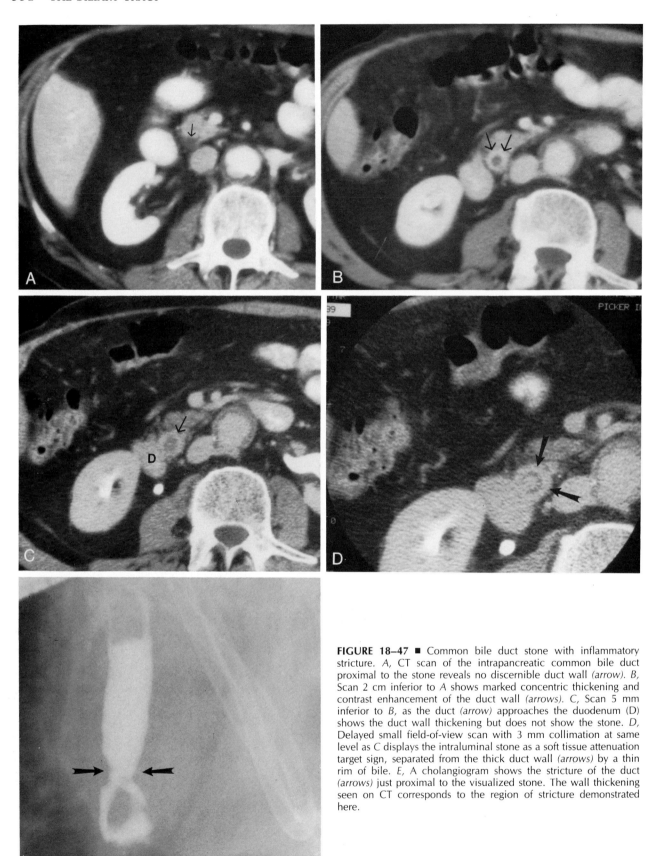

FIGURE 18–47 ■ Common bile duct stone with inflammatory stricture. *A*, CT scan of the intrapancreatic common bile duct proximal to the stone reveals no discernible duct wall *(arrow)*. *B*, Scan 2 cm inferior to *A* shows marked concentric thickening and contrast enhancement of the duct wall *(arrows)*. *C*, Scan 5 mm inferior to *B*, as the duct *(arrow)* approaches the duodenum (D) shows the duct wall thickening but does not show the stone. *D*, Delayed small field-of-view scan with 3 mm collimation at same level as C displays the intraluminal stone as a soft tissue attenuation target sign, separated from the thick duct wall *(arrows)* by a thin rim of bile. *E*, A cholangiogram shows the stricture of the duct *(arrows)* just proximal to the visualized stone. The wall thickening seen on CT corresponds to the region of stricture demonstrated here.

Biliary malignancies occurring in choledochal cysts. Radiology 173:389–392, 1989.

35. Pollack M, Shirkhoda A, Charnsangavej C: Computed tomography of choledochocele. J Comput Assist Tomogr 9:360–362, 1985.

36. Brodey PA, Fisch AE, Fertig S, Roberts GS: Computed tomography of choledochocele. J Comput Assist Tomogr 8:162–164, 1984.

37. Mall JC, Ghahremani GG, Boyer JL: Caroli's disease associated with congenital hepatic fibrosis and renal tubular ectasia. Gastroenterology 66:1029–1035, 1974.

38. Boyer JL: What is Caroli's disease? Gastroenterology 68:417–419, 1975.

39. Musante F, Derchi LE, Bonati P: CT cholangiography in suspected Caroli's disease. J Comput Assist Tomogr 6:482–485, 1982.

40. Choi BI, Yeon KM, Kim SH, Han MC: Caroli disease: central dot sign in CT. Radiology 174:161–163, 1990.

41. Jutras JA, Levesque HP: Adenomyoma and adenomyomatosis of the gallbladder; radiologic and pathologic correlations. Radiol Clin North Am 4:483–500, 1966.

42. Berk RN, van der Vegt JH, Lichtenstein JE: The hyperplastic cholecystoses: cholesterolosis and adenomyomatosis. Radiology 146:593–601, 1983.

43. Raghavendra BN, Subramanyam BR, Balthazar EJ, Horii SC, Megibow AJ, Hilton S: Sonography of adenomyomatosis of the gallbladder: radiologic-pathologic correlation. Radiology 146:747–752, 1983.

44. Boukadoum M, Siddiky MA, Zerhouni EA, Stitik RP: CT demonstration of adenomyomatosis of the gallbladder. J Comput Assist Tomogr 8:177–180, 1984.

45. Robbins SL, Cotran RS: Pathologic Basis of Disease. Philadelphia, WB Saunders Company, 1979.

46. Beltz WR, Condon RE: Primary carcinoma of the gallbladder. Ann Surg 180:180–184, 1974.

47. Thorsen MK, Quiroz F, Lawson TL, Smith DF, Foley WD, et al: Primary biliary carcinoma: CT evaluation. Radiology 152:479–483, 1984.

48. Do Carmo M, Perpetuo MO, Valdivieso M, Heilbrun LK, Nelson RS, Connor T, Bodey GP: Natural history study of gallbladder cancer. Cancer 42:330–335, 1978.

49. Yum HY, Fink AH: Sonography findings in primary carcinoma of the gallbladder. Radiology 134:693–696, 1980.

50. Polk HCJ: Carcinoma of the calcified gallbladder. Gastroenterology 50:582–585, 1966.

51. Kane RA, Jacobs R, Katz J, Costello P: Porcelain gallbladder: ultrasound and CT appearance. Radiology 152:137–141, 1984.

52. Orloff MG, Charters AC: Tumors of the gallbladder and bile ducts. In Bockus HL (ed): Gastroenterology, 3rd ed, Vol 3. Philadelphia, WB Saunders Company, 1976, pp 829–842.

53. Itai Y, Araki T, Yoshikawa K, Furui S, Yashiro N, et al: Computed tomography of gallbladder carcinoma. Radiology 137:713–718, 1980.

54. Weiner SN, Koenigsberg M, Morehouse H, Hoffman J: Sonography and computed tomography in the diagnosis of carcinoma of the gallbladder. AJR 142:735–739, 1984.

55. Lane J, Buck JL, Zeman RK: Primary carcinoma of the gallbladder: a pictorial essay. Radiographics 9:209–228, 1989.

56. Araki T, Hihara T, Karikomi M, Kachi K, Uchiyama G: Intraluminal papillary carcinoma of the gallbladder: prognostic value of computed tomography and sonography. Gastrointest Radiol 13:261–265, 1988.

57. Engels JT, Balfe DM, Lee JKT: Biliary carcinoma: CT evaluation of extrahepatic spread. Radiology 172:35–40, 1989.

58. Smathers R, Lee JKT, Heiken JP: Differentiation of complicated cholecystitis from gallbladder carcinoma by computed tomography. AJR 143:255–259, 1984.

59. Rossmann MD, Friedman AC, Radecki PD, Caroline DF: MR imaging of gallbladder carcinoma. AJR 148:143–144, 1987.

60. Willis RA: The Spread of Tumors in the Human Body. London, Butterworth's, 1952.

61. Baron RL, Rohrmann CA Jr, Lee SP, Shuman WP, Teefey SA: CT evaluation of gallstones in vitro: correlation with chemical analysis. AJR 151:1123–1128, 1988.

62. Barakos JA, Ralls PW, Lapin SA, et al: Cholelithiasis: evaluation with CT. Radiology 162:415–418, 1987.

63. Hickman MS, Schwesinger WH, Bova JD, Kurtin WE: Computed tomographic analysis of gallstones. Arch Surg 121:289–291, 1986.

64. Baron RL, Kuyper SJ, Lee SP, Rohrmann CA Jr, Shuman WP, et al: In vitro dissolution of gallstones with MTBE: correlation with characteristics at CT and MR imaging. Radiology 173:117–121, 1989.

65. Becker CD, Vock P: Appearance of gas-containing gallstones on sonography and computed tomography. Gastrointest Radiol 9:323–328, 1984.

66. Rajagopal S, Bills P, Keightley A, Murphy GM, Dowling RH: Predictive value of computed tomography (CT) scanning of the gall bladder in determining gallstone type. Gut 29:A1487, 1988.

67. Brakel K, Lameris JS, Nijs HGT, Terpstra OT, Steen G, et al: Predicting gallstone composition with CT: in vivo and in vitro analysis. Radiology 174:337–341, 1990.

68. Auteri AG, Malet PF: Radiographic imaging to predict gallstone dissolution: more than meets the eye. Gastroenterology 98:1715–1716, 1990.

69. van Sonnenberg E, Casola G, Zakko SF, Varney RR, Cox J, Wittich GR, Hoffman AF: Gallbladder and bile duct stones: percutaneous therapy with primary MTBE dissolution and mechanical methods. Radiology 169:505–509, 1988.

70. Valette PJ, Barkun AN, Ponchon P, Cathignol D: Radiologic variables that determine the success of in vitro solitary gallstone lithotripsy. Radiology 173(P):245, 1989.

71. Ell C, Schneider HT, Benninger, J et al: Significance of computed tomography for shockwave therapy of "radiolucent" gallbladder stones. Presented at the Third International Symposium on Biliary Lithotripsy, Munich, September 13–15, 1990.

72. Franke F, Holl J, Sackmann M, Pauletzki J, Paumgartner G, et al: Computed tomography (CT) does not improve the selection of radiolucent stones for extracorporeal shock wave lithotripsy (ESWL). Presented at the Third International Symposium on Biliary Lithotripsy, Munich, September 13–15, 1990.

73. Moriyasu F, Ban N, Nishida O, Nakamura T, Soh Y, Kawasaki T, Tamada T, Sakai M, Miyake T, Uchino H: Central signals of gallstones in magnetic resonance imaging. Am J Gastroenterol 82:139–142, 1987.

74. Terrier F, Becker CD, Stoller C, Triller JK: Computed tomography in complicated cholecystitis. J Comput Assist Tomogr 8:58–62, 1984.

75. Kane RA, Costello P, Duszlak E: Computed tomography in acute cholecystitis: new observations. AJR 141:697–701, 1983.

76. Jenkins PF, Golding RH, Cooperberg PL: Sonography and computed tomography of hemorrhagic cholecystitis. AJR 140:1197, 1983.

77. Solomon A, Kreel L, Pinto D: Contrast-computed tomography in diagnosis of acute cholecystitis. J Comput Assist Tomogr 3:585–588, 1979.

78. Somer K, Kivisaari L, Standertskjold-Nordenstam C-G, Kalima TV: Contrast-enhanced computed tomography of the gallbladder in acute pancreatitis. Gastrointest Radiol 9:31–34, 1984.

79. McMillin K: Computed tomography of emphysematous cholecystitis. J Comput Assist Tomogr 9:330, 1985.

80. Duber C, Storkel S, Wagner PK, Muller J: Xanthogranulomatous cholecystitis mimicking carcinoma of the gallbladder: CT findings. J Comput Assist Tomogr 8:1195–1198, 1984.

81. Cossi AF, Scholz FJ, Aretz HT, Larsen CR: Computed tomography of xanthogranulomatous cholecystitis. Gastrointest Radiol 12:212–214, 1987.

82. Hanada K, Nakata H, Nakayama T, Tsukamoto Y, Terashima H, Kuroda Y, Okuma R: Radiologic findings in xanthogranulomatous cholecystitis. AJR 148:727–730, 1987.

83. Loflin TG, Simeone JF, Mueller PR, et al: Gallbladder bile in cholecystitis: in vitro MR evaluation. Radiology 157:457–459, 1985.

84. Weissleder R, Stark D, Compton CC, Simeone JF, Ferrucci

JT: Cholecystitis: diagnosis by MR imaging. Magn Reson Imaging 6:345–348, 1988.

85. Berland LL, Doust BD, Foley WD: Acute hemorrhage into the gallbladder diagnosed by computerized tomography and ultrasonography. J Comput Assist Tomogr 4:260–262, 1980.

86. Krudy AG, Doppman JL, Bissonette MB, Girton M: Hemobilia: computed tomographic diagnosis. Radiology 148:785–789, 1983.

87. Nichols DA, MacCarty RL, Gaffey TA: Cholangiographic evaluation of bile duct carcinoma. AJR 141:1291–1294, 1983.

88. Todani T, Tabuchi K, Watanabe Y, Kobayashi T: Carcinoma arising in the wall of congenital bile duct cysts. Cancer 44:1134–1141, 1979.

89. Strohl EL, Reed WH, Diffenbaugh WG, Andersen RE: Carcinoma of the bile ducts. Arch Surg 87:567–577, 1963.

90. Van Heerden JA, Judd ES, Dockerty MB: Carcinoma of the extrahepatic bile ducts. A clinicopathologic study. Am J Surg 113:49–56, 1967.

91. Nesbit GM, Johnson CD, James EM, MacCarty RL, Nagorney DM, et al: Cholangiocarcinoma: diagnosis and evaluation of resectability by CT and sonography as procedures complementary to cholangiography. AJR 151:933–938, 1988.

92. Dennis MA, Pretorius DH, Manco-Johnson ML: CT detection of portal venous gas associated with suppurative cholangitis and cholecystitis. AJR 145:1017–1018, 1985.

93. MacCarty RL, LaRusso NF, May GR, et al: Cholangiocarcinoma complicating primary sclerosing cholangitis: cholangiographic appearances. Radiology 156:43–46, 1985.

94. Federle MP, Cello JP, Laing FC, Jeffrey RB Jr: Recurrent pyogenic cholangitis in Asian immigrants: use of ultrasonography, computed tomography, and cholangiography. Radiology 143:151–156, 1982.

95. Harrison-Levy A: The biliary obstruction syndrome of the Chinese. Br J Surg 49:674–685, 1962.

96. Stock FE, Fung JHT: Oriental cholangiohepatitis. Arch Surg 84:409–412, 1962.

97. Coehlo JC, Buffara M, Pozzobon CE, Altenburg FL, Artigas GV: Incidence of common bile duct stones in patients with acute and chronic cholecystitis. Surg Gynecol Obstet 158:76–80, 1984.

98. Sauerbrei EE: Ultrasound of the common bile duct. Ultrasound Annu 1–45, 1983.

99. Jeffrey RB Jr, Federle MP, Laing FC, Wall S, Rego J, et al: Computed tomography of choledocholithiasis. AJR 140:1179–1183, 1983.

100. Baron RL: Common bile duct stones: reassessment of criteria for CT diagnosis. Radiology 162:419–424, 1987.

101. Mitchell SE, Clark RA: Comparison of computed tomography and sonography in choledocholithiasis. AJR 142:729, 1984.

102. Cronan JJ, Mueller PR, Simeone JF, O'Connell RS, vanSonnenberg E, Wittenberg J, Ferrucci JT Jr.: Prospective diagnosis of choledocholithiasis. Radiology 146:467–469, 1983.

103. Gross BH, Harter LP, Gore RM, Allen PW, Filly RH, et al: Ultrasonic evaluation of common bile duct stones: prospective comparison with endoscopic retrograde cholangiopancreatography. Radiology 146:471, 1983.

104. Laing FC, Jeffrey RB: Choledocholithiasis and cystic duct obstruction: difficult ultrasonographic diagnosis. Radiology 146:475, 1983.

105. Baron RL: CT diagnosis of choledocholithiasis. Semin US CT MR 8:85–102, 1987.

106. Friedman AC, Sachs L, Birns M: Radiology of jaundice, including choledocholithiasis and biliary neoplasms. In Friedman AC (ed): Radiology of the Liver, Biliary Tract, Pancreas and Spleen. Baltimore, Williams & Wilkins, 1987, pp 497–548.

107. Montana MA, Rohrmann CA Jr: Cholangiocarcinoma in a choledochal cyst: preoperative diagnosis. AJR 147:516–517, 1986.

CHAPTER 19

THE PANCREAS

MICHAEL P. FEDERLE ▪ *HENRY I. GOLDBERG*

Anatomy

The pancreas is located in the most ventral of the three retroperitoneal compartments, the anterior pararenal space. This space is defined ventrally by the posterior parietal peritoneum and dorsally by the anterior renal (Gerota's) fascia. Laterally, the anterior pararenal space is separated from the posterior pararenal space by the lateral conal fascia (Fig. 19–1). In all but the thinnest or most emaciated patients, the pancreas is surrounded by fat that clearly defines its margins. In asthenic individuals and young children, peripancreatic fat is often minimal, making the margins difficult to discern, especially along the anterior margin of the pancreas.

The pancreas is commonly divided descriptively into the head, neck, body, and tail segments. The *head* is the broad right end of the gland lying within the curve of the duodenum. The uncinate process is the prolongation of the left and caudal borders of the head that extends to and behind the superior mesenteric vein. The *neck* is the constricted portion to the left of the head, lying ventral to the superior mesenteric vessels. The *body* lies behind the lesser sac (omental bursa) and stomach, and its dorsal surface is indented by the splenic vein, the course of which generally parallels that of the pancreatic body and tail. The pancreatic *tail* is usually at the same level or cephalic to the body of the pancreas and

follows the splenic vessels into the splenic hilum. The most distal part of the gland lies within the splenorenal ligament, where it becomes an intraperitoneal structure (Fig. 19–2).[1]

The position and configuration of the pancreas are quite variable, and these variations may simulate disease states.[2] For example, the pancreatic head is not fixed in position, though it almost invariably maintains a fixed relationship medial to the second portion of duodenum and lateral to the root of the superior mesenteric vessels, even if these structures are shifted to the left of midline. Although the splenic vein usually marks the dorsal margin of the body and tail, the tip of the gland may rarely curve dorsal to the splenic vein to simulate adrenal pathologic abnormality.[1, 3] Occasionally, even in normal persons, the pancreatic tail may lie anteromedial to the kidney, where it may appear as a pseudomass on excretory urography. Congenital or surgical absence of the left kidney alters the retroperitoneal compartments, and the pancreatic tail may be displaced into the empty renal fossa, simulating recurrent tumor or a primary retroperitoneal lesion.[2]

Several attempts have been made to determine normal limits of pancreatic size on axial computed tomographic (CT) sections in the expectation that this would permit more accurate determination of pathologic states such as pancreatitis, tumor, or atrophy. Using different scanners, Haaga and co-workers[4] and

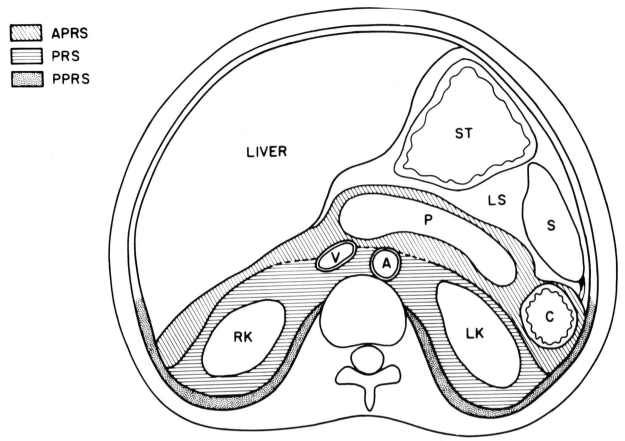

APRS
PRS
PPRS

FIGURE 19–1 ■ Retroperitoneal compartments. The pancreas (P) lies in the anterior pararenal space (APRS), the borders of which are the posterior parietal peritoneum ventrally, the anterior renal (Gerota's) fascia dorsally, and the lateral conal fascia laterally. Other important structures in the APRS are the duodenal loop (not shown) and the ascending and descending colon (C). A = Aorta; LS = lesser sac; PRS = pararenal space; PPRS = posterior pararenal space; RK and LK = right and left kidney; S = spleen; ST = stomach; V = vena cava.

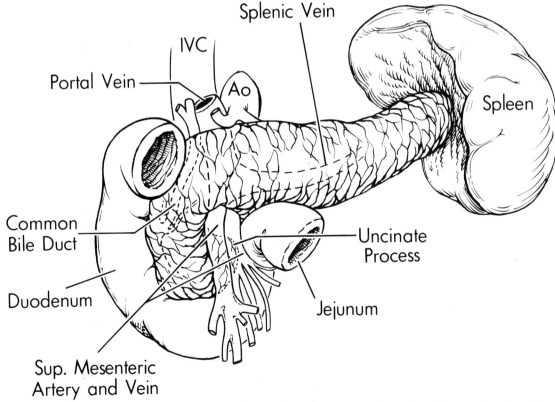

FIGURE 19–2 ■ Pancreatic anatomy. The pancreatic head lies between the superior mesenteric vessels and the second portion of the duodenum. The uncinate process lies behind the mesenteric vessels, and the neck lies ventral to them. The body lies ventral to the splenic vein. The tail constitutes the last few centimeters of the gland, lies intraperitoneally, and inserts into the splenic hilum within the leaves of the splenorenal ligament.

Stanley et al.[5] published somewhat different criteria, though each group related the anteroposterior diameter of the pancreas to the transverse diameter of the adjacent vertebral body. In general, the pancreatic head dimension does not exceed the width of the vertebral body, averaging about 0.7 when expressed as a ratio. The pancreatic body–to-vertebral ratio is usually about 0.33. However, these authors[4, 5] noted a broad overlap between the upper and lower limits of normal and the abnormal gland. Kreel and colleagues[6] published a set of in vivo and in vitro measurements of pancreatic dimensions and concluded that the "normal" diameter of the head was up to 3 cm; that of the neck and body, up to 2.5 cm; and that of the tail, up to 2 cm. In assessing these values, the authors noted the importance of assuring that adjacent structures such as the portal and splenic veins, superior mesenteric vein, and duodenum are not included in the measurements.

All experienced CT observers have noted that the size, shape, and position of the normal pancreas are highly variable. Rigid adherence to any ratio or absolute measurements, without consideration of other factors, will lead to interpretive error. In general, there is a gradual tapering from the head to the tail without abrupt alterations in size or contour. There is also gradual diminution in pancreatic size with advancing age, sometimes becoming quite marked beyond the seventh decade. The contour of the pancreas is smooth (Fig. 19–3) in about 80 per cent of cases and lobulated in 20 per cent.[6] Fatty lobulations are more commonly observed in obese and elderly subjects (Fig. 19–4). Such lobulations are not indicative of disease; to the contrary, the observation of evenly distributed lobulations may help exclude underlying inflammation or tumor.

Techniques of Examination

Because the pancreas has essentially the same attenuation coefficient as unopacified bowel and blood vessels, techniques of examination are mainly directed toward identifying all adjacent structures by use of oral and intravenous contrast media.

Oral contrast medium administration is almost always indicated, because the stomach, duodenum, and proximal small bowel must be distinguished from the pancreas and because these structures are commonly involved by pancreatic lesions. The two oral contrast agents in common use are dilute (one to three per cent) meglumine and sodium diatrizoate and barium. Preliminary attempts[7] to introduce a "negative" oral contrast medium, polyunsaturated oil, met with little enthusiasm because of poor patient acceptance and medical contraindications in pancreatitis, cholecystitis, and other conditions.

When the stomach is collapsed, jejunal segments are commonly interposed between the pancreas and stomach[8] and may simulate a tumor or lesser sac abnormality or result in a distorted impression of pancreatic size.[5] The fundus of the collapsed stomach may itself give rise to a pseudotumor in the pancreatic tail.[6, 9] Full distension of the stomach with dilute oral contrast medium effectively eliminates both these potential pitfalls by outlining the gastric lumen and displacing small bowel loops away from the ventral surface of the pancreatic body and tail.[10] Gastric distention serves the additional purpose of orienting the pancreas more transversely as a result of caudal displacement of the spleen, allowing complete visualization on several contiguous sections.

Intravenous contrast administration is useful to distinguish pancreatic parenchyma from adjacent blood vessels and to better delineate normal structures (e.g., pancreatic and common bile ducts) and abnormal conditions (pseudocysts, peripancreatic edema). An intense pancreatogram can be obtained by rapid bolus injection of 100 to 160 mL of 60 per cent contrast medium followed by rapid consecutive CT scanning. Following a bolus injection of contrast medium, the normal pancreas enhances uniformly (Fig. 19–5); during the brief pancreatogram phase (lasting less than 2 minutes), the distinction between normal pancreatic parenchyma and intrinsic or extrinsic lesions is more evident than with the drip infusion method of contrast administration.[11] Some investigators have suggested that the normal or "high" enhancement of the pancreas following bolus injection of contrast medium can be used to separate areas of necrotizing pancreatitis, that show "low" enhancement from viable pancreatic tissue.[12] Dynamic CT is also useful for diagnosing such specific entities as splenic vein occlusion, pseudoaneurysms, and vascular tumors.

The collimation and spacing of CT sections vary somewhat depending on the indication for the study and the findings on preliminary sections. For most purposes, 8- to 10-mm collimation (section thickness) is adequate, although 3- to 5-mm collimation through the pancreatic parenchyma is extremely useful in detecting small masses and abnormalities of the pancreatic and distal common bile ducts. Contiguous sections are usually obtained, although spacing can be increased to 15 or 20 mm through the pancreatic area in many cases of widespread inflammation.

Techniques for examination of the pancreas using magnetic resonance imaging (MRI) are in a state of transition as a result of rapid advancements in imaging the abdomen. Respiratory motion and intestinal peristalsis have produced artifacts that degrade pancreatic image quality. This has been particularly true on the long repetition time (TR) and long echo delay time (TE) T2-weighted images but also to some degree on T1-weighted images of standard spin-echo sequences. Increasing the signal averaging, decreasing TR and TE results in reduced-motion artifacts and improvement of signal-to-noise ratio and anatomic delineation of the pancreas.[13] Imaging time may also be reduced with use of partial flip angles,

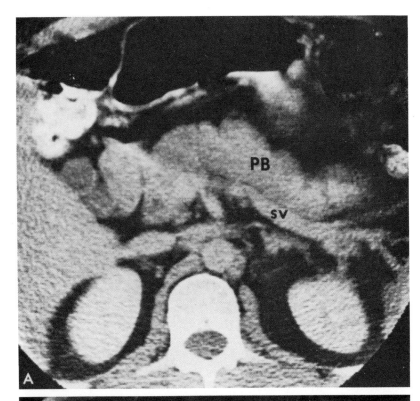

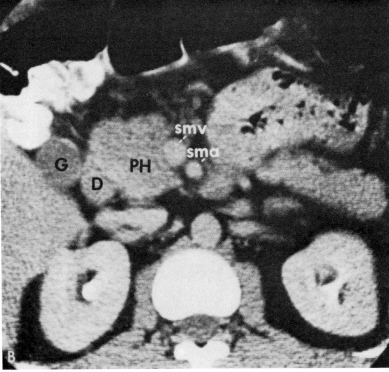

FIGURE 19–3 ■ Normal pancreas. Patient is a 30-year-old man. *A,* The pancreatic body (PB) lies just ventral to the splenic vein (sv). *B,* CT scan 2 cm caudal to *A.* Pancreatic head (PH) lies between the superior mesenteric vessels and second portion of duodenum. The uncinate process lies behind the superior mesenteric vein and has a beaklike medial margin. D = Duodenum; G = gallbladder; SMA = superior mesenteric artery; SMV = superior mesenteric vein.

because TR is reduced. The resultant images have improved signal-to-noise ratio and have resulted in less motion artifact.[14] The use of fast scan techniques permits imaging of the pancreas within the breath-holding capabilities of most patients. The use of body surface coils over the region of the pancreas has improved signal-to-noise ratios and pancreatic imaging quality.[15]

Adjacent stomach, duodenum and jejunum may be of signal intensity similar to that of the pancreas and may obscure the true boundaries of the pancreas. Some form of gastrointestinal MR contrast material

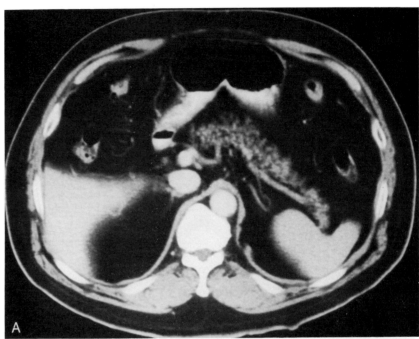

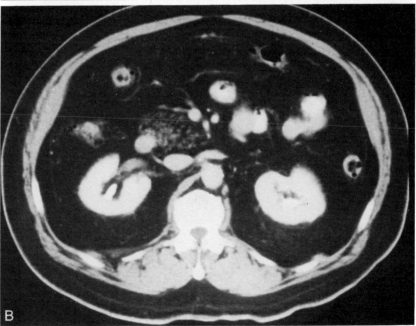

FIGURE 19–4 ■ *A* and *B,* Normal pancreas. Patient is a moderately obese 60-year-old man. The fatty infiltration and lobulation of the pancreas are normal findings, particularly with advanced age and obesity.

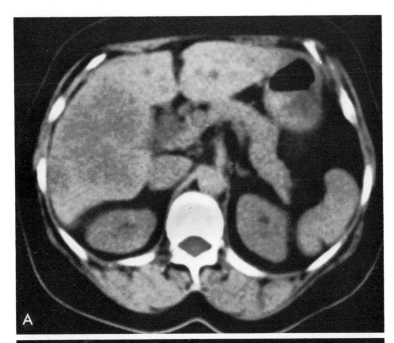

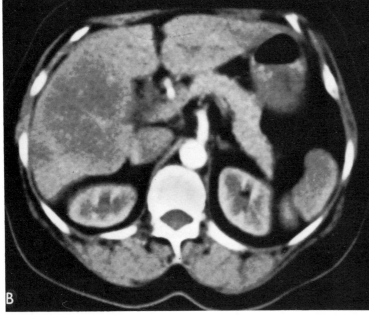

FIGURE 19–5 ■ Dynamic CT scans of a normal pancreas. *A*, Before intravenous injection of a bolus of 60 mL of iodinated contrast material. The CT scan shows a normal pancreas that had a CT density of 44 H. *B*, CT scan during maximum aortic enhancement. The pancreas has increased in CT density to 66 H. The aorta and celiac artery are enhanced, as are the hepatic artery and renal cortex.

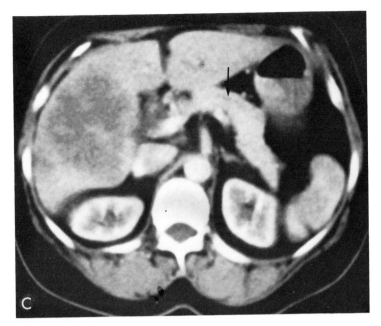

FIGURE 19–5 *Continued* ■ *C,* CT scan 10 seconds later; the pancreas has reached a CT density of 84 H. The faint outlines of the normal pancreatic duct *(arrow)* are evident; it is detected as the result of enhancement of surrounding pancreatic parenchyma.

is desirable to identify bowel and permit its distinction from pancreatic tissue. Orally administered ferric ammonium citrate solutions have been successfully utilized for this purpose.[16] Newer contrast agents being currently evaluated include iron oxide particles[17] and perfluorocytylbromide.[18] It appears that some form of contrast material in the gastrointestinal tract will be necessary to improve pancreatic imaging by MR.

The normal pancreas can be identified in almost all patients (Fig. 19–6). The intensity or brightness of the pancreas is approximately the same as that of the liver on both T1- and T2-weighted spin-echo and inversion recovery images. The splenic vein, portal vein, and their confluence with the mesenteric vein usually aid in identification of the tail, body, and head of the pancreas. Distention of the duodenum by air or contrast material further aids in defining the head of the pancreas. In all but very thin individuals, infants, and young children, the pancreas is surrounded by enough fat, with its bright signal, to permit recognition of the pancreatic boundaries. The use of intravenous glucagon to abate gastroduodenal and jejunal peristalsis further improves the image of both normal and abnormal pancreas by providing sharper delineation among bowel, fat, and pancreas.[19]

Pathology

Acute Pancreatitis

Acute pancreatitis may have one of numerous origins, including alcohol, trauma or surgery, cholelithiasis, penetrating peptic ulcer, hyperlipoproteinemia, hypercalcemia, and infection. Regardless of the origin, the pathologic and radiographic findings are similar and represent a spectrum of changes. It has not been established that acute and chronic pancreatitis are different stages of the same disease. The international symposium held at Marseilles in 1963 defined acute pancreatitis as inflammation with the potential for complete healing, whereas chronic pancreatitis is associated with residual permanent damage. Either form may be marked by relapses of acute inflammation. Duration of the disease is not considered in this classification.[20]

Acute pancreatitis can be subdivided into somewhat overlapping clinical categories reflecting the underlying process of interstitial (edematous) pancreatitis or hemorrhagic (necrotizing) pancreatitis. In some cases, however, it may be difficult to differentiate these two types of pancreatitis except by their clinical course, with a more prolonged complicated course thought to be indicative of hemorrhagic pancreatitis. Interstitial pancreatitis accounts for 75 to 95 per cent of cases, with most patients showing clinical improvement within 48 to 72 hours on supportive management. The incidence of hemorrhagic or necrotizing pancreatitis varies with the criteria for diagnosis, ranging from 5 to 25 per cent, but results in a disproportionate amount of morbidity and mortality.[21–23]

Ranson and Pasternak have defined a set of laboratory and clinical criteria that are commonly used to judge the severity of an attack of acute pancreatitis and have some prognostic significance in predicting complications, including abscess development and hemorrhage (Table 19–1).[24] Several investigators have recently reported using CT early in the course of pancreatitis as a predictor of outcome. In most reports the presence and extent of extrapancreatic abnormalities as detected by CT have correlated well with Ranson and Pasternak's criteria and the subsequent development of complications.[25–28]

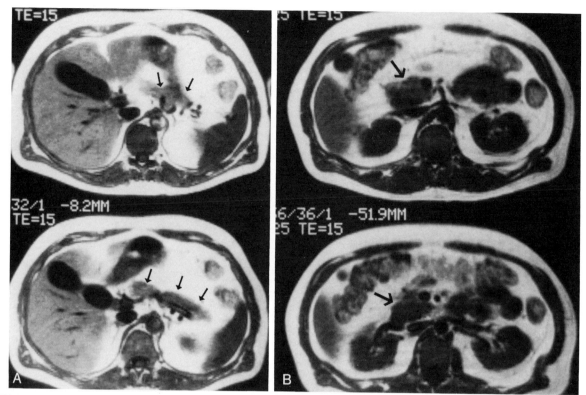

FIGURE 19–6 ■ Magnetic resonance images of the normal pancreas. *A,* On these T1-weighted images the tail of the pancreas and the body are well shown *(arrows, A and B),* because they are of intermediate signal intensity and are surrounded by high signal from retroperitoneal fat. *B,* The head of the pancreas and the uncinate process have a signal intensity similar to that of the liver and can be differentiated from the superior mesenteric artery and vein, which are black because of lack of signal from flowing blood.

INDICATIONS FOR CT

Some controversy remains concerning the indications for and predictive value of CT in acute pancreatitis, but a consensus can be reached at a practical level. The diagnosis of pancreatitis is made accurately in most cases with an appropriate patient history, symptoms, physical signs, and supporting laboratory determinations. When the inflammation is mild, symptoms usually regress spontaneously within 48 hours, and recovery is complete. CT in such cases may be normal or may detect glandular swelling and limited peripancreatic inflammation. In our opinion, however, CT is of little value in this setting, as it rarely influences the care of the patient with mild pancreatitis.

In patients with an uncertain diagnosis or patients who are suspected of having some complication of pancreatitis (such as hemorrhage, pseudocyst, or abscess), CT is of proven value. As noted previously, CT has been reported to be an accurate prognostic test, alone or along with Ranson and Pasternak's clinical criteria, in predicting which patients might suffer greater morbidity and mortality from acute pancreatitis.[25–27] In our experience, the extent of peripancreatic inflammation on early scanning correlates well with subsequent fluid replacement requirements and pseudocyst development, but we have had less success in predicting which patients will develop abscesses or other life-threatening complications.[28, 29]

Although acute pancreatitis is generally a clinical diagnosis made on the basis of patient history and physical examination, it has a wide range of manifestations, and the diagnosis may not be considered. Peterson and Brooks[30] noted that in 40 patients dying of severe pancreatitis, a premortem diagnosis was not made in 43 per cent. Other diseases may exactly simulate the clinical, laboratory, and radiographic manifestations of acute pancreatitis; these include acute cholecystitis, peptic ulcer disease, and bowel infarction. Patients may be subjected to nonthera-

TABLE 19–1 ■ Early Prognostic Signs of Acute Pancreatitis (Ranson and Pasternak's Criteria)

AT ADMISSION OR DIAGNOSIS	DURING INITIAL 48 HOURS
Age over 55 years	Hematocrit fall greater than 10 percentage points
White blood cell count over 16×10^3/mL	Blood urea nitrogen level rise more than 5 mg/dL
Blood glucose level over 200 mg/dL	Serum calcium level below 8 mg/dL
Serum lactic acid dehydrogenase level over 350 IU/L	Arterial P_{O_2} below 60 mg Hg
Serum glutamic-oxaloacetic transaminase level over 250 IU/dL	Base deficit greater than 4 mEq/L
	Estimated fluid sequestration more than 6000 mL

Source: Data compiled from Ranson JHC, Pasternak BS: J Surg Res 22:79, 1977.

peutic laparotomy because of misdiagnosis; laparotomy is generally contraindicated in acute interstitial pancreatitis. Even more serious is delaying surgical intervention in cases of bowel infarction misdiagnosed as acute pancreatitis.

CT FINDINGS

The manifestations of acute pancreatitis on CT are varied, and there is not a close correlation between the extent of disease as shown by CT and the clinical severity of the attack. One of the most common findings in acute interstitial pancreatitis is swelling of the gland, though this finding must be interpreted with caution in light of the normal variability of pancreatic size. The swelling is diffuse in the majority of cases, though focal swelling of the head and tail is seen in approximately 48 per cent of cases.[31] The pancreas does not have a firm capsule, and pancreatic secretions commonly break through the thin layer of connective tissue that surrounds the gland (Fig. 19–7). When pancreatic or peripancreatic fluid collections become loculated and fixed by a dense fibrous capsule, they are called *pseudocysts*.

Some authors[32] have chosen to designate as "fluid collections" all manifestations of extrapancreatic spread of inflammation. Most investigators prefer the term *phlegmon* to indicate an inflammatory mass arising from the pancreas or diffuse spreading inflammation that may go on to suppurate, liquefy, or resolve spontaneously (Fig. 19–8).[31, 33] Proof that pancreatic phlegmons are not fluid collections is obtained by sonography and the results of attempted needle aspiration. Although the attenuation value of a pancreatic phlegmon may be near 0 Hounsfield units (H), pathologically, phlegmons are boggy, edematous soft tissue masses composed of an admixture of inflammation, exudate, and retroperitoneal fat.

Phlegmonous extension is demonstrable in 18 per cent of unselected cases of pancreatitis[31] and well over 50 per cent of patients with more severe disease.[29, 32] The most common sites of involvement are the lesser sac and left anterior pararenal space; less frequently involved are the transverse mesocolon and small bowel mesentery.[33] Given the aggressive nature of pancreatic inflammation and enzymatic tissue necrosis, almost every area of the abdomen has been noted to harbor pancreatic inflammatory masses, including the perirenal spaces and peritoneal cavity.[33, 34]

Commonly encountered CT signs of pancreatitis are diffuse pancreatic enlargement, blurring of the pancreatic margins, and thickening of the renal (Gerota's) fascia (Figs. 19–9 through 19–12). Thickening of the renal fascia is a strong indicator of local inflammation and is not seen in normal individuals or those with focal intrapancreatic neoplasms.[35, 36] Infiltration of the pararenal spaces with sparing of the perirenal space can result in the "renal halo sign" on either plain radiographs or CT (see Figs. 19–8 through 19–10).[37] The perinephric space is uncommonly involved (see Fig. 19–11). Focal thickening of the gastric wall (see Fig. 19–9) is seen in 70 per cent of cases of acute pancreatitis in which accurate measurements are possible,[38] and although focal thickening has been described as a sign of gastric carcinoma or lymphoma, pancreatitis is a more common origin in some patient populations.

COMPLICATIONS

The morbidity and mortality associated with acute pancreatitis can be attributed largely to the development of hemorrhage, vascular complications, pseudocysts, or abscesses.

Hemorrhagic Pancreatitis ■ The diagnosis of hemorrhagic pancreatitis is based on clinical criteria such as a falling hematocrit, hypocalcemia, and failure to respond quickly to resuscitative measures. Significant hemorrhage occurs in two to five per cent of patients with acute pancreatitis. The mortality in cases of acute hemorrhagic pancreatitis varies from 33 to 100 per cent, depending on the criteria for diagnosis.[22, 23, 39, 40] Prompt surgical intervention has been advocated if intensive resuscitative efforts have failed.[39]

The accuracy of CT in detecting hemorrhagic pancreatitis is not known, but pancreatic hemorrhage is identified in about five per cent of cases of acute pancreatitis as a collection of high attenuation (greater than 60 H) in the pancreatic area (Fig. 19–13).[41] However, the CT diagnosis of hemorrhagic pancreatitis is not simple, because it is difficult to differentiate diffuse peripancreatic hemorrhage from hemorrhage into a preexisting pseudocyst; moreover, there is no correlation of CT evidence of hemorrhage with the clinical diagnosis of hemorrhagic pancreatitis.[41, 42] Because CT reveals hemorrhage in some patients with a benign clinical course, surgical management is not generally indicated unless clinical factors indicate otherwise.

Vascular Complications ■ Although hemorrhagic pancreatitis usually results from small vessel erosions, larger vessels may develop pseudoaneurysms or occlusions as a result of pancreatitis, usually complicating pseudocyst development or chronic relapsing pancreatitis. The histiolytic enzymes released during episodes of pancreatitis may erode vessel walls, leading to pseudoaneurysm or rupture of vessels in the pancreatic bed, including the splenic, gastroduodenal, and hepatic arteries. These may be presumptively diagnosed by bolus-enhanced CT as highly enhancing perivascular structures, usually within or adjacent to pseudocysts; definitive diagnosis (and therapy) requires angiography (Fig. 19–14).[43] Pseudocysts and chronic pancreatitis may also cause venous occlusions of any of the portal vein tributaries, with splenic vein thrombosis being most common. A bolus-enhanced CT scan may demonstrate the thrombosis along with complications such as gastric varices (Fig. 19–15).[44]

Pseudocysts ■ Data on the true incidence and natural history of pancreatic pseudocysts are difficult to compare because of varying criteria and modalities employed for diagnosis. We use the term *pseudocyst*

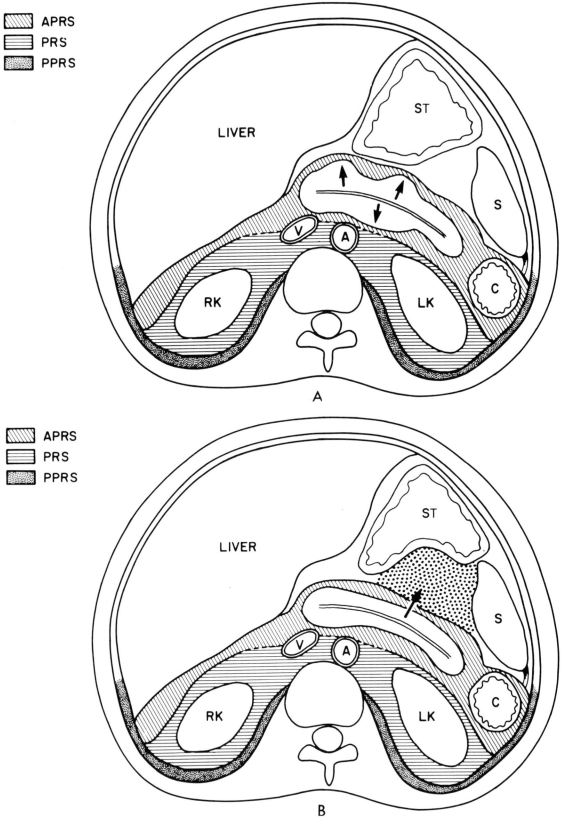

FIGURE 19–7 ■ Acute pancreatitis—pathways of spread. *A,* Mild pancreatitis causes glandular swelling limited by the thin capsule. More extensive inflammation commonly breaks through the capsule to spread within the lesser sac *(B),* anterior pararenal space *(C),* or both *(D).* (For key to abbreviations see legend for Figure 19–1.)

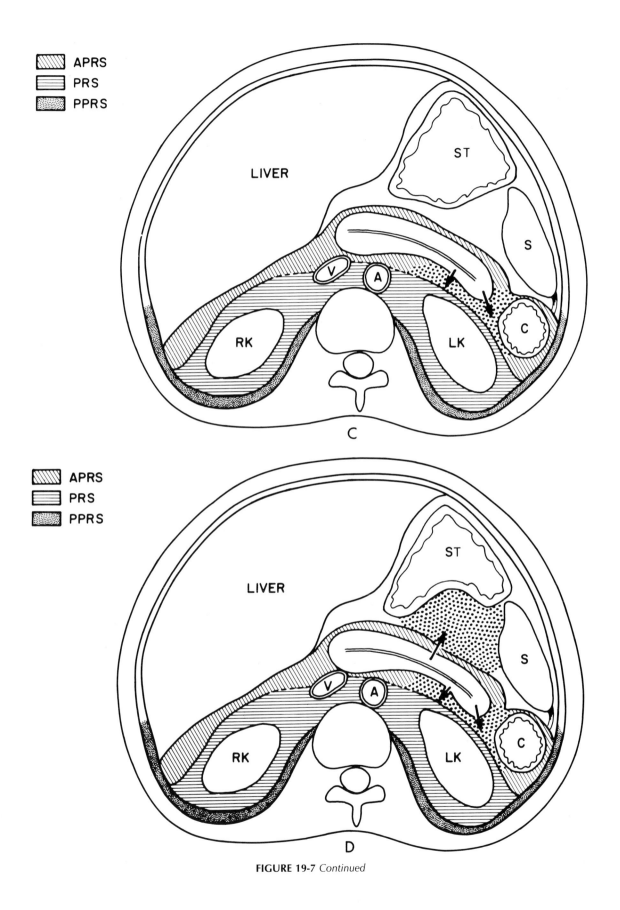

FIGURE 19-7 *Continued*

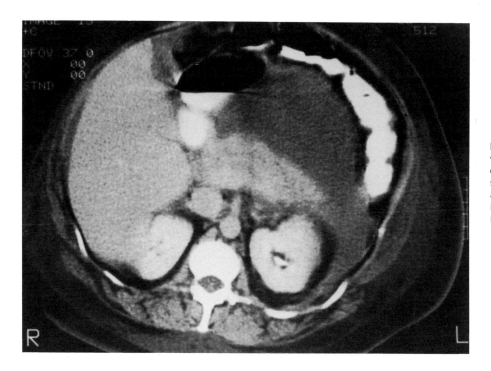

FIGURE 19–8 ■ Acute pancreatitis with large phlegmon. The pancreas is diffusely swollen. A large water-density mass extends into the mesentery and anterior pararenal space. This mass lacks a definite capsule and was not fluid-containing on ultrasound. Note sparing of the perirenal space.

to indicate a collection of necrotic tissue, old blood, and secretions that have escaped from the pancreas damaged by pancreatitis.[45] These secretions, rich in proteolytic enzymes, may become loculated in the lesser sac or may extend along retroperitoneal tissue planes in any direction. Pseudocysts may remain within the pancreatic capsule (Fig. 19–16), but more commonly they are found in an extrapancreatic location. They may dissect up into the mediastinum[46] as far as the neck or retroperitoneally until they reach the groin. Pseudocysts may burrow into the wall of the duodenum and simulate intramural or obstructing masses (Figs. 19–17 and 19–18),[47] or they may dissect into the liver or spleen (Fig. 19–19). Pseudocysts extending into the liver along portal tracts may simulate dilated bile ducts.[48]

The wall of the pseudocyst is initially formed by whatever tissue structures first limit its spread. Gradually the evoked inflammatory reaction encapsulates the contents of the pseudocyst with granulation tissue and then with a fibrous wall; when this has occurred, the pseudocyst is considered mature.[45, 49]

The incidence of pseudocyst following acute pancreatitis in the pre–ultrasound and CT era was estimated as only two to three per cent.[50, 51] However, using CT, Bradley and colleagues[52] found "fluid collections" in 56 per cent of patients with moderately severe pancreatitis, and Siegelman et al.[32] found "fluid collections" complicating pancreatitis in 54 per cent of patients. However, both these studies are somewhat misleading, because they grouped all peripancreatic exudates, whether phlegmonous or truly cystic, under the same designation and excluded patients with mild pancreatitis. In a prospective CT study of consecutive patients with pancreatitis, pseudocysts were detected in ten per cent and extrapan-

creatic phlegmons in 18 per cent,[31] figures that are comparable to those when sonography is used for diagnosis.[53]

It is important to understand the clinical implications of pancreatic inflammation, despite the differences in semantics used to describe pancreatic inflammatory lesions. A phlegmon is a pancreatic inflammatory mass or a spreading diffuse inflammation that may resolve completely or may go on to liquefy or suppurate. The inflammatory mass may be indistinguishable from neoplasm by CT,[54] but a presumptive diagnosis is usually possible when clinical and biochemical findings are considered. CT scans and sonography can demonstrate evolution of a phlegmon into a pseudocyst by showing a progressive liquefaction of the contents and development of a well-defined fibrous capsule. A pseudocyst may simulate a solid mass early in its formation, as blood and proteinaceous necrotic debris elevate the attenuation value. Ultrasonography is useful in confirming the fluid nature of the contents of the developing cyst.

The appearance of a pancreatic pseudocyst may be simulated by pancreatic tumors (cystadenocarcinoma, necrotic carcinoma, islet cell tumor) (Fig. 19–20), abscess, and even a dilated afferent loop.[55–57] The combination of CT findings and clinical information is usually sufficient for diagnosis. Patients with cystic fibrosis may develop pancreatic cysts and calcifications. These patients have pancreatic insufficiency but not pancreatitis.[58] If uncertainty remains, fine-needle aspiration from cysts can be checked for cytologic and bacteriologic abnormalities, amylase content, and carcinoembryonic antigen (CEA). An elevated CEA level appears to be specific for carcinoma.[59] The wall of a pseudocyst may calcify, usually

Text continued on page 889

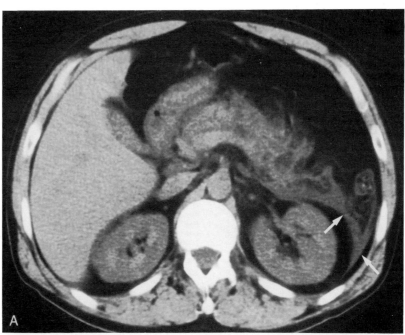

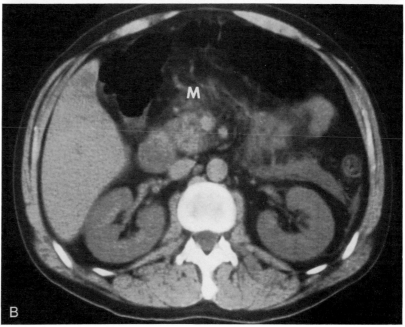

FIGURE 19–9 ■ Acute pancreatitis. Gland swelling is not obvious, but there is definite infiltration of peripancreatic fat planes, including the anterior pararenal space and mesentery (M). Note sharp demarcation by the renal and lateroconal fascia *(arrows),* sparing the perirenal space ("renal halo").

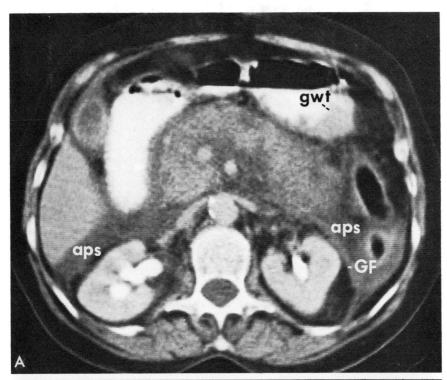

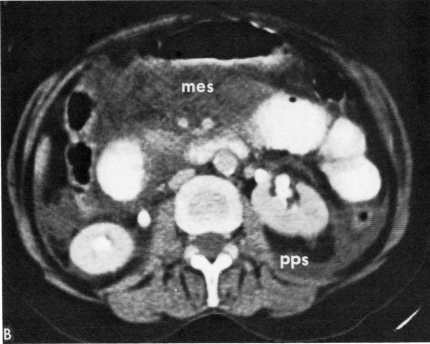

FIGURE 19–10 ■ Acute pancreatitis. Typical pathways of spread of pancreatic inflammation include the left and right anterior pararenal spaces (aps), transverse mesocolon, and small bowel mesentery (mes). Note also focal thickening of the gastric wall (gwt), thickening of Gerota's (anterior renal) fascia (GF), and involvement of the posterior pararenal space (pps) on the left, with sparing of the perinephric space. This is the origin of the "renal halo" sign.

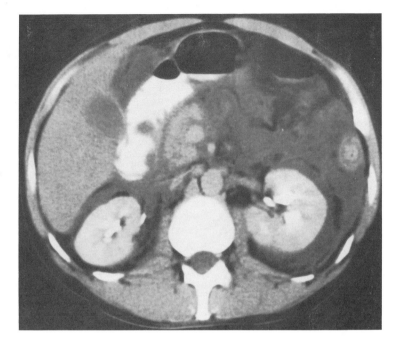

FIGURE 19–11 ■ Acute pancreatitis. The left perirenal space is infiltrated along with the more common areas such as mesentery and pararenal spaces.

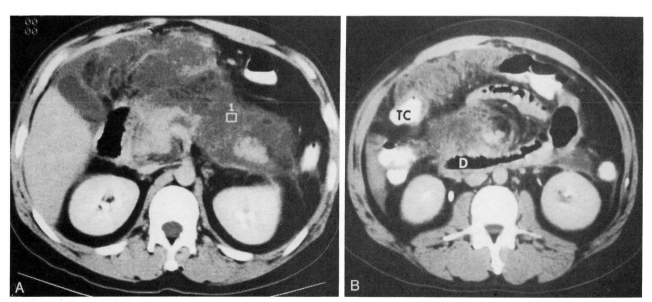

FIGURE 19–12 ■ Acute necrotic pancreatitis: bowel-mesenteric involvement. *A,* Diffuse spread of inflammation into the retroperitoneum and mesentery. A portion of the pancreatic body appears to be absent or necrotic. *B,* The transverse colon (TC) and duodenum (D) are encased by inflammation with wall thickening and luminal narrowing.

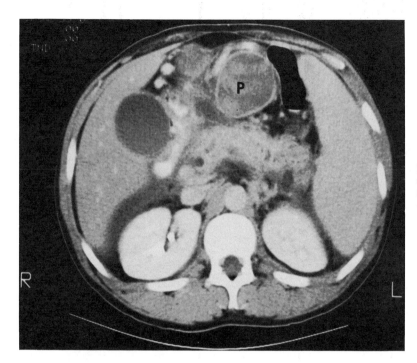

FIGURE 19–13 ■ Hemorrhagic pseudocyst. The pseudocyst (P) is well encapsulated, usually indicating some chronicity, but contains high-density fluid indicative of pus or hemorrhage.

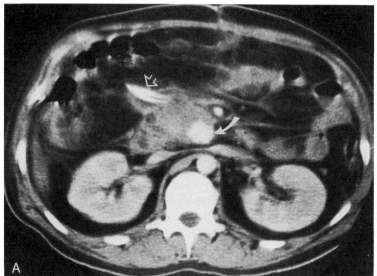

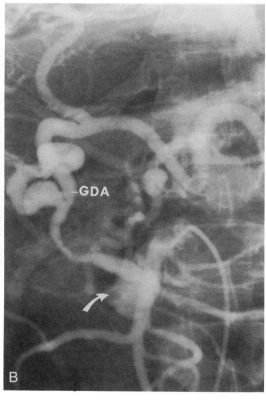

FIGURE 19–14 ■ Traumatic pancreatic pseudoaneurysm. A, CT after surgery revealed a pancreatic "contusion"; no fracture was identified by CT or surgery. Note surgical drain (open arrow). Abnormal enhancing structure in pancreatic head (curved arrow) has an arterial enhancement pattern on this bolus-enhanced scan. B, Superior mesenteric arteriogram. Retrograde filling of an occluded celiac trunk through a dilated gastroduodenal artery (GDA), part of which is spastic or stenotic. Note the pseudoaneurysm (curved arrow).

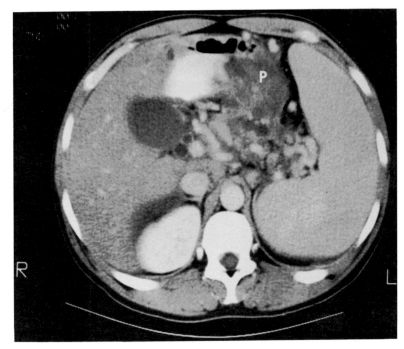

FIGURE 19–15 ■ Acute relapsing pancreatitis: splenic vein occlusion. CT demonstrates splenomegaly, pseudocyst, or phlegmon (P), and numerous varices in the gastric and pancreatic bed.

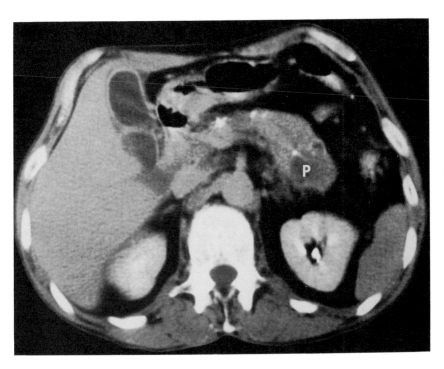

FIGURE 19–16 ■ Small pseudocyst (P), possibly intrapancreatic and associated with chronic pancreatitis.

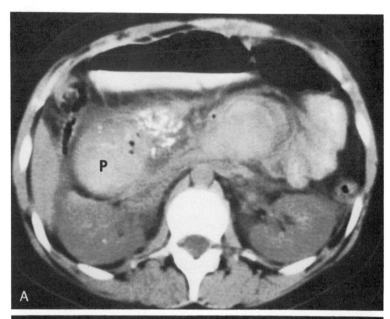

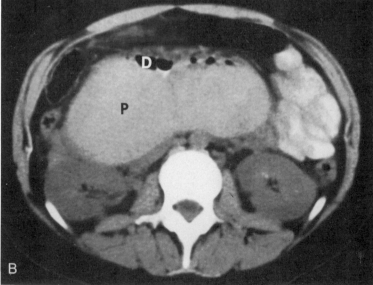

FIGURE 19–17 ■ *A,* Duodenal intramural pseudocyst. Calculi in head of pancreas and gastric distention are apparent. *B,* The duodenal lumen (D) is displaced and narrowed by an encapsulated, high-density (hemorrhagic) fluid collection (P) that parallels the second and third portions of duodenum.

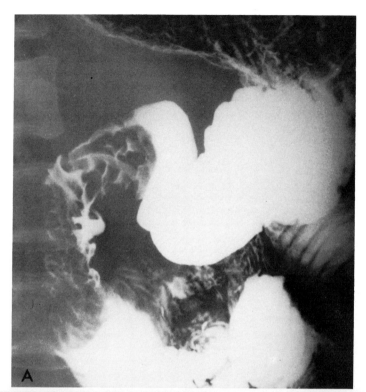

FIGURE 19–18 ■ Intramural pseudocyst of the duodenum. *A,* Upper gastrointestinal series shows an intramural mass in the duodenum producing thickening of the mucosal folds and a partial gastric outlet obstruction. *B,* CT scan demonstrates that the duodenum (D) is compressed medially by a pseudocyst (PC). The pancreatic head is enlarged, and peripancreatic inflammatory infiltrate is present *(arrow).*

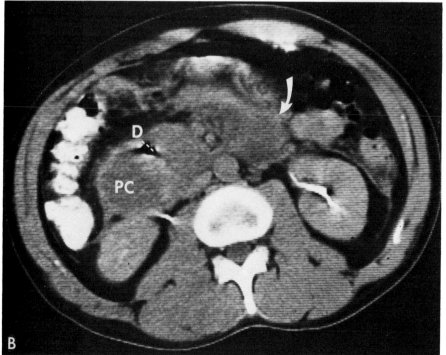

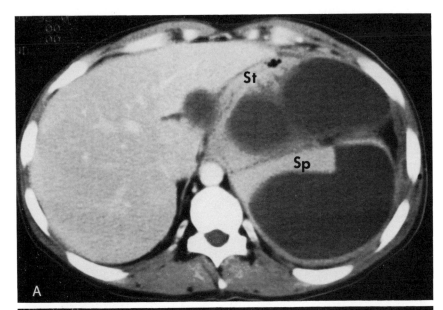

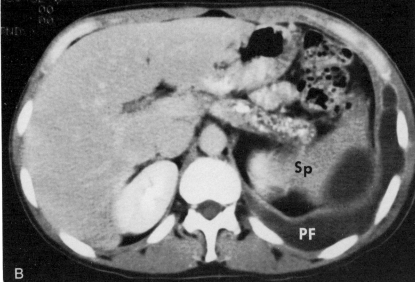

FIGURE 19–19 ■ Intrasplenic pseudocyst: chronic pancreatitis. Stomach (St) is displaced by a large pseudocyst. Spleen (Sp) is also displaced and deformed by a subcapsular pseudocyst. Pleural fluid (PF) is also noted.

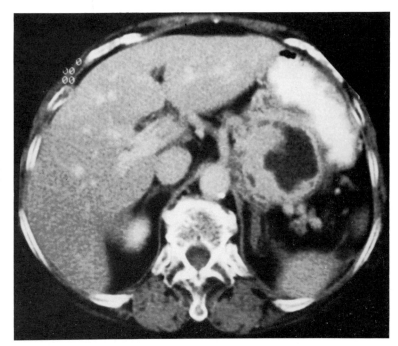

FIGURE 19–20 ■ A CT scan of a cystadenocarcinoma simulating a pancreatic pseudocyst. The mural nodularity and thickening are clues to the neoplastic nature of the mass.

in a chronic pseudocyst with prior complication of hemorrhage or infection.[60]

Both CT and ultrasonography are useful in following the course of phlegmons and pseudocysts. Twenty to 44 per cent of pseudocysts resolve spontaneously within 6 weeks,[51, 52] but beyond 6 weeks further resolution is rare, as a firm fibrous capsule has usually formed (Fig. 19–21). Although CT can be used to follow the maturation of a pseudocyst, sonography is preferred because of its low cost and lack of ionizing radiation. However, prior to surgery, a CT scan should be performed, as CT reveals the number, size, and location of cysts relative to pertinent gastrointestinal structures better than sonography.

Pseudocysts that fail to resolve by 6 weeks should be drained; in a prospective study of nonoperative management of pseudocysts, Bradley et al. reported complications in 41 per cent of patients and a mortality rate of 14 per cent.[52] Patients with pseudocysts can be separated into two distinct groups: those who are acutely ill, requiring urgent intervention, and those who are stable, allowing for elective intervention. Operative treatment of the acutely ill group of patients requires external pseudocyst drainage in 50 to 75 per cent of cases because of the immaturity of the cyst wall or the presence of infection. Morbidity and mortality in this group is high, with recurrence of pseudocysts in 28 per cent and death in 25 per cent.[61–63] Elective operative cyst drainage is usually performed as an internal drainage procedure, most often cystogastrostomy, and carries a much lower rate of cyst recurrence and mortality.

Percutaneous catheter drainage of pseudocysts can be accomplished with lower morbidity and mortality than operative drainage and with a cure rate of 70 to 80 per cent.[64, 65] Success rates are higher and the incidence of pancreatic cutaneous fistulas is lower if the cyst no longer communicates with the pancreatic duct. Percutaneous transgastric catheter drainage of pseudocysts is a further refinement that reduces the incidence of pancreatic-cutaneous fistula (Fig. 19–22).[66, 67] Prolonged catheter drainage creates a tract between the cyst and the posterior wall of the stomach, facilitating drainage even after the catheter has been removed and even if the cyst still communicates with the pancreatic duct.

Abscesses ■ Infectious complications of pancreatitis are uncommon but life threatening. No universally accepted definition of the different types of infectious complications has yet been adopted; different authors have grouped together such disparate entities as infected pseudocysts and infected pancreatic necrosis. These have a very different patient prognosis, making it very difficult to find a consensus on the incidence, diagnostic criteria, and therapy for "pancreatic abscesses."

Abscesses are said to occur in four per cent of all patients with acute pancreatitis,[68] but the incidence increases with the severity of the attack. Abscesses are found in 50 to 70 per cent of fatal cases of necrotizing pancreatitis.[68–70] Survival without drainage is rare, but newer techniques of diagnosis and therapy have markedly improved the prognosis for many patients.

Bittner and colleagues have helped to better characterize local septic complications of pancreatitis in an attempt to develop improved concepts for their prevention, early diagnosis, and treatment.[71] They clearly distinguish between two separate clinical entities, infected necrosis and pancreatic abscesses, based on morphologic, clinical, and laboratory criteria. They define infected necrosis as a diffuse bacterial inflammation of necrotic pancreatic and peripancre-

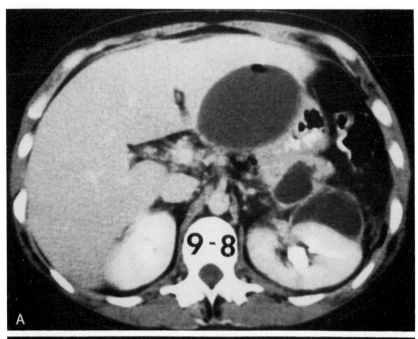

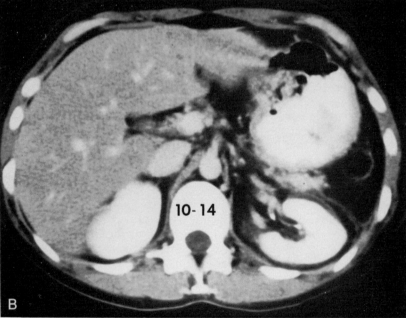

FIGURE 19–21 ■ Spontaneous resolution of pseudocysts. *A*, Multiple encapsulated pseudocysts are seen on the initial CT. Gas bubble in largest pseudocyst is the result of prior aspiration. Note left perinephric pseudocyst. *B*, Repeat CT 5 weeks later shows spontaneous resolution of cysts, even though they appeared to be relatively "mature" on an earlier study.

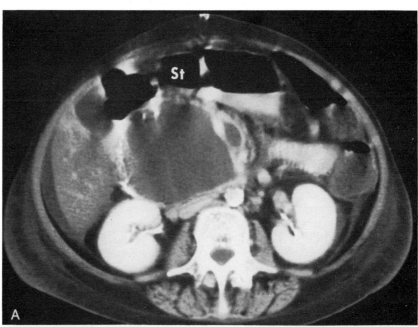

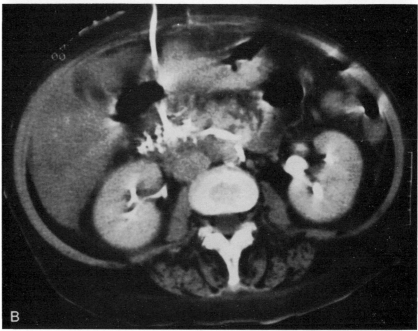

FIGURE 19–22 ■ Percutaneous drainage of pseudocyst. *A,* Large painful pseudocyst in the head of the pancreas displaces the stomach (St). Needle aspiration confirmed infection. *B,* CT-guided placement of a sump catheter completely drained the pseudocyst. The connection to the stomach helped prevent pancreatic cutaneous fistula.

atic tissue, but without significant pus collections. Pancreatic abscess is a localized collection of pus surrounded by a more or less distinct capsule. Infected necrosis becomes clinically evident during the early phase of acute pancreatitis, and patients show evidence of both sepsis and severe pancreatitis (e.g., amylasemia, hypocalcemia, and hyperglycemia). These patients have a fulminant course of pancreatitis, often complicated by pulmonary or renal insufficiency, and have a mortality of 32 per cent. Pancreatic abscess, however, was found to never occur before the fifth week after symptoms developed. In these patients, the clinical and laboratory signs of acute pancreatitis have generally subsided. Pulmonary and renal insufficiency are also less common, and mortality is 22 per cent. In the experience of Bittner et al., CT detected pancreatic abscesses readily, but diagnosis of infected necrosis was difficult.

Others have described additional criteria for distinguishing pancreatic necrosis from simple phlegmon, though considerable overlap may be found in the early phase of disease. Bolus enhancement with dynamic CT scanning appears to help distinguish devitalized, nonenhancing parenchyma from viable inflamed gland.[12, 12a] There appears to be a high correlation between the presence of pancreatic necrosis as determined by bolus-enhanced dynamic CT scans and the occurrence of significant complications and mortality. The greater the degree of pancreatic necrosis, the higher the morbidity.[12a]

There are a variety of CT findings in pancreatic abscesses,[72, 73] although the CT findings may not permit a specific diagnosis to be made in all cases. The most diagnostic CT finding is the demonstration of pancreatic or peripancreatic gas, which is usually produced by gas-forming coliform bacteria (Fig. 19–23). However, gas is found in only 30 to 50 per cent of proven abscesses,[72–75] and caution must be exercised to exclude extraneous sources of gas such as cutaneous or enteric fistulae, ruptured duodenum, or prior surgical intervention. If doubt exists, water-soluble contrast studies of the upper and lower gastrointestinal tract should be obtained, particularly in stable patients, to detect fistulous communications and to avoid unnecessary surgery. Spontaneous rupture of a pseudocyst into the stomach or duodenum may be associated with clinical improvement (Figs. 19–24 and 19–25), but spontaneous communication with the distal small bowel or colon usually results in bacterial contamination and necessitates surgery. Half of pseudocysts that rupture spontaneously do so into the peritoneal cavity; these patients have a reported mortality rate of 70 per cent,[76] although our own experience suggests that this is a more common and benign occurrence.

If gas is not present, abscesses are indistinguishable from noninfected phlegmons or pseudocysts (see Fig. 19–21).[72, 73] When persistent fever and leukocytosis are present in combination with the CT findings of an inflammatory mass or fluid collection, a percutaneous thin-needle aspiration of the fluid for bacteriologic studies is strongly recommended (Figs. 19–26 and 19–27).[77] CT or sonography is helpful in planning an approach that avoids needle puncture of bowel, thus minimizing the danger of contaminating a sterile collection.

The therapy for "pancreatic abscess" remains somewhat controversial.[78–81] There is general agreement that infected pseudocysts are best managed by percutaneous catheter drainage, a simple and effective alternative to surgical external drainage.[64, 78, 79] True pancreatic abscesses usually contain pockets of

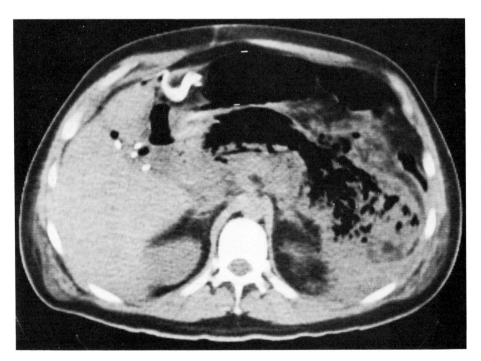

FIGURE 19–23 ■ Pancreatic abscess or infected necrosis. Pancreatic parenchyma is disrupted, and gas is present throughout the pancreatic bed. This patient had severe metabolic derangement, sepsis, and hypocalcemia early in the course of his illness. Such cases are rarely drained effectively by percutaneous catheters.

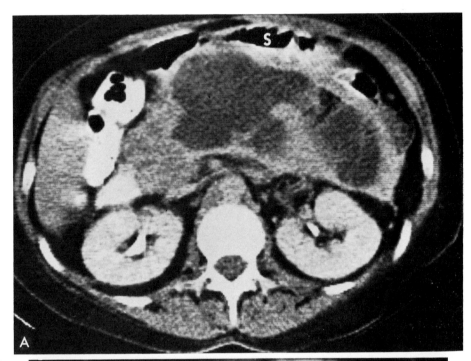

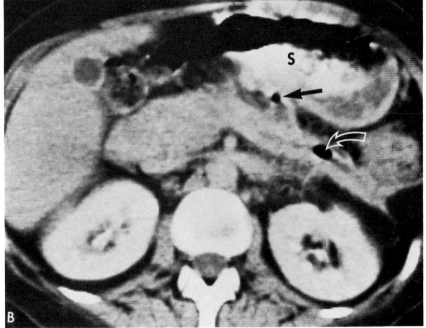

FIGURE 19–24 ■ Spontaneous rupture of pseudocyst into the stomach. *A,* A large pseudocyst in the lesser sac is displacing the stomach (S) forward. *B,* One day after a sonogram documented the existence of the large pseudocyst, the patient reported voluminous vomiting and diarrhea. The CT scan demonstrates decompression of the pseudocyst into the stomach. Gas bubbles are noted within a dilated pancreatic duct *(open arrow)* and within a fistula *(solid arrow)* between the pancreas and stomach. The patient had an uneventful recovery without surgery.

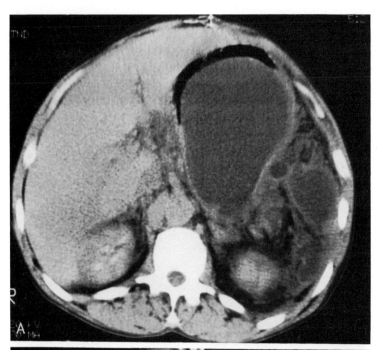

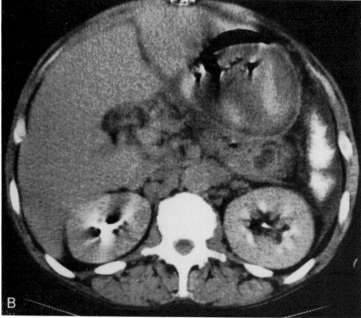

FIGURE 19–25 ■ Infected pseudocyst. *A*, Initial CT shows multiple pseudocysts including a large one in the retrogastric area (lesser sac). *B*, Repeat CT 9 days later. The cyst has decreased in size, presumably because of rupture into the stomach. The cyst contents, however, are heterogeneous, and gas bubbles are suspended within the viscid contents. Needle aspiration confirmed frank pus.

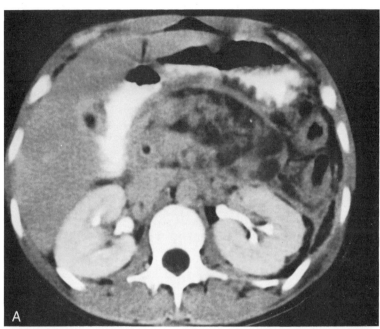

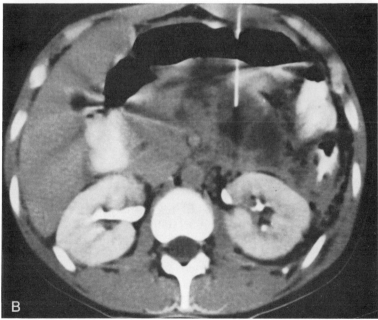

FIGURE 19–26 ■ Noninfected phlegmon. Patient was suspected to have a pancreatic abscess based on persistent fever, leukocytosis, and amylasemia. *A,* CT demonstrates heterogeneous pancreatic bed mass displacing the stomach and duodenum. *B,* Percutaneous aspiration was done through the stomach to avoid nonsterile bowel. Gram's stain and culture tests were negative for organisms.

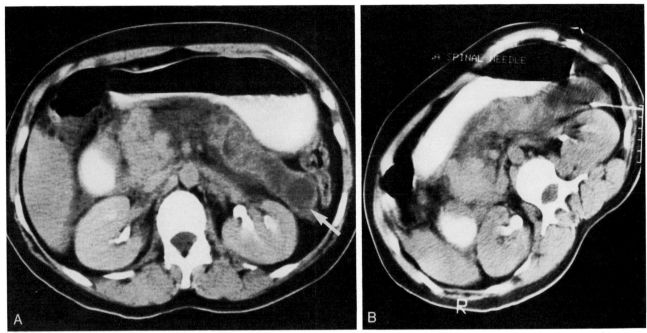

FIGURE 19–27 ■ Pancreatic abscess. Patient had an abrupt increase in fever, leukocyte count, and serum amylase after 10 days of slowly resolving pancreatitis. *A,* CT signs of pancreatitis including a small cystic area *(arrow)* near the descending colon. *B,* CT-guided aspiration yielded pus, which was drained by percutaneous catheter.

pus and necrotic tissue debris. The liquefied pus can be drained by catheter, but the solid tissue component must be debrided by hand at surgery. A combination of surgical and interventional radiologic therapy has been found to be the most effective management. Percutaneous catheter drainage may play a primary role (curative in 40 to 65 per cent of patients), a temporizing role before surgery, or a postsurgical role to drain missed or recurrent abscesses.[78–81]

Although the mortality rate from pancreatic abscesses has remained high in some recent series,[82] averaging about 40 per cent, we have achieved a mortality rate of 19 per cent during a recent 4-year period that we attribute to earlier diagnosis by CT and diagnostic needle aspiration, better antibiotic therapy, and more complete drainage of pus and debris.[81] Surgery remains the most definitive therapy in most cases, and repeated surgical intervention is frequently necessary.

Even when surgery is planned on the basis of a strong clinical suspicion of abscess, CT is available in demonstrating the full extent of spread.[55, 60] Multiple abscesses occur in about a third of patients and often are far removed from the pancreatic bed.[70, 82, 83] The preoperative information provided by CT can optimize surgical drainage.

CT scans of patients who have had previous surgical drainage for necrotizing pancreatitis or abscess are also useful. One third of patients require repeated operations for drainage of pancreatic abscesses, and recurrent infection is particularly difficult to diagnose in the postoperative patient. In our experience, CT has been accurate in postoperative patients in confirming the presence or absence of pancreatic abscess.

Chronic Pancreatitis

Chronic pancreatitis is an irreversible inflammatory disease of the pancreas associated with a number of predisposing factors. Although patients frequently give a history of multiple prior attacks of acute pancreatitis, some patients present with the metabolic, radiographic, and pathologic changes associated with chronic pancreatitis during their first acute attack or even without any episodes of pain.[84] Chronic pancreatitis may be clinically manifested as chronic abdominal pain, weight loss, steatorrhea, and diabetes. These clinical features and various laboratory determinations are nonspecific, and concern about possible pancreatic carcinoma or other pathologic abnormality often ultimately requires extensive, expensive, and invasive investigation.

CT FINDINGS

Standard radiographic modalities, including plain abdominal radiographs and barium studies, may reveal pancreatic calcifications or evidence of a mass. Calcifications strongly suggest a diagnosis of chronic alcohol-related pancreatitis, although other origins have been rarely implicated.[85] CT can detect calcifications not evident on plain radiographs, dilatation of the pancreatic and common bile duct, and atrophy of the gland and can better delineate and characterize pancreatic mass lesions (Figs. 19–28 and 19–29).[86]

The diameter of the main pancreatic duct is usually

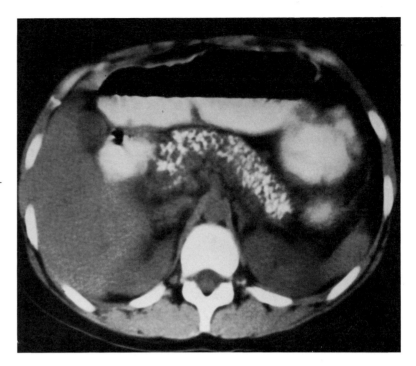

FIGURE 19–28 ■ Chronic pancreatitis; extensive calcification of pancreatic parenchyma.

maximum in the head of the pancreas, ranging from 2.0 to 6.5 mm (average 3.0 mm) and gradually decreasing in caliber toward the tail.[87] With the use of thin-section (5-mm) collimation and bolus contrast injection with rapid sequence scanning, normal-sized pancreatic ducts can be identified by CT in 70 per cent of pancreatic studies (see Fig. 19–5).[88] Using optimal CT technique, dilated pancreatic ducts are detectable in all instances.

Neither the diameter nor the degree of irregularity of the lumen of the pancreatic duct is a reliable distinguishing feature between benign and malignant causes of duct obstruction.[88–91] However, in our series of 73 cancers and 46 cases of chronic pancreatitis, the degree of dilatation was less with pancreatitis than with cancer, and the contour was more irregular.[92] Similarly, dilatation of both the pancreatic and common bile ducts (double duct sign) is found in both chronic pancreatitis and carcinoma (Fig. 19–30).[93] CT can display the anatomy of the pancreatic duct when it is obstructed to retrograde contrast injection and can disclose the underlying cause of ductal obstruction. When endoscopic retrograde cholangiopancreatography (ERCP) fails, CT is useful for determining whether the failure is technical or is the result of a distal duct obstruction.[65]

Several technical and anatomic points must be considered in interpretation of pancreatic duct pathology. CT is technically capable of detecting normal ducts, but streak artifacts may obscure a normal-sized duct. A low-attenuation linear structure mimicking a pancreatic duct may be produced by the margins between the pancreas and splenic vessels or by alignment of fatty septa within the gland.[94]

Atrophy of the pancreas is a common consequence of chronic inflammation of the pancreas. The CT diagnosis is somewhat subjective but can be suggested when the pancreas is small, the parenchyma is thin, and there are signs of chronic pancreatitis.

Pancreatic size and shape vary considerably between normal individuals, and there is a decrease in size with advancing age, sometimes becoming quite marked beyond the sixth decade.[95] Parenchymal atrophy is often accompanied by mild dilatation of the pancreatic duct. However, there is little correlation between the CT appearance of "senile atrophy" and clinical evidence of pancreatic insufficiency.

CT signs of chronic pancreatitis correlate well with the degree of pancreatic exocrine functional impairment.[96] Pancreatic calcifications may be found in patients with only mildly impaired exocrine function, whereas ductal dilatation and atrophy usually indicate severe pancreatic insufficiency.[97] Attempts to correlate morphologic changes, as detected by CT or ERCP, with chronic pain accompanying pancreatitis have been less successful, although CT may detect pseudocysts or marked ductal dilatation amenable to surgical decompression.[97] Celiac axis nerve block may offer pain relief and can be guided by CT.[98]

During an acute exacerbation of chronic pancreatitis, the gland may appear small, normal, or enlarged. Focal enlargements of the gland, accompanied by signs of duct dilatation, may closely mimic pancreatic carcinoma (see Fig. 19–30). Chronic pancreatitis and carcinoma coexist in two to five per cent of cases,[99] and accurate diagnosis by CT is rarely possible unless there is evidence of extrapancreatic spread of tumor.

The abilities of real-time ultrasonography and CT to detect normal or enlarged pancreatic ducts are similar. However, CT appears to detect other morphologic features such as duct calculi, parenchymal

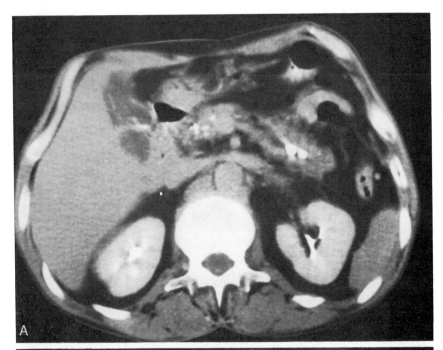

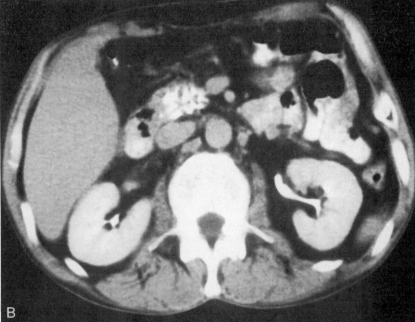

FIGURE 19–29 ■ Chronic pancreatitis. Glandular atrophy plus calcification in the pancreatic head. Two calculi appear to be within a dilated pancreatic duct.

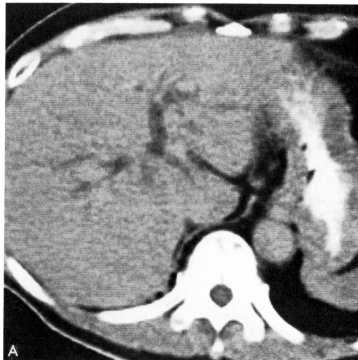

FIGURE 19–30 ■ Chronic pancreatitis simulating carcinoma. Patient is a 57-year-old man with painless jaundice and no history of alcohol abuse. *A,* CT scan demonstrating dilated intrahepatic ducts. *B,* CT scan at level of pancreatic head reveals the common bile duct *(arrow)* to be dilated as it enters the pancreas. The pancreatic body and tail appear normal.

Illustration continued on following page

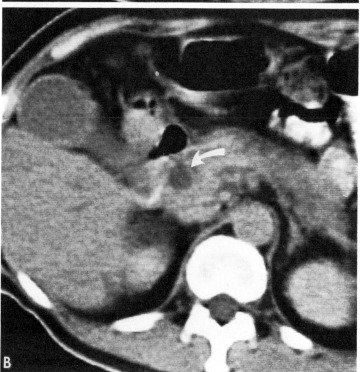

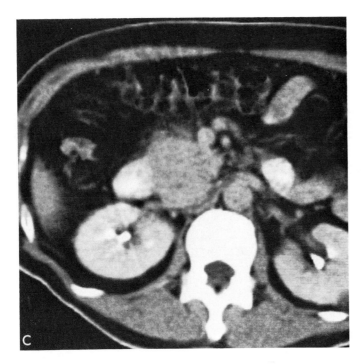

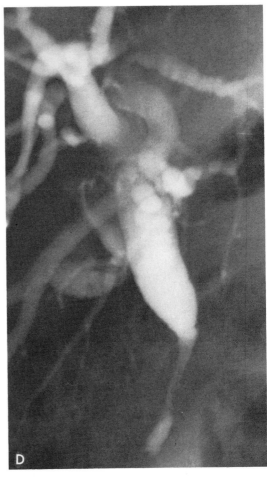

FIGURE 19–30 *Continued* ■ *C,* Focal enlargement of head and uncinate process of pancreas with obliteration of common bile duct. *D,* A transhepatic cholangiogram demonstrating a focal stricture and angulation of common bile duct within the pancreatic head, with proximal dilatation of the intrahepatic ducts. At surgery, a focal hard mass was found in the pancreatic head and a total pancreatectomy was performed. Multiple sections revealed only chronic inflammatory changes.

atrophy, and associated inflammatory or neoplastic masses to better advantage than sonography.[100] False-positive and false-negative studies for chronic pancreatitis occur with CT, ultrasonography, and ERCP. CT and ERCP are equally accurate in detecting an abnormality (95 per cent in one series) and in suggesting the correct diagnosis (70 per cent).[101] Currently, patients suspected of having chronic pancreatitis or pancreatic carcinoma are initially examined with CT. Further investigation by ERCP is indicated if CT is negative but a high clinical index of suspicion remains, or if CT reveals changes of chronic pancreatitis and surgical therapy is being considered.[101–103]

MRI FINDINGS

In acute pancreatitis, increase in tissue edema and later cellular infiltrate enlarge the pancreas and change its water content. These pathologic processes are reflected in the MR appearance of the pancreas in acute inflammation. Gland enlargement is readily detected (Fig. 19–31).[104–107] In experimental acute pancreatitis, influx of edema is correlated with prolongation of T1 and T2 relaxation times. This has been noted as changes in signal intensity on T1- and T2-weighted images.[108] When the pancreas becomes edematous and contains more organ water, it appears more like the signal intensity of the spleen, which is of lower intensity on T1 and higher intensity on T2-weighted images than the liver. This is often associated with infiltration of peripancreatic fat. This infiltrative process, best demonstrated on T1-weighted images, results in strands of low signal intensity replacing the high signal intensity of the peripancreatic fat. Thickening of the renal fascia may also be seen and is best detected on T1-weighted images.[108] Extensive phlegmonous infiltrates destroy the normal peripancreatic fat planes and alter the appearance of the anterior pararenal space in a manner similar to that seen on CT. Frequently the phlegmon has signal similar to that of the adjacent bowel, so it may be difficult to ascertain the true extent of the inflammatory process. To date, no information is available on the ability of MR to distinguish between edematous and hemorrhagic pancreatitis.

Some features of chronic pancreatitis have been detected by MR. Gland enlargement and pancreatic duct dilation may be detected. The dilated duct appears as a tubular structure with low signal intensity on T1-weighted images and increased signal intensity on T2-weighted images. Pancreatic pseudocysts appear as areas of well-circumscribed, relatively homogeneous fluid collections with low signal intensity on T1-weighted images and markedly increased signal intensity on T2-weighted images, re-

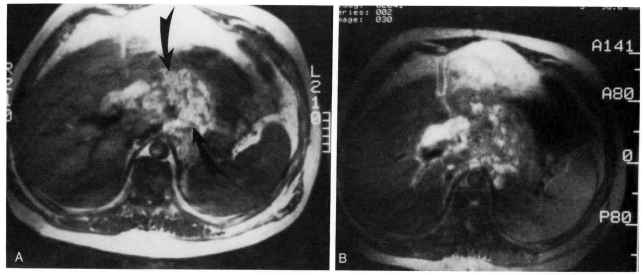

FIGURE 19–31 ■ MR scan of a nonalcoholic male with severe acute pancreatitis. *A,* T1-weighted image illustrates enlargement of the body of the pancreas *(arrows)* with inhomogeneous signal intensity generally higher than that of the liver and spleen. In ordinary edematous pancreatitis, the signal intensity is similar to that of the spleen and lower than that of the liver. Hemorrhagic changes in the inflamed pancreas might account for the higher signal from the pancreas in this patient. *B,* T2-weighted image shows marked signal inhomogeneity, indicating a complex inflammatory and possibly hemorrhagic process.

flecting prolonged T1 and T2 relaxation times of the cyst fluid.[104, 105, 108, 108a] Calcifications seen in the wall of pseudocysts in CT are not seen on MR images.

Neoplasms

The widespread availability of fast, high-resolution CT scanners has permitted the demonstration of finer details of the pancreas and surrounding tissues. The application of CT scanning and ultrasound to guidance of transabdominal needles for obtaining histologic and cytologic samples has provided new dimensions to the detection of pancreatic cancer. The development of rapid-sequence, contrast-enhanced scanning techniques has permitted evaluation of vasculature surrounding and supplying the pancreas, as well as vascularity of pancreatic tumors. Thus technological advances have resulted in greater potential for the detection of pancreatic tumors and have decreased false-negative determinations.[109]

INDICATIONS FOR CT

Symptoms or signs suggestive of cancer of the pancreas often reflect the location of the tumor. In cancer of the head of the pancreas, the most common features are jaundice and weight loss. If the tumor is confined to the tail or body, frequently no symptoms are present until the lesion is very large, at which time weight loss, back pain, and occasionally a palpable mass may be present. Peripheral thrombophlebitis may indicate an underlying carcinoma. In these clinical situations, CT scanning of the pancreas is indicated. Pancreatic CT scans are also indicated in the presence of a metastatic lesion detected in the lungs or liver, in the absence of a known primary site, and in patients with biochemical evidence of a functioning islet cell tumor. There is

evidence that although early detection of pancreatic carcinoma may not alter overall survival rate, dynamic CT of the pancreas has shortened the delay and expense of diagnosis, diminishing the need for exploratory laparotomy, angiography, and ERCP.[110]

PRIMARY PANCREATIC TUMORS

Pancreatic Adenocarcinoma ■ Change in the size and shape of the pancreas, along with abnormalities in CT attenuation values, obliteration of peripancreatic fat, loss of boundaries with surrounding structures, involvement of vessels and regional lymph nodes, pancreatic ductal dilatation, pancreatic cysts, and obstruction of the common bile duct are all features that indicate possible presence of a pancreatic malignancy.

Change in the Size of the Pancreas ■ Pancreatic cancer may produce either focal or diffuse pancreatic enlargement. Focal enlargement is most common and is usually confined to specific anatomic areas such as the tail, body, head, or uncinate process or at the interface between these boundaries. Diffuse enlargement of the pancreas resulting from an underlying cancer is uncommon and most often is the result of an associated pancreatitis rather than diffuse neoplastic infiltration. However, with cystic neoplasms of the pancreas, the majority of the pancreas may be diffusely involved.

Pancreatic enlargement is common in pancreatic carcinoma, and was seen in one series in 96 per cent of cases,[111] but enlargement is a nonspecific finding and cannot be used as the sole criterion to diagnose carcinoma because an enlarged pancreas can be due to an anatomic variation, inflammation, or benign disease. On the other hand, aging and chronic pancreatitis can result in an atrophic pancreas that may also harbor a small cancer. Measurements have not aided in the detection of small pancreatic masses because of the wide variation in size of the normal pancreas. Usually by the time the pancreatic width is abnormal, an advanced neoplasm is present, and other features of malignancy are evident (Fig. 19–32).

Change in Shape and Contour of the Pancreas ■ This feature is frequently more important than the actual size of the suspected mass. Pancreatic cancer may produce a focal, eccentric mass involving only one surface of the gland, focal rounding of the posterior and anterior surfaces, smooth or lobulated enlargement of the uncinate process, or diffuse enlargement of the head of the pancreas. Even in the absence of absolute enlargement of the head of the pancreas, a focal bulge on one surface may indicate an underlying tumor (Fig. 19–33).[109]

The most difficult area for detecting focal pancreatic enlargement is in the head of the pancreas, whereas such changes in shape and contour are most readily detected in the tail or anterior surface of the pancreatic body. Focal alterations in shape and contour are frequently encountered in the patient with pancreatic carcinoma, but occasionally focal lobulations prove to be normal anatomic variations. With high-resolution CT scanners, it is possible to detect the fatty interstices frequently seen in the normal pancreas (see Fig. 19–4). If fatty interstices enter an area of focal enlargement, then the underlying tissue is more likely to be normal, whereas if the focal enlargement is solid, without fatty lobulations, it is most likely to be abnormal and should be the subject of a CT-guided needle biopsy (Fig. 19–34). Diffuse enlargement of the head of the pancreas may result in either a smooth or lobulated contour. When the uncinate process is involved, the sharp, tonguelike contour of the process is lost and is replaced by a blunted enlargement projecting between the superior mesenteric vein and the renal vein or duodenum. Change in the size and change in the shape or contour together are the most frequent features of

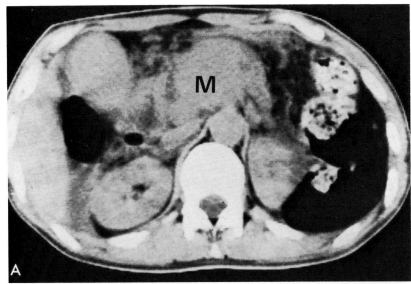

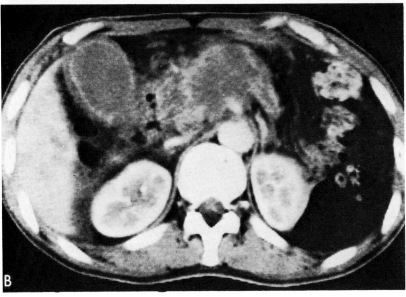

FIGURE 19–32 ■ Intravenous bolus injection of contrast material and dynamic scan technique for outlining pancreatic carcinoma. *A,* CT scan prior to intravenous contrast material administration demonstrates a homogeneous mass (M) in the body of the pancreas. *B,* CT scan after an intravenous bolus of contrast material. Sequential scans were obtained every 5 seconds for 1 minute. Scan at time of maximum aortic contrast reveals enhancement of the surrounding vascular structures and normal pancreatic parenchyma, whereas the pancreatic carcinoma remains unchanged and thereby appears as a low-density mass.

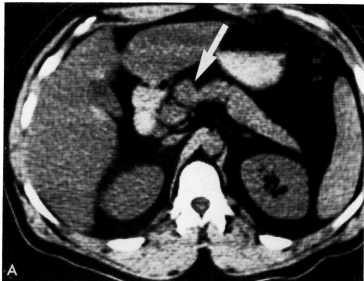

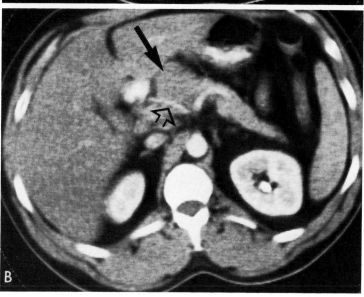

FIGURE 19–33 ■ Rapid growth of small pancreatic carcinoma. *A,* CT scan demonstrating a focal change in shape of the ventral contour of the pancreas at the junction of the body and head *(arrow).* No enlargement of pancreatic tissue is present. This was initially interpreted as representing an anatomic variation. *B,* Three months later, a repeat CT scan shows a focal tumor mass *(solid arrow)* in the location of the focal contour abnormality seen in *A.* A dynamic CT scan after intravenous bolus injection demonstrates splenic and hepatic arteries at the base of the tumor. The hepatic artery *(open arrow)* has an irregular contour. Arteriography showed encasement by tumor.

pancreatic cancer, occurring in 95 per cent of patients.[111, 112]

Abnormalities in CT Attenuation Values ■ The normal mean CT attenuation value of the pancreas ranges from 30 to 50 H,[6] and many pancreatic tumors do not have CT numbers significantly different from those of the surrounding pancreatic parenchyma (Fig. 19–35).[5, 9, 112] However, in one series, a central zone of diminished CT attenuation was seen in 83 per cent of patients with pancreatic tumors, but in only a small number was actual tumor necrosis responsible for low attenuation.[111] Pancreatic tumors undergoing necrosis have lower CT numbers, but usually the decrease in CT attenuation has an irregular distribution without sharply defined margins. However, in some cases a necrotic tumor simulates a pseudocyst by having well-defined borders and a uniform low density (Fig. 19–36). The term *pseudopseudocyst* has been used to describe these necrotic, cystic pancreatic carcinomas.[113] Necrotic pancreatic

carcinomas must be differentiated from true pseudocysts secondary to pancreatitis and from massively dilated pancreatic ducts containing mucin. Generally, necrotic pancreatic neoplasms have thicker walls and central attenuation values greater than that seen in inflammatory pseudocysts. However, a CT-guided biopsy may be needed to confirm or exclude the diagnosis of a necrotic pancreatic tumor.

The usefulness of intravenous contrast medium administration to detect pancreatic carcinoma is still being clarified. In one series of tumors studied before and after intravenous infusion of contrast material, the tumors were noted to enhance to the same degree as the normal pancreas.[114] However, by giving an intravenous bolus of 100 to 150 mL of contrast material and performing rapid-sequence scanning, some solid pancreatic tumors do not increase or increase less in density than the surrounding normal pancreatic parenchyma and thereby appear as relatively low-density lesions. The difference in CT attenuation

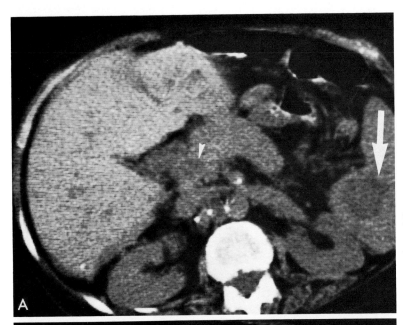

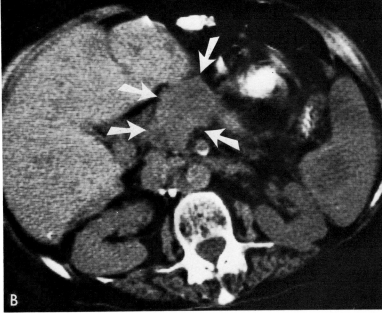

FIGURE 19–34 ■ Carcinoma of pancreatic head with CT-guided percutaneous needle biopsy. *A,* CT scan of the pancreas in a 38-year-old patient with weight loss and mild jaundice shows a normal body, with an ill-defined, low-density mass in the pancreatic head *(arrowhead).* A metastatic lesion is also present in the spleen *(arrow). B,* CT scan 2 cm caudal to *A.* Focal enlargement of the pancreatic head is seen *(arrows).*

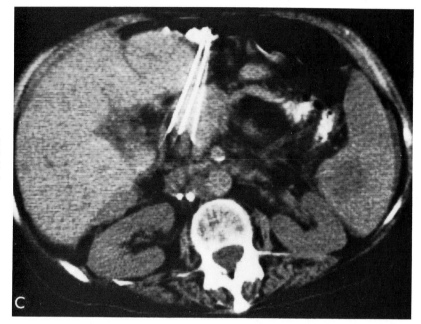

FIGURE 19–34 *Continued* ■ *C,* CT-guided percutaneous needle biopsy was performed using the tandem needle technique. CT scan documents placement of needles into the mass. Malignant cells were aspirated from the area of focal enlargement.

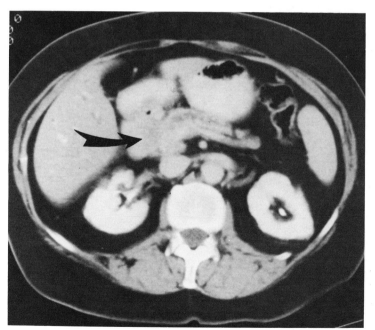

FIGURE 19–35 ■ A small low-density carcinoma of the head of the pancreas *(arrow)* has not enlarged the pancreas but has produced dilatation of the pancreatic duct distal to the tumor.

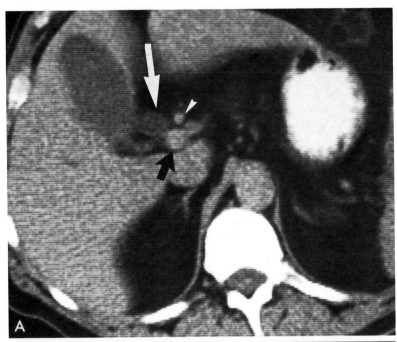

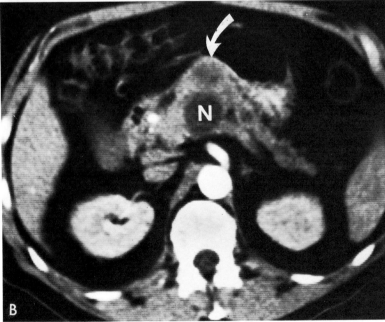

FIGURE 19–36 ■ Necrotic pancreatic carcinoma associated with cystic dilatation of the obstructed pancreatic duct. *A,* CT scan through the porta hepatis of a cirrhotic patient with jaundice and weight loss demonstrates a mildly dilated common hepatic duct *(white arrow),* with the portal vein *(black arrow)* and hepatic artery *(arrowhead)* just ventral to it. *B,* CT section through the body of the pancreas demonstrates a necrotic lesion (N) with a low-density area that simulates a pseudocyst. Ventral to the mass is the dilated pancreatic duct *(arrow),* which has a rounded appearance. The dilated duct in the tail of the pancreas is somewhat beaded in appearance.

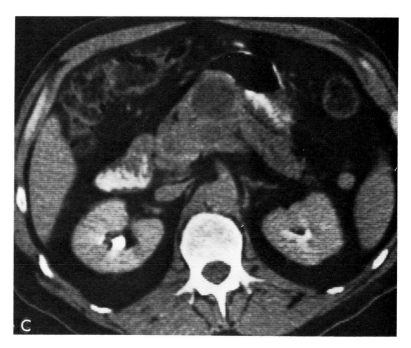

FIGURE 19–36 *Continued C,* The tumor has spread into the head of the gland. The obstructed pancreatic duct now also simulates a pancreatic pseudocyst. (*B* from Itai Y, Moss AA, Goldberg HI: J Comput Assist Tomogr 6:772, 1982. Used with permission.)

value of pancreatic tumor and normal pancreatic tissue can be very transient, as it is undetectable minutes after contrast agent injection. Our current procedure is to give a bolus injection of contrast media and perform a dynamic CT scan sequence through any area of suspected pancreatic abnormality (Fig. 19–37).

Obliteration of Peripancreatic Fat ■ As pancreatic carcinoma extends from the substance of the gland, peripancreatic fat is invaded, resulting in an increase in CT number and obliteration of the normally detected fat. Peripancreatic spread of carcinoma may take the form of subtle irregularity in the pancreatic margin, or it may be seen as a diffuse change in part or all of the peripancreatic fat. Obliteration of some portion of the fat is one of the most common findings in pancreatic cancer,[9, 112, 115] occurring in 84 per cent of one series,[112] and evidence of extension to fat and other structures was found in 92 per cent in another series.[111] Changes in the CT appearance of fat are almost always the result of tumor invasion.[5, 9] However, pancreatitis associated with cancer may contribute to the change in fat density.

Pancreatic carcinoma can extend to obliterate the fat planes between the pancreas and the spleen, splenic flexure of the colon, posterior gastric wall, gastric antrum, duodenum, transverse mesocolon, and porta hepatis (Figs. 19–38 through 19–40).[4, 5, 9,]

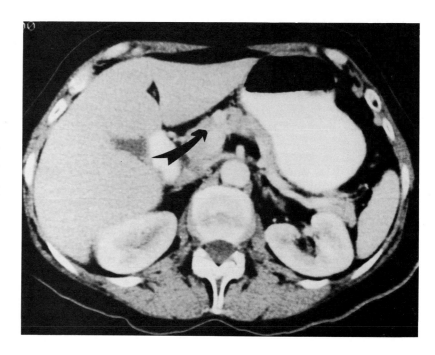

FIGURE 19–37 ■ A small glucagon-secreting islet cell carcinoma of the head of the pancreas *(arrow)* is well shown, because it enhances after a high-volume bolus of intravenous contrast material. Rapid sequence scanning and 5-mm-thick sections aid in demonstrating small vascular lesions of this type.

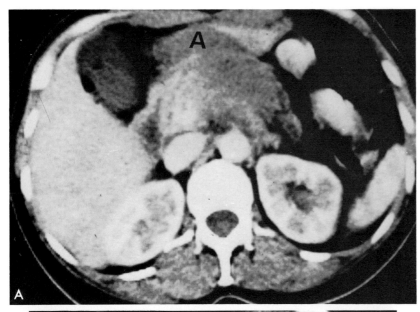

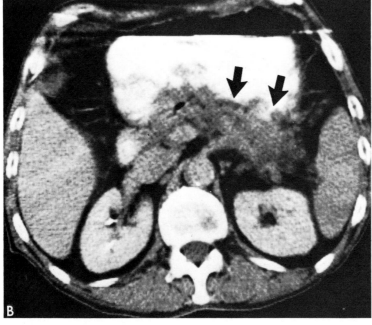

FIGURE 19–38 ■ Pancreatic carcinoma invading the stomach. *A,* There is invasion of the antrum of the stomach (A) by an adjacent pancreatic cancer, causing thickening of the antral wall and obliteration of fat between the antrum and pancreas. *B,* Direct invasion of the greater curvature of the stomach by pancreatic cancer originating in the body and tail *(arrows).* (From Itai Y, Moss AA, Goldberg HI: J Comput Assist Tomogr 6:772, 1982. Used with permission.)

[109, 115] Although a mass in the porta hepatis is readily detected on CT scans, extension of tumor along the gastrohepatic ligament may be difficult to detect.

When no fat plane is seen separating a pancreatic mass from an adjacent organ or structure, usually it is assumed that pancreatic tumor has invaded the adjacent organ by direct extension. However, obliteration of the peripancreatic fat plane indicates that the pancreatic mass is touching a surrounding organ, but it is not proof that the pancreatic mass has actually extended into the adjacent structures. Caution must therefore be exercised in reporting direct pancreatic invasion into adjacent structures unless the peripancreatic fat plane is obliterated and the pancreatic tumor is seen to directly replace or invade the parenchyma of nearby organs. Caution must also be exercised in interpreting preservation of the peri-

pancreatic fat planes as absolute proof that no direct extension has occurred, as microscopic invasion may occur without obliteration of peripancreatic fat.[111]

When a very thin fat plane exists between the mass and the organ, it is also possible that small fingerlike extensions of tumor may be present and not detected by CT scanning. Despite these limitations, evidence from studies on extension of rectal, gastric, and esophageal carcinoma to adjacent structures indicates that when tumor obliterates adjacent fat planes and appears on CT scans to extend into adjacent organs, tumor extension is confirmed by surgical examination.[116, 117]

When adjacent organs are directly invaded by pancreatic tumor, the CT number of the tumor may be the same as that of the involved organ, thereby rendering the actual amount of the tumor indistin-

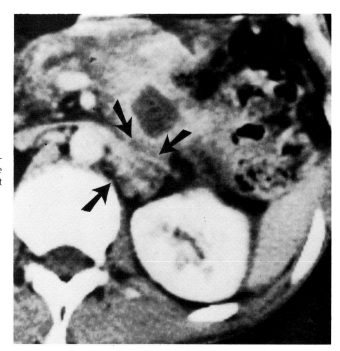

FIGURE 19–39 ■ Pancreatic carcinoma involving the renal vasculature. A CT scan demonstrates direct extension of carcinoma from the tail of the pancreas to the left renal vein and artery *(arrows)*. The fat ordinarily separating these structures has been obliterated.

guishable from the invaded tissue. In other instances, the tumor has a lower CT number than that of the involved organ and can readily be identified and distinguished from normal tissue. Intravenous contrast injections help to accentuate the difference between pancreatic tumor and surrounding normal tissue.

Involvement of Vessels and Regional Lymph Nodes ■ Pancreatic malignancies frequently extend to involve adjacent vascular structures. Angiographic techniques reveal that the splenic and portal vein, as well as the celiac, superior mesenteric, splenic, and hepatic arteries, can be narrowed, displaced, or occluded by pancreatic tumors (Figs. 19–33, 19–39, and 19–41). Computed tomography using bolus injection techniques can also demonstrate abrupt obstruction, narrowing, or displacement of peripancreatic vessels

(Figs. 19–33 and 19–42). Venous occlusion is often accompanied by collateral venous circulation, which is manifest on contrast-enhanced CT scans as a plethora of vessels located in and around the gastric wall and splenic hilum (Fig. 19–43). Loss of the perivascular fat plane around the celiac or superior mesenteric artery is evidence that a pancreatic tumor is probably unresectable.

Tumor spread to regional lymph nodes is frequently detected by CT scans. In a series of 73 cases reviewed at the University of California, San Francisco, 23 (32 per cent) had evidence of regional lymph node involvement, and in other series, 65 per cent and 28 per cent had lymph node enlargement.[111, 112]

Tumor commonly metastasizes to the group of lymph nodes around the celiac and superior mesenteric arteries. Ordinarily, lymph nodes occurring in

FIGURE 19–40 ■ Pancreatic carcinoma invading the porta hepatis. A CT scan demonstrates direct extension of carcinoma of the head of the pancreas into the porta hepatis *(small arrows)*, encasing the hepatic arteries and common bile duct *(large arrow)*. (Courtesy of General Electric Medical Systems Division, Milwaukee, WI.)

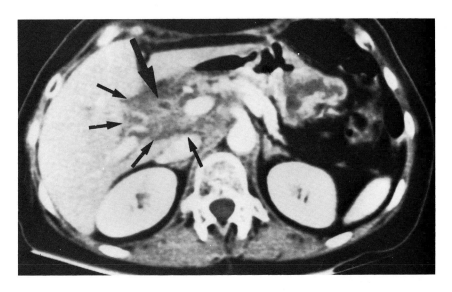

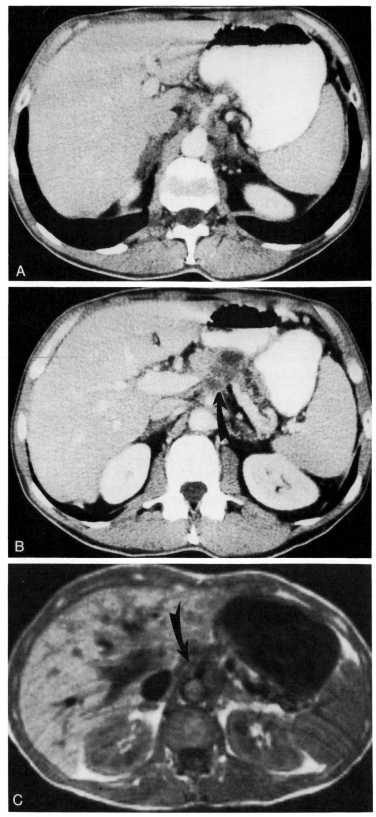

FIGURE 19–41 ■ Perivascular extension of pancreatic carcinoma seen on CT and MRI scans. *A,* Tumor surrounding the celiac artery and origin of the hepatic and splenic arteries on a high-volume, bolus contrast injection, rapid sequence, 5-mm-thick section CT scan. *B,* Necrotic tumor of the body of the pancreas with partial compression of the splenic vein *(arrow). C,* T1-weighted image of the same area as in *A* and *B,* demonstrating tumor surrounding the celiac artery *(arrow).* The tumor has low signal intensity and has replaced the fat that would ordinarily surround this vessel.

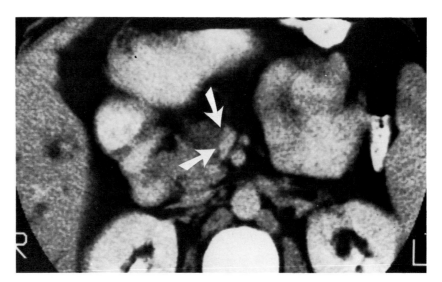

FIGURE 19–42 ■ Flattening of superior mesenteric vein *(arrows)* by a small pancreatic tumor.

this area are too small to produce significant soft tissue densities in the background of perivascular fat. However, when tumor is present, the fat surrounding the celiac or superior mesenteric artery becomes the same density as the unenhanced artery, producing a triangle of soft tissue density (Fig. 19–41). The increased density may be caused by enlargement of regional lymph nodes or by direct extension of tumor into the fat ordinarily surrounding these vessels. Angiography may demonstrate encasement of the involved artery when this finding is present on CT scans. Occasionally the appearance of a soft tissue density around the celiac and superior mesenteric arteries occurs in the absence of a definable pancreatic mass. In one study, obliteration of perivascular fat around these arteries was present in one third of patients with pancreatic cancer studied by CT scanning,[118] and in our series of 73 pancreatic cancers, 34 per cent had this finding. Involvement of peripancreatic arteries and veins was actually seen in 84 per cent of patients with pancreatic cancer in one series.[111] Enlargement of lymph nodes in the paraaortic, pericaval, retrocrural, and porta hepatis regions as a result of metastasis can also be detected on CT scans. The overall occurrence of regional lymph node spread has been reported to vary between 38 and 65 per cent.[112, 118]

Metastases to the liver are common in pancreatic cancer, occurring in 17 to 55 per cent of patients.[111, 112, 114] Hepatic metastases from pancreatic adenocarcinoma usually appear as low-density lesions in the unenhanced liver and only rarely dramatically enhance after administration of the intravenous contrast material. They may be isolated, single or multiple metastases and can occur in all lobes of the liver. Splenic metastases are rare (see Fig. 19–34A).

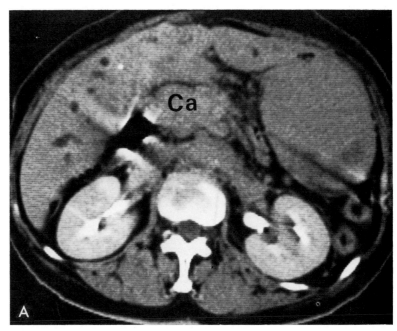

FIGURE 19–43 ■ Compression of splenic vein by tumor. *A,* A carcinoma of the head of the pancreas (Ca) producing obstructive jaundice.

Illustration continued on following page

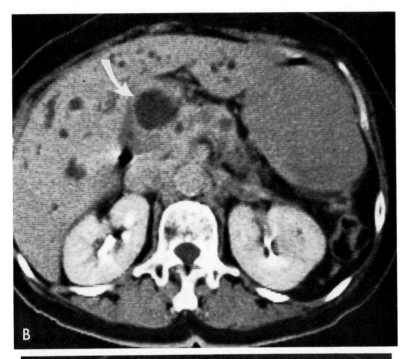

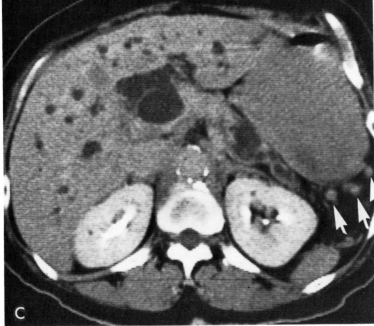

FIGURE 19–43 *Continued B,* CT scan at a higher level demonstrates pancreatic ductal dilatation and dilatation of the common bile duct *(arrow). C,* CT scan 2 cm cephalic to *B* reveals dilated gastric venous collaterals *(arrows)* resulting from splenic vein compression.

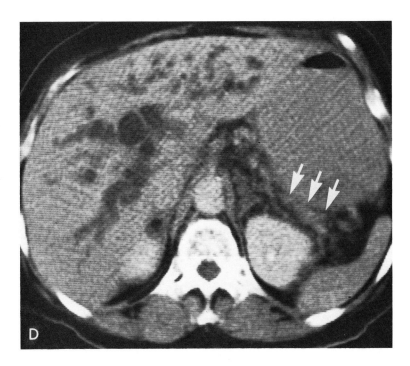

FIGURE 19–43 *Continued D,* CT scan 1 cm cephalic to C confirms patency of the splenic vein *(arrows).*

Association of Pancreatic Cancer with Pseudocysts, Pancreatic and Biliary Ductal Dilatation, and Chronic Pancreatitis ■ Pancreatic cancer, which invariably originates from ductal epithelium, often results in obstruction of the pancreatic duct with resultant dilatation.[88–90, 119–122] With the utilization of high-resolution, rapid-sequence CT scanning, dilated and normal pancreatic ducts can be readily detected (see Fig. 19–5).[88, 100] Sagittal and coronal reconstructed images can also aid in the evaluation of the pancreatic duct.[123] Using appropriate techniques, linear low-density structures of 3 mm are clearly seen in phantoms of the pancreas,[88] and short segments of normal pancreatic ducts can be identified in vivo (see Fig. 19–5).

The incidence of pancreatic ductal dilatation in the presence of pancreatic cancer is difficult to ascertain. In a study of 500 CT scans of the pancreas,[90] a dilated duct was found in ten patients (two per cent), and in half of these associated pancreatic cancer was present. In our series of 73 pancreatic cancers, the pancreatic duct was detected in 72 per cent of patients and was dilated in 66 per cent. In another series[115] of 15 cases of cancer of the pancreatic head, the duct was dilated in 11 patients (73 per cent), and in a third series, the duct was dilated in 68 per cent.[111] The size of the dilated duct resulting from pancreatic carcinoma ranged from 5 to 10 mm and was either smooth or beaded (Figs. 19–35, 19–44, and 19–45). The contour of the dilated duct in pancreatic cancer is more often smooth or beaded, whereas in chronic pancreatitis it is more often irregular. However, there is an overlap in these features.[111] It is important to detect ductal dilatation, because it may represent the major pancreatic abnormality in pancreatic cancer in which the tumor is too small to be identified by CT scanning. In our series, five of ten pancreatic carcinomas without a demonstrable mass had a dilated pancreatic duct. In another series, isolated pancreatic and bile duct dilatation was the only CT abnormality in 6 of 159 patients with pancreatic cancer.[111]

Pancreatic Cysts ■ Cystic lesions in the body and tail of the pancreas are occasionally found in association with carcinoma of the head of the pancreas. Although these cystic lesions may be pseudocysts associated with chronic pancreatitis, they can also represent cysts secondary to pancreatic cancer or small cystic mucinous cystadenomas or cystadenocarcinomas.[124] These secondary cysts are relatively uncommon, occurring in one series in eight per cent of 73 documented pancreatic cancers.[125] The cysts, which on CT scans may be indistinguishable from pseudocysts associated with pancreatitis, are always located distal to the tumor (Figs. 19–46 and 19–47). Differentiation of a secondary cyst from a true pseudocyst or a congenital cyst occurring as part of polycystic renal-liver disease or von Hippel–Lindau disease may depend on analysis of the fluid content after CT-guided needle aspiration. Even examination of pathologic specimens may not permit differentiation between true pseudocysts and retention cysts secondary to cancer. When a pseudocyst is encountered in a patient without a history of predisposing factors for pancreatitis, further investigation is necessary to determine whether an underlying tumor is present.

Association with Chronic Pancreatitis ■ An increased incidence of carcinoma of the pancreas has been noted in chronic calcific pancreatitis.[99, 126] However, the CT detection of carcinoma in a gland that has undergone the changes of chronic inflammation depends on whether the tumor is hypodense, is larger than the rest of the pancreas, has spread to adjacent lymph nodes and organs, or has metastasized to the liver. In the absence of these findings, the detection

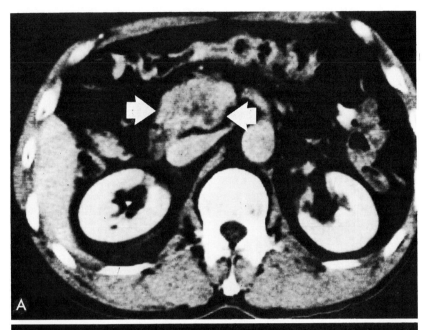

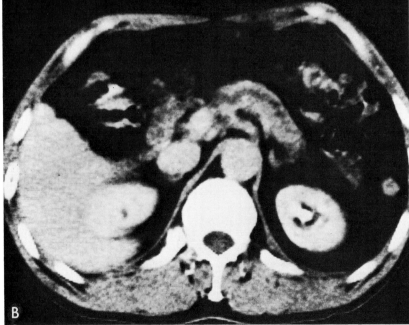

FIGURE 19–44 ■ Pancreatic duct dilatation produced by carcinoma in the head of the gland. *A*, Low-density focal carcinoma in the head of the pancreas *(arrows)*. *B*, The main pancreatic duct is dilated. The duct has a smooth contour in the body and a slightly irregular contour in the tail.

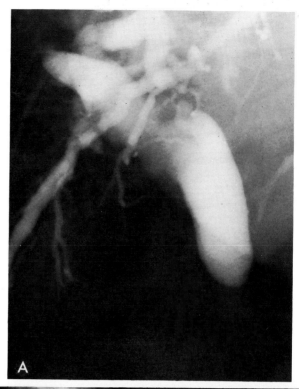

FIGURE 19–45 ■ Carcinoma of the papilla of Vater causing biliary and pancreatic duct dilatation. *A,* Percutaneous transhepatic cholangiogram demonstrates dilatation of the common bile duct with obstruction in the distal intrapancreatic portion. *B,* CT scan through the head of the pancreas and uncinate process shows no tumor mass and no common bile duct dilatation. *C,* CT scan 1 cm cephalic to *B* shows the dilated distal common bile duct *(arrow)* and defines the point of obstruction in the head of the pancreas. No tumor mass is demonstrated.

Illustration continued on following page

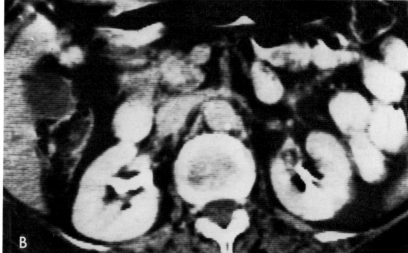

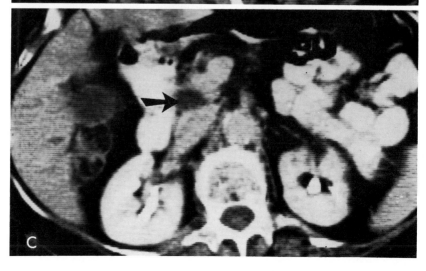

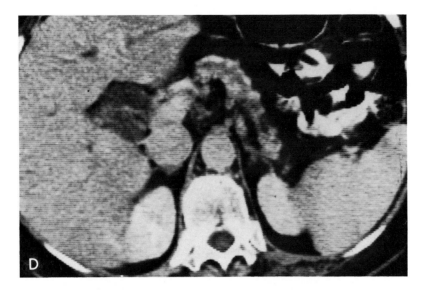

FIGURE 19–45 *Continued D,* The main pancreatic duct is dilated proximal to the papillary tumor. Although the contour is undulating, it does not have the beaded appearance typical of chronic pancreatitis.

ot a carcinoma is often not possible in the chronically inflamed, enlarged, inhomogeneous pancreas containing a dilated duct and calcification. Except for rare malignant islet cell tumors (Fig. 19–48)[127] most pancreatic cancers do not contain calcification. In pancreatitis with pancreatic atrophy, the presence of a tumor may be suggested by detection of a focal mass associated with pancreatic ductal dilatation. In some patients with pancreatitis and pancreatic carcinoma, CT-guided percutaneous needle aspiration biopsy of the pancreas has documented a pancreatic tumor. However, experience in detecting pancreatic cancer in the presence of chronic pancreatitis has not been encouraging unless signs of advanced malignancy are present.

Association with Dilatation of the Biliary Tract ■ Cancer of the head of the pancreas is frequently associated with obstructive jaundice. Biliary ductal dilatation was detected in 43 of 47 (91 per cent),[112] 8 of 17 (47 per cent),[114] 16 of 36 (44 per cent), and 92 of 159 (58 per cent) cases.[111, 128] Dilatation of the gallbladder, common bile duct, common hepatic duct, and intrahepatic ducts caused by cancer of the pancreas can be demonstrated (Figs. 19–43 and 19–45). When a large pancreatic mass causes the obstruction, it often displaces the common bile duct anteriorly and medially. When the tumor is small and located near the papilla of Vater, the dilated duct appears as a low-density, round structure medial to the duodenum in the region of the head of the pancreas (Fig. 19–45). Accuracy in detecting a malignant obstruction of the biliary tract by CT scanning ranges from 90 to 95 per cent.[129]

Ascites ■ Although malignant ascites occurs in some

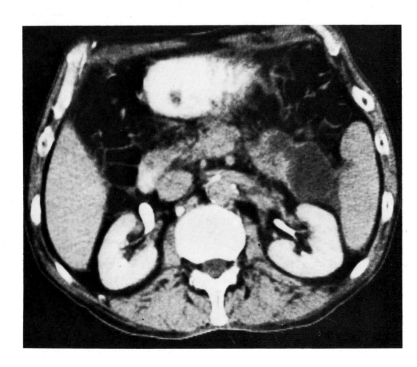

FIGURE 19–46 ■ Cystic changes in the tail of the pancreas occurring distal to the carcinoma of the body of the pancreas shown in Figure 14–38*B.* (From Itai Y, Moss AA, Goldberg HI: J Comput Assist Tomogr 6:772, 1982. Used with permission.)

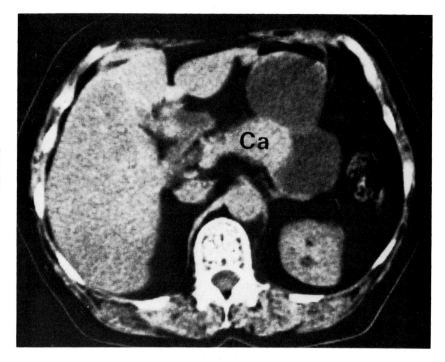

FIGURE 19–47 ■ Carcinoma of the body of the pancreas (Ca) with two large cysts distal to the tumor. (From Itai Y, Moss AA, Goldberg HI: J Comput Assist Tomogr 6:772, 1982. Used with permission.)

patients with pancreatic cancer, it is not a common feature. Ascites can be the result of spread of pancreatic cancer throughout the lesser sac with the induction of fluid or distant spread to the greater peritoneal cavity. In one series[112] ascites was found in 13 per cent of patients with pancreatic cancer, most frequently in patients with far advanced disease.

Detection of the Pancreatic Tumor 3 cm in Size or Less ■ By the time most pancreatic cancers are clinically suspected, the carcinoma is usually greater than 3 cm in size. Takekawa found only 3 of 24 (12.5 per cent),[114] and Levitt et al. reported only 3 of 18 (16.66 per cent)[109] pancreatic cancers were 3 cm or less in size. Functioning islet cell tumors of the pancreas are an exception to this rule, as many of

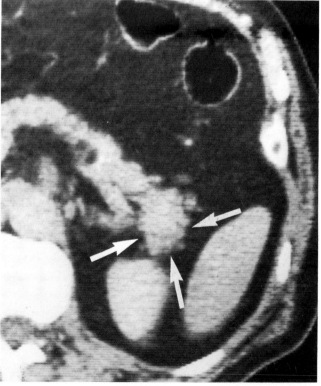

FIGURE 19–48 ■ Focal enlargement of the tail of the pancreas *(arrows)* is the result of the presence of an insulinoma. The lesion is isodense with the adjacent pancreatic tissue.

these are smaller than 3 cm in size.[130–132] In most instances, large tumors are inoperable.[130]

Rarely is a tumor less than 3 cm in diameter detected on the basis of an abnormality in size or shape of the pancreas.[133, 134] In Sager et al.'s series[130] only 50 per cent of small, operable tumors were detected by CT scans. A small lesion is more likely to be suspected because of secondary signs, such as metastasis to regional lymph nodes or liver, obliteration of a portion of the peripancreatic fat plane, dilatation of pancreatic duct, or obstructive jaundice.

In Ariyama's series,[135] 14 of 62 patients (22 per cent) with resectable pancreatic cancer had tumors 3 cm in size or less. Survival was prolonged in this group when compared with that in a group of patients who had resection of tumor larger than 3 cm, indicating that it is worthwhile to attempt to detect pancreatic tumors when they are small. However, the detection of a small lesion, even one in which no mass is seen and only secondary findings of ductal dilatation are present, does not assure prolongation of life as a result of resection.[111] Even though the tumor may be resectable, local spread to organs or metastasis to regional lymph nodes and the liver may already have occurred. In ten pancreatic cancers less than 3 cm in size diagnosed at the University of California, San Francisco, four already had evidence of metastasis. In five of seven patients with small, "resectable" pancreatic cancer, lymph node metastasis was found in the surgical specimens.[111] Nonetheless, a CT scan of the pancreas showing a dilated pancreatic or bile duct should stimulate further evaluation by ERCP and possibly angiography to detect small pancreatic tumors. Ariyama's experience indicates that when some small pancreatic tumors are resected, there is prolonged survival when such patients are compared with patients with large pancreatic tumors.[135]

Islet Cell Tumors of the Pancreas ■ Pancreatic islet cell tumors are either secretory or nonfunctioning. The tumors that actively secrete one or more hormones produce clinical and biochemical abnormalities that signal their underlying presence. The insulin-secreting tumors are the most common islet cell tumors and account for 60 to 75 per cent of all islet cell neoplasms.[136] Next in frequency (20 per cent) are the gastrin-secreting alpha-1 islet cell tumors that cause the Zollinger-Ellison syndrome. Rarer islet cell tumors are those producing glucagon (alpha-2 cell), vasoactive intestinal peptide (VIP) (non–beta cell), and somatostatin (delta cell).[137] In addition, APUDomas* of the pancreas are occasionally encountered, particularly in association with other endocrine-secreting tumors such as pituitary adenomas, pheochromocytomas, medullary carcinoma of the thyroid, and bronchial and intestinal carcinoids. APUDomas produce endocrine peptides of various types and are thought to originate from neural crest derivatives. These tumors in the pancreas produce adrenocorticotropic hormone (ACTH), antidiuretic hormone (ADH), and vasoactive intestinal polypeptide (VIP).[137] Because all secretory pancreatic islet cell tumors produce clinically apparent abnormalities as a result of excessive hormone secretion, they are often detected at a smaller size than nonfunctioning islet cell lesions or pancreatic adenocarcinomas. Because functioning islet cell tumors tend to be referred for diagnosis while tumors are small, CT demonstration of these tumors is often difficult.[132, 138]

No specific CT features consistently separate the islet cell tumors from ductal adenocarcinomas. The smaller islet cell lesions are usually isodense with the

---

*Tumors composed of *a*mine *p*recursor *u*ptake and *d*ecarboxylation cells.

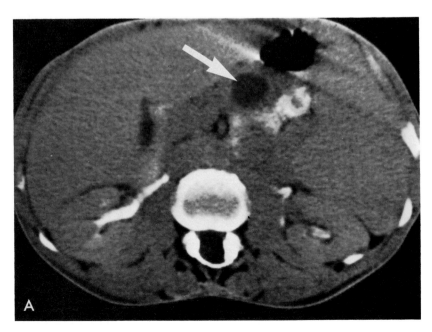

FIGURE 19–49 ■ Large gastrin-secreting islet cell tumor of the pancreas. *A,* The tumor occupies the entire body and tail of the pancreas and encases a segment of contrast-filled jejunum. An area of low density *(arrow)* is present in the tumor as a result of tumor necrosis.

uninvolved pancreas with conventional CT scanning technique (see Fig. 19–48). However, with high-volume bolus dynamic CT scans, even small gastrinomas and insulinomas may enhance, thus permitting their detection (see Fig. 19–37).[139, 140] Larger tumors can have low-density areas indicating foci of tumor necrosis (Fig. 19–49). The location of the tumor determines whether the common bile duct or pancreatic ducts are obstructed and which adjacent organ is likely to be involved. Calcification has been noted in both functioning and nonfunctioning islet cell tumors (Fig. 19–50),[127] a finding almost never seen in adenocarcinomas. Dense calcification may be seen in gastrinomas and glucagonomas (see Fig. 19–50). In a series of 27 cases of nonfunctioning islet cell tumors studied by CT, most of the lesions were large, some 10 cm in size. Calcification was present in 22 per cent.[141] Other findings include incomplete contrast enhancement and pancreatic and bile duct

dilatation—features similar to those in adenocarcinoma.

As a result of the small size of some primary tumors, it is frequently easier to detect evidence of metastatic disease than to locate the primary neoplasm. In one series of 25 patients, hepatic metastases were detected in 40 per cent, whereas the primary lesion was detected by CT in only 33 per cent.[132] In another series hepatic metastasis occurred in 56 per cent of 27 patients with malignant nonfunctioning islet cell carcinomas.[141] Moreover, the tumors detected by CT scanning were large, ranging from 4 to 10 cm in diameter. In another series of insulinomas studied by CT scanning,[131] only 6 of 14 tumors (43 per cent) were detected. However, both of these studies were carried out using second-generation 18-second CT scanners. Studies at the University of California, San Francisco, using high-resolution, fast scanners demonstrated that 70 per cent of 20 patients

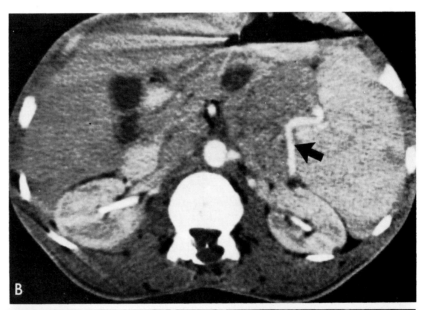

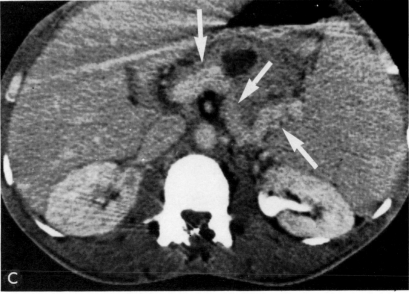

FIGURE 19–49 *Continued B,* CT scan from a dynamic scan sequence clearly shows the splenic artery *(arrow)* displaced by the tumor. *C,* CT scan obtained later in the dynamic scan sequence. Although the spleen is enlarged and the tumor is in a location to obstruct the splenic vein, the dynamic CT scan shows a large, patent splenic vein *(arrows)* surrounded by tumor.

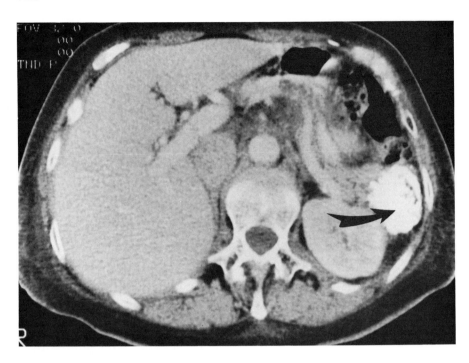

FIGURE 19–50 ■ Densely calcified glucagon-secreting islet cell tumor *(arrow)* of the tail of the pancreas.

with functioning islet cell tumors had tumors demonstrated by CT scans.[140] In general CT scanning is 50 per cent to 80 per cent accurate in detecting functioning islet cell tumors, and detection is size dependent.[142]

Cystic Pancreatic Neoplasms ■ Primary cystic neoplasms of the pancreas are categorized as nonmucinous, glycogen-rich microcystic or serous adenomas, and mucinous cystadenomas and cystadenocarcinomas. These two types of cystic neoplasms make up only about 10 to 15 per cent of all cystic pancreatic lesions[143, 143a–145] and account for only a few per cent of all pancreatic tumors.[143, 144]

Mucinous lesions arise from ductal epithelium and are either obviously malignant or, in the case of cystadenomas, considered to be premalignant.[143, 145] On the other hand, nonmucinous microcystic adenomas have no malignant potential.[143–145] Complete surgical resection is recommended for patients with any mucinous cystic pancreatic tumor, whereas microcystic adenomas may be safely followed or have local surgical resection.

Mucinous Cystic Tumors ■ The vast majority of mucinous cystic tumors occur in the body and tail of the pancreas,[143] whereas solid adenocarcinomas occur more frequently in the head of the pancreas. A new form of mucinous cystadenoma, the "ductectatic" type, has been reported and occurs in the

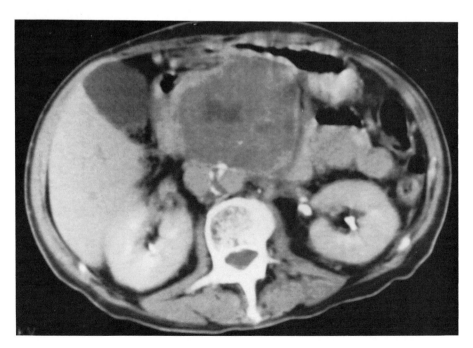

FIGURE 19–51 ■ A large cystic mass in the body of the pancreas containing material of two different CT densities. The mass is well circumscribed and contains a speck of calcification. This is the typical appearance of a cystadenomatous tumor, in this case a mucinous cystadenocarcinoma.

uncinate process.[124] Mucinous neoplasms are almost always greater than 2 cm in size, usually exhibiting areas of low CT density and appearing as fluid-filled cysts. As a result of their large size and low CT density, almost all cystic pancreatic neoplasms are readily detected by CT. Many tumors are multiloculated but usually contain less than ten cystic components (Fig. 19–51 and 19–52). The number of cysts (less than six) and the size of the majority of the cysts (2 cm or greater) is typical of mucinous cystic tumors in contrast to microcystic serous adenomas, which have more cysts that are smaller.[143a] Well-

defined margins are usually present, but in some, multiple, irregular cystic masses are surrounded by normal pancreatic tissue. In others, only a portion of the tumor is connected to the pancreas (Figs. 19–52 through 19–54). Cyst walls are often thin but may be thickened locally. The degree of thickening does not correlate with the presence of malignancy.[145] Septa and local projections into the cyst are frequently seen, and these undergo CT enhancement after delivery of contrast material (Figs. 19–52 and 19–55). Occasionally the septa contain small collections of calcification. In cystadenocarcinomas, typically there

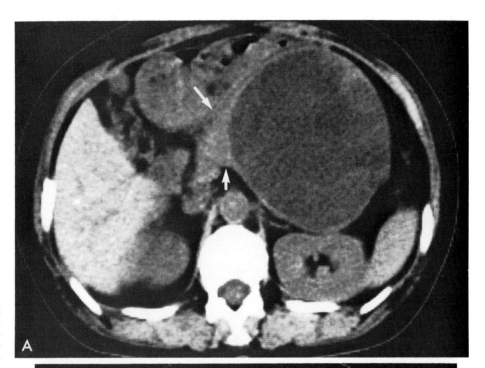

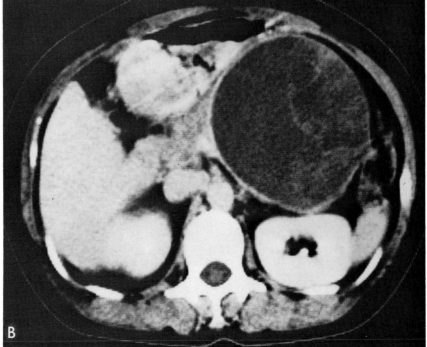

FIGURE 19–52 ■ Mucinous cystadenoma of the pancreas. A, A precontrast scan reveals a large, low-density, well-circumscribed mass in the left abdomen. Its pancreatic origin is shown by the extension of pancreatic tissue (arrows) over the medial border of the mass. B, After administration of intravenous contrast material, the capsule and the internal septa are shown more clearly. (From Itai Y, Moss AA, Ohtomo K: Radiology 145:419, 1982. Used with permission.)

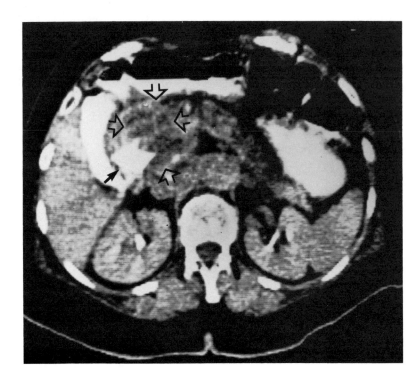

FIGURE 19–53 ■ Cystadenocarcinoma. A postcontrast scan reveals a large, lobulated mass in the head of the pancreas *(open arrows)* that has multiple irregular cystic portions. The dense area *(solid arrow)* is contrast material in a duodenal diverticulum. (From Itai Y, Moss AA, Ohtomo K: Radiology 145:419, 1982. Used with permission.)

FIGURE 19–54 ■ Mucinous macrocystic cystadenoma of the tail of the pancreas. A somewhat solid component *(arrow)* is accompanied by a large cystic component anteriorly. The cyst has a well-formed wall and contains internal structures.

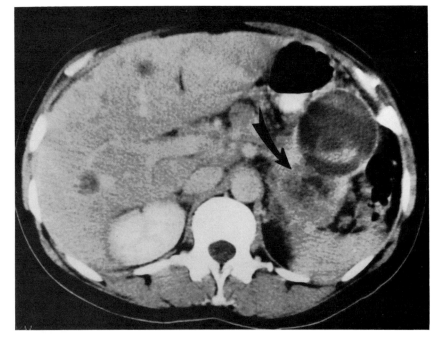

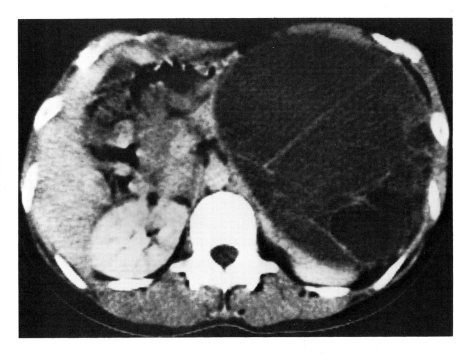

FIGURE 19–55 ■ Mucinous cystadenoma. Postcontrast scan demonstrates a large, rounded mass with thin straight and curvilinear septa. (From Itai Y, Moss AA, Ohtomo K: Radiology 145:419, 1982. Used with permission.)

is a large solid component to the tumor, along with small daughter cysts immediately adjacent to one of the large cystic masses (see Figs. 19–53 and 19–54). Although stomach, spleen, colon, and small bowel may be displaced by these large tumors, adjacent organs are not usually invaded.

Serous Cystic Tumors ■ Serous or microcystic adenomas occur in all areas of the pancreas and are usually made up of multiple small cysts less than 2 cm in size (Fig. 19–56).[144, 145] Often a mass that appears to be made up of many small cysts intermixed with solid portions is identified. These cysts may contain central connective tissue with radiating strands, giving a stellate or honeycomb appearance (Figs. 19–56 and 19–57),[144, 145] and foci of calcification may be seen in the center of the cyst. In one series, calcification was seen in 38 per cent of microcystic adenomas.[143a] Simple cysts of the pancreas are easily differentiated from serous cystic tumors, because although they may be multiple, as may occur in von Hippel–Lindau disease or polycystic disease, they are sharply outlined and have no internal architecture (Fig. 19–58). In some cases, the CT features of microcystic or serous adenomas appear to be sufficiently different from the mucinous cystadenoma-carcinoma to permit differentiation on the basis of CT scans alone. However, the premalignant cystadenoma cannot be distinguished from the frankly malignant cystadenocarcinoma by CT unless there is evidence of local invasion or metastatic lesions.

STAGING OF PANCREATIC CARCINOMA

The ability of CT to outline the margins of a pancreatic mass and evaluate peripancreatic fat and adjacent structures such as stomach, spleen, duodenum, peripancreatic vessels, regional lymph nodes, and the liver indicates that CT is an effective tool for aiding the surgeon in preoperative staging of pancreatic tumors.[111, 146] By demonstrating invasion of peripancreatic fat, encasement of superior mesenteric artery or vein, invasion of duodenum or stomach, presence of regional lymph node enlargement, abnormal tissue in the porta hepatis, or liver metastasis, surgical resection may be avoided. However, the absence of these findings on CT does not always indicate that a small pancreatic cancer may be resectable. In two series, patients with small pancreatic carcinomas thought by CT to be resectable were found at surgery to have local invasion in the duodenum and vessels and spread to lymph nodes.[111, 147] In one series, none of 42 tumors considered unresectable based on CT findings was resectable at surgery, whereas two of nine tumors judged to be resectable by CT findings were not resectable at time of surgery.[111] In five of seven that did undergo resection, microscopic tumor was found in the lymph nodes. Nevertheless, CT is a useful technique for aiding in preoperative staging of patients with pancreatic carcinoma.

METASTATIC TUMORS

As a result of its strategic location in the abdomen, the pancreas is susceptible to invasion or displacement by neoplasms from adjacent organs and lymph nodes. Carcinoma of the stomach, gallbladder, and liver may invade pancreatic tissue (Fig. 19–59). In these patients, CT scans demonstrate that the fat normally separating the pancreas from the stomach or the liver is obliterated, and tumor extends directly into the pancreatic substance, producing indistinct margins between pancreas and adjacent organs. In addition, lesions of the left adrenal gland and kidney may displace the tail of the pancreas, destroy surrounding fat, and occlude the splenic vein.

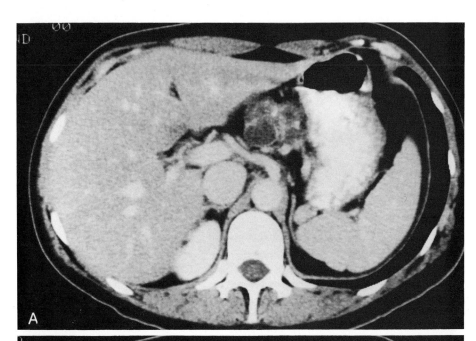

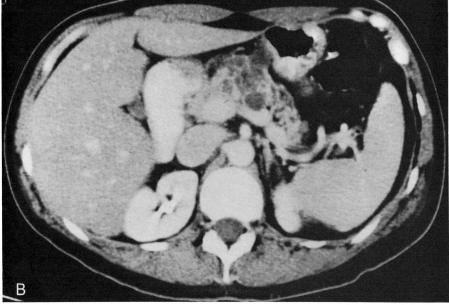

FIGURE 19–56 ■ Microcystic adenoma of the body of the pancreas. Note the multiple small cysts with thin-walled septa that make up the large part of this benign lesion.

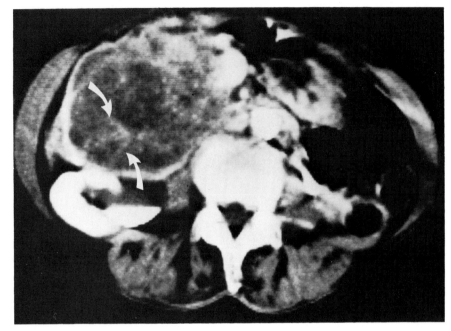

FIGURE 19–57 ■ Serous cystadenoma. Postcontrast scan reveals a large, well-defined mass in the head of the pancreas. The wall of the mass and internal septa *(arrows)* show marked contrast enhancement. (From Itai Y, Moss AA, Ohtomo K: Radiology 145:419, 1982. Used with permission.)

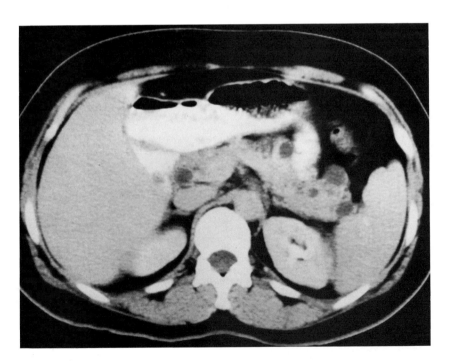

FIGURE 19–58 ■ Multiple simple cysts of the pancreas present in a patient with von Hippel-Lindau disease.

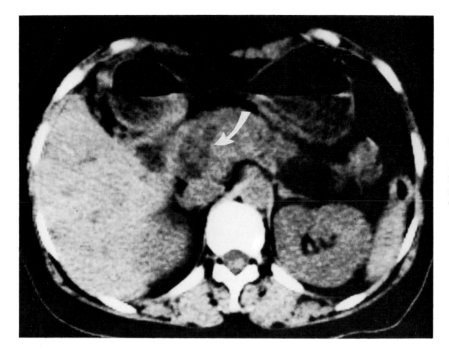

FIGURE 19–59 ■ Carcinoma of the gallbladder invading the pancreas. Scan demonstrates a mass in the head of the pancreas proven to be the result of spread from carcinoma of the gallbladder. The mass has caused pancreatic duct dilatation *(arrow)*.

Involvement of peripancreatic lymph nodes, particularly those in and around the celiac and mesenteric arteries, may simulate pancreatic tumors (Fig. 19–60). Enlargement of peripancreatic lymph nodes resulting from metastatic tumor, infection, or lymphoma can result in lobulated masses that impinge on the pancreas. Differentiating a primary pancreatic tumor from peripancreatic lymphadenopathy may not be possible if the fat planes are totally obliterated. However, if the fat planes are intact, a diagnosis of peripancreatic lymph node enlargement can be suggested on CT. Occasionally the differentiation between a lymph node mass simulating a lesion in the head and/or body of the pancreas and a true pancreatic mass is possible by enhancement of the pancreatic parenchyma as a result of an intravenous bolus of contrast material. A lymph node mass that does not enhance can be more clearly seen and the actual boundary between the lymph node mass and the pancreas more readily discerned.

ACCURACY IN DETECTION OF PANCREATIC CARCINOMA

The accuracy of computed tomography in detecting pancreatic cancer has been determined in several studies using various scanners and techniques (Table

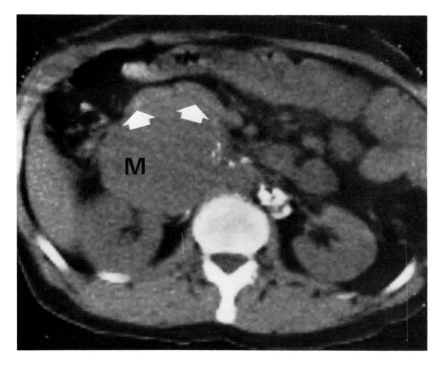

FIGURE 19–60 ■ Enlarged pericaval lymph nodes as a result of lymphoma simulating the CT appearance of a mass (M) in the head of the pancreas. Several contrast-enhanced lymph nodes are present as a result of a prior lymphangiogram. The pancreas is displaced and stretched over the top of the mass *(arrows)*.

19–2). In some studies, false-negative and false-positive results have also been reported, providing a measure of sensitivity and specificity. In a total of 696 cases of pancreatic tumor reported in Table 19–2, the overall CT accuracy ranged from 71 to 91 per cent, with a sensitivity of 71 to 95 per cent and specificity, when reported, of 83 to 90 per cent. The type of scanning equipment, technique, use of contrast material, amount of natural peripancreatic fat, and density of the pancreatic lesion all affect detection by CT techniques. To date, the few false-positive CT studies that have been reported were mostly the result of pancreatic lobulations, pancreatic cysts, chronic pancreatitis, or peripancreatic lymphoma.[111]

The use of fine-needle percutaneous CT-guided biopsy has greatly increased the overall accuracy of computed tomography in diagnosing pancreatic disease. This technique, discussed in an earlier chapter, has been applied effectively in establishing the presence of pancreatic cancer. In Mitty et al.'s series,[148] fine-needle aspiration of 43 patients with clinically diagnosed pancreatic carcinoma revealed cancer in 37, with six false-negative results, for an accuracy of 88.7 per cent. We achieved a 95 per cent accuracy in patients with pancreatic tumor biopsied by fine-needle aspiration technique. In our series of 32 needle biopsies performed because of the presence of either a pancreatic mass or peripancreatic lymph nodes, 21 gave true-positive and 28 gave true-negative results, with only one false-negative result and one inadequate sample.

Relationship of Imaging Modalities

In a hospital or clinical radiology department setting having modern radiographic, CT, ultrasound, and MRI equipment, several imaging techniques are available for evaluating pancreatic cancer. We first utilize a noninvasive technique and depend on invasive techniques such as ERCP, percutaneous transhepatic cholangiogram (PTC), and angiography only when CT scanning, ultrasound, or MRI fails to provide adequate diagnostic information.

Currently CT is considered the imaging procedure of choice for evaluating the pancreas for suspected pancreatic cancer. Pancreatic CT scanning is recommended in all patients with suspected pancreatic cancer on the basis of back and/or epigastric pain and weight loss. CT is ideally suited for patients with sufficient retroperitoneal fat because of its ability to outline abnormalities in the pancreas and other structures within the retroperitoneal fat. Emaciated patients, on the other hand, are studied best with ultrasound. CT scanners are almost always capable of imaging the entire pancreas and providing important information concerning peripancreatic spread and distant metastatic disease. MRI is currently used as an alternative to CT when patients have surgically placed metallic clips in or around the pancreas that degrade the CT image. In patients who have had severe reactions to intravenous contrast material, MRI may be used as an alternative to dynamic CT.

If a patient presents with jaundice and a pancreatic mass in the head or uncinate process is the suspected cause, ultrasound is usually performed as the initial imaging procedure. Ultrasonography and CT have identical rates of detection of dilated bile ducts and of lesions in the head of the pancreas.[138, 149] Ultrasonography is also the imaging procedure of choice in emaciated jaundiced patients. Overall, ultrasound detection rates for pancreatic carcinoma have been reported to be similar to those of CT scanning (85 to 94 per cent).[150–152] However, although overall detection rates for pancreatic cancer may be similar, CT better demonstrates peripancreatic tumor spread and more completely images the tail of the pancreas.

If a mass or definite contour abnormality is detected in the pancreas, fine-needle aspiration biopsy should be performed using either CT or ultrasound guidance. This additional technique greatly enhances the usefulness of CT or ultrasound, because direct cytologic or histologic confirmation may be obtained without resorting to further diagnostic imaging tests or exploratory laparotomy. If the mass detected proves to be adenocarcinoma, CT is used to stage the pancreatic carcinoma. If any question remains

TABLE 19–2 ■ Accuracy of CT in Detection of Pancreatic Cancer

AUTHOR	NO. CASES TUMOR/NORMAL	TP	TN	FP	FN	SENSITIVITY	SPECIFICITY	ACCURACY (%)
Foley[100]	7/13	5	—	—	2	—	0.71	71
Freeny[110]	77/146	62	135	17	15	0.82	0.88	88
Gmelin[153]	10	6	—	0	2	0.75	—	80
Haaga[4]	32/12	28	11	0	4	0.87	1.00	88
Haertel[112]	75	71	—		4	0.95	—	—
Hessel[156]	52	—	—	—	—	0.84	—	—
Inamoto[115]	43/235	37	195	40	6	0.86	0.83	83
Itai[119]	62	54	—	—	8	0.87	—	—
Lackner[150]	41	—	—	—	1	0.93	—	—
Levitt[109]	18/150	15	147	0	1	0.93	1.00	88
Moss[154]	8/32	6	27	1	1	0.85	0.90	84
Pistolesi[128]	36/39	33	—	—	3	0.84	—	—
Stanley[5]	52	36	—	4	12	0.75	—	—
Freeny[111]	159/15	159	0	13	2	0.91	—	91

Abbreviations: FN = False-negative; FP = false-positive; TN = true-negative; TP = true-positive.

about the extent of the tumor or if the tumor appears on the basis of CT scanning to be possibly resectable, selected pancreatic angiography is performed to provide information about encasement of adjacent vascular structures.[111, 138] If CT or ultrasonograms of the pancreas appear normal but a strong clinical suspicion of pancreatic disease remains, endoscopic retrograde pancreatography (ERP) should be performed. When the pancreatic duct is successfully cannulated, most studies show ERP to be more accurate than CT in detecting pancreatic cancer.[100, 153–155] However, because of cannulation failures, overall accuracy rates for ERP are lower than with CT or ultrasound.[154, 156]

The overall impact of CT scanning of the pancreas for suspected pancreatic disease was studied by Freeny and colleagues.[111] The study showed that when CT scanning was used in the evaluation of pancreatic disease, additional examinations such as ERP and angiography were not necessary in 74 per cent of cases. Using CT as the initial screening process, ERP utilization decreased 68 per cent and angiography 54 per cent. This indicates that ERP and angiography have important but secondary roles in the overall evaluation of suspected pancreatic cancer and should act as complementary studies to computed tomography whenever the CT findings are nonspecific or equivocal.

Because of respiratory motion artifacts and resolution limitations, MR was thought initially to be inferior to CT in imaging the pancreas to detect neoplasms.[104, 105] However, improved techniques, including highly T1-weighted spin-echo sequences and gradient-echo sequences, and rapid scan times within

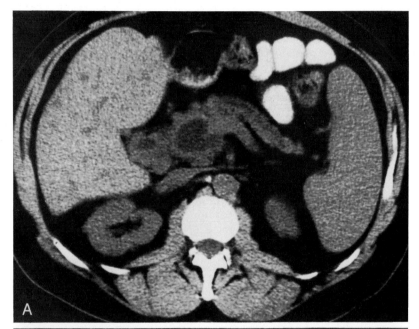

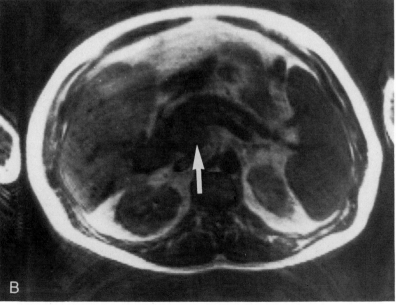

FIGURE 19–61 ■ *A,* A low-density mass is seen in the head of the pancreas and uncinate process on a noncontrast CT scan through the pancreas. *B,* On a T1-weighted MR image through the same area as *A,* the mass appears isointense with the rest of the pancreas but can be seen by virtue of its expansion of the uncinate process *(arrow).*

the breath-holding ability of a patient, have improved imaging of the pancreas. Therefore the features of pancreatic tumors may be more readily detected by MRI than in the past. The same criteria used for CT detection of pancreatic cancer may be used for MRI detection (e.g., size, inhomogeneity of signal, evidence of invasion of adjacent organs or vessels, and metastasis).

Changes in size and shape of the pancreas may be detected best on T1-weighted images (Fig. 19–61). Invasion of peripancreatic fat is also best evaluated on T1-weighted images (see Fig. 19–41).[108] In addition, obstruction of the pancreatic duct with ductal dilatation may be seen. Localized lymphadenopathy, hepatic metastasis, obstruction of the portal vein and splenic vein, and involvement of the superior mesenteric vein may be demonstrated.[108]

The signal intensity and T1 and T2 relaxation times of pancreatic cancer may vary in relation to the surrounding normal pancreas. In some instances, tumors are isointense with the pancreas on T1-weighted images,[108] and in others, particularly with utilization of short TR and short TE T1-weighted spin-echo techniques, the tumors are hypointense. On T2-weighted images, the tumors increase in signal intensity compared with the rest of the pancreas in some cases.[108] In one study[108] the mean T1 relaxation time of normal pancreas was 507 ± 98 ms, and the T1 relaxation time of tumor was 660 ± 115 ms; the T2 relaxation time of normal pancreas was 59 ± 9 ms, and the T2 of tumor was 67 ± 29 ms. Tumors with necrotic centers may have particularly low signal on T1-weighted images, providing additional tumor-to-pancreas contrast. Gadolinium DTPA given intravenously may prove useful as a means of defining pancreatic neoplasms, in that the signal enhancement of the normally perfused pancreas may provide improved contrast against the unenhanced tumor. Functioning islet cell carcinomas have been demonstrated by MR.[105, 106, 108] These have been large lesions and have had high signal intensity on T2-weighted images. However, smaller lesions have been reported to be detected by MRI[106] as well as missed by MRI.[108] It would appear that MRI may be more valuable for staging the extent and spread of pancreatic carcinoma than for detecting the primary lesions. In one study[108a] MRI was found to demonstrate the pancreatic neoplasm as well as CT. This study also found that heavily T1-weighted spin-echo images were the most useful for showing these lesions. However, very few cases have been analyzed by MRI along with other imaging modalities in the same patient. CT at this time remains the preferred method of searching for and staging pancreatic neoplasms.

References

1. Meyers MA: Dynamic Radiology of the Abdomen: Normal and Pathologic Anatomy. New York, Springer, 1976.
2. Neumann CH, Hessel S: CT of the pancreatic tail. AJR 135:741, 1980.
3. Callen PW, Breiman RS, Korobkin M, DeMartini WJ, Mani JR: Carcinoma of the tail of the pancreas: an unusual CT appearance. AJR 133:135, 1979.
4. Haaga JR, Alfidi RJ, Havrilla TR, Tubbs R, Gonzales L, et al: Definitive role of CT scanning of the pancreas: the second year's experience. Radiology 124:723, 1977.
5. Stanley RJ, Sagel SS, Levitt RG: Computed tomographic evaluation of the pancreas. Radiology 124:715, 1977.
6. Kreel L, Haertel M, Katy D: Computed tomography of the normal pancreas. J Comput Assist Tomogr 1:290, 1977.
7. Baldwin CN: Computed tomography of the pancreas: negative contrast medium. Radiology 128:827, 1978.
8. Jeffrey RB, Federle MP, Goodman PC: Computed tomography of the lesser peritoneal sac. Radiology 141:117, 1981.
9. Sheedy PF, Stephens DH, Hattery RR, MacCarty RL, Williamson B Jr: Computed tomography of the pancreas. Radiol Clin North Am 15:349, 1977.
10. Stuck KJ, Kuhns LR: Improved visualization of the pancreatic tail after maximum distention of the stomach. J Comput Assist Tomogr 5:509, 1981.
11. Marchal G, Baert AL, Wilms G: Intravenous pancreatography in computed tomography. J Comput Assist Tomogr 3:727, 1979.
12. Kivisarri L, Somer K, Standertskjold-Nordenstam CG, Schröder T, Kivilaakso E, et al: A new method for the diagnosis of acute hemorrhagic-necrotizing pancreatitis using contrast enhanced CT. Gastrointest Radiol 9:27, 1984.
12a. Balthazar EJ, Robinson DL, Migibow AJ, Ranson JHC: Acute pancreatitis: value of CT in establishing prognosis. Radiology 174:331–336, 1990.
13. Stark DD, Hendrick RE, Hahn PF, Ferrucci JT: Motion artifact reduction with fast spin echo imaging. Radiology 164:183–191, 1987.
14. Mills TC, Ortendahl DA, Hylton NM, Crooks LE, Carlson JW, Kaufman L: Partial flip angle MR imaging. Radiology 162:531–539, 1987.
15. Simeone JF, Edleman RR, Stark DD, Wittenberg J, White EM, et al: Surface coil imaging of abdominal viscera. Part III. The pancreas. Radiology 157:437–441, 1985.
16. Wesbey GE, Brasch RC, Englestad BL, Moss AA, Crooks LE, Brito AC: Nuclear magnetic resonance contrast enhancement study of the gastrointestinal tract of rats and a human volunteer using nontoxic oral iron solutions. Radiology 149:175–180, 1983.
17. Hahn PF, Stark DD, Saini S, Lewis JM, Wittenberg J, Ferrucci JT: Ferrite particles for bowel contrast in MR imaging: design issues and feasibility studies. Radiology 164:37–41, 1987.
18. Mattrey RF, Hajek PC, Gylys-Marin VM, Baker LL, Matin J, et al: Perfluorochemicals as gastrointestinal contrast agents for MR imaging: preliminary studies in rats and humans. AJR 148:1259–1263, 1987.
19. Winkler MR, Hricak H: Pelvis imaging with MR: technique for improvements. Radiology 159:123–126, 1986.
20. Etiology and pathological anatomy of chronic pancreatitis. Symposium of Marseilles, April 1963. Bibl Gastroenterol, 1965.
21. Spiro HM: Pancreatic disorders. In Spiro HM (ed): Clinical Gastroenterology, 1st ed. London, Macmillan, 1970, pp 813–823.
22. Jordan GL, Spjut HJ: Hemorrhagic pancreatitis. Arch Surg 104:489, 1972.
23. Lawson DW, Daggett WM, Givetta JM, Corry RJ, Bartlett MK: Surgical treatment of acute necrotizing pancreatitis. Ann Surg 172:605, 1970.
24. Ranson JHC, Pasternak BS: Statistical methods for quantifying the severity of clinical acute pancreatitis. J Surg Res 22:79, 1977.
25. Schroder T, Kivisaari L, Somer K, Standertskjöld-Nordenstam CG, Kivilaakso E, et al: Significance of extrapancreatic findings in computed tomography of acute pancreatitis. Eur J Radiol 5:273, 1985.
26. Balthazar EJ, Ranson JH, Naidich PD, Megibow AJ, Caccavale R, et al: Acute pancreatitis: predictive value of CT. Radiology 156:767, 1985.
27. Block S, Maier W, Bittner R, Büchler M, Malfertheiner P, et

al: Identification of pancreatic necrosis in severe acute pancreatitis: imaging procedures versus clinical staging. Gut 27:1035, 1986.

28. Vernacchia F, Jeffrey RB Jr, Federle MP, Grendell JH, Laing FC, et al: Pancreatic abscess: predictive value of early abdominal CT. Radiology 162:435, 1987.

29. Jeffrey RB, Federle MP, Cello JP, Crass RA: Early computed tomographic scanning in acute severe pancreatitis. Surg Gynecol Obstet 154:170, 1982.

30. Peterson LM, Brooks JR: Lethal pancreatitis, a diagnostic dilemma. Am J Surg 137:491, 1979.

31. Silverstein W, Isikoff MB, Hill MC, Barkin J: Diagnostic imaging of acute pancreatitis: prospective study using CT and sonography. AJR 137:497, 1981.

32. Siegelman SS, Copeland BE, Saba GP, Cameron JL, Sanders RC, Zerhouni EA: CT of fluid collections associated with pancreatitis. AJR 134:1121, 1980.

33. Jeffrey RB Jr, Federle MP, Laing FC: Computed tomography of mesenteric involvement in fulminant pancreatitis. Radiology 147:185, 1983.

34. Casolo F, Bianco R, Franceschelli N: Perirenal fluid collection complicating chronic pancreatitis: CT demonstration. Gastrointest Radiol 12:117, 1987.

35. Dembner AG, Jaffe CC, Simeone J, Walsh J: A new computed tomographic sign of pancreatitis. AJR 133:477, 1979.

36. Nicholson RL: Abnormalities of the perinephric fascia and fat in pancreatitis. Radiology 139:125, 1981.

37. Susman N, Hammerman AM, Cohen E: The renal halo sign in pancreatitis. Radiology 142:323, 1982.

38. Brown BM, Federle MP, Jeffrey RB: Gastric wall thickening and extragastric inflammatory processes. J Comput Assist Tomogr 6:762, 1982.

39. Baker RJ, Duarte B: The current status of recognition and treatment of severe necrotizing pancreatitis. Surg Annu 18:129, 1986.

40. Waterman NC, Walsky BA, Kasdan ML, Abrams BL: The treatment of acute hemorrhagic pancreatitis by sump drainage. Surg Gynecol Obstet 126:963, 1968.

41. Isikoff MB, Hill MC, Silverstein W, Barkin J: The clinical significance of acute pancreatic hemorrhage. AJR 136:679, 1981.

42. Hashimoto BE, Laing FC, Jeffrey RB Jr, Federle MP: Hemorrhagic pancreatic fluid collections examined by ultrasound. Radiology 150:813, 1984.

43. Burke JW, Erickson SJ, Kellum CP, Tegtmeyer CJ, Williamson BRJ, et al: Pseudoaneurysms complicating pancreatitis: detection by CT. Radiology 161:447, 1986.

44. Nishiyama T, Iwas N, Myose H, Okamoto T, Fujitomi Y, et al: Splenic vein thrombosis as a consequence of chronic pancreatitis: a study of three cases. Am J Gastroenterol 81:1193, 1986.

45. Warshaw AL: Inflammatory masses following acute pancreatitis. Surg Clin North Am 54:621, 1979.

46. Owens GR, Arger PH, Mulhern CB, Coleman BG, Gohel V: CT evaluation of mediastinal pseudocyst. J Comput Assist Tomogr 4:256, 1980.

47. McCowin MJ, Federle MP: Computed tomography of pancreatic pseudocysts of the duodenum. AJR 145:1003, 1985.

48. Nacianceno SE, Gross SC, Rajn JS, Song SH, Joseph RR: Pancreatic pseudocyst simulating dilated biliary duct system in computed tomography. Radiology 134:165, 1980.

49. Trapnel J: The natural history and management of acute pancreatitis. Clin Gastroenterol 1:147, 1972.

50. Rosenberg IK, Kahn JA, Walt JA: Surgical experience with pancreatic pseudocysts. Am J Surg 117:11, 1969.

51. Trapnel J: Management of the complication of acute pancreatitis. Ann R Coll Surg Engl 49:361, 1971.

52. Bradley EL III, Clements JL Jr, Gonzalez AC: The natural history of pancreatic pseudocysts: a unified concept of management. Am J Surg 137:135, 1979.

53. Sarti DA: Rapid development and spontaneous regression of pancreatic pseudocysts documented by ultrasound. Radiology 125:789, 1977.

54. Kolmannskog F, Kolbenstvedt A, Aakhus T: Computed to-

mography in inflammatory mass lesions following acute pancreatitis. J Comput Assist Tomogr 5:169, 1981.

55. Yellin JA: Cystlike lesions of the pancreatic region on computed tomography. Semin Roentgenol 22:82, 1987.

56. Stair JM, Schaefer RF, McCowan TC, Balachandran S: Cystic islet cell tumor of the pancreas. J Surg Oncol 32:46, 1986.

57. Sigirjonsson SU, Elberg O, Hjelmquist B, Nyman V: Acute afferent loop syndrome simulating pancreatic pseudocysts. ROFO 139:699, 1983.

58. Hernarz-Schulman M, Teele RL, Perex-Atayde A, Zollars L, Levine J, et al: Pancreatic cytosis in cystic fibrosis. Radiology 158:629, 1986.

59. Pinto MM, Kaye AD, Brogan DA, Crisuolo EH: Diagnosis of cystic lesions of the pancreas: a biochemical and cytologic analysis of material utilizing radiographic or intraoperative technique. Diagn Cytopathol 2:40, 1986.

60. Mann J, Altergott R, Prinz PA: Calcified pancreatic pseudocysts. Surgery 101:511, 1987.

61. Shatney CH, Lillehei RC: The timing of surgical treatment of pancreatic pseudocysts. Surg Gynecol Obstet 152:809, 1981.

62. Wade JW: Twenty-five year experience with pancreatic pseudocysts: are we making progress? Am J Surg 149:705, 1985.

63. Dranha GV, Prinz RA, Freeark RJ, Daniel MK, Herbert BG: Evaluation of therapeutic options of pancreatic pseudocysts. Arch Surg 117:717, 1982.

64. Van Sonnenberg E, Wittich GR, Casola G, Stauffer AE, Polansky AD, et al: Complicated pancreatic inflammatory disease: diagnostic and therapeutic role of interventional radiology. Radiology 155:335, 1985.

65. Jones WE, Evert MB, Baumgarten BR, Bernardino ME: Percutaneous aspiration and drainage of pancreatic pseudocysts. AJR 147:1007, 1986.

66. Nunez D Jr, Yrizarry JM, Russell E, Sadighi A, Casillas J, et al: Transgastric drainage of pancreatic fluid collections. AJR 145:815, 1985.

67. Matzinger FRK, Ho CS, Yee AC, Gray RR: Pancreatic pseudocysts drained through a percutaneous transgastric approach: further experience. Radiology 167:431, 1988.

68. Altemeier WA, Alexander JW: Pancreatic abscess: a study of 32 cases. Arch Surg 87:80, 1963.

69. Bolooki H, Jaffe B, Geidiman ML: Pancreatic abscesses and lesser omental sac collections. Surg Gynecol Obstet 126:1301, 1968.

70. Warshaw AL: Pancreatic abscess. N Engl J Med 287:1234, 1972.

71. Bittner R, Block S, Buckler M, Berger HG: Pancreatic abscess and infected pancreatic necrosis. Different local septic complications in acute pancreatitis. Diag Dis Sci 32:1082, 1987.

72. Federle MP, Jeffrey RB, Crass RA, Van Dalsem V: Computed tomography of pancreatic abscesses. AJR 136:879, 1981.

73. White EM, Wittenberg J, Mueller PR, Simeone JF, Butch RJ, et al: Pancreatic necrosis: CT manifestations. Radiology 158:343, 1986.

74. Mendez G, Isikoff MB: Significance of intrapancreatic gas demonstrated by CT: a review of nine cases. AJR 132:59, 1979.

75. Alexander ES, Clark RA, Federle MP: Pancreatic gas: indication of pancreatic fistula. AJR 139:1089, 1982.

76. Clements JL, Bradley EL, Eaton SB: Spontaneous internal drainage of pancreatic pseudocysts. AJR 126:985, 1976.

77. Gerzof SG, Banks PA, Robbins AH, Johnson WC, Spechler SJ, et al: Early diagnosis of pancreatic infection by computed tomography-guided aspiration. Gastroenterology 93:1315, 1987.

78. Karlson KB, Martin EC, Fankuchen EI, Mattern RF, Schultz RW, et al: Percutaneous drainage of pancreatic pseudocysts and abscesses. Radiology 142:619, 1982.

79. Freeny PC, Lewis GP, Traverso LW, Ryan JA: Infected pancreatic fluid collections: percutaneous catheter drainage. Radiology 167:435, 1988.

80. Steiner E, Mueller PR, Hahn PF, Saini S, Simeone JF, et al: Complicated pancreatic abscess: problems in interventional management. Radiology 167:443, 1988.

81. Jeffrey RB Jr, Grendell JH, Federle MP, Meyer AA, Wing

VW, et al: Improved survival with early CT diagnosis of pancreatic abscess. Gastrointest Radiol 12:26, 1987.

82. McClave SA, McAllister EW, Earl RC, Nord HJ: Pancreatic abscess: ten year experience at the University of South Florida. Am J Gastroenterol 81:180, 1986.

83. Hubbard TB Jr, Eilber FR, Okdroyd H: The retroperitoneal extension of necrotizing pancreatitis. Surg Gynecol Obstet 134:927, 1972.

84. Benson JA Jr: Chronic pancreatitis. In Sleisenger MH, Fordtran JS (eds): Gastrointestinal Disease. Philadelphia, WB Saunders, 1973, pp 1185–1197.

85. Ring EJ, Eaton SB, Ferrucci JT Jr, Short WF: Differential diagnosis of pancreatic calcification. AJR 117:446, 1973.

86. Ferrucci JT Jr, Wittenberg J, Black EB, Kirkpatrick RH, Hall DA: Computed body tomography in chronic pancreatitis. Radiology 130:175, 1979.

87. Ohto M, Ono T, Tsuchiya Y, Saisho H: Cholangiography and Pancreatography. Tokyo, Igaku-Shoin, 1978, p 82.

88. Berland LL, Lawson TL, Foley D, Greenan JE, Stewart ET: Computed tomography of the normal and abnormal pancreatic duct. Correlation with pancreatic ductography. Radiology 141:715, 1981.

89. Gold RP, Seaman WB: Computed tomography and the dilated pancreatic duct: an ominous sign. Gastrointest Radiol 6:35, 1981.

90. Fishman A, Isikoff MB, Barkin J, Friedland JT: Significance of dilated pancreatic duct on CT examination. AJR 133:225, 1979.

91. Hauser H, Bettikha JG, Wettstein P: Computed tomography of the dilated pancreatic duct. J Comput Assist Tomogr 4:53, 1980.

92. Karasawa E, Goldberg HI, Moss AA, Federle MP, London SS: CT pancreatogram in carcinoma of the pancreas and chronic pancreatitis. Radiology 148:489, 1983.

93. Freeny PC, Bilbao MK, Katon RM: "Blind" evaluation of endoscopic retrograde cholangiopancreatography (ERCP) in the evaluation of pancreatic carcinoma: the "double duct" and other signs. Radiology 119:271, 1976.

94. Seidelmann FE, Cohen WN, Bryan PJ, Brown J: CT demonstration of the splenic vein-pancreatic relationship: the pseudodilated pancreatic duct. AJR 129:17, 1977.

95. Kreel L, Sadin B: Changes in pancreatic morphology associated with aging. Gut 14:962, 1973.

96. Malfertheimer P, Buckler M, Stanescu A, Ditschuneit H: Exocrine pancreatic function in correlation to ductal and parenchymal morphology in chronic pancreatitis. Hepatogastroenterology 33:110, 1986.

97. Malfertheimer P, Buckle RM, Stanescu A, Ditschuneit H: Pancreatic morphology and function in relationship to pain in chronic pancreatitis. J Pancreatol 2:59, 1987.

98. Filshire J, Golding S, Robbie DS, Husband JE: Unilateral computerized tomography guided coeliac plexus block: a technique for pain relief. Anesthesia 38:498, 1983.

99. Johnson JR, Zintel HA: Pancreatic calcification and cancer of the pancreas. Surg Gynecol Obstet 117:585, 1963.

100. Foley WD, Steward ET, Lawson TL, Geenan J, Longuidice J, et al: Computed tomography, ultrasonography, and endoscopic retrograde cholangiopancreatography in the diagnosis of pancreatic disease: a comparative study. Gastrointest Radiol 5:29, 1980.

101. Tobin RS, Vogelzang RL, Gore RM, Keigley B: A comparative study of computed tomography and ERCP in pancreaticobiliary disease. J Comput Tomogr 11:261, 1987.

102. Jaffe MH, Glazer GM, Amendola AM, Nostrant T, Wilson JA: Endoscopic retrograde computed tomography of the pancreas. J Comput Assist Tomogr 8:63, 1984.

103. Swobodnik W, Meyer W, Brecht-Kraus D, Wechsler JC, Geiger S, et al: Ultrasound, computed tomography and endoscopic retrograde cholangiopancreatography in the morphologic diagnosis of pancreatic disease. Klin Wochenski 15:291, 1983.

104. Stark DD, Moss AA, Goldberg HI, Davis PL, Federle MP: Magnetic resonance and CT of the normal and diseased pancreas: a comparative study. Radiology 150:153–162, 1984.

105. Goldberg HI, Margulis AR, Moss AA, Stark DD: Imaging of the liver, gallbladder, spleen, pancreas, peritoneal cavity and alimentary tube. In James TL, Margulis AR (eds): Biomedical Magnetic Resonance. San Francisco, University of California Press, 1984.

106. Stark DD: The liver, pancreas and spleen. In Higgins CB, Hricak H (eds): Magnetic Resonance Imaging of the Body. New York, Raven Press, 1987.

107. Tsay DG, Neiderau C, Schmidt H, Goldberg H, Higgins CB, et al: Experimental acute pancreatitis. In vitro magnetic resonance characteristics. Invest Radiol 22:556–561, 1987.

108. Tscholakoff D, Hricak H, Thoeni R, Winkler ML, Margulis AR: MR imaging in the diagnosis of pancreatic disease. AJR 148:703–709, 1987.

108a. Steiner E, Stark DD, Hahn PF, Saini S, Simeone JF, et al: Imaging of pancreatic neoplasms: comparison of MR and CT. AJR 152:487–491, 1989.

109. Levitt RG, Stanley RJ, Sagel SS, Lee JKT, Weyman PJ: Computed tomography of the pancreas: 3 second scanning vs 18 second scanning. J Comput Assist Tomogr 6:259, 1982.

110. Freeny PC, Marks WM, Ball TJ: Impact of high-resolution computed tomography of the pancreas on utilization of endoscopic retrograde cholangiopancreatography and angiography. Radiology 142:35–39, 1982.

111. Freeny PC, Marks WM, Ryan JA, Traverso LW: Pancreatic ductal adenocarcinoma: diagnosis and staging with dynamic CT. Radiology 166:125–133, 1988.

112. Haertel M, Zaunbauer W, Fuchs WA: Die computertomographische morphologische. Morphologie des Pankreaskarzinoms. ROFO 133:1, 1980.

113. Kaylan JO, Isikoff MB, Barkin J, Livingstone AS: Necrotic carcinoma of the pancreas: "the pseudo-pseudocyst." J Comput Assist Tomogr 4:166, 1980.

114. Takekawa S: Comparison study in the diagnosis of pancreatic carcinoma by CT and angiography. Presented at 40th annual meeting of the Japanese Society of Radiology, Tokyo, 1981.

115. Inamoto K, Yamazaki H, Kuwata K, Okamoti E, Kotoura Y, Ishikawa Y: Computed tomography of carcinoma in the pancreatic head. Gastrointest Radiol 6:343, 1981.

116. Moss AA, Schnyder P, Marks W, Margulis AR: Gastric adenocarcinoma: a comparison of the accuracy and economics of staging by computed tomography and surgery. Gastroenterology 80:45, 1981.

117. Thoeni RF, Moss AA, Schnyder P, Margulis AR: Detection and staging of primary rectal and rectosigmoid cancer by computed tomography. Radiology 141:135, 1981.

118. Meyerbow AJ, Roxniak MA, Ambios MA, Berenbaum ER: Thickening of the celiac axis and/or superior mesenteric artery: a sign of pancreatic carcinoma on computed tomography. Radiology 141:449, 1981.

119. Itai Y: Progress of imaging diagnosis for cancer: computed tomography of abdominal malignancy. Jpn J Cancer Clin 26:1029, 1980.

120. Gosink BB, Leopold GR: The dilated pancreatic duct: ultrasonic evaluation. Radiology 126:475, 1978.

121. Weinstein DP, Weinstein BJ: Ultrasonic demonstration of the pancreatic duct: an analysis of 41 cases. Radiology 130:729, 1979.

122. Ohto M, Saoteme S, Saisho H, Tsuchiya Y, Ono T, et al: Real-time sonography of the pancreatic duct: application to percutaneous pancreatic ductography. AJR 134:647, 1980.

123. Foley DW, Lawson TL, Quiroz F: Sagittal and coronal image reconstruction: application in pancreatic computed tomography. J Comput Assist Tomogr 3:717, 1979.

124. Itai Y, Ohhashi K, Nagai H, Murakami Y, Kokubo T, et al: "Ductectatic" mucinous cystadenoma and cystadenocarcinoma of the pancreas. Radiology 161:697–700, 1986.

125. Itai Y, Moss AA, Goldberg HI: Pancreatic cysts caused by carcinoma of the pancreas: a pitfall in the diagnosis of pancreatic carcinoma. J Comput Assist Tomogr 6:772, 1982.

126. Paulino-Netto A, Dreiling DA, Baronofsky ID: The relationship between pancreatic calcification and cancer of the pancreas. Ann Surg 151:530, 1960.

127. Imhof H, Frank P: Pancreatic calcifications in malignant islet cell tumors. Radiology 122:333, 1977.

128. Pistolesi GF, Procacci C, Fugazzola C, Marzoli GP, Pederzoli P, Quarta Colosso P: Place of computed tomography in pancreatic disease: comparison with other radiological methods. Comput Tomogr 5:115, 1981.

129. Goldberg HI, Filly RA, Korobkin M, Moss AA, Kressel HY, Callen PW: Capability of CT body scanning and ultrasonography to demonstrate the status of the biliary ductal system in patients with jaundice. Radiology 129:731, 1978.

130. Sager WD, zur Nedden D, Lepuschütz H, Zalaudek G, Bodner E, et al: Computertomographische Diagnostik der Pankreatitis und des Pankreaskarzinoms. Computertomographie 1:52, 1981.

131. Dunnick NR, Long JA, Kridy A, Shawker TH, Doppman JL: Localizing insulinomas with combined radiographic methods. AJR 135:747, 1980.

132. Dunnick NR, Doppman JL, Mills SR, McCarthy DM: Computed tomographic detection of nonbeta pancreatic islet cell tumors. Radiology 135:117, 1980.

133. Stanley RJ, Sagel SS, Evens RG: The impact of new imaging methods on pancreatic arteriography. Radiology 136:251, 1980.

134. Levin DG, Wilson R, Abrams HL: The changing role of pancreatic arteriography in the era of computed tomography. Radiology 136:245, 1980.

135. Ariyama J: Radiology in Disorders of the Liver, Biliary Tract, and Pancreas. Tokyo, Igaku-Shoin, 1981, pp 147–149.

136. Arky RA, Knopf RH: Evaluation of islet-cell function in men. N Engl J Med 285:1130, 1971.

137. Tischler AS, Dichter MA, Bilaes B, Greene LA: Neuroendocrine neoplasms and their cells of origin. N Engl J Med 296:919, 1977.

138. Simeone JF, Wittenberg J, Ferrucci JT Jr: Modern concepts of imaging the pancreas. Invest Radiol 15:6, 1980.

139. Krudy AG, Doppman JL, Jensen RT, Norton JA, Collen MJ, et al: Localization of islet cell tumors by dynamic CT: comparison with plain CT, arteriography, sonography and venous sampling. AJR 143:585–589, 1984.

140. Stark DD, Moss AA, Goldberg HI, Deveney CW: CT of pancreatic islet cell tumors. Radiology 150:491–494, 1984.

141. Eelkema EA, Stephens DH, Ward EM, Sheedy PF: CT features of non-functioning islet cell carcinoma. AJR 143:943–948, 1984.

142. May G, Gardiner R: Clinical Imaging of the Pancreas. New York, Raven Press, 1987, pp 140–148.

143. Logan SE, Boet RL, Tompkins RK: The malignant potential of mucinous cysts of the pancreas. West J Med 136:157, 1982.

143a. Johnson CD, Stephens DH, Charboneau JW, Carpenter HA, Welch TJ: Cystic pancreatic tumors: CT and sonographic assessment. AJR 151:1133–1138, 1988.

144. Wolfman NT, Ramquest NA, Karstaedt N, Hopkins MB: Cystic neoplasms of the pancreas: CT and sonography. AJR 138:37, 1982.

145. Itai Y, Moss AA, Ohtomo K: Computed tomography of cystadenoma and cystadenocarcinoma of the pancreas. Radiology 145:419, 1982.

146. Itai Y, Araki T, Tasaka A, Maruyama M: Computed tomographic appearance of resectable pancreatic carcinoma. Radiology 143:719–726, 1982.

147. Tsuchiya R, Noda T, Horada N: Collective review of small carcinomas of the pancreas. Ann Surg 203:77–81, 1986.

148. Mitty HA, Efrimidis SC, Heh H-C: Impact of fine-needle biopsy on management of patients with carcinoma of the pancreas. AJR 137:1119, 1981.

149. Taylor KJW, Rosenfeld AT: Grey scale ultrasonography in the differential diagnosis of jaundice. Arch Surg 112:820, 1970.

150. Lackner K, Frommhold H, Grauthoff H, Modder I, Heuser L, et al: Wertigkeit der Computertomographie und der Sonographie innerhalb der Pankreasdiagnostik. ROFO 132:509, 1980.

151. Taylor KJW, Buchin PJ, Biscomi GN, Rosenfeld AT: Ultrasonographic scanning of the pancreas. Radiology 138:211, 1981.

152. Freeny PC, Ball TJ: Rapid diagnosis of pancreatic carcinoma. Radiology 127:627, 1978.

153. Gmelin Von E, Weiss HD, Fuchs HD, Reiser M: Vergleich der diagnostischen Treffsicherheit von Ultraschall, Computertomographie und ERPC bei der chronischen Pankreatitis und beim Pankreaskarzinom. ROFO 134:136, 1981.

154. Moss AA, Federle M, Shapiro H, Ohto M, Goldberg H, et al: The combined use of computed tomography and endoscopic retrograde cholangiopancreatography in the assessment of suspected pancreatic neoplasm: a blind clinical evaluation. Radiology 134:159, 1980.

155. Cotton PB, Denyer ME, Kreel L, Husband J, Meire HB, Lees W: Comparative clinical impact of endoscopic pancreatography, grey-scale ultrasonography and computed tomography (EMI scanning) in pancreatic diseases: preliminary report. Gut 19:679, 1978.

156. Hessel SJ, Siegelman SS, McNeil BJ, Sanders R, Adams DF, et al: A prospective evaluation of computed tomography and ultrasound of the pancreas. Radiology 143:129, 1982.

CHAPTER 20

THE KIDNEYS

ALBERT A. MOSS ▪ *WILLIAM H. BUSH*

Since its introduction and up to the present, computed tomography (CT) has provided valuable diagnostic information in various renal and ureteral lesions.[1-13] Although excretory urography is still the principal uroradiologic imaging procedure, CT has enlarged the capacity to image the genitourinary tract noninvasively. CT is a rapid, easily performed, safe diagnostic imaging procedure that can be performed independent of renal function, provides cross-sectional anatomic information, and is unsurpassed in evaluating lesions containing fat or calcium. The only complications are reactions to contrast media. The combination of unique information, safety, and high diagnostic yield make CT a vital component of uroradiologic diagnosis.

Anatomy

Basic to an understanding of the anatomy of the kidney and ureters is a detailed knowledge of the extraperitoneal fascial planes, which divide the retroperitoneal region into three compartments, and the relationships among the renal fascia, the retroperitoneal compartments, and the organs within the retroperitoneal region. By its ability to differentiate between fat and fascial tissue, CT demonstrates the three retroperitoneal compartments in all but the most emaciated patients.[2, 14-21]

The extraperitoneal region is divided into the anterior pararenal, the perinephric, and the posterior pararenal compartments by the anterior and posterior layers of renal fascia (Fig. 20–1).[14-21] The kidney and its blood vessels are surrounded by a mass of fatty tissue, or perinephric fat, which is enveloped by the dense, collagenous renal fascia. The renal fascia is connected to the kidney by numerous trabeculae that cross the fatty tissue.[21] The anterior and posterior layers of the renal fascia fuse behind the descending colon into the lateroconal fascia, which continues around the flank to blend with the posterior peritoneal reflection.[14, 15, 17, 19]

Anterior Pararenal Compartment

The anterior pararenal compartment lies between the anterior renal fascia and posterior parietal peritoneum (Figs. 20–1 and 20–2). The lateral border is defined by the lateroconal fascia, and the compartment is potentially contiguous across the midline.[14, 15, 22]

The anterior pararenal compartment contains the pancreas; the descending, horizontal, and terminal portions of the duodenum; the ascending and de-

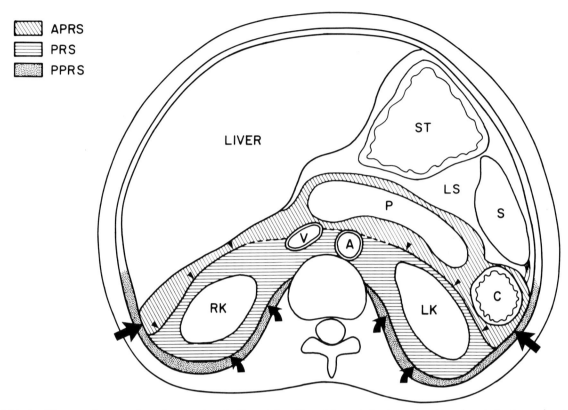

FIGURE 20–1 ■ Diagram of extraperitoneal compartments. The relationships of the anterior (*arrowheads*) and posterior (*curved arrows*) renal fascia to the anterior, perinephric, and posterior pararenal compartments are shown. Arrows = Lateroconal fascia; dashed lines = anterior renal fascia where debate exists over degree of fusion to great vessels; A = aorta; C = splenic flexure of colon; LS = lesser sac; P = pancreas; S = spleen; ST = stomach; V = inferior vena cava.

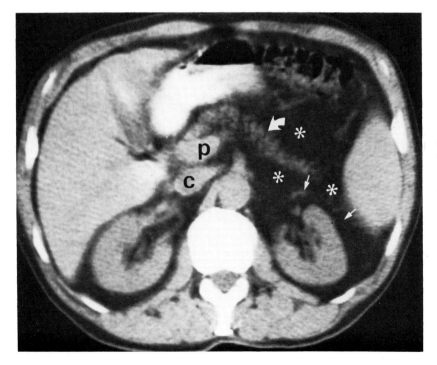

FIGURE 20–2 ■ CT scan through normal kidneys demonstrating that the pancreas (*curved arrow*) lies in the anterior pararenal compartment (*asterisk*). The posterior parietal peritoneum is not visible, but portions of the anterior renal fascia (*arrows*) are demonstrated. c = Inferior vena cava; p = portal vein.

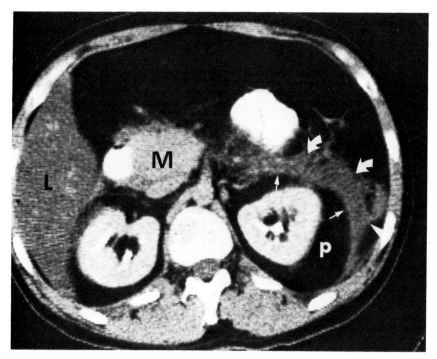

FIGURE 20–3 ■ Pancreatitis producing a mass (M) that simulates a pancreatic carcinoma. Pancreatitis also has caused a diffuse increase in density of fat in the anterior pararenal space (*curved arrows*). The anterior renal fascia (*arrows*) and lateroconal fascia (*arrowhead*) are also thickened. The perinephric space (p) is normal. The liver (L) contains excessive fat.

scending colon; and the splenic, hepatic, pancreatic, and duodenal vascular supply. Medially the second portion of the duodenum descends immediately in front of the right renal fascia, and inferiorly the extraperitoneal colon courses obliquely over the lower pole of the right kidney. The extraperitoneal left colon is adjacent to the anterior surface of the left renal fascia and medial to the lateroconal fascia formed by the fusion of the two layers of the renal fascia.

Abnormalities of any structures within the anterior pararenal compartment can produce thickening of the anterior renal and lateroconal fascia (Fig. 20–3).[14–17, 19, 23] The most common sources of abnormalities in the anterior pararenal space are lesions arising in the pancreas, colon, duodenum, or appendix. Only rarely are renal abnormalities the cause of anterior pararenal space lesions.

Perinephric Compartment

The perinephric compartment, also called *Gerota's space*, is limited by the cone of renal fascia formed by the fusion of the anterior renal fascia (Zuckerkandl's fascia) and the posterior renal fascia (Gerota's fascia) (Figs. 20–1, 20–3, and 20–4).[24] The renal fascia fuses superiorly with the diaphragmatic fascia and laterally with the lateroconal fascia; inferiorly the layers of

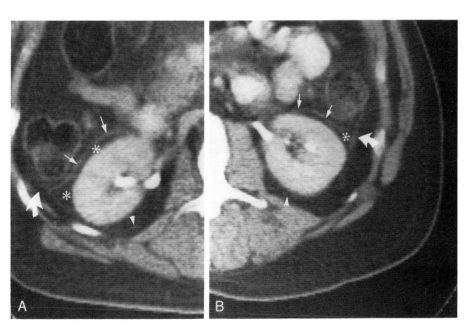

FIGURE 20–4 ■ Normal CT anatomy of the renal fascia and perinephric space. Scans through the right (A) and left (B) kidney demonstrate the anterior (*arrows*) and posterior (*arrowheads*) pararenal fasciae, which join to form the lateroconal fascia (*curved arrows*). The perinephric space (*asterisk*) contains fat and is limited by the renal fascia.

renal fascia fuse weakly with the iliac fascia and blend loosely with the periureteric connective tissue.[14–17, 19] The inferior apex of the compartment remains open toward the iliac fossa,[14, 15, 25] and the weakest point of the perinephric compartment through which urine or perinephric effusions escape most easily is at the inferomedial angle adjacent to the ureter.[14, 17, 26] The posterior renal fascia fuses medially with the psoas and the quadratus lumborum fascia.[3, 14, 17]

There is disagreement concerning the continuity of the perinephric space anteriorly. Meyers[14] claimed that the anterior renal fascia fused with the connective tissue around the great vessels in the root of the mesentery, prohibiting any "actual or potential direct communication" between the right and left perirenal compartments This conclusion was also reached by other investigators.[26] However, Gerota[27] reported that the anterior layer of the renal fascia continued across the midline to fuse with the fascia on the opposite side. Using CT, Somogyi and colleagues demonstrated a communication between the right and left perinephric compartments in a patient after blunt abdominal trauma.[25] More recently, Kneeland et al.,[22] using cadavers, showed unequivocally that the perinephric spaces may communicate across the midline, anterior to the vena cava.

The perinephric compartment contains the adrenal gland, the kidney, the renal vasculature, perinephric fat, and the proximal part of the renal collecting system. Abnormalities of these organs can extend into the perinephric compartment, thicken the renal fascia, and obliterate the perinephric fat (Fig. 20–5).[14]

Posterior Pararenal Compartment

The posterior pararenal compartment lies between the posterior renal fascia and the transversalis fascia (see Figs. 20–1 and 20–4). It contains only fatty tissue and continues laterally as the properitoneal fat strip. The space is open inferiorly at the iliac crest, but medially the transversalis fascia fuses with the psoas fascia and prevents communication between the right and left posterior pararenal compartments.

The posterior pararenal compartment contains no major organs; therefore diseases rarely arise there. Abnormalities of the posterior pararenal compartment are associated with diseases involving other retroperitoneal compartments or contiguous structures.[14, 20] Traumatic or spontaneous retroperitoneal hemorrhage, retroperitoneal lymphatic extravasation, posterior spread of pancreatitis, infection as a complication of rib or spinal osteomyelitis, or, rarely, a neoplasm can selectively involve the posterior pararenal compartment.[14, 19, 20] Also, pelvic lesions can spread upward to involve the posterior pararenal space because it is open inferiorly.

Intercompartmental Communcation

Although the three retroperitoneal compartments are anatomically well defined, there are pathways by which a process involving one space can spread to the others. Commonly a process originating caudally in the anterior pararenal space spreads around the inferior border of the cone of renal fascia and extends cephalad into the posterior pararenal compartment.[15, 19, 20] Pelvic disease can spread cephalad directly into

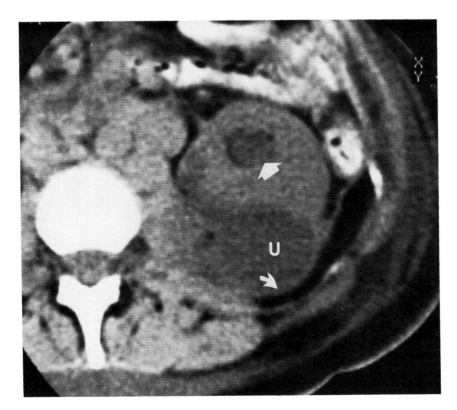

FIGURE 20–5 ■ Abnormal perinephric space. A urinoma (U) is present in the left perinephric space as a result of obstruction of the left ureter by a lymphomatous mass and spontaneous rupture of an obstructed calyx. A dilated hydronephrotic collecting structure is demonstrated (*arrow*). The posterior renal fascia (*curved arrow*) is thickened.

the three retroperitoneal compartments. Rectal and sigmoid diseases are particularly likely to spread into the retroperitoneal spaces. Abnormalities arising in any of the retroperitoneal compartments can spread directly through the lateroconal fascia or Gerota's fascia into the other retroperitoneal compartments, usually after pus, pancreatic enzymes, or tumors have eroded and destroyed the limiting fascial planes.[15]

Kidneys

CT directly displays axial cross-sectional renal anatomy and permits reconstruction of renal anatomy into coronal, sagittal, and oblique planes (Fig. 20–6). The kidneys are surrounded by abundant perinephric fat, which permits sharp delineation of the renal margins in almost every patient. The transverse contour of the kidneys is smooth, except where the vascular pedicle points anteromedially toward the aorta and the inferior vena cava.[1] The renal parenchyma in a given patient has a relatively uniform density of 30 to 50 Hounsfield units (H).[11] The cortex and medullary portions of the kidney cannot be distinguished by density differences on precontrast CT scans.[1] Segments of the urine-filled calices have the same CT attenuation value as water; fat in the perirenal space and renal hilum has a CT density less than that of water and can therefore be identified by density differences.

The size and volume of the kidneys can be measured by CT (Fig. 20–7). These measurements corre-

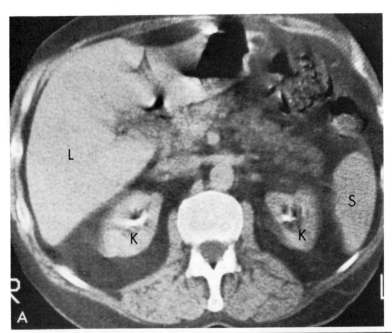

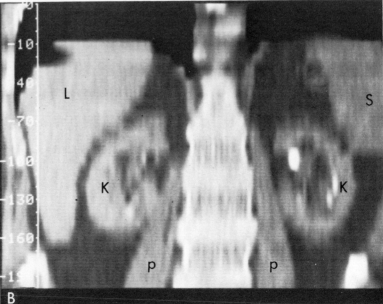

FIGURE 20–6 ■ Normal kidneys. Axial (A), coronal (B), and right sagittal.
Illustration continued on following page

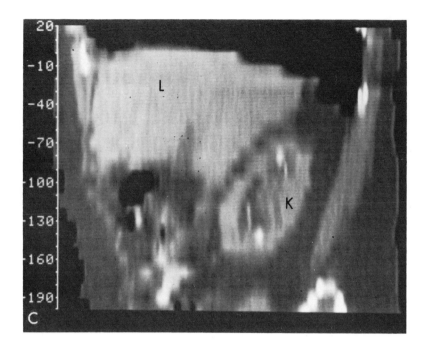

FIGURE 20–6 *Continued C*, CT scans demonstrate the relationships of the kidneys to adjacent organs. K = Kidney; L = liver; p = psoas muscle; S = spleen.

late closely with the direct measurements of resected specimens.[28] As patients age, there is a gradual decrease in thickness of the renal parenchyma.[29]

In most patients, the renal arteries and veins join the aorta or inferior vena cava (Fig. 20–8). The renal arteries arise posterior (dorsal) to the renal veins, and CT scans frequently demonstrate accessory renal arteries. The renal veins are usually larger than the corresponding artery, and the longer left renal vein crosses anterior to the aorta and enters the inferior vena cava at the level of the uncinate process of the pancreas (Figs. 20–8 and 20–9). The aorta and superior mesenteric artery may pinch the left renal vein, which causes the left renal vein to appear larger than the right.[30]

Identification of a retroaortic left renal vein, accessory retroaortic vein, or vena cava anomaly is important for the urologic surgeon. Accessory veins,

shown as rounded structures on CT, can simulate lymph nodes unless contrast-enhanced scans are carefully compared with precontrast CT images.[31]

The CT appearance of the renal parenchyma after the administration of contrast medium depends on the amount and concentration of the contrast injected, the rapidity of injection, and the timing of the scan. If a dynamic series of 10 to 15 CT scans is obtained after a bolus injection of contrast medium, the first CT images usually demonstrate the renal arteries or renal veins (Fig. 20–10). The contrast effect in the renal cortex increases rapidly and may reach a peak of 120 H at 30 to 50 seconds,[32, 33] permitting a clear differentiation of the renal cortex from the renal medulla (see Fig. 20–10). The thickness of the renal cortex measured by CT is 0.48 ± 0.02 cm and decreases with age.[29, 32]

Dynamic CT scans can display the change in atten-

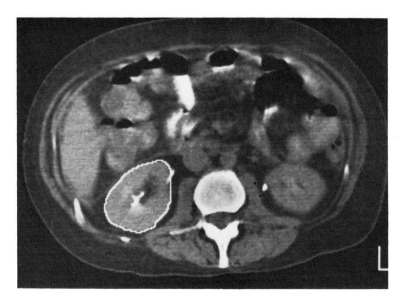

FIGURE 20–7 ■ Renal size and volume determination. The kidney margin has been traced, and the calculated area within the trace is 23.3 cm². The slice thickness is 1 cm, and thus a volume of 23.3 cm³ is contained within the outline of the kidney. Summation of individual slice volumes provides a measure of total renal volume.

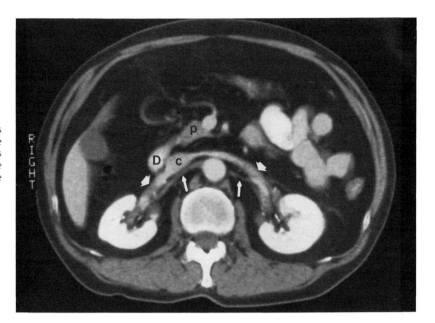

FIGURE 20–8 ■ Normal renal arterial and venous anatomy. The renal arteries (*small arrows*) arise from the aorta dorsal to the renal veins. In this patient, both the left and right renal veins (*large arrows*) are seen crossing over the aorta to join the inferior vena cava (C). D = Duodenum; p = uncinate process of the pancreas.

uation value versus time (time-density curves) in various portions of the kidney (Figs. 20–10 and 20–11). The attenuation value of the renal medulla increases more slowly but ultimately rises to a higher level than that of the renal cortex. The crossover of medullary and cortical values typically occurs about 65 seconds after a bolus injection of contrast medium. This component of the time-density curve, the corticomedullary junction, may reflect renal glomerular function.[32]

Following a bolus injection, prominent columns of Bertin are shown as structures having a density equal to that of the surrounding cortex (Fig. 20–12). The attenuation value of the medulla increases for 1 to 5 minutes; then the density of the renal parenchyma becomes uniform, and the calices and renal pelvis are sharply delineated. Following contrast administration, fetal lobulations are shown to have the same attenuation value as the rest of the functioning renal parenchyma.[1] After an intravenous infusion of contrast medium, renal parenchymal density increases uniformly, and the sharp delineation of the corticomedullary junction seen after a bolus injection is absent (Fig. 20–13).

Techniques of Examination

Ideally, every CT study should be monitored by a radiologist and modified to meet the clinical problem being addressed. Renal or ureteral CT is usually performed to clarify a suspected abnormality detected on an excretory urogram or an ultrasonogram.

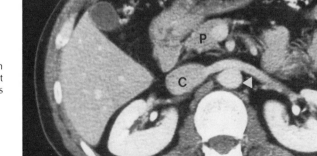

FIGURE 20–9 ■ The normal left renal vein (*arrowhead*) joins the inferior vena cava (C) at the level of the uncinate process of the pancreas (P).

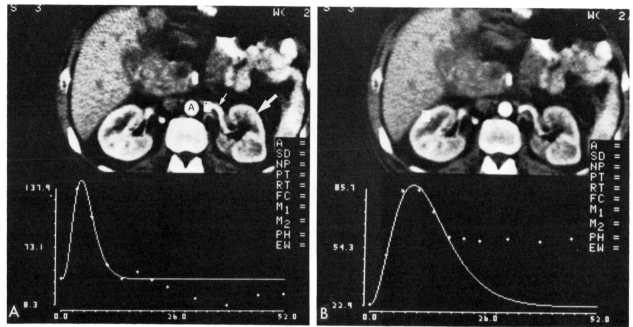

FIGURE 20–10 ■ Dynamic CT scan following a bolus injection of contrast material. *A*, The left renal artery (*small arrow*) is maximally opacified during peak aortic (*A*) contrast enhancement. The renal cortex (*large arrow*) is shown as a densely opacified peripheral zone. The time-density curve plots the increase in CT density with time and shows a rapid rise and fall in CT density of the left renal artery. *B*, Time-density plot of the right renal cortex. The curve demonstrates a rapid increase in the CT density of the renal cortex to 85.7 H and then a gradual decline. The rise in attenuation value of the cortex parallels that of the renal artery, but there is a slower rise to a lower peak and then a more gradual decline in CT density. The curve is not corrected for recirculation.

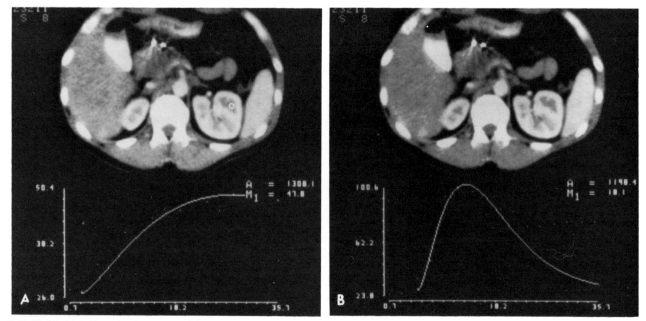

FIGURE 20–11 ■ Time-density curves of the renal cortex and medulla following a bolus injection of contrast material. *A*, The cursor ○ is in the renal medulla. There is a gradual increase in the CT density of the renal medulla to 50 H by 25 to 30 seconds and no evidence of a decline in attenuation value. *B*, The time-density plot of the renal cortex reveals a rapid increase to 100 H by 15 seconds, followed by a decline. The curve is not corrected for recirculation.

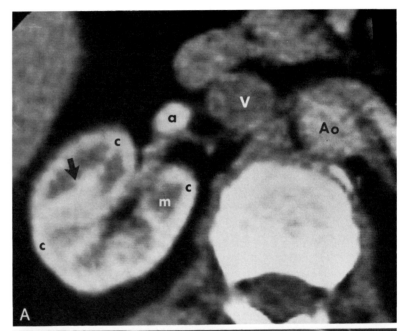

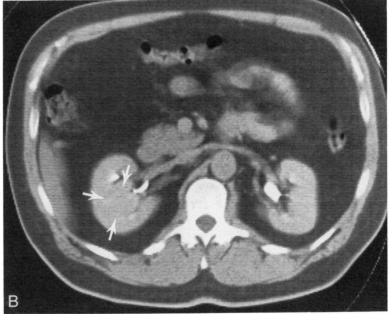

FIGURE 20–12 ■ Column of Bertin. *A,* This dynamic CT scan through the right kidney was obtained after a bolus injection of contrast material. There is sharp demarcation between the renal cortex (c) and renal medulla (m). The column of Bertin *(arrow)* has a density equal to that of the renal cortex and extends into the renal medulla. *B,* CT scan 5 minutes after administration of contrast reveals a prominent column of Bertin *(arrows)* that has the same CT attenuation value as the renal cortex. a = Renal artery; Ao = aorta; V = vena cava.

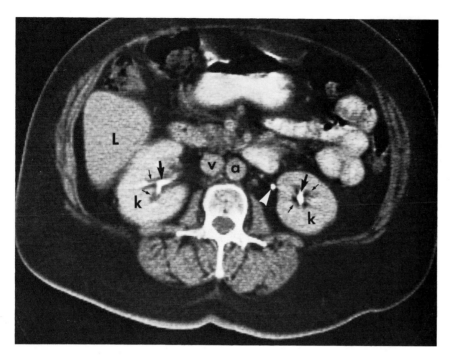

FIGURE 20–13 ■ Normal kidneys (k) following a drip infusion of contrast material. The renal parenchyma is homogeneous, without distinction of the renal cortex and medulla. The attenuation value of the kidneys is greater than that of the liver (L), aorta (a), or inferior vena cava (v). The renal pelvic collecting structures (*large arrows*) are surrounded by fat (*small arrows*). The left ureter (*arrowhead*) is shown as a dot of high density.

The usual anatomic location of the kidneys is from the T12 to L3 vertebrae, or roughly from the xiphoid to the umbilicus.[2] thus an initial CT scan should be performed at the level of the xiphoid process, with the technician adjusting the scan level according to the location of the kidneys on the scan. A trained and experienced technician can precisely position the patient for a renal CT by viewing the initial baseline CT scan or scout radiograph.

The entire kidney is routinely scanned using contiguous CT sections 1 cm thick during suspended respiration with the patient supine. Scans are continued down through the pelvis if a distal ureteral abnormality is suspected. Technical factors should be appropriate to the patient's size. Scan times are selected to ensure that high-resolution CT images are obtained, permitting the maximal amount of information to be extracted from the CT study. Oral contrast medium—480 mL of 1 per cent meglumine diatrizoate (Gastrografin) or barium sulfate given 30 minutes before the CT scan and another 240 mL 5 minutes before the examination—is administered to ensure that the gastrointestinal tract is adequately opacified. Adequate opacification is particularly important when the ureter is examined for expected abnormality, as unopacified bowel may simulate a solid periureteral mass lesion. Occasionally, prone or decubitus positioning is useful in evaluating juxtarenal pathologic abnormalities or obstructive uropathy.[3] Scanning in the prone position is often helpful in planning the best route for percutaneous access to the kidney for endourologic procedures such as lithotripsy or endopyelotomy.

CT scans less than 1.0 cm thick or overlapping scans can be used to better delineate small abnormalities. Reformatting axial CT images into coronal, sagittal, or various oblique planes provides additional information for evaluating the extent of renal abnormalities and may help to determine the organ from which a right upper abdominal mass lesion originates. However, closely applied organs with a common or contact surface that is oblique to the axial plane of the CT scan can be extremely difficult to separate, as the partial volume effect can make one organ "arise" out of the other. Although reformatting axial CT scans may help to avoid this "pitfall," magnetic resonance imaging (MRI) done in the coronal or sagittal plane is often a better way to solve this particular problem.

Scanning of the kidneys before and after administration of intravenous contrast medium[1–3] ensures the greatest diagnostic yield, but the patient receives twice the radiation exposure, the examination is longer, and frequently the precontrast scans provide no unique information.

Engelstad and co-workers[34] studied 176 patients to determine the role of precontrast CT scans of the kidney. All 152 mass lesions were detected, accurately classified as a simple cyst or a solid renal mass, and characterized as to size and extent from the contrast-enhanced CT scans alone. In no patient with a renal mass lesion, hydronephrosis, or polycystic disease was the diagnosis hindered by administration of contrast medium. Precontrast CT images added diagnostic information in only nine per cent of 176 patients (i.e., when contrast medium obscured calcification in the renal parenchyma or collecting system or in cases of renal or perinephric hemorrhage).

Unless CT is performed to detect renal calcification, extravasation of contrast medium, or perinephric hemorrhage, contrast-enhanced CT scans of the kidneys are obtained as the initial scan procedure. Intravenous contrast medium has been given as a drip infusion, a bolus injection, or as a combination of the two methods.[1-3, 34-36] Most commonly, either a 100 to 120 mL bolus of standard diatrizoic acid salts (Renografin-60 or Conray-60) or nonionic agents are administered as a bolus injection at a rate of 1.5 to 2 mL per second by a mechanical injector. Contrast is usually administered through an antecubital vein, and dynamic CT scanning is begun when half of the contrast medium has been administered.

Dynamic CT scanning permits sequential CT images of the kidneys and renal vasculature to be obtained rapidly.[32, 33, 35-37] After intravenous bolus injection, a series of dynamic CT scans can differentiate the renal cortex from the renal medulla (Figs. 20–10, 20–11, and 20–14).[2, 32, 33, 35-38] Dynamic renal CT scans can demonstrate renal vascular anatomy, the vascularity of mass lesions, the relationship of the great vessels to the ureters, and time-density curves of the renal cortex and medulla (see Figs. 20–8 through 20–11).[2, 32, 33, 35-38]

The best dynamic CT images are obtained when a bolus of contrast is given after a nonenhanced baseline CT study. If contrast medium has been administered, satisfactory results can be obtained by waiting 10 to 15 minutes and then injecting the contrast bolus. Repeated 40- to 50-mL bolus injections can be given to evaluate different anatomic regions of the kidney. It is important to allow enough time for the contrast medium to be excreted. A persistent nephrogram on subsequent CT scans may indicate a contrast-induced nephropathy has developed.[39]

Pathology

Renal Masses

CT has proved valuable for detecting, localizing, and characterizing renal mass lesions. CT has been used to determine the extent and stage of a renal tumor, to plan and evaluate the response to therapy, and to detect tumor recurrence after therapy.

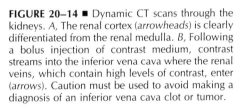

FIGURE 20–14 ■ Dynamic CT scans through the kidneys. *A,* The renal cortex (*arrowheads*) is clearly differentiated from the renal medulla. *B,* Following a bolus injection of contrast medium, contrast streams into the inferior vena cava where the renal veins, which contain high levels of contrast, enter (*arrows*). Caution must be used to avoid making a diagnosis of an inferior vena cava clot or tumor.

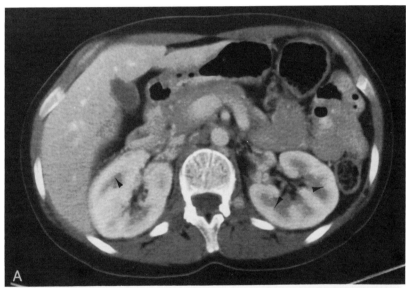

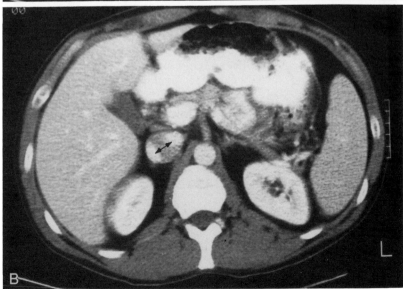

Renal masses are easily detected by CT for the following reasons:

1. They have an attenuation value different from that of normal renal parenchyma.
2. They alter the normal contour of the kidney.
3. They are enhanced to a different degree after intravenous contrast administration.
4. They distort the renal collecting structures.
5. They cause hydronephrosis.
6. They produce filling defects in the renal pelvis or caliceal system.

CYSTIC RENAL MASSES

Benign Renal Cysts ■ Simple cysts are extremely common lesions of the kidney. They are present in more than 50 per cent of patients older than 50 years[2, 40] and vary greatly in number, size, and location. The cause of renal cysts is unknown, although tubular obstruction or vascular compromise has been suggested.[41]

The simple renal cyst originates in the renal parenchyma and usually produces an abnormal renal outline that is readily detected by CT. A typical benign renal cyst has the following characteristics:

1. It is a round or slightly oval mass with a smooth outer margin.
2. The cyst wall has no measurable thickness.
3. The attenuation value is uniform and close to that of water and does not increase after intravenous contrast administration.
4. The interface with normal renal parenchyma is distinct and sharp.
5. It may abut but does not obliterate renal sinus fat.
6. It is confined wholly within the renal fascia and does not invade renal veins (Table 20–1 and Figs. 20–15 and 20–16).

When a renal mass meets all the criteria of a renal cyst, the accuracy of the CT diagnosis approaches 100 per cent.[1, 3, 42] Applying strict criteria, McClennan and associates[42] found no erroneous CT interpretations in 56 proved benign renal cysts; Sagel and associates[1] found none in 104 cysts, and Hattery's group[3] found none in 60 cysts in 20 patients. There is no convincing evidence that a renal lesion meeting all the CT criteria of a renal cyst has developed into a solid renal mass.[2] Because renal cysts are so common and the CT diagnosis so secure, further examination or follow-up to confirm the CT diagnosis of a simple renal cyst is not indicated.

Although CT can accurately detect and characterize a renal mass as a benign cyst, there are potential pitfalls to avoid. Depending on the size and location of a renal cyst, its measured attenuation value may be greater than that of water (Fig. 20–17). Unless a cyst occupies the entire thickness of the CT slice, partial volume averaging with the normal adjacent renal parenchyma will raise the displayed attenuation value of the renal cyst (Fig. 20–18). Cysts smaller in diameter than the CT slice thickness always undergo partial volume averaging, and multiloculated and parapelvic cysts may have elevated attenuation values resulting from adjacent cysts, septa, or hilar structures. The magnitude of partial volume averaging can be reduced or eliminated by using CT scan sections thinner than the renal cyst. In addition to increasing the measured CT attenuation of a simple renal cyst, partial volume averaging may make a simple cyst located at either renal pole appear to have a "thick wall" on axial CT scanning. This effect is created by axial sections through the peripherally encircling renal parenchyma toward the base of the cyst.[43]

High-density renal cysts are produced by a variety of conditions:

1. Hemorrhage into the cyst (Fig. 20–19).
2. Contrast medium leaking into the cyst by a communication with the collecting system[44, 45] or by diffusion[46] (Fig. 20–20).
3. Calcification of the cyst wall (Fig. 20–21).
4. Infection (Fig. 20–22).
5. High protein content of cyst fluid.[47, 48]

Infection can also produce thickening of the rim of a cyst and can cause the rim to dramatically enhance after contrast administration (see Fig. 20–22).

A CT diagnosis of a benign renal cyst should never be based solely on the attenuation value of the renal mass but only after all of the CT characteristics of the lesion have been appraised. If the attenuation value of a renal mass exceeds 15 H or if the mass has other atypical features, then it is considered to be indeterminate (Fig. 20–23), and additional studies are recommended to determine its true nature.

High-density cysts can be found anywhere in the kidney, from a peripheral, exophytic location, to the parapelvic area, where they may be multiple (see

Text continued on page 952

TABLE 20–1 ■ CT Differentiation of Renal Masses

CT FEATURE	CYST	NEOPLASM
Shape	Round, slightly oval	Irregular, lobulated
Margin	Smooth	Lobulated
Wall	Thin, no measurable thickness	Thick, can measure thickness
Interface with parenchyma	Sharp, distinct	Indistinct, irregular
Density	Homogeneous	Inhomogeneous
	Close to water (0–15 H)	Close to renal parenchyma (+30 H)
Contrast enhancement	No	Yes
Vascular invasion	No	Yes

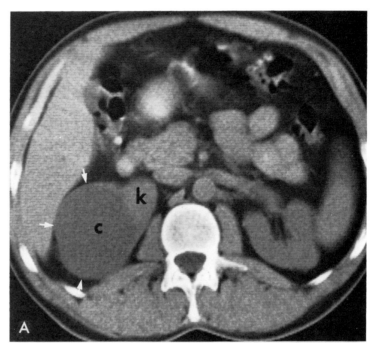

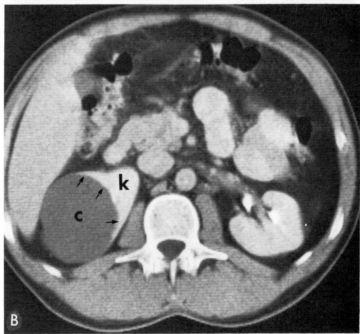

FIGURE 20–15 ■ Benign renal cyst. *A,* Precontrast CT scan demonstrates the cyst (c) to be round and to have a smooth outer margin (*arrows*). The density of the cyst is uniform and measures 2 H. *B,* Scan after contrast injection reveals the cyst (c) to have a sharp interface (*arrows*) with normal renal parenchyma, no increase in attenuation value, and a cyst wall that has no measurable thickness. k = Normal kidney.

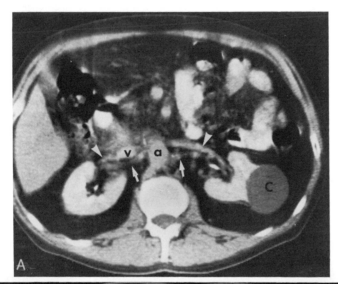

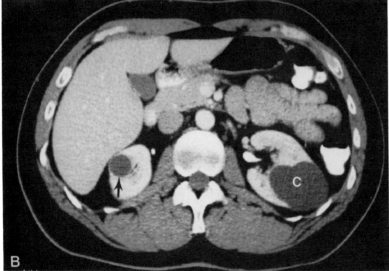

FIGURE 20–16 ■ Typical renal cysts following contrast injection. *A*, Peripheral cyst (C) of water density in the left kidney with a sharp cyst-parenchyma junction. Arrows = renal arteries; arrowheads = renal veins. a = aorta; v = vena cava. *B*, Large left renal cyst (C) extending close to the renal hilus and a small, round right renal cyst (*arrow*). Both cysts have the same CT density as the gallbladder (C).

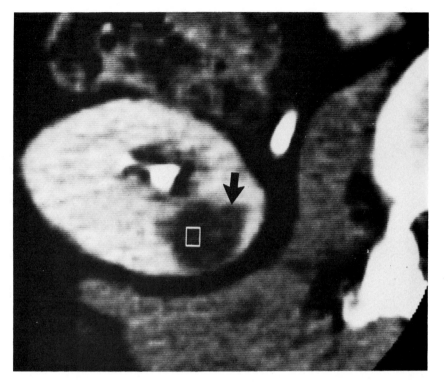

FIGURE 20–17 ■ Intrarenal cyst (*box*) which has slightly irregular margins (*arrow*) and a measured density of 24 H. Aspiration proved the lesion to be a simple cyst. Partial volume averaging was responsible for the spuriously high attenuation value.

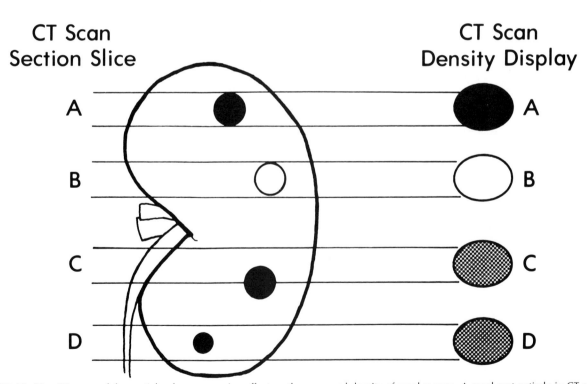

FIGURE 20–18 ■ Diagram of the partial volume averaging effect on the measured density of renal masses. A renal cyst entirely in CT section appears as low-density lesion (A). A solid renal mass entirely in the section of the scan appears as a mass of soft tissue density (B). A large renal cyst partially in the scan section and a renal cyst smaller than the slice thickness both have intermediate CT densities (C and D, respectively).

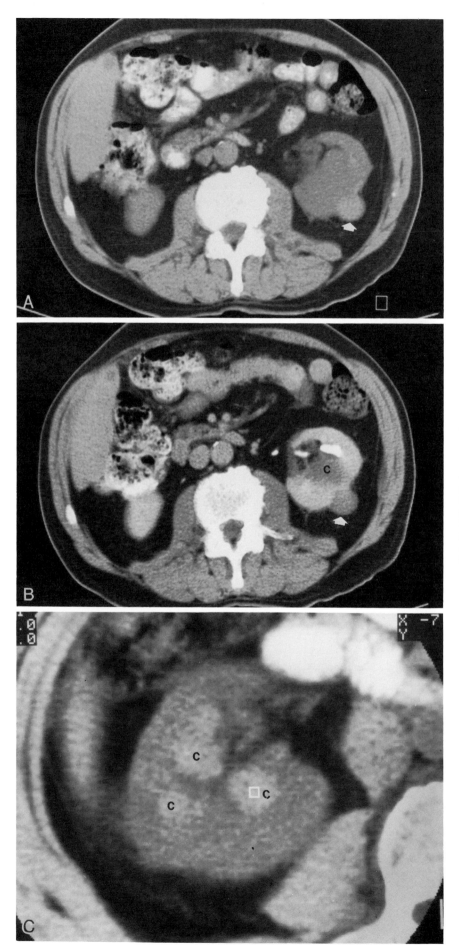

FIGURE 20–19 ■ High-density renal cyst caused by hemorrhage. *A,* Precontrast CT scan. A high-density round mass (*arrow*) is present in the peripheral portion of the left kidney and has a CT attenuation value of 42 H. *B,* Postcontrast CT scan. The renal parenchyma has increased in density so that the mass (*arrow*) now appears as a low-density lesion having the same characteristics as a simple renal cyst. A central renal cyst (C) is also present and has a CT density of 16 H. Aspiration revealed fresh hemorrhage.

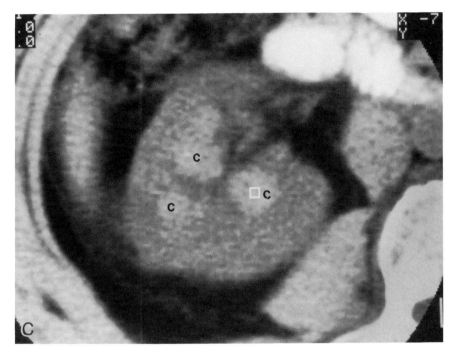

FIGURE 20–19 *Continued C,* Multiple high-density parapelvic cysts have a CT attenuation value of 63 H. This patient developed hematuria while on anticoagulation therapy.

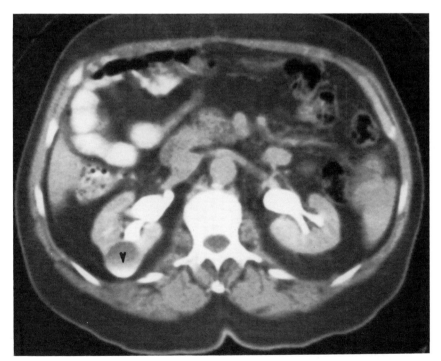

FIGURE 20–20 ■ High-density renal cyst with contrast layering in the dependent portion of the cyst (*arrowhead*). The cyst communicates with the renal collecting system.

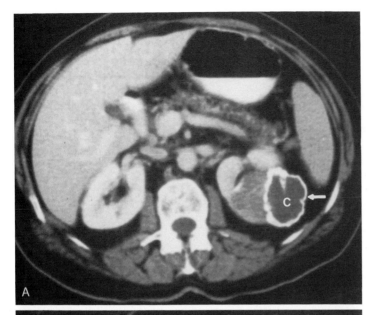

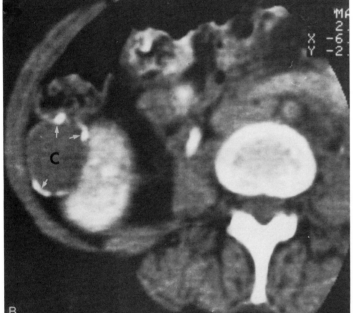

FIGURE 20–21 ■ Renal cysts with peripheral calcification. *A,* Posteriorly directed left renal cyst (C), which has a density of 6 H and a cyst wall that is totally calcified (*arrow*). *B,* Laterally positioned right renal cyst (C) with partial cyst wall calcification (*arrows*) and a CT density of 34 H. Diagnosis was simple cyst with recent hemorrhage. *C,* A large water-density right renal cyst with a calcified medial wall. Rim calcification is more common in cysts than in carcinoma but occurs in both.

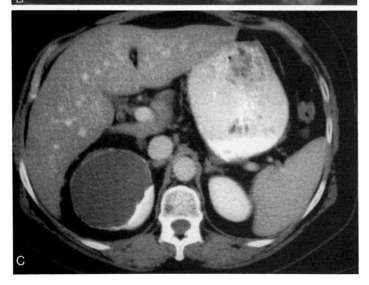

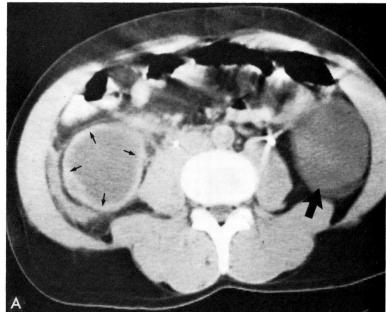

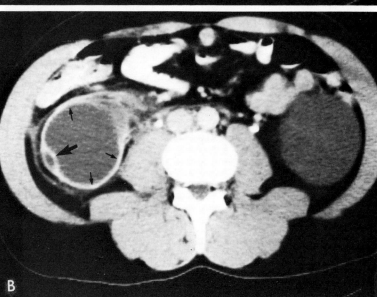

FIGURE 20–22 ■ Infected right renal cyst. *A,* CT scan after contrast infusion. A large left renal cyst (*large arrow*) is seen without a measurable cyst wall. A thick cyst wall (*small arrows*) is noted around a right renal cyst. The density of the right cyst is slightly higher than that of the left renal cyst. *B,* Dynamic CT study after a bolus injection of contrast material demonstrates marked contrast enhancement of the wall (*small arrows*) of the right renal cyst. The cyst also contains a septation (*large arrow*). The wall of the left renal cyst did not enhance.

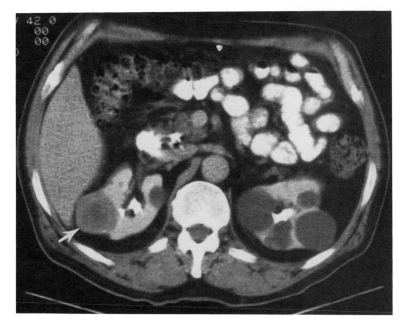

FIGURE 20–23 ■ CT scan in a patient with multiple simple renal cysts and an indeterminate right renal cyst. Multiple left renal cysts all have a CT density of less than 10 H and no discernable rim. A cystic right renal mass (*arrows*) measured 30 H and had a thick rim. Surgery revealed a cystic right renal cell carcinoma.

Fig. 20–19). The high density is best appreciated on unenhanced scans, where the cyst density may range from 60 to 80 H or higher.[49, 50] Following intravenous contrast, these high-density cysts have the relative density of a "solid" mass. The size, location, uniformity, and other CT findings characteristic of cysts may provide clues leading to an unenhanced CT scan or ultrasound recommendation. The most frequent component of a high-density cyst is hemorrhage or proteinaceous material.[47–52]

Parapelvic Cysts ■ Parapelvic cysts have all the features of simple benign renal parenchymal cysts but are located adjacent to the renal sinus. Parapelvic cysts have an attenuation value close to that of water but may be difficult to distinguish from a dilated or an extrarenal pelvis on nonenhanced CT scans. After contrast medium is administered, the unenhanced parapelvic cyst is readily detected adjacent to the contrast-filled hilar collecting structures (Fig. 20–24A). The average size of parapelvic cysts is 4 × 3 cm; the largest reported was 6 × 4 cm. CT can easily distinguish between a parapelvic cyst and pelvic fibrolipomatosis (Fig. 20–24B).[54] The attenuation value of fibrolipomatous tissue ranges from −5 to −100 H and is always less than that of a parapelvic cyst.

Polycystic Disease ■ Polycystic disease is commonly classified into infantile and adult types. In the infantile form, the kidneys are bilaterally large but retain a reniform shape. Cystic lesions in the liver, spleen, and pancreas are common. The kidneys are riddled with small cysts a few millimeters in size that usually do not produce caliceal or pelvic distortion.[41, 55] Renal function is poor, and most infants die shortly after birth. Other children survive into young adult life with signs of renal insufficiency, chronic pyelonephritis, portal hypertension, progressive portal fibrosis, and gastroesophageal varices.

Adult polycystic kidney disease is an inherited disorder genetically transmitted as an autosomal dominant trait that is characterized by multiple cysts of varying sizes in both the cortex and medulla.[51, 52, 55, 56] Both kidneys are involved but usually not symmetrically. The intervening renal tissue appears grossly normal but contains numerous very small renal cysts. Cysts are often present in the liver and less frequently in the spleen, lung, and pancreas.[56] Progressive renal failure and hypertension usually become evident in the fourth decade, but the adult form of polycystic renal disease may also be seen in children and young adults.[41]

The CT appearance of adult polycystic disease consists of bilateral renal enlargement, splaying and distortion of the collecting system, and multiple renal cysts (Fig. 20–25).[1, 51, 52, 56] The renal contour is lobulated and a multitude of small and large cysts that appear benign give the kidneys a honeycomb or "Swiss cheese" appearance. In one third of patients, CT also demonstrates hepatic or pancreatic cystic disease (see Fig. 20–25B, C). The CT diagnosis of polycystic kidney is usually straightforward; confu-

sion occurs only in distinguishing patients with multiple simple cysts (Fig. 20–26) from those with polycystic disease. Patients with multiple simple renal cysts usually have fewer renal cysts, show no family history of polycystic renal or liver disease, and are not predisposed to hypertension and renal failure.

CT is particularly valuable in examining patients with polycystic kidney disease who have hematuria and are suspected of having a renal malignancy. CT can readily distinguish a mass with a high attenuation value from multiple renal cysts, which have an attenuation value close to that of water. However, the presence of a mass with high attenuation value does not necessarily imply the presence of a tumor. Hemorrhage or infection can increase the attenuation value of a cyst and thereby simulate a solid mass lesion (Figs. 20–19, 20–21B, and 20–25B).

Multicystic Kidney ■ Multicystic kidney is a dysplastic condition characterized by severe structural disorganization, incomplete corticomedullary differentiation, primitive ducts, and multiple cysts of various sizes.[41] Multicystic kidney is a frequent cause of a palpable abdominal mass in an otherwise healthy infant or child.[41, 57, 58] The entire kidney is usually involved, but the disease may be segmental.[59] A plain abdominal film may show a flank mass, but excretory urography will fail to reveal any renal function.[57, 58] CT shows that the entire kidney consists of numerous cystic masses that vary in size and have attenuation values similar to that of water. No functioning renal parenchyma is detectable after contrast administration, and the collecting structures cannot be distinguished from the mass. Multilocular cystic nephromas and unilateral polycystic disease may produce similar clinical findings but can be excluded if CT demonstrates the absence of functioning renal parenchyma.[57, 58]

Multilocular Renal Cysts (Multilocular Cystic Nephroma) ■ A multilocular renal cyst is a "densely encapsulated solitary intrarenal mass composed of a myriad of noncommunicating cysts of varying size."[60] The multiple cysts have thick walls and septa that do not contain normal renal tissue. The external surface of the mass is smooth, but the lack of normal renal tissue in the septa clearly distinguishes the multilocular cyst from contiguous benign renal cysts and most other congenital cystic diseases. Of the reported cases of multilocular renal cysts, about half are in children and half in adults.[60]

The origin and pathogenesis of multilocular renal cysts are unclear.[60–63] In children, these cysts appear to be congenital; they manifested as an abdominal mass in children younger than 5 years (mean age, 17 months).[61, 64] In adults, multilocular renal cysts are usually discovered as an incidental finding during excretory urography in women 40 to 70 years old.[60, 62] The lack of reported cases in the intervening years suggests an acquired origin in adult cases.

Because of the spectrum of histologic features and theories of cause and pathogenesis, multilocular renal cysts have been called by many names, includ-

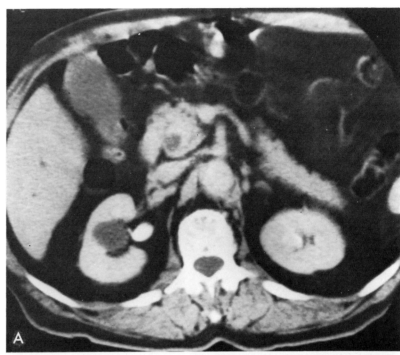

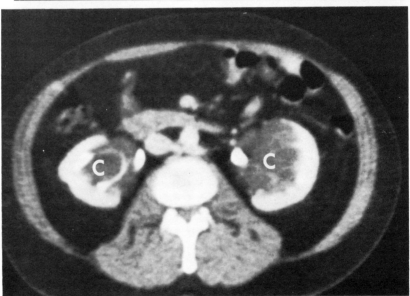

FIGURE 20–24 ■ Parapelvic cysts. *A,* A single cystic structure of water density adjacent to the renal sinus is seen. *B,* CT scan reveals bilateral parapelvic cysts (C) without evidence of polycystic disease or renal pelvic fibrolipomatosis.

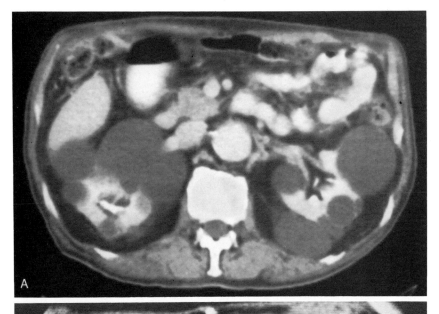

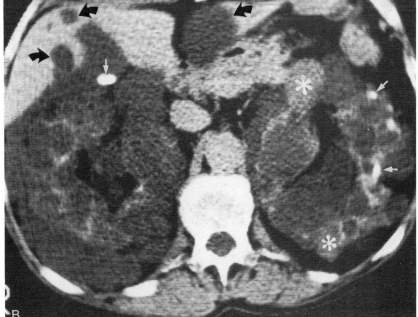

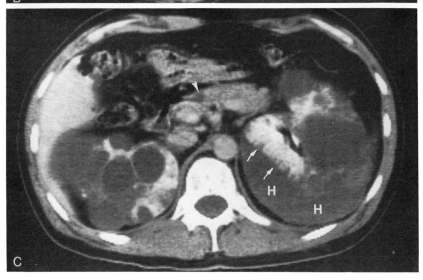

FIGURE 20–25 ■ Various CT appearances of polycystic kidney disease. *A,* Numerous bilateral renal cysts of varying sizes are identified in kidneys that are otherwise normal in size and exhibit normal renal function. *B,* Bilateral renal enlargement caused by multiple renal cysts. There are foci of calcification (*arrows*) and marked renal contour distortion. Several cysts (*asterisk*) have a high CT density as a result of hemorrhage. Multiple hepatic cysts (*curved arrows*) are also present. *C,* Bilaterally enlarged kidneys containing multiple cysts. An old left subcapsular hematoma (H) is seen to enlarge the left renal contour. The hematoma has a low CT density, indicating that it is not of recent origin. It flattens the medial portion of the left kidney (*arrows*) and a small pancreatic cyst (*arrowhead*).

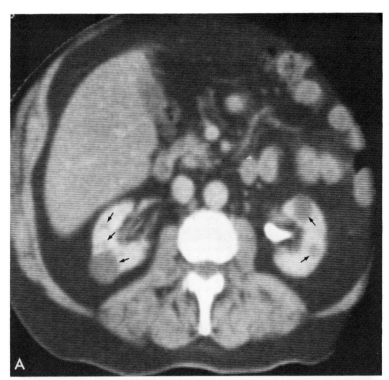

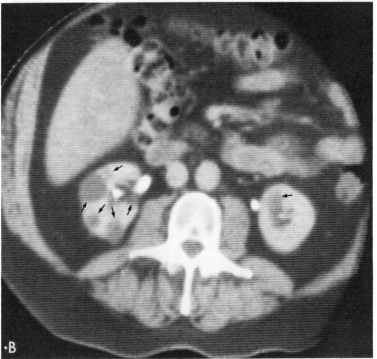

FIGURE 20–26 ■ Multiple renal cysts. *A,* Scan through the level of the midportion of both kidneys demonstrates multiple renal cysts (*arrows*) of varying size in each kidney. *B,* Scan at a lower level more clearly delineates multiple right renal cysts (*arrows*). The kidneys are not enlarged and function normally. No liver or pancreatic cysts are present.

ing cystic adenoma, cystic lymphangioma, cystic hamartoma, cystadenoma, multilocular cystadenoma, cystic Wilms' tumor, polycystic nephroblastoma, cystic differentiated nephroblastoma, segmental polycystic kidney, segmental multicystic kidney, Perlmann's tumor, multilocular cystic nephroma, and adenomatous polycystic kidney tumor.[60-62] The great variety of names has produced confusion as to the true incidence of these cysts. The term *multilocular cystic nephroma* appears to have become the preferred term to describe these multilocular renal cysts.[63, 64]

The CT appearance is that of single and multiple fluid-filled cysts separated by thick septa and sharply demarcated from the normal renal parenchyma (Fig. 20–27). Peripheral or central calcification is present in 10 to 50 per cent of cases and may have a circular, stellate, flocculent, or granular pattern.[60, 64] The attenuation values of multilocular cysts range from 2 to 40 H after contrast administration.[61] The sonographic appearance of multilocular renal cysts is that of multiple cystic masses separated by highly echogenic septa. Thus the CT or ultrasonic features alone may be confusing, but the combined CT and ultrasonic features often are sufficiently characteristic and suggest a preoperative diagnosis of multilocular cystic nephroma and permit a partial rather than a total nephrectomy to be performed.

SOLID RENAL TUMORS

Solid renal masses can be benign, malignant, neoplastic, infectious, congenital, or traumatic in origin. The most common solid renal masses are malignant tumors arising from the renal parenchyma or from the epithelium of the renal pelvis.

Various benign and malignant tumors originate in the kidney. Primary renal tumors may arise from the renal capsule, mature and immature renal parenchyma, renal mesenchymal derivatives, and the renal pelvis; various malignant lesions can secondarily involve the kidney. Malignant tumors of the kidney account for approximately two per cent of all neoplasms. Adenocarcinoma constitutes about 83 per cent of all renal malignancies; carcinoma of the renal pelvis, eight per cent; nephroblastoma, six per cent; and other varieties, approximately three per cent.[65]

Renal Cell Carcinoma (Adenocarcinoma) ■ Adenocarcinoma is the most common malignant renal tumor. It is three times more frequent in males than in females and is rare in children and young adults.[65] Gross hematuria occurs in approximately 60 per cent of patients, and about 50 per cent of patients have flank pain. However, less than 15 per cent of patients have the classic triad of renal carcinoma: gross hematuria, back pain, and flank mass.[65] Renal carcinoma occasionally produces hypertension and hyperparathyroidism. Spontaneous hemorrhage from a kidney without evidence of a vasculopathy or bleeding disorder is highly suggestive of an underlying renal cell carcinoma, which may be small and difficult to detect (Fig. 20–28).[66] A much more unusual origin is spontaneous renal hemorrhage resulting from cyst rupture.[67]

Renal vein thrombosis without apparent cause in an otherwise apparently healthy individual can be a premonitory sign of an occult tumor.[68] Familial occurrences are uncommon except in patients with von Hippel–Lindau disease, 12 to 83 per cent of whom develop adenocarcinoma.[69, 70]

The characteristic CT appearance of a renal adenocarcinoma is a solid renal lesion that produces a mass or an abnormality of the renal contour (Fig. 20–29).[1-4, 7, 35, 36, 71-74] The tumor is frequently irregularly shaped and has a lobulated or ill-defined outer margin. In contrast to renal cysts, the demarcation between the tumor mass and normal renal parenchyma is usually ill defined; the attenuation value of the tumor on precontrast CT scans is close to that of normal renal parenchyma, and although the density of the tumor may be homogeneous, necrosis commonly causes part of the tumor to have a inhomogeneous CT density (Figs. 20–23, 20–29, and 20–30). Recent intratumoral hemorrhage may cause areas of the tumor to have higher attenuation values than those of adjacent normal renal parenchyma (see Fig. 20–28B). Central renal sinus fat is often partially obliterated (Fig. 20–31).

Administration of intravenous contrast medium accentuates the difference in CT density between normal parenchyma and tumor (see Figs. 20–28 through 20–31). The density of the normal renal parenchyma increases 80 to 120 H, whereas density of the tumor, which lacks functioning tubular elements, increases less and only in proportion to the pooling of contrast medium in the tumor's vascular and extravascular compartments. Dynamic CT studies after a bolus injection of contrast medium may detect an early peak that corresponds to the early hypervascular phase on renal angiograms (Figs. 20–29 and 20–32).[35, 36] Scans performed minutes after contrast administration do not demonstrate the early hypervascular phase of renal cell carcinomas but clearly demonstrate the interface between tumor and normal renal parenchyma.

If the CT attenuation values of a renal lesion are between that of a simple renal cyst and that of a solid mass lesion, the mass should be considered indeterminate, as it may represent a tumor (Figs. 20–23, 20–33, and 20–34) or benign renal cysts (see Figs. 20–21 and 20–22). Benign cysts may be septated and have higher attenuation values because of hemorrhage, inflammation, contrast administration, proteinaceous content, or calcification (see Fig. 20–21).[75, 76]

Solid renal masses may have lower CT densities or contain cystic components as a result of necrosis, infection, or a high fat content in the lesion. In a series of 78 renal cell carcinomas, 17 (22 per cent) had some features suggesting a simple renal cyst, but none fulfilled all of the CT criteria of a simple renal cyst.[72] Calcification in malignant solid renal tumors is most often central and associated with a soft tissue mass, but the calcification may be peripheral.[65, 77] The presence of central calcification or rim calcification is reason to classify the renal mass as indeterminate.

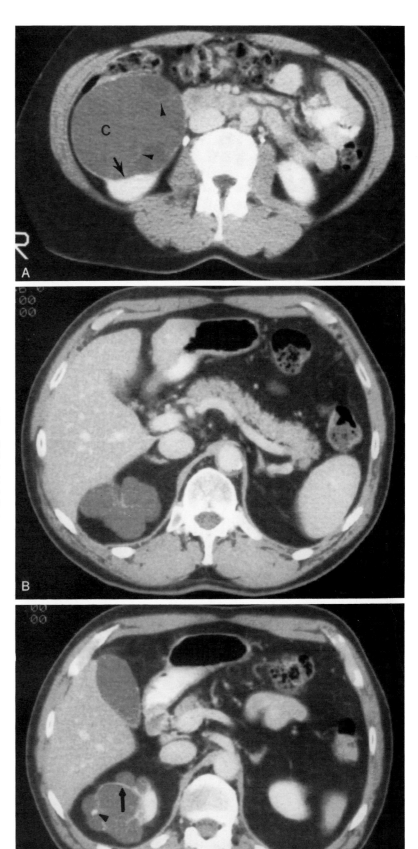

FIGURE 20–27 ■ Multilocular cystic nephroma. *A,* CT scan demonstrates a large cystic mass (C) that displaces (*arrow*) but does not invade the adjacent, normally functioning renal parenchyma. There are multiple septations (*arrowheads*) within the cystic mass. *B,* CT scan reveals multiple water-density cystic masses arising in the upper pole of the right kidney. *C,* CT scan at a lower level demonstrates foci of calcification (*arrowhead*), thick septations (*arrow*) between multiple cysts, and sharp demarcation of the cystic mass from normal renal tissue.

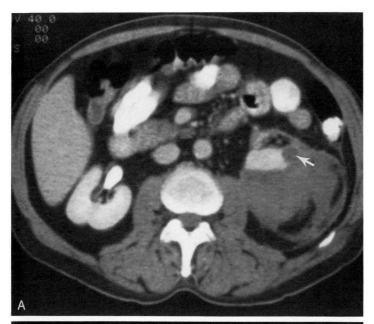

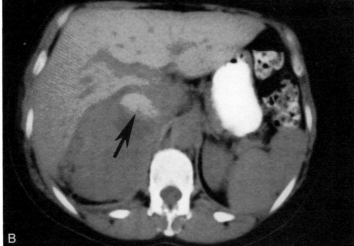

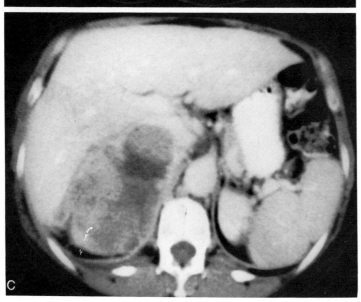

FIGURE 20–28 ■ Renal cell carcinoma presenting with spontaneous hemorrhage. *A,* A small renal cell carcinoma (*arrow*) has hemorrhaged into the left perinephric space and displaced the kidney anteriorly. *B,* A precontrast CT scan demonstrates a large mass with a focal area of high CT density (*arrow*) caused by recent hemorrhage. *C,* Following intravenous contrast injection, the full extent of the renal call carcinoma is better demonstrated, but the region of hemorrhage cannot be distinguished from solid tumor.

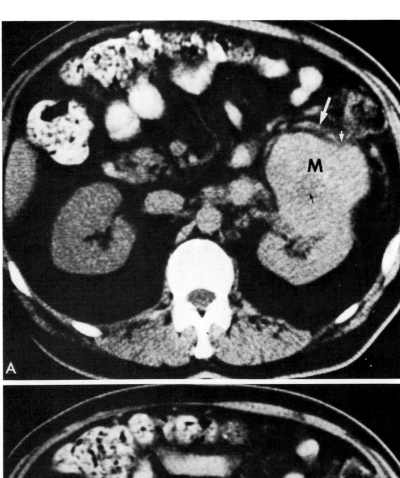

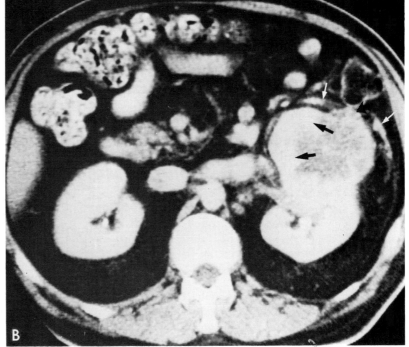

FIGURE 20–29 ■ Renal cell carcinoma. *A,* Non–contrast-enhanced CT scan demonstrates a large solid mass (M) arising from the ventral surface of the left kidney. The outer contour is lobulated, and demarcation from normal renal parenchyma is poor. The center of the tumor (*black arrow*) has a slightly decreased attenuation compared with the periphery of the tumor. The tumor has extended into the perinephric space (*small arrow*) and has thickened the anterior renal fascia (*large arrow*). *B,* CT scan after bolus injection of contrast material. The renal cell carcinoma shows areas of marked contrast enhancement (*black arrows*) and areas of lesser enhancement. The anterior renal fascia (*white arrows*) is thickened and enhances after contrast injection. Perinephric extension (*curved arrow*) is more clearly demonstrated.

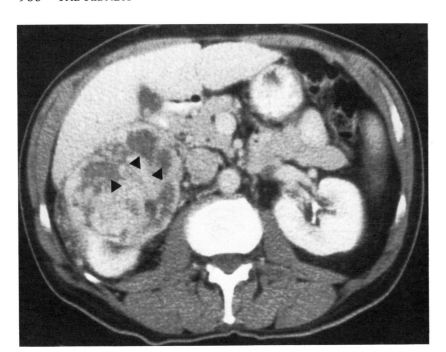

FIGURE 20–30 ■ Renal cell carcinoma. A CT scan after a bolus injection of contrast demonstrates a large, lobulated right renal mass containing regions of high attenuation (*arrowheads*) and areas of low CT density. Angiography revealed a hypervascular renal cell carcinoma. Surgery demonstrated areas of tumor necrosis corresponding to the regions of low CT attenuation value.

When an indeterminate renal mass is diagnosed, additional studies such as ultrasonography, angiography, MRI, or aspiration biopsy are indicated to further clarify the nature of the renal mass.[78, 79] In our experience, the majority of indeterminate masses are benign, but atypical malignancies are also encountered.

Pathologically, renal carcinoma can be divided into four stages (Table 20–2)[2, 80–82]:

1. Stage I tumors are wholly confined within the renal capsule (see Figs. 20–32 and 20–34*A*).
2. Stage II tumors extend through the renal capsule and invade the perinephric fat but do not extend beyond Gerota's fascia (Figs. 20–27 through 20–29, 20–31, 20–33, and 20–35).
3. Stage III tumors involve the renal veins or lymph nodes (Fig. 20–36).
4. Stage IV tumors extend through Gerota's fascia and involve adjacent organs or have metastasized to distant organs.

Refinements to the staging system include dividing stage III lesions into IIIA, IIIB, and IIIC, depending on involvement of vessels, nodes, or both, and separating stage IV tumors on the basis of local or distant organ spread (see Table 20–2).

The overall prognosis is affected by the stage and histologic pattern of the renal tumor at the time of diagnosis. The 10-year survival rate for stage I and II adenocarcinoma is 60 to 67 per cent and for stage III lesions is only 38 per cent. Stage IV tumors have a less than five per cent 5-year survival rate.[2] Because renal cell carcinomas within any particular stage may exhibit different biologic behavior, histologic pattern appears to be a better parameter than size in predicting prognosis.[83, 84] The group having a papillary pattern consisting of vascularized connective tissue stalks lined by a single layer of neoplastic cells (5 to 15 per cent of tumors) and showing less vascularity on angiography or CT has a better prognosis.[83, 84] Nonpapillary tumors have neoplastic cells arranged in cords, tubules, or sarcomatoid or spindle-shaped patterns; are more vascular; are invasive; and have a poor prognosis.[84, 85]

The surgical approach largely depends on preoperative assessment of the tumor's stage. All stage I tumors can be approached from the retroperitoneum, but radical nephrectomy and resection of stage IV tumors require an abdominal approach. A thoracoabdominal incision is required if the tumor invades the inferior vena cava. Radical nephrectomy increases the survival rate in patients with stage II and III renal tumors. In this operation, the kidney and all of the perinephric fatty tissues are removed together, thereby reducing the chance of incomplete tumor resection or local seeding of tumor cells.

CT is an excellent method to detect and stage renal cell carcinoma. CT can diagnose renal cell carcinoma with greater than 90 per cent accuracy and also has a greater than 90 per cent accuracy in staging renal

Text continued on page 967

TABLE 20–2 ■ **Staging Renal Cell Carcinoma**

ROBSON	PATHOLOGY	TNM
I	Small intrarenal tumor	T1
	Large intrarenal tumor	T2
II	Tumor into perinephric fat contained in Gerota's fascia	T3a
IIIA	Tumor to inferior vena cava or renal vein	T3b
IIIB	Tumor to local nodes	N1–N3
IIIC	Tumor to local nodes and vessels	T3b, N1–N3
IVA	Tumor to adjacent organs	T4
IVB	Distant metastasis	M1 and N4

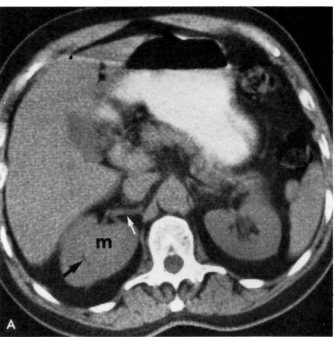

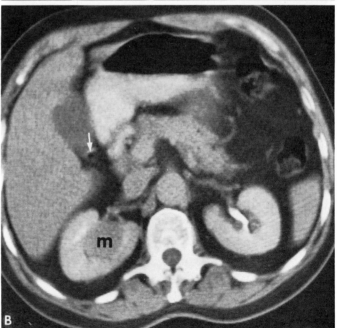

FIGURE 20–31 ■ Central renal cell carcinoma. *A,* Precontrast CT scan appears normal except for obliteration of the central renal sinus fat (*arrow*) by a mass (m) that has the same density as the adjacent kidney parenchyma. White arrow = Renal artery. *B,* Postcontrast scan. The difference between the tumor mass (m) and the renal parenchyma is accentuated. The tumor has obliterated the renal sinus fat. White arrow = Low-density gallstone.

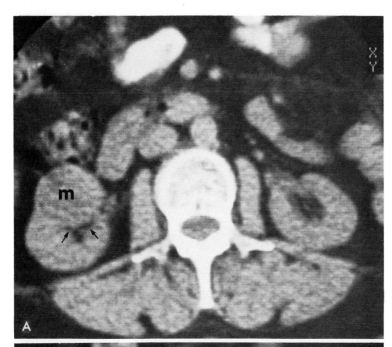

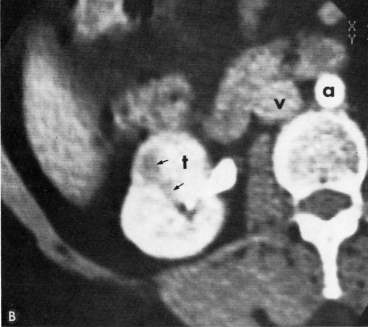

FIGURE 20–32 ■ Hypervascular stage I renal cell carcinoma—dynamic CT study. *A,* Precontrast scan reveals a small rounded mass (m) confined to the renal parenchyma with a density similar to that of the normal kidney. The central renal fat (*arrows*) is preserved. *B,* Scan during maximum arterial contrast. A portion of the tumor (t) greatly enhances, whereas other parts (*arrows*) are little enhanced. a = Aorta; v = inferior vena cava.

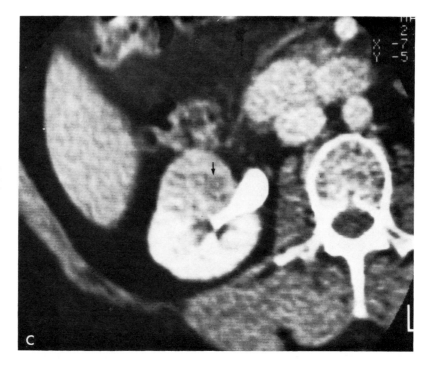

FIGURE 20–32 *Continued C,* Scan 45 seconds after injection. The central portion of the hypervascular tumor (*arrow*) now appears to be slightly lower in density than the remaining areas of tumor.

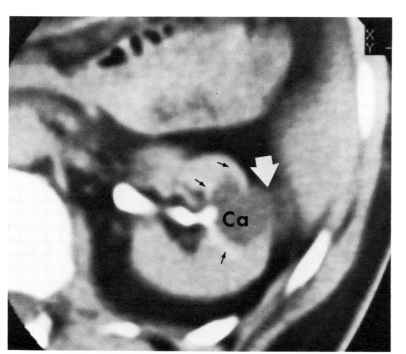

FIGURE 20–33 ■ Stage II renal cell carcinoma. A cystic renal cell carcinoma (Ca) extends through the renal capsule into the perinephric space (*large arrow*). The density of the central portion of the carcinoma was 18 H, whereas the peripheral portion of the tumor demonstrated a higher density rim (*small arrows*).

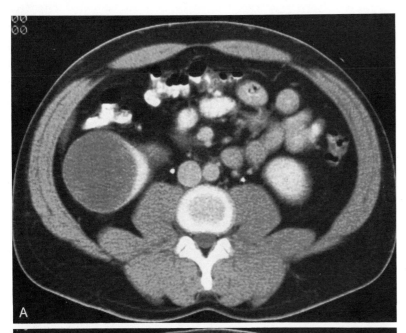

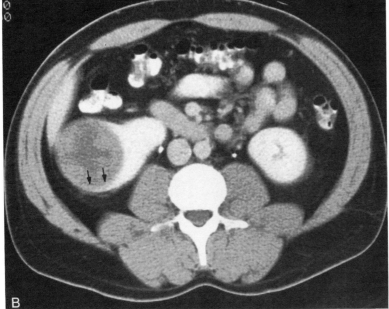

FIGURE 20–34 ■ Cystic renal cell carcinoma. *A,* A large right renal mass appears homogeneous and is sharply demarcated from normal-functioning renal parenchyma. *B,* A CT scan at a higher level reveals the mass to be heterogeneous and to have a thick rim (*arrows*).

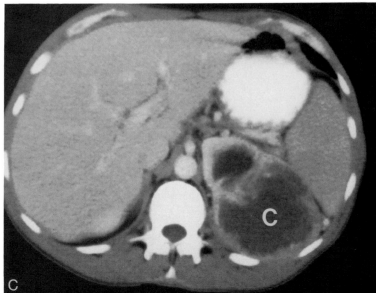

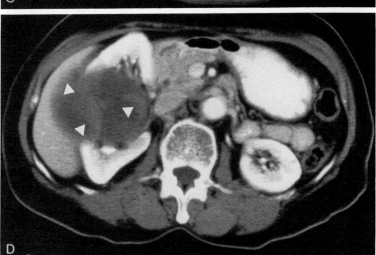

FIGURE 20–34 *Continued C,* Cystic carcinoma having a thick, irregular rim and an ill-defined interface with the normal portion of the kidney. *D,* A large central cystic mass containing areas of slightly elevated attenuation value (*arrowheads*).

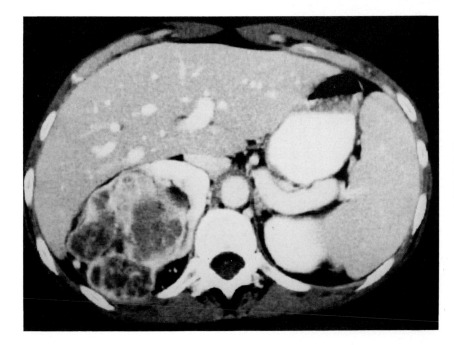

FIGURE 20–35 ■ Dynamic CT scan of stage II renal cell carcinoma. A large right renal tumor exhibits foci of high and low attenuation. The neoplasm extends into the perinephric space but does not involve vascular structures or lymph nodes.

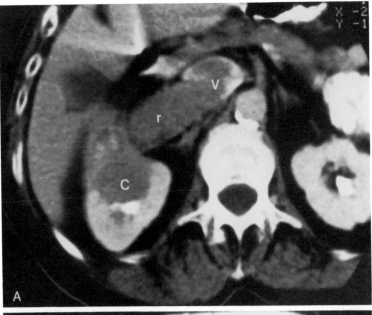

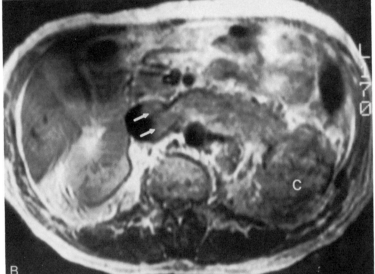

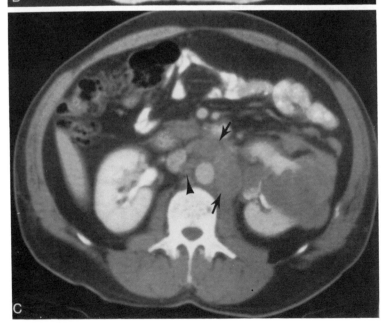

FIGURE 20–36 ■ Stage III renal cell carcinoma. *A*, A CT scan demonstrates a large right renal mass (C) that has extended into the right renal vein (r) and inferior vena cava (v). *B*. T1-weighted MR image reveals a large left renal cell carcinoma (C) with a mixed signal intensity. The tumor extends into the left renal vein and inferior vena cava (*arrows*). *C*, A large left renal cell carcinoma has spread to involve the paraaortic (*arrow*) and aortocaval lymph nodes (*arrowhead*).

cell carcinoma.[1-4, 7, 35, 36, 73, 74, 86] Tumoral invasion of the inferior vena cava or main renal vein can be diagnosed with a 78 to 93 per cent accuracy.[7, 35, 87, 88] Tumor extension produces hazy tumor margins, thickens the renal capsule, and obliterates the perinephric fat. Perinephric extension into adjacent organs is detected in about 80 per cent of pathologically proved cases.[7, 15, 71, 77, 80, 87] False-negative interpretations are usually the result of microscopic invasion, and false-positive CT scans are caused by necrosis of perirenal fat or perinephric hematomas. Lymph node involvement is demonstrated by enlarged perinephric, paraaortic, paracaval, or retrocrural lymph nodes (see Fig. 20–36C). Perinephric extension, lymph node involvement, and metastatic disease are detected with greater accuracy by CT than by angiography, and renal vein or caval involvement is identified with equal or greater accuracy.[7, 35, 71, 87, 89] Because of the high accuracy of CT in diagnosing and staging renal cell carcinoma, preoperative angiography is no longer performed in every patient with renal cell carcinoma. This has led to a reduction in the cost of evaluating renal mass lesions, as angiography is performed only in patients in whom the CT findings are uncertain or when a complete depiction of renal vascular anatomy is required (Fig. 20–37).[90]

Magnetic resonance imaging has also been advocated as an accurate technique to diagnose, characterize, and stage renal mass lesions.[78, 79, 91–93] However, MRI using conventional T1- and T2-weighted spin-echo sequences has shown that small renal tumors are often isointense with normal renal parenchyma,[91, 94, 95] and thus the diagnosis of renal cell carcinoma on MR scans can be made with confidence only when a mass deforms the renal contour, disrupts the corticomedullary junction, or has a signal

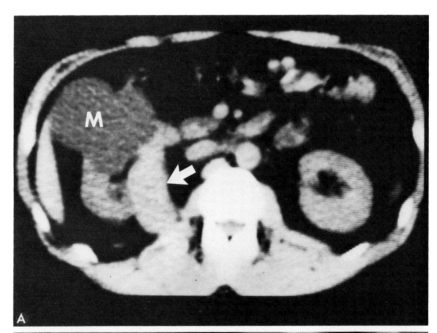

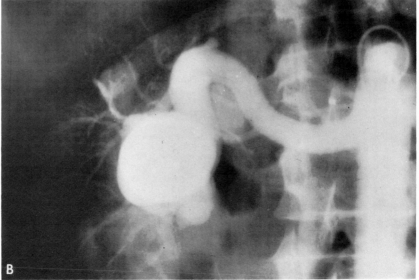

FIGURE 20–37 ■ Renal cell carcinoma producing an arteriovenous fistula. *A*, A precontrast CT scan demonstrates a large low-density mass (M) arising from the right kidney and a higher density mass (*arrow*) medial to the kidney, which has the same attenuation value as the aorta. *B*, An aortogram reveals a tremendously enlarged right renal artery feeding a large arteriovenous fistula.

intensity between that of the cortex and that of the medulla on T1 weighting and becomes hyperintense on T2-weighted sequences (Figs. 20–36B and 20–38).[79, 91, 95] Despite initial enthusiasm, MRI does not appear to be able to accurately characterize cystic lesions as either benign or malignant,[79, 94, 96] cannot reliably differentiate stage I from stage II neoplasms,[91, 95] and cannot distinguish among various types of renal tumors.[94, 79] However, MR does provide better definition of venous structures, and by being able to image in the coronal and sagittal planes, MR can precisely identify renal vein and vena caval involvement and extent of tumor thrombus growth more readily than can CT (see Fig. 20–36B).[91, 92]

Overall it appears that MRI, as currently performed, offers little diagnostic advantage over CT. The ability of MRI to stage renal cell carcinoma is slightly lower than that of CT, but the ability of MR to provide useful information about vascular invasion and its multidimensional assessment of tumor extent may be important in certain patients (Fig. 20–39). The advent of contrast-enhanced MR imaging may improve the accuracy of MR in diagnosing renal cell carcinoma.[93]

Von Hippel-Lindau Syndrome ■ Patients with von Hippel-Lindau syndrome are at increased risk of developing renal cell carcinoma. In these patients, the carcinoma is frequently bilateral and multicentric (Fig. 20–40).[65, 69, 70] Multiple renal cysts and small solid tumors are also frequently present (Figs. 20–41 and 21–42), making the diagnosis of small tumors difficult by urographic, angiographic, and ultrasonic techniques.[97] Pancreatic cysts are commonly present (see Figs. 20–41 and 20–42).

CT has been able to detect and distinguish between renal cysts and small solid mass lesions in patients with von Hippel–Lindau syndrome (see Fig. 20–42).[70] Solid mass lesions and cysts less than 2 cm in diameter are best evaluated by using finely collimated CT scans. Solid mass lesions larger than 3 cm are all classified as renal carcinomas, whereas solid lesions less than 3 cm are often classified as benign "adenomas," although histologically they cannot be distinguished from renal cell carcinoma. Recently the concept of an "adenoma" has been challenged, and the current thinking is that all solid lesions should be considered renal cell carcinomas.[73, 74, 98]

CT is recommended as the primary renal screening procedure in all patients suspected of having von Hippel-Lindau syndrome.[70, 99] Relatives of patients with known von Hippel-Lindau syndrome should probably be studied. CT detection of a small, noninvasive tumor permits a wide local resection rather than a radical nephrectomy to be performed, thereby preserving renal function.[70, 99]

Nephroblastoma (Wilms' Tumor) ■ Nephroblastoma, or Wilms' tumor, arises from immature renal parenchyma and occurs most frequently in children 1 to 5 years old.[100] It constitutes six per cent of all renal malignancies and is the most common abdominal malignant tumor in children (see Chapter 26). Approximately 25 per cent of Wilms' tumors occur in infants younger than 1 year; less than five per cent occur after the age of 6 years.[65, 100] Bilateral involvement occurs but is less frequent (1 to 13 per cent) than in neuroblastoma. Pathologically, nephroblastomas often show areas of necrosis or hemorrhage, and renal vein invasion is common (30 to 40 per cent).[70] Metastasis to lungs is frequent, but metastasis to bones, liver, and lymph nodes is uncommon.

Clinical presentation includes a palpable abdomi-

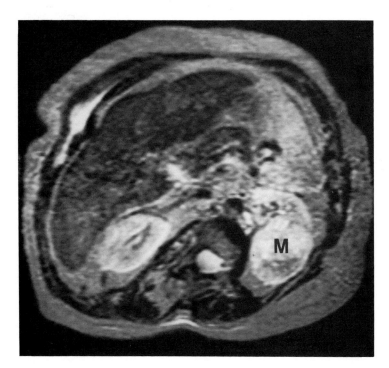

FIGURE 20–38 ■ Renal cell carcinoma. A T2-weighted MR scan demonstrates a hyperintense left kidney mass (M) that appears to be confined to the kidney. Surgery revealed stage I renal cell carcinoma.

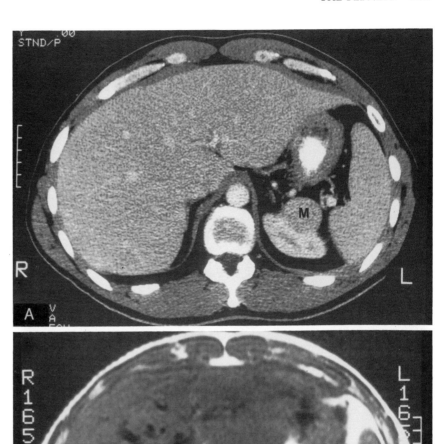

FIGURE 20–39 ■ Suspected renal cell carcinoma. *A,* CT scan demonstrates an apparent mass (M) arising from the left kidney. *B.* A T1-weighted spin-echo scan reveals the mass to have the same intensity as the spleen. *C,* A T2-weighted spin-echo scan shows the mass to be isointense with the spleen. Diagnosis was splenic lobulation appearing as renal pseudotumor.

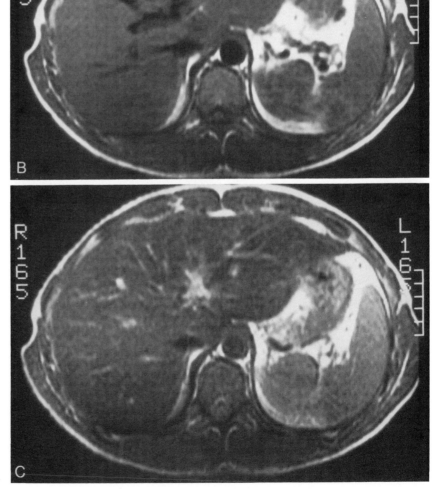

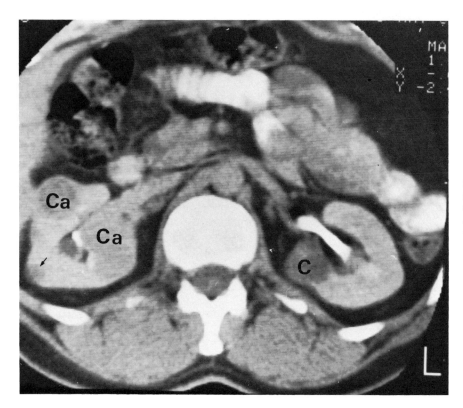

FIGURE 20–40 ■ Von Hippel–Lindau syndrome. There is a multicentric renal cell carcinoma (Ca) and a small adenoma (*arrow*) of the right kidney. A left renal cyst (C) is also present.

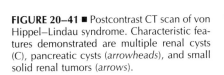 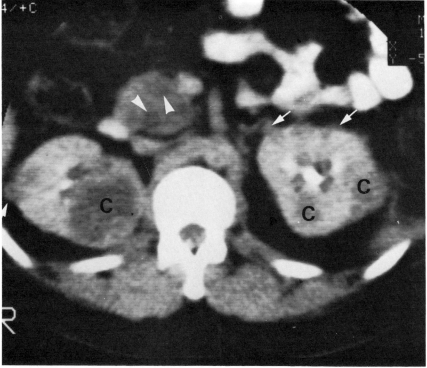

FIGURE 20–41 ■ Postcontrast CT scan of von Hippel–Lindau syndrome. Characteristic features demonstrated are multiple renal cysts (C), pancreatic cysts (*arrowheads*), and small solid renal tumors (*arrows*).

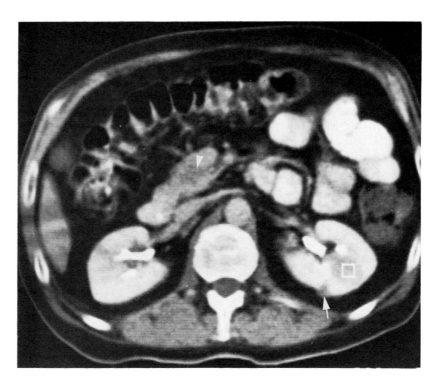

FIGURE 20–42 ■ Von Hippel–Lindau syndrome. The postcontrast CT scan findings demonstrated include a small peripheral left renal cyst (*arrow*). A central solid mass (*box*) measuring 56 H proved to be a renal cell carcinoma. A cyst in the head of the pancreas (*arrowhead*) is also shown.

nal mass (60 per cent incidence) and a low-grade fever (50 per cent incidence). Hypertension is frequent, but hematuria is the presenting complaint in less than 20 per cent of cases.[70] The incidence of aniridia and hemihypertrophy is increased in patients with Wilms' tumor.

Nephroblastoma is most frequently demonstrated by CT to be a noncalcified (90 per cent), inhomogeneous solid mass lesion arising in the kidney (Fig. 20–43).[100–102] Rarely will a Wilms' tumor present as a botryoid renal pelvicaliceal mass.[103]

The CT appearance of a nephroblastoma is similar to that of an adult renal cell carcinoma. Similarly, initial MR studies have shown Wilms' tumor to have prolonged T1 and T2 relaxation times in the same range as adult renal cell carcinoma.[104] The MR signal is often variable because of tumor necrosis and hemorrhage, and thus MR is not able to differentiate Wilms' tumor from other neoplasms.[104]

Angiomyolipoma ■ The renal angiomyolipoma is a fairly common benign renal tumor usually classified as a hamartoma and is composed of various propor-

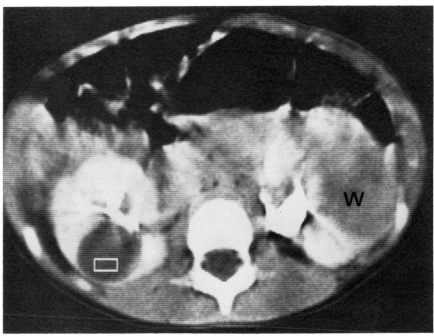

FIGURE 20–43 ■ Bilateral Wilms' tumors. CT scan demonstrates a large left solid renal mass (W) and a smaller, more cystic-appearing right renal mass (*box*). At surgery the right tumor was found to contain a large amount of fatty tissue.

tions of smooth muscle, blood vessels, and fat.[105] The term *angiomyolipoma* is used to describe the complete lesion; terms such as *angiomyoma* or *myolipoma* have been used when other tissues predominate.

Angiomyolipomas occur in two distinct groups of patients. Forty to eighty per cent of patients with tuberous sclerosis have angiomyolipomas (Fig. 20–44).[106] The tumors in these patients are usually small, asymptomatic, bilateral, tend to occur in childhood or early adulthood, and are equally distributed between the sexes.[65] Angiomyolipomas found in patients without tuberous sclerosis tend to be larger, symptomatic, single, occur in middle age, and have a 4:1 female predominance.[65]

Pathologically, the lesions are identical in the two groups. Angiomyolipomas are nonencapsulated, grow slowly, and tend to enlarge in an expansile fashion, replacing the renal parenchyma and distorting but not destroying the pelvicaliceal system. Some tumors (25 per cent) have a predominantly extrarenal growth pattern that extends to, or even through, the renal capsule into the perinephric compartment.[107] Because the prominent tumor vessels lack an internal elastic lining, intratumoral and perinephric hemorrhage is common, causing hematuria, flank pain, or a palpable mass.[107]

The CT findings in angiomyolipomas are so distinctive that a histologic diagnosis may be suggested in virtually every case.[107–112] Single or multiple renal masses have zones of different density ranging from −150 H (fat) to +150 H (calcification) Because fat is present in nearly all angiomyolipomas, there is usually at least one region with a CT density of at least −20 H (Figs. 20–44 and 20–45). The detection of even a small amount of fat in renal mass is important, as it confirms the diagnosis of angiomyolipoma.[105] In angiomyolipomas composed mainly of vascular tissue and muscle or in those in which recent hemorrhage has occurred, the majority of the tumor may

have CT density values greater than 20 H (Fig. 20–46).[110, 112, 113]

Angiomyolipomas typically join the normal renal tissue at an acute angle, rarely obstruct the caliceal system, and range in size from less than 2 cm to more than 8 cm when detected.[105, 107, 114] After contrast medium injection, portions of the tumor may be enhanced, but fatty tissue and areas of necrosis do not increase in density (see Fig. 20–46). Dynamic CT may reveal an early hypervascular phase, which reflects the increased vascularity found at angiography. If an angiomyolipoma is suspected, but contrast enhancement has elevated tissue density measurements, a repeat study through the mass should be done without contrast enhancement. Even though angiomyolipomas may invade the perinephric compartment or adjacent structures such as the inferior vena cava,[115] no evidence of distant metastatic disease will be evident.

Although the CT diagnosis of angiomyolipoma is highly specific, renal lipoma, liposarcoma, or retroperitoneal liposarcomas invading the kidney cannot be absolutely excluded. CT has also demonstrated fatty tissue in cases of Wilms' tumor.[116] It is also important to be certain that renal sinus fat, which can be enveloped by renal tumors, is not mistaken for the intrinsic fat within an angiomyolipoma.[105, 117] The diagnosis may be difficult in small lesions, as partial volume averaging can erroneously elevate the measured CT density to that of water or solid tissue. The use of thinner CT scan sections and performing the CT study without intravenous contrast will help avoid this diagnostic pitfall.[105] If the diagnosis is still in doubt, ultrasonography or MRI (Fig. 20–47) can help establish the diagnosis by demonstrating foci that are characteristic of fat rather than fluid or nonfatty solid tissue.[111, 118]

Renal Oncocytoma ■ Oncocytomas are rare, benign, solid renal tumors, always at least partially encap-

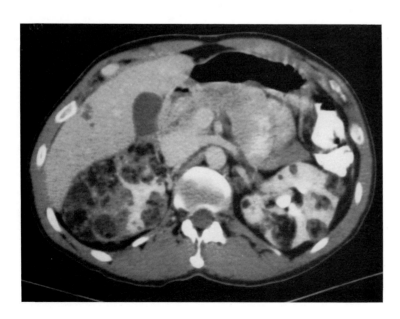

FIGURE 20–44 ■ Bilateral angiomyolipomas in a patient with tuberous sclerosis. CT scan demonstrates multiple bilateral, small renal masses having a CT density ranging from +40 H to −40 H.

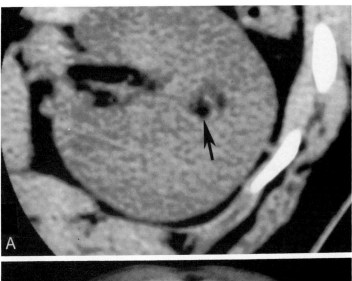

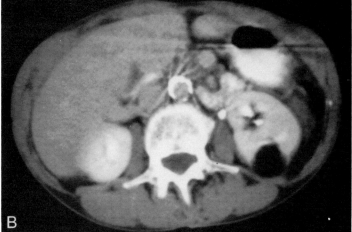

FIGURE 20–45 ■ Various CT appearances of angiomyolipoma. *A,* A small foci of fat (*arrow*) is shown in the central portion of the left kidney. The CT density was −30 H. *B,* A rounded, 3-cm peripheral mass having a CT density of −150 H. *C,* A solid mass of mixed density that showed considerable contrast enhancement. Only one focus of minimal fatty density remained after contrast injection. Region of interest (ROI) was −20 H.

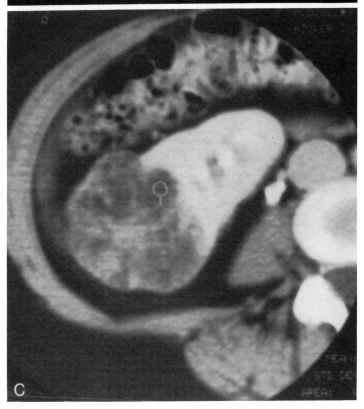

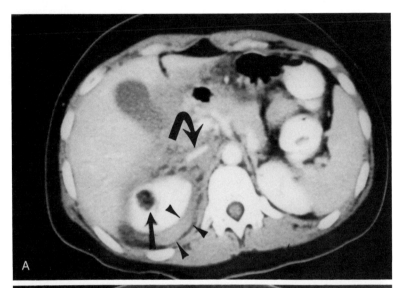

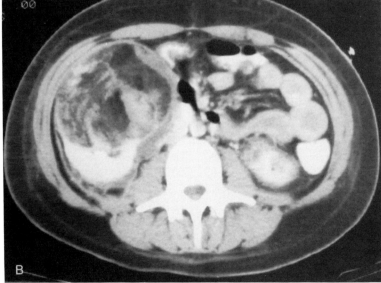

FIGURE 20–46 ■ Angiomyolipoma with hemorrhage. *A,* CT scan demonstrates a small fat-containing intrarenal tumor (*arrow*). There has been hemorrhage into the perinephric space (*arrowheads*), which has extended to displace and flatten the inferior vena cava (*curved arrow*). *B,* A large angiomyolipoma of the right kidney has hemorrhaged into the perinephric space and has thickened Gerota's fascia. The tumor shows areas of contrast enhancement and regions of nonenhanced fatty tissue.

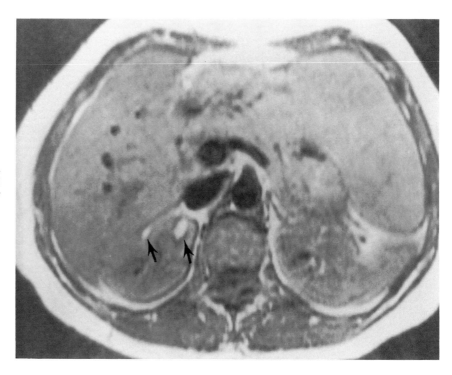

FIGURE 20–47 ■ Angiomyolipoma. A T1-weighted MR scan demonstrates two small hyperintense foci (*arrows*) in the right kidney that have the same characteristics as fat.

sulated, that are thought to originate from proximal tubular epithelial cells.[65, 119–126] Microscopically, the oncocytes are large cells that have an eosinophilic, finely granular cytoplasm containing numerous mitochondria.[123, 125]

Oncocytomas are usually asymptomatic, may be single or multiple, account for approximately three to five per cent of renal parenchymal neoplasms, and are often larger than 2 cm when discovered.[119–126] Distinction from renal cell carcinoma is difficult by conventional radiologic methods. Angiographically, a spokes-on-a-wheel configuration of vessels, a homogeneous nephrogram, and a sharp interface with normal parenchyma have been described as characteristic of oncocytomas.[119, 123] However, the same pattern has been described in renal cell carcinoma.[123]

The typical CT appearance of oncocytoma is a homogeneous solid renal mass that may be only slightly less dense than the renal parenchyma after intravenous injection of contrast medium (Fig. 20–48*A*). Oncocytomas may also appear as low-density masses after administration of contrast (see Fig. 20–48*B*). The tumor mass is sharply separated from the normal cortex and does not invade the caliceal system or adjacent structures.[119, 120, 123] A central star-shaped scar of lower density than the otherwise homogeneous mass is seen in approximately 33 per cent of cases and is highly suggestive of oncocytoma.[123] Although renal cell carcinomas do not have a central scar, a similar pattern may be mimicked by a renal cell carcinoma with an area of central necrosis.[123]

Oncocytomas are only rarely calcified,[121] infrequently are bilateral, rarely occur with a concomitant renal cell carcinoma,[122] and have been known to grow to a weight of greater than 4 kg.[126]

Unusual Renal Tumors ■ Tumors of the renal capsule, such as fibromas, leiomyomas, lipomas, hemangioendothelioma (Fig. 20–49), and angiomas, are rare and can be benign or malignant.[65] Renal tumors arising from mesenchymal derivatives; muscle; and connective, adipose, lymphatic, or vascular tissue are also rare.[65, 127, 128] Together, these rare tumors account for less than one per cent of renal tumors. The CT findings of only a few of these tumors has been reported, and it is unlikely that a specific CT diagnosis will be made except perhaps in cases of tumors of fatty tissue or in rare primary osteogenic sarcoma. MR may be helpful in identifying a medullary fibroma because of its low signal intensity on T1- and T2-weighted pulse sequences.[128]

SECONDARY RENAL TUMORS

Renal Lymphoma ■ Renal involvement by lymphoma is commonly found at postmortem examination (30 to 50 per cent) but is seldom detected by conventional urographic studies.[65, 129, 130] The most common manifestation of renal lymphoma is multiple parenchymal nodules (61 per cent), whereas invasion from perirenal disease (11 per cent), solitary nodules (seven per cent), large single lesions (six per cent), and diffuse infiltration (six per cent) are less frequent features.[129–132] Bilateral involvement is three times as common as unilateral involvement.[129, 131]

Urography may demonstrate diffuse or focal renal enlargement and indirectly detect extrarenal disease by ureteral obstruction or displacement. However, Lalli[130] reported that lymphomas produce lesions that are usually too small to be recognized by conventional roentgenographic methods.

CT has been able to detect a variety of abnormali-

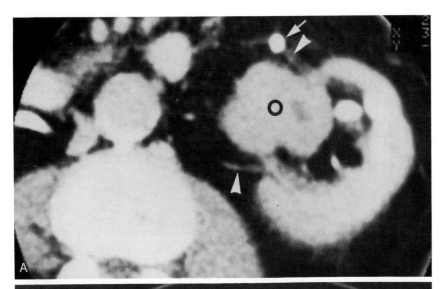

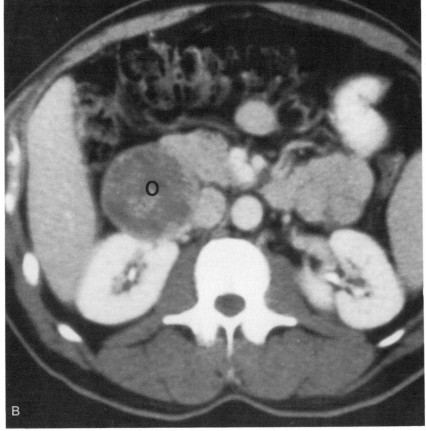

FIGURE 20–48 ■ Oncocytoma. *A*, CT scan after injection of contrast material. A lobulated oncocytoma (o), seen as a homogeneous solid mass, is slightly less dense than functioning renal parenchyma. The CT number of the tumor was 70 H. The ureter (*arrow*) and renal vessels (*arrowheads*) are displaced by the tumor, but there is no evidence of obstruction of collecting structures, invasion of perirenal fat, or vascular occlusion. The tumor had been present for more than 10 years. *B*, CT scan showing rounded right renal mass (o) of mixed CT density. Notice that the tumor does not invade the caliceal system or adjacent structures.

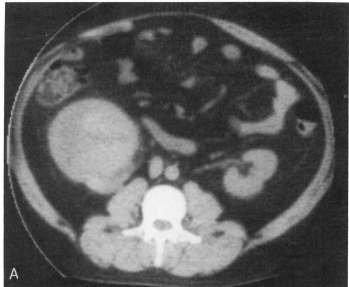

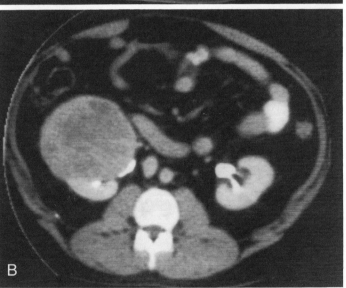

FIGURE 20–49 ■ Renal hemangioendothelioma. *A*, Precontrast CT scan demonstrates a large exophytic right renal mass containing foci of high density (*arrowhead*) representing fresh hemorrhage. *B*, CT scan after contrast injection more clearly delineates the tumor. The CT appearance cannot be distinguished from that of a renal cell carcinoma.

ties in patients with renal lymphoma. The CT manifestations of lymphomatous infiltration of the kidneys are varied and include the following[129, 132–136]:

1. Bilaterally enlarged kidneys without demonstrable masses.

2. Enlarged or normal kidneys with multiple focal, nodular, solid masses of various sizes that have decreased density on postcontrast scans (Fig. 20–50*A, B*).

3. Solitary focal, irregular, solid intrarenal mass lesions (see Fig. 20–50*B*).

4. Retroperitoneal disease that extends into the renal pelvis (see Fig. 20–50*C*).

5. Infiltration of intrarenal collecting structures produced by diffuse interstitial infiltration of the kidneys. The kidney maintains its reniform shape (see Fig. 20–50*B*).

6. Kidney nonfunction (see Fig. 20–50*B, C*).

It is not possible to distinguish among the various

forms of lymphoma or to differentiate lymphoma from other solid intrarenal masses by CT. However, when CT reveals coexisting retroperitoneal adenopathy, splenomegaly, or mesenteric adenopathy, renal lymphoma should be considered as the most likely cause of solid renal mass.

Renal lymphoma is more common after renal transplantation.[137] It appears as a bulky, poorly marginated mass with inhomogeneous CT density. Posttransplant lymphomas primarily affect the central nervous system, but outside the central nervous system the transplanted kidney is the organ most often infiltrated by posttransplant lymphoma.[137, 138]

Hodgkin's disease, or histiocytic lymphoma, occurring in a patient with chronic lymphocytic leukemia is known as Richter's syndrome[139] and occurs in three to ten per cent of patients with chronic lymphocytic leukemia.[139] Several cases of solitary hyperdense nodular lymphomatous masses have been reported.

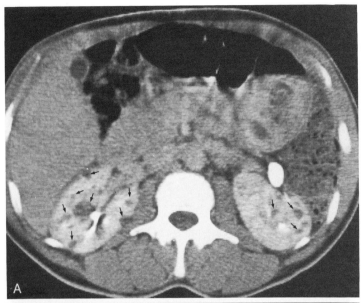

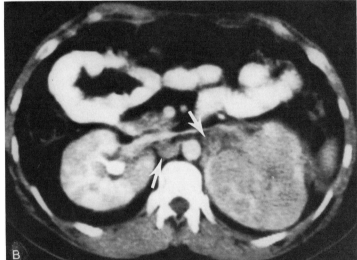

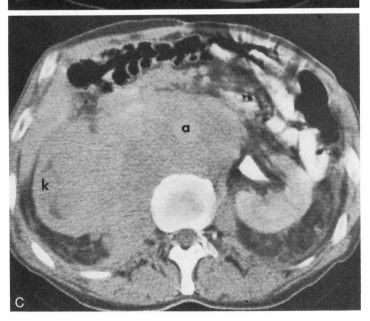

FIGURE 20–50 ■ CT features of lymphoma involving the kidneys. *A,* Multiple bilateral focal, nodular masses (*arrows*) of various sizes are seen scattered throughout the renal parenchyma in a patient with Hodgkin's disease. *B,* The right kidney has multiple parenchymal solid masses but has normal function. The left kidney is markedly enlarged by a large solid mass. The kidney maintains its renoform shape and is nonfunctioning except for a small amount of preserved tissue at the periphery of the kidney. Arrows = Paraaortic and aortocaval enlarged lymph nodes. *C,* Nonfunction of the right kidney (k) as a result of invasion by a large retroperitoneal lymphomatous mass. a = Aorta.

Renal Metastasis ■ Leukemia infiltration of the kidneys can produce bilateral renal enlargement and intrarenal masses.[65] Tumors from the lung (Fig. 20–51), breast, stomach, colon, cervix, skin, and pancreas frequently metastasize to the kidneys, but most metastases are small and do not produce symptoms of renal failure, hydronephrosis, or hemorrhage.[140, 141] The CT appearance of a solitary renal metastasis is that of a solid mass lesion that is indistinguishable from a primary renal malignancy. Renal metastasis is the likely diagnosis when small, multiple renal masses are present with metastatic disease elsewhere in the body. Colon metastasis tend to be large (>4 cm) and may be calcified if from a mucinous adenocarcinoma.[140] Melanoma tends to infiltrate the perinephric space, and lung, breast, and head and neck carcinoma typically are manifest by multiple small nodules.[140, 141]

TUMORS OF THE RENAL PELVIS

Transitional cell carcinoma is the most common (82 per cent to 90 per cent) epithelial tumor of the renal pelvis.[10, 65] Transitional cell carcinoma is often multiple (20 per cent to 44 per cent); similar tumors affect the bladder (ten per cent), ipsilateral ureter (17 per cent), or bladder and ureter (15 per cent). More than 85 per cent of transitional cell carcinomas are of the papillary type (i.e., low-grade malignancies that are slow to infiltrate, late to metastasize, and follow a relatively benign course).[10, 142] The nonpapillary form of transitional cell carcinoma is a more aggressive malignancy; direct extension and metastasis occur early, resulting in a 5-year survival rate of less than ten per cent.[10, 65, 142] Transitional cell carcinoma is three to four times more common in males than in females, and about 70 per cent of patients are more than 60 years old at the time of presentation.[142]

A number of azo dyes and pigments used in the textile, printing, and plastics industries have been implicated as etiologic agents for transitional cell carcinoma. Thorotrast has also been found to cause transitional cell carcinoma. The compound spreads subepithelially during retrograde pyelography, and after a latent period of 20 to 35 years, transitional call carcinoma occurs in 50 per cent of patients.[142–144]

Squamous cell carcinoma constitutes approximately 15 per cent of tumors of the renal pelvis and is frequently associated with chronic leukoplakia. Calculi are present in 50 per cent of patients, and extrarenal spread at the time of diagnosis is the rule rather than the exception. Hematuria and flank pain are common presenting symptoms, as the tumor is usually well advanced and has extended deeply into the adjacent tissues by the time the diagnosis is made. There is no sex predilection, and the mean age of patients is greater than 60 years. The prognosis is very poor; the average survival is 1 to 1½ years, and there are almost no long-term survivors.[65]

The diagnosis of a pelvic tumor is usually suggested when an excretory urogram demonstrates hydronephrosis or a filling defect within the renal pelvis.[142] Differentiation of renal pelvic tumors from filling defects caused by nonopaque calculi, blood clots, polyps, aberrant or hypertrophied renal papillae, vascular impressions, prominent renal columns, or inflammatory conditions is frequently difficult by conventional urography and angiography.[142, 145]

The CT appearance of renal pelvic tumors is varied. Small pelvic tumors that do not produce hydronephrosis or invade the peripelvic fat are usually not detected on precontrast CT scans.[142, 145] After intravenous contrast injection, pelvic neoplasms are detected as pelvic filling defects that have a smooth, lobulated, or irregular margin (Fig. 20–52).[142, 145] Tumors may prevent contrast from filling the dependent portion of the renal collection structures (Fig. 20–53). CT density values typically range from 8 to 40 H and do not dramatically increase after contrast medium administration. Rarely, a transitional cell carcinoma may be calcified.[146] The peripelvic fat stripe is pre-

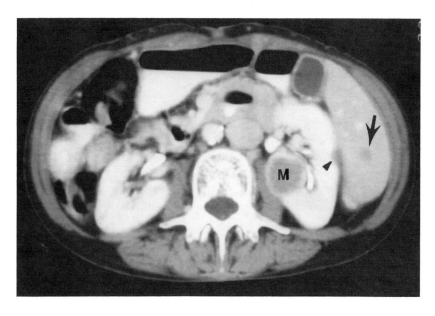

FIGURE 20–51 ■ Metastatic carcinoma to the right kidney. A rounded mass (M) has a thick enhancing rim and a necrotic center resulting from metastatic lung carcinoma. A liver metastasis (*arrow*) and another small renal metastasis (*arrowhead*) are also shown.

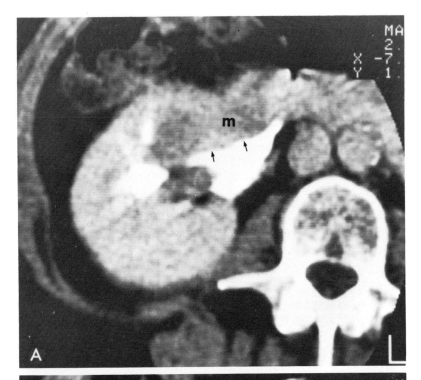

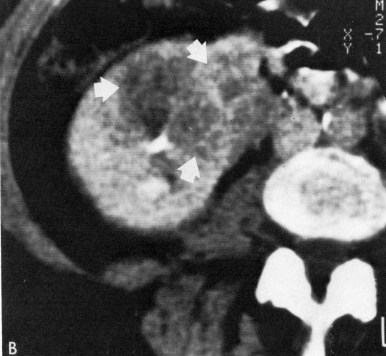

FIGURE 20–52 ■ Transitional cell carcinoma of the renal pelvis. *A,* The carcinoma has produced a pelvic mass (m), which has a slightly irregular inferior margin (*arrows*). *B,* CT scan at a more caudal level demonstrates the mass to have invaded through the renal pelvis into the renal parenchyma (*arrows*).

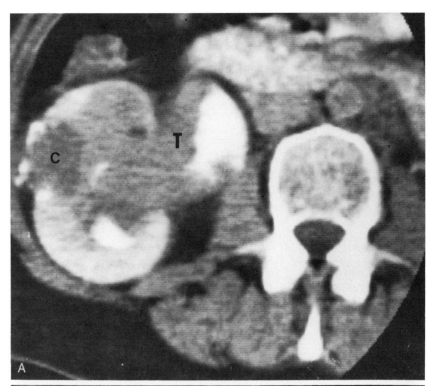

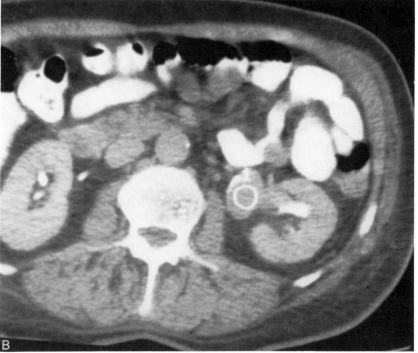

FIGURE 20–53 ■ Transitional cell carcinoma. *A,* CT scan through the renal pelvis demonstrates a large tumor (T), which partially fills the renal pelvis, preventing contrast material from filling the dependent portion of the collecting structure. The tumor has extended into the renal parenchyma, obliterating the peripelvic fat. c = Calcified renal cyst. *B,* A small left pelvic tumor (o) measuring 30 H that almost completely fills the renal pelvis. The tumor prevents contrast from reaching the dependent portion of the renal pelvis.

served when tumors are confined to the renal pelvis (Figs. 20–53B and 20–54) but obliterated when extrapelvic extension has occurred (Figs. 20–52 and 20–55). Larger tumors produce hydronephrosis, invade renal parenchymal or vascular structures, and are a cause of a nonfunctioning kidney (see Fig. 20–55).[142, 145, 147]

Distinguishing between transitional cell and squamous cell carcinoma by CT is usually not possible except when the pelvic filling defect has a frondlike appearance (papillary transitional cell carcinoma) or is associated with a pelvic calculus (squamous cell carcinoma). Nonopaque renal calculi have higher attenuation values than pelvic tumors,[145] and blood clots tend to be round, smooth, and dependently positioned within the renal pelvis, whereas tumors are frequently irregular, nondependent renal pelvic masses (Fig. 20–56). Whenever a renal pelvic tumor is detected, the entire ureter and bladder should be examined to exclude synchronous uroepithelial tumors.[10, 142]

TUMORS OF THE URETER

The ureter has the same epithelium as the renal pelvis and bladder; therefore ureteral tumors are of cell types similar to those of the renal collecting system and bladder. Of malignant ureteral tumors, transitional cell carcinoma occurs most frequently (85 per cent), but squamous cell carcinoma accounts for 15 per cent of ureteral malignancies.[65] Hematuria (80 per cent), pain (60 per cent), and flank mass (40 per cent) constitute the most frequent clinical presentation.[8, 65, 142, 148] Urography may reveal a nonfunctioning kidney (46 per cent), hydronephrosis (34 per cent), delayed renal excretion of contrast, or hydroureter with or without a ureteral filling defect or stenosis.

In cases of ureteral tumor, CT typically demonstrates delayed renal excretion of contrast, hydronephrosis, and the obstructed ureter down to the level of the tumor. Ureteral neoplasms appear as soft tissue filling defects within the ureter or as thickening of the ureteral wall.[142] If a periureteral mass is present, CT usually cannot differentiate a primary ureteral neoplasm from direct ureteral involvement by metastasis from the cervix, rectum, bladder, prostate, or ovary.[149, 150] However, CT can distinguish ureteral obstruction resulting from calculi that are nonopaque by conventional radiography from ureteral tumors. All nonopaque calculi have a high CT density (50 + H) that permits ready distinction from tumors which have a soft tissue density.[145, 150, 151]

Non-Neoplastic Disease

RENAL AND URETERAL CALCULI

CT detects radiodense calculi in the ureters, renal pelvis, or caliceal collecting structures,[150, 151] and renal parenchymal calcifications also are frequently demonstrated during CT examinations performed for other clinical problems.[1–3, 34] Although CT is not the primary diagnostic technique for evaluating urinary calculi, when it is employed, it should be performed without intravenous contrast injection, as contrast material obscures the diagnosis in more than 75 per cent of instances (Fig. 20–57).[34] The slice thickness should be the same or thinner than the sought-after calculus to avoid the effect of partial volume averaging.

Approximately five to eight per cent of calculi are nonopaque, consisting mostly of pure uric acid, xanthine, or matrix calculi.[132, 151, 153] Stones containing a mixture of components are also found; uric acid is often combined with calcium oxalate, which makes

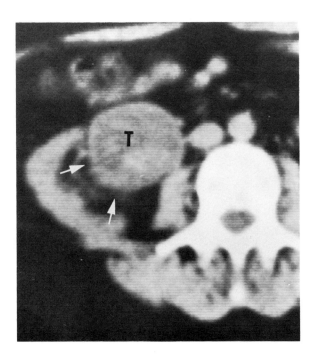

FIGURE 20–54 ■ A transitional cell carcinoma (T) causing marked enlargement of the extrarenal pelvis. The tumor is completely contained within the pelvis, and the peripelvic fat planes (*arrows*) are preserved.

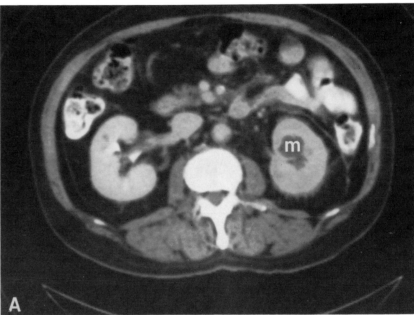

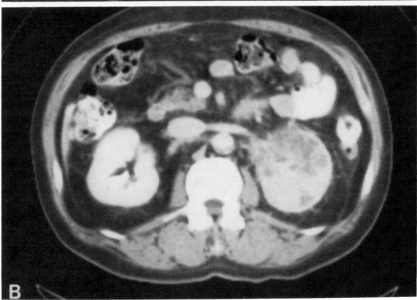

FIGURE 20–55 ■ Transitional cell carcinoma of the left kidney. *A,* CT scan through the midportion of the left kidney demonstrates a central soft tissue mass (m) obliterating the renal sinus fat. Left renal function is diminished. *B,* A very large tumor mass that has enlarged and infiltrated the left kidney is seen at a higher level. There is no functioning renal tissue at this level.

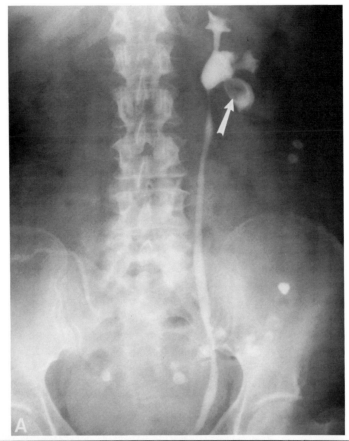

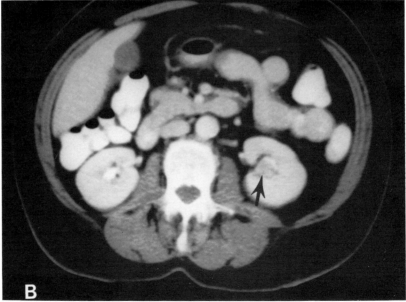

FIGURE 20–56 ■ Small transitional cell carcinoma. *A,* Retrograde pyelogram reveals an oval, smooth, filling defect in the lower pole calix (*arrow*) of the left kidney. *B,* CT scan demonstrates a small mass (*arrow*) contained within the lower pole calix. It had a CT density of 32 H, thus excluding a nonopaque calculus or blood clot. Contrast does not layer dependently.

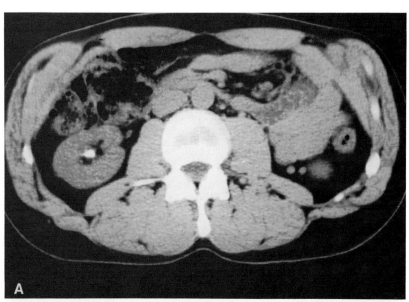

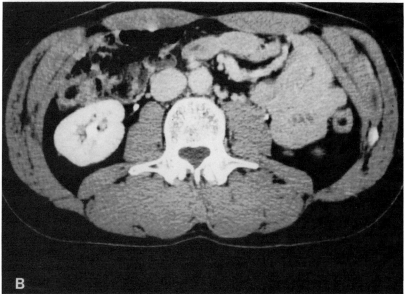

FIGURE 20–57 ■ Nonopaque renal calculi. *A,* Precontrast CT scan reveals a small high-density calculus in the right renal pelvis. *B,* Postcontrast CT scan obscures the renal calculi. Diagnosis was uric acid calculi.

the stone mildly opaque.[151–153] The usual appearance of a nonopaque calculus is a negative filling defect in the urinary collecting structures during excretory urography (Fig. 20–58A). Urographic differentiation is difficult, because tumors, blood clots, papillomas, and nonopaque calculi produce similar urographic findings.

All reported nonopaque urinary calculi examined by CT have been of high density (see Figs. 20–57 and 20–58B).[145, 151, 154] Calculi in the renal collecting structures and ureter are readily identified as dense filling defects on nonenhanced CT scans. Differentiation among calculi of various compositions has been attempted by CT analysis, but because the CT densities of different calculi overlap, differentiation has not proven to be reliable.[5, 152, 155]

The increased CT density of nonopaque calculi is directly related to the increased physical density of the calculus[154] and does not indicate calcium content.[152] Calculi exposed to urographic contrast material can show an increased density because of their absorption of contrast.[152] Thus the detected CT density of calculi reflects a combination of inherent physical density and contrast effect on the calculi, if the CT study is performed after administration of contrast medium.

CT can distinguish calculi from other nonopaque filling defects in almost every instance. Tumors of all types have soft tissue attenuation values (30 to 50 H), and although blood clots may have a higher density than unopacified urine or renal parenchyma, their density does not approach that of urinary tract calculi.[145, 151, 152, 156] Contiguous thin (5 mm or less) CT sections through the region of the suspected calculi

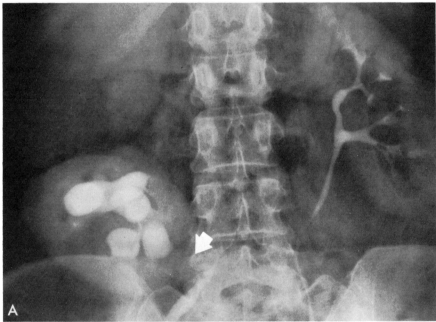

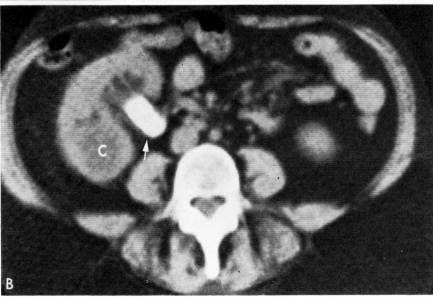

FIGURE 20–58 ■ Uric acid calculus. A, Excretory urogram. There is a hydronephrotic, distorted, and rotated right kidney. A nonopaque filling defect is present in the renal pelvis (arrow). B, Non–contrast-enhanced CT scan. A high-density calculus (arrow) fills the renal pelvis. A lower pole renal cyst (C) is present. The CT number of the uric acid calculus was +150 H.

permit calculi as small as 2 to 3 mm to be detected and ensure that small calculi are not missed because of partial volume averaging.

RENAL TRAUMA

CT findings can be used to diagnose and depict the extent of renal traumatic injuries.[157–162] Urography is a sensitive screening procedure, but it does not accurately reflect the type and extent of renal injury.[157, 160] Based on CT findings, renal injuries have been grouped into various categories.[157, 158, 160, 162–166]

Subcapsular hematoma is a frequent finding after blunt or penetrating renal trauma.[157–160, 167–169] It is diagnosed when fluid is confined to the immediate extrarenal area and separated from Gerota's fascia by fat (Fig. 20–59). The collection of fluid is usually lenticular in shape and may flatten the adjacent renal parenchyma.[157–159, 167, 170] Subcapsular hematomas occur in approximately 28 per cent of patients after percutaneous renal biopsy.[168] CT scans shortly after injury often show the subcapsular hematoma to have a higher density than the surrounding kidney (see Fig. 20–59A); follow-up scans show that the hematoma diminishes in density as it liquifies.[159, 168] CT scans after contrast medium administration demonstrate the hematoma to have a lower attenuation value than that of the functioning renal parenchyma (see Fig. 20–59B). Isolated subcapsular hematomas are minor injuries that can be managed conservatively.[157–160, 170] Subcapsular hematomas are commonly present (15 per cent) after extracorporeal shock wave lithotripsy.[167]

Perinephric hematomas are larger fluid collections extending to and confined to Gerota's fascia (Fig. 20–60).[157–160, 162, 168] A perinephric hematoma can be an isolated injury confined to the anterior or posterior perinephric space, but usually there is an associated subcapsular hematoma. Hemorrhage into the perinephric space occurs in more than 95 per cent of patients following renal biopsy.[168]

Renal contusion (intrarenal hematoma) is a focal renal parenchymal injury that prevents normal enhancement of the kidney after intravenous contrast administration.[160] The nephrogram is less dense than normal, and the calices fill poorly, but no renal fracture is identified. The injury produces interstitial edema and extravasation of blood and urine into the renal interstitial space. The result is transient vasospasm, which resolves with conservative, nonsurgical management.[157, 158, 160]

More severe renal injuries are diagnosed whenever there is a renal laceration, renal fracture, or shattered kidney (Figs. 20–61 and 20–62). The term *renal laceration* indicates a focal renal parenchymal tear that extends into the renal parenchyma and over the collecting system and usually results in extravasation of urine and blood. *Renal fracture* describes a single transection of the kidney into two poles, accompanied by extravasation of urine and blood; *shattered kidney* indicates the presence of renal fractures.[157, 158] Surgery is usually indicated in cases of renal fracture, shattered kidney, or injuries to the vascular pedicles, but the role of surgery in simple renal lacerations is still debated.[157, 160] CT can accurately determine the extent of renal injury preoperatively and may reduce the number of exploratory laparotomies performed to evaluate kidney trauma. However, it appears that reliable CT criteria for the diagnosis of renal vascular

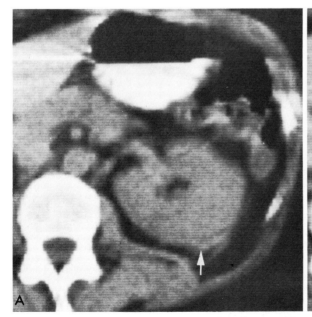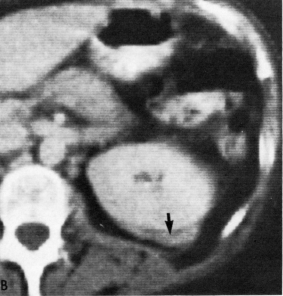

FIGURE 20–59 ■ Subcapsular renal hematoma resulting from renal biopsy. *A,* Precontrast CT scan. A slight irregularity posterior to the kidney is present (*arrow*). The hematoma has a slightly greater density than that of the kidney. *B,* Postcontrast CT scan. The renal parenchyma increases greatly in attenuation value, whereas the hematoma does not. This permits the subcapsular hematoma (*arrow*) to be seen as a lenticular low-density mass.

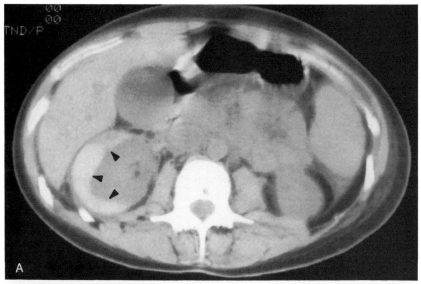

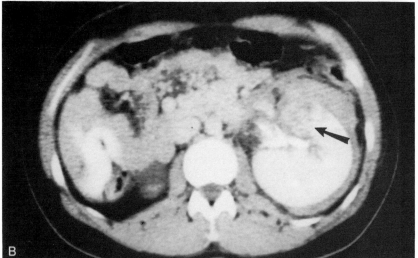

FIGURE 20–60 ■ Perinephric hematoma from a variety of causes. *A,* Precontrast CT scan demonstrates a large lenticular perinephric hematoma (*arrowheads*) that has a high CT attenuation value. The cause was renal biopsy. *B,* Postcontrast CT scan following blunt trauma reveals a perinephric hematoma extending to Gerota's fascia and a laceration of the left kidney (*arrow*). *C,* A large perinephric hematoma (H) containing foci of high CT density (*arrows*), caused by spontaneous hemorrhage from a renal cell carcinoma. The tumor (T) has a calcified rim that simulates a renal cyst.

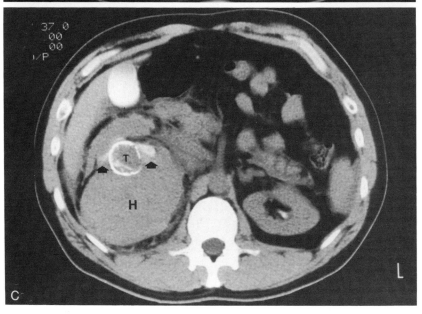

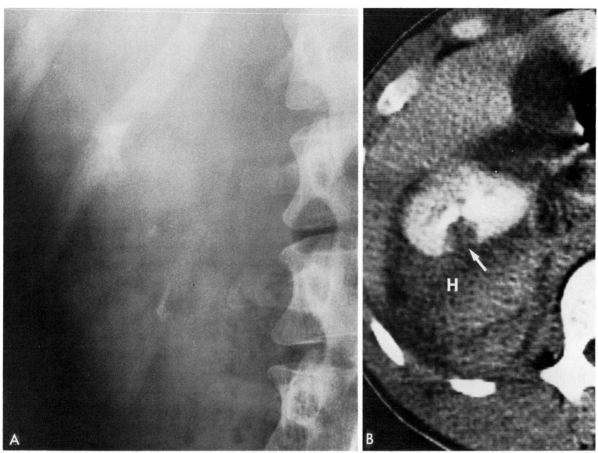

FIGURE 20–61 ■ Renal laceration following blunt trauma. *A,* Poor renal function is shown on the excretory urogram, but the extent of injury cannot be adequately assessed. *B,* A focal laceration (*arrow*) resulting in a large perinephric hematoma (H) is present. The kidney is displaced but has good function. No extravasation of contrast material has occurred. The patient was successfully treated by conservative methods. (From Federle MP: In Federle MP, Brant-Zawadski M (eds): Computed Tomography in the Evaluation of Trauma. © by Williams & Wilkins, Baltimore, 1982. Used with permission.)

FIGURE 20–62 ■ A CT scan following blunt trauma reveals extensive perinephric hemorrhage (H) and extension of the blood into the anterior and posterior pararenal space (*arrows*). There is preservation of renal function, but multiple renal lacerations are present (*arrowheads*).

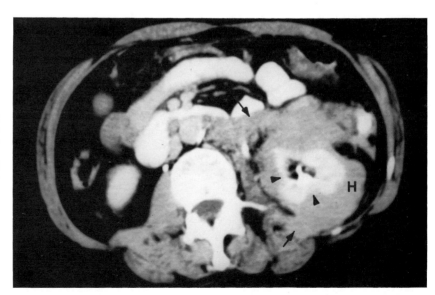

injury are lacking, and thus when renal vascular injury is suspected, an arteriogram should be performed.[160]

INFECTION

Acute renal infection usually produces fever, chills, flank pain, sepsis, nausea, and vomiting. When the renal inflammation primarily affects the connective tissues, it is called *pyelonephritis* to distinguish it from glomerulonephritis.[171] Pathologically, acute pyelonephritis produces kidneys enlarged by edema and "containing foci of intense inflammation."[171] There are microabscesses and white blood cell infiltration throughout the involved interstitial tissue.[171] The process is usually focal, with intervening areas of normal kidney parenchyma.[171, 172]

In acute pyelonephritis, the urographic findings may be normal; minimal and nonspecific abnormalities are identified in only 24 to 28 per cent of patients.[171–173] Caliceal dilatation; diminished ureteral peristalsis; decreased density of nephrogram; delayed caliceal appearance time; generalized enlargement; and focal, patchy, or parenchymal opacification have been reported.[173–178] When the acute infection is more severe, a focal mass demonstrated by excretory urography may represent a frank abscess[171] or a mass without drainable pus (acute focal bacterial nephritis).[171, 179]

The CT findings in acute pyelonephritis depend on the severity of the infection. In most cases, precontrast scans are normal[172] (Fig. 20–63A) or reveal an area of slightly lower density in the renal parenchyma. Postcontrast CT scans demonstrate patchy, linear, radially oriented low-density areas in the renal parenchyma (Figs. 20–63B, C and 20–64) that are absent on the precontrast studies.[172, 178, 179] These focal abnormal zones of renal parenchyma enhancement correspond to similar findings on excretory urography and are thought to represent nonfunctioning nephrons resulting from obstruction or vascular compromise (see Fig. 20–63C).[178–181]

More severe renal infection may extend into the perinephric space, produce a focal renal mass, or develop into a frank abscess (Figs. 20–65 and 20–66). Perinephric extension of infection causes increased density in the perinephric fat, thickens Gerota's fascia, and displaces the kidney. Gas-forming renal infections can result in pelvicaliceal air, gas within a mass (Fig. 20–67A), subcapsular gas (Fig. 20–67B, C), or gas that has extended through the renal capsule into Gerota's fascia or the retroperitoneum.[182, 183] Renal gas must not be equated with infection in patients after embolization of renal tumors, as intratumoral gas can occur in infarcted tissues without evidence of infection.[184, 185]

The term *acute focal bacterial nephritis* is used to describe focal renal enlargement in the clinical setting of acute pyelonephritis.[171, 179] Acute focal bacterial nephritis has also been called *severe acute pyelonephritis*,[175] *focal* or *suppurative pyelonephritis*,[33] acute lobar nephronia,[180] and acute bacterial nephritis.[174] Acute

focal bacterial nephritis produces a solid renal mass with an attenuation value similar to or slightly lower than that of normal parenchyma on precontrast CT scans. The mass is enhanced in a patchy, nonhomogeneous manner after contrast medium injection (see Figs. 20–63 and 20–64). No capsule is demonstrated, and the margin with adjacent renal parenchyma may be poorly defined. The adjacent renal fascia may be thickened, but perinephric extension is absent.[179] Although most of these "masses" heal without residual scarring, focal contour and caliceal abnormalities have been reported.[171]

Although difficult to differentiate by clinical examination and urography, acute focal bacterial nephritis and renal abscess can usually be differentiated by CT. Renal abscesses frequently have a lower attenuation value than normal renal parenchyma on noncontrast scans and either fail to enhance or enhance in a patchy, nonhomogeneous fashion after contrast medium administration (Fig. 20–68). The abscess is often well delineated from the renal parenchyma and may have a thick, irregular wall or an ill-defined margin with adjacent parenchyma. The wall of the abscess may be enhanced after contrast medium injection, but the liquified central part of the abscess does not enhance. Perinephric extension, extension into the renal pelvis, and thickening of the renal fascia are more common in renal abscess than in acute focal bacterial nephritis.[171] Focal scarring and caliceal abnormalities are common after healing.

Although CT distinction between abscess and acute focal bacterial nephritis is usually straightforward, the appearance of either is not pathognomonic. If confirmation is required, a needle aspiration for culture can be safely guided by ultrasound or CT.[186]

Acute diffuse bacterial nephritis is a more severe form of pyelonephritis that frequently occurs in diabetics and immunocompromised patients.[171, 178, 182] In diabetic patients, the CT findings are those of acute pyelonephritis and, rarely, emphysematous pyelonephritis.[182, 183] In patients with leukemia, multiple small renal abscesses caused by fungal infections (Fig. 20–69) can be seen. These small abscesses are best demonstrated by enhanced CT scans and are often associated with similar lesions in the liver and spleen.[187] CT scans after treatment demonstrate resolution of the abscesses.

Aspergillosis[188] and *Torulopsis glabrata*[189] can produce pelvic filling defects, and *Mycobacterium tuberculosis*,[190, 191] *Echinococcus*,[192, 193] and *Actinomyces israelii*[194] can produce renal mass lesions. Renal tuberculosis is often accompanied by renal calcifications or evidence of tuberculosis elsewhere in the chest or abdomen,[190, 194] but absolute distinction from a solid tumor is often not possible by CT alone. CT in xanthogranulomatous pyelonephritis usually demonstrates poor or absent renal function, renal calculi, a mass with an attenuation value similar to that of surrounding kidney, and extension into the perinephric fat (Fig. 20–70).[1, 195–197] By CT criteria alone, xanthogranulomatous pyelonephritis cannot be ab-

Text continued on page 999

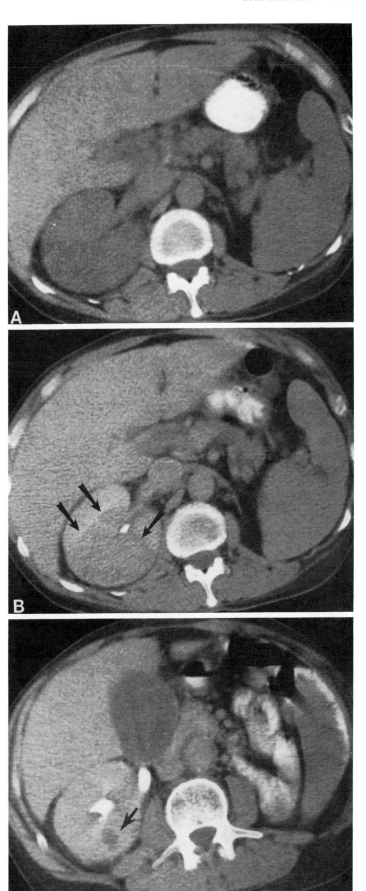

FIGURE 20–63 ■ Acute pyelonephritis. *A,* Precontrast CT scan demonstrates a slightly enlarged right kidney, but no focal abnormalities are seen. *B,* CT scan at the same level demonstrates a focal pie-shaped zone of slightly decreased density (*arrows*). *C,* CT scan at a lower level reveals a focal area of low attenuation (*arrow*) that developed into a renal abscess.

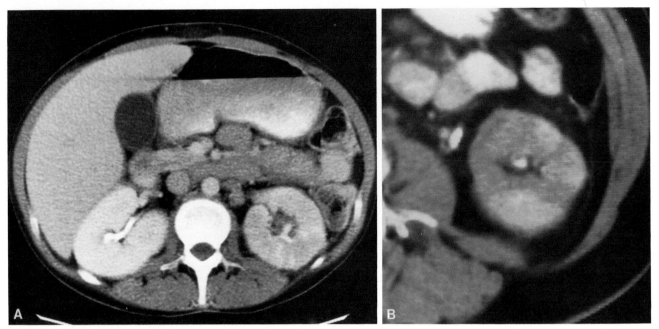

FIGURE 20–64 ■ Acute pyelonephritis affecting the left kidney. *A,* Postcontrast CT scan reveals decreased renal function and patchy, linear, radially oriented low-density areas in the renal parenchyma. *B,* Postcontrast CT scan in another patient clearly demonstrates the patchy, radially oriented zones of decreased attenuation.

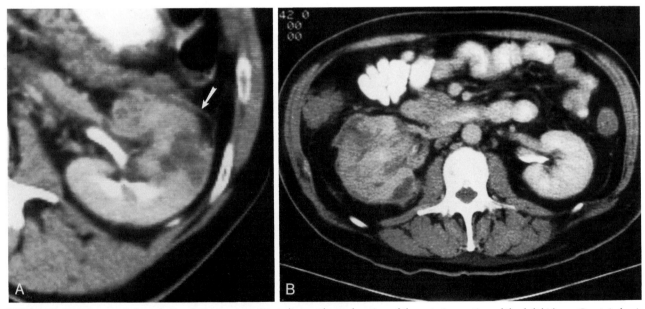

FIGURE 20–65 ■ Severe pyelonephritis. *A,* Postcontrast CT study reveals nonfunction of the anterior portion of the left kidney. Gerota's fascia is thickened (*arrow*), and multiple low-density masses are scattered throughout the renal parenchyma. *B,* Postcontrast CT scan demonstrates enlargement of the right kidney, which has essentially no renal function. Focal low-density areas cannot be distinguished from abscesses.

FIGURE 20–66 ■ Acute bilateral pyelonephritis and renal abscess. There are patchy, triangular areas of decreased renal function radiating into zones of normal renal function (*black arrows*). Some of the hypofunctioning areas of renal parenchyma appear as linear areas, which are radially oriented (*white arrow*). A focal renal abscess (A) is seen as a large low-density mass in the right kidney.

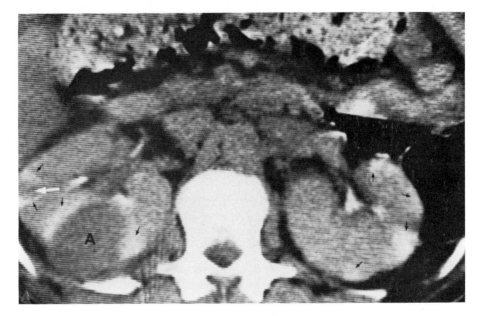

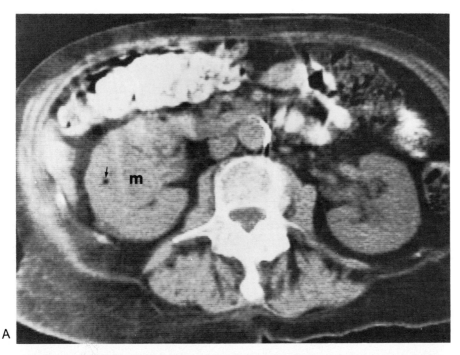

A

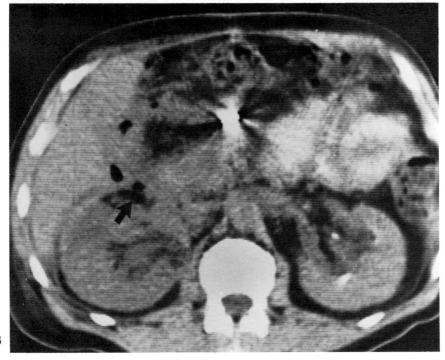

B

FIGURE 20–67 ■ Gas-forming renal abscess. *A,* Precontrast CT scan. There is gross enlargement of the right kidney and a mass (m) obliterating the renal sinus fat, which contains a focus of gas (*arrow*). *B,* Renal abscess with subcapsular gas. Postinfusion CT scan shows an enlarged, poorly functioning right kidney with a collection of gas (*arrow*) in the renal subcapsular space.

FIGURE 20–67 *Continued C,* CT scan during the venous phase. The left renal vein is patent (*white arrow*), but the right renal vein is thrombosed. A renal abscess (A) and a focal area of hypofunction (*arrowhead*) are seen. Subcapsular gas is present (*black arrow*).

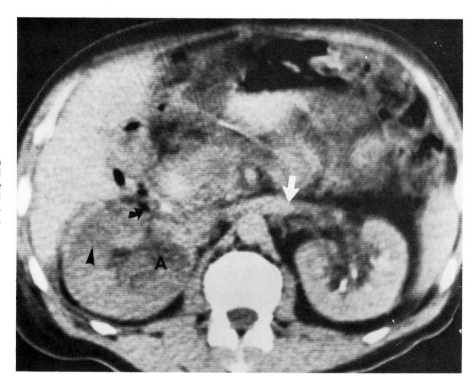

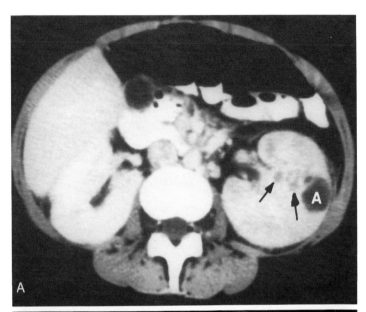

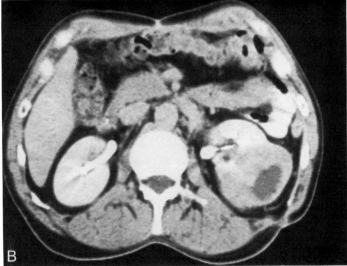

FIGURE 20–68 ■ Renal abscesses. *A*, CT scan demonstrates an enlarged left kidney with a patchy decrease in attenuation value after administration of contrast. There are several small, focal, low-density masses (*arrows*) and one large mass that proved to be an abscess (A). *B*, A large left renal abscess (A) with a thick, irregular wall and a necrotic low-density center. The margin between the abscess and normal renal parenchyma is ill defined.

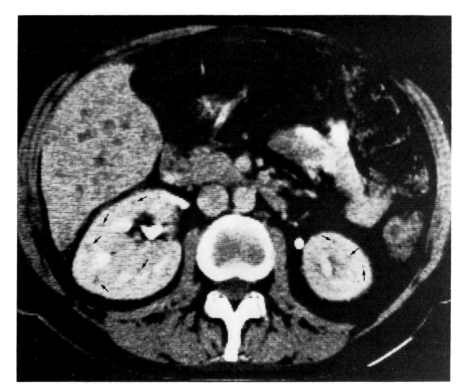

FIGURE 20–69 ■ Fungal infection of the kidneys. Multiple small, rounded, low-density lesions (*arrows*) in both kidneys were proved to be fungal abscesses in an immunosuppressed patient with leukemia. Similar lesions were present in the liver.

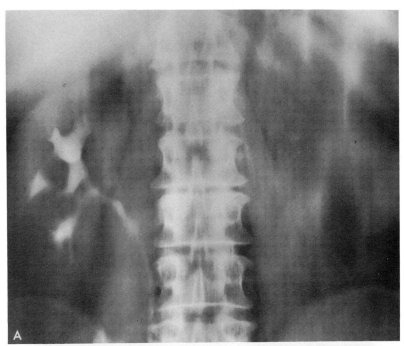

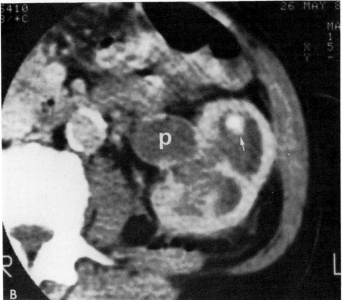

FIGURE 20–70 ■ Xanthogranulomatous pyelone-phritis, global and focal. *A,* Excretory urogram demonstrates nonfunction of the left kidney. *B,* CT scan in global type. There is prolonged opacification of the left renal cortex. The renal pelvis (p) is filled with pus, as are the intrarenal collecting structures. The high-density focus (*arrow*) is a renal calculus. At surgery, xanthogranulomatous pyelonephritis with ureteral obstruction was found.

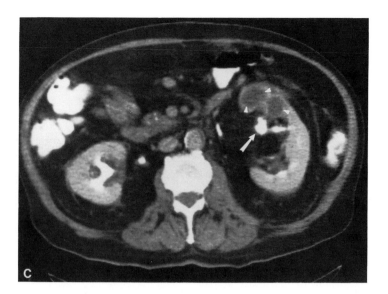

FIGURE 20–70 *Continued C*, CT scan in focal type. An upper pole calculus (*arrow*) is causing focal obstruction of the intrarenal collecting system (*arrowhead*). The posterior portion of the kidney is normal.

solutely distinguished from a renal malignancy or abscess.[198, 199]

Renal echinococcal infection occurs in two per cent of patients with systemic hydatid disease[193] and produces renal cystic lesions with calcification of the cyst wall and daughter cysts of different density within the larger cysts.[192, 193] The fibroblastic wall of the cyst is enhanced after intravenous contrast administration, and the identification of daughter cysts distinguishes hydatid renal disease from simple renal cysts or polycystic renal disease. The most common presentation is a patient with a flank mass; pain and hydatiduria occur when a cyst ruptures into the renal collecting system. Associated findings are liver and lung echinococcal disease.

OBSTRUCTIVE UROPATHY

Obstructive uropathy can result in diminished or absent renal function on excretory urography.[200] Hydronephrosis is readily detected by CT, as the dilated renal collection structures and ureter on nonenhanced scans are low-density structures with attenuation values that approximate that of water.[1, 3, 34, 200] After intravenous contrast is injected, the CT appearance of the collecting system depends on the degree of renal function remaining and the volume and concentration of contrast in the collecting system. Scans usually reveal delayed function on the affected side and little excretion into the renal collecting structures (Fig. 20–71), or there may be an interface between urine and contrast medium, with the contrast medium layering in the dependent portions of the collecting structures. Urinary milk of calcium may occur secondary to chronic urinary tract obstruction. The obstruction may be at the ureteropelvic junction or may be caused by a caliceal diverticulum, pyelogenic cyst, or staghorn calculus.[201, 202] Precontrast CT studies show the high-density milk of calcium in the dependent portion of a dilated urinary collecting system.[201, 202]

The level of obstruction is located by identifying a dilated collecting system down to the site of obstruction.[203] Ureteropelvic junction obstructions result in dilated upper collecting systems and a normal-size ureter, whereas distal ureteral obstructions result in a dilated ureter down to the obstructing lesion (see Fig. 20–71). Nonopaque calculi, fibrosis, and retroperitoneal or pelvic tumors can be correctly diagnosed by CT as the cause of hydronephrosis (see Fig. 20–71).

As obstruction becomes chronic, the renal parenchyma atrophies, caliceal dilatation progresses, and the kidney appears to be little more than a fluid-filled cyst with a thin rim of solid renal tissue (Fig. 20–72). At this stage, renal function is usually very poor or absent and cannot be restored.

CT detects hydronephrosis with a reported accuracy of virtually 100 per cent.[1, 34, 133, 200] However, it may be difficult to detect very early hydronephrosis, because no definite criteria for demonstrating slight degrees of caliceal dilatation have been established.[204]

RENAL FAILURE

Chronic Pyelonephritis ▪ On CT, chronic pyelonephritis is usually manifested by small, contracted kidneys that have broad-based inflammatory scars opposite deformed calices. The scars cause the renal outline to be irregular but do not cause dilatation of the collecting system (Fig. 20–73). Chronic pyelonephritis may affect one kidney predominantly and result in a small, marginally functioning kidney and a scarred cortex as a result of severe focal parenchymal atrophy (Fig. 20–73).

Renal Failure From Miscellaneous Causes ▪ Diffuse parenchymal atrophy, which uniformly involves the entire kidney and results in a small kidney, can occur as a result of renal artery stenosis, glomerulonephritis, or obstructive uropathy. The renal outline is smooth, and there is an apparent increase in the proportion of renal sinus and perinephric fat (Fig. 20–74).[3] The calices are normal in renal artery stenosis and glomerulonephritis but are dilated in atrophy

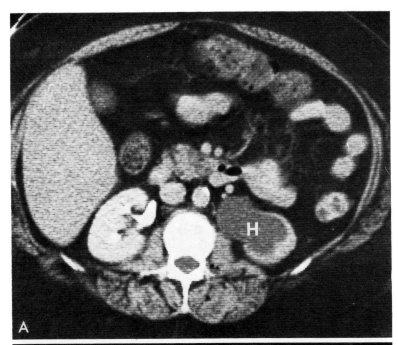

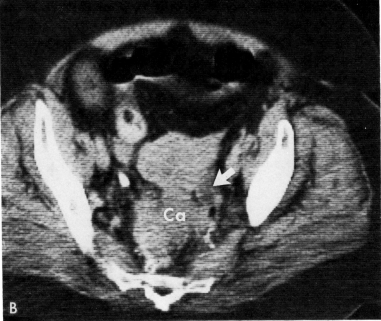

FIGURE 20–71 ■ Chronic ureteral obstruction. *A,* Marked hydronephrosis (H) of the left kidney has resulted in atrophy of the kidney, manifested by cortical thinning, diminished function, and small size. *B,* A dilated left ureter (*arrow*) is seen extending into the pelvis, where it was obstructed by a recurrent carcinoma of the colon (Ca).

FIGURE 20–72 ■ Chronic hydronephrosis, the result of an aortic pseudoaneurysm. The hydronephrotic, poorly functioning left kidney (H) appears as a large urine-filled sac surrounded by a thin rim of atrophied renal cortex (*small arrows*). There has been back-pressure rupture of the collecting system with leak of urine into the perinephric space (*large arrow*). At this stage, irreversible renal damage has occurred.

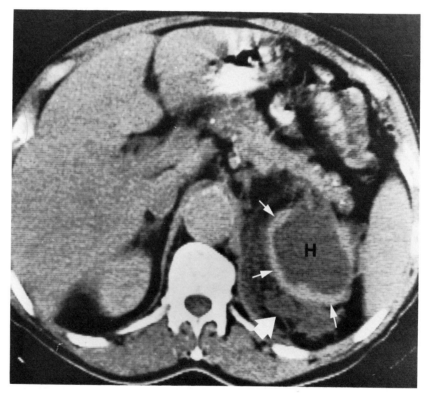

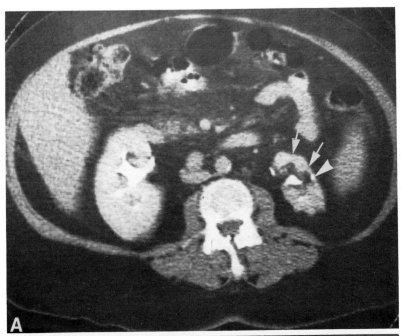

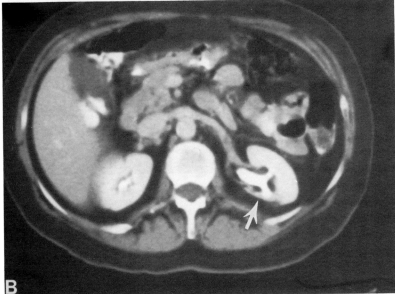

FIGURE 20–73 ■ Chronic pyelonephritis. *A,* The left kidney is small, with marked cortical thinning (*arrows*). Renal function is poor, as evidenced by a diminished nephrogram compared with that for the right kidney. A focus of parenchymal calcification (*arrowhead*) is present in the region of maximal cortical atrophy. No hydronephrosis is noted. The pyelonephritis has been present long enough for the right kidney to hypertrophy. *B,* The left kidney has a broad-based posterior scar (*arrow*), which has resulted in loss of the renal cortex in this region.

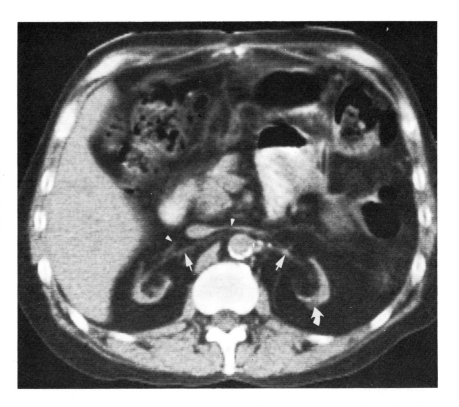

FIGURE 20–74 ■ Glomerulonephritis. Bilateral small, poorly functioning kidneys with a smooth outline are seen; there is also an increase in renal sinus and perinephric fat. Renal arteries (*arrows*) and veins (*arrowheads*) are patent. There is no evidence of hydronephrosis. A small left renal cyst (*curved arrow*) is present.

because of chronic obstruction (see Fig. 20–71). Glomerulonephritis involves both kidneys, but renal artery stenosis and obstructive uropathy can be unilateral or bilateral. Compensating hypertrophy of the involved kidney frequently accompanies unilateral renal atrophy.

Differentiating renal agenesis from a small, nonfunctioning kidney, the result of pyelonephritis, is difficult with urographic techniques. Identification of renal vascular structures is vital (see Fig. 20–71). In right renal agenesis, the right renal vein receives no tributaries and thus does not develop. Identifying the right renal vein by CT excludes a diagnosis of right renal agenesis. On the left side, the left renal vein receives inflow from the left adrenal and gonadal veins; therefore in left renal agenesis, a small vein is always demonstrated as it crosses in front of the aorta and enters the inferior vena cava.[133, 205]

RENAL ISCHEMIA

Renal ischemia resulting from renal parenchymal compression by a perinephric hematoma can cause hypertension. This clinical entity has been called the *Page kidney*,[206] because Page[207] demonstrated that hypertension could be produced in dogs by wrapping the kidney in cellophane.

A perinephric hematoma can result following biopsy, lithotripsy, trauma, or surgery, but infection, arterial diseases, blood disorders, and renal calculi have also been implicated as etiologic factors.[167, 206, 208–210] CT has demonstrated enlargement of the affected kidney and a surrounding perinephric mass of fluid or soft tissue density.[208] Postcontrast scans

show decreased renal function and nonenhancement of a fibrotic band of crescent-shaped perinephric fluid collection. Extensive perinephric adhesions and concentric fibrosis extending to involve the contracted scarred kidney beneath the renal capsule are found at surgery.[20]

Regional renal infarction produced by segmental vascular occlusion produces wedge-shaped areas of decreased density in the renal cortex after contrast medium administration (Fig. 20–75).[211] The low attenuation values are caused in part by nonperfusion of the infarcted tissue by contrast-filled blood and in part by tissue edema. *Global renal infarction* indicates an entire kidney or region of a kidney is infarcted. CT reveals a thin rim of high-attenuation tissue surrounding a central zone of diminished density (Fig. 20–76). The high-density rim represents perfusion of the preserved outer rim of cortex by collateral vessels in the presence of renal artery occlusion.[212]

Polyarteritis nodosa is a focal inflammatory process that predominantly affects small and medium-size arteries. The kidneys are involved in more than 85 per cent of patients, with multiple areas of infarction, arterial aneurysms, and glomerulonephritis being the most common pathologic finding.[213–215] Aneurysms can rupture, resulting in perinephric intrarenal subcapsular or retroperitoneal hemorrhage. On CT, multiple wedge-shaped areas of ischemia or infarction can often be seen.[213, 214] CT also reliably demonstrates the location of spontaneous hemorrhage resulting from aneurysm rupture[214] and also can depict the multiple aneurysms that are the hallmark of the disease.[215] Multiple intrarenal arterial aneurysms can

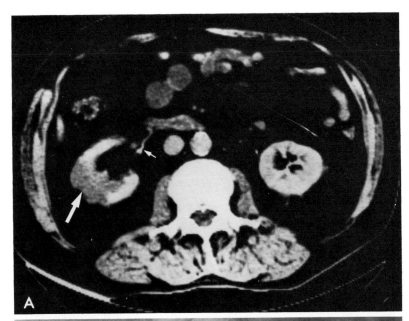

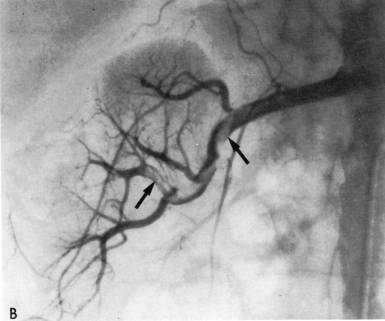

FIGURE 20–75 ■ Renal artery thrombosis following coronary arteriography. *A,* CT scan. A central area of the right kidney (*large arrow*) has no function, whereas other parts of the right kidney function normally. The kidney is not enlarged, the inferior vena cava is patent, and the renal artery (*small arrow*) is small. *B,* Right renal arteriogram demonstrates multiple renal artery filling defects (*arrows*), which proved to be emboli at surgery.

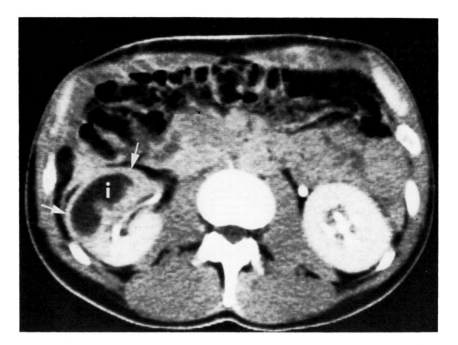

FIGURE 20–76 ■ Global renal infarction. CT scan after contrast medium injection reveals a thin rim of high-attenuation tissue (*arrows*), which surrounds an infarcted area (i) of absent function having an attenuation value near that of water. The high-density rim is thought to be cortex preserved by capsular arteries and collateral vessels.

also be found in drug users and in patients with lupus erythematosis, bacterial endocarditis, Wegener's granulomatosis, and atrial myxoma emboli.[215]

Acute renal cortical necrosis is a rare cause of renal failure in which the renal medulla is spared, but the renal cortex undergoes necrosis. Sepsis, shock, transfusion reactions, toxins, and severe dehydration are the usual clinical problems that produce renal cortical vasoconstriction leading to necrosis of the renal cortex. CT demonstrates a thin rim of tissue with a low attenuation value between the thin capsule and adjacent medulla.[216] If contrast has been administered, it may remain in the medullary space for a long period of time (Fig. 20–77). A persistent nephrogram

may be seen in less severe forms of acute renal failure (Fig. 20–78). These CT findings correlate well with the pathologic features of the disease; thus CT is valuable in confirming the clinical diagnosis and determining the extent of involvement.[216, 217]

Renal vein thrombosis can be produced by a variety of neoplastic, infectious, or metabolic disorders.[218, 219] In animals, acute renal vein thrombosis causes edema and hemorrhage, which produces an enlarged, poorly functioning or nonfunctioning kidney that on follow-up examination shows shrinkage and marked loss of parenchymal tissue.[178, 220] In patients, CT demonstrates an enlarged renal vein containing a filling defect on enhanced CT scans (Figs. 20–36 and

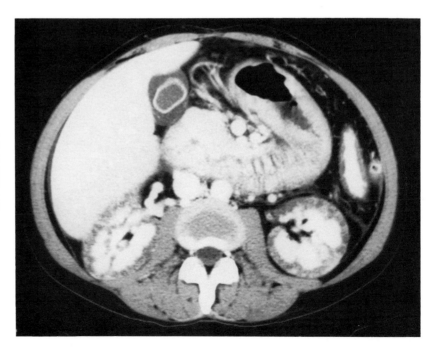

FIGURE 20–77 ■ Acute cortical necrosis occurring in a patient with severe congestive heart failure and dehydration. CT scan reveals contrast remaining in the renal medullary space collecting system and vessels 15 minutes after contrast administration. The cortex has a low CT density. Note the edematous gut with persistent contrast in vascular branches.

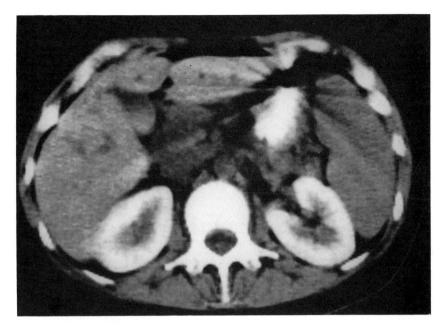

FIGURE 20–78 ■ Acute renal failure. CT scan 45 minutes after intravenous contrast administration reveals a persistent nephrogram, which has a striated appearance. Patient had acute tubular necrosis, and contrast was given inadvertently.

20–79). The thrombosis may be the result of direct tumor extension or nontumorous causes. Idiopathic deep vein thrombosis in an apparently healthy patient can be an early sign of an occult carcinoma.[68] On CT, renal vein thrombosis can produce notching of the ureters by periureteral collateral veins,[221] distention of perinephric veins leading to perinephric "cobwebs," and thickening of the renal fascia.[222]

CONGENITAL LESIONS

Congenital variation in the size, shape, and location of the kidneys is common. Pelvic kidney (Fig. 20–80A); "horseshoe" kidneys (see Fig. 20–80B);[2] intrathoracic kidney;[223] and crossed, fused ectopia are readily detected by CT (Fig. 20–81). Pathologic enlargement of the left kidney can be simulated by splenic compression of the left kidney and by an

ectopic pancreas (see Fig. 20–39).[224] Unexpected motility of the kidneys and alterations in the location of the colon, small bowel, and duodenum can result in malposition of the kidney, which simulates renal displacement by a mass lesion (Figs. 20–82 and 20–83).[224]

Fetal lobulation and compensatory hypertrophy of normal renal parenchyma can produce focal enlargment of the kidney, which simulates a tumor on excretory urography. If the "mass" is the result of fetal lobulation or focal renal hypertrophy (column of Bertin) (see Fig. 20–12), enhanced scans will show the "mass" to be functioning renal parenchyma. If the renal mass is caused by peripelvic lipomatosis, CT will demonstrate the fatty composition of the mass. If the peripelvic tissue contains enough fibrous tissue to raise the density above that of fat, differ-

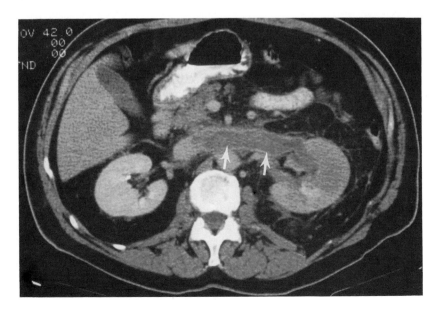

FIGURE 20–79 ■ Renal vein thrombosis resulting from hypercoagulopathy. CT scan after injection of contrast material shows an enlarged left renal view, which contains a large thrombus. There is severely delayed left renal function.

FIGURE 20–80 ■ Congenital variations in renal position or fusion. *A,* A normally functioning pelvic kidney. *B,* A horseshoe kidney fusing anterior to the great vessels in a thin isthmus of renal parenchyma.

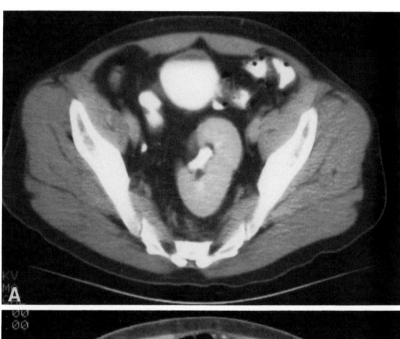

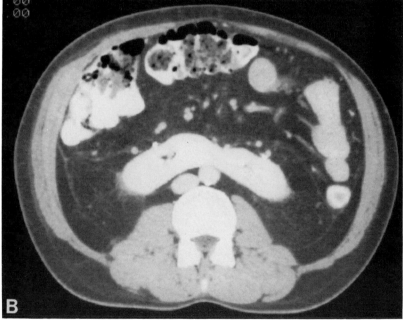

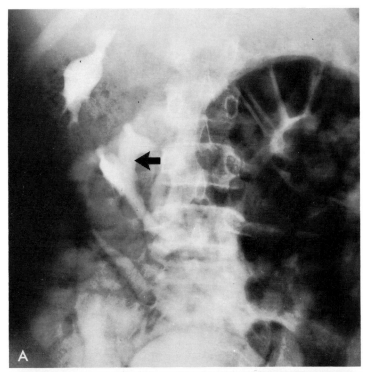

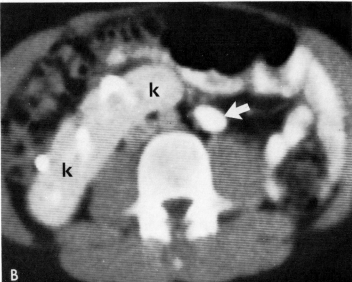

FIGURE 20–81 ■ Crossed-fused renal ectopia in a child with a palpable mass. *A,* Excretory urogram showing the left kidney (*arrow*) to be positioned in the right abdomen. It is not possible to determine whether the left kidney is fused to the lower pole of the right kidney. *B,* CT scan clearly shows the kidneys (k) to be fused. Despite the ectopic position of the left kidney, the left ureter (*arrow*) is in normal position.

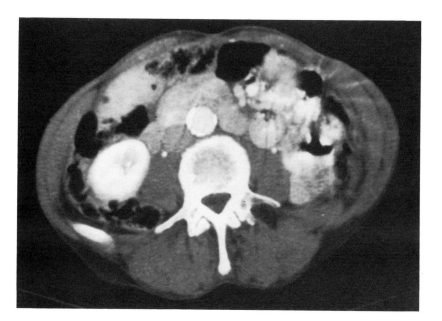

FIGURE 20–82 ■ Colon positioned behind the right kidney. CT scan reveals a gas-filled colon surrounding the right kidney. A blind renal biopsy would be very hazardous in this patient.

entiation from a solid peripelvic mass is difficult. Replacement lipomatosis of the kidney[225] is a sequela of chronic calculous disease and inflammation. There is marked renal atrophy and a marked increase in renal sinus fat, which makes the kidney appear as if it has been replaced by fat.[225] Unlike xanthogranulomatous pyelonephritis, in which the increased lipid content is located in inflammatory foam cells, in replacement lipomatosis there is proliferation of normal fat cells in the renal sinus, hilus, and perinephric space.[225]

Unusual congenital variations of the ureter can be detected by CT scanning. The circumcaval ureter[226] is an anomaly in which the proximal right ureter courses medially behind and then anterior to the inferior vena cava, partially encircling it. Circumcaval

ureter occurs in about one of every 1000 persons, and males are affected two to three times more frequently than females. Ureteral obstruction in varying degrees can be produced, but it is frequently an incidental autopsy finding. CT can demonstrate the retrocaval position of the ureter and the dilated proximal ureter without the need for retrograde urography or an inferior vena cavogram.[226]

CT is useful in determining the cause of ureteral deviations or irregularities, readily demonstrating those that result from congenital variations in location, enlarged psoas muscles, tumors, retroperitoneal fibrosis (Fig. 20–84), aortic aneurysms, lymphadenopathy, or retroperitoneal lipomatosis.[226, 227] Duplications of the ureter are identified as two high-density, rounded structures following contrast ma-

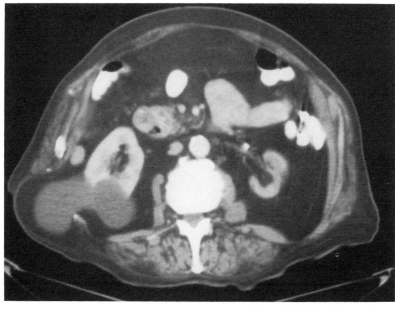

FIGURE 20–83 ■ A congenital defect in the muscular wall of the posterior chest permits herniation of a renal cyst into the flank. The left kidney is atrophic.

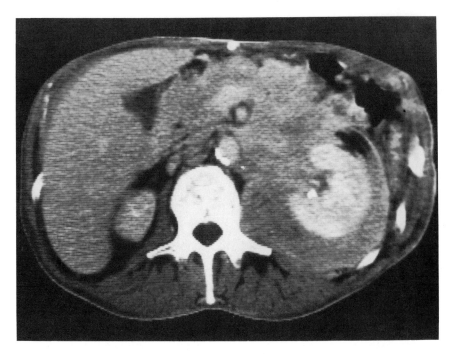

FIGURE 20–84 ■ Retroperitoneal fibrosis. A CT scan demonstrates encasement of the left kidney by a fibrotic mass that extends throughout the perinephric space and into the anterior pararenal space. There is a persistent nephrogram on the left, indicating poor renal function, probably as a result of encasement of the left renal vein and ureter.

terial injection. If one ureter is obstructed, the hydronephrotic part of the kidney (usually the upper pole) is shown on CT (Fig. 20–85) as a water-density mass and the ectopic ureter as a round defect in the urinary bladder.[203] In patients with a bifid renal pelvis or complete duplication of the renal collecting system, an axial CT scan at the juncture zone of the upper and lower poles may reveal a normal-size kidney without any vascular or collecting system elements.[228] Hulnick and Bosniak[228] have termed this appearance the *faceless kidney.*

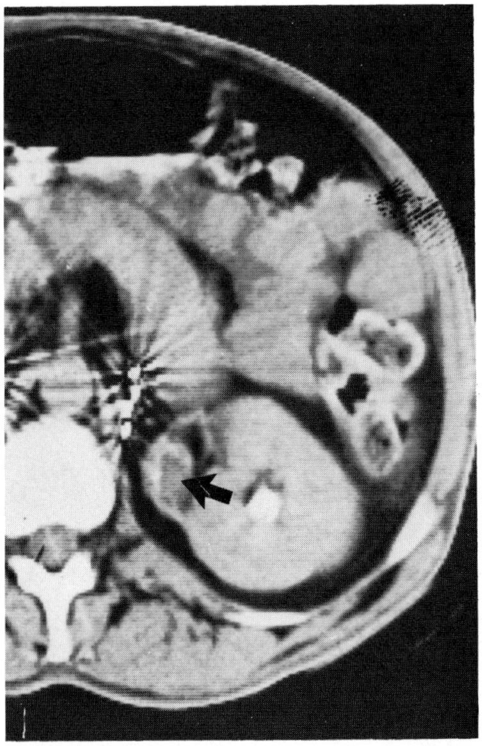

Postsurgical Evaluation

Postnephrectomy

Interpretation of CT scans after nephrectomy demands a knowledge of postnephrectomy anatomy and enough time for postoperative changes to take place. Postoperative complications include hematoma or abscess (Fig. 20–86). Their occurrence must be diagnosed or excluded in the immediate postoperative period. After nephrectomy, small collections of retroperitoneal gas may be detected for a week or more without indicating abscess formation.[229] More important than the mere presence of retroperitoneal gas is whether the quantity of gas is increasing or decreasing. An increase in retroperitoneal gas is more indicative of abscess than the absolute volume of air or the time elapsed since surgery.[229]

After right nephrectomy, the liver and colon shift to occupy the nephrectomy site; the second duodenum becomes located more posteriorly than usual and must not be mistaken for a paracaval tumor mass or recurrent renal neoplasm.[230, 231] After left nephrectomy, the stomach and small bowel fill the renal bed, and the tail of the pancreas falls posteriorly and medially to lie next to the left psoas muscle and aorta, giving the normal pancreas an inverted U shape. Bowel in the empty renal fossa is common,

FIGURE 20–85 ■ Duplicated ureter with obstructed upper pole collecting system. The obstructed collecting system is demonstrated as an oval, small, low-density mass (*arrow*) surrounded by cortical tissue. The nonobstructed portion of the kidney is shown lateral to the obstructed segment. Clip artifacts are present from prior adrenalectomy.

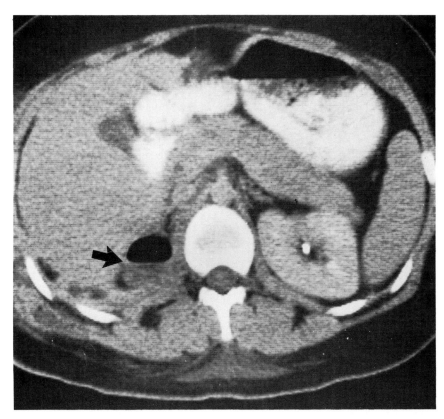

FIGURE 20–86 ■ Postnephrectomy abscess (*arrow*) presents as a mass with an air-fluid level in the right renal fossa.

and unopacified bowel must not be interpreted as an abscess.

Postoperatively, the psoas margins are usually symmetric and are neither enlarged nor irregular.[230] Asymmetry, irregularity, or enlargement of the psoas muscle on the side of the nephrectomy is an important sign of recurrent or residual tumor involvement. Postoperative scar tissue occurs in less than ten per cent of patients who undergo radical nephrectomy,[231] and thus a solid mass in the renal bed must be considered tumorous until proved otherwise (Fig. 20–87).

Following surgical excision of a renal cortical mass, retroperitoneal fat is commonly used to pack the renal defect.[232] The fat used to fill the renal cortical wedge defect can appear as a mass on ultrasonography and requires CT to demonstrate that the "mass" represents only retroperitoneal fat.[232] When a mass is detected, a CT-guided needle biopsy can be used to document or exclude recurrent neoplasm.

Ureteral injury can result from retroperitoneal or pelvic surgery and cause a variety of abnormalities depending on the nature and location of the injury. A ureteroarterial fistula following surgery has been shown to produce an enlarged ureter with a fluid-fluid level in which the dependent layer is hyperdense on noncontrast CT scans, suggesting hemorrhage into the ureter.[233]

Ureteral disruption as a result of pelvic surgery can be shown on CT as hyperdense ascites following contrast administration,[234] whereas in traumatic ureteral disruption the contrast medium extravasation is confined to the medial perinephric space.[235]

Renal Transplants

Although potential complications of renal transplants are best evaluated initially by ultrasonography and radionuclide imaging techniques, CT and MRI can provide additional information in certain patients.[236–239] Urinoma, hematoma, lymphocele, and abscess can be diagnosed (Fig. 20–88) and the relationship of the abnormality to the transplanted kidney accurately demonstrated.[240] Perinephric fluid collections are common in the early posttransplantation period. Lymphoceles are the most common peritransplant fluid collections, typically seen within 2 to 3 weeks of transplantation.[237] The typical location is medial or inferior to the lower pole of the transplanted kidney. Lymphoceles tend to be large and may be septated (see Fig. 20–88). Urinomas occurring shortly after transplantation require some type of surgical or radiologic intervention.[237] Urinomas can result from anastomotic leaks or ureteral leaks caused by vascular injury. Abscesses are less frequent and have no specific features unless gas is detected in a complex fluid collection. Hematomas are found in a subcapsular or perinephric location and have a high CT attenuation value when acute.[237]

Ultrasonography, CT, and MR have been used in an attempt to specifically characterize posttransplant perinephric fluid collections. Urinomas and lympho-

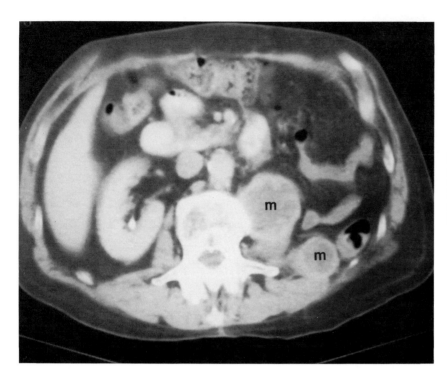

FIGURE 20–87 ■ Recurrent left renal cell carcinoma producing two cystic-appearing masses (m) in the left renal fossa. The tumor recurrence has a thick, slightly hypervascular rim. Nephrectomy had been performed 13 months previously.

FIGURE 20–88 ■ Post–renal transplant lymphocele. The CT scan demonstrates two lymphoceles (L) as homogeneous water-density masses surrounding a normally functioning transplanted kidney (K). The lateral lymphocele protrudes through the abdominal flank muscles.

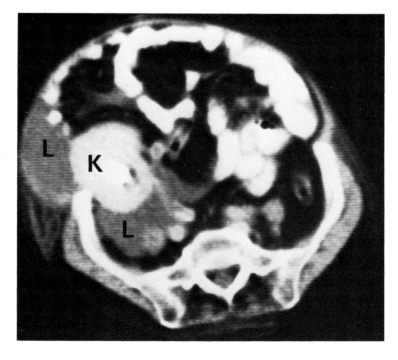

celes have uniform low CT density, are simple fluid collections on ultrasonography, and have low T1 and high T2 values. Abscesses and hematomas are sonographically complex, have mixed CT attenuation values, and tend to have high T1 and T2 values.[237] Although these appearances may be relatively specific, significant overlap occurs, and often a percutaneous aspiration must be performed to confirm a specific diagnosis.

Hydronephrosis shortly after transplantation can be the result of edema at the ureteric implantation site, extrinsic compression of the ureter by a perinephric fluid collection, ureteric blood clots, or calculi. Late ureteric strictures can result from rejection or vascular insufficiency.[237]

Diagnosing transplant rejection is both important and extremely difficult. Many types of rejection occur. Temporally, rejection ranges from hyperacute to chronic (Fig. 20–89), whereas histologic analysis describes vascular and interstitial varieties.[237] The hope that CT, Doppler sonography, or MRI would prove specific in diagnosing rejection reactions and vascular insufficiency (Fig. 20–90) and in separating them from acute tubular necrosis and cyclosporin-induced nephrotoxicity has unfortunately not yet occurred.

Although a variety of sonographic findings in acute rejection have been reported, the specificity and sensitivity of each is still incompletely understood. Early reports of MRI were encouraging, with loss of the corticomedullary junction on T1-weighted images being heralded as highly diagnostic of acute rejection.[238, 239] However, further investigations have demonstrated considerable overlap of diagnostic results.[237, 241–244] Consequently, more investigation is needed to better define the role of MRI, MR spectroscopy, and Doppler ultrasonography in the diagnosis of transplant rejection.

End-Stage Kidney Disease

Because of advances in dialysis technology and renal transplantation, patients with end-stage renal failure commonly survive for long periods of time. The native kidneys of some patients maintained on dialysis or transplantation have been found to undergo marked changes. Multiple renal cysts develop in 27 to 47 per cent of patients on long-term dialysis, a condition termed *acquired cystic disease*.[13, 245, 247] These cysts involve primarily the renal cortex, and most are less than 2 cm in diameter. Solid renal tumors, often multiple, occur in 10 to 20 per cent of patients, and although most of these appear benign, some have a definite malignant behavior.[13, 245–247] Hughson et al. reported a 5.8 per cent incidence of renal cell carcinoma in patients with acquired cystic disease,[248] but renal cell carcinoma also occurs without cystic change (Fig. 20–91). Spontaneous subcapsular and perinephric hemorrhage has also been found to be an unexpected complication of acquired cystic disease in patients with end-stage kidney disease.[13, 245–247] These patients usually present with flank pain, and CT readily confirms the diagnosis of acute hemorrhage. CT also demonstrates the underlying cystic disease and may detect an underlying renal malignancy. Another complication of long-term dialysis or renal transplant rejection is diffuse cortical

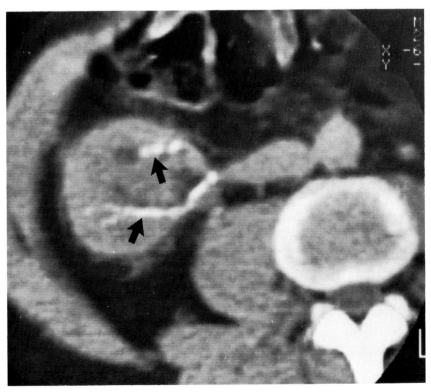

FIGURE 20–89 ■ Long-standing renal transplant failure. CT scan following bolus injection of contrast material demonstrates no function of the right renal transplant. There is extensive calcification of the renal arteries (*arrows*).

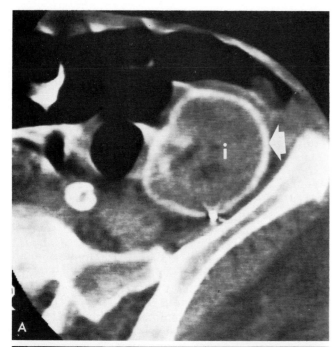

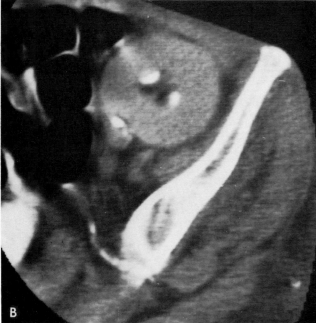

FIGURE 20–90 ■ Vascular insufficiency resulting in regional infarction of transplanted kidney. *A,* CT scan demonstrates a thin rim of tissue having a high attenuation value (*arrow*) surrounding an area of renal infarction (i) that has a CT density of water in the upper pole of the transplanted kidney. *B,* The lower pole of the transplant functions normally. Total occlusion of the arterial branch to the upper pole of the kidney was found at surgery.

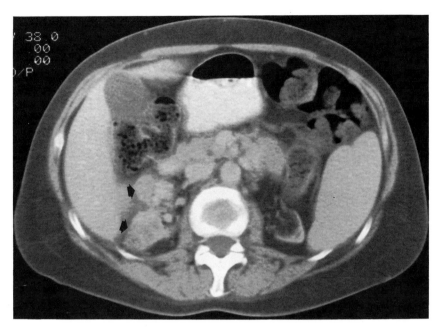

FIGURE 20–91 ■ Renal cell carcinoma in native right kidney after renal transplantation. CT scan reveals a multilobulated right renal mass (*arrows*) proven to be renal cell carcinoma. Note the small, nonfunctioning left kidney and lack of cystic changes following transplantation.

calcification.[249, 250] The calcification is the result of oxalate crystal deposition in the cortical tubules.[249, 250] A similar finding has been reported after methoxyflurane administration,[251] congenital oxalosis,[251–253] cortical glomerulonephritis, cortical necrosis, Alport's syndrome, Fabry's disease, sickle cell disease, and the nail-patella syndrome.[254] The appearance of diffuse cortical calcification must be differentiated from the delayed, markedly dense, striated nephrogram seen on CT in patients with impending acute renal failure (see Fig. 20–78).[255]

References

1. Sagel SS, Stanley RJ, Levitt RG, Geisse G: Computed tomography of the kidney. Radiology 124:359, 1977.
2. Love L, Reynes CJ, Churchill R, Moncada R: Third generation CT scanning in renal disease. Radiol Clin North Am 17:77, 1979.
3. Hattery RR, Williamson B, Stephens DH, Sheedy PF II, Hartman GW: Computed tomography of renal abnormalities. Radiol Clin North Am 15:401, 1977.
4. Williamson B, Hattery RR, Stephens DS, Sheedy PF: Computed tomography of the kidneys. Semin Roentgenol 13:249, 1978.
5. Newhouse JH, Prien EL, Amis ES Jr, Dretter SP, Pfister RC: Computed tomographic analysis of urinary calculi. AJR 142:545–548, 1984.
6. Gatewood OMB, Fishman EK, Burrow CR, Walker WG, Goldman SM, Siegelman SS: Renal vein thrombosis in patients with nephrotic syndrome: CT diagnosis. Radiology 159:117–122, 1986.
7. Johnson CD, Dunnick NR, Cohan RH, Illescas FF: Renal adenocarcinoma: CT staging of 100 tumors. AJR 148:59–63, 1987.
8. Kenney PJ, Stanley RJ: Computed tomography of ureteral tumors. J Comput Assist Tomogr 11(1):102–107, 1987.
9. Federle MP, Brown TR, McAninch JW: Penetrating renal trauma: CT evaluation. J Comput Assist Tomogr 11(6):1026–1030, 1987.
10. Yousem DM, Gatewood OMG, Goldman SM, Marshall FF: Synchronous and metachronous transitional cell carcinoma of the urinary tract: prevalence, incidence, and radiographic detection. Radiology 167:613–618, 1988.
11. Sacks D, Banner MP, Meranze SG, Burke DR, Robinson M, McLean GK: Renal and related retroperitoneal abscesses: percutaneous drainage. Radiology 167:447–451, 1988.
12. Birnbaum BA, Bosniak MA, Megibow AJ, Lubat E, Gordon RB: Observations on the growth of renal neoplasms. Radiology 176:695–701, 1990.
13. Levine E, Slusher SL, Grantham JJ, Wetzel LH: Natural history of acquired renal cystic disease in dialysis patients: a prospective longitudinal CT study. AJR 156:501–506, 1991.
14. Meyers MA: Dynamic Radiology of the Abdomen in Normal and Pathologic Anatomy. Heidelberg, Springer, 1976, pp 113–194.
15. Love L, Meyers MA, Churchill RJ, Reynes CJ, Moncada R, Gibson D: Computed tomography of extraperitoneal spaces. AJR 136:781, 1981.
16. Parienty RA, Pradel J, Picard JD, Ducellier R, Lubrano JM, Smolarski N: Visibility and thickening of the renal fascia on computed tomograms. Radiology 139:119, 1981.
17. Raptopoulos V, Kleinman PK, Marks S, Snyder M, Silverman PM: Renal fascial pathway: posterior extension of pancreatic effusions within the anterior pararenal space. Radiology 158:367–374, 1986.
18. McClennan BL, Lee JKT, Peterson RR. Anatomy of the perirenal area. Radiology 158:555–557, 1986.
19. Dodds WJ, Darweesh RMA, Lawson TL, Stewart ET, Foley WD, et al: The retroperitoneal spaces revisited. AJR 147:1155–1161, 1986.
20. Love L, Demos TC, Posniak H: CT of retrorenal fluid collections. AJR 145:87–91, 1985.
21. Kunin M: Bridging septa of the perinephric space: anatomic, pathologic, and diagnostic considerations. Radiology 158:361–365, 1986.
22. Kneeland JB, Auh YH, Rubenstein WA, Zirinsky K, Morrison H, et al: Perirenal spaces: CT evidence for communication across the midline. Radiology 16:657–664, 1986.
23. Siegelman SS, Copeland BE, Saba BE, Cameron JL, Sanders RC, Zerhouni EA: CT of fluid collections associated with pancreatitis. AJR 134:1121, 1980.
24. Chesbrough RM, Burkhard TK, Martinez AJ, Burks DD: Gerota versus Zuckerkandl: the renal fascia revisited. Radiology 173:845–846, 1989.
25. Somogyi J, Cohne WN, Omar MM, Makhuli Z: Communication of right and left perirenal spaces demonstrated by computed tomography. J Comput Assist Tomogr 3:270, 1979.
26. Mitchell GAG: Renal fascia. Br J Surg 37:257, 1950.

27. Gerota D: Beiträge zur Kenntniss des Befestigungsapparates der Niere. Arch f Anat u Entwicklungsgesch Leipz, 1895, pp 265–285.

28. Moss AA, Cann CE, Friedman MA, Brito AC: Determination of liver, kidney and spleen volumes by computed tomography: an experimental study in dogs. J Comput Assist Tomogr 5:12, 1981.

29. Gourtsoyiannis H, Prassopoulos P, Cavouras D, Pantelidis H: The thickness of the renal parenchyma decreases with age: a CT study of 360 patients. AJR 155:541–544, 1990.

30. Buschi AJ, Harrison RB, Brenbridge ANAG, Williamson BRJ, Gentry RR, Cole R: Distended left renal vein: CT/sonographic normal variant. AJR 135:339, 1980.

31. Royal SA, Callen PW: CT evaluation of anomalies of the inferior vena cava and left renal vein. AJR 132:759–763, 1979.

32. Ishikawa I, Onouchi Z, Saito Y, Kitada H, Shinoda A, et al: Renal cortex visualization and analysis of dynamic CT curves of the kidney. J Comput Assist Tomogr 5:695, 1981.

33. Heinz ER, Dubois PJ, Drayer BP, Hill R: A preliminary investigation of the role of dynamic computed tomography in renovascular hypertension. J Comput Assist Tomogr 4:63, 1980.

34. Engelstad BL, McClennan BL, Levitt RG, Stanley RJ, Sagel SS: The role of pre-contrast images in computed tomography of the kidney. Radiology 136:153, 1980.

35. Zeman RK, Cronan JJ, Rosenfield AT, Lynch JH, Jaffe MH, Clark LR: Renal cell carcinoma: dynamic thin-section CT assessment of vascular invasion and tumor vascularity. Radiology 167:393–396, 1988.

36. Lang EK: Angio-computed tomography and dynamic computed tomography in staging of renal cell carcinoma. Radiology 151:149–155, 1984.

37. Turner RJ, Young SW, Castellino RA: Dynamic continuous computed tomography: study of retroaortic left renal vein. J Comput Assist Tomogr 4:109, 1980.

38. Brennan RE, Curtis JA, Pollack HM, Weinberg I: Sequential changes in the CT numbers of the normal canine kidney following intravenous contrast administration: II. The renal medulla. Invest Radiol 14:239, 1979.

39. Love L, Lind JA, Olson MC: Persistent CT nephrogram: significance in the diagnosis of contrast nephropathy. Radiology 172:125–129, 1989.

40. Kissane JM: The morphology of renal cystic disease. Perspect Nephrol Hypertension 4:31, 1976.

41. Elkin M: Renal cystic disease. In Elkin M (ed): Radiology of the Urinary System. Boston, Little, Brown & Company, 1980, pp 912–966.

42. McClennan BL, Stanley RJ, Nelson GL, Levitt RG, Sagel SS: CT of the renal cyst: is cyst aspiration necessary? AJR 133:671, 1979.

43. Segal AJ, Spitzer RM: Pseudo thick-walled renal cyst by CT. AJR 132:827, 1979.

44. Papanicolaou N, Pfister RC, Yoder IC: Spontaneous and traumatic rupture of renal cysts: diagnosis and outcome. Radiology 160:99–103, 1986.

45. Mayer DP, Baron RL, Pollack HM: Increase in CT attenuation values of parapelvic renal cysts after retrograde pyelography. AJR 139:991–993, 1982.

46. Shanser JD, Hedgcock MW, Korobkin M: Transit of contrast material into renal cysts following urography or arteriography. Abstract. AJR 130:584, 1978.

47. Fishman MC, Pollack HM, Arger PH, Banner MP: High protein content: another cause of CT hyperdense benign renal cyst. J Comput Assist Tomogr 7(6):1103–1106, 1983.

48. Dunnick NR, Korobkin M, Silverman PM, Forster WL: Computed tomography of high density renal cysts. J Comput Assist Tomogr 8(3):458–461, 1984.

49. Nussbaum A, Hunter TB, Stables DP: Spontaneous cyst rupture on renal CT. AJR 142:751–752, 1984.

50. Sussman S, Cochran ST, Pagani JJ, McArdle C, Wong W, et al: Hyperdense renal masses: a CT manifestation of hemorrhagic renal cysts. Radiology 150:207–211, 1984.

51. Levine E, Grantham JJ: High-density renal cysts in autosomal dominant polycystic kidney disease demonstrated by CT. Radiology 154:477–482, 1985.

52. Meziane MA, Fishman EK, Goldman SM, Friedman AC, Siegelman SS: Computed tomography of high density renal cysts in adult polycystic kidney disease. J Comput Assist Tomogr 10(5):767–770, 1986.

53. Morag B, Rubinstein ZJ, Hertz M, Soloman A: Computed tomography in the diagnosis of renal parapelvic cysts. J Comput Assist Tomogr 7(5):833–836, 1983.

54. Ambos MA, Bosniak MA, Gordon R, Madayag MA: Replacement lipomatosis of the kidney. AJR 130:1087, 1978.

55. Bosniak MA: The current radiological approach to renal cysts. Radiology 158:1–10, 1986.

56. Segal AJ, Spataro RF: Computed tomography of adult polycystic disease. J Comput Assist Tomogr 6(4):777–780, 1982.

57. Takao R, Amamoto Y, Matsunaga N, Tasaki T, Kakimoto S, et al: Computed tomography of multicystic kidney. J Comput Assist Tomogr 4:548, 1980.

58. Hayden CK, Swischuk LE, Smith TH, Armstrong EA: Renal cystic disease in childhood. RadioGraphics 6:97–116, 1986.

59. Nussbaum AR, Hartman DS, Whitley N, McCauley RGK, Sanders RC: Multicystic dysplasia and crossed renal ectopia. AJR 149:407–410, 1987.

60. Banner MP, Pollack HM, Chatlen J, Witzleben C: Multilocular renal cysts: radiologic pathologic correlation. AJR 136:239, 1981.

61. Parienty RA, Pradel J, Imbert MC, Picard JD, Savart P: Computed tomography of multilocular cystic nephroma. Radiology 140:135, 1981.

62. Carlson DH, Carlson D, Simon H: Benign multilocal cystic nephroma AJR 131:621, 1978.

63. Hartman DS, Davis CJ, Sanders RC, Maj TTJ, Smirniotopoulos J, Goldman SM: The multiloculated renal mass: considerations and differential features. RadioGraphics 7(1):29–52, 1987.

64. Madewell JE, Goldman SM, Davis CJ, Hartman DS, Feigin DS, Lichtenstein JE: Multilocular cystic nephroma: a radiologic-pathologic correlation of 58 patients. Radiology 146:309–321, 1983.

65. Elkin M: Tumors of the kidney. In Elkin M (ed): Radiology of the Urinary System. Boston, Little, Brown & Company, 1980, pp 296–397.

66. Belville JS, Morgentaler A, Loughlin KR, Tumeh SS: Spontaneous perinephric and subcapsular renal hemorrhage: evaluation with CT, US, and angiography. Radiology 172:733–738, 1989.

67. Davis JM, McLaughlin AP: Spontaneous renal hemorrhage due to cyst rupture: CT findings. AJR 148:763–764, 1987.

68. Aderka D, Brown A, Zelikovski A, Pinkhas J: Idiopathic deep vein thrombosis in an apparently healthy patient as a premonitory sign of occult cancer. Cancer 57:1846–1849, 1986.

69. Fill WL, Lamiell JM, Polk NO: The radiographic manifestations of von Hippel-Lindau disease. Radiology 133:289, 1979.

70. Levine E, Lee KR, Weigel JW, Farber B: Computed tomography in the diagnosis of renal carcinoma complicating von Hippel-Lindau syndrome. Radiology 130:703, 1979.

71. Levine E, Leek KR, Weigel J: Preoperative determination of abdominal extent of renal cell carcinoma by computed tomography. Radiology 132:395, 1979.

72. Zagoria RJ, Wolfman NT, Karstaedt N, Hinn GC, Dyer RB, Chen YM: CT features of renal cell carcinoma with emphasis on relation to tumor size. Invest Radiol 25:261–266, 1990.

73. Smith SJ, Bosniak MA, Megibow AJ, Hulnick DH, Horii SC, Raghavendra BJ: Renal cell carcinoma: earlier discovery and increased detection. Radiology 170:699–703, 1989.

74. Curry NS, Schabel SI, Betsill WL: Small renal neoplasms: diagnostic imaging, pathologic features, and clinical course. Radiology 158:113–117, 1986.

75. Coleman BG, Arger PH, Mintz MC, Pollack HM, Banner MP: Hyperdense renal masses: a computed tomographic dilemma. AJR 143:291–294, 1984.

76. Rosenberg ER, Korobkin M, Foster W, Silverman PM, Bowie JD, Dunnick NR: The significance of septations in a renal cyst. AJR 144:593–595, 1985.

77. Weymen PJ, McClennan BL, Lee JKT, Stanley RJ: CT of calcified renal masses. AJR 138:1095, 1982.

78. Sussman SK, Glickstein MF, Krzymowski MD: Hypointense

renal cell carcinoma: MR imaging with pathologic correlation. Radiology 177:495–497, 1990.

79. Quint LE, Glazer GM, Chenevert TI: In vivo and in vitro MR imaging of renal tumors: histopathologic correlation and pulse sequence optimization. Radiology 169:359–362, 1988.

80. Love L, Churchill R, Reynes C: Computed tomography staging of renal carcinoma. Urol Radiol 1:3, 1979.

81. Robson CJ: The results of radical nephrectomy for renal cell carcinoma. J Urol 146:1173–1177, 1969.

82. McClennan BL: Computed tomography in the diagnosis and staging of renal cell carcinoma. Semin Urol 3:111–131, 1985.

83. Reis M, Fario V: Renal carcinoma: reevaluation of prognostic factors. Cancer 61:1192–1199, 1988.

84. Press GA, McClennan BL, Melson GL, Weyman PJ, Mauro MA, Lee JKT: Papillary renal cell carcinoma: CT and sonographic evaluation. AJR 143:1005–1009, 1984.

85. Shirkhoda A, Lewis E: Renal sarcoma and sarcomatoid renal cell carcinoma: CT and angiographic features. Radiology 162:353–357, 1987.

86. Amendola MA, Bree RL, Pollack HM, Francis IRF, Glazer GM, et al: Small renal cell carcinomas: resolving a diagnostic dilemma. Radiology 166:637–641, 1988.

87. Weyman PJ, McClennan BL, Stanley RJ, Levitt RG, Sagel SS: Comparison of computed tomography and angiography in the evaluation of renal cell carcinoma. Radiology 137:417, 1980.

88. Thomas JL, Bernardino ME: Neoplastic-induced renal vein enlargement: sonographic detection. AJR 136:75, 1981.

89. Winfield AC, Gerlock AJ Jr, Shaff MI: Perirenal cobwebs: a CT sign of renal vein thrombosis. J Comput Assist Tomogr 5:705, 1981.

90. Zimmer WD, Williamson B, Hartman GW, Hattery RR, O'Brien PC: Changing patterns in the evaluation of renal masses: economic implications. AJR 143:285–289, 1984.

91. Fein AB, Lee JKT, Balfe DM, Heiken JP, Ling D, et al: Diagnosis and staging of renal cell carcinoma: a comparison of MR imaging and CT. AJR 148:749–753, 1987.

92. Patel SK, Stack CM, Turner DA: Magnetic resonance imaging in staging of renal cell carcinoma. RadioGraphics 7:703–728, 1987.

93. Eilenberg SS, Lee JKT, Brown JJ, Mirowitz SA, Tartar VM: Renal masses: evaluation with gradient-echo Gd-DTPA-enhanced dynamic MR imaging. Radiology 176:333–338, 1990.

94. Choyke PL: MR imaging in renal cell carcinoma. Radiology 169:2:572–578, 1988.

95. Hricak H, Thoeni RF, Carroll PR, Demas BE, Marotti M, Tanagho EA: Detection and staging of renal neoplasms: a reassessment of MR imaging. Radiology 166:643–649, 1988.

96. Marotti M, Hricak H, Fritzsche P, Crooks LE, Hedgcock MW, Tanagho EA: Complex and simple renal cysts: comparative evaluation with MR imaging. Radiology 162:679–684, 1987.

97. Lee KR, Wulfsberg E, Kepes JJ: Some important radiologic aspects of the kidney in Hippel-Lindau syndrome: the value of prospective study in an affected family. Radiology 122:649, 1977.

98. Levine E, Huntrakoon M, Wetzel LH: Small renal neoplasms: clinical, pathologic and imaging features. AJR 153:69–73, 1989.

99. Choyke PL, Filling-Katz MR, Shawker TH, Gorin MB, Travis WD, et al: Von Hippel-Lindau disease: radiologic screening for visceral manifestations. Radiology 174:815–820, 1990.

100. Reiman RAH, Siegal MJ, Shackelford GD: Wilms' tumor in children: abdominal CT and ultrasound evaluation. Radiology 160:501–505, 1986.

101. Cohen MD: Kidneys. In Siegel MJ (ed): Pediatric Body CT. New York, Churchill Livingstone, 1988, pp 135–175.

102. Fishman EK, Hartman DS, Goldman SM, Siegelman SS: The CT appearance of Wilms tumor. J Comput Assist Tomogr 7:659–665, 1983.

103. Johnson KM, Horvath LJ, Gaisie G, Mesrobian HG, Koepke JF, Askin FB: Wilms tumor occurring as a botryoid renal pelvicalyceal mass. Radiology 163:385–386, 1987.

104. Belt TG, Cohen ME, Smith JA, Cory DA, McKenna S, Weetman R: MRI of Wilms' tumor: promise as the primary imaging method. AJR 146:955–961, 1986.

105. Bosniak MA, Megibow AJ, Hulnick DH, Horii S, Raghavendra BN: CT diagnosis of renal angiomyolipoma: the importance of detecting small amounts of fat. AJR 151:497–501, 1988.

106. Lipman JC, Loughlin K, Tumeh SS: Bilateral renal masses in a pregnant patient with tuberous sclerosis. Invest Radiol 22(11):912–915, 1987.

107. Farrow GM, Harrison EG Jr, Utz DC, Jones DR: Renal angiomyolipomas: a clinical pathologic study of 32 cases. Cancer 22:564, 1968.

108. Bosniak MA: Angiomyolipoma (hamartoma) of the kidney: a preoperative diagnosis is possible in virtually every case. Urol Radiol 3:135–138, 1981.

109. Bret PM, Bretagnolle M, Gaillard D, Plauchu H, Labadie M, et al: Small, asymptomatic angiomyolipomas of the kidney. Radiology 154:7–12, 1985.

110. Hansen GC, Hoffman RB, Sample WF, Becker R: Computed tomography diagnosis of renal angiomyolipoma. Radiology 128:789, 1978.

111. Totty WG, McClennan BL, Nelson GL, Patel R: Relative value of computed tomography and ultrasonography in the assessment of renal angiomyolipoma. J Comput Assist Tomogr 5:173, 1981.

112. Frija J, Larde D, Belloir C, Botto H, Martin N, Vasile N: Computed tomography diagnosis of renal angiomyolipoma. J Comput Assist Tomogr 4:843, 1980.

113. Gentry LR, Gould HR, Alter AJ, Wegenke JD, Atwell DT: Hemorrhagic angiomyolipoma: demonstration by computed tomography. J Comput Assist Tomogr 5:861, 1981.

114. Pitts WR Jr, Kazam E, Gray G, Vaughan ED Jr: Ultrasonography, computed transaxial tomography and pathology of angiomyolipoma of the kidney: solution to diagnostic dilemma. J Urol 124:907, 1980.

115. Kutcher R, Rosenblatt R, Mitsudo SM, Goldman M, Kogan S: Renal angiomyolipoma with sonographic demonstration of extension into the inferior vena cava. Radiology 143:755, 1982.

116. Parvey LS, Warner RM, Calliham TR, Magill HL: CT demonstration of fat tissue in malignant renal neoplasms: atypical Wilms' tumors. J Comput Assist Tomogr 5:851, 1981.

117. Curry MS, Schabel SI, Garvin AJ, Fish G: Intratumoral fat in a renal oncocytoma mimicking angiomyolipoma. AJR 154:307–308, 1990.

118. Hartman DS, Goldman SM, Friedman AC, Davis CJ, Madewell JE, Sherman JL: Angiomyolipoma: ultrasonic-pathologic correlation. Radiology 139:451, 1981.

119. Lautin FM, Gordon PM, Friedman AC, McCormick JF, Fromowitz FB, et al: Radionuclide imaging and computed tomography in renal oncocytoma. Radiology 138:185, 1981.

120. Levine E, Huntrakoon M: Computed tomography of renal oncocytoma. AJR 141:741–746, 1983.

121. Wasserman NF, Ewing SL: Calcified renal oncocytoma. AJR 141:747–749, 1983.

122. Velasquez G, Glass TA, D'Souze JD, Formanek AG: Multiple oncocytomas and renal carcinoma. AJR 142:123–124, 1984.

123. Quinn MJ, Hartman DS, Friedman AC, Sherman JL, Lautin EM, et al: Renal oncocytoma: new observations. Radiology 153:49–53, 1984.

124. Goiney RC, Goldenberg L, Cooperberg PL, Charboneau JW, Rosenfield AT, et al: Renal oncocytoma: sonographic analysis of 14 cases. AJR 143:1001–1004, 1984.

125. Scully RE, Mark EJ, McNeely BU: Case records of the Massachusetts General Hospital. N Engl J Med 313:1596–1603, 1985.

126. Demos TC, Malone AJ: Computed tomography of a giant renal oncocytoma. J Comput Assist Tomogr 12:889–890, 1988.

127. Jacobs JE, Sussman SK, Glickstein MF: Renal lymphangiomyoma—a rare cause of a multiloculated renal mass. AJR 152:307–308, 1989.

128. Cornimier P, Patel SK, Turner DA, Hoeksema J: MR imaging findings in renal medullary fibroma. AJR 153:83–84, 1989.

129. Rubin BE: Computed tomography in the evaluation of renal lymphoma. J Comput Assist Tomogr 3:759, 1979.

130. Lalli AF: Lymphoma and the urinary tract. Radiology 93:1051, 1969.

131. Richmond J, Sherman RS, Diamond HD, Craver LF: Renal lesions associated with malignant lymphomas. Am J Med 32:184, 1962.
132. Hartman DS, Davidson AJ, Davis CJ, Goldman SM: Infiltrative renal lesions: CT-sonographic-pathologic correlation. AJR 150:1061–1064, 1988.
133. Forbes W St C, Isherwood I, Fawcitt RA: Computed tomography in the evaluation of the solitary or unilateral nonfunctioning kidney. J Comput Assist Tomogr 2:389, 1978.
134. Jafri SZH, Bree RL, Amendoke MA, Glazer GM, Schwab RE, et al: CT of renal and perirenal non-Hodgkin lymphoma. AJR 138:1101, 1982.
135. Weinberger E, Rosenbaum DM, Pendergrass TW: Renal involvement in children with lymphoma: comparison of CT with sonography. AJR 155:346–349, 1990.
136. Cohan RH, Dunnick NR, Leder RA, Baker ME: Computed tomography of renal lymphoma. J Comput Assist Tomogr 14:933–938, 1990.
137. Frick MP, Salomonowitz E, Hanto DW, Gedgaudas-McClees K: CT of the abdominal lymphoma after renal transplantation. AJR 142:97–99, 1984.
138. Tubman DE, Frick MP, Hanto DW: Lymphoma after organ transplantation: radiologic manifestations in the central nervous system, thorax and abdomen. Radiology 149:625–631, 1983.
139. Olson M, Posniak H: CT characteristics of a hyperdense renal mass due to Richter syndrome. J Comput Assist Tomogr 12(4):669–670, 1988.
140. Choyke PL, White EM, Zeman RK, Jaffe MH, Clark LR: Renal metastases: clinicopathologic and radiologic correlation. Radiology 162:359–363, 1987.
141. Mitnick JS, Bosniak MA, Rothberg M, Megibow AJ, Raghavendra BN, Subramanyam BR: Metastatic neoplasm to the kidney studied by computed tomography and sonography. Comput Assist Tomogr 9(1):43–49, 1985.
142. Leder RA, Dunnick NR: Transitional cell carcinoma of the pelvicalices and ureter. AJR 155:713–722, 1990.
143. Oyen RH, Gielen JL, Van Poppel HP, Verbeken EK, Van Damme BJ, et al: Renal thorium deposition associated with transitional cell carcinoma: radiologic demonstration in two patients. Radiology 169:705–707, 1988.
144. Kauzlaric D, Barmeir E, Luscieti P, Binek J, Ramelli F, Petrovic M: Renal carcinoma after retrograde pyelography with thorotrast. AJR 148:897–898, 1987.
145. Pollack HM, Arger PH, Banner MP, Mulhern CB, Coleman BG: Computed tomography of renal pelvic filling defects. Radiology 138:645–651, 1981.
146. Dinsmore BJ, Pollack HM, Banner MP: Calcified transitional cell carcinoma of the renal pelvis. Radiology 167:401–404, 1988.
147. Bree RL, Schultz SR, Hayes R: Large infiltrating renal transitional cell carcinomas: CT and ultrasound features. J Comput Assist Tomogr 14:381–385, 1990.
148. Baron RL, McClennan BL, Lee JK, Lawson TL: Computed tomography of transitional cell carcinoma of the renal pelvis and ureter. Radiology 144:125–130, 1982.
149. Mieza M, Rotstein JM, Geffen A: CT demonstration of periureteral fibrosis of malignant etiology. J Comput Assist Tomogr 6:290, 1982.
150. Bosniak MA, Megibow AJ, Ambos MA, Mitnick JS, Lefleur RS, Gordon R: Computed tomography of ureteral obstruction. AJR 138:1107, 1982.
151. Segal AJ, Spataro RF, Linke CA, Frank IN, Rabinowitz R: Diagnosis of nonopaque calculi by computed tomography. Radiology 129:447, 1978.
152. Federle MP, McAninch JW, Kaiser JA, Goodman PC, Roberts J, Mall JC: Computed tomography of urinary calculi. AJR 136:255, 1981.
153. Herring LC: Observations on the analysis of ten thousand urinary calculi. J Urol 88:545, 1962.
154. Brown RC, Loening SA, Ehrhardt JC, Hawtrey CE: Cystine calculi are radiopaque. AJR 135:565, 1980.
155. Hillman BJ, Drach GW, Tracey P, Gaines JA: Computed tomographic analysis of renal calculi. AJR 142:549–552, 1984.
156. Tessler AN, Ghazi MR: Case profile: computerized tomographic assistance in diagnosis of radiolucent calculi. Urology 6:672, 1979.
157. Federle MP, Kaiser JA, McAninch JW, Jeffrey RB, Mall JC: The role of computed tomography in renal trauma. Radiology 141:455, 1981.
158. Sandler CM, Toombs BD: Computed tomographic evaluation of blunt renal injuries. Radiology 141:461, 1981.
159. Schaner EG, Balow JE, Doppman JL: Computed tomography in the diagnosis of subcapsular and perirenal hematoma. AJR 129:83, 1977.
160. Lang EK, Sullivan J, Frentz G: Renal trauma: radiological studies. Radiology 154:1–6, 1985.
161. Wing VW, Federle MP, Morris JA, Jeffrey RB, Bluth R: The clinical impact of CT for blunt abdominal trauma. AJR 145:1191–1194, 1985.
162. Yale-Loehr AJ, Kramer SS, Quinlan DM, LaFrance ND, Mitchell SE, Gearhart JP: CT of severe renal trauma in children: evaluation and course of healing with conservative therapy. AJR 152:109–113, 1989.
163. Siegel MJ, Balfe DM: Blunt renal and ureteral trauma in childhood: CT patterns of fluid collections. AJR 152:1043–1047, 1989.
164. Lupetin AR, Mainwaring BL, Daffner RH: CT diagnosis of renal artery injury caused by blunt abdominal trauma. AJR 153:1065–1068, 1989.
165. Bretan PH, McAninch JW, Federle MP, Jeffrey RB: Computerized tomographic staging of renal trauma: 85 consecutive patients. J Urol 136:561–565, 1986.
166. Pollack HM, Wein AJ: Imaging of renal trauma. Radiology 172:297–308, 1989.
167. Rubin JI, Arger PH, Pollack HM, Banner MP, Coleman BG, et al: Kidney changes after extracorporeal shock wave lithotripsy: CT evaluation. Radiology 162:21–24, 1987.
168. Ralls PW, Barakos JA, Kaptein EM, Friedman PE, Fouladian G, et al: Renal biopsy-related hemorrhage: frequency and comparison of CT and sonography. J Comput Assist Tomogr 11(6):1031–1034, 1987.
169. Cronan JJ, Dorfman GS, Amis ES, Denny DF: Retroperitoneal hemorrhage after percutaneous nephrostomy. AJR 144:801–803, 1985.
170. Rosenbaum R, Hoffsten PE, Stanley RJ, Klahr S: Use of computerized tomography to diagnose complications of percutaneous renal biopsy. Kidney Int 14:87, 1978.
171. Gold RP, McClennan BL, Rottenberg RR: CT appearance of acute inflammatory disease of the renal interstitium. AJR 141:343–349, 1983.
172. Evans JA, Meyers MA, Bosniak MA: Acute renal and perirenal infections. Semin Roentgenol 6:274, 1971.
173. Little PJ, McPherson DR, de Wardener HE: The appearance of the intravenous pyelogram during and after acute pyelonephritis. Lancet 1:1186, 1965.
174. Davidson AJ, Talner LB: Urographic and angiographic abnormalities in adult-onset of acute bacterial nephritis. Radiology 106:249, 1973.
175. Silver TM, Kass EJ, Thornbury JR, Konnak JW, Wolfman MG: The radiological spectrum of acute pyelonephritis in adults and adolescents. Radiology 118:65, 1976.
176. Rauschkolb EN, Sandler CM, Patel S, Childs TL: Computed tomography of renal inflammatory disease. J Comput Assist Tomogr 6:502, 1982.
177. Bigongiari LR, Patel SK, Appelman H, Thornbury JR: Medullary rays: visualization during excretory urography. AJR 125:795, 1975.
178. Hoffman EP, Mindelzun RE, Anderson RU: Computed tomography in acute pyelonephritis associated with diabetes. Radiology 135:691, 1980.
179. Lee JKT, McClennan BL, Nelson GL, Stanley RJ: Acute focal bacterial nephritis: emphasis on gray scale sonography and computed tomography. AJR 135:87, 1980.
180. Rosenfield AT, Glickman MG, Taylor KJW, Crade M, Hodson J: Acute focal bacterial nephritis (acute lobar nephronia). Radiology 132:553, 1979.
181. Rigsby CM, Rosenfield AT, Glickman MG, Hodson J: Hemorrhagic focal bacterial nephritis: findings on gray-scale sonography and CT. AJR 146:1173–1177, 1986.

182. Kim DS, Woesner ME, Howard TF, Oson LK: Emphysematous pyelonephritis demonstrated by computed tomography. AJR 132:287, 1979.

183. Potter JL, Sullivan BM, Flournoy JG, Gerza C: Emphysema in the renal allograft. Radiology 155:51–52, 1985.

184. Wilms G, Baert AL, Marchal G, Bruneel M: CT demonstration of gas formation after renal tumor embolization. J Comput Assist Tomogr 3:838, 1979.

185. Marks WM, Filly RA: Computed tomographic demonstration of intra-arterial air following hepatic artery ligation. Radiology 132:665, 1979.

186. Schneider M, Becker JA, Staiano S, Campos E: Sonographic-radiographic correlation of renal and perirenal infections. AJR 127:1007, 1976.

187. Callen PW, Filly RA, Marcus FS: Ultrasonography and computed tomography in the evaluation of hepatic microabscesses in the immunosuppressed patient. Radiology 136:433, 1980.

188. Flechner SM, McAninch JW: Aspergillosis of the urinary tract: ascending route of infection and evolving patterns of disease. J Urol 125:598, 1981.

189. Doemeny JM, Banner MP, Shapiro MJ, Amendola MA, Pollack HM: Percutaneous extraction of renal fungus ball. AJR 150:1331–1332, 1988.

190. Elkin ME: Radiology of the urinary system. In Elkin M (ed): Computed Tomography of the Urinary Tract. Boston, Little, Brown & Company, 1980, pp 1114–1139.

191. Goldman SM, Fishman EK, Hartman DS, Kim YC, Siegelman SS: Computed tomography of renal tuberculosis and its pathological correlates. J Comput Assist Tomogr 9(4):771–776, 1985.

192. Petrillo G, Tomaselli S, Greco S: Renal ecchinococcus. J Comput Assist Tomogr 5:912, 1981.

193. Gilzanz V, Lozano F, Jimenez J: Renal hydatid cysts: communicating with collecting system. AJR 135:357, 1980.

194. Allen HA, Scatarige JC, Kim MH: Actinomycosis: CT findings in six patients. AJR 149:1255–1258, 1987.

195. Merine D, Fishman EK, Siegelman SS: Renal xanthogranulomatosis: radiological, clinical and pathological features in two cases. J Comput Assist Tomogr 11(5):785–789, 1987.

196. Sussman SK, Gallmann WH, Cohan RH, Saeed M, Lawton JS: CT findings in xanthogranulomatous pyelonephritis with coexistent renocolic fistula. J Comput Assist Tomogr 11(6):1088–1090, 1987.

197. Goldman SM, Hartman DS, Fishman EK, Finizo JP, Gatewood OMB, Siegelman SS: CT of xanthogranulomatous pyelonephritis: radiologic-pathologic correlation. AJR 142:963–969, 1984.

198. Morgan WR, Nyberg LM: Perinephric and intrarenal abscesses. Urology 26:529–536, 1985.

199. Shah M, Haaga JR: Focal xanthogranulomatous pyelonephritis simulating a renal tumor: CT characteristics. J Comput Assist Tomogr 13:712–713, 1989.

200. Karasick SR, Herring W: Computed tomography evaluation of the poorly or nonvisualized kidney. Comput Tomogr 4:39, 1980.

201. Patriquin H, Lafortune M, Filiatrault D: Urinary milk of calcium in children and adults: use of gravity-dependent sonography. AJR 144:407–413, 1985.

202. Sussman SK, Goldberg RP, Griscom NT: Milk-of-calcium hydronephrosis in patients with paraplegia and urinary-enteric diversion: CT demonstration. J Comput Assist Tomogr 10:257–259, 1986.

203. Cronan JJ, Amis ES, Zeman RK, Dorfman GS: Obstruction of the upper-pole moiety in renal duplication in adults: CT evaluation. Radiology 161:17–21, 1986.

204. Amis ES, Cronan JJ, Pfister RC: Pseudohydronephrosis on noncontrast computed tomography. J Comput Assist Tomogr 6:511, 1982.

205. Pozzo GD, Bozza A, Martorana G: Use of computed tomography in kidney agenesis. XTract 5:27, 1979.

206. Chamorro HA, Forbes TW, Padkowsky GO, Wholey MH: Multiimaging approach to the diagnosis of Page kidney. AJR 136:620, 1981.

207. Page IH: The production of persistent arterial hypertension by cellophane perinephritis. JAMA 113:2046, 1939.

208. Takahaski M, Tamakawa Y, Shibata A, Fukushima Y: Computed tomography of "Page" kidney. J Comput Assist Tomogr 1:344, 1977.

209. Hellebusch AA, Simmons JL, Holland N: Renal ischemia and hypertension from a constrictive perirenal hematoma. JAMA 214:757, 1970.

210. McKay A, Proctor LD, Roome NW: Hypertension after removal of renal calculus. Can Med Assoc J 50:328, 1944.

211. Haaga JR, Morrison SC: CT appearance of renal infarct. J Comput Assist Tomogr 4:246, 1980.

212. Glazer GM, London SS: CT appearance of global renal infarction. J Comput Assist Tomogr 5:847, 1981.

213. Pope TL Jr, Buschi AJ, Moore TS, Williamson BRJ, Brenbridge ANAG: CT features of polyarteritis nodosa. AJR 136:986, 1981.

214. Hekali P, Kivisaari L, Standertskjold-Nordenstam C-G, Pajari R, Turto H: Renal complications of polyarteritis nodosa: CT findings. J Comput Assist Tomogr 9(2):333–338, 1985.

215. Wilms G, Oyen R, Waer M, Baert AL, Michielsen P: CT demonstration of aneurysms in polyarteritis nodosa. J Comput Assist Tomogr 10:513–515, 1986.

216. Goergen TG, Lindstrom RR, Tan H, Lille Y: CT appearance of acute renal cortical necrosis. AJR 137:176, 1981.

217. Jordan J, Low R, Jeffrey RB: CT findings in acute cortical necrosis. J Comput Assist Tomogr 14:155–156, 1990.

218. Rosenfield AT, Zeman RK, Cronan JJ, Taylor KJW: Ultrasound in experimental and clinical renal vein thrombosis. Radiology 137:735, 1980.

219. Starinsky R, Graif M, Lotan D, Kessler A: Thrombus calcification of renal vein in neonate: ultrasound and CT diagnosis. J Comput Assist Tomogr 13:545–546, 1989.

220. Hricak H, Sandler MA, Madrozo BL, Eyler WR, Sy GS: Sonographic manifestations of acute renal vein thrombosis: an experimental study. Invest Radiol 16:30, 1981.

221. Bjorgvinsson E, Friedman AC: Notching of the ureter: CT demonstration of periureteral collaterals. J Comput Assist Tomogr 8(6):1215–1216, 1984.

222. Lien HH, Lund G, Talle K: Collateral veins in left renal vein stenosis demonstrated via CT. Eur J Radiol 3:29–32, 1983.

223. Nishitani H, Nakata H, Kowo J: Intrathoracic kidney. J Comput Assist Tomogr 3:409, 1979.

224. Sandler CM, Conley SB, Fogel SR, Brewer ED: Splenic compression of the left kidney simulating pathologic unilateral renal enlargement. J Comput Assist Tomogr 4:248, 1980.

225. Subramanyam BR, Bosniak MA, Horii SC, Megibow AJ, Balthazar EJ: Replacement lipomatosis of the kidney: diagnosis by computed tomography and sonography. Radiology 148:791–792, 1983.

226. Gefter WB, Arger PH, Mulhern CB, Pollack HM, Wein AJ: Computed tomography of circumcaval ureter. AJR 131:1086, 1978.

227. Chen HH, Panella JS, Rochester D, Ignatoff JM, McVary KT: Non-Hodgkin lymphoma of ureteral wall: CT findings. J Comput Assist Tomogr 12(1):157–158, 1988.

228. Hulnick DH, Bosniak MA: "Faceless kidney": CT sign of renal duplicity. J Comput Assist Tomogr 10(5):771–772, 1986.

229. McDonald JE, Lee JKT, McClennan BL, Melzer JS, Sicard GA, et al: Natural history of extraperitoneal gas after renal transplantation CT demonstration. J Comput Assist Tomogr 6:507, 1982.

230. Bernardino ME, de Santos LA, Johnson DE, Bracken RB: Computed tomography in the evaluation of postnephrectomy patients. Radiology 130:183, 1979.

231. Alter AJ, Vehling DT, Zwiebel WJ: Computed tomography of the retroperitoneum following nephrectomy. Radiology 133:663, 1979.

232. Papanicolaou N, Harbury OL, Pfister RC: Fat-filled postoperative renal cortical defects: sonographic and CT appearance. AJR 151:503–505, 1988.

233. Baum ML, Baum RD, Plaine L, Bosniak MA: Computed tomography in the diagnosis of fistula between the ureter and iliac artery. J Comput Assist Tomogr 11(4):719–721, 1987.

234. Hirsch M: Enhanced ascities: CT sign of ureteral fistula. J Comput Assist Tomogr 9(4):825–826, 1985.
235. Kenney PJ, Panicek DM, Witanowski LS: Computed tomography of ureteral disruption. J Comput Assist Tomogr 11(3):480–484, 1987.
236. Kittredge RD, Brensilver J, Pierce JC: Computed tomography in renal transplants. Radiology 127:165, 1978.
237. Letourneau JG, Day DL, Ascher NL, Zuniga WRC: Imaging of renal transplants. AJR 150:833–838, 1988.
238. Hricak H, Terrier F, Demles BE: Renal allografts: evaluation by MR imaging. Radiology 159:435–441, 1986.
239. Geisinger MA, Risius B, Jordan ML: Magnetic resonance imaging of renal transplants. Radiology 148:407–412, 1983.
240. Nakstad P, Kilmannskog F, Kolbenstvedt A, Sodal G: Computed tomography in surgical complications following renal transplant. J Comput Assist Tomogr 6:286, 1982.
241. Steinberg HV, Nelson RC, Murphy FB, Chezmar JL, Baumgartner BR, et al: Renal allograft rejection: evaluation by Doppler US and MR imaging. Radiology 162:337–342, 1987.
242. Hricak H, Terrier F, Marotti M, Engelstad BL, Filly RA, et al: Posttransplant renal rejection: Comparison of quantitative scintigraphy, US, and MR imaging. Radiology 162:685–688, 1987.
243. Baumgartner BR, Nelson RC, Ball TI, Wyly JB, Bourke E, et al: MR imaging of renal transplants. AJR 147:949–953, 1986.
244. Terrier F, Hricak H, Revel D, Alpers C, Bretan P, et al: Magnetic resonance imaging in the diagnosis of acute renal allograft rejection and its differentiation from acute tubular necrosis: experimental study in the dog. Invest Radiol 20:617–624, 1985.
245. Levine E, Grantham JJ, Slusher SL, Greathouse JL, Krohn BP: CT of acquired cystic kidney disease and renal tumors in long-term dialysis patients. AJR 142:125–131, 1984.
246. Levine E, Grantham JJ, MacDougall ML: Spontaneous subcapsular and perinephric hemorrhage in end-stage kidney disease: clinical and CT findings. AJR 148:755–758, 1987.
247. Siegel SC, Sandler MA, Alpern MB, Pearlberg JL: CT of renal cell carcinoma in patients on chronic hemodialysis. AJR 150:583–585, 1988.
248. Hughson MD, Buchwald D, Fox M: Renal neoplasia and acquired cystic kidney disease in patients receiving long term dialysis. Arch Pathol Lab Med 110:592–601, 1986.
249. Fayemi AO, Ali M, Braun EV: Oxalosis in neurodialysis patients: a pathologic study of 80 cases. Arch Pathol Lab Med 103:58–62, 1979.
250. Lamkin N, Raval B, Carey LS: CT appearance of long-term renal transplant rejection. Comput Tomogr 5:340–342, 1981.
251. Brennan RP, Pearlstein AE, Miller SA: Computed tomography of the kidneys in a patient with methoxyflurane abuse. J Comput Assist Tomogr 12(1):155–156, 1988.
252. Day DL, Scheinman JI, Mahan J: Radiological aspects of primary hyperoxaluria. AJR 146:395–401, 1986.
253. Luers PR, Lester PD, Siegler RL: CT demonstration of cortical nephrocalcinosis in congenital oxalosis. Pediatr Radiol 10:116–118, 1980.
254. Lalli A: Renal parenchymal calcifications: Semin Roentgenol 17:101–112, 1982.
255. Mangano FA, Zaontz M, Pahira JJ, Clark LR, Jaffe MHJ, et al: Computed tomography of acute renal failure secondary to rhabdomyolysis. J Comput Assist Tomogr 9(4):77–779, 1985.

CHAPTER 21

THE ADRENAL GLANDS

WILLIAM P. SHUMAN ▪ *ALBERT A. MOSS*

Imaging of the adrenals is usually performed for one of three reasons: to evaluate abnormal adrenal function, to search for metastases in a patient with a known primary malignancy, or to further characterize an incidentally found adrenal mass. In abnormalities of adrenal function, laboratory tests coupled with imaging studies have proven useful in determining the nature and location of adrenal abnormality. Detection of mass lesions and some degree of tissue characterization of adrenal masses has been accomplished using both computed tomography (CT) and magnetic resonance imaging (MRI).

CT has revolutionized the imaging of adrenal glands. Normal adrenal glands can be imaged in almost every patient, and virtually all adrenal tumors larger than 0.5 cm can be detected if meticulous CT techniques are employed.[1-6] The superiority of CT over ultrasound for detecting adrenal masses has been convincingly demonstrated using receiver operating characteristic (ROC) analysis.[7] Thus because of its greater overall sensitivity, CT has become the imaging procedure of choice to evaluate patients with suspected adrenal tumors.

The main limitation of adrenal CT is its lack of specificity. Although fat-containing adrenal tumors and simple adrenal cysts have characteristic CT appearances, the majority of tumors have similar appearances and cannot be characterized beyond size and location.

Magnetic resonance imaging has offered the hope of better adrenal tissue characterization. The reported sensitivity of MRI has been comparable to that of CT in the detection of adrenal masses larger than 1 cm,[8] but magnetic resonance has also been found to provide some distinction among malignancies, hyperfunctioning tumors, and nonmalignant or hypofunctioning tumors when intensity and T2 criteria are used.[8-13] Combining MR information with adrenal cortical scintigraphy may permit a further improvement in tissue characterization of adrenal masses.[9]

Techniques of Examination

Computed Tomography

In all but the most emaciated adults, the adrenal glands are readily identified by CT, as they are surrounded by retroperitoneal fat, a great natural CT contrast material. However, to prevent confusion between gut and adrenal tissue, oral contrast should be administered prior to CT scanning. Adult patients are given 500 to 750 mL of a two per cent solution of sodium diatrizoate or a two per cent solution of barium sulfate over the 1 hour prior to the examination; an additional 250 mL are given immediately before scanning. This regimen opacifies stomach, small bowel, and duodenum and permits the adrenal glands to be easily differentiated from adjacent gut structures. When CT scan times longer than 5 sec are employed, glucagon (0.5 mg) administered intravenously is useful to reduce artifacts caused by intestinal motility. The risks of glucagon administration are small, but the use of glucagon in patients with a pheochromocytoma may induce a hypertensive crisis. If a patient with a suspected pheochromocytoma requires glucagon administration, the risk can be obviated by injecting propantheline bromide prior to giving the glucagon.

In many patients, imaging of the adrenal glands can be satisfactorily accomplished without the use of intravenous contrast material. However, intravenous contrast should be used in patients with a paucity of retroperitoneal fat, when the vascularity of an adrenal mass is in question, or in instances when the adrenal gland must be distinguished from the upper

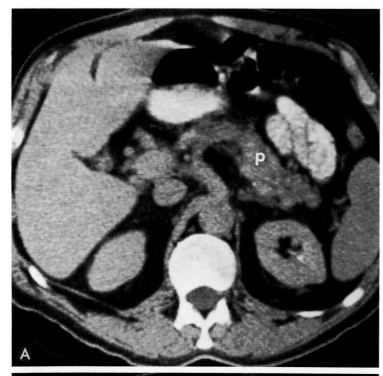

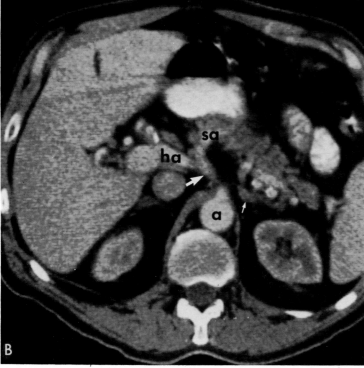

FIGURE 21–1 ■ *A,* CT scan performed after a slow contrast infusion demonstrates the tail of the pancreas (p), but the left adrenal cannot be easily separated from splenic vessels. *B,* CT scan taken during bolus injection of contrast showing aorta (a), celiac axis *(large arrow),* hepatic artery (ha), and splenic artery (sa). The left adrenal *(small arrow)* is now clearly identified.

pole of the kidney or other adjacent organ. Administration of intravenous contrast opacifies adjacent vessels and may cause enhancement of adrenal tumors, thus improving the interface between tumor and surrounding normal tissue (Fig. 21–1). Intravenous contrast is best administered as a rapid bolus injection (1.5 to 2 mL/sec) of 150 to 180 mL of 60 per cent diatrizoate meglumine or a nonionic agent. The use of a power injector results in more predictable flow rates and enables a single technologist to control both injection and scanning.[14] CT scanning is begun 30 to 50 sec after the start of the contrast injection and continued through the adrenal gland in a dynamic fashion.

CT scans of the adrenal glands are obtained with the patient supine and the CT gantry at 0° of angulation. Scans are usually done at resting expiration, as this phase of the respiratory cycle is most reproducible. Milliampere (mA) and peak kilovolt (kVp) values are chosen to allow adequate photon flux without excessive radiation exposure, depending on the type of scanner used. Contiguous 3 to 5-mm-thick scans are usually employed, but occasionally,

ultrathin sections (1.5-mm) through the region of the adrenals prove useful when scanning to detect small tumor masses such as aldosterinomas. Scans should extend from 2 to 3 cm above the adrenal glands to an equal amount below the glands to ensure that the entire adrenal region is encompassed. Adrenal images are best displayed axially, but occasionally, reformatting of axial CT images into coronal or sagittal configurations provides additional information (Fig. 21–2). Adrenal images are best displayed at a moderately wide window (300 to 500 Hounsfield units [H]) and at soft tissue levels (40 to 80 H).

CT has been widely used to guide adrenal biopsies.[15-18] On the right, a transhepatic approach is commonly used, although larger lesions may be approached posteriorly. On the left, a posterior approach is more commonly used, although a transsplenic approach has been described.[17] Posterior approaches usually require an angled technique in which the biopsy needle is inserted inferior to the adrenal and then angled superiorly to avoid passing through the lung. When using the posterior approach, the ipsilateral decubitus position may occa-

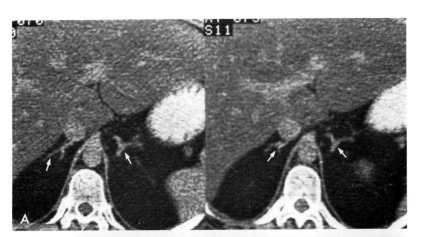
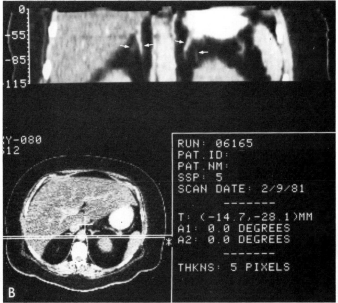

FIGURE 21–2 ■ A, CT scan of normal adrenal glands (arrows) in axial plane. Slice thickness is 5 mm. B, Coronal reformatting of serial contiguous 5-mm-thick slices. The plane of reformation is indicated by parallel lines. Both limbs of each adrenal are shown (arrows).

sionally be useful, as it elevates the diaphragm and decreases respiratory motion on the dependent side (Fig. 21–3).[16]

Magnetic Resonance

We currently perform adrenal MRI using respiratory gating and gradient moment nulling to help decrease motion artifact. Saturation pulses are placed superior and inferior to the adrenals to reduce artifact from blood flow in adjacent vessels. An initial T1-weighted sequence is performed in the coronal plane to localize the adrenals. Axial T1- and T2-weighted sequences are then obtained through the adrenals using a repetition time/echo delay time (TR/TE) of 600/20 for the T1 sequence and either a TR/TE of 2000/80 or a double-echo sequence (2000/20/80) for the T2 sequence. Adrenal MR images are reconstructed using a matrix of 128 × 256, and the field of view is adjusted for the patient's size. Most commonly, MR scans are obtained using two repetitions and a 5-mm slice thickness, with a 2- to 3-mm skip between the slices. Large adrenal masses can be scanned using 10-mm-thick slices. The frequency and phase encoding directions are selected so that any residual artifact from the great vessels does not pass across the adrenals. This usually requires the phase direction to run from top to bottom on axial images, but use of more than one imaging plane is frequently helpful. Sagittal or coronal images are particularly useful in determining the superior and inferior margins of large adrenal tumors.

In addition to T1- and T2-weighted spin-echo pulse sequences, MR scans using short T1 inversion recovery (STIR) have been employed in an attempt to improve sensitivity for focal abnormality in the adrenals.[19] The adrenal STIR technique involves obtaining 5-mm-thick slices with a 3-mm gap between scans using a TR/TI/TE of 2000/160/40. To date, additional sensitivity of the STIR technique when compared with spin-echo techniques has not been proven in the adrenal glands, although it has been demonstrated in other areas of the body.[19] The use of intravenous gadolinium in conjunction with fast gradient-echo MR imaging of the adrenals during suspended respiration offers promise of providing additional information in delineation and differentiation of adrenal masses.[11] Fast gradient-echo techniques also shorten examination time and improve image quality compared with spin-echo techniques.[11]

There probably is no single pulse sequence that is optimal for all adrenal imaging. Generally it is important to obtain T1- and T2-weighted sequences that are optimized for the MR instrument being used. T1 and T2 values can be measured on most MR systems, but such two-point measurements may not reflect accurate tissue T1 and T2 values. However, these measurements can prove useful in comparing different tissue types if the measurements are performed on a single scanner of a particular field strength. When obtaining T1 and T2 measurements, it is important to minimize the amount of motion-induced noise so that the measurements reflect true tissue values rather than noise.

The spatial resolution of modern MRI is such that normal adrenal glands can be imaged in up to 97 per cent of patients (Fig. 21–4).[8,20] Using routine body coil imaging, 100 per cent of left adrenals and 86 per

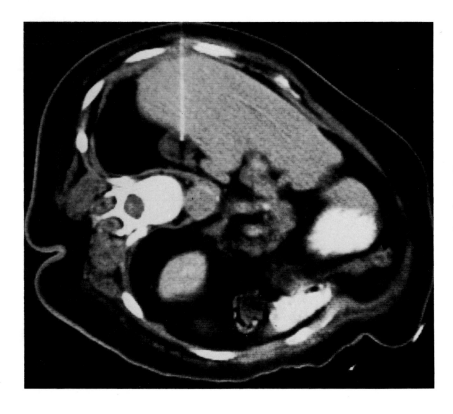

FIGURE 21–3 ■ *A,* CT-directed aspiration needle biopsy of a right adrenal mass, which proved to be metastatic vulvar carcinoma. The decubitus position and the transhepatic approach were used to avoid the posterior sulcus of the pleura.

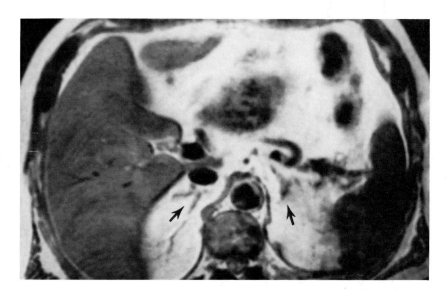

FIGURE 21–4 ■ T1-weighted MR scan demonstrates normal adrenal glands *(arrows)* to be hypointense relative to surrounding fat. The shape of the adrenal glands is similar to that seen on CT scans.

cent of right adrenals can be depicted,[20] and rectangular surface coils placed behind the patient can further improve spatial resolution. Newly designed butterfly pairs or planar pairs of loop-gap resonator surface coils appear to be superior for adrenal MRI, as they are intrinsically decoupled from a transmitted field of arbitrary orientation.[21] Using such resonators, local high-resolution images can be obtained with a 3-mm slice thickness, resulting in a pixel size of 0.6 × 0.6 mm.

Anatomy

Each adrenal gland lies within Gerota's fascia in the perinephric space, embedded in adipose tissue and surrounded by a tough fibroelastic tissue capsule that penetrates the cortex and divides the gland into columns.[22] The upper pole of each adrenal gland is firmly anchored to the top portion of Gerota's fascia by fibrous bands. Embryologically the cortex and medulla of the adrenal gland are derived from two separate sources. The cortex is formed in the sixth week of life from a proliferation of mesodermal coelomic epithelial cells medial to the mesonephros. One week later the medulla is formed by ectodermal neural crest migrating from sympathetic ganglia. Once formed, the adrenals descend caudally to meet the ascending kidney.

Location

RIGHT ADRENAL GLAND

The right adrenal gland is located just dorsal to the inferior vena cava at the level of its intra- and extrahepatic portions (Fig. 21–5). The right adrenal vein is very short and drains directly into the inferior vena cava. Laterally the gland is separated from the posteromedial portion of the right lobe of the liver by a variable amount of retroperitoneal fat. Medially the crus of the right diaphragm runs a course roughly parallel to the medial border of the gland. If there is a paucity of retroperitoneal fat, it can be difficult to separate the right adrenal gland from adjacent liver or crus of the diaphragm.

Most right adrenal glands are positioned 1 to 2 cm superior to the upper pole of the right kidney and just cephalic to the left adrenal. The most caudal extent of the right adrenal gland is always cephalic to the renal vessels. The right adrenal is usually located about 1 cm lateral to the vertebral body and between 0.5 cm and 1 cm posterior to the anterior margin of the vertebral body.[3]

LEFT ADRENAL GLAND

The medial portion of the left adrenal gland is positioned lateral to the crus of the left diaphragm, but its course is usually not as parallel to the diaphragm as that of the right adrenal gland. Almost all left adrenal glands are anterior to the anterior vertebral margin and posterior to the anterior aorta.[3] The lower portion of the left adrenal gland and the superior pole of the left kidney are usually seen on the same section, because the inferior portion of the left adrenal touches the left kidney (see Fig. 21–5A).[22] The upper margin of the right adrenal is cephalic to (34 per cent), at the same level as (51 per cent), or lower than (15 per cent) the upper pole of the left adrenal.[5] The lower pole of the left gland is cephalic to the renal vessels, but because the left adrenal arteries are shorter than the right, it is closer than the right adrenal to the aorta and renal vascular pedicle.

The tail of the pancreas is located anterior and/or slightly lateral to the left adrenal gland (see Fig. 21–5B). The tail of the pancreas is seen on at least one section with the left adrenal gland in more than 95 per cent of patients and serves as a good marker for identification of the left gland. The splenic vessels are just dorsal to the lateral limb of the left adrenal. The most cephalic portion of the left adrenal may be related to the dorsal border of the stomach.

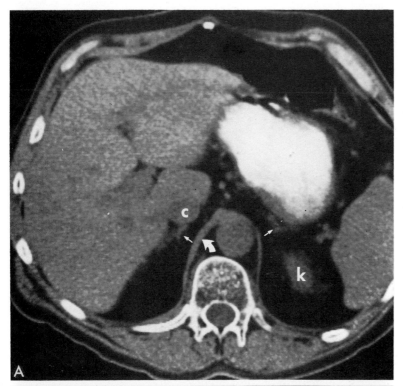

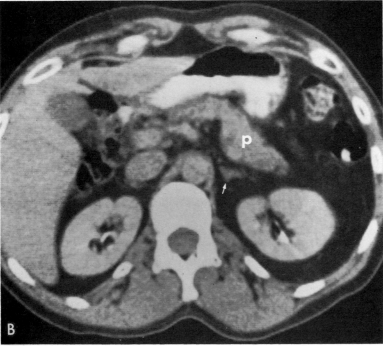

FIGURE 21–5 ■ Normal position of adrenal glands. *A,* The right gland *(small arrow)* is just dorsal to the inferior vena cava (c). Retroperitoneal fat separates the medial margin of the liver from the right adrenal gland. The right adrenal lies above the upper pole of the right kidney and courses parallel to the crus of the diaphragm *(curved arrow).* The left adrenal *(small arrow)* is seen in the same section as the upper pole of the left kidney (k) and is closely related to the dorsal margin of the stomach. *B,* The left adrenal *(arrow)* is positioned just dorsal to the tail of the pancreas (p).

Despite the close position of the adrenals and the kidney, the two organs have different embryologic backgrounds. The kidney develops in the pelvis of the embryo, whereas the adrenal cortex develops at the lower thoracic level, and the adrenal medulla comes from neural crest cells. For this reason, patients with congenital renal anomalies almost always have normally positioned adrenal glands, although the shape of the adrenal can be affected. When there is unilateral renal agenesis, inferior renal ectopy, or cross-fused ectopy, the ipsilateral adrenal is usually present in its normal location but frequently is disk shaped rather than linear or cross shaped.[23]

Morphology

RIGHT ADRENAL GLAND

The right adrenal gland has a variety of cross-sectional configurations (Fig. 21–6). CT usually depicts the right adrenal gland as linear, with a course parallel to the diaphragmatic crura. High-resolution CT often shows the body of the right adrenal to be split into medial and lateral limbs, giving it an inverted V shape. The lateral limb is frequently shorter than the medial limb; it usually courses parallel to the medial limb but may be directed a little more laterally at an angle to the body of the adrenal gland. The right adrenal gland can also appear as a horizontal linear structure or have a K configuration (Fig. 21–7).[5]

LEFT ADRENAL GLAND

The shape of the left adrenal gland varies considerably (see Fig. 21–6). Most frequently it has an inverted V or Y shape but can appear linear, triangular, crescentic, or V shaped. The body of the left adrenal usually splits at an acute angle into medial and lateral limbs of equal length. If the two limbs are unequal in length, the lateral limb is usually longer.

Because the adrenal glands are polymorphic in shape at different levels, the CT appearance of the adrenal gland varies greatly depending on the level of the CT section (see Fig. 21–7).[1] The margins of all normal adrenal glands are smooth, although accessory cortical bodies can give a normal gland a slightly nodular configuration.[3]

Size

Adrenal length, width, and thickness can be measured according to the method of Montagne et al.[5] The length of each gland is determined by counting the number of contiguous CT scans in which the gland is identified. The thickness of the gland is the greatest dimension perpendicular to the long axis of the gland or to one of its limbs (Fig. 21–8A). The greatest thickness is usually at the junction of the body of the adrenal with its medial and lateral limbs. The width of the gland is measured by determining the greatest ventral-dorsal dimension of the gland (see Fig. 21–8B).

Montagne et al.[5] found that 92 per cent of the right and 96 per cent of the left adrenal glands were between 2 and 3.5 cm in length. The width of the adrenal glands varies between 2 and 2.5 cm in about 80 per cent of patients, but normal adrenal glands up to 3 cm in width can be found. Except for triangular left adrenal glands, the thickness of each adrenal gland is usually 1 cm or less, with the left adrenal usually slightly thicker than the right.

The measurements of adrenal gland size are in close agreement with measurements from pathologic specimens and indicate that CT is an accurate method for quantifying adrenal size and volume.[5,22,24] Rather than measuring adrenal thickness, the thickness of the adrenal glands can be readily compared with the adjacent diaphragmatic crus. In most instances, the adrenal gland is no thicker than the maximal thickness of the crura at the same level on the side of the gland being evaluated.

Pathology

The appearance of an adrenal mass may be simulated by an appropriately located vasculature struc-

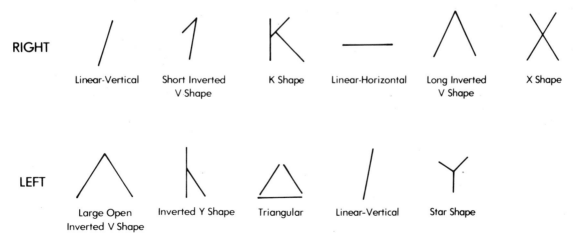

FIGURE 21–6 ■ Diagram of some of the various adrenal shapes as seen on computed tomography. (From Moss AA: CT of the adrenal glands. In Noy C, Friedenberg RM [eds]: Radiographic Atlas of the Genitourinary System. Philadelphia, JB Lippincott, 1981.)

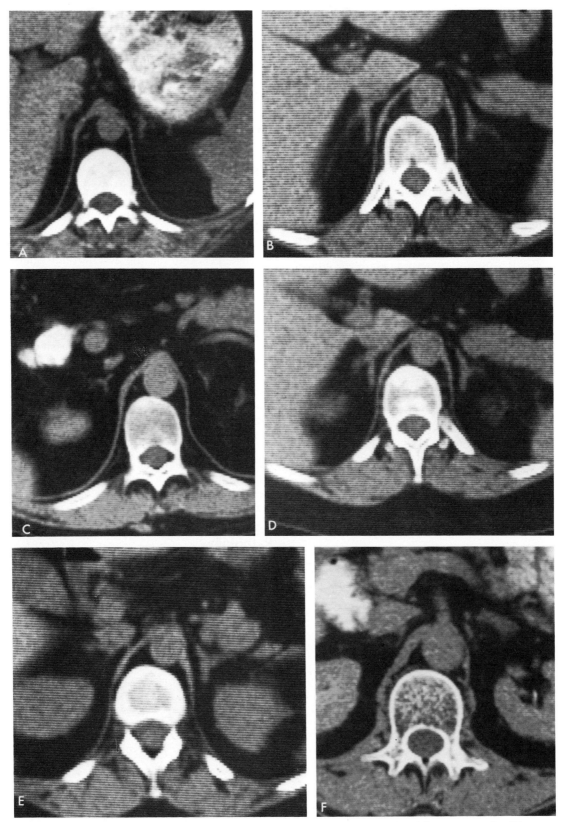

FIGURE 21–7 ■ A range of different shapes of the adrenal glands demonstrated in different patients by CT.

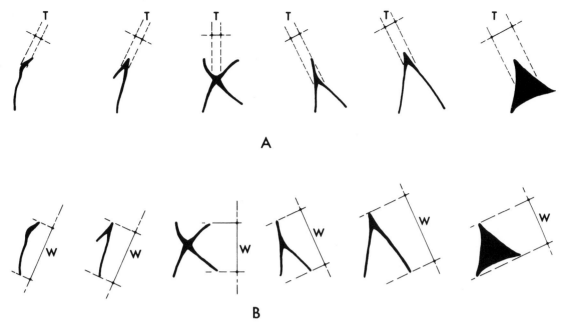

FIGURE 21–8 ■ Diagrams of the method of measuring adrenal thickness *(A)* and width *(B)*.

ture, portion of the gastrointestinal tract, or adjacent organ. On the right, a tortuous renal artery, masses projecting off the right kidney or the liver, and/or interposition of normal colon between the liver and kidney can simulate an adrenal tumor.[25] On the left, adrenal pseudotumors may be caused by varices arising from the left inferior phrenic vein, which passes anterior to the left adrenal gland, or by a tortuous splenic artery.[26,27] Left-sided adrenal pseudomasses can also be produced by the tail of the pancreas (Fig. 21–9) or by a medial lobulation of the spleen (Fig. 21–10). Small bowel, a gastric diverticulum, or a posteriorly positioned gastric fundus can also produce a left adrenal pseudotumor. Injection of intravenous contrast material and use of oral contrast usually makes the diagnosis of an adrenal pseudotumor readily apparent. Occasionally MRI can

be used to establish the vascular nature of an adrenal pseudomass.

Interpretation of adrenal appearances on cross-sectional imaging is best done in conjunction with information from biochemical studies, as well as from other imaging modalities. Although CT or MR findings may indicate nonspecific tumor or hyperplasia, biochemical information and information from radionuclide studies or ultrasound may make it possible to suggest the specific pathologic entity.

Cortical Abnormalities

CUSHING'S SYNDROME

Patients with Cushing's syndrome have a constellation of symptoms and physical findings produced by elevated plasma corticosteroid levels. Physical

FIGURE 21–9 ■ CT of adrenal pseudomass produced by the tail of the pancreas *(straight arrow)*. The left adrenal gland *(curved arrow)* is seen just lateral to the left diaphragmatic crus.

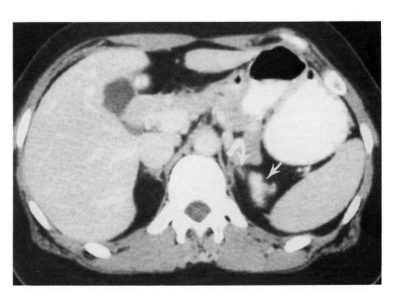

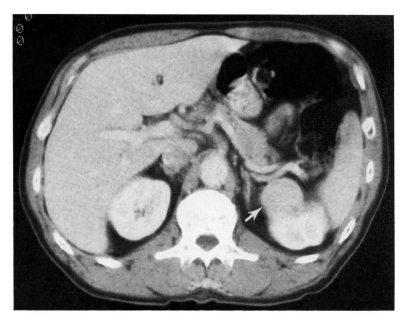

FIGURE 21–10 ■ An adrenal pseudomass produced by a medial lobulation of the spleen *(arrow)*.

findings include truncal and facial obesity with increased intraabdominal fat. Hypertension may be present, along with oligomenorrhea, easy bruiseability, acne, and generalized weakness.[28] The diagnosis is confirmed biochemically by documenting an absence of corticosteroid response to insulin-produced hypoglycemia, loss of normal steroid circadian rhythm, and resistance to steroid suppression by low-dose dexamethasone.[29] Cushing's syndrome is three to four times as common in females as in males and occurs most frequently in patients between the ages of 25 and 35.[30]

Cushing's syndrome can be produced by excessive pituitary adrenocorticotropic hormone (ACTH) production, which results in adrenal cortical hyperplasia. In addition, Cushing's syndrome can result from excessive ACTH production by nonpituitary sources, such as nonendocrine tumors, adrenal tumors, or adrenal nodular hyperplasia, or from exogenous administration of ACTH.[28,30,31] Many tumors are capable of producing ACTH; these include bronchial and thymic carcinoma, medullary thyroid carcinoma, islet cell tumor of the pancreas, pheochromocytoma, paraganglioma, chemodectoma, and small cell carcinoma of the lung.[32] Cushing's syndrome is caused by pituitary overstimulation of the adrenal gland in 80 per cent of patients, hyperfunctioning adrenal adenoma in 18 per cent, hyperfunctioning adrenal carcinoma in one per cent, and ectopic ACTH production by nonadrenal tumor in one per cent.[32] CT is useful in detecting many of these tumors, although CT scans of both the chest and abdomen may be required.

In approximately 20 per cent of patients, biochemical studies cannot separate patients with Cushing's syndrome caused by an adrenal steroid–producing neoplasm from those with Cushing's syndrome caused by excessive ACTH production, which stimulates the adrenals to produce excessive steroids.[33]

When blood chemistry levels are abnormal, CT may be able to differentiate among diffuse hyperplasia, nodular hyperplasia, benign adenoma, and malignant carcinoma.[34]

A benign cortical adenoma is present in 10 to 15 per cent of patients with Cushing's syndrome, and adrenal carcinoma is present in an additional five per cent.[35] Functioning adrenal adenomas usually appear as unilateral (90 per cent), solid, well-defined, homogenous mass lesions at least 2 cm in diameter,[36] although they can be larger and have an inhomogenous appearance (Fig. 21–11). Although the usual CT density of adrenal adenomas ranges between 30 and 50 H, some cortical adenomas have lower values because of high lipid content.[37] At times, ultrasound may be necessary to distinguish a well-defined, low-density adenoma from a simple adrenal cyst. CT distinction between adrenal adenoma and carcinoma is possible only when metastases are found or local invasion of vascular structures is demonstrated.[38] Neither the enhancement pattern after intravenous contrast nor the presence of calcification can absolutely separate adenoma from carcinoma.

In patients with Cushing's syndrome, the most frequent CT finding is normal adrenal glands, as the basic pathologic abnormality present is microscopic hyperplasia.[36] Diffuse bilateral adrenal enlargement with preservation of shape is the next most frequent finding in ACTH-dependent Cushing's syndrome (Fig. 21–12).[36] Absolute measurements have not been helpful in defining whether adrenal hyperplasia is present.[32] In most cases, hyperplastic glands have smooth outlines but may occasionally have a nodular or lumpy appearance (Fig. 21–13).[32] The macronodular form of bilateral adrenal hyperplasia can be diagnosed by identifying one or more nodules in a diffusely enlarged gland.[39] Macronodular hyperplasia may evolve into an autonomous adrenal adenoma,[39] and when nodular hyperplasia presents as a single

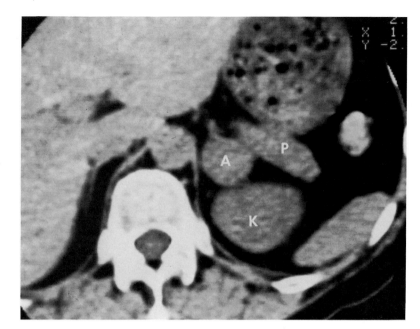

FIGURE 21–11 ■ Cushing's syndrome. CT scan demonstrates a solid, left functioning left adrenal adenoma (A) 2 × 3 cm in size. The relationship of the adenoma to the kidney (K), pancreas (P), and aorta is demonstrated.

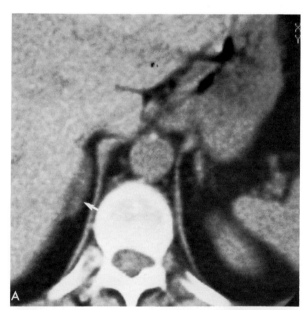

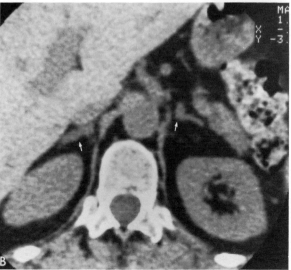

FIGURE 21–12 ■ Cushing's syndrome secondary to overproduction of corticotropin. A, CT scan at the level of the right adrenal gland. The right adrenal is thickened (arrow) but maintains its normal shape. Note that the adrenal is thicker than the diaphragmatic crus. B, CT scan at a lower level shows that both adrenals (arrows) are diffusely thickened.

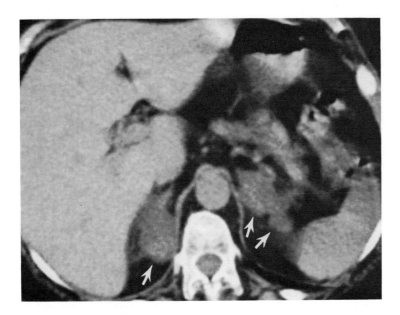

FIGURE 21–13 ■ Cushing's syndrome associated with adrenal nodular hyperplasia. Both adrenals are enlarged and contain multiple nodules *(arrows)*.

dominant nodule, it is usually impossible to distinguish the hyperplastic nodule from an adrenal adenoma. Adrenal CT shows hyperplasia more frequently in patients with ectopic ACTH than in patients with ACTH produced by a pituitary adenoma.[32] When ectopic ACTH production arises from a pheochromocytoma, bilateral hyperplasia may be associated with a unilateral mass. Although CT can never exclude a diagnosis of hyperplasia, it can separate Cushing's syndrome caused by ACTH-dependent hyperplasia from Cushing's syndrome caused by adrenal neoplasm in 90 per cent of cases.[6,36,37]

Adrenal cortical carcinoma and adenoma are both readily detected by CT. Carcinomas usually range in size from 6 to 20 cm[38] and frequently contain areas of necrosis or calcification (Fig. 21–14). Less frequently, functioning adrenal carcinoma is demonstrated as a homogenous mass less than 5 cm in size that simulates an adenoma.[40] Associated CT findings in patients with Cushing's syndrome are an abnormally low attenuation value of the liver (resulting

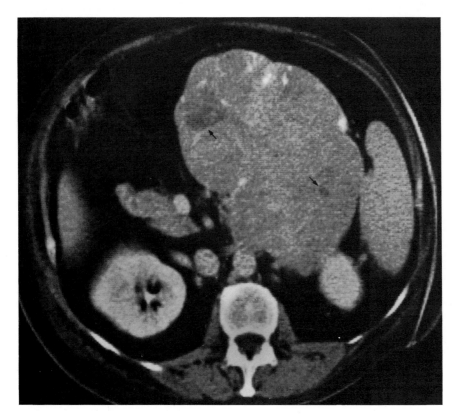

FIGURE 21–14 ■ Cushing's syndrome secondary to a large, functioning adrenal carcinoma that contains foci of calcification and necrosis *(arrows)*.

from hepatic fat deposition) and an increase in the amount of retroperitoneal, intraabdominal, and subcutaneous fat. CT usually does not demonstrate contralateral adrenal atrophy in patients with unilateral hyperfunctioning adrenal neoplasms, but it can document reduction in hyperplastic glands after pituitary surgery.

The roles of MRI and CT in Cushing's syndrome are complementary. Anatomic delineation of the adrenal glands and adrenal tumors by MRI is comparable to that of CT, but MRI may be capable of providing additional tissue specificity. MR scanning reveals benign hyperfunctioning adrenal cortical tumors to have low signal intensity on both T1- and T2-weighted images and T2 relaxation times of less than 60 ms.[10] Malignant hyperfunctioning adrenal cortical carcinomas typically have T2 values greater than 60 ms and become hyperintense on T2-weighted images.[10] The underlying basis for this difference is not definitely understood, but it may result in part from the fact that malignant hyperfunctioning tumors contain less fat and more water than do benign neoplasms. Despite general MRI differences between benign and malignant adrenal masses, adrenal masses that become hyperintense on T2-weighted sequences are not always malignant.[10, 41–44] Hemorrhage into a benign adrenal adenoma can produce a hyperintense mass that appears similar to adrenal malignancy.[44–46]

CONGENITAL ADRENAL CORTICAL HYPERPLASIA

Virilizing congenital adrenal cortical hyperplasia results from an inborn enzyme deficiency that produces a complete block of adrenal cortical steroid synthesis. The absence of steroid synthesis induces chronic overproduction of ACTH by the pituitary gland, causing adrenal hyperplasia and excessive production of steroid precursors. High levels of circulatory steroid precursors produce in utero virilization of females and precocious puberty of males. CT scans of these patients later in life may demonstrate benign tumorous transformation of hyperplastic adrenal glands.[47] The benign tumors found in patients with congenital adrenal cortical hyperplasia may have calcification, necrosis, and hemorrhage and thus be indistinguishable from an adrenal malignancy.[47]

PRIMARY ALDOSTERONISM (CONN'S SYNDROME)

Primary aldosteronism (Conn's syndrome) results from excessive production of aldosterone and is characterized by mild hypertension, hypokalemia, headache, sodium retention, and reduced or absent plasma renin.[35,48] Primary aldosteronism is the cause of hypertension in approximately one per cent of patients with elevated blood pressure. Males are affected twice as often as females, and the patient's age at onset is usually between 30 and 50 years.[35]

Approximately 80 per cent of patients with Conn's syndrome have a unilateral adrenal cortical adenoma, located twice as frequently on the right as on the left, which rarely exceeds 4 cm in diameter and is often less than 2 cm in greatest dimension.[2,35] The remaining 20 per cent of adult patients have idiopathic hyperaldosteronism resulting from nodular bilateral adrenal hyperplasia.[49] In pediatric patients the situation is reversed: bilateral nodular hyperplasia is more common than functioning adenomas.[35] The diagnosis of nodular hyperplasia is based on the identification of multiple adrenal nodules, although any single nodule may be indistinguishable from an aldosteronoma.[50] Carcinoma very rarely causes primary aldosteronism.[35]

Primary aldosteronism is diagnosed by finding an elevated rate of aldosterone secretion and a clinical response to spironolactone therapy. Aldosteronomas tend to produce higher than normal urinary and plasma aldosterone levels, but biochemical distinction between adenoma and hyperplasia is often unclear.[2] However, this distinction is important, as therapy for the two entities is different. Resection of a solitary adenoma cures a patient's hypertension, but adrenal surgery, even bilateral adrenalectomy, will not cure hypertension caused by idiopathic hyperaldosteronism.[2,6,50]

The presence and location of an adenoma may be confirmed by arteriography or venography and adrenal venous sampling.[51] However, because CT is easy to perform, noninvasive, and greater than 80 per cent accurate even in the detection of small (0.5 cm) adenomas, it has replaced more invasive techniques.[2,6,36,37] To detect tiny adrenal nodules, 1.5- to 3-mm contiguous CT scans through the entire adrenal glands must be performed. In patients with negative CT results, adrenal venography, venous sampling, and NP 59 scintigraphy have proven helpful.[51,52]

On CT scans, aldosteronomas can appear homogenous and have an attenuation value similar to that of other solid organs, or they may have low CT attenuation values, because they can contain as much as 5.1 per cent lipid (Fig. 21–15A).[37] Less frequently, aldosteronomas contain calcium and thus have CT high attenuation values (Fig. 21–15B). Intravenous administration of contrast material usually does not greatly enhance the aldosteronoma, but contrast may make the lesion more apparent because of enhancement of normal adrenal tissue.[32] In more than 90 per cent of cases, CT can distinguish aldosterone-producing adenoma from hyperplasia and thus determine the most effective mode of therapy.[2]

The exact role of MRI in the diagnosis of aldosteronomas is yet to be determined. Because of the small size of aldosteronomas, MR will likely be less sensitive than CT until improved scanning techniques are available. Aldosterone-producing adenomas and aldosterone-producing nodular hyperplasia have both been reported to be isointense with liver and produce a low signal on T1- and T2-weighted images (Fig. 21–16).[13] Thus compared with CT, MR has not demonstrated an increased sensitivity or specificity in the evaluation of patients with hyperaldosteronism.

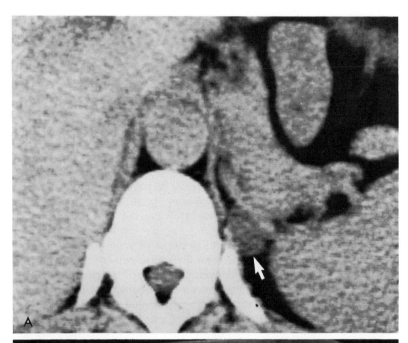

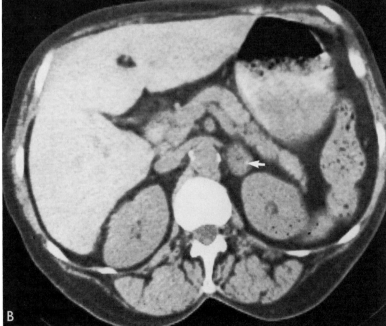

FIGURE 21–15 ■ Variation in CT density of aldosteronomas. *A,* Left aldosteronoma *(arrow)* with low density resulting from its high fat content. *B,* Higher density left aldosteronoma containing a focus of calcification *(arrow).*

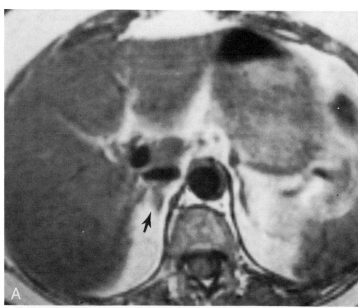

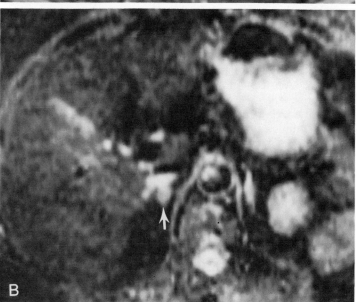

FIGURE 21–16 ■ MR scan of a small aldosteronoma. *A,* T1-weighted image shows a relatively dark, small mass projecting off posterior medial limb of right adrenal *(arrow).* *B,* STIR image depicts the adrenal glands as hyperintense. A small bright mass is projected off the right adrenal *(arrow).*

HYPOADRENALISM (ADDISON'S DISEASE)

At least 90 per cent of the adrenal cortex must be destroyed before Addison's disease becomes evident.[32] Prior to the eradication of tuberculosis, granulomatous disorders were the most common cause of Addison's disease. At the current time, idiopathic atrophy of the adrenal glands probably is the most common cause. Hemorrhage secondary to trauma, stress, or anticoagulation therapy can produce Addison's disease.[53–55] Rare causes of Addison's disease include secondary hemochromatosis, histoplasmosis, blastomycosis, lymphoma, bilateral metastases, and absence of ACTH production because of destruction of the pituitary gland (Fig. 21–17).[32,55–59]

The CT findings in patients with hypoadrenalism vary with the underlying origin. Idiopathic hypoadrenalism produces bilaterally atrophic adrenals. Calcification of the adrenals indicates prior infection by fungus or tuberculosis or old hemorrhage.[32] Acute hemorrhage produces bilaterally enlarged adrenal glands that have a rounded or oval shape, with focal areas of hyperdensity.[46,53,55] The adrenals in patients with Addison's disease may be enlarged and have low-density centers as a result of ongoing infection, metastases, or lymphoma.[56–59]

MRI has only a small role to play in the diagnosis of Addison's disease, as it may miss calcifications suggestive of prior granulomatous infection. However, MRI should be considered the imaging procedure of choice whenever hemorrhage is suspected as the cause of Addison's disease. MRI not only demonstrates the presence of adrenal masses, but also provides tissue characterization strongly suggesting the presence of blood.

MRI can distinguish hemorrhagic lesions from other masses by their short T1 and long T2 relaxation times.[43,46] Acute hemorrhage typically results in hyperintense masses on T1 images, which become markedly hyperintense on T2-weighted images.[43,46] On T1 images, subacute adrenal hemorrhage typically has a center of intermediate intensity surrounded by an outer ring of high intensity and either an inhomogeneous high signal or a central intermediate and peripheral high intensity on T2 images.[43,46] Follow-up T1 and T2 scans demonstrate smaller adrenal glands with high-intensity centers surrounded by peripheral hypointense rings.[46]

The early MR findings are best explained as resulting from the paramagnetic effects of the free methemoglobin (Fe^{3+}) produced by the oxidation of hemoglobin (Fe^{2+}) as the hemorrhage ages. The high-intensity center on the late MR scans presumably reflects the high concentration of free methemoglobin.[46] The hypointense ring is thought to represent hemosiderin-laden macrophages and a fibrous capsule.[46] MR is useful for both diagnosis and follow-up of adrenal hemorrhage, as it is capable of imaging the biochemical changes occurring at the time and during the healing process.

Nonfunctioning Adrenal Adenoma and Carcinoma

The adrenal cortical adenoma is usually unilateral, 2 to 5 cm in diameter, and of variable density. About half have a soft tissue density, and the remainder demonstrate decreased attenuation, presumably because of high lipid content (Fig. 21–18).[32] Adrenal adenomas occur in 12 to 15 per cent of patients with renal cell carcinoma but in less than three per cent of the general population.[60] Calcification is more common in carcinoma, but adenomas can also contain calcification. Ten per cent of patients with benign adrenal cortical adenomas have bilateral neoplasms.

Adrenal cortical carcinoma typically is a slow-growing tumor that can become extremely large before producing symptoms. Although 50 per cent of adrenal cortical carcinomas are nonfunctioning, hormonally active carcinoma is twice as common in women, and nonfunctioning adrenal carcinoma is more common in men.[32]

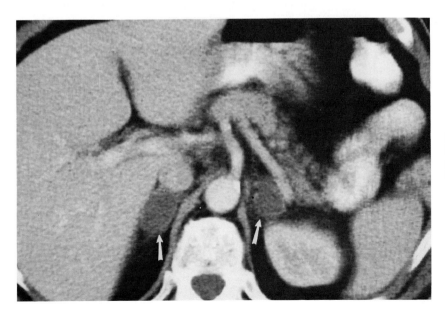

FIGURE 21–17 ■ Addison's disease caused by bilateral adrenal hemorrhages secondary to anticoagulant therapy. CT scan demonstrates enlarged, low-density adrenal glands (arrows).

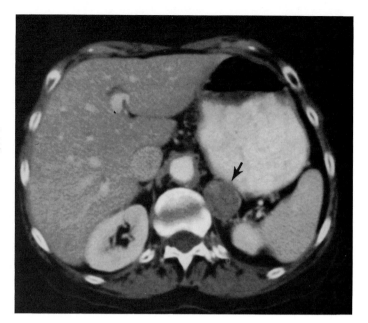

FIGURE 21–18 ■ CT scan of nonfunctioning left adrenal adenoma *(arrow)*. Attenuation of the adenoma is mixed as a result of high fat content. The scan was performed during injection of contrast.

Frequently the CT features alone cannot distinguish whether a solid adrenal mass is benign or malignant. CT findings of adrenal cortical carcinoma include areas of central low attenuation, irregular contrast enhancement, calcification, and a thin capsule rim surrounding the tumor (Fig. 21–19). However, adrenal cortical carcinoma may also produce a smooth homogenous mass.[40] When diagnosed, adrenal carcinomas are usually large (8 to 10 cm in diameter) and contain a region of central necrosis (Fig. 21–20). When a right adrenal mass becomes very large, it may be difficult to determine from axial scans alone whether the mass is hepatic, renal, or adrenal in origin. Reformatting the axial CT images in the coronal or sagittal plane may help determine the organ of origin. CT has proven useful in detecting recurrence of adrenal carcinoma after resection. To prevent confusing postoperative fibrosis and scarring with recurrent disease, baseline CT scans are recommended at 3 to 6 months after surgery.

On MR examination, nonfunctioning adenomas appear low in signal intensity on both T1- and T2-weighted images (Fig. 21–21).[41] Adrenal carcinomas often have a mixed signal intensity on T1-weighted images, but typically become hyperintense on T2-weighted images (Fig. 21–22).[42,61] Gadolinium enhancement may be helpful in detecting intravenous extension of adrenal cortical carcinoma[62] and in permitting improved visualization of the tissue interfaces between tumor and adjacent organs.

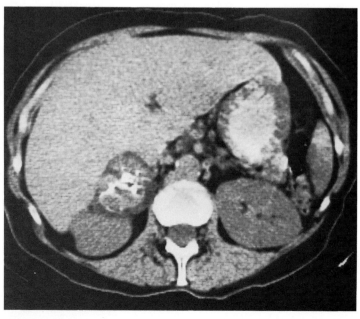

FIGURE 21–19 ■ CT scan of small, calcified, nonfunctioning adrenal carcinoma.

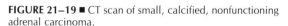

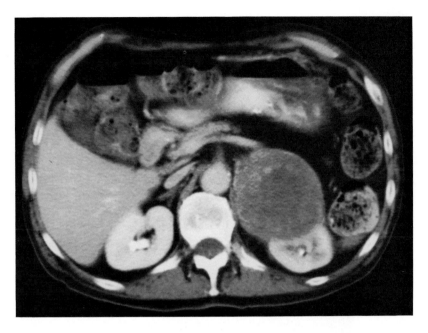

FIGURE 21–20 ■ CT scan of larger, noncalcified, nonfunctioning adrenal carcinoma invading the left kidney.

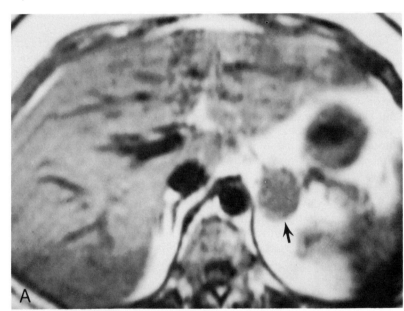

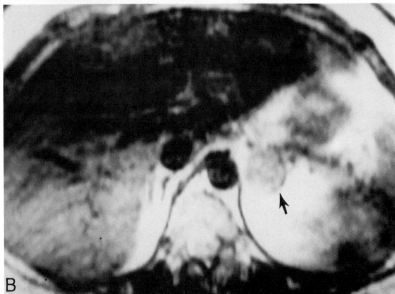

FIGURE 21–21 ■ MR scan of nonfunctioning left adrenal adenoma. *A,* T1-weighted image shows adenoma *(arrow)* isointense with liver. *B,* T2-weighted image shows adenoma *(arrow)* is similar in intensity to the posterior portion of the liver. Darkening of the anterior aspect of the liver is the result of a metal object on the patient's abdomen.

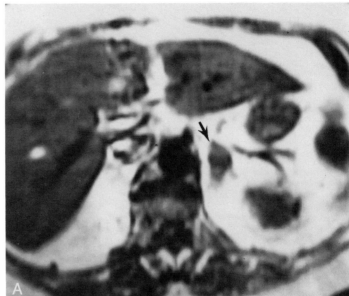

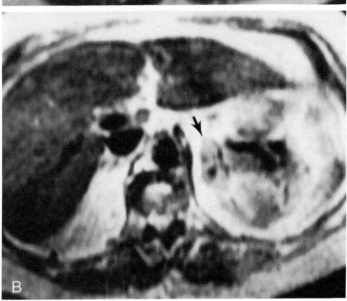

FIGURE 21–22 ■ MR scan of nonfunctioning left adrenal carcinoma. *A,* T1-weighted image shows a mass *(arrow)* that is isointense with the liver. *B,* T2-weighted image shows the same mass *(arrow),* this time more intense than the liver.

Myelolipoma

The adrenal myelolipoma is an uncommon tumor of the adrenal cortex that is found in 0.08 per cent to 0.2 per cent of patients at autopsy.[63] The tumor contains varying proportions of bone marrow elements, and fat or calcification occurs in approximately 20 per cent of cases.[63–65] The tumorous cells are thought to arise from a common precursor stem cell that resides within the adrenal gland.[64] The stimulus for metaplasia of reticulum cells in the adrenal cortex to produce a myelolipoma is unknown, but the result is a mixture of hematopoietic and lipoid cells with coexistent reticulum cells in the fatty areas of the tumor. The presence of myeloid precursors, specifically megakaryocytes, in a biopsy specimen allows the specific diagnosis of myelolipoma to be made.[64]

Most adrenal myelolipomas are asymptomatic, although hemorrhage and necrosis within the tumor and/or compression of surrounding structures may cause flank or upper abdominal pain.[65] No correlation has been found between adrenal myelolipomas and anemia or extramedullary hematopoiesis, but occasionally myelolipoma has been associated with endocrine abnormalities such as Conn's syndrome. The tumors are most often unilateral, affect the right and left gland equally, and although usually less than 5 cm, may become as large as 12 cm.[65]

Myelolipomas are readily diagnosed by CT as well-circumscribed adrenal mass lesions that have attenuation values in the −30- to −140-H range and frequently (20 per cent) contain foci of calcification (Figs. 21–23 and 21–24).[66,67] In some instances, hemorrhage, calcification, and/or myeloid material may occupy the majority of the volume of the tumor, resulting in the lesion having a soft tissue density. In these patients, the myelolipoma is indistinguishable from any other solid adrenal mass.[66, 67]

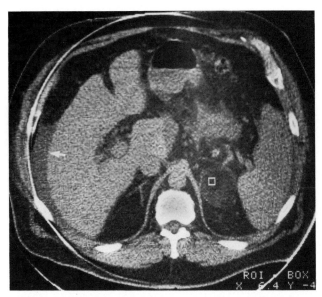

FIGURE 21-23 ■ CT scan of myelolipoma of the left adrenal. CT density measurement (*square*) is −38 H, indicating fat. Note the normal right adrenal. Ascites is present (*arrow*).

The CT demonstration of fat in an adrenal tumor should not be considered pathognomonic for a myelolipoma, as both cortical adenomas and aldosteronomas can have low attenuation values because of high fat content.[37] If a myelolipoma is small, asymptomatic, and has the CT appearance of mature fat, surgical removal may not be necessary, although follow-up should be obtained to ensure that the character of the lesion does not change.[54] The differential diagnosis of a suprarenal fatty mass includes angiomyolipoma of the kidney, retroperitoneal lipoma, liposarcoma, and unusual metastatic disease. Metastatic lung carcinoma to the adrenal gland may simulate a myelolipoma on CT, as the malignant metastatic cells engulf adjacent retroperitoneal fat and form a suprarenal fatty mass.[68]

The MR appearance of myelolipoma depends predominantly on the amount of fat within the tumor. Typically myelolipomas have MR imaging characteristics similar to those of retroperitoneal fat and are hyperintense on spin-echo pulse sequences but suppress and become hypointense on STIR sequences. Myelolipomas with predominantly soft tissue rather than fat elements will appear like other solid nonfunctioning adrenal tumors on MR scans.[8]

Medullary Abnormalities

PHEOCHROMOCYTOMA

Pheochromocytomas are derived from mature neural crest cells in the adrenal medulla called *pheochromocytes*,[69] from chromaffin cell nests anywhere along the autonomic ganglia chain, or from chromaffin bodies such as the organ of Zukerkandl. Although 90 per cent of pheochromocytomas are located in the adrenal glands, they can be located anywhere along the axial skeleton from the base of the skull to the lower rectum.[70–72]

Pheochromocytomas secrete abnormal amounts of catecholamines, which are responsible for the paroxysmal attacks characterized by hypertension, diaphoresis, tachycardia, and anxiety.[73] Although only about 1 of 3000 hypertensive patients has a pheochromocytoma,[69] episodic uncontrolled hypertension in a middle-aged patient should alert the clinician to the possibility of a pheochromocytoma. The prevalence of pheochromocytoma is roughly equal in adult males and females, although prior to puberty it is more common in males.[69] Hypertension may be precipitated by exercise, palpation of the tumor, or biopsy.[74,75] Because about 15 per cent of pheochromocytomas have an atypical clinical presentation, the possibility of catastrophe should be kept in mind

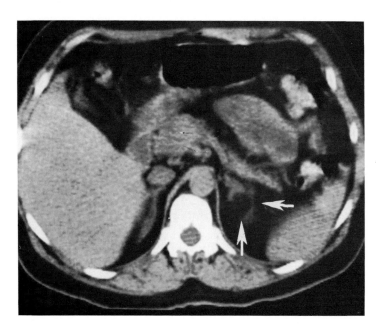

FIGURE 21-24 ■ CT scan of myelolipoma of the left adrenal (*arrows*). The CT density of the mass is similar to that of subcutaneous and retroperitoneal fat.

during biopsy of any adrenal lesion. Treatment of an acute hypertensive crisis includes the administration of 1 mg of phentolamine followed by intravenous titration of blood pressure with 20 mg of phentolamine diluted in 500 mg of five per cent dextrose in water.[75]

Prior to imaging studies, there should be laboratory documentation of elevated catecholamine levels. Evaluating all hypertensive patients with imaging is expensive, unwarranted, and unproductive unless there is laboratory evidence of elevation of urinary metanephrine or vanillylmandelic acid (VMA) levels.[69]

Adult pheochromocytomas are usually solitary and are more frequently located on the right; approximately ten per cent are bilateral, ten per cent are extraadrenal, and 10 to 13 per cent are malignant.[72,76] In children, however, the right-to-left predominance increases to 2:1; 24 per cent are bilateral, 30 per cent have extraadrenal tumors, and eight per cent have both adrenal and extraadrenal tumors.[70,71] Forty per cent of extraadrenal pheochromocytomas are malignant. The most common location of an extraadrenal pheochromocytoma is in the organ of Zuckerkandl.

Pheochromocytomas are associated with neuroectodermal disorders such as tuberous sclerosis, neurofibromatosis, and von Hippel-Lindau syndrome and are also associated with the multiple endocrine neoplasia (MEN) type IIa (50 per cent) and type IIb (90 per cent).[77–79] MEN IIa is characterized by medullary thyroid carcinoma, parathyroid hyperplasia, and pheochromocytoma. Patients with MEN IIb have multiple mucosal neuromas, gastrointestinal ganglioneuromatosis, a marfanoid body habitus, medullary thyroid carcinoma, and pheochromocytoma.[77] Pheochromocytomas in the MEN syndromes are bilateral in 65 per cent, are frequently asymptomatic, and are more often malignant.[77]

The overall accuracy of CT in detecting pheochromocytoma is greater than 95 per cent.[80] Most frequently, CT identifies a unilateral homogeneous adrenal mass greater than 2 cm in diameter and of soft tissue density. However, pheochromocytomas may be entirely solid, contain both cystic and solid components, or be almost entirely cystic (Figs. 21–25 through 21–28).[50] Calcification occurs in seven per cent.[69] Pheochromocytomas enhance markedly after administration of intravenous contrast material, to the point of becoming briefly isodense with adjacent vascular structures (see Fig. 21–27).[80] A low-density central area after intravenous contrast administration usually represents central necrosis or hemorrhage.

Radionuclide imaging has proven useful as an adjunct to CT in the detection of pheochromocytoma.[80] Metaiodobenzylguanidine (MIBG), an analogue of norepinephrine, is taken up by adrenal chromaffin tissue, thus permitting the detection of pheochromocytoma in 90 per cent of cases (see Fig. 21–28B).[81,82] MIBG has proven particularly useful in the detection of extraadrenal or recurrent pheochromocytoma, situations in which CT accuracy is less than 60 per cent.[50] Extraadrenal, recurrent, and meta-

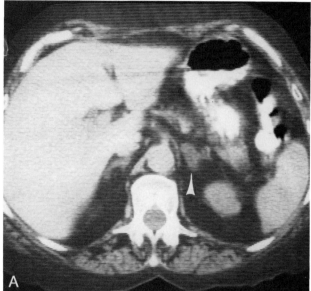

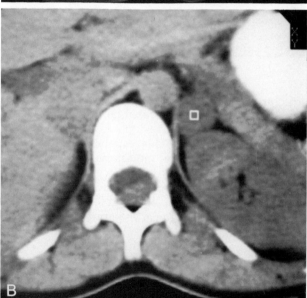

FIGURE 21–25 ■ CT scan of two small, surgically proven pheochromocytomas. *A*, Pheochromocytoma *(arrowhead)* arising from the medial limb of the left adrenal has a mottled attenuation during contrast injection. *B*, Small (2-cm), round, left pheochromocytoma *(square)*, isodense with the kidney on the unenhanced CT scan.

static pheochromocytomas are probably best initially evaluated with MIBG I 123 or MIBG I 131.[80–82] MIBG imaging can be followed by CT if more precise spatial localization of abnormalities is required.

In 37 cases of proven pheochromocytoma evaluated by MRI, all but one was clearly delineated.[10,11,43,83,84] Overall accuracy of MRI is comparable to that of CT in detecting primary adrenal pheochromocytoma, but MRI had a higher sensitivity in the detection of extraadrenal, recurrent, and metastatic pheochromocytomas.[82,85,86] Local tumor recurrence can be accurately evaluated by MRI despite the presence of multiple metallic clips, and MRI is particularly useful in delineating tumors from vascular

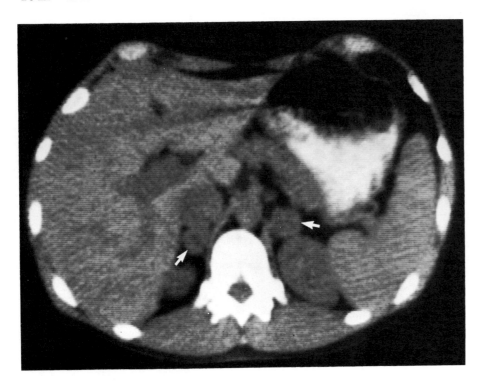

FIGURE 21–26 ■ CT scan of bilateral pheochromocytomas *(arrows)* in a patient with MEN II syndrome. The patient had familial medullary carcinoma of the thyroid.

structures and adjacent organs. The ability of MRI to directly image in the coronal and sagittal planes permits large anatomic regions to be imaged in a short period of time. This capability is useful in screening the body for metastasis, as well as in searching for ectopic pheochromocytomas.

Pheochromocytomas have long T2 relaxation times (>60 ms), and thus on T2-weighted images, most pheochromocytomas appear hyperintense relative to the liver parenchyma (Fig. 21–29A),[43,85] and some appear to be more intense than fat (Fig. 21–29B).[84] Pheochromocytomas have been reported to have a higher signal intensity than nonfunctioning adrenal gland adenomas.[85]

NEUROBLASTOMA

Neuroblastoma is the most common extracranial solid malignant neoplasm of childhood, accounting for approximately ten per cent of all pediatric neoplasms.[69] Approximately 80 per cent occur in children younger than 3 years, and more than 50 per cent of children with neuroblastoma have metastases at the time of diagnosis.[87] The histologic features range from highly malignant (sympathicogonioma) to

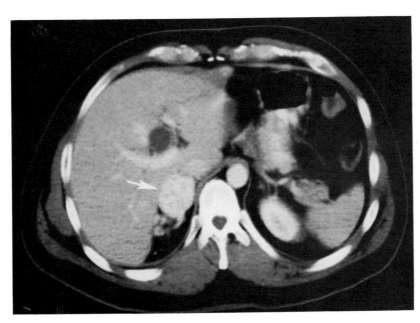

FIGURE 21–27 ■ CT scan of a right pheochromocytoma *(arrows)*, which strongly enhances following intravenous contrast. The tumor *(arrow)* is isointense with aorta. The patient has von Hippel–Lindau disease.

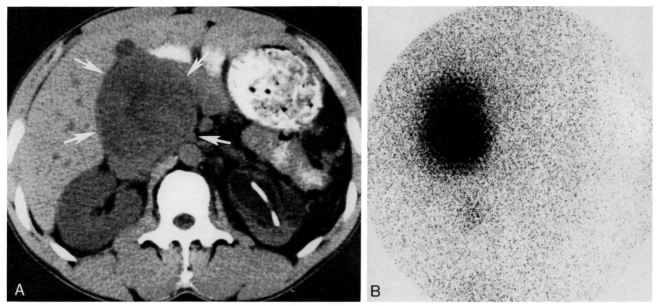

FIGURE 21–28 ■ CT scan of a large right pheochromocytoma. *A,* The tumor *(arrows)* has an attenuation value lower than that of liver, and there is an area of central necrosis. Nephrostomy stent is seen in the left kidney. *B,* MIBG scan shows intense uptake in the pheochromocytoma.

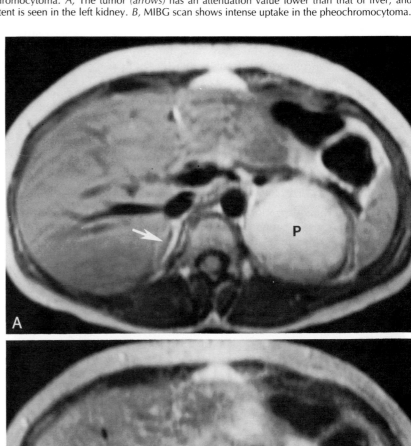

FIGURE 21–29 ■ MR scan of a large left pheochromocytoma in a patient with MEN II syndrome. *A,* Mixed-weighted image shows a homogenous mass (P) with a signal intensity greater than that of liver. Note the normal-appearing right adrenal *(arrow). B,* T2-weighted image shows a mass (P) that is intensely bright. Normal right adrenal *(arrow)* is still dark.

slightly less malignant (neuroblastoma) to benign (ganglioneuroma). The term *neuroblastoma* is commonly used to refer to various malignant grades and *ganglioneuroma* to the more benign forms. Neuroblastomas occasionally can spontaneously regress from malignant to benign.[87]

Neuroblastomas arise from the sympathic ganglia and the adrenal medulla.[30] Neuroblastomas most frequently originate from the adrenal glands (35 per cent to 50 per cent), elsewhere in the abdomen (24 per cent to 40 per cent), or rarely in the chest.[69,88] Extraadrenal tumors most often are located in sympathetic ganglion cells or paraaortic bodies near the adrenal glands. Approximately 15 per cent of neuroblastomas arise in the organ of Zuckerkandl and five per cent in the pelvis. Neuroblastomas are more frequent on the left side of the body. Skeletal, lymph node, and hepatic metastases are most common. Pulmonary metastases are present in only 11 per cent of patients at the initial diagnosis.[87]

A neuroblastoma most commonly presents as a painless abdominal mass, although weight loss, liver enlargement, and/or bone pain may be the first clinical sign. An elevated urinary VMA level is present in approximately 75 per cent of patients and confirms the diagnosis. Evaluating the extent of tumor is clinically important, because tumors that extend beyond the midline or have remote metastases are not treated surgically. Tumors confined to a single organ and/or extending only to adjacent lymph nodes are treated surgically, with a 60 to 90 per cent cure rate.[69]

CT has become the primary diagnostic imaging modality in the evaluation of neuroblastoma, as it provides information regarding tumor size, position, and the relationship of the tumor to surrounding structures. CT readily detects calcification that is not apparent on conventional radiographs and accurately determines the extent of tumor spread.

On CT, neuroblastomas typically appear as irregularly shaped, solid masses of predominantly soft tissue density that frequently contain areas of necrosis, hemorrhage, and/or calcification (Fig. 21–30). Punctate calcification is most frequently observed, but the calcification may be solid, ringlike, or confluent and become more dense after chemotherapy (Figs. 21–31 and 21–32).[89] Neuroblastomas can also appear as noncalcified masses of soft tissue or fat density with or without cystic components. When noncalcified neuroblastomas invade the adjacent kidney, it is difficult to differentiate a neuroblastoma from a Wilms' tumor.

One limitation of CT is its detection of skeletal metastases. CT has proven less accurate than bone scintigraphy in detecting spread of disease to bone marrow, and thus bone scintigraphy remains the primary procedure for detecting bone metastases from neuroblastomas.

MRI has been useful in evaluating patients for the presence and extent of neuroblastoma.[90,91] It has proven particularly helpful in defining the relationship between a neuroblastoma and adjacent abdominal vessels, without requiring an intravenous contrast injection.[91,92] Neuroblastoma typically appears slightly more intense than adjacent muscle on T1 images but is significantly more intense on T2-weighted images (Fig. 21–33). The ability of MRI to image in the coronal plane has proven more useful than axial CT imaging in determining the extent of disease, organ of origin, presence of bone marrow metastases, spinal cord extension, or vascular invasion.[91–93] However, MRI misses small areas of calcification and thus is less specific than CT in making the diagnosis of neuroblastoma.

Secondary Tumors

The adrenal glands are the fourth most frequently involved site of blood-borne metastatic disease. Metastasis from carcinoma of the lung is most common,

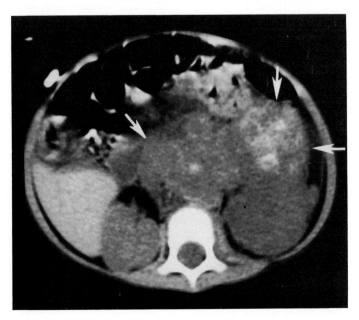

FIGURE 21–30 ■ CT scan of a neuroblastoma *(arrows)* in a 3-year-old child. Note multiple areas of calcification, vascular encasement of the aorta, and tumor crossing the midline.

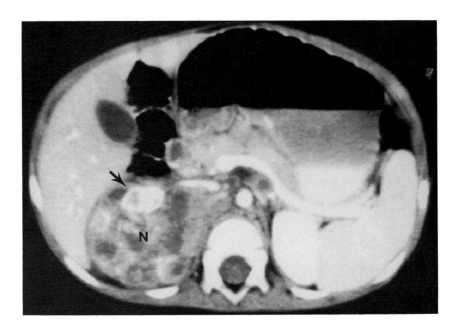

FIGURE 21–31 ■ CT scan of a large right neuroblastoma (N) following chemotherapy. The lesion contains an area of dense calcification *(arrow)* and areas of low density and does not cross the midline.

followed in order by metastasis from breast, thyroid, and colon carcinoma and melanoma.[94] Rarely, metastatic disease may be associated with hypoadrenalism (Addison's disease), but usually adrenal metastases produce no symptoms.

In patients with a known primary malignancy, an adrenal mass is equally as likely to be a nonfunctioning adenoma as an adrenal metastasis. A needle biopsy is often needed to confirm or exclude metastatic disease because of the high incidence of nonfunctioning adenomas (eight per cent) and the inability to separate benign adenomas from metastases by imaging methods. The adrenal is the only site of metastatic disease in 15 per cent of patients with bronchogenic carcinoma,[95–98] and confirmation of ad-

renal metastases will preclude attempts at curative lung resection. In patients with non-Hodgkin's lymphoma, adrenal metastases are usually bilateral, producing diffusely enlarged rather than nodular glands.[36,57] Occasionally the adrenal glands are the only site of involvement with lymphoma.[99]

Metastases produce unilateral or, more often, bilateral circumscribed masses that alter the normal adrenal gland contours (Fig. 21–34). Metastases produce masses that have soft tissue attenuation unless central necrosis, hemorrhage, or calcification is present (Fig. 21–35).[57] Adrenal metastases are usually small but can be enormous. There are no characteristics that permit CT to separate metastases from other adrenal masses. Microscopic foci of metastatic

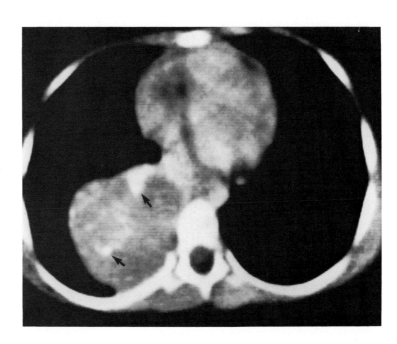

FIGURE 21–32 ■ CT scan of a supradiaphragmatic neuroblastoma that has foci of calcification *(arrows)*.

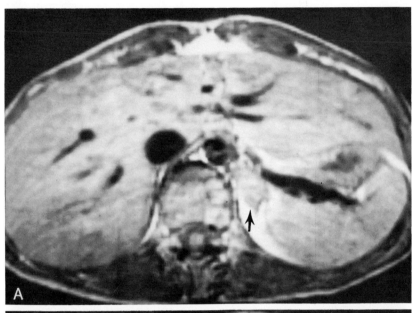

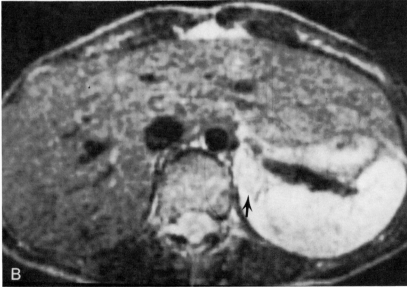

FIGURE 21–33 ■ MR scan of a small left ganglioneuroma. *A,* Mixed-weighted image demonstrates a mass *(arrow)* that is more intense than adjacent muscle and isointense with liver. *B,* On a T2-weighted image, the mass *(arrow)* becomes much brighter than liver or muscle.

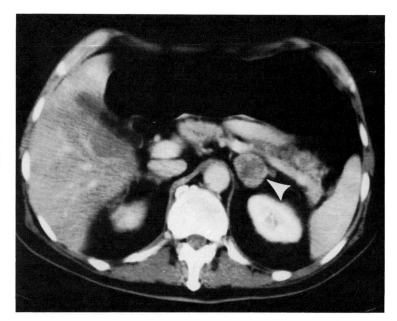

FIGURE 21–34 ■ Colon cancer metastatic to the left adrenal gland *(arrow)*. The contours of the adrenal are rounded, and the metastasis undergoes mixed enhancement during contrast administration.

disease are common, and thus the CT appearance of a normal adrenal gland can never absolutely exclude disease.

The MRI appearance of adrenal metastases has been widely reported.[10,11,42,43,61,100] Typically, adrenal metastasis have an intensity below or close to that of liver on T1-weighted sequences but become hyperintense relative to liver on T2-weighted sequences (Fig. 21–36). Hemorrhagic metastasis produce masses that have a high signal intensity on T1 images. Nonfunctional adrenal adenomas are usually less intense than adrenal metastases on T2-weighted pulse sequences,[42,43,61,100] possibly because nonfunctioning adenomas can contain bound intracellular cholesterol, which has a shorter T2 time than lipid.[50]

Glazer et al. reported that optimal adrenal tissue characterization using midfield MR systems was obtained using a pulse sequence with a TR of 2 sec and a TE of 50 ms.[42,100] Whenever the calculated lesion-liver intensity ratio was less than 1.2, the adrenal mass was found to be an adenoma. An intensity ratio greater than 1.4 was highly indicative of metastatic disease (Fig. 21–37).[42] However, the adrenal lesion-liver ratio has proven insufficient to accurately separate benign from malignant disease, as 21 to 31 per cent of adrenal masses have intensity ratios between 1.2 and 1.4.[10,42,43,61,100] Recent studies have found the calculated T2 relaxation time to be more accurate at 1.5 T than lesion-to-liver intensity ratios.[10] All adrenal masses with a T2 less than 60 ms were adenomas, whereas longer T2 relaxation times were found in metastatic disease and in a variety of func-

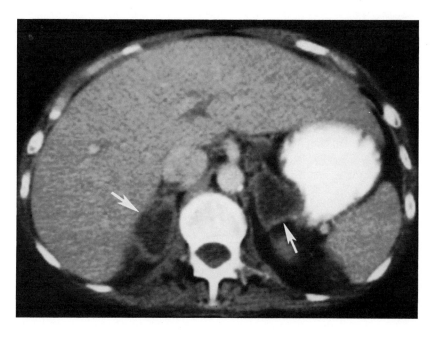

FIGURE 21–35 ■ CT scan of bilateral adrenal metastases *(arrows)* from lung carcinoma. The central low attenuation is a result of extensive tumor necrosis.

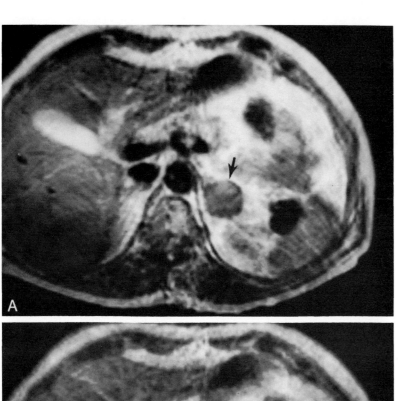

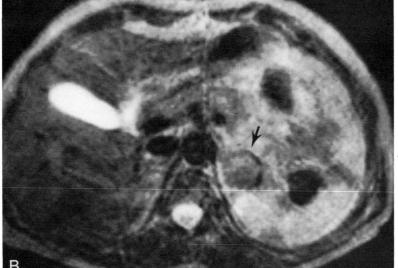

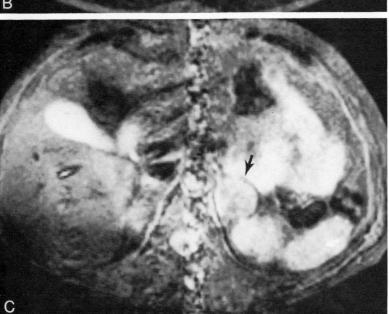

FIGURE 21–36 ■ MR scan of left adrenal metastasis from lung carcinoma. *A,* T1-weighted image shows the metastasis *(arrow)* to be isointense with liver. *B,* T2-weighted image demonstrates the metastasis to be slightly more intense than liver. *C,* STIR image (T1 plus T2 weighting) reveals the metastasis *(arrow)* to be much brighter than liver. Note darkening of subcutaneous fat by this fat suppression sequence.

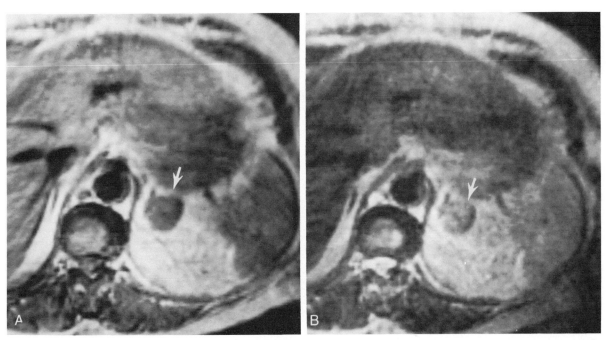

FIGURE 21–37 ■ MR scan of focal adrenal non-Hodgkin's lymphoma. *A,* T1-weighted image reveals the left adrenal mass *(arrow)* to be slightly lower in intensity than liver. *B,* T2-weighted image demonstrates the lymphoma to become slightly higher in intensity than liver.

tioning and nonfunctioning adrenal tumors.[10] However, other reports have documented metastases to have low intensity on T2 images, and high-intensity adenomas have also been reported.[50]

Unusual Primary Adrenal Tumors

Tumors can originate from any of the cellular components of the adrenal gland. Benign tumors such as lymphangiomas, hemangiomas, fibromas, neurofibromas, myomas, and hamartomas, as well as malignant degeneration of these tumors, can occur.[35,101] Adrenal hemangioma can appear as a low-density mass with scattered calcifications centrally and peripherally.[101]

Adrenal Cysts

Adrenal cysts are classified as parasitic, epithelial, endothelial (lymphangiectatic, angiomatous and hamartomatous), and pseudocystic (resulting from degenerative necrosis and hemorrhage into normal glands or into an adrenal mass).[102–104] Pseudocysts and endothelial cysts are most common, but only about 250 adrenal cysts of all types have been reported.[103]

Adrenal cysts typically produce rounded, low-density masses with a smooth, well-defined contour (Fig. 21–38).[12,103] Cysts range in size from small to very large, are usually (85 per cent) unilateral, and are asymptomatic. A rim of calcification is present in 15 per cent of cases,[105,106] particularly when the cyst has resulted from hemorrhage (Fig. 21–39). The MRI appearance of an adrenal cyst is that of a rounded adrenal lesion that has the MRI characteristics of water: hypointense on T1-weighted images and

markedly hyperintense on T2-weighted images.[104,107] Direct sagittal and coronal images have been helpful in localizing cystic masses to the adrenal gland.

Miscellaneous Abnormalities

INFECTIONS

Tuberculosis, histoplasmosis, blastomycosis, meningococcus, and echinococcus are the most frequent infectious agents affecting the adrenal glands.[58,108–111]

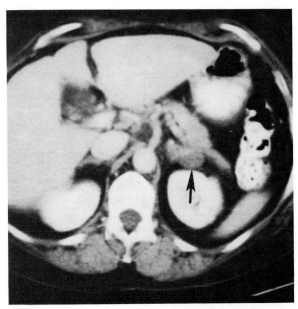

FIGURE 21–38 ■ CT scan of left adrenal cyst *(arrow)* confirmed by ultrasound. The cyst is homogenous, has a well-defined contour, and does not enhance after contrast administration.

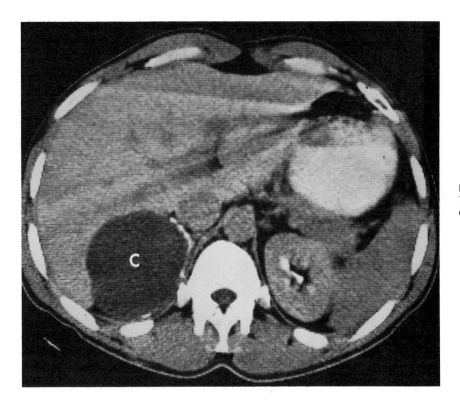

FIGURE 21–39 ■ Large right adrenal cyst (C). The cyst has a uniform density close to that of water and a partially calcified rim.

Infection can result in adrenal calcification or solid or cystic masses and may be either unilateral or bilateral. Tuberculosis has been reported to produce bilateral adrenal enlargement with hypodense regions caused by necrosis[54] or dense calcification of the adrenal gland.[109a] When tuberculous involvement of the adrenals is present, characteristic lung lesions may not be present, and pulmonary cultures may be negative.[108] Adrenal calcification without evidence of a soft tissue mass should suggest inflammatory disease rather than tumor.

The changes caused by histoplasmosis are usually bilateral and symmetric, with preservation of the shape of the adrenal gland (Fig. 21–40).[58,110] Central necrosis is common, but calcification occurs only in a minority of patients.[58] Adrenal histoplasmosis frequently results in adrenal insufficiency, and thus CT evaluation should be considered in patients with

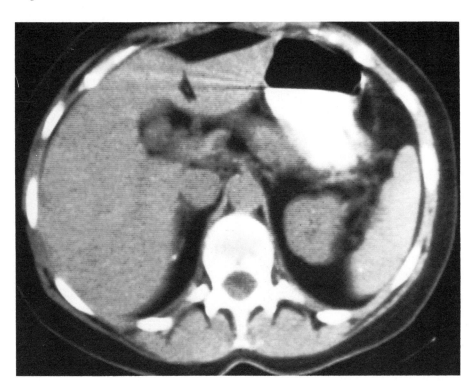

FIGURE 21–40 ■ CT scan of adrenal histoplasmosis producing linear calcification in the right adrenal. A calcified granuloma is also present in the spleen.

onset of Addison's disease who live in endemic areas.[58]

Adrenal abscesses caused by bacterial infection are uncommon in adults[111] but occur more frequently in neonates.[112] Neonatal adrenal abscesses can be unilateral or bilateral and are caused by either hematogenous bacterial seeding of normal adrenal glands or seeding of a neonatal adrenal hemorrhage with subsequent abscess formation.[112] In cases of adrenal infection, the diagnosis may be confirmed by needle aspiration and culture.

The MRI appearance of adrenal infection is nonspecific.[44] Infectious tuberculosis adrenal lesions are slightly more intense than liver on T1-weighted images and markedly more intense on T2-weighted images.[44]

HEMORRHAGE

Adrenal hemorrhage in the adult is uncommon but may lead to acute adrenal insufficiency, which, if not properly diagnosed, can be fatal. Although adrenal hemorrhage often occurs in situations of severe stress such as sepsis, trauma, hypotension, or surgery, the most common cause of bilateral adrenal hemorrhage is anticoagulation therapy.[113] Adrenal hemorrhage is most common during the first 3 weeks of treatment and can occur despite clotting factors being within the therapeutic range. CT demonstrates bilateral adrenal masses as having a density equal to or slightly greater than that of soft tissue. As the hemorrhage resolves, CT demonstrates a progressive decrease in adrenal size and the development of areas of decreased attenuation.

Posttraumatic adrenal hemorrhage is frequently unilateral and is more common on the right.[114,115] The right side predominance is the result of traumatic compression of the inferior vena cava, producing a pressure wave that is transmitted through the short right adrenal vein directly into the right adrenal gland.[115] Right adrenal gland hemorrhage has also been reported as a complication of liver transplantation,[116] possibly because during transplantation surgery, the right adrenal vein is often sacrificed, resulting in vascular congestion and hemorrhage into the right adrenal gland.[116]

The MRI appearance of adrenal hemorrhage secondary to trauma has been reported to be an enlarged adrenal gland that is isointense with liver on T1-weighted images and of increased intensity on T2 pulse sequences.[115]

OTHER ABNORMALITIES

The adrenal glands in acromegalic patients are larger than normal, although they do have normal shape and function. In patients with severe hemochromatosis, the adrenal gland may be slightly greater in attenuation, a finding that is also seen in the liver and spleen. In extramedullary hematopoiesis CT shows bilateral asymmetric enlargement.[117] Nonspecific enlargement of the adrenal glands may also be seen in hyperthyroidism and in diabetes mellitus.

The Incidentally Discovered Adrenal Mass

A patient with no evidence of adrenal hyperfunction and who has an adrenal mass incidentally discovered by CT is a difficult management problem, particularly if the patient has a known primary malignancy that can metastasize to the adrenal. Benign adrenal masses are typically sharply marginated, have an absent or thin rim, maintain a normal adrenal configuration, have a homogeneous CT density approximately equal to that of muscle, and undergo punctate contrast enhancement (Fig. 21–41).[118–121] Ad-

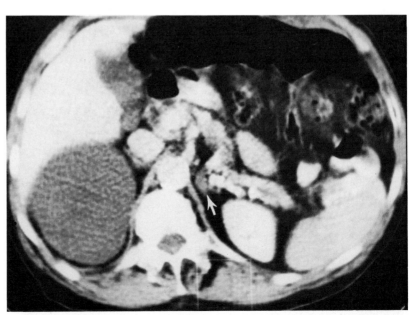

FIGURE 21–41 ■ CT scan of small, nonfunctioning, left adrenal adenoma *(arrow)*, which has a low CT density. CT cannot distinguish benign from malignant lesions of this size.

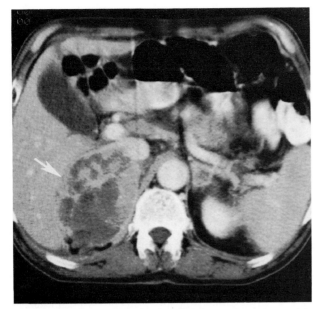

FIGURE 21–42 ■ CT scan of right adrenal mass *(arrow)* caused by metastatic melanoma. The mass is separated and inhomogeneous and has poorly defined margins and an enhancing rim.

masses. Clinical history is of little help, as even in patients with carcinoma of the lung, an adrenal mass is more likely to be an adenoma rather than a metastatic deposit.[120] In patients with small cell carcinoma of the lung, 17 per cent of normal-appearing adrenal glands have malignant cells.[122] This dilemma has led to the liberal use of CT-guided percutaneous biopsy to confirm or exclude a diagnosis of malignancy.[122–125]

In patients with no known malignancy, an incidentally discovered adrenal mass is usually either a nonfunctioning adenoma or an adrenal carcinoma. Adrenal carcinomas are extremely rare (1 per 1 million population),[32] and two thirds are biologically active. Asymptomatic, hormonally inactive adrenal masses less than 5 cm in diameter should undergo follow-up at 6-month intervals (see Fig. 21–41).[123] Lesions that remain stable over a period of 1 year can safely be considered benign.[32] Adrenal masses greater than 5 cm in diameter may warrant surgery, as needle biopsy may be inaccurate as a result of sampling error.

The role of MRI in separating benign from malignant adrenal masses is still evolving. Most investigations have attempted to use T2-weighted pulse sequences to separate adrenal adenomas from adrenal metastases.[42,43,61,84,100] Adrenal metastases as a group have longer T2 relaxation times than adenomas and therefore are usually more intense than adenomas on T2-weighted images (Figs. 21–44 and 21–45). Measuring the adrenal lesion-to-liver intensity ratios on T2-weighted images can help separate an adrenal adenoma from a malignancy.[50,61] Lesion-to-liver intensity ratios of less than 1.2 tend to correlate with adenoma and ratios greater than 1.4 with malignancy.[50,61] The usefulness of this technique has been limited, because more than 20 per cent of adrenal masses have lesion-to-liver intensity ratios between 1.2 and 1.4.[44,50,61]

renal masses with a thick enhancing rim, poorly defined margins, and inhomogeneous attenuation are more likely to be malignant (Figs. 21–42 and 21–43). When these criteria are strictly applied, the positive predictive value of a malignant diagnosis is only 72 per cent, although the positive predictive value of a benign diagnosis is more than 90 per cent.[118]

There is no single CT feature that is totally reliable in distinguishing metastases from benign adenomas. Size, tissue density, homogeneity, and the degree and nature of contrast enhancement do not accurately separate benign from malignant adrenal

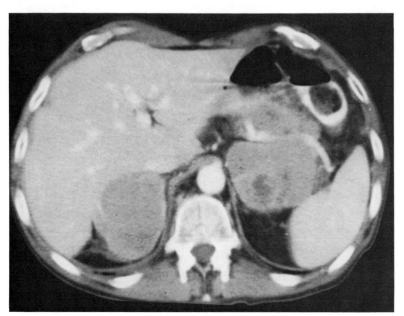

FIGURE 21–43 ■ CT scan of bilateral adrenal metastases from lung carcinoma. There is a thick enhancing rim and inhomogeneous attenuation following contrast administration. The left adrenal metastasis has a foci of tumor necrosis.

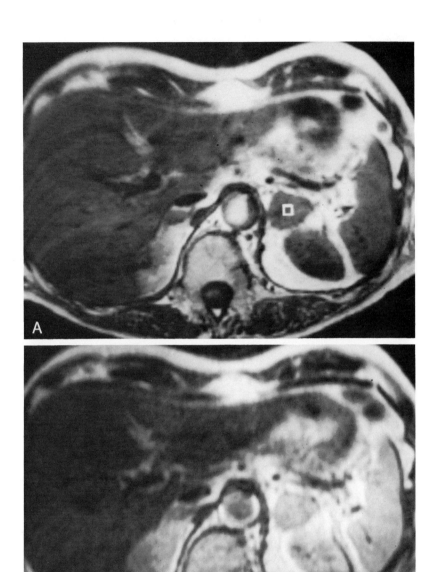

FIGURE 21–44 ■ MR scan of adrenal metastasis from esophageal carcinoma. *A*, T1-weighted image of the mass *(square)* demonstrates the metastasis to be isointense with liver. *B*, The mass becomes hyperintense relative to liver on T2-weighted images. The lesion-liver intensity ratio was 1.6.

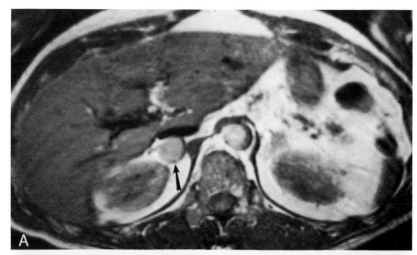

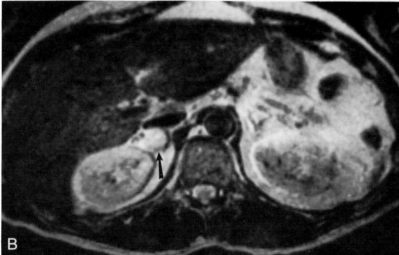

FIGURE 21–45 ■ MR scan of right adrenal metastasis from breast carcinoma. *A,* Mixed-weighted image reveals the adrenal mass *(arrow)* to be slightly more intense than liver. *B,* T2-weighted image shows marked brightening of metastatic deposit.

Calculation of adrenal mass-to-fat intensity ratios on T1-weighted images has also been tried as a method to separate benign from malignant adrenal masses.[125] Benign adrenal masses tend to have a ratio of 0.42 or greater, whereas a ratio of 0.35 or lower was indicative of malignancy.[124] However, more than 30 per cent of masses were judged to be indeterminate using this method.

Currently no MR technique can accurately separate benign from malignant adrenal disease. However, MRI offers the advantage of being better able to identify the adrenal epicenter of a large mass because of its ability to image in multiple planes. In patients who have had previous surgery, MRI may better characterize adrenal masses, because artifacts from surgical clips degrade the CT image more than the MR image.[41]

References

1. Wilms G, Baert A, Marchal G, Goddeeris P: Computed tomography of the normal adrenal glands: correlative study with autopsy specimens. J Comput Assist Tomogr 3:467–469, 1979.
2. White EA, Schambelan M, Rost CR, Biglieri EG, Moss AA, Korobkin M: Use of computed tomography in diagnosing the cause of primary aldosteronism. N Engl J Med 303:1503–1507, 1980.
3. Brownlie K, Kreel L: Computer assisted tomography of normal suprarenal glands. J Comput Assist Tomogr 2:1–20, 1978.
4. Buck J, Reiser U, Hevok F: Computed tomography of the adrenal glands. Eur J Radiol 2:52–59, 1982.
5. Montagne JP, Kressel HY, Korobkin M, Moss AA: Computed tomography of the normal adrenal glands. AJR 130:963–996, 1978.
6. Eghrari M, McLoughlin MJ, Rosen IE, St Louis EL, Wilson SR, et al: The role of computed tomography in the assessment of tumoral pathology of the adrenal glands. J Comput Assist Tomogr 4:71–77, 1980.
7. Abrams HL, Siegelman SS, Adams DF, Sanders R, Finberg HJ, et al: Computed tomography versus ultrasound of the adrenal gland: a prospective study. Radiology 143:121–128, 1982.
8. Schultz CL, Haaga JR, Fletcher BJ, Alfidi RJ, Schultz MA: Magnetic resonance imaging of the adrenal glands: a comparison with computed tomography. AJR 143:1235–1240, 1984.
9. Francis IR, Smid A, Gross MD, Shapiro B, Naylor B, Glazer GM: Adrenal masses in oncologic patients: functional and morphologic evaluation. Radiology 166:353–356, 1988.
10. Kier R, McCarthy S: MR characterization of adrenal masses: field strength and pulse sequence considerations. Radiology 171:671–674, 1989.
11. Krestin GP, Steinbrich W, Friedmann G: Adrenal masses: evaluation with fast gradient echo MR imaging and Gd-

DTPA-enhanced dynamic studies. Radiology 171:675–680, 1989.

12. Tung GA, Pfister RC, Papanicolaou N, Yoder IC: Adrenal cysts: imaging and percutaneous aspiration. Radiology 173:107–110, 1989.

13. Remer EM, Weinfeld RM, Glazer GM, Quint LE, Francis IR, et al: Hyperfunctioning and nonhyperfunctioning benign adrenal cortical lesions: characterization and comparison with MR imaging. Radiology 171:681–685, 1989.

14. Shuman WP, Adam JL, Schoenecker SA, Tazioli PK, Moss AA: Use of a power injector during dynamic computed tomography. J Comput Assist Tomogr 10:1000–1002, 1986.

15. Bernardino ME, Walther MM, Phillips VM, Graham SD Jr, Sewell CW, et al: CT guided adrenal biopsy: accuracy, safety, and indications. AJR 144:67–69, 1984.

16. Heiberg E, Wolverson MK: Ipsilateral decubitus position for percutaneous CT-guided adrenal biopsy. J Comput Assist Tomogr 9:217–218, 1985.

17. Luning M, Neuser D, Kursawe R, Potschke B: CT guided percutaneous fine needle biopsy in the diagnosis of small adrenal tumors. Eur J Radiol 3:308–384, 1983.

18. Heaston DK, Handel DB, Ashton PR, Korobken M: Narrow-gauge needle aspiration of solid adrenal masses. AJR 138:1143–1148, 1982.

19. Shuman WP, Baron RL, Peters MJ, Tazioli PK: Comparison of STIR and spin-echo MR imaging at 1.5T in 90 lesions of the chest, liver, and pelvis. AJR 152:853–859, 1989 .

20. Moon KL, Hricak H, Crooks LE, Gooding CA, Moss AA, et al: Nuclear magnetic resonance imaging of the adrenal gland: a preliminary report. Radiology 147:155–160, 1983.

21. Kneeland JB, Jesmanowicz AJ, Froncisz W, Grist TM, Hyde JS: High resolution MR imaging using loop-gap resonators. Radiology 158:247–250, 1986.

22. Meschan I: Synopsis of Radiologic Anatomy With Computed Tomography. Philadelphia, WB Saunders, 1978, pp 534–538.

23. Kenney PJ, Robbins GL, Ellis DA, Spirt BA: Adrenal glands in patients with congenital renal anomalies: CT appearance. Radiology 155:181–182, 1985.

24. Herbut PA: Urologic Pathology, Vol 2. Philadelphia, Lea & Febiger, 1952, pp 693–696.

25. Schwartz JM, Bosniak MA, Megibow AJ, Hulnick DH: Right adrenal pseudotumor caused by colon: CT demonstration. J Comput Assist Tomogr 12:153–154, 1988.

26. Brady TM, Gross BH, Glazer GM, Williams DM: Adrenal pseudomass due to varices: angiographic-CT-MRI-pathologic correlation. AJR 145:301–304, 1985.

27. Mitty HA, Cohen BA, Sprayregen S, Schwartz K: Adrenal pseudotumors on CT due to dilated portosystemic veins. AJR 141:727–730, 1983.

28. Soffer LS: Diseases of the Endocrine Glands. Philadelphia, Lea & Febiger, 1951, pp 693–696.

29. Besser GM, Edwards CRW: Cushing's syndrome. Clin Endocrinol Metab 1:451, 1972.

30. McAlister WH, Koehler PR: Diseases of the adrenal. Radiol Clin North Am 2:205, 1967.

31. Pojunas KW, Daniels DL, Williams AL, Thorsen MK, Haughton VM: Pituitary and adrenal CT of Cushing syndrome. AJR 146:1235–1238, 1986.

32. Johnson CM, Sheedy PF, Welch TJ, Hattery RR: CT of the adrenal cortex. Semin Ultra CT MR 6:241–260, 1985.

33. Pojunas KW, Daniels DL, Williams AL, Thorsen MK, Haughton VM: Pituitary and adrenal CT of Cushing syndrome. AJR 146:1235–1238, 1986.

34. Huebener KH, Treugut H: Adrenal cortex dysfunction: CT findings. Radiology 150:195–199, 1984.

35. Bethune JE: The Adrenal Cortex. Kalamazoo, MI, Upjohn Company, 1974.

36. Korobkin M, White EA, Kresel HY, Moss AA, Montagne JP: Computed tomography in the diagnosis of adrenal disease. AJR 132:231–238, 1979.

37. Schaner EG, Dunnick NR, Doppman JL, Stroh CA, Gill JR Jr, Javadpour N: Adrenal cortical tumors with low attenuation coefficients: a pitfall in computed tomography diagnosis. J Comput Assist Tomogr 2:11–15, 1978.

38. Dunnick NR, Heaston D, Halvorsen R, Moore AV, Korobkin M: CT appearance of adrenal cortical carcinoma. J Comput Assist Tomogr 6:978–982, 1982.

39. Doppmen JL, Miller DL, Dwyer AJ, Loughlin T, Nieman L, et al: Macronodular adrenal hyperplasia in Cushing disease. Radiology 166:347–352, 1988.

40. Fishman EK, Deutch BM, Hartman DS, Goldman SM, Zerhouni EA, Siegelman SS: Primary adrenocortical carcinoma: CT evaluation with clinical correlation. AJR 148:531–535, 1987.

41. Reinig JW, Doppmen JL, Dwyer AJ, Johnson AR, Knop RH: Distinction between adrenal adenomas and metastases using MR imaging. J Comput Assist Tomogr 9:898–901, 1985.

42. Chang A, Glazer HS, Lee JKT, Ling D, Heiken JP: Adrenal gland: MR imaging. Radiology 163:123–128, 1987.

43. Reinig JW, Doppmen JL, Dwyer AJ, Johnson AR, Knop RH: Adrenal masses differentiated by MR. Radiology 158:81–84, 1986.

44. Baker ME, Spritzer C, Blinder R, Herfkins RJ, Leight GS, Dunnick NR: Benign adrenal lesions mimicking malignancy on MR imaging: Report of two cases. Radiology 163:669–671, 1987.

45. Koch KJ, Cory DA: Simultaneous renal vein thrombosis and bilateral adrenal hemorrhage: MR demonstration. J Comput Assist Tomogr 10:681–683, 1986.

46. Itoh K, Yamashita K, Satoh Y, Sawada H: MR imaging of bilateral adrenal hemorrhage. J Comput Assist Tomogr 12:1054–1056, 1988.

47. Falke THM, van Seters AP, Schaberg A, Moolenaar AJ: Computed tomography in untreated adults with virilising congenital adrenal cortical hyperplasia. Clin Radiol 37:155–160, 1986.

48. Conn JW: Presidential address: part I: painting background. Part II: primary aldosteronism, a new clinical syndrome. J Lab Clin Med 45:3–17, 1955.

49. Roberts L, Dunnick NR, Thompson WM, Foster WL Jr, Halvorsen RA, et al: Primary aldosteronism due to bilateral nodular hyperplasia: CT demonstration. J Comput Assist Tomogr 9:1125–1127, 1985.

50. Glazer GM, Francis IR, Quint LE: Imaging of the adrenal glands. Invest Radiol 23:3–11, 1988.

51. Geisinger MA, Zelch MG, Bravo EL, Risius BF, O'Donovan PB, Barkowski GP: Primary hyperaldosteronism: comparison of CT, adrenal venography, and venous sampling. AJR 141:299–302, 1983.

52. Machida K, Nishikawa J: Computed tomography and scintigraphy of aldosteronoma. A comparative study. Clin Nucl Med 8:610–612, 1983.

53. Wolverson MK, Kannegiesser H: CT of bilateral adrenal hemorrhage with acute adrenal insufficiency in the adult. AJR 142:311–314, 1984.

54. Schultz CL: CT and MR of the adrenal glands. Semin Ultra CT MR 7:219–233, 1986.

55. Shah HR, Love L, Williams MR, Buckner BC, Ferris EJ: Hemorrhagic adrenal metastasis: CT findings. J Comput Assist Tomogr 13:77–81, 1989.

56. Paling MR, Williamson BRJ: Adrenal involvement in non-Hodgkin lymphoma. AJR 141:303–305, 1983.

57. Jafri SZH, Francis IR, Glazer GM, Bree RL, Amendola MA: CT detection of adrenal lymphoma. J Comput Assist Tomogr 7:254–256, 1983.

58. Wilson DA, Muchmore HG, Tisdal RG, Fahmy A, Pitha JV: Histoplasmosis of the adrenal glands studied by CT. Radiology 150:779–783, 1984.

59. Doppman JL, Gill JR Jr, Nienhuis AW, Earll JM, Long JA Jr: CT findings in Addison's disease. J Comput Assist Tomogr 6:757–761, 1982.

60. Ambos MA, Bosniak MA, Lefleur RS, Mitty HA: Adrenal adenoma associated with renal cell carcinoma. AJR 136:81–84, 1981.

61. Reinig JW, Doppman JL, Dwyer AJ, Frank J: MRI of indeterminate adrenal masses. AJR 147:493–496, 1986.

62. Falke THM, Peetoom JJ, Roos AD, Velde CJH, Mazer M: Gadolinium DTPA enhanced MR imaging of intravenous extension of adrenocortical carcinoma. J Comput Assist Tomogr 12:331–334, 1988.

63. Olsson CA, Krane RJ, Klugo RC: Adrenal myelolipoma. Surgery 73:665, 1973.

64. Gould JD, Mitty HA, Pertsemlidis D, Szporn AH: Adrenal myelolipoma: diagnosis by fine needle aspiration. AJR 148:921–922, 1987.

65. Fink DW, Wurtzebach LR: Symptomatic myelolipoma of the adrenal. Radiology 134:451–452, 1980.

66. Vick CW, Zeman RK, Mannes E, Cronan JJ, Walsh JW: Adrenal myelolipoma: CT and ultrasound findings. Urol Radiol 6:7–13, 1984.

67. Musante F, Derchi LE, Zappasodi F, Bazzocchi M, Riviezzo GC, et al: Myelolipoma of the adrenal gland: sonographic and CT features. AJR 151:961–964, 1988.

68. Greene KM, Brantly PN, Thompson WR: Adenocarcinoma metastatic to the adrenal gland simulation myelolipoma: CT evaluation. J Comput Assist Tomogr 9:820–821, 1985.

69. Johnson CM, Welch TJ, Hattery RR, Sheedy PF: CT of the adrenal medulla. Semin Ultra CT MR 6:219–240, 1985.

70. Manger WM, Gifford RW Jr, Hoffman BB: Pheochromocytoma: a clinical and experimental overview. Curr Probl Cancer 9:1–89, 1985.

71. Radin DR, Ralls PN, Boswell WD, Colletti PM, Lapiw SA, et al: Pheochromocytoma detection by unenhanced CT. AJR 146:741–744, 1986.

72. Thomas JL, Bernardino ME, Samaan VA, Hickey RC: CT of pheochromocytoma. AJR 135:477, 1980.

73. Engleman K: Phaeochromocytoma. Clin Endocrinol Metab 6:709, 1977.

74. Casola G, Nicolet V, vanSonnenberg E, Withers C, Bretagnolle M, et al: Unsuspected pheochromocytoma: risk of blood-pressure alterations during percutaneous adrenal biopsy. Radiology 159:733–735, 1986.

75. McCorkell SJ, Niles NL: Fine needle aspiration of catecholamine-producing adrenal masses: a possibly fatal mistake. AJR 145:113–114, 1985.

76. Sheps SG, van Heerden JA, Sheedy PF: Current approaches to the diagnosis of pheochromocytoma. In Glaufox MD, Branchi C (eds): Secondary Form of Hypertension. Orlando, FL, Grune & Stratton, 1981, p 11.

77. Brunt LM, Wells SA Jr: The multiple endocrine neoplasia syndromes. Invest Radiol 20:916–927, 1985.

78. Mathieu E, Despres E, Delepine N, Taieb A: MR imaging of the adrenal gland in Sipple disease. J Comput Assist Tomogr 11:790–794, 1987.

79. Thomas JL, Bernardino ME: Pheochromocytoma in multiple endocrine adenomatosis: efficacy of computed tomography. JAMA 245:1467, 1981.

80. Francis IR, Glazer GM, Shapiro B, Sisson JC, Gross BH: Complementary roles of CT and I 131 MIBG scintigraphy in diagnosing pheochromocytoma. AJR 141:719, 1983.

81. Lynn MD, Shapiro B, Sisson JC, Beierwaltes WH, Meyers LJ, et al: Pheochromocytoma and the normal adrenal medulla: improved visualization with I-123 MIBG scintigraphy. Radiology 156:789–792, 1985.

82. Quint LE, Glazer GM, Francis IR, Shapiro B, Chenevert TL: Pheochromocytoma and paraganglioma: comparison of MR imaging with CT and I-131 MIBG scintigraphy. Radiology 165:89–93, 1987.

83. Fink IJ, Reinig JW, Dwyer AJ, Doppman JL, Linehan WM, Keiser HR: MR imaging of pheochromocytomas. J Comput Assist Tomogr 9:454–458, 1985.

84. Falke THM, Strake LT, Shaff MI, Sandler P, Kulkarni MV, et al: MR imaging of the adrenals: correlation with computed tomography. J Comput Assist Tomogr 10:242–253, 1986.

85. Glazer GM: MR imaging of the liver, kidneys, and adrenal glands. Radiology 166:303–312, 1988.

86. Welch TJ, Sheedy PF, van Heerden JA, Sheps SG, Hattery RR, Stephens DH: Pheochromocytoma: value of computed tomography. Radiology 148:501–503, 1983.

87. Dominick HC, Bachmann KD: Neuroblastoma. In Lohr E (ed): Renal and Adrenal Tumors. Berlin, Springer-Verlag, 1987, pp 241–249.

88. Brasch RC, Korobkin M, Gooding CA: Computed body tomography in children: evaluation of 45 patients. AJR 131:21, 1978.

89. Stark DD, Moss AA, Brasch RC, deLorimier AA, Ablin AR, et al: Neuroblastoma: diagnostic imaging and staging. Radiology 148:101, 1983.

90. Cohen MD, Weetmen R, Provisor A, McGuire W, McKenna S, et al: Magnetic resonance imaging of neuroblastoma. AJR 143:1241–1248, 1984.

91. Daneman A: Adrenal neoplasms in children. Semin Roentgenol 23:205–215, 1988.

92. Dietrich RB, Kangarloo H, Lenarsky C, Feig SA: Neuroblastoma: the role of MR imaging. AJR 148:937–942, 1987.

93. Fletcher BD, Kopiwoda SY, Strandjord SE, Nelson AD, Pickering SP: Abdominal neuroblastoma: magnetic resonance imaging and tissue characterization. Radiology 155:699–703, 1985.

94. Reynes CJ, Curchill R, Moncada R, Love L: Computed tomography of the adrenal glands. Radiol Clin North Am 17:91–104, 1979.

95. Vas W, Zylak CJ, Mather D, Figueredo A: The value of abdominal computed tomography in the pre-treatment assessment of small cell carcinoma of the lung. Radiology 138:417–418, 1981.

96. Sandler MA, Pearlberg JL, Gitschlag KF, Gross SC: Computed tomographic evaluation of the adrenal gland in the preoperative assessment of bronchogenic carcinoma. Radiology 145:733–736, 1982.

97. Nielsen ME, Heaston DK, Dunnick NR, Korobkin M: Preoperative CT evaluation of adrenal glands in non–small cell bronchogenic carcinoma. AJR 139:317–320, 1982.

98. Oliver TW, Bernardino ME, Miller JI, Mansour K, Greene D, Davis WA: Isolated adrenal masses in non–small cell bronchogenic carcinoma. Radiology 153:217–218, 1984.

99. Vicks BS, Perusek M, Johnson J, Tio F: Primary adrenal lymphoma: CT and sonographic appearances. J Clin Ultrasound 15:135–139, 1987.

100. Glazer GM, Woolsey EJ, Borrello J, Francis IR, Aisen AM, et al: Adrenal tissue characterization using MR imaging. Radiology 158:73–79, 1986.

101. Lee WJ, Weinneb J, Kumari S, Phillips G, Pochaczevsky R, Pillari G: Adrenal hemangioma. J Comput Assist Tomogr 6:392–394, 1982.

102. Foster DG: Adrenal cysts. Review of literature and report of case. Arch Surg 92:131–143, 1966.

103. Johnson CD, Baker ME, Dunnick NR: CT demonstration of an adrenal pseudocyst. J Comput Assist Tomogr 9:817–819, 1985.

104. Pastakia B, Miller I, Wolfman M, Cutler GB, Doppman JL: MR imaging of a large adrenal cyst. J Comput Assist Tomogr 10:710–711, 1986.

105. Polubinskas AJ, Christensen WR, Harrison JH, Sosman MC: Calcified adrenal cyst. AJR 82:853, 1959.

106. Daffener RH: Evaluation of Suprarenal Mass. CT/T Clinical Symposium, Vol 1, No 3. Milwaukee, General Electric Company, 1979.

107. Pastakia B, Miller I, Wolfman M, Cutler GB Jr, Doppman JL: MR imaging of a large adrenal cyst. J Comput Assist Tomogr 10:710–711, 1986.

108. Sawczuk IS, Reitelman C, Libby C, Grant D, Vita J, et al: CT findings in Addison's disease caused by tuberculosis. Urol Radiol 8:44–45, 1986.

109. Hauser H, Gurret JP: Miliary tuberculosis associated with adrenal enlargement: CT appearance. J Comput Assist Tomogr 10:254–256, 1986.

109a. Wilms GE, Baert AL, Kint E, Pringot JH, Goddeeris PC: Computed tomographic findings in bilateral adrenal tuberculosis. Radiology 140:729–730, 1983.

110. Wilson DA, Muchmore HC, Tisdal RG, Fahmy A, Pitha JV: Histoplasmosis of the adrenal glands studied by CT. Radiology 150:779–783, 1984.

111. O'Brien WM, Choyke PL, Copeland J, Klappenbach RS, Lynch JH: Computed tomography of adrenal abscess. J Comput Assist Tomogr 11:550–551, 1987.

112. Atkinson GO, Kodroff MB, Gay BB, Ricketts RR: Adrenal abscess in the neonate. Radiology 155:101–104, 1985.

113. Ling D, Korobkin M, Silverman PM, Dunnick NR: CT demonstration of bilateral adrenal hemorrhage. AJR 141:307–308, 1983.

114. Wilms G, Marchal G, Baert A, Adisoejoso B, Mangkuwerdojo

S: CT and ultrasound features of post-traumatic adrenal hemorrhage. J Comput Assist Tomogr 11:112–115, 1987.

115. Murphy BJ, Casillas J, Yrizarry JM: Traumatic adrenal hemorrhage: Radiologic findings. Radiology 169:701–703, 1988.

116. Solomon N, Sumkin J: Right adrenal gland hemorrhage as a complication of liver transplantation: CT appearance. J Comput Assist Tomogr 12:95–97, 1988.

117. King BF, Kopecky KK, Baker MK, Clark SA: Extramedullary hematopoiesis in the adrenal glands: CT characteristics. J Comput Assist Tomogr 11:342–343, 1987.

118. Berland LL, Koslin DB, Kenney PJ, Stanley RJ, Lee JY: Differentiation between small benign and malignant adrenal masses with dynamic incremented CT. AJR 151:95–101, 1988.

119. Mitnick JS, Bosniak MA, Megibow AJ, Naidich DP: Nonfunctioning adrenal adenomas discovered incidentally on computed tomography. Radiology 148:495–499, 1983.

120. Glazer HS, Weyman PJ, Sagel SS, Levitt RG, McClennan BL: Nonfunctioning adrenal masses: incidental discovery on computed tomography. AJR 139:81–85, 1982.

121. Hussain S, Belldegrun A, Seltzer SE, Richie JP, Gittes RF, Abrams HL: Differentiation of malignant from benign adrenal masses: predictive indices on computed tomography. AJR 144:61–65, 1985.

122. Pagani JJ: Normal adrenal glands in small cell lung carcinoma: CT guided biopsy. AJR 140:949–951, 1983.

123. Bernardino ME: Management of the asymptomatic patient with a unilateral adrenal mass. Radiology 166:121–123, 1988.

124. Chezmar JL, Robbins SM, Nelson RC, Steinberg HV, Torres WE, Bernardino ME: Adrenal masses: characterization with T1-weighted MR imaging. Radiology 166:357–359, 1988.

125. Heaston DK, Handel DB, Ashton PR, Korobkin M: Narrow gauge needle aspiration of solid adrenal masses. AJR 138:1143–1148, 1982.

CHAPTER 22

THE SPLEEN

MICHAEL P. FEDERLE

COMPUTED TOMOGRAPHY

Techniques of Examination

The spleen is not often the primary organ of interest when abdominal computed tomographic (CT) scans are obtained. However, a wide variety of splenic variations and abnormalities may be detected on abdominal scans designed to evaluate the liver, pancreas, or retroperitoneum.[1]

In most instances, the spleen is evaluated as part of a scan of the liver or upper abdomen; only in a few instances is a direct CT study of the spleen requested. CT scans 1 cm thick taken at 1-cm intervals are adequate to evaluate the spleen. Precontrast CT scans add little information except in some cases of trauma. Splenic CT studies thus can be performed only after administration of intravenous contrast material.

Selective Splenic Enhancement

In rare instances, it may be difficult to separate the spleen from contiguous structures such as the kidney or pancreas on CT scans, and in such cases, renal or pancreatic tumors may be simulated. Experimental studies using intravenous liposoluble contrast material have demonstrated a preferential increase in the attenuation of liver and spleen parenchyma (Fig. 22–1).[2–6] Experimental contrast material has been produced using phospholiposomes to carry standard diatrizoic acid salts,[4] and Lauteala et al. developed an injected specific liver-spleen contrast agent of particulate iodipamide ethyl ester.[7] Such agents may ultimately prove clinically useful in a variety of hepatic and splenic pathologic processes, including evaluation of space-occupying lesions and separation of spleen from contiguous organs or masses. However, these agents are still classified as investigational and have not yet been approved for general clinical use.

Dynamic CT Scanning

Dynamic CT scanning during an intravenous bolus of 100 to 180 mL of meglumine diatrizoate injected at 1 to 2 mL/sec is useful to assess splenic vasculature and parasplenic masses. Ionic and nonionic agents produce similar degrees of contrast enhancement.[8] The splenic artery will be clearly shown, and delayed CT scans will determine patency of the splenic vein (Fig. 22–2).

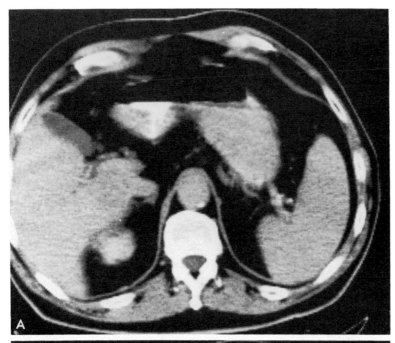

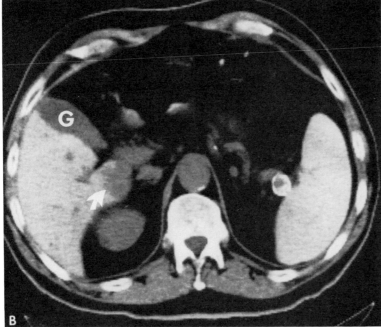

FIGURE 22–1 ■ Use of liposoluble contrast material. *A,* CT scan through the liver and spleen following an intravenous infusion of diatrizoate meglumine (Renografin-60) reveals a questionable lesion in the caudate lobe. *B,* Following intravenous infusion of iodinated oil, areas of normal reticuloendothelial cells in the liver and spleen become densely opacified. The questionable metastasis in the caudate lobe *(arrow)* is now obvious. G = Gallbladder.

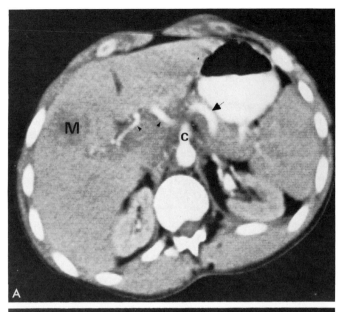

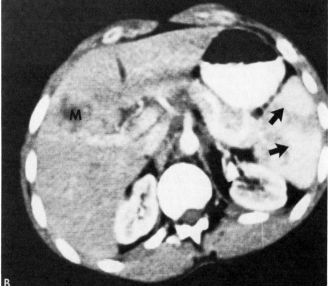

FIGURE 22–2 ■ Dynamic CT section of normal spleen following intravenous bolus of contrast medium. *A*, Early arterial phase. The splenic artery *(arrow)* arises from the celiac trunk (c). Arrowheads = Hepatic artery. *B*, Capillary phase. There are areas of high density *(arrows)* separated by low-density clefts. The spleen enhances in a mottled pattern as a result of variable rates of blood flow in the red pulp of the spleen. *C*, Venous phase. The splenic parenchyma gradually becomes more homogeneous. The splenic (s) and portal (p) veins are patent. M = Hepatic metastasis. (From Federle MP, Moss AA: CRC Crit Rev Diagn Imaging 19:1, 1983.)

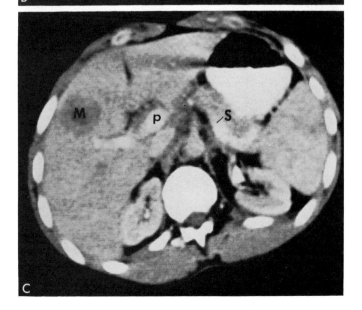

Dynamic CT studies are helpful for separating the spleen from adjacent organs and demonstrating abnormal vascular structures such as gastroesophageal varices, collateral vessels, and splenic artery aneurysms. However, dynamic CT scanning of the spleen has not been as useful as dynamic scans of other solid parenchymal organs such as the liver or kidney. This is primarily because of the inhomogeneous pattern of contrast enhancement seen in about half of normal spleens (see Fig. 22–2).[9, 10] The inhomogeneous contrast enhancement is the result of variable rates of blood flow through the cords of the red pulp of the spleen.[9] Because the normal spleen often appears mottled on dynamic scans obtained during the first 1 to 2 minutes of contrast injection, the diagnosis of small intrasplenic masses should be confirmed on delayed CT images.

Anatomy

Shape

The lateral border of the spleen along the abdominal wall and diaphragm has a smooth, convex margin. The visceral surface is usually lobulated, having a variety of notches, indentations, and ridges in its contour (Fig. 22–3). On axial CT sections, the appearance of the spleen varies depending on the level of the CT scan (Figs. 22–3 and 22–4). An indentation or fossa is usually formed by the left kidney, and there may also be a less discrete fossa for the gastric fundus. Occasionally a prominent notch appears as a complete transection through the splenic parenchyma and simulates a splenic laceration (Fig. 22–5).

A prominent ridge or bulge is commonly seen along the visceral surface or occasionally appears as a discrete lobulation between the tail of the pancreas and the left kidney (Figs. 22–4B and 22–6). This variant may simulate a pancreatic mass on ultrasonography[11] or a pararenal mass on excretory urography,[12, 13] but it is easily recognized as a splenic variation by CT. It is more common with splenomegaly but can occur with normal-sized spleens. Sometimes an enlarged spleen almost encircles the kidney, displacing it anteriorly, posteriorly, or inferiorly (Fig. 22–7).[14] Compression of the kidney by an enlarged spleen may rarely impair renal function.[15]

Size

The spleen varies considerably in size among individuals and even within the same person according to age, state of nutrition, and body habitus. The average adult spleen weighs about 150 g (range, 100 to 250 g) and measures about 12 cm in length, 7 cm in breadth, and 3 to 4 cm in thickness.[15] Because of the variable size of the normal spleen, splenomegaly must be diagnosed with some reservation. From a

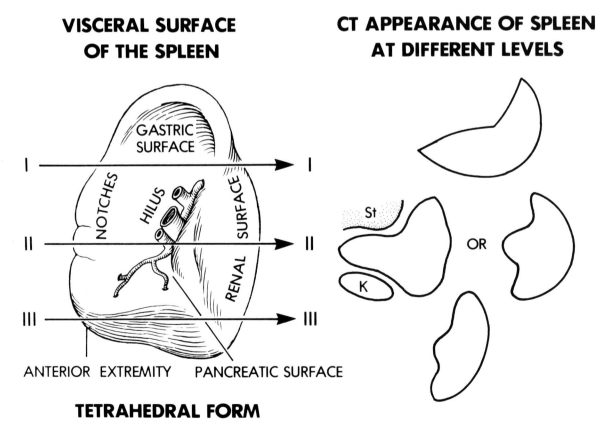

VISCERAL SURFACE OF THE SPLEEN

CT APPEARANCE OF SPLEEN AT DIFFERENT LEVELS

TETRAHEDRAL FORM

FIGURE 22–3 ■ Diagram of the visceral surface of the spleen (tetrahedral form) with the corresponding axial CT appearance. Note the variable appearance at the level of the hilum, where a prominent ridge or lobulation is frequently seen. K = Kidney; St = stomach. (From Piekarski J, Federle MP, Moss AA, London SS: Radiology 135:683, 1983. Reprinted by permission.)

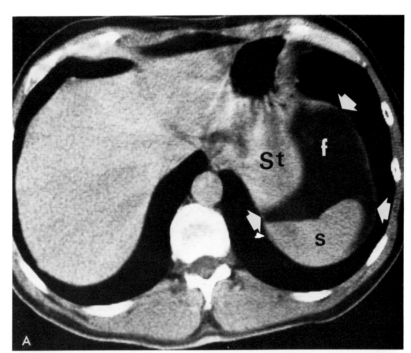

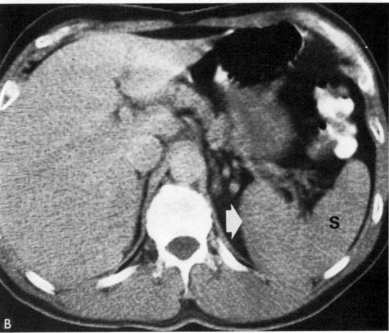

FIGURE 22–4 ■ Variation in shape of normal spleen at different levels in the same patient. *A,* The upper portion of the spleen (s) is semilunar in shape, surrounded by fat (f), and closely related to the diaphragm *(arrows)* and stomach (St). *B,* The midportion of the spleen (s) has a prominent medial bulge *(arrow),* which should not be interpreted as a splenic mass.

Illustration continued on following page

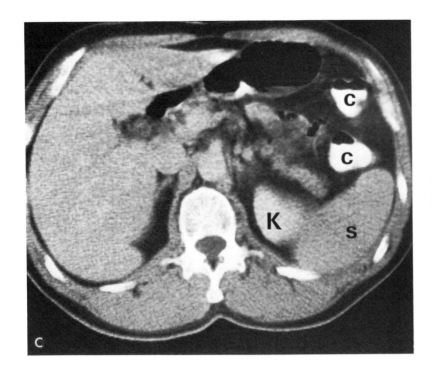

FIGURE 22–4 *Continued* ■ C, The lower portion of the spleen (s) is related to the left kidney (K) and the splenic flexure of the colon (c), and it has a more vertical, elongated shape.

practical standpoint, most experienced observers are able to judge splenic volume as smaller or larger than normal by a simple review of the CT scans. In general, the length of the normal spleen is less than 15 cm, and the splenic tip does not extend caudally as far as the tip of the right lobe of the liver. The anterior edge of the spleen usually does not extend beyond the midaxillary line, although thin crescentic spleens may do so.

When indicated, CT can be used to accurately measure splenic volume. Contiguous scans are obtained through the spleen, and the area occupied by the spleen on each CT section is calculated using the computer program and trackball system available on

most CT scanners (Fig. 22–8). Because each CT section is of known thickness, the volume of the organ is determined by a simple addition of the volumes displayed on each section. In experimental studies, splenic volume determination by CT has been found to be accurate to ±5 per cent of the organ volume measured by water displacement.[16–18] CT changes in spleen volume following distal splenorenal shunt surgery have been quantitated and correlated with shunt patency. Reductions in size of up to 23 per cent have been found in patients with patent shunts, but failure of the spleen to shrink, particularly early after surgery, does not indicate that the shunt is occluded.[19]

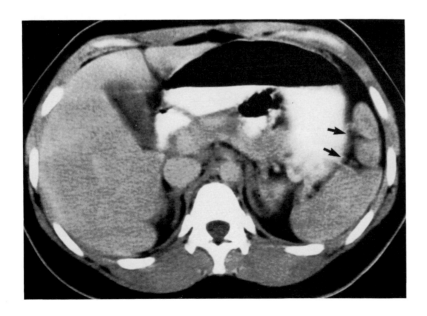

FIGURE 22–5 ■ Pseudofracture of the spleen. Prominent splenic notches or clefts *(arrows)* simulate lacerations of the spleen. Absence of perisplenic blood aids in identification of this common anatomic variant.

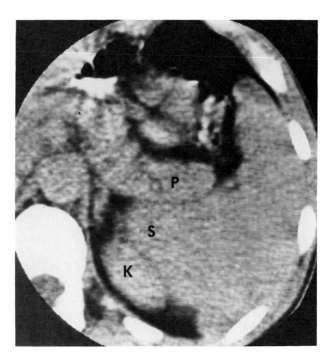

FIGURE 22–6 ■ Prominent splenic lobulation (S) interposed between the pancreas (P) and the left kidney (K). (From Federle MP, Moss AA: CRC Crit Rev Diagn Imaging 19:1, 1983.)

CT Density

The absolute attenuation value of the spleen is variable within any patient population, although it is stable and reproducible within a given individual. Piekarski and colleagues[20] reported a mean CT number of 42.2 Hounsfeld units (H) (range, 29.8 to 68.6 H) with a standard deviation of 8.2 H. Other authors,[21, 22] using different CT scanners, have reported a somewhat different range of attenuation values.

The wide range of CT numbers is largely the result of technical factors such as beam-hardening artifacts, patient size and shape, varying kilovolt peak [kV(p)] of the anode, and intermittent software revisions in scanner systems. However, in the normal patient, the liver and spleen maintain a concordant relationship in attenuation values, with the liver almost always slightly more dense than the spleen (Fig. 22–9). Within the first minute following an intravenous bolus of contrast material, the spleen is often tran-

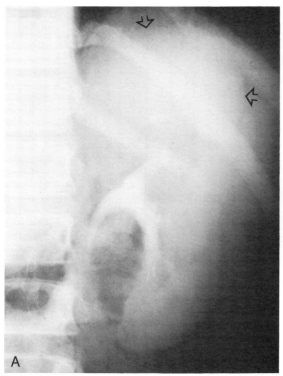

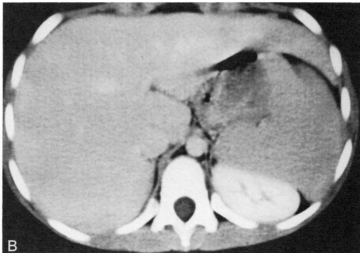

FIGURE 22–7 ■ A, Excretory urogram in a 9-year-old girl demonstrates an apparent mass in the upper pole of the left kidney (arrows). B, CT scan shows compression of the normal kidney by an enlarged spleen with a prominent medial lobulation.

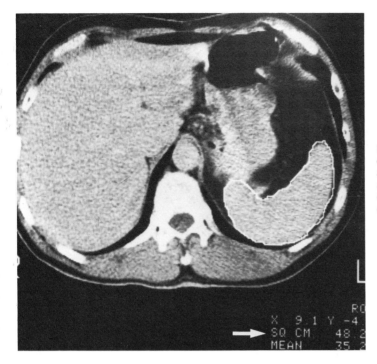

FIGURE 22–8 ■ Splenic volume measurement. An electronic cursor was used to trace the outline of the spleen. The enclosed area is 48.2 cm² *(arrow)*. Because the CT slice is 1 cm thick, a volume of 48.2 cm³ is displayed. Volumes measured on contiguous 1-cm sections through spleen are then added to determine the total splenic volume.

siently more dense than the liver because of prompt enhancement of the splenic pulp and delayed enhancement of the liver by way of the portal vein. Because the spleen is relatively inactive metabolically, large fluctuations of chemical content do not usually occur. Therefore alterations in the concordant relationship between the liver and spleen CT numbers are usually the result of changes in liver composition (e.g., fat, glycogen, or iron deposition) rather than changes in the attenuation value of the spleen. However, the spleen may demonstrate increased attenuation as a result of hemosiderin deposition in

β-thalassemic patients after multiple blood transfusions and changes in T1 and T2 relaxation times, but the spleen is usually of normal density and has normal T1 and T2 values in primary hemochromatosis.[23, 24]

Congenital Variations

Accessory Spleen

Accessory spleens are found in 10 to 30 per cent of unselected autopsy cases.[25, 26] They consist of

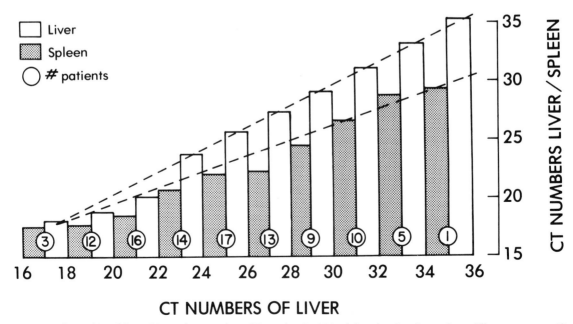

FIGURE 22–9 ■ Relationship of liver CT number to spleen CT number in 100 adults, showing liver-spleen differences at specific liver CT numbers. Scale, +500 to −500 H. (From Piekarski J, Goldberg HI, Royal SA, Axel L, Moss AA: Radiology 137:727, 1980. Reprinted by permission.)

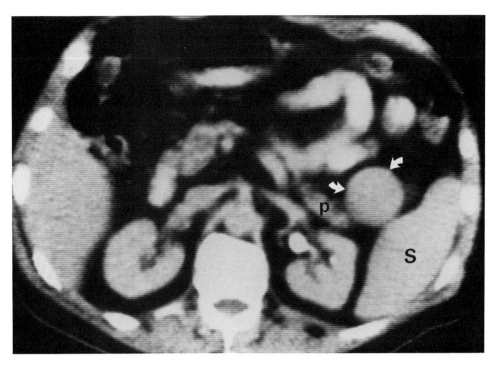

FIGURE 22–10 ■ An accessory spleen *(arrows)* is located near the hilum of the spleen and displaces the tail of the pancreas (p). Despite the large size of this accessory spleen, it maintains a round shape and has the same density as the spleen (S). (From Piekarski J, Federle MP, Moss AA, London SS: Radiology 135:683, 1980. Reprinted by permission.)

nodules of normal splenic tissue and vary from a few millimeters to several centimeters in diameter. They occur most frequently in the hilar region and may be completely isolated from the spleen or connected to it by thin bands of tissue (Fig. 22–10). Most are small and of no clinical significance, going undetected on routine radiographic studies. However, occasionally they are sufficiently large or atypical in location to resemble a tumor on ultrasonography or excretory urography.[12, 13, 27–29] Following splenectomy, the accessory spleen ("splenules") may enlarge dramatically, sometimes presenting as a left upper quadrant mass or causing recurrence of clinical problems in patients who have had splenectomy for hematologic or other disorders (Fig. 22–11).[26, 28, 30]

CT is an accurate method of diagnosing both symptomatic and asymptomatic accessory spleens.[16, 31–33] A round to oval mass in or near the hilum, having the same attenuation as a normal spleen both before and after intravenous contrast material, is virtually pathognomonic. If the CT diagnosis is still in doubt, technetium Tc 99m sulphur colloid images of the liver and spleen may be obtained.

Splenosis is the autotransplantation of splenic tissue that occurs rarely following splenic trauma.[34] The disrupted fragments of splenic tissue may seed the

FIGURE 22–11 ■ Accessory spleens. These splenic remnants have enlarged following splenectomy for trauma 2 years earlier.

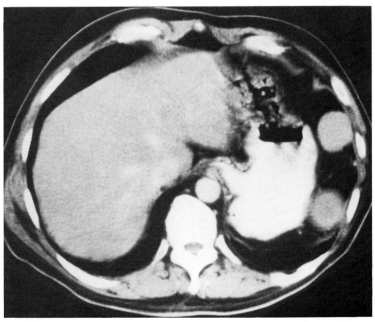
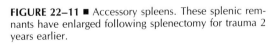

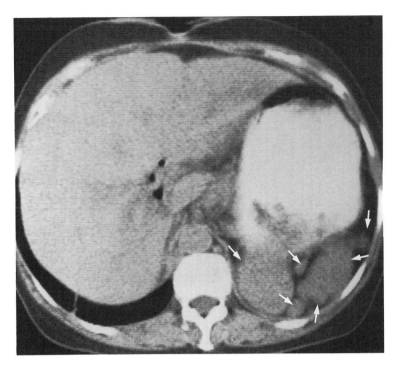

FIGURE 22–12 ■ Polysplenia. CT scan showing multiple spleens *(arrows)* in a patient with azygous continuation of the inferior vena cava.

omentum or peritoneum and may enlarge after acquiring a vascular supply.[34, 35] These may serve a useful purpose in preserving splenic function after surgical removal of the traumatized spleen but may be confused with other causes of peritoneal masses.

Polysplenia and Asplenia

The syndrome of polysplenia consists of multiple ectopic spleens associated with cardiovascular and visceral anomalies.[36-38] The multiple spleens are usually right-sided but may be bilateral. There is no normal-sized spleen as there is in patients having one or more small accessory spleens. Asplenia and polyspenia may occur as isolated anomalies but are frequently associated with various other congenital abnormalities, including partial or total failure of rotation of the intestinal tract, a midline mesentery, cardiac abnormalities, and occasional absence of the gallbladder. The right and left lobes of the liver are of equal size, and there is absence or hypoplasia[39] of the hepatic segment of the inferior vena cava and continuity of the cava with the azygos and hemiazygos veins.[36-40] A possible association between poly-

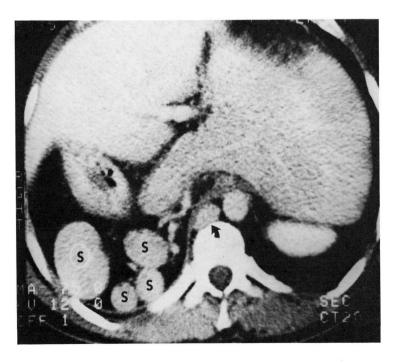

FIGURE 22–13 ■ Polysplenia. This CT scan demonstrates abdominal situs inversus. The liver is located centrally, and splenic silhouette is absent. Several rounded masses (S) in the right hypochondrium are multiple spleens. Note the retrocrural vascular structure *(arrow)*, which is an enlarged hemiazygous vein. The inferior vena cava is absent. (From J Comput Assist Tomogr 5:104, 1981. Reprinted with permission.)

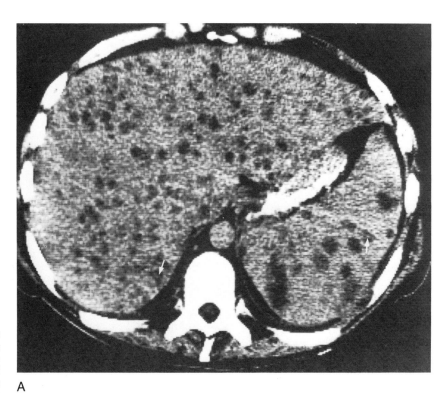

A

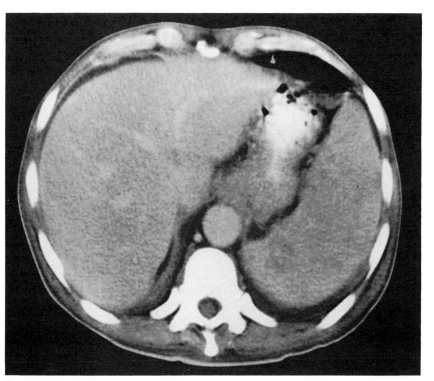

B

FIGURE 22–20 ■ *A,* Fungal abscesses. Multiple splenic and hepatic fungal abscesses in a young man with acute myelogenous leukemia. Several of the abscesses have a central core of higher density *(arrow),* giving the abscesses a target appearance. *B,* Acquired immunodeficiency syndrome patient with splenomegaly and multiple poorly defined focal splenic lesions. These proved to be poorly formed granuloma and abscesses from atypical mycobacteria. (*A* from Piekarski J, Federle MP, Moss AA, London SS: Radiology 135:683, 1980. Reprinted by permission.)

the contents can quickly determine whether fungi are responsible for a splenic abscess.

Following treatment with antifungal agents, CT scans may show a decrease in the number of microabscesses or punctate calcifications representing residual treated candidiasis.[65] However, in some patients, despite successful therapy, the low-density foci do not resolve. Biopsy in these cases has revealed focal areas of fibrosis or granuloma compatible with healing.[65, 66]

Patients with acquired immune deficiency syndrome (AIDS) only uncommonly develop the fungal microabscesses encountered in leukemic and transplant patients. More often the finding of several hypodense small splenic foci is the result of granulomas or abscesses caused by mycobacteria[67] (see Fig. 22–20B) or *Pneumocystis carinii*.[68–71]

Disseminated *P. carinii* in patients with AIDS commonly involves the liver and spleen.[68–71] The appearance can include splenomegaly without focal defects,[69] several scattered punctate calcifications, innumerable calcifications scattered throughout the spleen, or virtually total splenic calcification.[68–71] The liver, kidneys, adrenal glands, and abdominal lymph nodes are also commonly calcified. Calcifications may appear following therapy but also occur in the absence of treatment.

The low-density and calcified lesions represent different manifestations of extrapulmonary infection, rather than active and healed phases as in disseminated candidiasis. Both calcified and noncalcified splenic lesions can progress, and culture results are positive in both phases of the disease. Biopsy has yielded necrotizing granulomas with *P. carinii* organisms and dystrophic calcifications.[68–71]

Disseminated *P. carinii* infection occurs in patients with a history of *P. carinii* pneumonia and may produce few extrapulmonary symptoms. The incidence of disseminated *P. carinii* infection is estimated to be three to five per cent of those with AIDS and *P. carinii* pneumonia.[70]

Certain viral and bacterial illnesses, such as mononucleosis, typhoid fever, and bacterial endocarditis, can produce mild to marked splenomegaly without frank abscess formation. CT in such cases usually reveals only nonspecific splenomegaly.[1] Occasionally there may be intrasplenic hemorrhages or associated findings of enlarged retroperitoneal lymph nodes.

Infarction

Acute and chronic forms of splenic infarction are both detectable by CT.[72–74] Acute splenic infarction usually produces wedge-shaped areas of decreased attenuation extending to the capsule of the spleen that do not enhance after administration of intravenous contrast medium (Fig. 22–21). Renal infarction is frequently diagnosed at the same study. The CT diagnosis of splenic infarction is usually straightforward, but care must be taken not to interpret the nonhomogeneous areas of contrast enhancement during the initial portion of a dynamic CT study as resulting from infarcted tissue. Chronic splenic infarction, as seen in sickle cell anemia, frequently produces a spleen with areas of calcification (Fig. 22–22).[75] Adults with homozygous sickle cell disease usually have small densely calcified spleens, whereas heterozygous hemoglobinopathies often demonstrate enlarged spleens with subcapsular calcification (Fig. 22–23).[76] AIDS patients are also prone to spontaneous acute splenic infarctions (Fig. 22–24).

Non-neoplastic Masses

Splenic cysts were initially regarded as rare but have been recognized more frequently as ultrasound

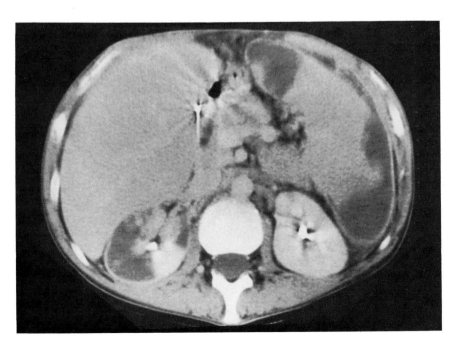

FIGURE 22–21 ■ Acute splenic and renal infarctions in an intravenous drug abuser with subacute bacterial endocarditis. Infarction in both organs is detected as areas of peripheral, often wedge-shaped, nonenhancing parenchyma extending to the "cortical rim" of enhancing capsular tissue supplied by collateral vessels.

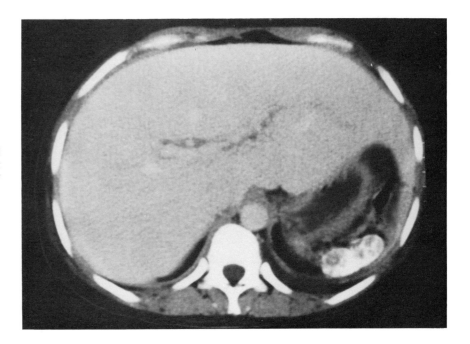

FIGURE 22–22 ■ Twenty-five-year-old woman with sickle cell anemia. Chronic splenic infarction is seen as a small, densely calcified spleen ("autosplenectomy").

and CT have come into greater use.[77–79] Splenic cysts may be parasitic, congenital, or traumatic in origin. They are usually asymptomatic but may cause pain or an enlarging left upper quadrant mass.

PARASITIC CYSTS

Parasitic splenic cysts are almost always caused by an *Echinococcus* tapeworm. The most common organism is *E. granulosus,* which tends to produce a round to oval mass of near-water density and having sharp margins. CT reveals a nonhomogeneous mass with sharp edges that may have foci of calcification (Fig. 22–25). The cyst wall may or may not contain foci of calcification. Noncalcified portions of the cyst wall enhance after contrast injection, and daughter cysts

budding from the outer cyst wall often give a multi-loculated appearance to the cyst.

NONPARASITIC CYSTS

Nonparasitic splenic cysts are usually either congenital or traumatic in origin.[80] Congenital, or true, splenic cysts have a secreting epithelial lining denoting a developmental origin. False cysts, which account for 80 per cent of splenic cysts, lack an epithelial lining and are usually the result of cystic degeneration of a splenic hematoma. Infarcts and infection may rarely lead to cyst development. True and false splenic cysts appear identical on CT: both are characteristically unilocular, homogeneous, water-density lesions having pencil-thin margins that

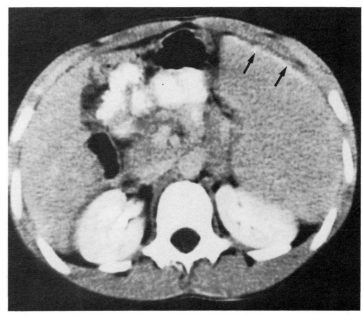

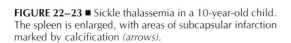

FIGURE 22–23 ■ Sickle thalassemia in a 10-year-old child. The spleen is enlarged, with areas of subcapsular infarction marked by calcification *(arrows)*.

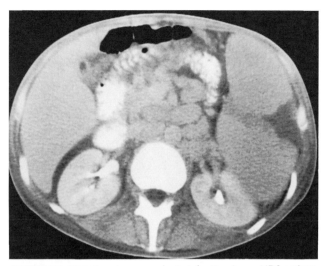

FIGURE 22–24 ■ Spontaneous splenic infarction in an AIDS patient. The splenic parenchymal defect simulates a laceration, which may be difficult to distinguish except for the absence of hemoperitoneum. (Enlarged lymph nodes are the result of opportunistic infection from *Mycobacterium avium–intracellulare*.)

do not enhance after contrast administration (Fig. 22–26). Although calcification in the wall of a splenic cyst is suggestive of *Echinococcus*, it also can occur in posttraumatic and true congenital splenic cysts. However, the history of trauma is often minimal or nonexistent, and it is only after pathologic examination demonstrates the lack of a cellular epithelial lining and absence of *Echinococcus* that a diagnosis of traumatic, partially calcified splenic cyst can be made with certainty.

A rare cause of a nonparasitic splenic cyst is pancreatitis. In these patients, dissection of enzymes into the spleen results in an intrasplenic pseudocyst (Fig. 22–27).[81, 82] In the absence of other CT criteria indicating pancreatitis, it may be difficult or impos-

sible to differentiate an intrasplenic pseudocyst from a congenital or traumatic splenic cyst.

Neoplastic Masses

Hemangioma, although rare, is the most common primary neoplasm of the spleen.[83–85] Hemangiomas produce either single or multiple solid, homogeneous, hypodense or multicystic splenic masses that often contain foci of speckled or snowflakelike calcification. These predominantly cystic lesions enhance after intravenous contrast administration and may become isodense with normal splenic tissue. Splenic hemangiomas are usually asymptomatic unless splenomegaly or rupture develops. Splenic hemangioma has been found to be a part of the Klippel-Trenaunay-Weber syndrome of port-wine cutaneous hemangiomas, superficial venous varicosities, hemangiomas of the bowel and soft tissue, and bony hypertrophy of an extremity (usually unilateral and usually the lower extremity).[84, 85]

Hamartomas, desmoid tumors, and lymphangiomas also can produce predominantly optic splenic masses. Lymphangiomas are malformations consisting of multiple endothelium-lined cysts containing lymph.[86–89] Capillary, cavernous, and cystic forms have been described, depending on the size of the lymphatic spaces.[86–89] CT reveals multiple low-density, nonenhancing, sharply margined, thin-walled cysts that may have foci of curvelinear calcification (Fig. 22–28).[88]

MALIGNANT TUMORS
Primary Neoplasms ■ Although the spleen is a rare site of primary cancer, malignant tumors do arise within the spleen. Splenic angiosarcoma can present with fever, malaise, ascites, hepatosplenomegaly, and hematologic abnormalities such as anemia, leukopenia, and thrombocytopenia.[90] These tumors can

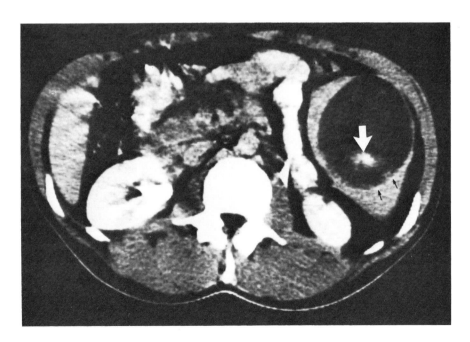

FIGURE 22–25 ■ Echinococcal cyst of the spleen presenting as an intrasplenic rounded mass having an attenuation value of 0 H, an area of intracyst calcification (*large arrow*), pencil-sharp margins, and a rim (*small arrows*) that enhances after contrast injection. (From Piekarski J, Federle MP, Moss AA, London SS: Radiology 135:683, 1980. Reprinted by permission.)

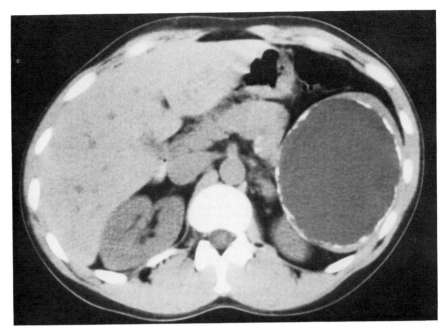

FIGURE 22–26 ■ Posttraumatic splenic cyst with an attenuation value of 0 H and a partially calcified wall. A true congenital cyst has an epithelial lining but can have an identical appearance, although usually without calcification of the cyst wall.

grow rapidly and metastasize early. The CT pattern is that of a nonhomogeneous complex mass of cystic and solid components that has a variable degree of tumor vascularity following contrast medium injection (Fig. 22–29).

Metastatic Neoplasms ■ The spleen is a relatively uncommon site of metastases, in spite of its large mass of lymphoid tissue and its filtration of systemic blood. Splenic metastasis are typically small and, when present, are grossly visible at autopsy in only 67 per cent of cases.[91, 92] Thus although CT can be expected to detect some splenic metastases, a normal spleen CT examination can never be used to exclude metastatic disease to the spleen.

CT demonstrates splenic metastases as ill-defined hypodense areas or well-delineated cystic lesions (Figs. 22–30 and 22–31). The spleen may or may not be enlarged, and the metastasis may appear unilocular (see Fig. 22–30) or contain multiple septations (see Fig. 22–31). Splenic metastases have been reported from melanoma and from ovarian, pancreatic, colon, breast, and endometrial carcinoma, as well as from chondrosarcoma and gastric lymphoma. In our experience, ovarian carcinoma and melanoma have been the most frequent primary malignancies to metastasize to the spleen.[1] Differentiation of a cystic splenic metastasis from a benign cystic lesion of the spleen is often difficult. The CT density and other

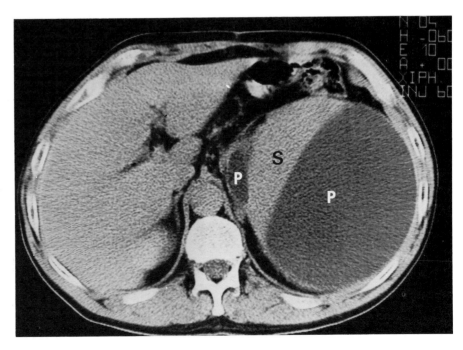

FIGURE 22–27 ■ Intrasplenic pseudocysts. The normal spleen (S) is sandwiched between two well-defined fluid collections of water density proved to be intrasplenic pseudocysts (P) in a patient with a history of pancreatitis. (Courtesy of Pierre A. Schnyder, Lausanne, Switzerland).

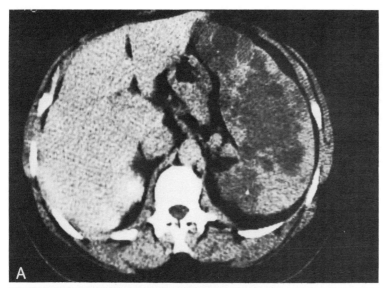

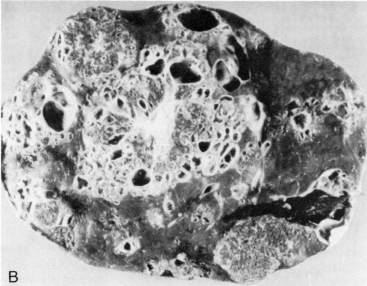

FIGURE 22–28 ■ Lymphangiomatosis. *A,* CT scan shows nonenhancing cystic areas within an enlarged spleen. *B,* Cut surface of spleen shows multiple cysts of varying sizes. (From AJR 150:121, 1988. © 1988, American Roentgen Ray Society.)

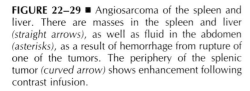

FIGURE 22–29 ■ Angiosarcoma of the spleen and liver. There are masses in the spleen and liver *(straight arrows),* as well as fluid in the abdomen *(asterisks),* as a result of hemorrhage from rupture of one of the tumors. The periphery of the splenic tumor *(curved arrow)* shows enhancement following contrast infusion.

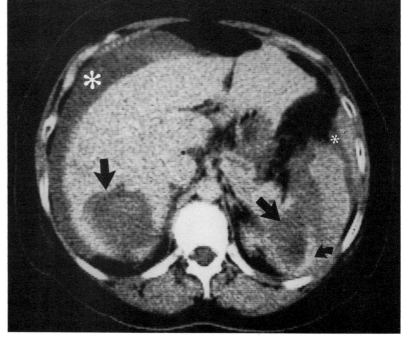

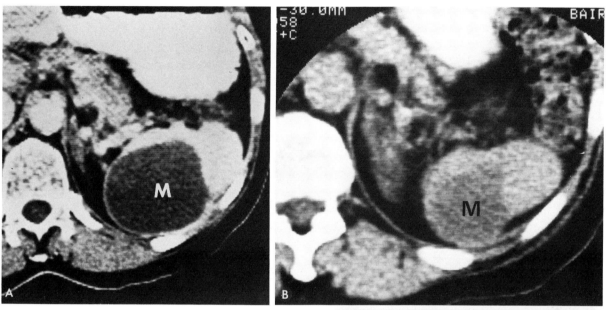

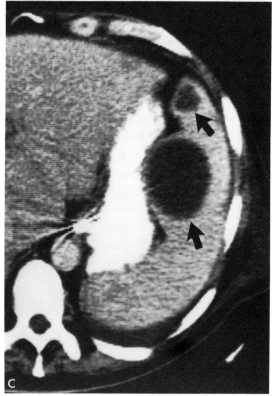

FIGURE 22–30 ■ Splenic metastasis. *A,* Sharply defined mass of water density (M) in the spleen proved to be endometrial carcinoma. CT number = 5 H. *B,* Ill-defined splenic mass (M) having a CT number (20 H) higher than that of a simple cyst. The diagnosis was metastatic endometrial carcinoma. *C,* Multiple unilocular cystic metastases *(arrows)* in an enlarged spleen, resulting from ovarian carcinoma. CT number = 4 H.

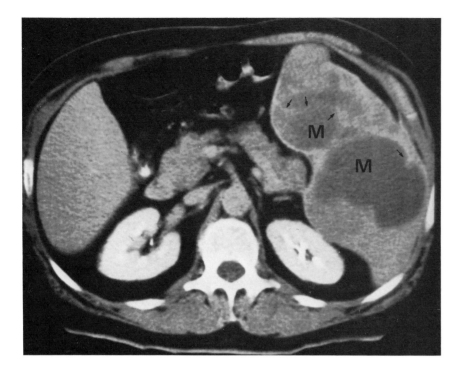

FIGURE 22–31 ■ Metastatic malignant melanoma. CT scan shows multiple, irregularly shaped cystic masses (M). Internal septations are present (arrows).

CT features of cystic splenic metastasis can be identical to those of a benign cyst, and therefore the use of cyst puncture should be employed to document the nature of suspicious cystic lesions of the spleen.[93, 94]

While splenic metastases usually have been believed to occur only in the setting of widespread tumor dissemination, CT has documented several instances of isolated splenic metastases.[1] In particular, CT has detected splenic lesions without any evidence of hepatic metastasis. Such findings may have important clinical implications, as CT detection of splenic involvement with tumor in the absence of other detectable metastatic foci may lead to initiation of focused therapy to the spleen, rather than systemic therapy.

Lymphoma ■ CT has been shown to play an important role in detecting paraaortic, paracaval, mesenteric, hilar, and mediastinal lymph node involvement in patients with lymphoma, but it has not proven to be an accurate method for determining splenic involvement with Hodgkin's disease or other lymphomas.

Although CT is a reliable indicator of splenic size, splenic size alone is of limited diagnostic value in determining splenic involvement with lymphoma. If

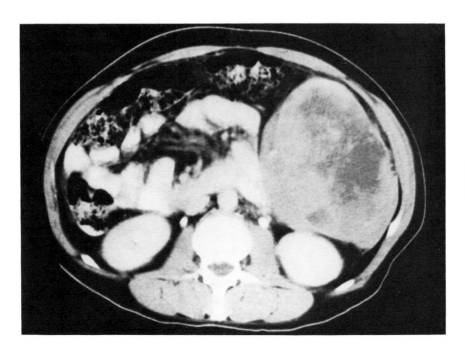

FIGURE 22–32 ■ Non-Hodgkin's lymphoma demonstrated as splenomegaly with a large nodular hypodense mass.

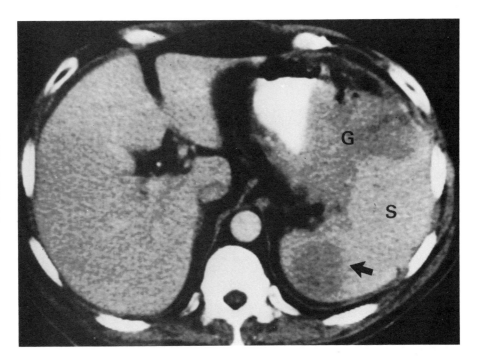

FIGURE 22–33 ■ Gastric lymphoma (G) invading the spleen (S) and obliterating the fat plane between the spleen and the greater curvature of the stomach. A focus of lymphomatous tissue *(arrow)* is also noted in the tip of the spleen. (From Buy J-N, Moss AA: AJR 138:859, 1982. © 1982, American Roentgen Ray Society. Used with permission).

massive splenomegaly is detected in a patient with non-Hodgkin's lymphoma, there is a high probability of lymphomatous involvement.[95] On the other hand, splenomegaly alone is not a reliable indicator of Hodgkin's disease, because a third of such patients do not have pathologic splenic involvement; in addition, a third of the patients with Hodgkin's and non-Hodgkin's lymphoma have normal-sized spleens but still harbor lymphoma.[96–99]

Occasionally lymphoma may take the form of nodular implants in the spleen or liver. When these nodules have a lower attenuation value than the surrounding parenchyma, they can be detected by CT if they are greater than 1.0 to 1.5 cm in diameter (Fig. 22–32). However, only a minority of patients with splenic lymphoma have such a pattern; the usual pattern is a spleen with a completely homogeneous CT density. Splenic involvement can rarely occur from direct invasion by lymphoma originating in the stomach or colon (Fig. 22–33).

The use of water-soluble contrast agents has not aided in the detection of splenic lymphoma, but iodinated lipsoluble contrast agents, which selectively increase the attenuation of normal hepatic and splenic parenchyma, probably aid in the detection of subtle nodular implants of lymphoma.[2, 96] However, the common pattern of microsopic infiltrates will still escape CT detection, and thus CT probably will not become the ultimate method of detecting splenic lymphoma.

Leukemia

The spleen in patients with leukemia can be markedly enlarged but usually maintains a homogeneous, normal CT attenuation value (Fig. 22–34); often there is evidence of lymphadenopathy elsewhere. No difference in the CT appearance of the spleen has been noted among the various forms of leukemia. Spontaneous rupture of the leukemic spleen is known to occur (Fig. 22–35).

Portal Hypertension

Portal hypertension is a frequent cause of splenomegaly. Associated CT findings commonly include a nodular liver, ascites, collateral vascular channels, and prominent caudate lobe (Fig. 22–36). The presence of gastroesophageal varices and collateral vascular channels about the spleen is best demonstrated by dynamic CT scanning techniques. Dynamic CT scanning can also demonstrate splenic vein thrombosis, and in many patients it can suggest the underlying cause (e.g., pancreatitis or pancreatic carcinoma).

Sarcoidosis

Splenomegaly occurs in 11 to 42 per cent of patients with sarcoidosis.[100] The CT appearance is that of homogeneous splenomegaly on non–contrast-enhanced CT scans, but following contrast injection, the appearance may become heterogeneous.[100] Just as different patterns of splenic sarcoidosis are seen after technetium Tc 99m liver spleen scanning, varying CT patterns are also likely to be encountered.

Amyloidosis

Splenic amyloidosis has been reported in patients having either primary amyloidosis or secondary amyloidosis resulting from chronic ulcerative colitis or

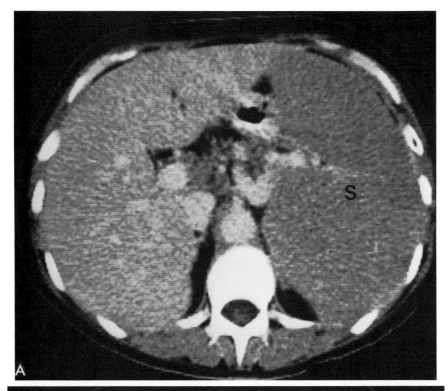

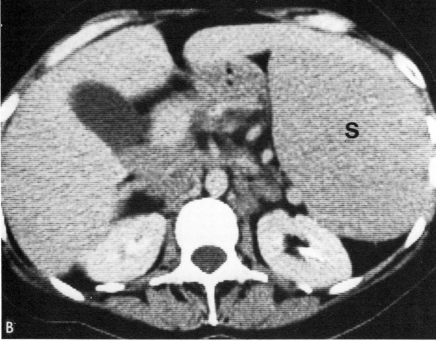

FIGURE 22–34 ■ Splenic enlargement from leukemia. *A*, Chronic lymphocytic leukemia producing marked splenomegaly without focal areas of decreased density. *B*, Chronic myelogenous leukemia with an identical appearance. S = Spleen.

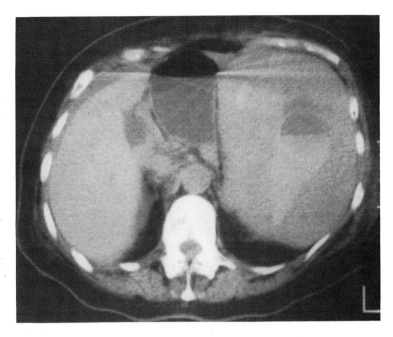

FIGURE 22–35 ■ Chronic myelogeneous leukemia presenting clinically as spontaneous rupture of an enlarged spleen. Note free blood around the spleen and liver and the fluid-fluid level ("hematocrit effect") indicative of coagulopathy. (Courtesy of Vincent McCormick, MD, Modesto, California.)

Crohn's disease.[101, 102] Two patterns of splenic amyloid have been reported: multiple discrete, low-attenuation masses, which may produce splenomegally,[102] and a pattern of diffuse, low CT attenuation and poor contrast enhancement.[101]

MAGNETIC RESONANCE IMAGING

Techniques of Examination

The spleen is routinely well visualized on magnetic resonance imaging (MRI) as a lobulated organ having a smooth contour and longer T1 and T2 relaxation times than normal liver.[103] Thus the spleen typically has a lower signal intensity than liver on T1-weighted images and a higher signal on T2-weighted scans. (Fig. 22–37).

T1- and T2-weighted spin-echo imaging sequences are routinely employed to scan the liver, upper abdomen, and spleen. Respiratory and cardiac gating techniques improve image quality and are frequently used. Short time inversion recovery (STIR) imaging has been shown to have superior sensitivity in the detection of liver and splenic lesions.[104] STIR is an inversion-recovery MR sequence that uses a 180° pulse followed by a 90° pulse and then another 180° pulse to produce an echo. The time between the first 180° pulse and the 90° pulse is termed *TI* and is made relatively short (100 to 170 ms) to produce fat suppression, resulting in fat appearing dark on STIR images. The effects of T1 and T2 tissue differences are additive on STIR images, thus enhancing differences in water content of tissues and improving detection of disease.[104]

Contrast Agents

Particulate contrast agents that localize to the reticuloendothelial tissue of the spleen have great potential as MR splenic contrast agents.[105–107] Ferrite (iron oxide) particles dramatically shorten the T2 of normal liver and spleen without affecting the relaxation parameters of tumors or other focal splenic lesions.[105–109] Following intravenous administration of ferrite particles, the spleen becomes markedly hypodense, thereby increasing lesion conspicuity and detection. Animal studies and preliminary studies in humans have confirmed enhanced tumor detection without toxic effects or histologic alterations in liver or splenic tissue.[105–109]

Pathology

Splenic Lesions

BENIGN LESIONS

Splenic cysts are round, low-intensity masses on T1-weighted images and have a high signal intensity on T2-weighted scans and a low signal on inversion recovery scans. Hemangiomas can have a similar appearance on non–contrast-enhanced images (Fig. 22–38). Injection of Gd-DPTA has no effect on a splenic cyst but increases the signal intensity of a hemangioma on T1 images.

Hematomas have longer T2 relaxation times than normal spleen and thus are easily demonstrated by MRI. The appearance of a splenic hematoma varies as blood undergoes breakdown into deoxyhemoglobin, methemoglobin, and other various paramagnetic products.[110] T1 images may show an acute hematoma to be isointense with spleen, have a high signal intensity days after hematoma formation, and become hypointense as the hematoma liquifies. T2

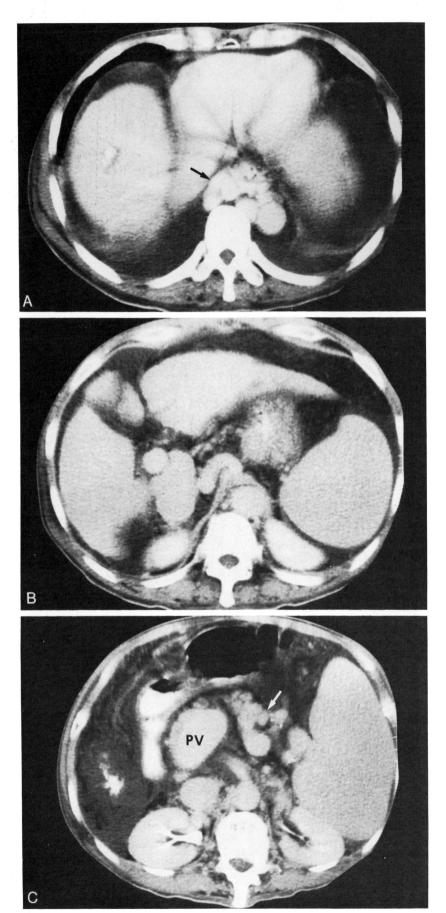

FIGURE 22–36 ■ Alcoholic cirrhosis with portal hypertension and splenomegaly. *A,* Large esophageal varices *(arrows).* *B,* Cirrhotic liver with enlarged left and caudate lobes and deep fissures. *C,* Splenomegaly, varices *(arrow),* and a massively enlarged portal vein (PV) are noted, along with ascites.

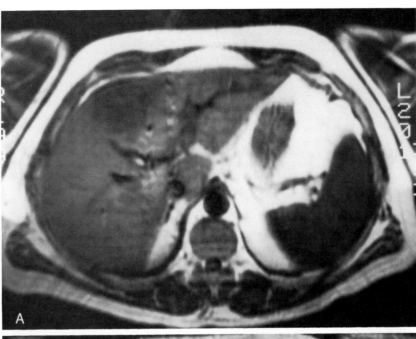

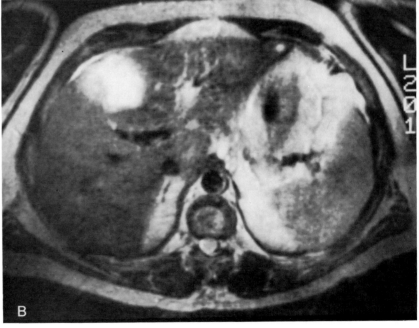

FIGURE 22–37 ■ *A,* Normal Spleen. A T1-weighted spin-echo image (TR, 300; TE, 25) demonstrates the spleen to have a lower signal intensity than the liver. A large liver metastasis is seen as a low-intensity lesion in the medial segment of the left hepatic lobe. *B,* Normal Spleen. A T2-weighted scan (TR, 2000; TE, 80) demonstrates the spleen to have a slightly higher intensity than the liver. The liver metastasis is seen as an extremely high intensity mass lesion.

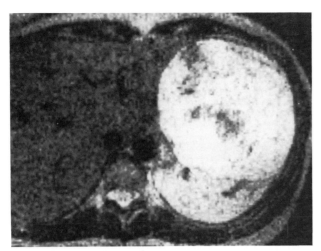

FIGURE 22–38 ■ Giant splenic hemangioma. A T2-weighted spin-echo image demonstrates a very large, hyperintense splenic mass with scattered areas of lower intensity in the center and periphery of the lesion. The low-intensity areas are seen in regions of fibrosis and scar formation, whereas the high-intensity mass represents nonfibrosed hemagioma.

imaging typically reveals an acute hematoma to be hyperintense; later the central clot may have a lower signal intensity, reflecting the T2-shortening effects of the concentrated paramagnetic materials. Old liquified hematomas exhibit high signal intensity.

MALIGNANT LESIONS

Malignant neoplasms have T1 and T2 values that differ on average by only 9 to 11 per cent from those of normal spleen, and as a result tumor signal intensities usually differ only slightly on most spin-echo pulse sequences (Fig. 22–39).[102] Thus non–contrast-enhanced MRI has been found to be less sensitive for detecting focal splenic malignancy than for de-

tecting focal hepatic lesions. However, the use of ferrite particle, STIR, and fast imaging techniques has the potential for increasing detection of splenic malignancy.[104, 105, 107, 109] Using new techniques, MRI will likely become the method of choice to detect focal splenic tumors, as CT has not proven to be a sensitive method to detect splenic lymphoma or metastatic disease. Although MRI may be highly sensitive, it is unlikely that current methods of MRI will prove to be highly specific in determining the nature of splenic lesions.

Splenomegaly

The spleen in patients with splenic enlargement caused by a variety of hematologic disorders has not been shown to have either a specific pattern or signal intensity change. The T1 and T2 relaxation times are typically unchanged. In a few patients with portal hypertension and splenomegaly, the T1 and T2 values of the spleen have been reported to be higher, resulting in a mild increase in signal intensity on T2-weighted images.[111]

Iron Overload

Patients with hemolysis and hematologic disorders that require multiple transfusions experience chronic iron overload and deposition of excess iron in the liver and spleen (Fig. 22–40).[76, 112] A similar process occurs in hereditary hemochromatosis, but the iron deposition is preferentially directed to the liver (Figs. 22–41 and 22–42).[110, 112]

The iron produces marked shortening of splenic T2 and thus greatly reduces signal intensity. The reduction in signal intensity is thought to be a result of the heterogeneous distribution of ferritin and hemosiderin within the reticuloendothelial cells.[110]

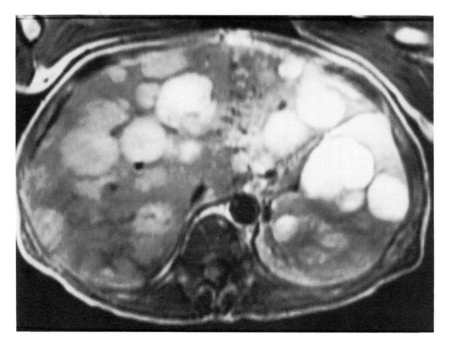

FIGURE 22–39 ■ Melanoma metastatic to liver and spleen. A T2-weighted spin-echo image demonstrates multiple high-intensity lesions scattered throughout the liver and spleen, proven later to be metastatic melanoma. Metastatic melanoma to the spleen has been particularly well demonstrated by MR techniques.

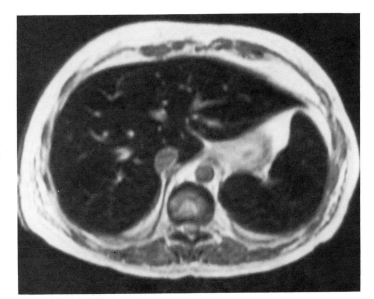

FIGURE 22–40 ■ Hemosiderosis. A spin-echo image (TR, 2200; TE, 30) demonstrates markedly reduced signal intensity in the liver and spleen. The patient had leukemia and had received multiple transfusions.

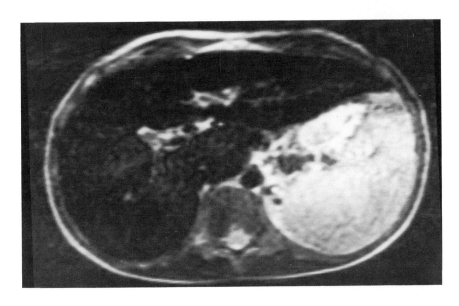

FIGURE 22–41 ■ Hereditary hemochromatosis. A T2-weighted spin-echo image demonstrates marked signal loss in the liver and a relatively normal spleen intensity.

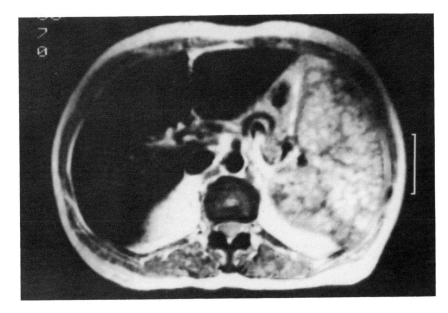

FIGURE 22–42 ■ Hereditary hemochromatosis with extramedullary hematopoiesis occurring in the spleen. A T2-weighted spin-echo image demonstrates marked loss of signal intensity in the liver and an enlarged spleen with multiple focal areas of high signal intensity. A biopsy proved this to represent splenic extramedullary hematopoiesis.

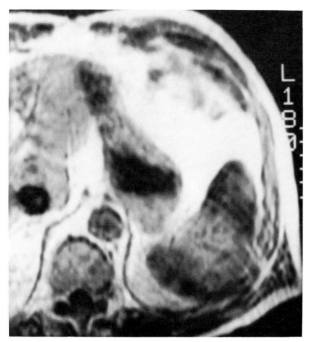

FIGURE 22–43 ■ Splenic infarction. Splenic infarction is demonstrated as focal zones of hyperintensity relative to the normal spleen on this spin-echo image (TR, 2000; TE, 25).

In patients with sickle cell anemia, regions of relative hyperintensity may be produced by splenic infarction without calcification or residual foci of hypertropical splenic tissue with lesion deposition (Fig. 22–43).[76]

References

1. Pierkarski J, Federle MP, Moss AA, London SS: Computed tomography of the spleen. Radiology 135:683, 1980.
2. Vermess M, Doppman JL, Sugarbaker P, Fisher RI, Chatterjee DC, et al: Clinical trial with a new intravenous liposoluble contrast material for computed tomography of the liver and spleen. Radiology 137:217, 1980.
3. Vermess M, Javadpour N, Blayney DW: Post-splenectomy demonstration of splenic tissue by computed tomography with liposoluble contrast material. J Comput Assist Tomogr 5:106, 1981.
4. Payne NI, Whitehouse GH: Delineation of the spleen by a combination of prolipsomes with water soluble contrast media: an experimental study using computed tomography. Br J Radiol 60:535, 1987.
5. Hauron A, Seltzer SE, David MA, Shulkin P: Radiopaque liposomes: a promising new contrast material for computed tomography of the spleen. Radiology 140:507, 1981.
6. Miller DL, Vermess M, Doppman JL, Simon PM, Sugarbaker PH, et al: CT of the liver and spleen with EOE-13: review of 225 examinations. AJR 143:235, 1984.
7. Lauteala L, Kormano M, Violante MR: Uptake and dissolution of particulate iodipamide ethyl ester in the spleen: a morphologic study. Invest Radiol 22:829–835, 1987.
8. Nelson RC, Chezman JL, Peterson JE, Bernardino ME: Contrast enhanced CT of the liver and spleen: comparison of ionic and nonionic contrast agents. AJR 153:973–976, 1989.
9. Glazer G, Axel L, Goldberg HI, Moss AA: Dynamic CT of the normal spleen. AJR 137:343, 1981.
10. Partaman K, Soimakallio K, Kivimaki T, Syrjanen K, Kormano M: Dynamic topography of the contrast enhancement of the spleen. Eur J Radiol 4:101, 1984.
11. Gooding GAW: The ultrasonic and computed tomographic appearance of splenic lobulations: a consideration of the ultrasonic differential of masses adjacent to the left kidney. Radiology 126:719, 1978.
12. Madayag M, Bosniak MA, Bernbaum E, Becker J: Renal and suprarenal pseudotumors caused by variations of the spleen. Radiology 105:43, 1972.
13. Roa AKR, Silver TM: Normal pancreas and splenic variants simulating suprarenal and renal tumors. AJR 126:530, 1976.
14. Requard CK: Retroperitoneal spleen mimicking suprarenal mass in association with malpositioned left kidney: embryologic theory. J Comput Assist Tomogr 5:443, 1981.
15. Goss CM (ed): Gray's Anatomy of the Human Body, 28th ed. Philadelphia, Lea & Febiger, 1966, p 772.
16. Moss AA, Friedman MA, Brito AC: Determination of liver, kidney and spleen volumes by computed tomography: an experimental study in dogs. J Comput Assist Tomogr 5:12, 1981.
17. Brieman RS, Beck JW, Korobkin M, Glenny R, Akwari OE, et al: Volume determination by computed tomography. AJR 138:329, 1982.
18. Heymsfeld SB, Fulenwider R, Nordlinger B, Barlow R, Sones P, Kutner M: Accurate measurement of liver, kidney and spleen volume and mass by computerized axial tomography. Ann Intern Med 90:185, 1979.
19. Hendersen JM, Heymsfeld SB, Horowitz J, Kutner MH: Measurement of liver and spleen volume by computed tomography. Radiology 141:525, 1981.
20. Piekarski J, Goldberg HI, Royal SA, Axel L, Moss AA: Difference between liver and spleen CT numbers in the normal adult: its usefulness in predicting the presence of diffuse liver disease. Radiology 137:727, 1980.
21. Babiker MA, Patel PJ, Karrar ZA, Hafeez MH: Comparison between serum ferritin and computed tomographic densities of liver, spleen, kidney and pancreas in beta-thalassemia major. Scand J Clin Lab Invest 47:715, 1987.
22. Mategrano VC, Petasnick J, Clark J, Bin AC, Weinsteins R: Attenuation values in computed tomography of the abdomen. Radiology 125:135, 1977.
23. Gomori JM, Grossman RI, Drott HR. MR relaxation times and iron content of thalassemic spleens: an in vitro study. AJR 150:567–569, 1988.
24. Long JA, Doppman JL, Nienhus AW, Mills SR: Computed tomographic analysis of beta-thalassemic syndromes with hemochromatosis: pathologic findings with clinical and laboratory correlation. J Comput Assist Tomogr 4:159, 1980.
25. Michaels NA: The variational anatomy of the spleen and splenic artery. Am J Anat 70:21, 1942.
26. Halpert B, Gyorkey F: Lesions observed in accessory spleens of 311 patients. Am J Clin Pathol 332:165, 1959.
27. Rosenkranz W, Kahmi B, Horowitz M: Retroperitoneal accessory spleen simulating a suprarenal mass. Br J Radiol 42:939, 1969.
28. Nishitani H, Hayashi T, Onitsuka H, Kawahira K, Itonda H, et al: Computed tomography of accessory spleens. Radiat Med 2:222, 1984.
29. Appel MF, Bart JB: The surgical and hematologic significance of accessory spleens. Surg Gynecol Obstet 143:191, 1976.
30. Ambriz P, Munoz R, Quintanara E, Sigler L, Avilés A, et al: Accessory spleen compromising response to splenectomy for idiopathic thrombocytopenic purpura. Radiology 155:793, 1985.
31. Stiris MB: Accessory spleen versus left adrenal tumor: computed tomographic and abdominal angiographic evaluation. J Comput Assist Tomogr 4:543, 1980.
32. Beahrs JR, Stephens DH: Enlarged accessory spleens: CT appearance in post-splenectomy patients. AJR 135:483, 1980.
33. Mostbeck G, Sonner G, Haller J, Herold C, Jaeger U, et al: Accessory spleen: presentation as a large abdominal mass in an asymptomatic young woman. Gastrointest Radiol 12:337, 1987.
34. Gentry LR, Brown JM, Lindgren RD: Splenosis: CT demonstration of heterotopic autotransplantation of splenic tissue. J Comput Assist Tomogr 5:1184, 1982.
35. Mendleson DS, Cohen BA, Armas RR: CT appearance of splenosis. J Comput Assist Tomogr 6:1188, 1982.

36. Vaughn T, Hawkins J, Elliot L: Diagnosis of polysplenia syndrome. Diagn Radiol 101:551, 1971.

37. Rose V, Izuhawa T, Moes CAF: Syndromes of asplenia and polysplenia. Br Heart J 37:840, 1975.

38. DeMaeyer P, Wilms G, Baert AL: Polysplenia. J Comput Assist Tomogr 5:104, 1981.

39. Shadle CA, Scott ME, Ritchie DJ, Seliger G: Spontaneous splenic infarction in polysplenia syndrome. J Comput Assist Tomogr 6:177, 1982.

40. Hirohata S, Isobe H, Mitamura T, Yoshinoya S, Miyamoto T, et al: Situs ambiguous with polysplenia complicated by renal adenocarcinoma. Arch Intern Med 145:1134, 1985.

41. Liu P, Daneman A: Unusual position of the spleen: a report of two patients. J Can Assoc Radiol 36:163, 1985.

42. Scicolone G, Contin I, Bano A, Motteran F, Zen F, et al: "Wandering spleen": preoperative diagnosis by echotomography of the abdomen. Chir Ital 38:72, 1986.

43. Stivelman RL, Glaubitz JP, Crampton RS: Laceration of the spleen due to nonpenetrating trauma: one hundred cases. Am J Surg 106:888, 1963.

44. Kelly J, Raptopoulos V, Davidoff A, Waite R, Norton P: The value of non-contrast-enhanced CT in blunt abdominal trauma. AJR 152:41–46, 1989.

45. Jeffrey RB, Laing FC, Federle MP, Goodman PC: Computed tomography of splenic trauma. Radiology 141:729, 1981.

46. Kaufman RA, Toubin R, Babcock DS, Gelfand MJ, Gaice KS, et al: Upper abdominal trauma in children: imaging evaluation. AJR 142:449, 1984.

47. Goldstein AS, Sclafani SJA, Kupferstein NH, Bass I, Lewis T, et al: The diagnostic superiority of computerized tomography. J Trauma 25:938, 1985.

48. Federle MP, Griffiths B, Minagi H, Jeffrey RB Jr: Splenic trauma: evaluation by CT. Radiology 162:69, 1987.

49. Pappas D, Mirvis SE, Crepps JT: Splenic trauma: false-negative CT diagnosis in cases of delayed rupture. AJR 149:727–728, 1987.

50. Fabian TC, Mangiante EC, White TJ, Patterson CR, Boldreghni RN, Britt LG: A prospective study of 91 patients undergoing both computed tomography and peritoneal lavage following blunt abdominal trauma. J Trauma 26:602–607, 1986.

51. Fagelman D, Hertz MA, Ross AS: Delayed development of splenic subcapsular hematoma: CT evaluation. J Comput Assist Tomogr 9:815–816, 1985.

52. Taylor CR, Rosenfield AT: Limitations of computed tomography in the recognition of delayed splenic rupture. J Comput Assist Tomogr 9:1205–1207, 1984.

53. Cholankeril JV, Zamora BO, Ketzer S: Left lobe of the liver draping around the spleen: a pitfall in computed tomography diagnosis of perisplenic hematoma. J Comput Tomogr 8:261, 1984.

54. Berland LL, Van Dyke JA: Decreased splenic enhancement on CT in traumatized hypotensive patients. Radiology 156:469, 1985.

55. Berger PE, Kuhn JP: CT of blunt abdominal trauma in childhood. AJR 136:105, 1981.

56. Brick SH, Taylor GA, Potter BM, Eichelberger MR: Hepatic and splenic injury in children: role of CT in the decision for laparotomy. Radiology 165:643, 1987.

57. Mucha P. Changing attitudes toward the management of blunt splenic trauma in adults. Mayo Clin Proc 61:472–744, 1986.

58. Rice LJ, Rosenstein R, Swikert NC: Splenic abscess: review of the literature and report of case. J Ky Med Assoc 75:375, 1977.

59. Lawhorne TW Jr, Zuidema GO: Splenic abscess. Surgery 79:686, 1976.

60. Faer MJ, Lynch RD, Lichtenstein JE, Feigin DS: Traumatic splenic cysts RPC from the AFIP. Radiology 134:371, 1980.

61. Balthazar EJ, Hilton S, Maidich D, Megibow A, Levine R: CT of splenic and perisplenic abnormalities in septic patients. AJR 144:53, 1985.

62. Callen PW, Filly RA, Marcus FS: Ultrasonography and computed tomography in the evaluation of hepatic microabscesses in the immunosuppressed patient. Radiology 136:433, 1980.

63. Grant E, Mertens MA, Mascatello VJ: Splenic abscess: comparison of four imaging methods. AJR 132:465, 1979.

64. Moss ML, Kirschner LP, Peereboom G, Ferris RA: CT demonstration of splenic abscess not evident at surgery. AJR 135:159, 1980.

65. Shirkhoda A, Lopez-Berestein G, Holbert JM, Luna MA: Hepatosplenic fungal infection: CT and pathologic evaluation after treatment with liposomal amphotericin B. Radiology 159:349–353, 1986.

66. Shirkoda A: CT findings in hepatosplenic and renal candidiosis. J Comput Assist Tomogr 11:795–798, 1987.

67. Jeffrey RB Jr, Nyberg DA, Bottles K, Abrams DI, Federle MP, et al: Abdominal CT in acquired immunodeficiency syndrome. AJR 146:7, 1986.

68. Feverstein IM, Francis P, Raffeld M, Pluda J: Widespread visceral calcification in disseminated *Pneumocystis carinii* infection: CT characteristics. J Comput Assist Tomogr 14:149–151, 1990.

69. Fishman EK, Magid D, Kuhlman JE: *Pneumocystis carinii* involvement of the liver and spleen: CT demonstration. J Comput Assist Tomogr 14:146–148, 1990.

70. Radin DR, Baker EL, Klatt EC, Balthazar EJ, Jeffrey RB Jr, et al: Visceral and nodal calcification in patients with AIDS-related *Pneumocystis carinii* infection. AJR 154:27–31, 1990.

71. Lubat E, Megibow AJ, Balthazar EJ, Goldenberg AS, Birnbaum BA, Bosniak MA: Extrapulmonary *Pneumocystis carinii* infection in AIDS: CT findings. Radiology 174:157–160, 1990.

72. Magid D, Fishman EK, Siegelman SS: Computed tomography of the spleen and liver in sickle cell disease. AJR 143:245–249, 1984.

73. Haft JI, Alteri J, Smith LG, Herskowitz M: Computed tomography of the abdomen in the diagnosis of splenic emboli. Arch Intern Med 148:193, 1988.

74. Balcar I, Seltzer SE, Davis S, Geller S: CT patterns of splenic infection: a clinical and experimental study. Radiology 151:723, 1984.

75. Magid D, Fishman EK, Charache S, Siegelman SS: Abdominal pain in sickle cell disease: the role of CT. Radiology 163:325–328, 1987.

76. Adler DD, Glazer GM, Aisen AM: MRI of the spleen: normal appearance and findings in sickle-cell anemia. AJR 147:843–845, 1986.

77. Graves JW, Tayiem AK: Splenic cysts. J Kansas Med Soc 74:332, 1973.

78. Ghimji DS, Soopeberg PL, Maiman S, Morrison RT, Shergill P: Ultrasound diagnosis of splenic cysts. Radiology 122:787, 1977.

79. Dachman AH, Ros PR, Murai PJH, Olmstead WW, Lichtenstein JE: Nonparasitic splenic cysts: a report of 52 cases with radiologic-pathologic correlation. AJR 147:537, 1986.

80. Garvin DF, King FM: Cysts of the nonlymphomatous tumors of the spleen. Pathol Annu 16:61–80, 1981.

81. Vick CW, Simeone JF, Ferrucci JT Jr, Wittenberg J, Meuller PR: Pancreatitis-associated fluid collections involving the spleen. Sonographic and computed tomographic appearance. Gastrointest Radiol 6:247, 1981.

82. Vyborny CJ, Merrill TN, Reda J, Geurkiwk RE, Smith SJ: Subacute subcapsular hematoma of the spleen complicating pancreatitis: successful percutaneous drainage. Radiology 169:161–162, 1988.

83. Ros PR, Moser RP, Dachman AH, Murari PJ, Olmstead WW: Hemangioma of the spleen: radiologic-pathologic correlation in ten cases. Radiology 162:73–77, 1987.

84. Pakter RL, Fishman EK, Nussbaum A, Giargiana FA, Zerhouni EA: CT findings in splenic hemangiomas in the Klippel-Trenavnay-Weber syndrome. J Comput Assist Tomogr 11:88–91, 1987.

85. Levine E, Wetzel LH, Neff JR: MR imaging and CT of extrahepatic cavernous hemangioma. AJR 147:1299–1304, 1986.

86. Pyatt RS, Williams ED, Clark M, Gasking R: CT diagnosis of splenic cystic lymphangiomatosis. J Comput Assist Tomogr 5:446, 1981.

87. Conraglia-Ferris P, Perlino GF, Barbaino A, Soave F, Oliva L: A pediatric case of cystic lymphangioma of the spleen. J Comput Assist Tomogr 5:449, 1981.

88. Pistoia F, Markowitz SK: Splenic lymphangiomatosis: CT diagnosis. AJR 150:121, 1988.
89. Tutle RJ, Minielly JA: Splenic cystic lymphangiomatosis: an unusual cause of massive splenomegaly. Radiology 126:47–48, 1978.
90. Mahoney B, Jeffrey RB, Federle MP: Spontaneous rupture of hepatic and splenic angiosarcoma demonstrated by CT. AJR 138:965, 1982.
91. Marmont JG Jr, Gross S: Patterns of metastatic cancer in the spleen. Am J Clin Pathol 40:58, 1963.
92. Warren S, Davis AH: Studies on tumor metastasis: the metastases of carcinoma to the spleen. Am J Cancer 21:517, 1981.
93. Federle MP, Filly RA, Moss AA: Cystic hepatic neoplasms: complementary roles of CT and sonography. AJR 135:345, 1981.
94. Newmark H III: Breast cancer metastasizing to the spleen: seminar on computerized tomography. Comput Radiol 6:53, 1982.
95. Dautenhahn LW, Rona G, Saperstein ML, Williams CD, Vermess M: Lymphoma in a pelvic spleen: CT features. J Comput Assist Tomogr 13:1081–1082, 1989.
96. Vermess M, Bernadino ME, Doppman JL, Fisher RI, Thomas JL, et al: Use of intravenous liposoluble contrast material for the examination of the liver and spleen in lymphoma. J Comp Assist Tomogr 5:709, 1981.
97. Strijk SP, Wagener DJ, Bogman NL, DePauw BE, Wobbes T: The spleen in Hodgkin disease: diagnostic value of CT. Radiology 154:753, 1985.
98. Gilbert T, Castellino RA: The spleen in Hodgkin disease: diagnostic value of CT. Crit Rev Invest Radiol 21:437, 1986.
99. Wobbes T, Lubbers EJC, dePauw BE: Results and complications of staging laparotomy in Hodgkin's disease. J Surg Oncol 26:135–137, 1984.
100. Mathieu D, Vanderstigel M, Schaeffer A, Vasile N: Computed tomography of splenic sarcoidosis. J Comput Assist Tomogr 10:679–680, 1986.
101. Suzuki S, Takizawa K, Nakajima Y, Katayama M, Sagawa F: CT findings in hepatic and splenic amyloidosis. J Comput Assist Tomogr 10:332–334, 1986.
102. Edwards P, Cooper DA, Turner J, O'Connor TJ, Byrnes DJ: Resolution of amyloidosis (AA type) complicating chronic ulcerative colitis. Gastroenterology 95:810–815, 1988.
103. Hahn PF, Weissleder R, Stark DD, Saini S, Elizondo G, Ferrucci JT: MR imaging of focal splenic tumors. AJR 150:823–827, 1988.
104. Shuman WP, Baron RL, Peters MJ, Tazioli PK: Comparison of STIR and spin-echo MR imaging at 1.5T in 90 lesions of the chest, liver, and pelvis. AJR 152:853–859, 1989.
105. Weissler R, Hahn PF, Stark DD, Elizondo G, Saini S, et al: Supraparamagnetic iron oxide: enhanced detection of focal splenic tumors with MR imaging. Radiology 169:399–403, 1988.
106. Weissleder R, Stark DD, Rummeny EJ, Compton CC, Ferrucci JT Jr: Splenic lymphoma: ferrite-enhanced MR imaging in rats. Radiology 166:423–430, 1988.
107. Hess CF, Griebel J, Schmiedl U, Kurtz B, Koelbel G, Jaehde E: Focal lesions of the spleen: preliminary results with fast MR imaging at 1.5T. J Comput Assist Tomogr 12:569–574, 1988.
108. Weissleder R, Hahn PF, Stark DD, Rummeny E, Saini S, et al: MR imaging of splenic metastases: ferrite-enhanced detection in rats. AJR 149:723–726, 1987.
109. Weissleder R, Elizondo G, Stark DD, Hahn PF, Marfil J, et al: The diagnosis of splenic lymphoma by MR imaging: value of superparamagnetic iron oxide. AJR 152:175–180, 1989.
110. Stark DD: Biliary system, pancreas, spleen and alimentary tract. In Stark DD, Bradley WG Jr (eds): Magnetic Resonance Imaging. St Louis, CV Mosby, 1988, pp 1114–1123.
111. Stark DD, Goldberg HF, Moss AA, Bass NM: Chronic liver disease: evaluation by magnetic resonance. Radiology 150:149–151, 1984.
112. Gomori JM, Grossman RI, Drott HR: MR relaxation times and iron content of thalassemic spleens: an in vitro study. AJR 130:567–569, 1988.

CHAPTER 23

RETROPERITONEUM AND LYMPHOVASCULAR STRUCTURES

RANDALL M. PATTEN · WILLIAM P. SHUMAN · R. BROOKE JEFFREY, JR.

Lymphatic Structures

Both computed tomography (CT) and magnetic resonance imaging (MRI) are capable of evaluating abdominal and pelvic lymph nodes. Both imaging modalities are noninvasive, well tolerated, simple to perform, and capable of directly imaging nodal areas not routinely visualized during bipedal lymphangiography. The demonstration of pelvic or retroperitoneal adenopathy by either technique (particularly when confirmed by directed biopsy) may obviate the need for more invasive procedures such as lymphangiography or lymph node dissection.

MRI is comparable to CT in its ability to detect retroperitoneal lymphadenopathy and has several advantages.[1-3] Chief among these advantages is the ability to display vascular anatomy without the need for intravascular contrast agents. Tortuous blood vessels or vascular anomalies that may simulate lymphadenopathy on non–contrast-enhanced CT scans are easily depicted as vascular structures on MR scans because of the lack of signal in rapidly flowing blood. Additional advantages of MRI include multiplanar imaging capability, superior soft tissue contrast resolution, and in some cases, reduced artifact from adjacent metallic wires, clips, and prostheses. Whereas CT images may be significantly compromised by such metallic streak artifacts, these artifacts are often less significant on MR scans, thereby allowing more confident evaluation of nodal regions.

However, MRI also has several significant limitations when compared with CT. Poorer spatial resolution may compromise visualization of normal or minimally enlarged lymph nodes. Similarly, a cluster of normal-sized lymph nodes that are readily defined by CT as discrete structures may appear as a solitary enlarged node on MR. Third, because an optimal MR oral contrast agent has not yet been developed, differentiating lymphadenopathy from bowel loops may be difficult, especially in a thin or cachectic patient. Fourth, because longer acquisition times are needed for MR imaging, artifacts from patient movement and peristaltic and respiratory motion may compromise the examination. Last but not least in importance, MRI is more expensive and generally less available than CT. For these reasons, contrast-enhanced CT remains the procedure of choice for initial evaluation of retroperitoneal and pelvic lymphadenopathy. MR is used in those cases in which CT findings are equivocal or when there is a contraindication to the use of iodinated contrast.

Lymph node enlargement is the only criterion for abnormality when using either CT or MRI. No characteristic signal intensity or attenuation coefficients can reliably predict malignancy. Although initial reports of tissue-specific MR relaxation differences between malignant and benign lymph nodes suggested some hope for in vivo tissue characterization based on T1 and T2 values,[4] such characterization is not yet possible.[3, 5] Lymph nodes that are normal in size but diffusely infiltrated by tumor may not be recognized as abnormal (Fig. 23–1). Moreover, in patients with lymphadenopathy caused by reactive hyperplasia or benign disease, neither CT nor MR is able to exclude malignancy as a cause for lymph node enlargement. CT-guided percutaneous needle biopsy of enlarged lymph nodes may be important in these cases to establish a histologic diagnosis. In addition, alternative diagnostic techniques such as lymphangiography will probably continue to hold an important ancillary role in the staging of lymphatic malignancy.

Anatomy

Normal pelvic and retroperitoneal lymph nodes are detected on cross-sectional imaging studies as small soft tissue densities ranging in size from 3 to 10 mm, often identified by their characteristic relationship to normal abdominal and pelvic vessels (Fig. 23–2). Within the pelvis, the external iliac nodes may be subdivided into three separate nodal chains—the external (lateral), internal (medial), and middle chains—designated by their relationship to the external iliac artery and vein (Fig. 23–3).[6] The external group is composed of three to four nodes along the lateral aspect of the external iliac artery, whereas

internal iliac nodes are related to the hypogastric artery. Lymph nodes in the middle chain are often referred to as the *obturator nodes* and are located along the lateral pelvic sidewalls medial to the obturator internus muscle and inferior to the external iliac vein (Fig. 23–4). Obturator nodes are frequently the first to be involved in carcinomas of the cervix, bladder, or prostate (Fig. 23–5). Identification of a lymph node group along the posterior iliac crest, parallel to the course of the deep circumflex iliac artery and vein, has also been described.[7]

Inguinal nodes are located at the upper part of the femoral triangle and are usually divided into superficial and subinguinal groups.[6] The superficial nodes are immediately anterior to the femoral vessels (Figs. 23–6 and 23–7). The lumbar lymph nodes are also commonly divided into three separate nodal chains. These include nodes that are anterior, posterior, and lateral to the aorta (paraaortic); similar nodes positioned adjacent to the inferior vena cava (paracaval); and nodes between the aorta and the cava (aortocaval) (Fig. 23–8). In the lumbar region, lymphadenopathy characteristically obscures the fat planes between the aorta and cava. When lymphadenopathy is massive, all three nodal chains merge to form a bulky mantle of lymphadenopathy that may deviate the aorta and inferior vena cava anteriorly (Fig. 23–9). Lesser degrees of lymphadenopathy can cause asymmetry of muscular contours and distortion of vascular structures.[8]

Retrocrural nodes are located beneath the reflections of the diaphragmatic crura (Fig. 23–10). They can be differentiated from vascular structures (the azygos and hemiazygos veins) by absence of vascular flow (the "flow void" phenomenon) on MR scans and by their lack of enhancement with intravenous contrast material on CT.

Pancreatic, celiac, and superior mesenteric lymph

Text continued on page 1097

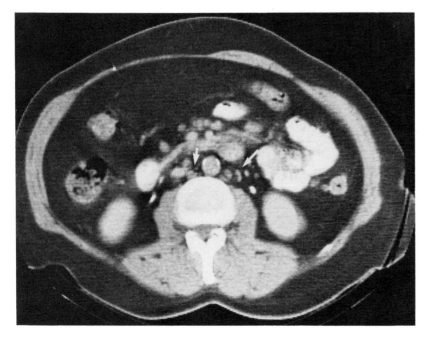

FIGURE 23–1 ■ CT scan demonstrating a cluster of paraaortic lymph nodes *(arrows)*, all less than 1 cm in diameter, that contained foci of metastatic prostatic carcinoma.

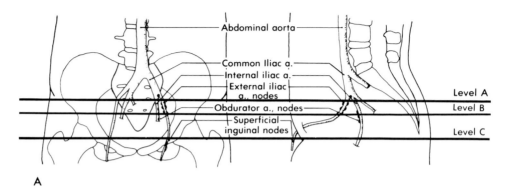

A

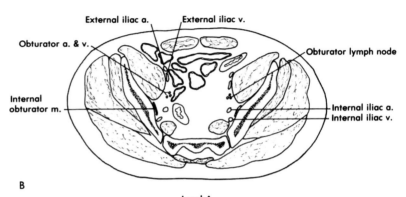

B

Level A

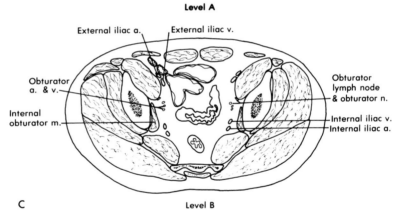

C

Level B

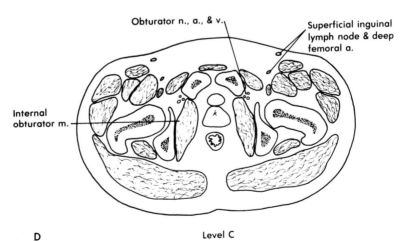

D

Level C

FIGURE 23–2 ■ *A,* Diagram of frontal and lateral projections displaying the relationships of pelvic lymph nodes to pelvic vascular structures. *B–D,* Cross-sectional diagrams depicting anatomic relationships at levels A, B, and C. (Modified from Walsh JW, Amendola MA, Konerding KF, Tinsnado J, Hazra TA: Radiology 137:157, 1980.)

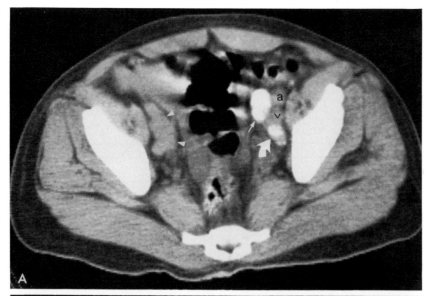

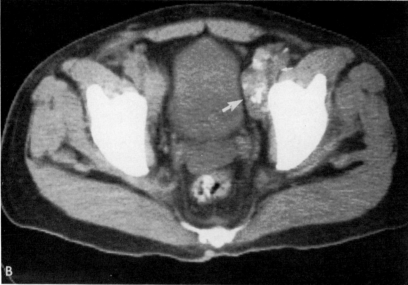

FIGURE 23–3 ■ CT scan following lymphangiogram in a patient with lymphoma. *A*, Enlarged external (lateral) *(straight arrow)* and middle (obturator) *(curved arrow)* nodes of the external iliac nodal group filled with lymphangiographic contrast material from left foot injection. Enlarged nonopacified external and obturator nodes *(arrowheads)* are present on the right side. Internal iliac nodes are also enlarged bilaterally. a = External iliac artery; v = external iliac vein. *B*, Middle chain *(large arrow)* of external iliac nodes enlarged and partially filled with contrast material. Small arrow = External iliac vein.

FIGURE 23–4 ■ Bulky nodal metastases to obturator (middle) (O) and external (lateral) iliac nodes (E) from prostatic carcinoma.

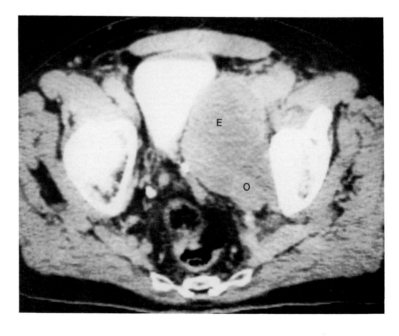

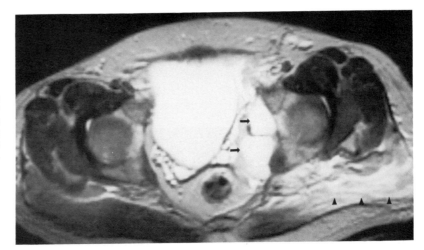

FIGURE 23–5 ■ T2-weighted axial scan (TR, 2000; TE, 80) shows enlarged inflammatory left obturator nodes *(arrows)* deviating the bladder toward the right. This 43-year-old man had a tuberculous abscess of the left hip. Note the inflammatory changes in the left gluteal musculature *(arrowheads)*.

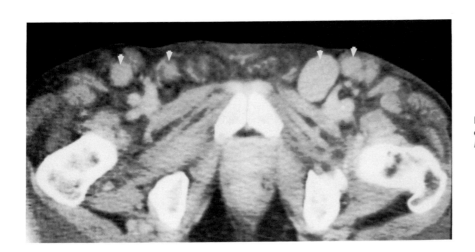

FIGURE 23–6 ■ CT scan shows multiple enlarged superficial inguinal nodes *(arrowheads)* secondary to T-cell lymphoma.

FIGURE 23–7 ■ Proton density–weighted coronal image (TR, 2000; TE, 20) shows the superficial nature of enlarged inguinal nodes *(arrows)* in a patient with lymphoma.

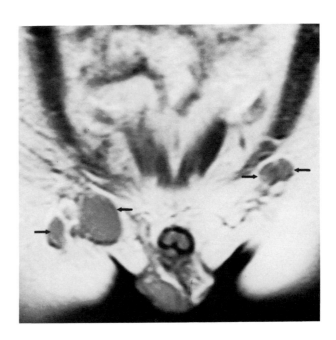

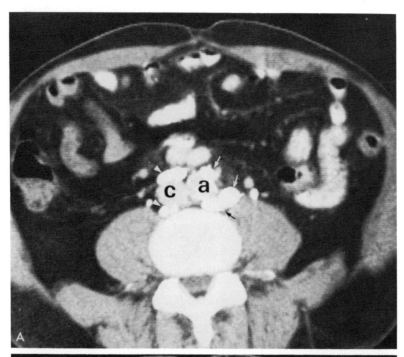

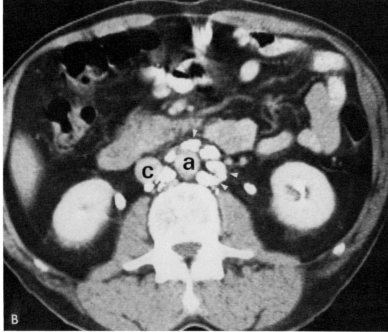

FIGURE 23–8 ■ Anatomy of lumbar lymph nodes in a patient with poorly differentiated nodular lymphoma. *A,* Lymph nodes in the paraaortic *(arrows)* and paracaval nodal chains *(arrowheads)* are slightly enlarged and contain lymphangiographic contrast material. a = Aorta; c = inferior vena cava. *B,* Scan at higher level demonstrates enlarged aortocaval *(arrows)* and paraaortic nodes *(arrowheads).* a = Aorta; c = inferior vena cava.

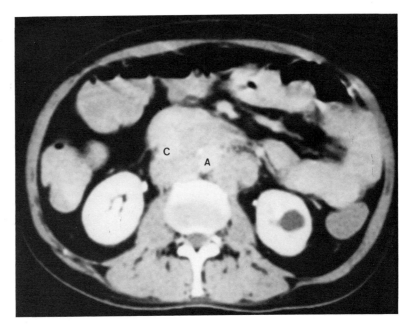

FIGURE 23–9 ■ Massive adenopathy in the paraaortic region forms a mantle of tissue encasing the aorta and displacing the inferior vena cava anteriorly. A = Aorta; C = inferior vena cava. A small left renal cyst is incidentally noted.

nodes are usually not identified with confidence unless they are enlarged or imaged against a background of a fatty mesentery. The anatomy and pathology of mesenteric nodes are discussed in Chapter 24.

Lymphadenopathy may present as multiple discrete soft tissue nodules or as a large, amorphous, confluent mass (Fig. 23–11). In the abdomen and pelvis, lymph nodes larger than 1.5 cm in cross-sectional diameter are considered abnormal, whereas retrocrural nodes are considered abnormal if larger than 6 mm in diameter.[9] A solitary pelvic or abdominal lymph node between 1 and 1.5 cm in size is regarded with suspicion, and a cluster of multiple small nodes is also suspect. Percutaneous biopsy with CT guidance may be helpful in equivocal cases.

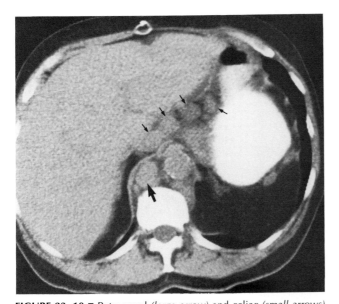

FIGURE 23–10 ■ Retrocrural *(large arrow)* and celiac *(small arrows)* lymphadenopathy in a patient with non-Hodgkin's lymphoma.

Techniques of Examination

Accurate CT or MR diagnosis of pelvic and retroperitoneal adenopathy depends on both anatomic and technical factors. Enlarged lymph nodes are most readily identified in patients who have ample pelvic and retroperitoneal fat; the preservation of fat planes surrounding the paraaortic and pelvic vessels is an important finding in excluding lymphadenopathy. The detection of nodal enlargement in children and in thin adults is often considerably more difficult because of a lack of perivascular and retroperitoneal fat.

Fluid-filled bowel loops can mimic adenopathy, and differentiation will remain a significant problem for MRI until a suitable bowel contrast is available. With CT, adequate bowel opacification with dilute contrast medium is also essential but is more easily accomplished. Administration of 800 mL of a one to two per cent meglumine diatrizoate (Gastrografin) or barium solution 60 minutes prior to the CT study, followed by an additional 400 mL of solution 30 minutes prior to examination and 250 mL immediately prior to examination is usually sufficient to opacify both the proximal and distal small bowel. If the pelvis is to be scanned, a 300- to 400-mL enema of one per cent diatrizoate sodium (Hypaque) is also administered. In selected patients having either slow or very rapid transit of contrast material, additional oral contrast and delayed scans may be required to avoid diagnostic errors.

Techniques developed for rapid administration of contrast material, including dynamic scanning with a power injector, have been adopted as routine for all contrast-enhanced abdominal studies at many centers. Usually 150 to 180 mL of contrast material are rapidly injected during dynamic scanning of the liver to optimize conspicuity of intrahepatic lesions and to optimally display upper abdominal vasculature. When performing combined abdomen-pelvis

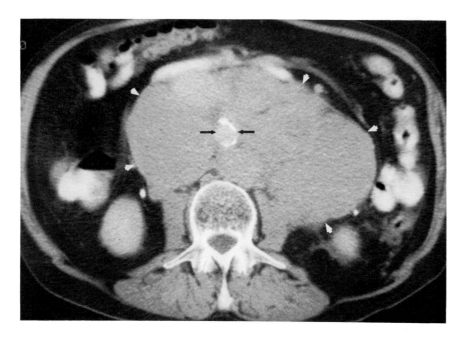

FIGURE 23–11 ■ Massive lymphadenopathy from non-Hodgkin's lymphoma is seen on this CT scan as a confluent mass *(arrowheads)* surrounding the calcified aorta *(arrows)*.

CT scanning, Platt and Glazer advocate intravenous administration of contrast material using a split-bolus technique—an initial bolus at the level of the liver, followed by a second bolus at the level of the iliac crest.[10] However, another report suggests that the split-bolus technique may be unnecessary for optimal CT examination of the pelvis.[11] Teefey et al. found that delayed pelvic scans obtained 3 to 7 minutes after initialization of the primary bolus provided maximum venous enhancement and allowed differentiation of pelvic veins from pelvic lymph nodes without the need for a second bolus dose.[11] In patients with ample pelvic and retroperitoneal fat, intravenous contrast injection is not routinely necessary for CT diagnosis; however, in patients with a

paucity of retroperitoneal fat, intravenous contrast injection is often helpful to identify the retroperitoneal and pelvic vascular structures. On occasion, tortuous iliac vessels, varices, aneurysms, and normal variants, such as a prominent left gonadal vein or duplicated inferior vena cava, may simulate lymphadenopathy on noncontrast scans (Fig. 23–12).[12]

CT scanning protocols can be modified to best evaluate for suspected pathology. For example, in the evaluation of lymphoma or testicular neoplasm, patients can be scanned throughout the abdomen at 2-cm intervals without loss of diagnostic accuracy.[13] However, because pelvic carcinomas may present with only minimal pelvic nodal enlargement, patients

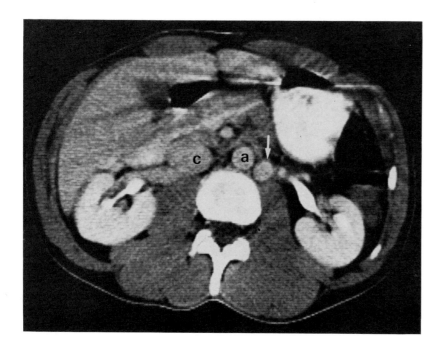

FIGURE 23–12 ■ Prominent left gonadal vein *(arrow)* demonstrated by bolus injection enhances to the same degree as the aorta (a) and inferior vena cava (c). On nonenhanced scans, the unopacified gonadal vein can mimic an enlarged lymph node.

evaluated for pelvic malignancies are usually studied throughout the pelvis at 1-cm intervals.

Lee et al. have found that a single intermediate-weighted MR sequence (repetition time [TR], 900 to 1000; echo delay time [TE], 30 to 35) accurately demonstrates lymphadenopathy and may be used to rapidly survey the pelvis and retroperitoneum.[3] In contrast, Dooms et al. advocate the use of both T1- and T2-weighted imaging sequences for optimal evaluation of lymphadenopathy.[1] Because the T1 relaxation time of lymph nodes is similar to that of muscle and longer than that of fat, lymph nodes are readily distinguished from surrounding fat on T1-weighted (short TR, short TE) imaging sequences. On the other hand, T2-weighted (long TR, long TE) imaging sequences can readily distinguish lymph nodes from surrounding muscle but may decrease the conspicuity of lymph nodes surrounded by fat. Short T1 inversion recovery (STIR) produces both fat suppression and the additive effect of T1 and T2 mechanisms on tissue brightening, and therefore STIR sequences may improve MRI sensitivity in detecting focal pathology (Fig. 23–13).[14] However, the use of the STIR technique for detection of lymphadenopathy has not been extensively studied.

In general, axial scans are sufficient for detection of lymphadenopathy, and sagittal or coronal planes of section do not add substantial clinical information. Whereas lymph nodes usually appear homogeneous on spin-echo pulse sequences, nodes that are partially calcified or filled with lymphangiographic contrast may be heterogeneous or indistinguishable from surrounding fat.[15] Weissleder and co-workers[16] have reported preliminary experience with MR lymphography following interstitial administration of superparamagnetic iron oxide particles into the footpads of mice. Experimental results suggest that MR lymphography may potentially increase the sensitivity

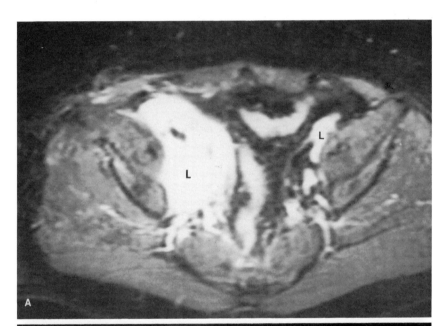

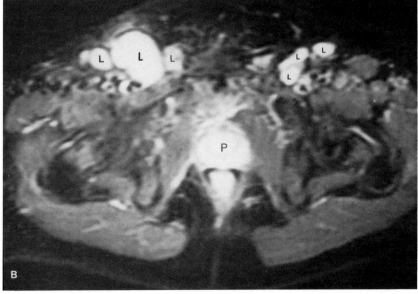

FIGURE 23–13 ■ Detection of lymphadenopathy on STIR image. *A*, Axial scan (TR, 2000; TE, 43; TI, 165) at the level of the iliac wings shows marked brightening of signal from right external iliac and obturator lymphadenopathy (L). Smaller lymph nodes are seen on the left. *B*, Bilateral inguinal lymphadenopathy is also identified by STIR imaging. Patient had non-Hodgkin's lymphoma. P = Prostate.

of MR imaging in the detection of lymphatic malignancy.

Pathology

LYMPHOMA

Accurate staging in both Hodgkin's and non-Hodgkin's lymphoma is vital for determining appropriate therapy and patient prognosis. Patients therefore usually undergo a rigorous diagnostic evaluation including bipedal lymphangiography and, frequently, a staging laparotomy.[17] Whereas lymphangiography has been in clinical use for years and has an 85 to 90 per cent accuracy in the staging of lymphoma,[18, 19] lymphangiography alone is unable to evaluate mesenteric, high paraaortic, and internal iliac nodal chains and may underestimate the extent of disease beyond points of lymphatic obstruction. Moreover, lymphangiography is an invasive, time-consuming procedure that requires considerable skill to perform and interpret.

CT does not provide any information concerning intranodal architecture, but it can detect abnormally enlarged lymph nodes in areas not visualized by lymphangiography. CT therefore may demonstrate the true degree of nodal involvement and permit more accurate planning of radiation therapy. CT routinely detects retrocrural, mesenteric, and peripancreatic adenopathy, as well as enlarged nodes involving the splenic, renal, and hepatic hila (Fig. 23–14). At times CT may demonstrate lymphomatous involvement of solid organs that is clinically unsuspected. When compared with the results of lymphangiography and staging laparotomies, CT has proved to be an accurate noninvasive method of detecting abdominal lymphadenopathy, with overall accuracy rates ranging from 72 to 90 per cent.[17-19]

The precise role of CT and lymphangiography in the staging and follow-up of lymphomas varies among institutions. Some oncologic centers consider the studies complementary and routinely perform both CT and lymphangiography.[17] However, most use CT as the initial screening examination. This is particularly true when evaluating patients with non-Hodgkin's lymphoma, a disease in which more than 50 per cent of patients have mesenteric nodal involvement undetectable by bipedal lymphangiography. Our current approach is to use CT to evaluate the patient with newly diagnosed lymphoma. If widespread lymphadenopathy is present, no further staging procedures are necessary. However, if CT studies are negative or equivocal, lymphangiography is performed to evaluate intranodal architecture of normal sized nodes. A CT-directed biopsy is useful whenever an isolated lymph node is enlarged or when lymphangiographic findings are equivocal (Fig. 23–15).

Following the initial diagnosis of lymphoma, CT scans may be used to monitor the effect of therapy and detect recurrent disease.[20, 21] If lymphangiography has been performed as part of the diagnostic workup, then abdominal radiographs are also useful for monitoring periaortic nodes, as long as such nodes contain sufficient lymphangiographic contrast material.[22] Follow-up using abdominal radiography alone reduces cost and radiation dosage for the individual patient. However, approximately 50 per cent of clinical relapses in lymphoma occur between 1½ and 5 years after diagnosis, and few patients retain adequate lymphangiographic contrast material for that period of time. Lee and co-workers[21] compared postlymphangiogram plain films with CT in patients with lymphoma. In 16 per cent of patients with apparent adequate residual contrast material, plain films failed to demonstrate the extent of disease adequately (Fig. 23–16). For this reason, and because plain films cannot detect disease appearing in those areas not opacified by lymphangiography, we follow

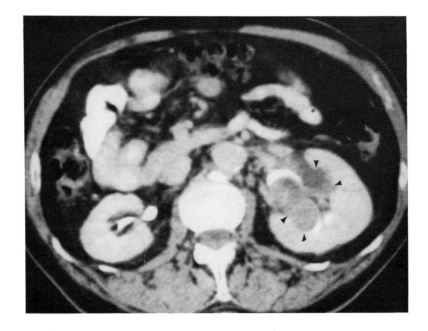

FIGURE 23–14 ■ CT scan demonstrates adenopathy extending into the left renal hilum *(arrowheads)* in a patient with metastatic prostate carcinoma.

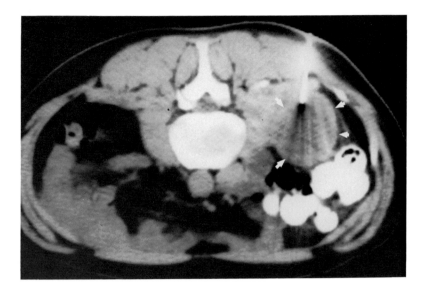

FIGURE 23–15 ■ CT-guided percutaneous biopsy of a retroperitoneal soft tissue mass *(arrows)* with a large-bore cutting needle yielded the histologic diagnosis of undifferentiated sarcoma. Tissue sampling with a large-bore needle is important to preserve histologic architecture and thereby assist tissue characterization.

the majority of lymphoma patients by CT rather than by abdominal and pelvic radiography.

Although MRI is comparable to CT for the detection of lymphadenopathy, the precise role of MR imaging in the evaluation of the patient with lymphoma has yet to be established. One report suggests, however, that because certain lymphangiographic contrast agents may reduce the T1 time and prolong the T2 relaxation time of opacified lymph nodes, abnormal nodes may be indistinguishable from surrounding fat on standard spin-echo MR pulse sequences.[15] Such a potential pitfall may be avoided by performing MR studies prior to lymphangiography.

TESTICULAR NEOPLASMS

Testicular tumors account for one to two per cent of malignancies in males and are the most common malignancy in men aged 20 to 34 years. The choice and success of therapy depend on both histologic classification and the extent of tumor dissemination. About 95 per cent of testicular cancers are of germ cell origin, with 40 per cent of these being pure seminoma;[23] nonseminomatous tumors are classified as embryonal cell, teratocarcinoma, choriocarcinoma, or mixed-element tumors on the basis of the predominant cellular component. Survival rates greater than 90 per cent at 10 years have been achieved with radiotherapy of early-stage seminoma, decreasing to

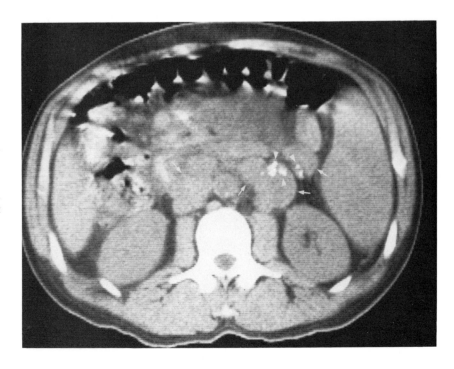

FIGURE 23–16 ■ Recurrent lymphoma following therapy. A small amount of residual contrast material *(arrowheads)* is present in several "normal-sized" paraaortic lymph nodes. The CT scan reveals extensive lymphadenopathy, which does not contain contrast material *(arrows)*.

60 to 70 per cent for advanced disease.[24] In contrast, only 62 per cent of patients with teratoma, 55 per cent of patients with mixed tumors, 39 per cent of patients with embryonal cell carcinoma, and 26 per cent of patients with choriocarcinoma will be disease free after 3 years.[25]

Testicular tumors tend to spread by way of the lymphatics rather than hematogenously. Lymphatics from the involved testis follow the course of the ipsilateral gonadal vein and drain into "sentinel nodes" located predominantly between the T11 and L4 levels.[25–27] Because these nodes are not characteristically opacified from bipedal lymphangiography, and because neoplastic involvement of the more frequently opacified medial lumbar paraaortic nodes occurs relatively late in the course of the disease, noninvasive staging of testicular neoplasm by CT or MRI is important to detect early spread of malignancy (Fig. 23–17).

Several studies have compared the use of CT with lymphangiography in the staging of testicular neoplasms.[25, 27–30] Despite overall accuracy rates that are approximately equal, CT appears to be superior for delineating the true extent of disease and influencing therapeutic decisions.[25, 27, 29, 30] CT has an advantage in detecting early metastases to sentinel lymph nodes, can better delineate the extent of tumor mass, and can detect metastases to extralymphatic sites. Additionally, in the majority of patients, metastases from testicular tumors produce, instead of focal metastatic deposits in normal-sized nodes, large, bulky, low-density retroperitoneal adenopathy, which is easily detectable by CT (Fig. 23–18). In one study, enlarged nodes with CT attenuation values close to those of a cyst—ranging from 10 to 30 Hounsfield units (H)—were found in 48 per cent of patients with testicular metastases.[27] For these reasons, most centers now use CT as the initial staging examination

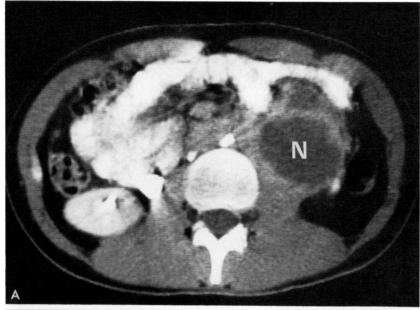

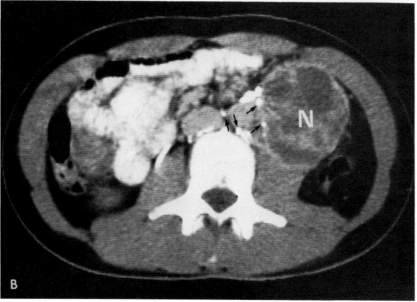

FIGURE 23–17 ■ Metastatic seminoma. *A,* CT scan demonstrating a huge, low-density, unopacified paraaortic nodal metastasis (N) from left testicular seminoma. *B,* CT scan at a lower level demonstrates multiple, normal-sized opacified lymph nodes *(arrows)* medial to the large, unopacified nodule metastasis (N).

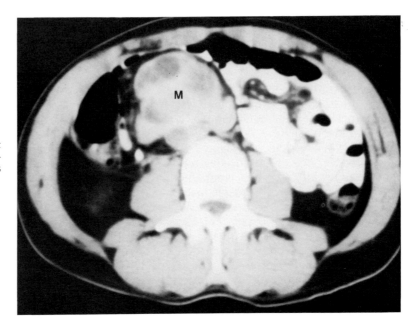

FIGURE 23–18 ■ CT scan in a patient with metastatic teratoma shows a large bulky mass (M) of lymphadenopathy in the paraaortic region. The mass contains several areas of low attenuation.

for patients with newly diagnosed testicular carcinoma, reserving lymphangiography for those patients in whom CT results are negative or equivocal.

MRI can also be used to detect metastatic retroperitoneal lymphadenopathy. A report by Ellis et al. compared CT with MRI in the evaluation of metastatic retroperitoneal adenopathy from testicular carcinoma and found the two modalities comparable (Fig. 23–19).[31] The presence or absence of lymphadenopathy was correctly predicted by CT in 88 per cent of cases and by MRI in 84 per cent; overall staging accuracy was 84 per cent for CT and 80 per cent for MRI.[31] CT did prove to be slightly superior to MRI for detecting extralymphatic abdominal abnormalities, although to some degree this finding may have reflected a lack of experience with MRI.

As with lymphoma, postlymphangiographic radiographs may be inadequate to detect recurrent disease following diagnosis and treatment.[26, 27, 32] The use of CT and serum tumor-marker assays are alternative, complementary methods to follow the effectiveness of therapy.[32, 33] However, posttreatment changes in the CT appearance of metastases must be interpreted cautiously. Although a decrease in mean CT attenuation value after chemotherapy may indicate favorable treatment response, foci of active malignancy may still be demonstrable at pathologic examination.[34] Conversely, residual retroperitoneal masses on CT scans should not be equated with therapeutic failure. After successful therapy, residual fibrosis or necrosis can result in paraaortic masses that are indistinguishable from recurrent or residual tumor.[35] In these patients, a fine-needle aspiration biopsy may be a safe and accurate method to determine whether viable tumor is present. Alternatively, T2-weighted MR images may be useful to differentiate the low signal of fibrosis from the high signal of edema and tumor.

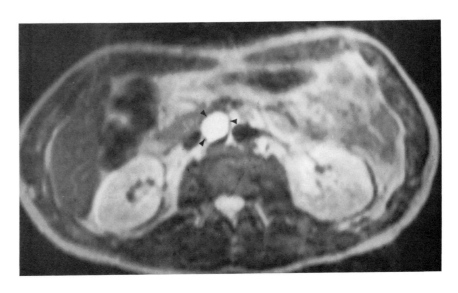

FIGURE 23–19 ■ Axial T2-weighted scan (TR, 2000; TE, 80) at the level of the kidneys demonstrates a single bright, enlarged node in the aortocaval space (arrowheads). Biopsy revealed metastatic embryonal cell carcinoma.

PELVIC MALIGNANCIES

CT is a useful imaging modality in preoperative staging and postoperative treatment of patients with a variety of pelvic neoplasms, including cervical, prostatic, bladder, uterine, and ovarian carcinoma. However, studies have revealed CT to be less accurate in the diagnosis of nodal metastasis from pelvic malignancies than in the staging of lymphoma and testicular neoplasms.[6, 8, 36, 37] This is because of the inability of CT to detect metastases to normal-sized lymph nodes. Lee and associates reported a 73 per cent accuracy of CT when compared with staging laparotomy in a variety of pelvic malignancies,[36] and similar results were obtained by Walsh and colleagues, who noted a 77 per cent accuracy of CT in histologically confirmed cases.[38] However, only nodes larger than 2 cm were considered abnormal,[38] and therefore the lower accuracy of CT in detecting pelvic lymphatic metastases may be related in part to the size criterion of normal pelvic lymph nodes.

In a study by Levine and co-workers[39] comparing the accuracy of CT and lymphangiography in detecting metastasis from prostatic carcinoma, CT achieved an overall accuracy of 93 per cent. In this study, deep pelvic nodes (hypogastric or obturator nodes) were considered abnormal if they were greater than 1.2 cm. Koss and colleagues,[40] using 1.5 cm as the upper limit for normal pelvic lymph nodes, demonstrated 92 per cent accuracy for CT in detecting bladder carcinoma.

In a comparison study of CT and lymphangiography in carcinoma of the cervix, Ginaldi and associates[8] emphasized the complementary role of CT and lymphography. CT has a greater diagnostic yield and more accurately reflects the true extent of disease in relatively advanced stages, whereas lymphangiography remains of considerable value in detecting subtle changes in nodal architecture produced by early metastases. We currently employ CT as the initial diagnostic procedure, followed by lymphan-giography only if CT is negative or equivocal. CT-guided needle aspiration biopsy of nodes that are equivocally enlarged is likely to aid significantly in detecting pelvic metastases.

BENIGN LYMPHADENOPATHY

Neither CT nor MRI can reliably differentiate between benign and malignant causes of lymphadenopathy. A CT study evaluating lymph node size, contour, density, and location found no distinctive features to separate a benign process from a malignant one,[41] and similar difficulties are experienced by MRI because of the overlap in signal characteristics between benign and malignant adenopathy.[1] Certainly the presence of enlarged retroperitoneal lymph nodes is not diagnostic of malignancy, even in a patient with a known primary tumor. A variety of inflammatory, hyperplastic, and granulomatous diseases may demonstrate abdominal or retroperitoneal lymphadenopathy, rendering the CT or MR differentiation from malignancy difficult without lymphangiography and/or tissue sampling (Fig. 23–20). This dilemma is particularly evident in patients with acquired immunodeficiency syndrome (AIDS), in which lymphadenopathy may represent lymphoma, Kaposi's sarcoma, tuberculosis, or benign reactive disease (lymph node syndrome).

In the immunocompromised patient, abdominal manifestations of tuberculosis may complicate pulmonary disease in 6 to 38 per cent of cases[42] and may be secondary to either *Mycobacterium tuberculosis* or *Mycobacterium avium–intracellulare*.[42] Tuberculous lymphadenopathy primarily involves mesenteric and peripancreatic lymph nodes, and characteristic CT features include central areas of low attenuation and inflammatory rim enhancement following intravenous contrast.[43] Lymphadenopathy with central areas of low density (caused by deposition of fat and fatty acids) is also characteristic of Whipple's disease, and may be seen with Crohn's disease, treated lym-

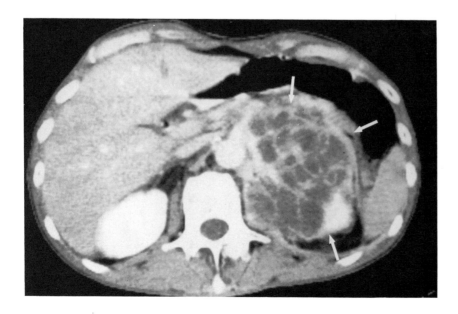

FIGURE 23–20 ■ Contrast-enhanced CT scan demonstrates a large, multiseptated, low-attenuation retroperitoneal mass with enhancing margins (*arrows*). The mass simulates a malignant retroperitoneal sarcoma or metastatic testicular malignancy. However, aspiration biopsy revealed this to be a *Nocardia* abscess in an immunosuppressed patient.

phoma, metastases from testicular neoplasms, and malignant necrosis.[41] Occasionally, benign fatty replacement of normal-sized nodes can be recognized by CT as a normal finding.

Abdominal and retroperitoneal lymphadenopathy from sarcoidosis has been reported in up to 75 per cent of chronic cases, occurring rarely in the absence of pulmonary involvement.[44] Because hepatosplenomegaly typically accompanies retroperitoneal nodal involvement, differentiating sarcoidosis from lymphoma is difficult without biopsy. Retroperitoneal lymphadenopathy may also be detected by cross-sectional imaging techniques in a host of infectious conditions and in patients with amyloidosis[45] or in those with localized and widespread Castleman's disease.[46, 47]

Lymphoceles are abnormal, masslike collections of lymphatic fluid that occur after renal transplantation or following pelvic or retroperitoneal lymphadenectomy. Typically occurring several weeks after lymphatic disruption, uncomplicated lymphoceles appear as homogeneous low-attenuation masses on CT scans (Fig. 23–21). Negative CT attenuation values indicate fat and are highly suggestive of simple lymphoceles; complicated lymphoceles or those secondarily infected may have higher CT numbers.[48] Lymphoceles demonstrate signal characteristics typical of fluid on MRI (long T1 and T2 relaxation times) and are hypoechoic to anechoic on sonography, occasionally containing internal septa and debris (Fig. 23–22).[48]

Although the characteristic appearance, clinical course, and postsurgical time interval usually help to differentiate lymphoceles from abscess, seroma, hematoma, and urinoma, diagnostic needle aspiration may be necessary in equivocal cases. Symptomatic or infected lymphoceles may be effectively drained by percutaneous radiologic techniques.[48]

Abdominal Aorta

Anatomy

The normal abdominal aorta measures less than 3 cm in diameter and tapers gradually in caliber before bifurcating into the common iliac arteries at the L3-4 level. Because its margins are usually well outlined by fat, the abdominal aorta is readily seen by either CT or MRI. Origins of the renal arteries, celiac axis, superior and inferior mesenteric arteries, and common vascular variants are routinely demonstrated.

Techniques of Examination

The abdominal aorta can be visualized on both contrast and noncontrast CT scans. Screening examinations for aortic size and appearance may be performed without intravenous contrast by using 1-cm collimated axial scans at 1.5- to 2-cm intervals from the diaphragm to the aortic bifurcation. Such noncontrast scans may be helpful in detecting displaced intimal calcifications in aortic dissection.[49] However, to better evaluate the aortic lumen for extent of thrombus, atherosclerotic plaque, dissection, or complications of surgery, dynamic CT scanning during a bolus injection of 150 mL of contrast media is recommended with contiguous 1-cm collimation scans. Five-millimeter collimated images may be performed through specific regions of interest to clarify equivocal findings.

MRI is also a useful technique for evaluation of the abdominal aorta.[50] Flowing blood within the aorta and its major branches emits no intraluminal signal—a "flow void" that can be clearly distinguished from surrounding retroperitoneal fat and muscle on both T1- and T2-weighted imaging sequences (Fig. 23–23). Vascular and anatomic relationships are therefore

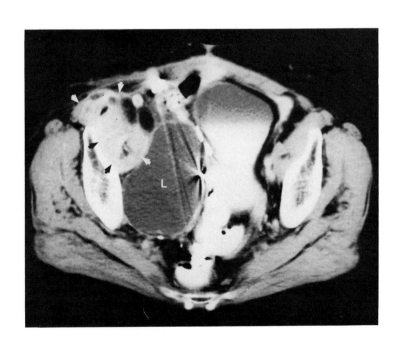

FIGURE 23–21 ■ CT scan shows a large, low-attenuation lymphocele (L) following right external iliac lymphadenectomy. The patient's primary malignancy was a liposarcoma, a segment of which can be identified anterior to the right ilium (arrowheads).

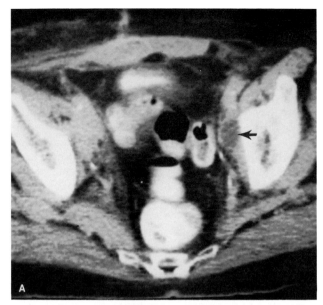

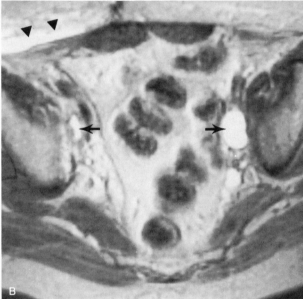

FIGURE 23–22 ■ Small bilateral lymphoceles in a patient with prostatic carcinoma. *A*, CT scan demonstrates small, low-attenuation lymphocele in the left external iliac region *(arrow)*. *B*, T2-weighted MR scan (TR, 2000; TE, 80) reveals small bilateral lymphoceles *(arrows)*, as well as lymphedema in the right anterior subcutaneous space *(arrowheads)*.

bus. Three-dimensional reconstruction of information from standard abdominal transaxial MR images has been reported and correlates well with angiographic findings in large vessel disease.[51]

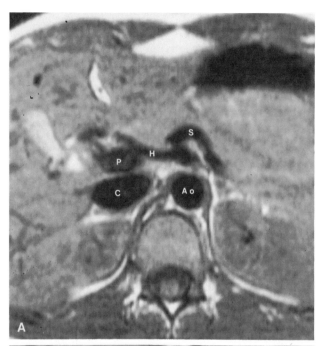

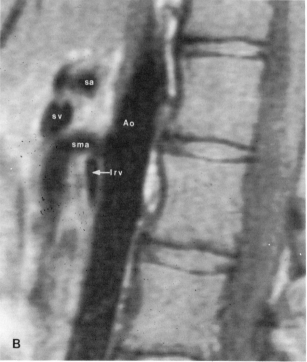

FIGURE 23–23 ■ Normal abdominal aortic anatomy. *A*, Axial T1-weighted scan (TR, 800; TE, 20) shows hepatic (H) and splenic (S) arteries arising from celiac trunk and aorta (Ao). Arterial lumen is well seen without the need for intravascular contrast material because of "flow void" from rapidly flowing blood. C = Inferior vena cava; P = portal vein. *B*, Multiplanar capacity of MR allows for sagittal depiction of vascular relationships. Ao = Aorta; lrv = left renal vein; sa = splenic artery; sma = superior mesenteric artery; sv = splenic vein.

clearly defined by MR and optimally displayed on images obtained in the axial plane. However, axial images obtained with a multislice technique may demonstrate artifactual signal within the aortic lumen related to entry-slice phenomenon, flow-related enhancement, or even-echo rephasing. Coronal and sagittal images may occasionally provide useful information to clarify flow phenomena and to further define anatomic relationships of the aorta to surrounding structures. However, gradient reversal imaging (flow sequence of TR, 40; TE, 13; flip angle, <40°) is probably the most important MR sequence to assist in differentiating flow artifact from throm-

Pathology

ATHEROSCLEROSIS

Almost all older patients have atherosclerotic changes of the abdominal aorta evident on CT scans. CT findings include increased vessel tortuosity, intimal calcification, and atheromatous plaque and thrombus formation. Contrast-enhanced CT has been shown to be as accurate as angiography in depiction of aortic stenosis, occlusion, and ectasia, but it is less sensitive for detection of iliac disease.[52]

Aortic manifestations of atherosclerotic disease may also be seen by MRI, although intimal calcifications may not be as readily identified. Both aortic thrombus and slow-flowing blood may result in intraluminal MR signal. Differentiation of clot from flow phenomena may best be achieved with phase-sensitive imaging or comparison of signal intensities on first and second echo images. Slow flow demonstrates an increase in absolute signal intensity on the second, or even, echo, whereas the signal from thrombus decreases in intensity.[53]

AORTIC ANEURYSM

Abdominal aortic aneurysms are focal areas of saccular or fusiform aortic dilatation, characteristically larger than 3 cm. They are common in the Western population, with an incidence of one to three per cent, and typically are secondary to atherosclerosis. Although many aneurysms may be asymptomatic, larger aneurysms may present as pulsatile abdominal masses with a significant risk of rupture. The risk of rupture varies directly with aneurysm size, and elective aortic aneurysm resection is advocated for patients with aneurysms larger than 5 cm in diameter.[54] Although clinical evaluation of patients with suspected abdominal aortic aneurysms frequently is unreliable and misleading, sonography is highly accurate for detecting and measuring these aneurysms. Therefore ultrasound has become an important study for primary screening and follow-up of patients with suspected aortic aneurysm. However, sonography may be technically difficult to perform in obese patients or in those with excessive bowel gas and may not reliably define the proximal and distal extent of the lesion or its relationship to the renal and iliac arteries.[55, 56]

Because of the limitations of sonography, both CT and MRI have been used to provide preoperative assessment of abdominal aortic aneurysms. CT can accurately identify the aneurysm and produces accurate measurements of outer wall diameter. The origin and length of the aneurysm and its relationship to the renal arteries and aortic bifurcation may be assessed by following contiguous axial images or by employing coronal or sagittal reconstructions. Following intravenous contrast administration, CT may identify the vascular lumen and distinguish lumen from thrombus or plaque formation (Figs. 23–24 and 23–25). CT is also better than sonography for evaluating the retroperitoneum, allowing for detection of unexpected abdominal pathology, evaluation

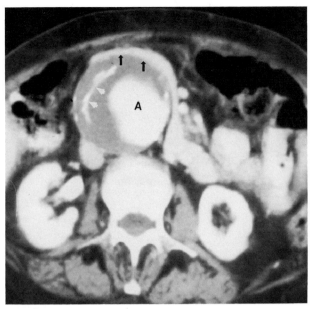

FIGURE 23–24 ■ Abdominal aortic aneurysm. A large saccular aneurysm of the abdominal aorta (A) elevating and stretching the third portion of the duodenum *(arrows)*. Intravenous contrast opacifies the vascular lumen. Heavy semilunar calcification *(arrowheads)* is seen within the low-density, partially circumferential chronic thrombus.

of clinically undetected pseudoaneurysm or aneurysmal leak, and assessment of possible periaortic inflammation.[55]

MRI has been shown to be as accurate as CT and sonography for evaluating the size of aortic aneurysms[56–58] and is more accurate than aortography for the detection of aortic thrombus.[56] However, because of its expense and longer examination time, MRI plays a secondary role to CT for the evaluation of abdominal aortic aneurysms. As with CT, axial MR images are adequate to detect and measure an abdominal aortic aneurysm. However, the multiplanar capabilities of MRI may occasionally prove helpful in better defining the craniocaudal extent of the aneurysm and the relationship of the aneurysm to the renal and iliac arteries.[57, 58] MRI therefore may be useful when there is a contraindication to intravenous contrast or when the CT study is confusing or equivocal.

CT is also the modality of choice in evaluating patients suspected of having rupture of an abdominal aortic aneurysm (Fig. 23–26).[54, 59] Because of the limitations of MRI for imaging the critically ill patient, the MR appearance of abdominal aortic aneurysm rupture has not yet been described. All six symptomatic patients studied with CT by Rosen et al. had large aortic aneurysms with high-density retroperitoneal hematoma tracking into the extracapsular perinephric space.[54] Focal indistinctness or frank discontinuity of the wall of the aneurysm and obscuration of the periaortic fat planes may also be seen.[54, 59]

The presence of a circumferential mass surrounding an abdominal aneurysm does not always mean

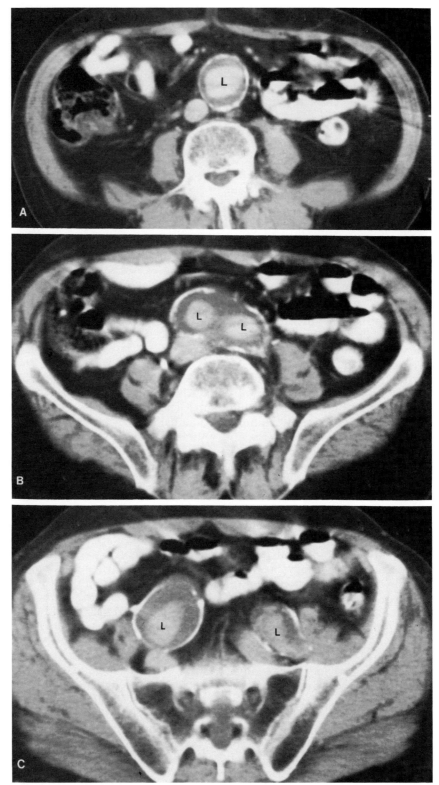

FIGURE 23–25 ■ Abdominal aortic aneurysm and bilateral iliac aneurysms. *A,* Axial CT scan through the lower abdomen demonstrates aneurysmal enlargement of the abdominal aorta. The aortic wall is calcified, and there is circumferential thrombus. The lumen of the aorta enhances with intravenous contrast (L). *B,* Scan at the level of the bifurcation demonstrates aneurysmal enlargement of the proximal common iliac arteries, again showing circumferential thrombus and central lumenal enhancement (L). *C,* Scan at a lower level shows bilateral iliac artery aneurysms (L).

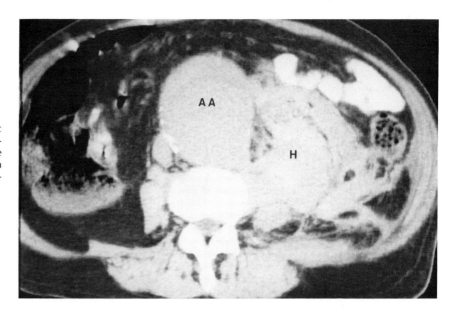

FIGURE 23-26 ■ Leaking abdominal aortic aneurysm. A large abdominal aortic aneurysm (AA) is seen, along with a soft tissue density representing hemorrhage (H), which extends to the left of the aneurysm and obscures the paraaortic fat planes.

that an aortic leak has occurred. In asymptomatic patients with abdominal aortic aneurysms, CT may demonstrate a thickened, often calcified, aortic wall and a diffuse mantle of inflammatory perianeurysmal fibrosis (Fig. 23–27).[60] Although the exact origin of this tissue is unknown, the lack of hemosiderin within the fibrotic mass suggests that it is not related to hemorrhage.[61] Nevertheless, following administration of intravenous contrast, the attenuation value of this tissue may dramatically increase and thereby simulate a periaortic hemorrhage. It is important to recognize this entity so as not to interpret this intense perianeurysmal inflammatory increase in CT density as representing a life-threatening aortic hemorrhage. Furthermore, because surgical repair of inflammatory aneurysms is associated with a higher morbidity and mortality than repair of simple aortic aneurysms, demonstration of these CT features may necessitate

modifications in surgical technique. Perianeurysmal fibrosis can also simulate idiopathic retroperitoneal fibrosis by encasing the ureter and causing hydronephrosis.[61]

AORTIC DISSECTION

The accuracy of CT in detecting both abdominal aortic dissection and extension of thoracic dissection into the abdomen is high, comparable to that of aortography.[62] In many institutions, CT has largely replaced aortography as the initial diagnostic procedure, except in patients in whom an immediate operation is warranted or in whom opacification of all aortic branch vessels is needed.

Initial noncontrast CT scans may be helpful to detect medial displacement of intimal calcification; however, the definitive CT finding of aortic dissection is a contrast-filled double channel with an inter-

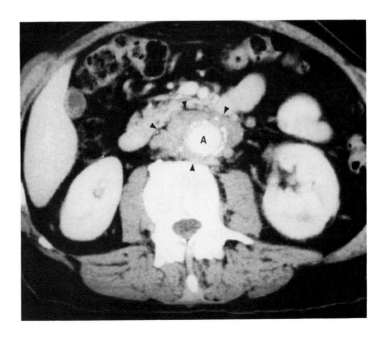

FIGURE 23-27 ■ Perianeurysmal fibrosis. This asymptomatic patient with a small abdominal aortic aneurysm (A) had a thickened perianeurysmal mass of tissue *(arrowheads)* that enhanced slightly following administration of an intravenous contrast agent. CT findings have been stable over a 3-year period.

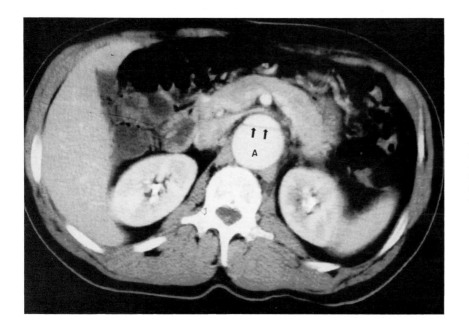

FIGURE 23–28 ■ Aortic dissection. CT scan at the level of the mid kidney shows a small aortic aneurysm (A), with nice depiction of an intimal flap separating both the true and false lumen in an aortic dissection (arrows). Contrast enhancement is seen within both the true and false lumina.

vening intimal flap (Fig. 23–28). Dynamic sequential scanning is preferred to diagnose differential opacification of the true and false lumen and to optimally detect the presence of the intimal flap. If one channel is completely thrombosed, differentiating a dissection from a fusiform aneurysm with adherent clot may be difficult. Associated findings in dissection are intraluminal thrombosis, dilatation of the aorta with compression of the true lumen, irregular contour of the contrast-filled part of the aorta, and differential flow to the kidneys.

MRI is also highly sensitive and specific for the diagnosis of aortic dissection[63] and appears to be at least as accurate as CT and aortography.[64, 65] Furthermore, the diagnosis can be made reliably without the use of iodinated intravenous contrast material—an important advantage for the patient with compro-

mised renal function. The intimal flap can be readily shown because of the inherent contrast between flowing blood and vascular structures (Fig. 23–29). In addition, MRI may enable differentiation of true and false channels, based on slower flow and greater amounts of thrombus in the false lumen. Such a distinction may be enhanced by use of gradient reversal imaging or a phase-shift technique (Fig. 23–30).[66] However, MR artifacts caused by slow-flow phenomena occasionally may be problematic; accurate diagnosis of dissection requires familiarity with these artifacts.[63]

Transaxial images are optimal for demonstrating the intimal flap of aortic dissection, but imaging in sagittal and coronal planes may assist in assessing branch vessel involvement.[63] The noninvasive character of MRI allows serial evaluation of both nonop-

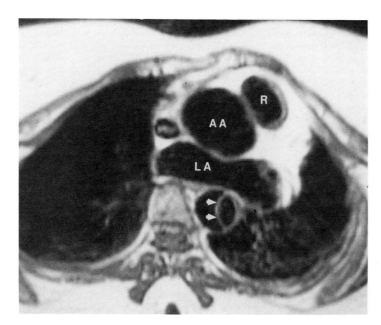

FIGURE 23–29 ■ Aortic dissection. Axial spin-density MR image (TR, 1000; TE, 25) shows the intimal flap (arrowheads) of an aortic dissection within the descending thoracic aorta. The flap is nicely seen because of flow void from rapidly flowing blood within both the true and false lumina. AA = Ascending aorta; LA = left atrium; R = right ventricular outflow tract.

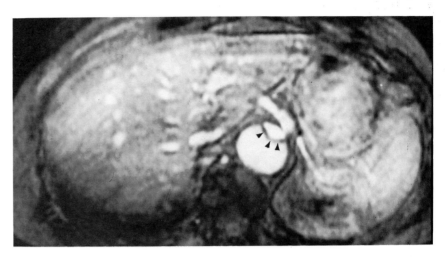

FIGURE 23–30 ■ Abdominal aortic dissection. Single breath-hold gradient-recalled acquisition in the steady state (GRASS) image (TR, 40; TE, 13; flip angle, 30°) shows the intimal flap *(arrowheads)* as a dark line against the high signal from flowing blood within both the true and false lumina.

erated and operated patients to determine disease progression or complications.

AORTIC SURGERY

Computed tomography and MRI are both capable of accurately displaying postsurgical anatomy and diagnosing a variety of complications following aortoiliac surgery (e.g., thrombosis, hemorrhage, infection, pseudoaneurysm, aortoenteric fistula, and ureteral obstruction) (Figs. 23–31 through 23–33).[67–70] In general, either imaging modality can be employed as the initial diagnostic procedure, reserving arteriography for those patients requiring surgery or further delineation of vascular anatomy. A number of factors, including the stability of the patient, the patient's renal function, the type of complication, and the cost and availability of the examination, may dictate whether CT or MRI is the examination of choice. For example, MRI may be the better choice for the patient with suspected thrombosis of an aortic graft. Although CT can suggest this diagnosis by depicting a low-density vascular lumen that does not enhance following intravenous contrast administration, MRI may directly show intraluminal thrombosis without subjecting the patient to the risk of contrast-induced nephrotoxicity. Similarly, although the CT findings in a postoperative patient with a chronic perigraft hematoma may be nonspecific and indistinguishable from seroma, lymphocele, or perigraft abscess, the tissue characteristics of chronic hematoma may be much more diagnostic on standard MR pulse sequences.[71, 72] On the other hand, if the clinical concern is of acute perigraft hematoma, noncontrast CT may be more sensitive and specific than MRI.

Cross-sectional imaging has been of particular value in the workup of suspected graft infections, helping to differentiate isolated groin infections, which may be managed with local therapy, from those infections that have spread to involve the intraabdominal graft and therefore require removal of the graft (Fig. 23–34). Anterior collections of perigraft gas and fluid may be normal postoperative findings, but retroperitoneal gas collections seen 2 to 3 weeks after surgery are considered to be pathologically abnormal.[73] In patients with infected grafts, CT usually demonstrates an irregular, septated periaortic fluid or gas collection (Fig. 23–35).[67, 68] On MR scans, the finding of an eccentric fluid collection of low-to-moderate signal intensity on T1-weighted images and high signal intensity on T2-weighted images more than 3 months after surgery is highly suggestive of an abscess, particularly if there is also inflammatory edema in the surrounding soft tissue.[74] However, MRI, because of its relative insensitivity for detection of small collections of gas, may be less sensitive for the diagnosis of abscess than CT. Because gas emits no MR signal, bubbles of gas may be undetected or indistinguishable from other signal voids such as calcification, flowing blood, or the graft material itself. Moreover, differentiation among abscess, noninfected perigraft fluid, and blood clots may be difficult because of overlapping T1 and T2 relaxation times.[69, 74] In equivocal cases, CT-guided aspiration can be performed to document the infection and to obtain specimens for culture.

Pseudoaneurysms, another complication of aortic surgery, occur at the site of anastomosis and are shown by CT as mass lesions of fluid density. These often contain septations and have rim enhancement after contrast administration. On MR scans, pseudoaneurysms show variable signal intensities, depending on residual blood flow and extent of thrombus formation.[70] Aortoduodenal fistulae are suggested by CT when gas is present in the retroperitoneal region near the level of the anastomosis (Fig. 23–36). A fluid level may or may not be seen. Loss of the normal fat plane between the aorta and duodenum may be an important but nonspecific finding (Fig. 23–37). No specific MR findings were seen in two cases of aortoenteric fistulae reported by Auffermann and colleagues.[70]

Inferior Vena Cava

Anatomy

The inferior vena cava (IVC), formed by the junction of right and left common iliac veins, originates
Text continued on page 1116

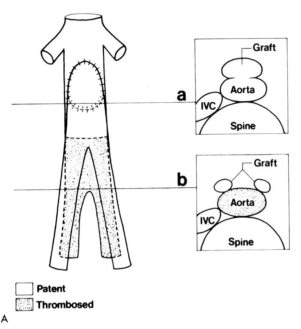

□ Patent
░ Thrombosed

A

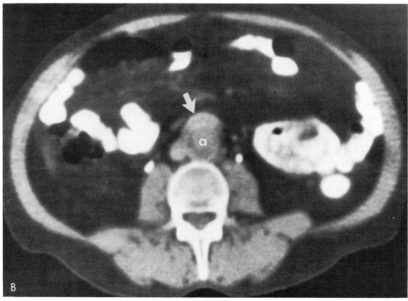

B

FIGURE 23–31 ■ *A*, Diagram of end-to-side aortic graft anastomosis. The graft is positioned ventral to the native aorta and usually bifurcates above the native bifurcation. Insets *(a and b)* demonstrate cross-sectional anatomy of the graft in relation to the native aorta. *B*, CT scan of a patent normal graft *(arrow)* located above the thrombosed native aorta (a). (*A* from Mark A, Moss AA, Lusby R, Kaiser JA: Radiology 145:409, 1982.)

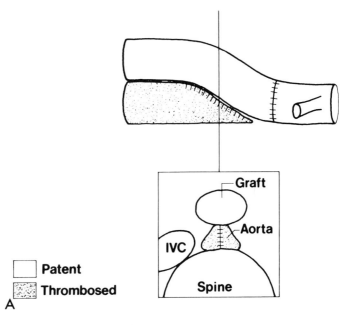

FIGURE 23–32 ■ *A*, Diagram of end-to-end aortic graft anastomosis (lateral and cross-sectional views). *B*, CT scan demonstrates a patent graft (G) and a small clotted native aorta *(arrow)* between the graft and the spine. The native aorta is slightly more ventral than is usually seen. c = Inferior vena cava. (*A* from Mark A, Moss AA, Lusby R, Kaiser JA: Radiology 145:409, 1982.)

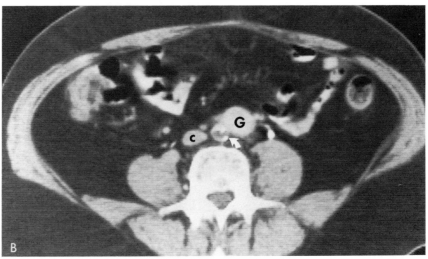

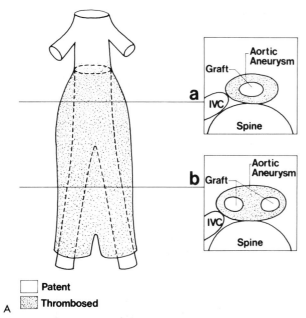

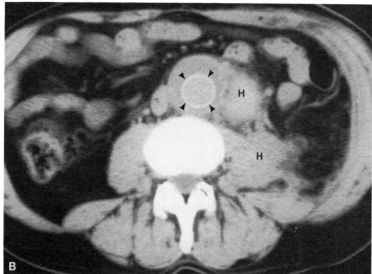

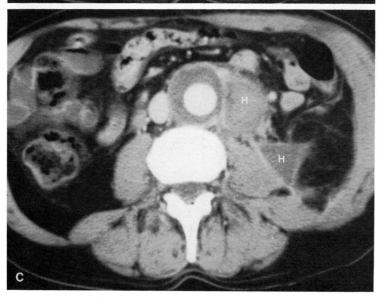

FIGURE 23–33 ■ *A,* Diagram of graft and native aorta after aortic graft placement in a patient with aortic aneurysm. The graft is positioned within the aneurysm, which is sutured around the graft. Inserts *(a and b)* demonstrate cross-sectional anatomy of the graft in relation to the native aorta. *B,* Non–contrast-enhanced CT study shows the aortic graft *(arrowheads)* within the thrombosed abdominal aortic aneurysm. C, Following intravenous contrast administration, there is normal opacification of the aortic graft lumen. Left periaortic fluid collection (H) was related to postsurgical hemorrhage. (*A* from Mark A, Moss AA, Lusby R, Kaiser JA: Radiology 145:409, 1982.)

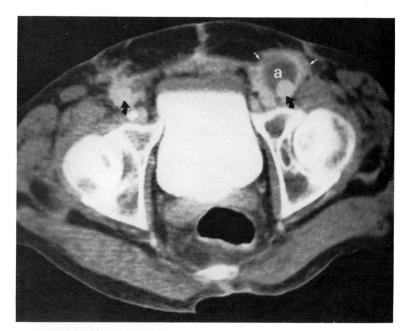

FIGURE 23–34 ■ Localized perigraft abscess. A patent, well-incorporated right iliac graft *(black arrow)* is surrounded by fibrosis but has no fluid collection. The patent left iliac graft *(black arrow)* is partially surrounded by a fluid collection, which proved to be a localized perigraft abscess (a). The abscess is surrounded by a thick enhancing rim *(white arrows)*.

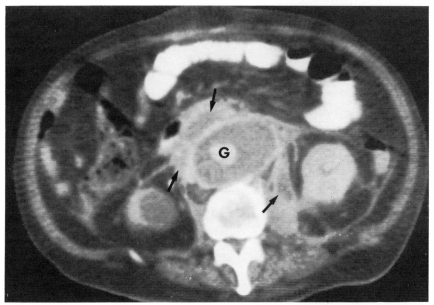

FIGURE 23–35 ■ Perigraft infection following aortoiliac graft surgery. Perigraft fluid collection *(arrows)*, without gas, proved to be abscess. The patent graft (G) is wrapped by an aortic aneurysm and surrounded by clot.

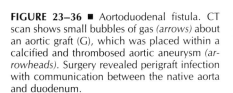

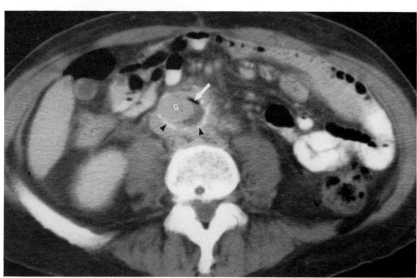

FIGURE 23–36 ■ Aortoduodenal fistula. CT scan shows small bubbles of gas *(arrows)* about an aortic graft (G), which was placed within a calcified and thrombosed aortic aneurysm *(arrowheads)*. Surgery revealed perigraft infection with communication between the native aorta and duodenum.

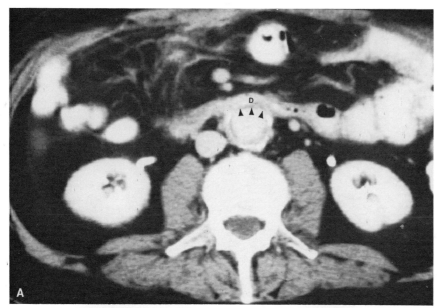

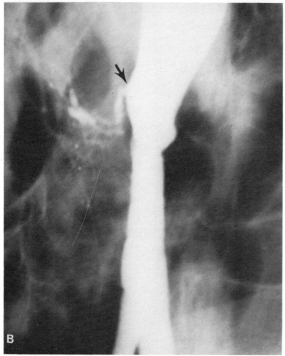

FIGURE 23–37 ■ Aortoduodenal fistula. *A,* CT scan reveals loss of fat planes and interruption of intimal calcification between aorta and duodenum (D). *B,* Aortogram shows aortoenteric leak *(arrow)* just proximal to anastomosis.

at the L4 or L5 level just caudal to the aortic bifurcation. From its origin, the normal IVC ascends to the right of the abdominal aorta, through the diaphragmatic hiatus, and ends in the right atrium. The IVC varies in size and shape from a rounded vessel 2 to 3 cm in diameter to a small slitlike structure that is barely detectable. The size is somewhat dependent on the phase of respiration and can vary from scan to scan within the same patient. A collapsed IVC seen at multiple levels may indicate severe hypovolemia.[75]

The IVC, portal vein, and major tributaries can be reliably imaged by both CT and MRI. Noncontrast CT may be sufficient to depict vascular anatomy, although occasionally a bolus of intravenous contrast

agent is necessary to delineate vascular anatomy and confirm vascular patency. On standard MR spin-echo images, the normal IVC demonstrates no intraluminal signal, a phenomenon that results in excellent vessel–soft tissue contrast and eliminates the need for intravascular contrast material. However, as in the aorta, flow-related enhancement secondary to slowly moving blood, even-echo rephasing, or entry slice artifacts may produce a signal in the IVC when transverse images are obtained.

Congenital Anomalies

The retroperitoneal veins evolve from three embryologic venous systems that develop in chronologic order within the first trimester: the posterior cardinal, subcardinal, and supracardinal systems. In approximately 97 per cent of the population, these paired embryonic veins undergo a complicated but orderly process of development, fusion, selective regression, and anastomosis to form the normal single right-sided IVC and its major tributaries.[76] The subcardinal system gives rise to the suprarenal segment of the IVC; the anastomosis between subcardinal and supracardinal systems forms the renal vein segment; and the supracardinal system forms the infrarenal IVC, azygos, and hemiazygos veins. Failure of normal embryogenesis may result in various anomalies of the IVC that can be reliably detected by CT[76, 77] and MRI[78] (Fig. 23–38).

CAVAL TRANSPOSITION

Caval transposition occurs rarely, with an incidence of 0.2 to 0.5 per cent.[76] In this anomaly, the left supracardinal venous system fails to regress normally, the right supracardinal vein involutes, and a single left-sided IVC develops. On transverse MR and CT images, a single venous structure is seen to the left of the aorta on caudal sections, crossing to the right side either anterior or posterior to the aorta at the level of the renal veins to continue superiorly to the right atrium (Fig. 23–39).

DUPLICATION OF THE IVC

Duplication of the IVC, seen in 0.2 to 3 per cent of the population,[77] results from persistence of both the left and right supracardinal veins. A second, left-sided IVC originates from the left common iliac vein

and ascends to the level of the renal veins, where a variety of anomalous vascular communications, representing intersubcardinal venous anastomoses, may link the left-sided IVC with the normally positioned vena cava (Fig. 23–40). A duplicated IVC may be differentiated from a prominent left gonadal vein by observing the course of the vessel on more caudal axial images. A dilated left gonadal vein can be traced to the level of the inguinal canal or ovary, but a duplicated IVC ends at the level of the left common iliac vein.[77]

ANOMALIES OF THE LEFT RENAL VEIN

CT and MRI may also diagnose congenital anomalies of the left renal vein, including circumaortic (incidence, 1.5 to 8.7 per cent) and retroaortic left renal vein (incidence, 1.8 to 2.4 per cent) (Figs. 23–41 and 23–42). During embryogenesis, the renal segment of the IVC originates as both a dorsal and a ventral intersubcardinal anastomosis, with eventual regression of the dorsal limb and persistence of the ventral limb to form the normal adult left renal vein. If, however, the dorsal limb fails to regress, a true circumaortic venous ring remains, comprising both preaortic and retroaortic components. If the dorsal limb persists and the ventral limb involutes, a single left renal vein courses posterior to the aorta to enter the IVC.

Rarely, a retrocaval ureter can be recognized (incidence, 0.09 per cent). Embryologically, this anomaly results when the right posterior cardinal venous system fails to involute and instead forms a portion of the infrarenal segment of the IVC. The posterior

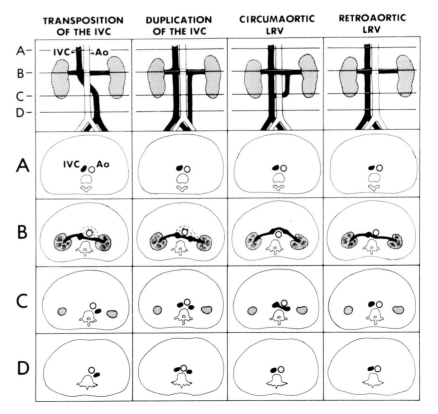

FIGURE 23–38 ■ Diagram of axial CT appearance of inferior vena cava and left renal vein anomalies. (From Royal SA, Callen PW: AJR 132:759, 1979, © 1979, Am. Roentgen Ray Soc.)

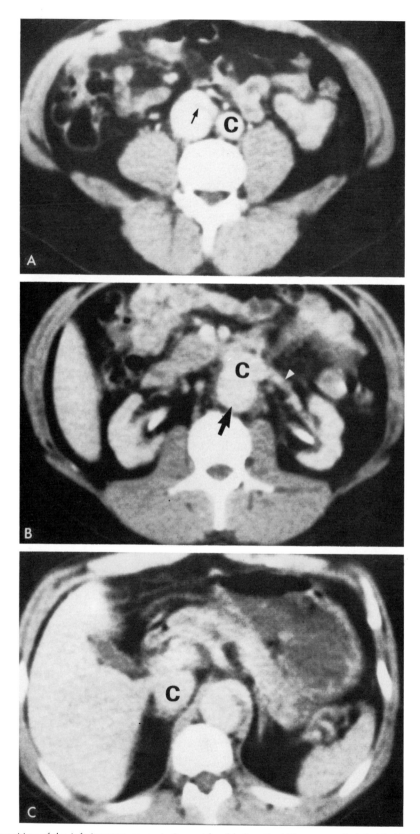

FIGURE 23–39 ■ Transposition of the inferior vena cava. *A,* Scan at level below the kidneys reveals left-sided inferior vena cava (C) and an aortic dissection *(arrow). B,* Scan at level of the midportion of kidneys. The inferior vena cava *(arrow)* has moved to lie directly ventral to the aorta. The left renal vein *(arrowhead)* enters the inferior vena cava (C) at this level. *C,* Scan at level above the kidneys demonstrates that the inferior vena cava (C) has crossed over to the right side of the abdomen.

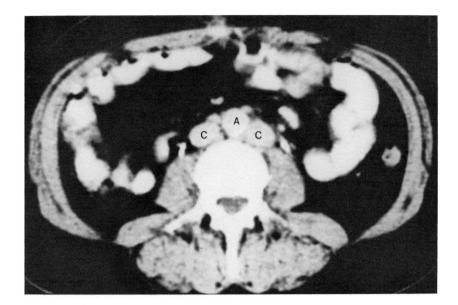

FIGURE 23–40 ■ CT scan just caudal to renal veins showing duplicated inferior vena cava (C), which appears as a large, paired vascular structure along either side of the aorta (A).

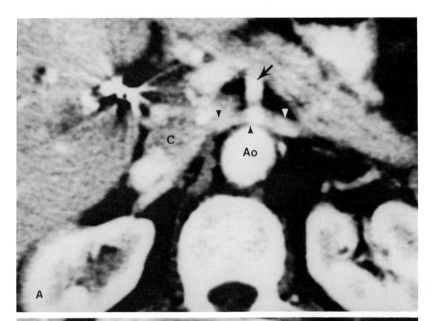

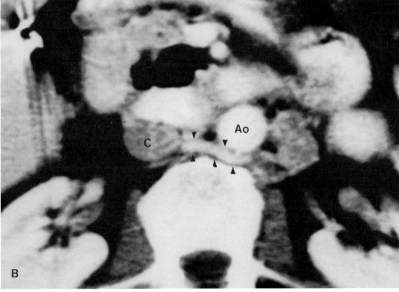

FIGURE 23–41 ■ Circumaortic left renal vein. *A,* CT scan at the level of the superior mesenteric artery *(arrow)* shows normal course of the left renal vein *(arrowheads)* ventral to the aorta (Ao). *B,* Scan 2 cm caudal to *A* demonstrates an anomalous retroaortic left renal vein *(arrowheads)*. C = Inferior vena cava.

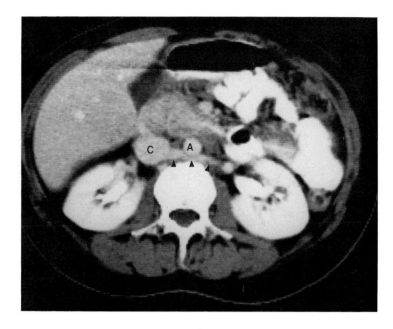

FIGURE 23–42 ■ Retroaortic left renal vein. CT scan demonstrates the left renal vein *(arrowheads)* coursing dorsal to the aorta (A) to join the inferior vena cava (C).

cardinal vein, located posterior and lateral to the developing ureter, drags the descending ureter medially as it migrates to form the IVC.[79] CT and MR scans demonstrate an abnormally positioned IVC or periureteric venous ring causing proximal ureteral dilatation and medial and posterior displacement of the mid right ureter. Patients with retrocaval ureter may be asymptomatic or may develop symptoms related to nephrolithiasis, ureteral compression, or repeated urinary tract infections.

INTRAHEPATIC IVC ANOMALIES

Infrahepatic interruption of the IVC occurs if, during the sixth embryologic week, the right subcardinal veins fail to unite with the hepatic veins. In this situation, the normal intrahepatic IVC does not form,

and therefore, in order to return to the heart, blood from the postrenal system must pass through the azygos or hemiazygos veins (supracardinal system).[80, 81] Detection of azygos continuation (incidence, 0.2 to 4.3 per cent) depends on identification of an enlarged azygos vein in the retrocrural space.[80, 81] On MR or CT scans, the dilated collateral vein can be seen as a tubular structure on multiple contiguous axial scans, demonstrating either flow void or marked contrast enhancement. Although azygos continuation may occasionally present as an isolated anomaly, congenital heart disease is present in 85 per cent of patients with this abnormality. Left pulmonary isomerism, polysplenia, dextrocardia, intracardiac defects, and transposed abdominal viscera are commonly associated.[81]

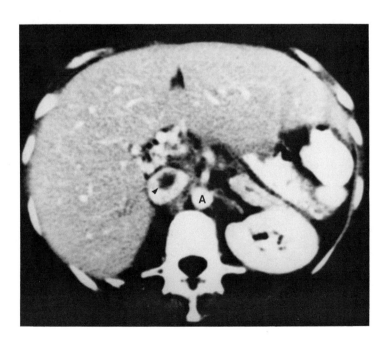

FIGURE 23–43 ■ Inferior vena cava thrombus secondary to thrombophlebitis. Scan after bolus injection of contrast material clearly outlines a thrombus *(arrowhead)* in the inferior vena cava. A = Aorta.

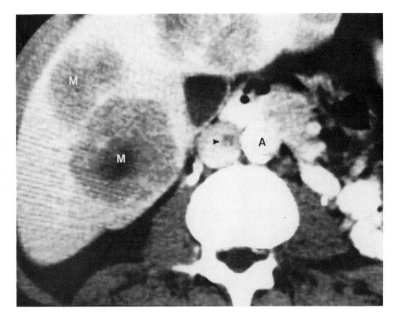

FIGURE 23–44 ■ Pseudothrombosis of the inferior vena cava. Axial scan demonstrates apparent filling defect within the inferior vena cava *(arrowhead)* in this patient with melanoma metastatic to the liver (M). This apparent filling defect simply represented unopacified blood from the right renal vein. A = Aorta.

Pathology

THROMBOSIS

Both intrinsic and extrinsic lesions of the IVC are readily identified by CT. Thrombus formation within the IVC may be secondary to tumor extension or the result of a bland or septic thrombosis.[82–88] Characteristic CT features of IVC thrombosis include focal caval enlargement resulting from intraluminal clot or neoplasm, a low-density intraluminal filling defect, and a rim of high density produced by contrast material surrounding the lower density thrombus (Fig. 23–43).[82–87] A false-positive diagnosis of IVC thrombosis may occasionally result from laminar flow phenomenon and incomplete mixing of unopacified blood from adjacent venous branches during foot injection[86] or from rapid upper arm vein contrast injection,[89] especially if a power injector is used (Fig. 23–44).[90] Such an error could be easily avoided by the acquisition of repeated images through the area in question. Fresh thrombus within the IVC may be isodense with other vascular structures, making detection of thrombus difficult on non–contrast-enhanced scans. With time, however, the density of the thrombus usually decreases; a chronic caval thrombus may calcify. Venous collateral channels may be recognized if caval obstruction is complete (Fig. 23–45).[91]

A specific diagnosis of septic thrombosis of the IVC can be made on CT when multiple gas bubbles are identified within a low-attenuation intraluminal caval filling defect (Fig. 23–46).[87] Inflammatory

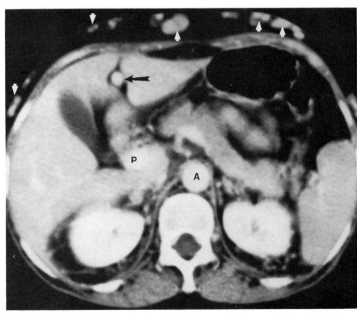

FIGURE 23–45 ■ Infrarenal occlusion of inferior vena cava. Axial scan at the level of the porta hepatis shows multiple subcutaneous venous collaterals *(arrowheads)* and patent umbilical vein *(arrow)*. A = Aorta; P = portal vein.

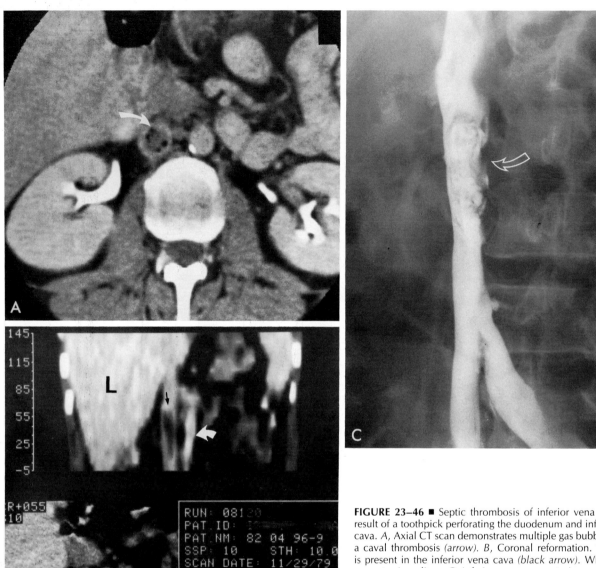

FIGURE 23–46 ■ Septic thrombosis of inferior vena cava, the result of a toothpick perforating the duodenum and inferior vena cava. *A*, Axial CT scan demonstrates multiple gas bubbles within a caval thrombosis *(arrow)*. *B*, Coronal reformation. Thrombus is present in the inferior vena cava *(black arrow)*. White arrow = aorta; L = liver. *C*, Inferior vena cava arteriogram confirms thrombus *(arrow)*. (From Schmitz L, Jeffrey RB, Palubinskas AJ, Moss AA: J Comput Assist Tomogr 5:259, 1981.)

changes around the occluded vein may also be seen.[92] CT may effectively guide percutaneous aspiration of septic thrombi to establish the causative organism.[93]

Distinction between tumor thrombus and a bland nontumor thrombus is problematic,[82–84, 88] although tumoral thrombus may be hypervascular on bolus dynamic CT.[94] CT is also relatively inaccurate in detection of IVC wall invasion when tumor thrombus is confined to the vessel lumen.[88] Although irregularity and inflammatory reaction of the venous wall are suggestive, the only reliable sign of vascular wall invasion is identification of tumor extension beyond the limits of the vessel.[88]

The CT demonstration of tumor extension into the IVC lumen is an important prognostic sign in patients with primary carcinoma of the liver, adrenal gland, or kidney and in some patients with primary retroperitoneal sarcomas.[85, 86, 88] Comparison studies of CT and angiography in patients with hypernephromas have demonstrated CT to be an accurate method of diagnosing tumor extension into the main renal vein and IVC.[85] In a study[95] utilizing dynamic CT scanning, bolus contrast injection, and 5- to 6-mm thin-section collimation, the ipsilateral renal vein was identified in 99 per cent of patients, and extension of tumor to the renal vein or IVC was correctly detected in 95 per cent. Detection of isolated invasion of intrarenal veins is unlikely to alter surgical therapy and therefore has less prognostic significance.[85]

In addition to demonstrating intrinsic involvement

of the inferior vena cava, CT can also diagnose extrinsic displacement and compression of the IVC by primary hepatic or retroperitoneal masses such as lymphadenopathy, primary retroperitoneal tumors, abscesses, or hemorrhage. CT can also be used to evaluate the patency of portacaval and mesocaval shunts (Fig. 23–47). Documentation of contrast medium flowing through the shunt confirms patency, and the time course of filling provides information concerning the hemodynamics of the shunt. CT may also be a valuable adjunct with which to monitor patients with inferior vena caval filters (Fig. 23–48).[96]

MR imaging has also been used to accurately identify intraluminal thrombus, to differentiate thrombus from high intraluminal signal caused by slow flow, and to demonstrate venous collaterals.[97] The increased signal from intraluminal thrombus may be readily differentiated from the flow void phenomenon seen with rapidly flowing blood. However, as discussed earlier, persistent intraluminal signal mimicking thrombus may occur with standard spin-echo imaging and is related to slow flow, phase-encoding artifact, and various flow phenomena. These entities may be differentiated most readily by use of gradient reversal imaging sequences or by comparing intraluminal signal intensities and appearances on first and second spin-echo images (Fig. 23–49).[97, 98] With flow-related phenomena, the absolute signal intensity of slowly flowing blood should increase from first to second spin-echo sequences.

Advantages of MRI include its noninvasiveness, absence of ionizing radiation, and its ability to image without iodinated intravascular contrast agent. The multiplanar imaging capability of MRI may allow accurate definition of the superior extent of tumor thrombus and allow for a more confident surgical approach.[97] With caval thrombosis, focal dilatation of the IVC and the presence of venous collaterals can be readily identified. MRI has also shown some potential for evaluating tumoral invasion of the caval wall and differentiating tumor from bland thrombus.[97]

Several reports have discussed the role of MRI in studying patients with intravascular stents, filters, and other devices.[99, 100] As the use of both intravascular devices and MR imaging expand, evaluation of MR imaging safety and artifacts assumes increased importance.[99] Preliminary reports document that MRI can be safely used to image patients with intravascular filters and stents and to evaluate for potential complications from these devices. Artifacts appear to be reduced when devices are made from beta-3-titanium alloy.[99]

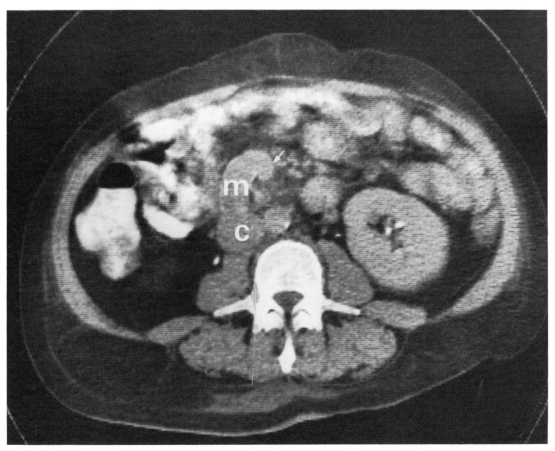

FIGURE 23–47 ■ Patent mesocaval shunt. The shunt (m) is shown to connect a mesenteric venous vessel (arrow) with the inferior vena cava (c). Contrast material is seen to flow through the shunt, demonstrating patency.

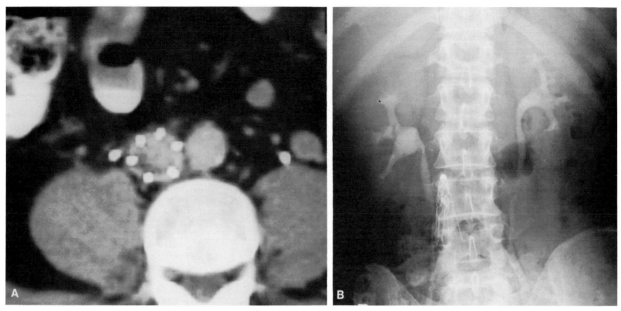

FIGURE 23–48 ■ Inferior vena cava filter. *A,* CT scan shows normal appearance of a Greenfield filter within the lumen of the inferior vena cava. Six arms of the distal portion of the filter are circumferentially placed on the lumen of the vessel. *B,* Corresponding plain film.

Retroperitoneum

Retroperitoneal Fibrosis

Retroperitoneal fibrosis (RPF) is a well-described but incompletely understood entity characterized by proliferation of both fibrous and inflammatory tissue within the retroperitoneum.[101] Seen in patients aged 8 to 80 years, RPF has a peak incidence in the fifth and sixth decades of life, affecting men twice as frequently as women.[102] Patients with idiopathic RPF develop a retractile and plaquelike mantle of inflammatory and fibrous tissue that encases the periaortic areas and envelops, compresses, and constricts retroperitoneal structures.[102, 103] The ureters are characteristically affected, although the biliary tract, duodenum, IVC, aorta, pancreas, mesenteric vessels, bladder, and rectosigmoid colon can also be involved.[101–103] Symptoms may be nonspecific, and the patient may complain of back, flank, or abdominal

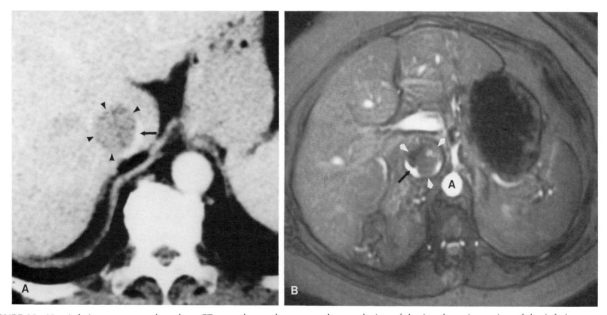

FIGURE 23–49 ■ Inferior vena cava thrombus. CT scan shows almost complete occlusion of the intrahepatic portion of the inferior vena cava by a large circular thrombus *(arrowheads).* Only a small rim of intravenous contrast agent is seen along the left lateral aspect of the thrombus *(arrow). B,* Single breath-hold gradient reversal image at a slightly lower level demonstrates the thrombus *(arrowheads)* within the dilated intrahepatic portion of the inferior vena cava. The area of flowing blood is seen as bright signal *(arrow).* A = Aorta.

pain, weight loss, vomiting, nausea, and malaise.[102] The etiology of RPF is obscure and is labeled idiopathic in 70 per cent of cases. In many of these cases, an immunologically mediated response to aortic atheroma is hypothesized.[104] Secondary forms may result from retroperitoneal trauma and hemorrhage, pancreatitis, urine extravasation, regional enteritis, vasculitis, radiation, or ingestion of methysergide or ergotamine tartrate.[101] A malignant form of RPF may be identified when primary malignancies or metastatic deposits infiltrate the retroperitoneal space, stimulating a desmoplastic response that is morphologically indistinguishable from the idiopathic form of the disease.[105] Treatment for nonmalignant RPF consists of corticosteroid therapy or surgical ureterolysis, and spontaneous regression of the disease has been reported.[106] On the other hand, patient prognosis for malignant RPF is poor. Mean patient survival following diagnosis is only 3 to 6 months.[107]

The CT findings in RPF are nonspecific and are variably described as a fibrous sheet or as a bulky or plaquelike mass located centrally and in the paravertebral regions, extending from kidneys to sacrum. The mass tends to envelop the aorta, inferior vena cava, iliac vessels, and ureters but does not cause significant displacement of these structures (Fig. 23–50).[102, 108] The anterior margin of the mass is usually sharply defined; the posterior margin is poorly delineated. Attenuation value on noncontrast CT scans approximates that of muscle, but after contrast administration, the mass may dramatically increase in attenuation. The degree of contrast enhancement reportedly correlates with the activity of the disease process.[108] Computed tomography has been advocated as the method of choice to assess the response of RPF to therapy.[106]

MRI has also been used to evaluate RPF in a limited number of patients.[109–111] The ability of MRI to depict perivascular relationships of the fibrotic process without intravenous contrast agents is a definite advantage and avoids the risk of contrast-induced nephrotoxicity in these patients, many of whom have impaired renal function.[110] In addition, direct coronal and sagittal imaging may occasionally provide a clearer anatomic delineation of the fibrosis. Although CT findings in RPF are relatively nonspecific and similar to those found with other forms of retroperitoneal pathology (including lymphoma, sarcoma, and metastatic neoplasm), the varied echo sequences available with MRI may permit more accurate tissue differentiation by identifying areas of proton-poor fibrosis.[111] Differentiation between malignant and nonmalignant RPF also may be possible based on differences in signal characteristics and homogeneity on T2-weighted images.[107]

Hemorrhage

CT and MR are both accurate, noninvasive modalities to detect, localize, and quantitate retroperitoneal hemorrhage. Cross-sectional imaging modalities are important for diagnosis, as clinical findings may be ambiguous and plain radiographs lack both sensitivity and specificity. Significant retroperitoneal hemorrhage may occur spontaneously or secondary to trauma, vascular tumors, leaking aneurysms, blood dyscrasias, anticoagulation, and long-term hemodialysis.[112]

Retroperitoneal hemorrhage can be detected on CT as an abnormal soft tissue mass with resultant obscuration, compression, or distortion of normal retroperitoneal structures.[113] Acute hematoma may demonstrate increased attenuation values secondary to clot formation and retraction, decreasing in CT density as the clot liquefies (Fig. 23–51). Subacute hemorrhage may thus present as a heterogeneous mass with central higher density and a more lucent periphery (Fig. 23–52), whereas chronic hematomas may present as a nonspecific low-attenuation mass with a thickened or calcific rim. Retroperitoneal hem-

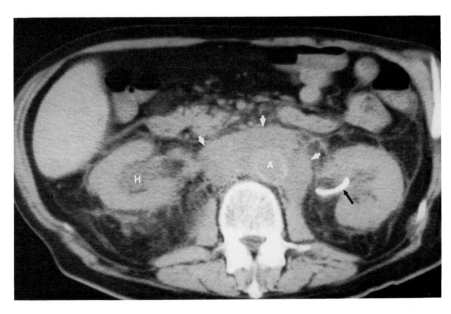

FIGURE 23–50 ■ Retroperitoneal fibrosis. CT scan at the level of the mid kidneys demonstrates a bulky retroperitoneal mass *(arrowheads)* encasing the calcified aorta (A). Hydronephrosis is noted within the right kidney (H) on this non–contrast-enhanced scan. The proximal end of a ureteral stent is seen within the left renal pelvis *(arrow).*

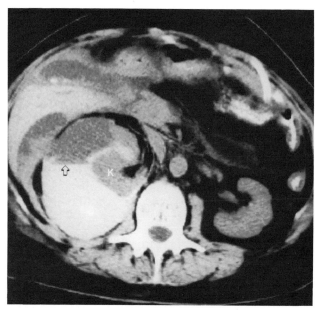

FIGURE 23–51 ■ Acute retroperitoneal hematoma. CT scan in a woman with ovarian carcinoma and disseminated intravascular coagulation shows a large perirenal hematoma that displaces and compresses the right kidney (K). Sedimentation effect is seen with a fluid level *(arrow)* defining interface between the hyperdense sedimented red cells and the hypodense serum.

T2-weighted images performed at mid and high field strength, respectively.[71, 72, 114] The paramagnetic effects of deoxyhemoglobin are enhanced at high magnetic field strength and lead to preferential T2 proton relaxation.[72]

In general, because of the T1 shortening effects of methemoglobin, the signal intensity of a hematoma increases with its age on T1-weighted images at both low and high field strengths. Unlike on CT, in which the periphery of the subacute hematoma is of low attenuation, the peripheral area demonstrates hyperintense signal on both T1- and T2-weighted MR imaging sequences. On the other hand, the central portion of the hematoma, which demonstrates increased attenuation value on CT scans, remains relatively hypointense on MR images. However, as the hematoma ages, this central area gradually converts to an area of homogeneous hyperintense MR signal. More chronic hematomas may develop a surrounding hypointense rim, seen best on T2-weighted images, that is thought to be secondary to hemosiderin-laden macrophages at the periphery of the hematoma.

Because CT has an advantage in the diagnosis of acute hematoma and MR may offer improved tissue characterization in the chronic hematoma, both MR and CT are viewed as complementary modalities for the diagnosis of retroperitoneal hemorrhage.

orrhage frequently is contained within well-defined muscle groups and usually resolves spontaneously over the course of several days.

The MR appearance of extracranial hematomas is variable and is dependent not only on the age of the hematoma, but also on the pulse sequence employed and the magnetic field strength. Acute hemorrhage may not have a specific MR appearance and has been variably described as hypointense, hyperintense, or isointense to muscle on T1-weighted images and slightly hyperintense or markedly hypointense on

Abscess

The most common causes of retroperitoneal abscess include colonic perforation, pancreatic abscess, unsuspected duodenal perforation, and surgical contamination. The CT appearance of a retroperitoneal abscess is identical to that of an intraperitoneal abscess, typically presenting as a well-defined mass of fluid density that may contain bubbles of gas. Following intravenous contrast, the rim of the abscess enhances in 30 to 40 per cent of patients. Failure of

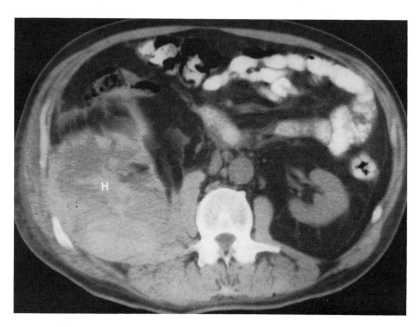

FIGURE 23–52 ■ Subacute retroperitoneal hematoma. Subacute retroperitoneal hemorrhage presents as an inhomogeneous mass (H) in the posterior pararenal space.

MRI to detect small quantities of gas (gas emits no MR signal and thus may be undetected or confused with other MR "signal voids" such as calcium or flowing blood) may limit the utility of MRI in the diagnosis of retroperitoneal abscess when compared with CT. CT-guided percutaneous aspiration and drainage of infected fluid collections have been shown to be effective in the diagnosis and treatment of retroperitoneal abscess (Fig. 23–53).[115–117]

Retroperitoneal Neoplasm

Computed tomography is the imaging method of choice in the evaluation of primary retroperitoneal neoplasms.[118, 119] These are rare neoplasms, accounting for only 0.2 per cent of all tumors arising in the retroperitoneal space. The vast majority of primary retroperitoneal neoplasms (77 to 90 per cent) are malignant and of mesodermal origin.[120] Typically these tumors present late in their course, growing unimpeded to great size in the potentially large retroperitoneal space before they are discovered (Fig. 23–54). Liposarcoma, leiomyosarcoma, malignant fibrous histiocytoma, fibrosarcoma, and malignant teratoma are the tumor types most frequently encountered. Metastatic retroperitoneal tumors are usually lymphomas or lymph node metastases from pelvic, testicular, lung, or gastrointestinal malignancy (Fig. 23–55). Benign retroperitoneal neoplasms are uncommon and include lipomas, paragangliomas, hemangiomas, lymphangiomas, benign teratomas, and neurogenic tumors (Fig. 23–56).

Liposarcomas are one of the more common primary retroperitoneal malignancies (Fig. 23–57). These tumors demonstrate a variety of histologic subtypes related to the anaplasia of the fat cells and

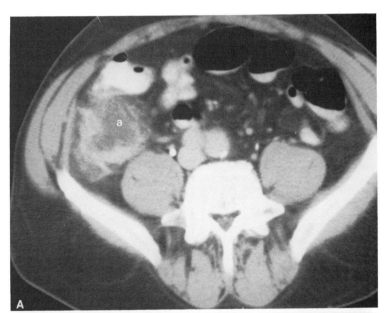
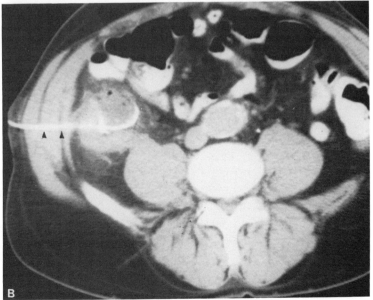

FIGURE 23–53 ■ Retroperitoneal abscess. *A,* CT scan shows complex soft tissue and fluid collection in the right lower quadrant compatible with abscess (a). *B,* CT was used to help guide percutaneous drainage of the abscess by a large-bore catheter *(arrowheads).* The abscess formed from a perforated appendix.

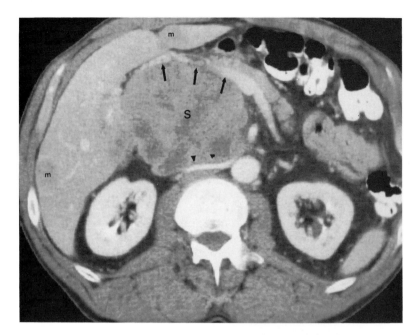

FIGURE 23–54 ■ Large retroperitoneal sarcoma (S) flattens the inferior vena cava *(arrowheads)* and displaces the duodenum anteriorly *(arrows)*. Note also the hepatic metastases (m).

FIGURE 23–55 ■ Retroperitoneal metastasis. Large inhomogeneous and necrotic tumor mass from squamous cell carcinoma of the lung has destroyed a portion of the L3 vertebral body *(open arrow)* and extends into the spinal canal and paravertebral musculature *(white arrowheads)*.

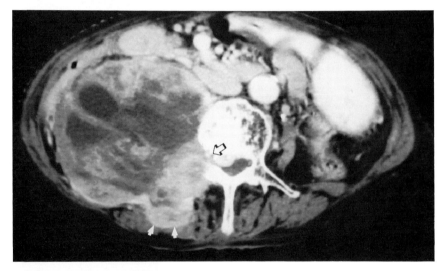

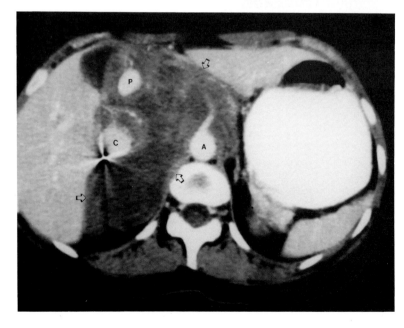

FIGURE 23–56 ■ CT scan shows a large, heterogeneous, low-attenuation, infiltrating retroperitoneal mass *(open arrows)* that separates the aorta (A) and inferior vena cava (C) and displaces the portal vein anteriorly (P). The histologic diagnosis of benign ganglioneuroma was confirmed at surgery.

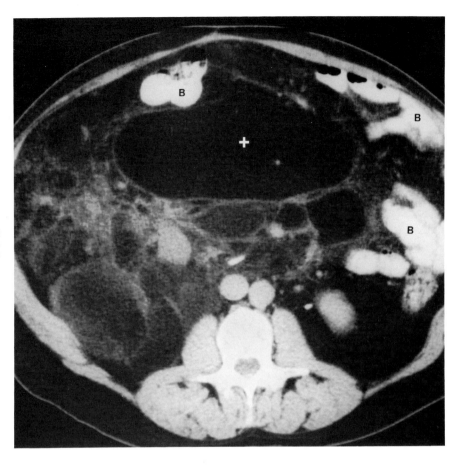

FIGURE 23–57 ■ Retroperitoneal liposarcoma. CT scan shows an extensive mass in the retroperitoneum that displaces small bowel loops (B) laterally and anteriorly. The mass has regions of relatively homogeneous fat (+) but also displays areas of nodularity and streaky soft tissue density.

the degree of admixture of fibrous or mucinous tissues.[118, 121, 122] As noted by Waligore and co-workers,[121] liposarcomas may be classified histologically into lipogenic, myxoid, or pleomorphic varieties, with the myxoid subtype being the most common. Lipogenic liposarcomas contain primarily lipid elements; myxoid varieties have varying degrees of mucinous and fibrous tissues; and pleomorphic subtypes contain little mucin or lipid. Friedman and associates[122] emphasized that liposarcomas had three distinct CT patterns: solid, mixed, and pseudocystic. In poorly differentiated liposarcomas, little fat is apparent, and the lesion has a solid CT appearance (CT attenuation coefficients greater than 20 H). Mixed lesions demonstrate focal fatty areas with attenuation values in the −40- to −20-H range. In the third CT subtype, because partial volume averaging of fatty and solid elements creates a pseudocystic appearance, such tumors present as a homogeneous mass having a density close to that of water. In general, even well-differentiated liposarcomas demonstrate CT attenuation coefficients that are higher than those for normal retroperitoneal fat, which ranges from −80 to −120 H. When evaluating a solid retroperitoneal mass, recognition that even a small part of the mass has a negative CT attenuation value is strong evidence that the mass is a liposarcoma. Detection of areas of fat signal intensity within a bulky retroperitoneal neoplasm may also allow the diagnosis of leiomyosarcoma by MRI,[123] although, like CT, the MRI features may depend on the degree of cellularity

and relative amount of intracellular mucin and lipid.[121] Moreover, areas of tumoral hemorrhage may demonstrate short T1 and long T2 relaxation times, simulating fat on some MR imaging sequences and thereby confounding attempts at tissue characterization.

CT can usually differentiate primary retroperitoneal malignancy from retroperitoneal lymphoma.[120] Primary retroperitoneal neoplasms tend to be heterogeneous on CT, whereas lymphomas are usually homogeneous.[120] However, except for liposarcomas, it may be impossible to distinguish between the different types of primary retroperitoneal tumors by CT or MR analysis. All of these tumors produce bulky, solid retroperitoneal masses, typically larger than 10 cm in diameter and with nonspecific tissue characteristics (Fig. 23–58). Because surgery is performed for evaluation and treatment on all patients with primary retroperitoneal neoplasm, regardless of the histology, the inability of CT and MRI to differentiate among most cell types probably is not clinically important.[120] Nevertheless, if histologic characterization is necessary prior to surgery, percutaneous biopsy is easily performed and readily distinguishes among the various entities.

Undescended Testes

The testes originate as paired retroperitoneal structures, arising from the gonadal ridge of the medial aspect of the mesonephros and descending into the

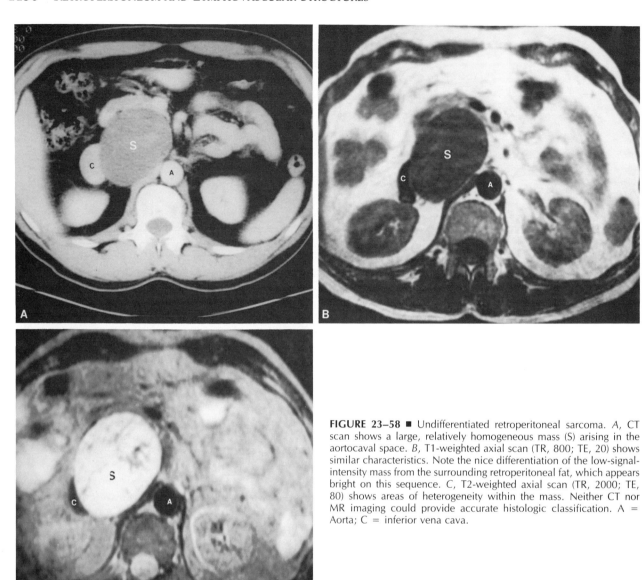

FIGURE 23–58 ■ Undifferentiated retroperitoneal sarcoma. *A*, CT scan shows a large, relatively homogeneous mass (S) arising in the aortocaval space. *B*, T1-weighted axial scan (TR, 800; TE, 20) shows similar characteristics. Note the nice differentiation of the low-signal-intensity mass from the surrounding retroperitoneal fat, which appears bright on this sequence. *C*, T2-weighted axial scan (TR, 2000; TE, 80) shows areas of heterogeneity within the mass. Neither CT nor MR imaging could provide accurate histologic classification. A = Aorta; C = inferior vena cava.

scrotum during the eighth month of gestation. Normal testicular descent, however, may be arrested at any point along a path extending from the renal hilum to the scrotum. Recognition of altered testicular descent is important, as undescended testes are 12 to 40 times more likely to harbor foci of malignancy (Fig. 23–59). Because 80 per cent of maldescended testes are found distal to the internal inguinal ring,[124] detection and localization of the incompletely descended testis is usually straightforward. Orchiopexy is performed by age 6 to preserve fertility and to monitor the testis for malignant transformation.

In 20 per cent of those with undescended testes, the testis is not palpable and it is congenitally absent in four per cent of patients in whom it is impalpable.[124] In patients with an impalpable testis, the standard surgical approach is to explore the inguinal canal and, if no testis is located, to further explore the retroperitoneal space from the inguinal region

along the course of the gonadal vein to the renal hilum. Several small series have suggested that both CT and MRI are sensitive techniques for preoperative localization of low undescended testes.[125–127] Preoperative localization of the testes aids the surgeon in operative planning, limits the extent of surgical dissection, and reduces anesthesia time.

With CT, Lee and co-workers[125] reported 100 per cent accuracy in eight patients, whereas Wolverson's group[126] found only one incorrect localization in 15 impalpable testes. Accurate CT localization requires careful attention to the pelvic anatomy, as the undescended testis is typically smaller and more elliptical than the normally descended testis. Atrophic and dysplastic testes appear as small foci of soft tissue similar in density to the adjacent abdominal wall or thigh musculature; these are difficult to identify by CT.[125, 126]

The multiplanar imaging capabilities and improved

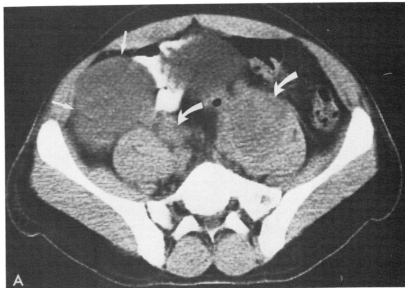

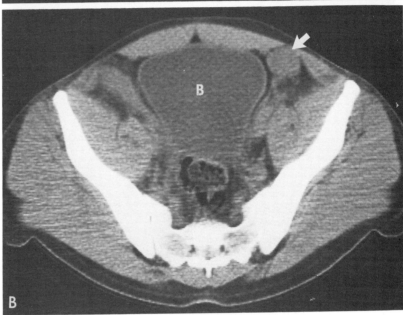

FIGURE 23–59 ■ Bilateral undescended testes. *A*, The undescended testis is enlarged by a mass *(straight arrows)*, which proved to be an embryonal cell carcinoma. The tumor has metastasized to the lymph nodes *(curved arrows)*, which are enlarged. *B*, The nontumorous intraabdominal left testis *(arrow)* is demonstrated as a smaller, rounded structure adjacent to the bladder (B).

contrast resolution of MRI may provide distinct advantages over CT scanning for identification and localization of undescended testes. Although studies comparing the accuracy of CT and MRI have not been performed, Fritzsche et al. correctly identified 15 of 16 undescended testes using standard MR spin-echo sequences at either 0.35 T or 1.5 T.[127] Contiguous transverse 5- to 10-mm-thick sections with minimal interslice gaps through the region of the inguinal canal may be optimal for identification of the undescended testis; coronal imaging planes may also be helpful to depict the intracanalicular testis. Both T1- and T2-weighted sequences are important for lesion detection. The atrophic, fibrotic undescended testes may frequently demonstrate abnormally low signal intensity on both imaging sequences.[127]

With both CT and MR imaging, physician monitoring is important, as the atrophic undescended testis may be difficult to identify, especially when

the testis is located outside the inguinal canal. Despite the accuracy of CT and MRI for detection of the low-lying undescended testis, neither imaging technique has proven reliable in identification of the high or intraabdominal testis.[128] An intraabdominal testis is most often located near the internal inguinal ring adjacent to the iliac vessels. If no testis is found along the usual pathway, ectopic locations such as the anterior abdominal wall, femoral triangle, perineum, and root of the penis should be examined.

Psoas Muscle

Anatomy

The psoas major muscles are paired muscle groups arising from the anterior and inferior surfaces of the transverse process of T12 to L5. These bulky paravertebral muscles extend inferiorly to merge with the iliacus muscles at approximately L5 to S2 before traversing the inguinal ligament to insert on the lesser trocanter of the femur. The psoas minor muscles, absent in up to 70 per cent of individuals,[129] originate from the lateral T12 and L1 vertebral bodies, lie anterior to the psoas major, and insert on the pectineal eminence of the ilium. Together, the psoas major, psoas minor, and iliac muscles constitute a bulky group of flexors responsible for flexion of the hip and thigh.

CT demonstrates the normal psoas major muscles as paired symmetric paraspinal structures, roughly triangular in shape superiorly, and more rounded and bulkier on caudal images. The psoas major reaches its largest axial diameter at approximately L3-4 and is usually surrounded by low-density fat laterally. Anteriorly, the psoas muscle has close relationship with the pancreas, aorta, IVC, and lymph nodes. The psoas minor muscle may occasionally be seen as a small tubular soft tissue mass anterior to the psoas major and should not be confused with lymphadenopathy.

With MRI, the normal anatomy of the psoas compartment can also be well delineated,[130] with the muscle groups appearing low to intermediate in signal intensity because of their relatively long T1 and short T2 relaxation times. In general, T1-weighted images provide optimal contrast between muscles and adjacent tissue, whereas T2-weighted images are more useful to detect pathologic changes in the muscles themselves.[130]

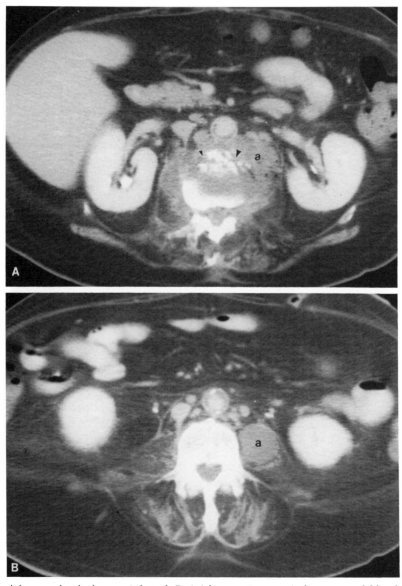

FIGURE 23–60 ■ Extensive left psoas sheath abscess. *A* through *D*, Axial scans at progressively more caudal levels show the extent of a large left psoas abscess (a) extending from L1 to the left hip. There is destruction of the anterior aspect of the L1 vertebral body *(arrowheads)* and extension of the inflammatory fluid collection inferiorly to the lesser trochanter of the left femur (L).

Pathology

Pathologic change in the iliopsoas muscle group may be insidious in onset, presenting with obscure signs and symptoms that are easily confused with other disease processes. Neoplasm, inflammation, and hemorrhage can all involve the psoas group, which, because of its anatomic extent, may allow the disease process to track from mediastinum to thigh (Fig. 23–60).[131] Plain radiographic findings may be nonspecific or misleading. Noninvasive cross-sectional imaging is frequently necessary to establish the diagnosis.

Primary neoplasm of the psoas muscle is rare; however, the psoas compartment is not infrequently involved by lymphoma, lymphatic metastasis, and extension of retroperitoneal malignancy. Neoplastic disease may affect the psoas by either total replacement or by medial or lateral displacement from enlarged nodal groups (Fig. 23–61).[132] Whereas CT may demonstrate asymmetric enlargement, obscur-

ation, or inhomogeneity of the psoas, MRI may detect increased signal intensity within the involved muscle on both T1- and T2-weighted imaging sequences. However, neither modality can reliably differentiate actual tumoral invasion from mere displacement by contiguous tumor.

Inflammatory processes account for approximately one third to one half of CT-detected psoas masses,[129] and such inflammation typically spreads from adjacent infection of the spine, kidneys, pancreas, or bowel. Asymmetric enlargement of the iliacus or psoas muscle bellies and focal areas of low density or gas frequently can be identified by CT,[129] and multiloculated fluid collections can be seen by MRI (Fig. 23–62). Selective administration of an intravenous contrast agent may improve visualization of the inflammatory process or demonstrate irregular rim enhancement of an abscess. CT-guided aspiration biopsy and percutaneous catheter drainage may be necessary to both diagnose and treat iliopsoas abscess.[129]

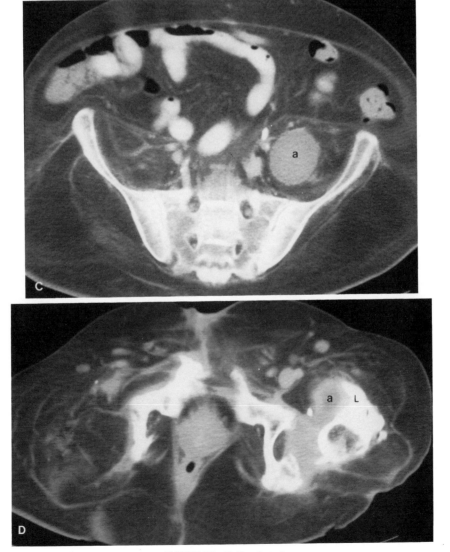

FIGURE 23–60 *Continued*

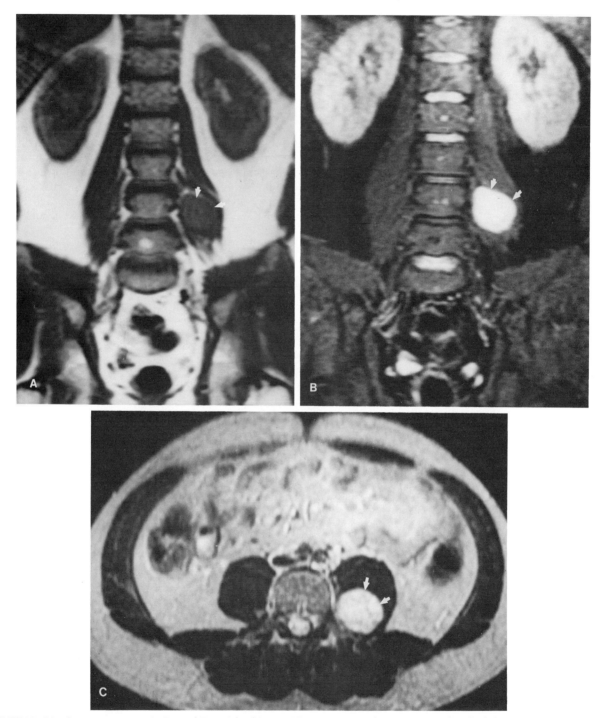

FIGURE 23–61 ■ Psoas metastases. *A,* Coronal T1-weighted image (TR, 800; TE, 20) shows a mass within the left psoas muscle *(arrowheads)* that is essentially isointense with muscle. *B,* Coronal STIR image (TR, 2000; TE, 43; TI, 160) shows the mass *(arrowheads)* to be markedly hyperintense compared with muscle. *C,* Axial T2-weighted scan (TR, 2000; TE, 80) further defines the position of this mass *(arrowheads)*. Biopsy revealed this mass to be a metastasis from the patient's known lung carcinoma.

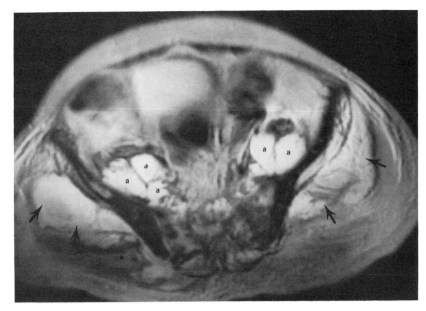

FIGURE 23–62 ■ Bilateral iliopsoas abscesses. Patient with known tuberculosis presented with tuberculous abscesses extending within bilateral iliopsoas muscle groups. T2-weighted scan (TR, 2000; TE, 80) at the level of the iliac wings demonstrates bilateral multiloculated abscesses (a) within the distribution of the iliopsoas muscle groups. Also note inflammatory changes and abscess formation in the gluteal region bilaterally *(arrows)*.

As with retroperitoneal hemorrhage in general, hemorrhage in and around the iliopsoas compartment is seen almost exclusively in patients with blood dyscrasias, excessive anticoagulation, leaking aortic aneurysms, trauma, or angiographic complications. Hemorrhage tends to be contained within well-defined borders, tracking between, but not through, fascial planes (Fig. 23–63). If the hemorrhage is acute, CT may detect an enlarged and hyperdense psoas muscle. Occasionally, fluid-fluid levels corresponding to areas of erythrocyte sedimentation may be seen. With time, the hematoma becomes progres-

sively less dense, and CT findings become less specific.

The MR appearance of hematoma varies both with time and magnetic field strength.[71] Whereas iliopsoas hemorrhage may demonstrate nonspecific features in the acute stage, the subacute or chronic hematoma may have more characteristic and diagnostic MR appearances.

Unfortunately, neither CT nor MRI can always reliably differentiate among the various pathologic processes that may involve the iliopsoas. Neoplastic, inflammatory, and hemorrhagic psoas masses are

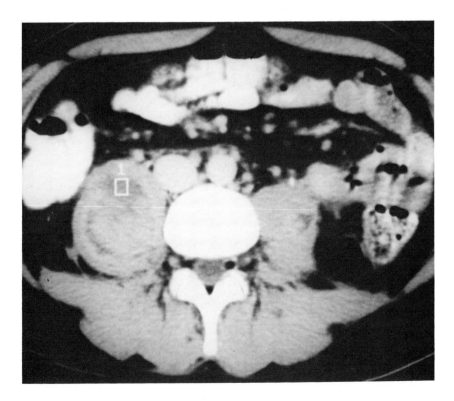

FIGURE 23–63 ■ CT scan reveals asymmetric enlargement and heterogeneity of the right psoas (square) compared with the left in this patient with subacute idiopathic psoas hemorrhage.

often indistinguishable by their CT appearances, and there is a similar overlap between benign and malignant MR signal characteristics. Reliance on clinical history and ancillary imaging studies alone may fail to provide a specific diagnosis in up to 20 per cent of patients,[131] thus necessitating needle aspiration biopsy. The few reports[130, 132] comparing CT and MRI in evaluation of pathologic abnormalities of the iliopsoas compartment suggest that MRI affords no definite advantage over CT in terms of sensitivity or specificity of diagnosis. At present, because of its shorter imaging time and more ready availability, CT appears to be the better screening modality to evaluate suspected disease of the iliopsoas.

References

1. Dooms GC, Hricak H, Crooks LE, Higgins CB: Magnetic resonance imaging of the lymph nodes: comparison with CT. Radiology 153:719, 1984.
2. Ellis JH, Bies JR, Kopecky KK, Klatte EC, Rowland RG, Donohue JP: Comparison of NMR and CT imaging in the evaluation of metastatic retroperitoneal lymphadenopathy from testicular carcinoma. J Comput Assist Tomogr 8:709, 1984.
3. Lee JKT, Heiken JP, Ling D, Glazer HS, Balfe DM, et al: Magnetic resonance imaging of abdominal and pelvic lymphadenopathy. Radiology 153:181, 1984.
4. Weiner JI, Chako AC, Merten CW, Gross S, Coffey EL, Stein HL: Breast and axillary MRI imaging: correlation of signal intensities and relaxation times with pathologic findings. Radiology 160:299, 1986.
5. Dooms GC, Hricak H, Moseley ME, Bottles K, Fisher M, Higgins CB: Characterization of lymphadenopathy by magnetic resonance relaxation times: preliminary results. Radiology 155:691, 1985.
6. Walsh JW, Amendola MA, Konerding KF, Tisnado J, Hazra TA: Computed tomographic detection of pelvic and inguinal lymph node metastasis from primary and recurrent pelvic malignant disease. Radiology 137:157, 1980.
7. Castellino RA: Lymph nodes of the posterior iliac crest: CT and lymphographic observations. Radiology 175:687, 1990.
8. Ginaldi S, Wallace S, Jing BS, Bernardino ME: Carcinoma of the cervix: Lymphangiography and computed tomography. AJR 136:1087, 1981.
9. Callen PW, Korobkin M, Isherwood I: Computed tomographic evaluation of the retrocrural prevertebral space. AJR 129:907, 1977.
10. Platt JF, Glazer GM: IV contrast material for abdominal CT: comparison of three methods of administration. AJR 151:275, 1988.
11. Teefey SA, Baron RL, Schulte SJ, Shuman WP: Differentiating pelvic veins and enlarged lymph nodes: optimal CT techniques. Radiology 175:683, 1990.
12. Koehler R, Mancuso AA: Pitfalls in the diagnosis of retroperitoneal lymphadenopathy. J Can Assoc Radiol 33:197, 1982.
13. Glazer GM, Goldberg HI, Moss AA, Axel L: Computed tomographic detection of retroperitoneal adenopathy. Radiology 143:147, 1982.
14. Shuman WP, Baron RL, Peters MJ, Tazioli PK: Comparison of STIR and spin-echo MR imaging at 1.5 T in 90 lesions of the chest, liver, and pelvis. AJR 152:853, 1989.
15. Buckwalter KA, Ellis JH, Baker DE, Borello JA, Glazer GM: Pitfall in MR imaging of lymphadenopathy after lymphangiography. Radiology 161:831, 1986.
16. Weissleder R, Elizondo G, Josephson L, Compton CC, Fretz CJ, et al: Experimental lymph node metastases: enhanced detection with MR lymphography. Radiology 171:835–839, 1989.
17. Breiman RS, Castellino RA, Harrell GS, Marshall WH, Glat-stein E, Kaplan HS: CT-pathologic correlations in Hodgkin's disease and non-Hodgkin's lymphomas. Radiology 126:159, 1978.
18. Castellino RA, Billingham M, Dorfman RF: Lymphographic accuracy in Hodgkin's disease and malignant lymphoma with a note on the "reactive" lymph node as a cause of most false-positive lymphograms. Invest Radiol 9:155, 1974.
19. Marglin SI, Castellino R: Lymphographic accuracy in 632 consecutive previously untreated cases of Hodgkin's disease and non-Hodgkin's lymphoma. Radiology 140:351, 1981.
20. Thomas JL, Barnes PA, Bernardino ME, Hagemeister FB: Limited CT studies in monitoring treatment of lymphoma. AJR 138:537, 1982.
21. Lee JKT, Stanley RJ, Sagel SS, Melson GT, Koehler RE: Limitations of the post-lymphangiogram plain abdominal radiograph as an indicator of recurrent lymphoma: comparison to computed tomography. Radiology 134:155, 1980.
22. Pera A, Capek M, Shirkhoda A: Lymphangiography and CT in the follow-up of patients with lymphoma. Radiology 164:631, 1987.
23. Garnick MB, Prout GR, Cannellos GP: Germinal tumors of the testis. In Holland JF, Frei I III (eds): Cancer Medicine, 2nd ed. Philadelphia, Lea & Febiger, 1982, pp 1937–1956.
24. Stomper PC, Jochelson MS, Friedman EL, Garnick MB, Richie JP: CT evaluation of advanced seminoma treated with chemotherapy. AJR 146:745, 1986.
25. Thomas JS, Bernardino VWF, Bracken RB: Staging of testicular carcinoma: comparison of CT and lymphangiography. AJR 137:991, 1981.
26. Lee JKT, McClennan BL, Stanley RJ, Sagel SS: Computed tomography in the staging of testicular neoplasm. Radiology 130:387, 1979.
27. Husband JE, Peckham MJ, MacDonald JS: The role of abdominal computed tomography in the management of testicular tumors. Comput Tomogr 4:1, 1980.
28. Dunnick NR, Javadpour N: Value of CT and lymphography: distinguishing retroperitoneal metastasis from nonseminomatous testicular tumors. AJR 136:1092, 1981.
29. Tesoro-Tess JD, Pizzocaro G, Zanoni F, Musumeci R: Lymphangiography and computerized tomography in testicular carcinoma: how accurate in early stage disease? J Urol 133:967, 1985.
30. Taylor RE, Duncan W, Best JJK: Influence of computed tomographic scanning and lymphography on the management of testicular germ-cell tumors. Clin Radiol 37:539, 1986.
31. Ellis HH: Comparison of NMR and CT imaging in the evaluation of metastatic retroperitoneal lymphadenopathy from testicular carcinoma. J Comput Assist Tomogr 8:709, 1984.
32. Williams MP, Husband JE, Heron CW: Stage 1 nonseminomatous germ cell tumors of the testis: radiologic follow-up after orchiectomy. Radiology 164:671, 1987.
33. Stomper PC, Socinski MA, Kaplan WD, Garnick MB: Failure patterns of nonseminomatous germ-cell testicular tumors: radiographic analysis of 51 cases. Radiology 167:641, 1988.
34. Scatarige JC, Fishman EK, Kuhajda FP, Taylor GA, Siegelman SS: Low attenuation nodal metastases in testicular carcinoma. J Comput Assist Tomogr 7:682, 1983.
35. Soo CS, Bernardino ME, Chuang VP, Ordonez N: Pitfalls of CT findings in post-therapy testicular carcinoma. J Comput Assist Tomogr 5:39, 1981.
36. Lee JKT, Stanley RJ, Sagel SS, McClennan BL: Accuracy of CT in detecting intraabdominal and pelvic lymph node metastases from pelvic cancers. AJR 131:675, 1978.
37. Walsh JW, Goplerud DR: Prospective comparison between clinical and CT staging in primary cervical carcinoma. AJR 137:997, 1981.
38. Walsh JW, Amendola MA, Hall DJ, Tisnado J, Goplerud DR: Recurrent carcinoma of the cervix: CT diagnosis. AJR 136:117, 1981.
39. Levine MS, Arger PH, Coleman BG, Mulhern CB, Pollock HM, Wein AJ: Detecting lymphatic metastases from prostatic carcinoma: superiority of CT. AJR 137:207, 1981.
40. Koss JC, Arger PH, Coleman BG, Mulhern CB, Pollock HM, Wein AJ: CT staging of bladder carcinoma. AJR 137:359, 1981.

41. Deutch SJ, Sandler MA, Alpern MB: Abdominal lymphadenopathy in benign disease: CT detection. Radiology 163:335, 1987.

42. Goldberg HI, Reeder MM: Infections and infestations of the gastrointestinal tract. In Margulis AR, Burhenne HJ (eds): Alimentary Tract Roentgenology. St Louis, CV Mosby, 1973, pp 1575–1607.

43. Meranze S, Coleman B, Arger P, Mintz M, Markowitz L: Retroperitoneal manifestations of sarcoidosis on computed tomography. J Comput Assist Tomogr 9:50, 1985.

44. Hulnick DH, Megibow AJ, Naidich DP, Hilton S, Cho KC, Balthazar EJ: Abdominal tuberculosis: CT evaluation. Radiology 157:199, 1985.

45. Glynn TP Jr, Kreipke DL, Irons JM: Amyloidosis: diffuse involvement of the retroperitoneum. Radiology 170:726, 1989.

46. Joseph N, Vogelzang RL, Hidvegi D, Neiman HL: Computed tomography of retroperitoneal Castleman disease (plasma cell type) with sonographic and angiographic correlation. J Comput Assist Tomogr 9:570, 1985.

47. Libson E, Fields S, Strauss S, Bloom RA, Okon E, et al: Widespread Castleman disease: CT and US findings. Radiology 166:753, 1988.

48. van Sonnenberg E, Wittich GR, Casola G, Wing VW, Halasz NA, et al: Lymphoceles: imaging characteristics and percutaneous management. Radiology 161:593, 1986.

49. Demos TC, Posniak HV, Churchill RJ: Detection of the intimal flap of aortic dissection on unenhanced CT images. AJR 146:601, 1986.

50. Amparo EG, Higgins CB, Hoddick W, Hricak H, Kerlan RK, et al: Magnetic resonance imaging of aortic disease: preliminary results. AJR 143:1203, 1984.

51. Valk PE, Hale JD, Crooks LE, Kaufman L, Higgins CB: MR imaging of aortoiliac atherosclerosis with 3D image reconstruction. J Comput Assist Tomogr 10:439, 1986.

52. Limpert JD, Vogelzang RL, Yao JST: Computed tomography of aortoiliac atherosclerosis. J Vasc Surg 5:814, 1987.

53. Bradley WG, Waluch V: Blood flow: magnetic resonance imaging. Radiology 154:443, 1985.

54. Rosen A, Korobkin M, Silverman PM, Moore AV Jr, Dunnick NR: CT diagnosis of ruptured abdominal aortic aneurysm. AJR 143:265, 1984.

55. Papanicolau N, Wittenberg J, Ferrucci JT Jr, Stauffen AE, Waltman AC, et al: Preoperative evaluation of abdominal aortic aneurysms by computed tomography. AJR 146:711, 1986.

56. Evancho AM, Osbakken M, Weidner W: Comparison of NMR imaging and aortography for preoperative evaluation of abdominal aortic aneurysms. Magn Reson Med 2:41, 1985.

57. Flak B, Li DKB, Ho BYB, Knickerbocker WJ, Fache S, et al: Magnetic resonance imaging of aneurysms of the abdominal aorta. AJR 144:991, 1985.

58. Lee JKT, Ling D, Heiken JP, Glazer HS, Sicard GA, et al: Magnetic resonance imaging of abdominal aortic aneurysms. AJR 143:1197, 1984.

59. Raptopoulos V, Cummings T, Smith EH: Computed tomography of life-threatening complications of abdominal aortic aneurysm: the disrupted aortic wall. Invest Radiol 22:372, 1987.

60. Cullenward MJ, Scanlan KA, Pozniak MA, Archer CA: Inflammatory aortic aneurysm (periaortic fibrosis): radiologic imaging. Radiology 159:75, 1986.

61. Vinton VC, Usselman JA, Warmath MA, Dilley RB: Aortic perianeurysmal fibrosis: CT density enhancement and ureteral obstruction. AJR 134:577, 1980.

62. Oudkerk M, Overbosch E, Dee P: CT recognition of acute aortic dissection. AJR 141:671, 1983.

63. Kersting-Sommerhoff BA, Higgins CB, White RD, Sommerhoff CP, Lipton MJ: Aortic dissection: sensitivity and specificity of MR imaging. Radiology 166:651, 1988.

64. Amparo EG, Higgins CB, Hricak H, Sollitto R: Aortic dissection: magnetic resonance imaging. Radiology 155:399, 1985.

65. Geisinger MA, Risius B, O'Donnell JA, Zelch MG, Moodie DS, et al: Thoracic aortic dissections: magnetic resonance imaging. Radiology 155:407, 1985.

66. Dinsmore RE, Wedeen VJ, Miller SW, Rosen BR, Fifer M, et al: MRI of dissection of the aorta: recognition of the intimal tear and differential flow velocities. AJR 146:1286, 1986.

67. Mark A, Moss AA, Lusby R, Kaiser JA: CT evaluation of the complications of abdominal aortic surgery. Radiology 145:409, 1982.

68. Haaga JR, Baldwin GN, Reich NB, Beven E, Kramer A, et al: CT detection of infected synthetic grafts: preliminary report of a new sign. AJR 131:317, 1978.

69. Justich E, Amparo EG, Hricak H, Higgins CB: Infected aortoiliac grafts: magnetic resonance imaging. Radiology 154:133, 1985.

70. Auffermann W, Olofsson PA, Stoney RJ, Higgins CB: MR imaging of complications of aortic surgery. J Comput Axial Tomogr 11:982, 1987.

71. Unger EC, Glazer HS, Lee JKT, Ling D: MRI of extracranial hematomas: preliminary observations. AJR 46:403, 1986.

72. Rubin JI, Gomori JM, Grossman RI, Gefter WB, Kressel HY: High-field MR imaging of extracranial hematomas. AJR 148:813, 1987.

73. O'Hara PJ, Borkowski GP, Hertzer NR, O'Donovan PB, Brigham SL, Beven EG: Natural history of periprosthetic air on computerized axial tomographic examination of the abdomen following abdominal aortic aneurysm repair. J Vasc Surg 1:429, 1984.

74. Auffermann W, Olofsson PA, Rabahie GN, Tavares NJ, Stoney RJ, Higgins CB: Incorporation versus infection of retroperitoneal aortic grafts: MR imaging features. Radiology 172:359, 1989.

75. Jeffrey RB Jr, Federle MP: The collapsed inferior vena cava: CT evidence of hypovolemia. AJR 150:431, 1988.

76. Mayo J, Gray R, St Louis E, Grosman H, McLoughlin M, Wise D: Anomalies of the inferior vena cava. AJR 140:339, 1983.

77. Royal SA, Callen PW: CT evaluation of anomalies of the inferior vena cava and left renal vein. AJR 132:759, 1979.

78. Fisher MR, Hricak H, Higgins CB: Magnetic resonance imaging of developmental venous anomalies. AJR 145:705, 1985.

79. Kellman GM, Alpern MB, Sandler MA, Craig BM: Computed tomography of vena caval anomalies with embryologic correlation. Radiographics 8:533, 1986.

80. Ginaldi S, Chuang VP, Wallace S: Absence of hepatic segment of the inferior vena cava with azygos continuation. J Comput Assist Tomogr 4:112, 1980.

81. Churchill RJ, Wesbey G III, Marsan RE, Moncada R, Reynes CJ, Love L: Computed tomographic demonstration of anomalous inferior vena cava with azygos continuation. J Comput Assist Tomogr 4:398, 1980.

82. Zerhouni EA, Barth KH, Siegelman SS: Demonstration of venous thrombosis by computed tomography. AJR 134:753, 1980.

83. Steele JR, Sones PJ, Heffner LT: The detection of inferior vena caval thrombosis with computed tomography. Radiology 128:385, 1978.

84. Marks WM, Korobkin M, Callen PW, Kaiser JA: CT diagnosis of tumor thrombosis of the renal vein and inferior vena cava. AJR 131:843, 1978.

85. Weyman PJ, McClennan BL, Stanley RJ, Levitt GR, Sagel SS: Comparison of computed tomography and angiography in the evaluation of renal cell carcinoma. Radiology 137:417, 1980.

86. Glazer GM, Callen PW, Parker JJ: CT diagnosis of tumor thrombus in the inferior vena cava: avoiding false positive diagnosis. AJR 137:1265, 1981.

87. Schmitz L, Jeffrey RB, Palubinskas AJ, Moss AA: CT demonstration of septic thrombosis of the inferior vena cava. J Comput Assist Tomogr 5:259, 1981.

88. Didier D, Racle A, Etievent JP, Weill F: Tumor thrombus of the inferior vena cava secondary to malignant abdominal neoplasms: US and CT evaluation. Radiology 162:83, 1987.

89. Vogelzang RL, Gore RM, Neiman HL, Smith SJ, Deschler TW, Vrla RF: Inferior vena cava CT pseudothrombus produced by rapid arm-vein contrast infusion. AJR 144:843, 1985.

90. Fagelman D, Lawrence LP, Black KS, Javors BR: Inferior vena

cava pseudothrombus in computed tomography using a contrast medium power injector: a potential pitfall. J Comput Assist Tomogr 11:1042, 1987.

91. Pagani JJ, Thomas JL, Bernadino ME: Computed tomographic manifestations of abdominal and pelvic venous collaterals. Radiology 142:415, 1982.

92. Shaffer PB, Johnson JC, Bryan D, Fabri PJ: Diagnosis of ovarian vein thrombophlebitis by computed tomography. J Comput Assist Tomogr 5:436, 1981.

93. Miner DG, Cohan RH, Davis WK, Braun SD: CT-guided percutaneous aspiration of septic thrombosis of the inferior vena cava. AJR 148:1213, 1987.

94. Lang EK: Angio-computed tomography and dynamic computed tomography in staging of renal cell carcinoma. Radiology 151:149, 1984.

95. Zeman RK, Cronan JJ, Rosenfield AT, Lynch JH, Jaffe MH, Clark LR: Renal cell carcinoma: dynamic thin-section CT assessment of vascular invasion and tumor vascularity. Radiology 167:393, 1988.

96. Miller CL, Wechsler RJ: CT evaluation of Kimray-Greenfield filter complications. AJR 147:45, 1986.

97. Hricak H, Amparo E, Fisher MR, Crooks L, Higgins CB: Abdominal venous system: assessment using MR. Radiology 156:415, 1985.

98. von Schulthess GK, Augustiny N: Calculation of T2 values versus phase imaging for the distinction between flow and thrombus in MR imaging. Radiology 164:549, 1987.

99. Teitlebaum GP, Bradley WG Jr, Klein BD: MR imaging artifacts, ferromagnetism, and magnetic torque of intravascular filters, stents, and coils. Radiology 166:657, 1988.

100. Liebman CE, Messersmith RN, Levin DN, Lu C-T: MR imaging of inferior vena cava filters: safety and artifacts. AJR 150:1174, 1988.

101. Hulnick DH, Chatson GP, Megibow AJ, Bosniak MA, Ruoff M: Retroperitoneal fibrosis presenting as colonic dysfunction: CT diagnosis. J Comput Assist Tomogr 12:159, 1988.

102. Fagan CJ, Larrieu AJ, Amparo EG: Retroperitoneal fibrosis: ultrasound and CT features. AJR 133:239, 1979.

103. Renner IG, Ponto GC, Savage WT II, Boswell WD: Idiopathic retroperitoneal fibrosis producing common bile duct and pancreatic duct obstruction. Gastroenterology 79:348, 1980.

104. Mitchinson MJ: Retroperitoneal fibrosis revisited. Arch Pathol Lab Med 110:784, 1986.

105. Usher SM, Brendler H, Ciavarra VA: Retroperitoneal fibrosis secondary to metastatic neoplasm. Urology 9:191, 1977.

106. Brooks AP, Reznek RH, Webb JAW, Baker LRI: Computed tomography in the follow-up of retroperitoneal fibrosis. Clin Radiol 38:597, 1987.

107. Arrivé L, Hricak H, Tavares NJ, Miller TR: Malignant versus nonmalignant retroperitoneal fibrosis: differentiation with MR imaging. Radiology 172:139, 1989.

108. Dalla-Palma L, Rocca-Rossetti S, Pozzi-Mucelli RS, Rizzatto G: Computed tomography in the diagnosis of retroperitoneal fibrosis. Urol Radiol 3:77, 1981.

109. Hricak H, Higgins CB, Williams RD: Nuclear magnetic resonance imaging in retroperitoneal fibrosis. AJR 141:35, 1983.

110. Mulligan SA, Holley HC, Koehler RE, Koslin DB, Rubin E, et al: CT and MR imaging in the evaluation of retroperitoneal fibrosis. J Comput Assist Tomogr 13:277, 1989.

111. Yancey JM, Kaude JV: Diagnosis of perirenal fibrosis by MR imaging. J Comput Assist Tomogr 12:335, 1988.

112. Illescas FF, Baker ME, McCann R, Cohan RH, Silverman PM, Dunnick NR: CT evaluation of retroperitoneal hemorrhage associated with femoral arteriography. AJR 146:1289, 1986.

113. Sagel SS, Siegel MJ, Stanley RJ, Jost RG: Detection of retroperitoneal hemorrhage by computed tomography. AJR 129:403, 1977.

114. Swensen SJ, Keller PL, Berquist TH, McLeod RA, Stephens DH: Magnetic resonance imaging of hemorrhage. AJR 145:921, 1985.

115. van Sonnenberg E, Mueller PR, Ferrucci JT Jr: Percutaneous drainage of 250 abdominal abscesses and fluid collections. I. Results, failures, and complications. Radiology 151:337, 1984.

116. Gordon DH, Machia RJ, Glanz S, Koser MW, Laungani GB: Percutaneous management of retroperitoneal abscesses. Urology 30:299, 1987.

117. Sacks D, Banner MP, Meranze SG, Burke DR, Robinson M, McLean GK: Renal and related retroperitoneal abscesses: percutaneous drainage. Radiology 167:447, 1988.

118. Stephens DH, Sheedy PF, Hattery RR, Williamson B: Diagnosis and evaluation of retroperitoneal tumors by computed tomography. AJR 129:395, 1977.

119. Lane RH, Stephens DH, Reiman HM: Primary retroperitoneal neoplasms: CT findings in 90 cases with clinical and pathologic correlation. AJR 152:83, 1989.

120. Cohan RH, Baker ME, Cooper C, Moore JO, Saeed M, Dunnick NR: Computed tomography of primary retroperitoneal malignancies. J Comput Assist Tomogr 12:804, 1988.

121. Waligore MP, Stephens DH, Soule EH, MacLeod RA: Lipomatous tumors of the abdominal cavity: CT appearance and pathologic correlation. AJR 137:539, 1981.

122. Friedman AC, Hartman DS, Sherman J, Lautin EM, Goldman M: Computed tomography of abdominal fatty masses. Radiology 139:415, 1981.

123. Dooms GC, Hricak H, Margulis AR, de Geer G: MR imaging of fat. Radiology 158:51, 1986.

124. Kogan SJ, Gill B, Bennett B, Smey P, Reda EF, Levitt SG: Human monorchism: a clinicopathological study of unilateral absent testes in 65 boys. J Urol 135:758, 1986.

125. Lee JKT, McClennan BL, Stanley RJ, Sagel SS: Utility of computed tomography in the localization of the undescended testis. Radiology 135:121, 1980.

126. Wolverson MK, Houttuin E, Heiberg E, Sundaram M, Shields JB: Comparison of computed tomography with high-resolution real-time ultrasound in the localization of impalpable undescended testis. Radiology 146:133, 1983.

127. Fritzsche PJ, Hricak H, Kogan BA, Winkler ML, Tanagho EA: Undescended testis: value of MR imaging. Radiology 164:169, 1987.

128. Friedland GW, Chang P: The role of imaging in the management of the impalpable undescended testis. AJR 151:1107, 1988.

129. Mueller PR, Ferucci JT Jr, Wittenberg J, Simeone JF, Butch RJ: Iliopsoas abscess: treatment by CT-guided percutaneous catheter drainage. AJR 142:359, 1984.

130. Weinreb JC, Cohen JM, Maravilla KR: Iliopsoas muscles: MR study of normal anatomy and disease. Radiology 156:435, 1985.

131. Feldberg MAM, Koehler PR, van Waes PFGM: Psoas compartment disease studied by computed tomography. Radiology 148:505, 1983.

132. Lee JKT, Glazer HS: Psoas muscle disorders: MR imaging. Radiology 160:683, 1986.

CHAPTER 24

THE PERITONEAL CAVITY AND MESENTERY

R. BROOKE JEFFREY, JR.

Peritoneal Cavity

Anatomy

Much of our recent understanding of the radiologic anatomy of the peritoneal cavity and the spread of intraperitoneal disease processes comes from the anatomic-radiologic correlations pioneered by Meyers.[1-4] The peritoneal cavity may be divided into the pelvis, upper abdomen, and the lesser peritoneal sac (Figs. 24–1 and 24–2). The pelvic cul de sac is the most dependent portion of the peritoneal cavity (Fig. 24–3) and often is the initial location of intraperitoneal fluid collections such as abscesses, hematomas, or ascites. Extending from the midline cul de sac, the paravesical fossae are in direct continuity with both the right and left paracolic gutters. Pelvic fluid collections preferentially extend into the upper abdomen by way of the right paracolic gutter, as it is broader and deeper than the left, and also because an anatomic barrier is created by the phrenicocolic ligament (Fig. 24–4). On computed tomographic (CT) scans, fluid in the paracolic gutters is seen to displace the colon medially (Fig. 24–5); however, the extraperitoneal attachment along the posterior aspect of the ascending and descending colon is preserved.

In the upper abdomen, the transverse mesocolon divides the peritoneal cavity into supramesocolic and inframesocolic compartments (Fig. 24–6). In the right upper quadrant, the peritoneum reflects over the diaphragm and liver to create a right subphrenic and right subhepatic space (Fig. 24–7). The right subphrenic space extends beneath the dome of the diaphragm to the edge of the coronary ligament, which suspends the right lobe of the liver from the diaphragm posteriorly. On CT scans, subphrenic fluid may be distinguished from a pleural effusion by its location anterior to the diaphragm (Fig. 24–8A). On occasion, it may be difficult to differentiate a subphrenic from an intrahepatic fluid collection in the transverse plane. Sagittal and coronal reformations are often helpful in clarifying the location of fluid collections near the dome of the diaphragm (Fig. 24–8B,C).

The peritoneal reflections along the undersurface of the liver form an anterior and posterior subhepatic space roughly separated by the origin of the transverse mesocolon. The posterior subhepatic space, or Morrisons's pouch (see Figs. 23–1 and 23–7), is bounded by the peritoneal reflections between the posterior aspect of the right lobe of the liver and the right kidney. Morrison's pouch is the most dependent portion of the peritoneal cavity in the right upper quadrant and is frequently the site of postop-

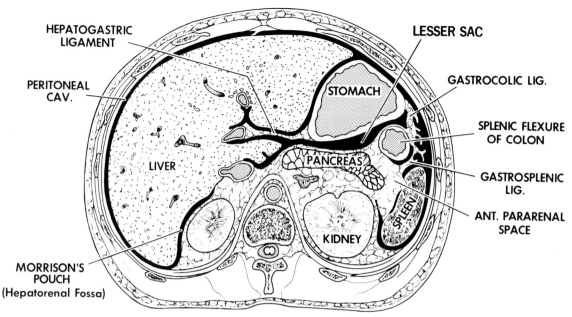

FIGURE 24–1 ■ Diagram of transverse section of upper abdomen demonstrating peritoneal cavity, Morrison's pouch, and the lesser sac. The relationships between the lesser sac, pancreas, colon, stomach, and liver are shown. The upper abdominal portion of the peritoneal cavity surrounds the liver, spleen, and lateral portion of the splenic flexure of the colon.

erative abdominal abscesses. As stressed by Meyers,[1] intraperitoneal fluid extending from the pelvis up the right paracolic gutter initially localizes into the posterior subhepatic space (Fig. 23–9; see also Fig. 23–4). With increasing volumes, intraperitoneal fluid extends from Morrison's pouch to the lateral peritoneal surface of the liver and finally into the subphrenic spaces. In patients with cirrhosis and other forms of hepatocellular disease, it is not unusual to identify varying amounts of ascitic fluid around the lateral aspects of the liver (see Fig. 23–9). In addition, the lateral peritoneal surface is an important site for the diagnosis of peritoneal implants in patients with abdominal malignancies.

The falciform ligament separates the right and left subphrenic spaces. Both the right and left subphrenic space, as well as the subhepatic space, communicate freely along the edges of the falciform ligament. The left coronary ligament attaches more anteriorly than the right coronary ligament, and therefore the left

Text continued on page 1144

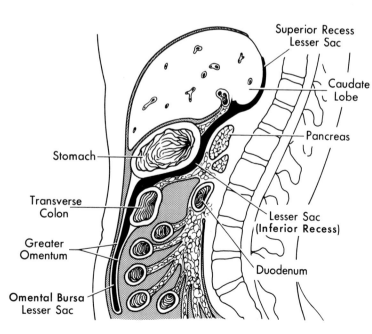

FIGURE 24–2 ■ Sagittal section of upper abdomen through the region of the lesser sac. Note the superior and inferior recesses of the lesser sac. The drawing demonstrates that in some patients a well-defined omental bursa is present between the reflections of the greater omentum. In most patients, the caudal extent of the lesser sac is at the level of the transverse mesocolon. (From Jeffrey RB, Federle MP, Goodman PC: Radiology 141:117, 1981.)

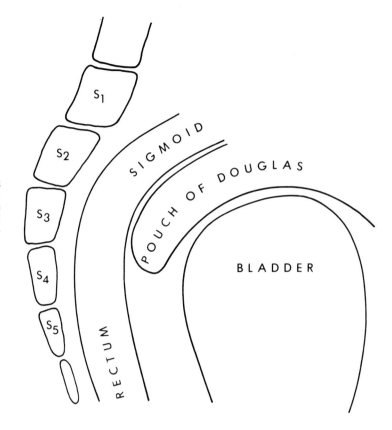

FIGURE 24–3 ■ Sagittal section through the pelvis depicting the relationship of the pouch of Douglas to the rectum, sigmoid colon, and urinary bladder. The pouch of Douglas extends to the top of S4 at the junction of the rectum and sigmoid colon. (Modified from Meyers MA: Dynamic Radiology of the Abdomen. Normal and Pathologic Anatomy. New York, Springer-Verlag, 1976.)

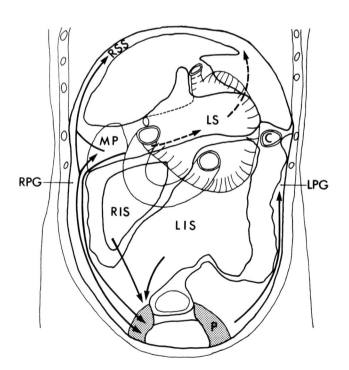

FIGURE 24–4 ■ Diagram of flow patterns of intraperitoneal fluid. Dashed arrows indicated spread anterior to the stomach into the left subphrenic area. C = Colon; LIS = Left intracolic space; LPG = Left paracolic gutter; LS = lesser sac; MP = Morrison's pouch; P = Pelvic cul de sac; RIS = Right infracolic space; RPG = Right paracolic gutter; RSS = Right subphrenic space. (Modified from Meyers MA: Dynamic Radiology of the Abdomen. Normal and Pathologic Anatomy. New York, Springer-Verlag, 1976.)

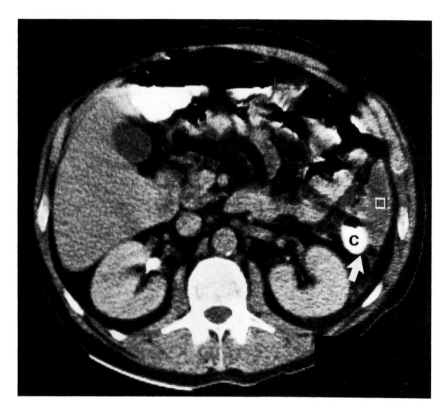

FIGURE 24–5 ■ Free intraperitoneal fluid *(box)* displaces the contrast-filled colon (C) medially. The extraperitoneal attachment of the colon in the anterior pararenal space is preserved *(arrow)*.

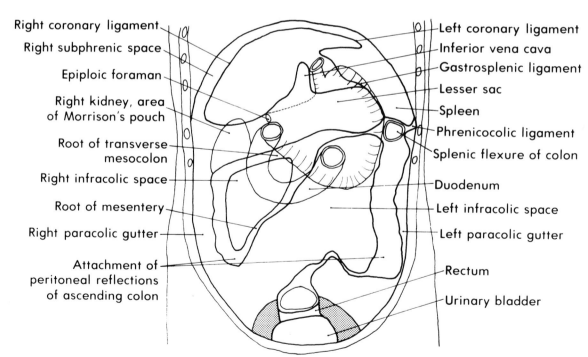

Right coronary ligament
Right subphrenic space
Epiploic foramen
Right kidney, area of Morrison's pouch
Root of transverse mesocolon
Right infracolic space
Root of mesentery
Right paracolic gutter
Attachment of peritoneal reflections of ascending colon

Left coronary ligament
Inferior vena cava
Gastrosplenic ligament
Lesser sac
Spleen
Phrenicocolic ligament
Splenic flexure of colon
Duodenum
Left infracolic space
Left paracolic gutter
Rectum
Urinary bladder

FIGURE 24–6 ■ Diagram of posterior peritoneal reflections and recesses dividing the peritoneal cavity into supramesocolic and inframesocolic compartments. (Modified from Meyers MA: Dynamic Radiology of the Abdomen. Normal and Pathologic Anatomy. New York, Springer-Verlag, 1976.)

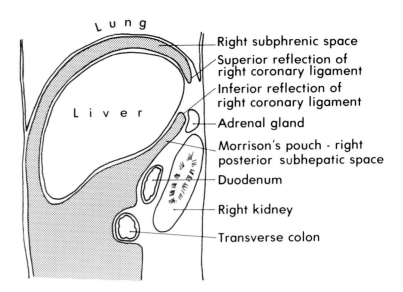

FIGURE 24–7 ■ Right parasagittal section. The right subphrenic space extends beneath the dome of the diaphragm to the superior edge of the coronary ligament. The right subhepatic space has both an anterior and posterior (Morrison's pouch) compartment and is contiguous with the reflections of the coronary ligament. (Modified from Meyers MA: Dynamic Radiology of the Abdomen. Normal and Pathologic Anatomy. New York, Springer-Verlag, 1976.)

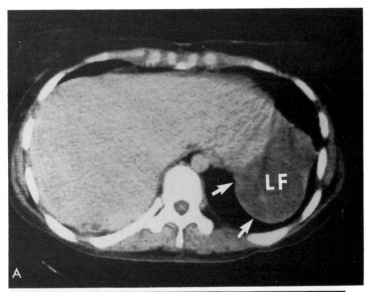

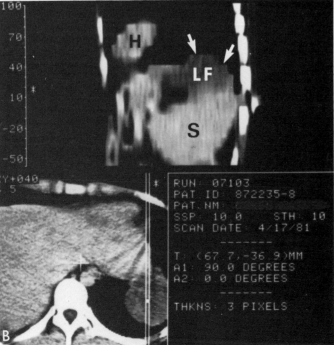

FIGURE 24–8 Bilateral subphrenic abscesses. A, Transverse CT scan reveals fluid collection (LF) in left subphrenic space above the diaphragm (arrows). B, Sagittal reformation more clearly demonstrates relationship of left subphrenic fluid (LF) to diaphragm (arrows) and spleen (S). H = Heart.

Illustration continued on following page

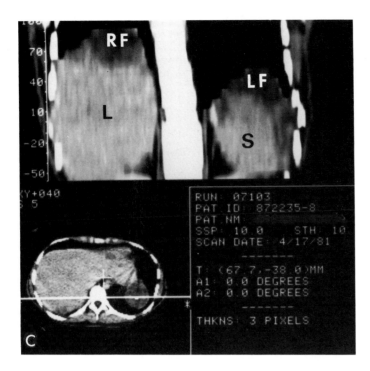

FIGURE 24–8 *Continued C,* Coronal reformation reveals left (LF) and right (RF) subphrenic fluid collections. L = Liver; S = spleen.

subphrenic space does not extend as far posterior as the right (Fig. 24–10).

The lesser sac lies behind the lesser omentum, stomach, duodenum, and gastric ligament and communicates with peritoneal cavity via the foramen of Winslow (see Figs. 24–1, 24–2, and 24–10). Superiorly the lesser sac extends to the diaphragm. The reflection of the parietal peritoneum off the gastrophrenic ligament extends to the gastric fundus and is contiguous inferiorly with the gastrosplenic ligament and

the splenorenal ligament, which form the left lateral caudate lobe of the liver. This extends superiorly to form the superior recess of the lesser sac. In most individuals the transverse mesocolon is the caudal extent of the lesser sac. However, in some patients there is a well-developed omental recess of the lesser sac between the reflections of the greater omentum (see Fig. 24–2). The anterior boundary of the lesser sac is formed by the posterior aspect of the stomach, the lesser omentum (gastrohepatic ligament), and

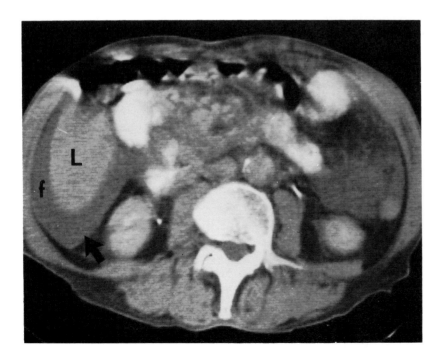

FIGURE 24–9 ■ Fluid (f) located lateral to the liver (L) and in Morrison's pouch *(arrow).* Small amounts of intraperitoneal fluid are often detectable in the right subhepatic space.

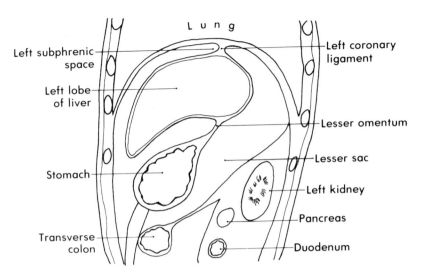

FIGURE 24–10 ■ Parasagittal section through the left lobe of the liver. The coronary ligament attaches more anteriorly than the right and limits the posterior extent of the left subphrenic space. At this level the perihepatic spaces are freely continuous. The lesser sac remains a separate space. (Modified from Meyers MA: Dynamic Radiology of the Abdomen. Normal and Pathologic Anatomy. New York, Springer-Verlag, 1976.)

the anterior reflection of the greater omentum. Posteriorly the lesser sac is bounded by the peritoneal reflection over the pancreas and left adrenal.

The lesser sac is divided into two main compartments, the superior and inferior recesses, by reflections of peritoneum over the left gastric artery.[5] The superior recess lies immediately adjacent to the caudate lobe of the liver and extends into the fissure for the ligamentum venosum. The gastrohepatic ligament, containing the left gastric artery, separates the superior recess from the left subhepatic space. The larger inferior recess of the lesser sac lies posterior to the stomach and anterior to the pancreas. It is bounded anteriorly by the gastrosplenic ligament and posteriorly by the splenorenal ligament. It may communicate caudally with the omental bursa by way of the leaves of the greater omentum.

To better visualize the complex three-dimensional relationships of the lesser sac Dodds and co-workers[6] used the analogy of a closed hand with an outstretched thumb to visualize the various recesses of the lesser sac. With the wrist positioned at the foramen of Winslow, the cranially outstretched thumb lies within the superior recess of the lesser sac (see Fig. 24–6). The closed fingers lie within the inferior recess. Along the thenar crease of the palm lies the posterior peritoneal reflection over the left gastric artery.

Reflections of the peritoneum containing fat, lymph nodes, and vascular structures create intraabdominal ligaments that are important pathways for the dissemination of peritoneal malignancies and inflammatory lesions.[1,4] Neoplasms can spread directly by ligamentous invasion. The gastrohepatic ligament of the lesser omentum suspends the lesser curvature of the stomach from the left lobe of the liver and creates a pathway for spread of either gastric or hepatic carcinoma. The gastrocolic ligament (i.e., the upper portion of the greater omentum) suspends the transverse colon from the greater cur-

vature of the stomach. Thus it permits direct invasion of gastric carcinoma along the superior margin of the transverse colon. Less commonly, carcinoma of the transverse colon may spread to the greater curvature of the stomach. Pancreatic carcinoma may directly invade either the splenic hilum via the splenorenal ligament or the splenic flexure via the phrenicolic ligament.

Scanning Technique

Scanning techniques used in evaluating suspected abnormalities of the peritoneal cavity must be individualized according to the clinical setting. Patients with possible intraperitoneal or pelvic abscesses are usually studied at 1- or 2-cm intervals from diaphragm to pelvis following oral and during an intravenous bolus injection of 150 ml of 60 per cent diatrizoate sodium (Renografin). In the evaluation of pelvic fluid collections or masses, rectal contrast is also given to help clarify the relationship of the mass to the colon. In patients evaluated for ascites and abdominal malignancies, scans are most frequently obtained at 1- to 2-cm intervals. However, in patients with known or suspected malignancies that may produce peritoneal implants or hepatic metastases, the liver and upper abdomen are scanned at 0.5- to 1-cm intervals and the lower abdomen and pelvis at 1- to 1.5-cm intervals.

Dunnick et al.[7] performed CT scans following injection of dilute contrast media through intraperitoneal catheters and found the technique to be of value in selected cases of peritoneal metastasis, in demonstrating the distribution of intraperitoneal fluid, and in diagnosing the presence of adhesions. However, because of the invasiveness of the procedure, it has not gained wide acceptance. Image reformation is not routinely performed in abdominal CT but has proved helpful in distinguishing subphrenic from intrahepatic fluid collections.

Pathology

INTRAPERITONEAL FLUID

Intraperitoneal fluid collections may occur as either a primary or a secondary manifestation of a variety of pathologic disorders, including peritonitis, trauma, and metastatic disease, as well as cardiac, hepatic, or renal failure. CT can accurately diagnose and precisely delineate the location of even small quantities of intraperitoneal fluid. Furthermore, it can distinguish between intraperitoneal and extraperitoneal fluid.[1] Fluid in the supramesocolic compartment of the peritoneal cavity often initially collects in Morrison's pouch or in the posterior hepatorenal fossa and is demonstrated as a water-density collection (0 to 10 Hounsfield units [H]) around the posterior edge of the right lobe of the liver (see Fig. 24–9). In the inframesocolic compartment, fluid initially collects in the cul de sac and then extends from the paravesical fossae into the paracolic gutters. Intraperitoneal fluid in the paracolic gutters may be readily distinguished from extraperitoneal fluid by the preservation of the extraperitoneal fat posterior to the colon in the anterior pararenal space. Extraperitoneal inflammatory processes such as pancreatitis often obliterate the fat plane posterior and medial to the colon in the anterior pararenal space (Fig. 24–11).

In patients with significant amounts of free ascites, the bowel loops are centrally positioned in the abdomen and the mesentery is clearly delineated (Fig. 24–12). Cystic masses can usually be distinguished from free intraperitoneal fluid by the presence of a mass effect that displaces adjacent bowel loops in a focal manner. However, at times differentiation of a cystic mass from loculated ascites can be difficult, and in patients with very tense ascites, bowel loops can be displaced from the central portion of the abdomen in the absence of an intraperitoneal mass.[8]

Loculated ascites is an important CT finding indicating benign or malignant adhesions. Adhesions may be secondary to prior surgery, peritonitis, or metastatic seeding in the peritoneum. The bowel loops in patients with loculated ascites do not float in the central abdomen but are displaced by the loculated ascitic fluid. Loculated fluid that is infected often exhibits focal mass effect on adjacent bowel loops (Fig. 24–13) and in patients with infected ascites, peritonitis or generalized thickening of the peritoneum can be readily diagnosed by CT (Fig. 24–14). Focal thickening of the peritoneum, particularly if nodular, is generally more indicative of metastatic malignancy rather than infection.

The CT attenuation values of benign and malignant ascites have not proven to be sufficiently different to permit differentiation. However, the distribution of ascitic fluid can be a clue as to whether the ascitic fluid is benign or malignant. Gore et al.[9] found that benign ascitic fluid was found free within the intraperitoneal compartment and usually did not enter the lesser sac. When present in the lesser sac, it was found in relatively small amounts (Fig. 24–15). Malignant ascites resulting from peritoneal seeding was usually present in the lesser sac to a degree matching its presence in the peritoneal cavity. Fluid confined only to the lesser sac indicated a local etiologic factor such as pancreatitis, lesser sac abscess, or pancreatic carcinoma. This distinction between benign and malignant ascites on the basis of distribution is not entirely reliable but is sufficiently accurate to warrant careful evaluation of the distribution of ascitic fluid in every patient with ascites.

In addition to serous ascites, other pathologic water-density intraperitoneal fluid collections, including bile, urine, or chyle, can be demonstrated by CT. Bile peritonitis generally results from trauma to the liver or biliary tree or perforation of a gangrenous gallbladder. In patients with blunt trauma to the gallbladder, a hematoma may be detected in the gallbladder lumen or gallbladder fossa. A useful clue on CT scans of a laceration of the gallbladder fundus

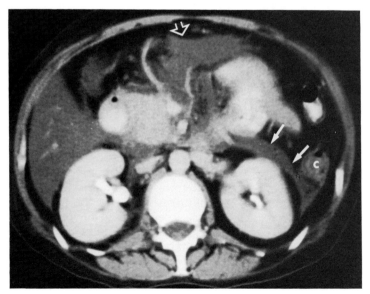

FIGURE 24–11 ■ Extraperitoneal effusion in acute pancreatitis. An inflammatory reaction in the left anterior pararenal space *(solid arrows)* obliterates the extraperitoneal fat planes posterior and medial to the descending colon (c). Note extensive inflammatory exudate in transverse mesocolon *(open arrow)*.

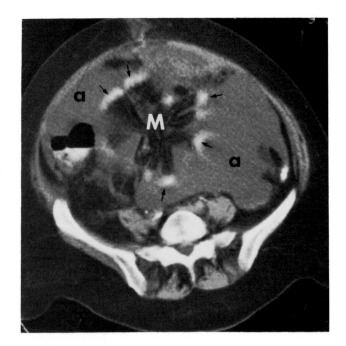

FIGURE 24–12 ■ Massive ascites (a) causing the small bowel *(arrows)* and mesentery (m) to float in the central abdomen. The fat content of the normal mesentery is particularly well delineated against the background of ascitic fluid.

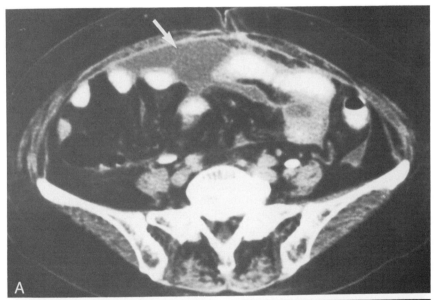

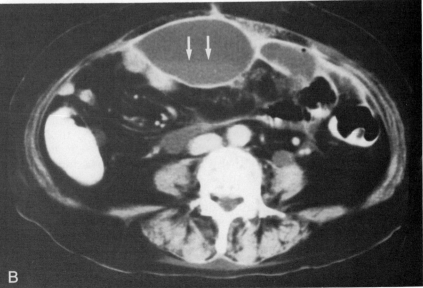

FIGURE 24–13 ■ Loculated peritoneal fluid collections. *A,* Loculated ascites *(arrow)* in a patient with postoperative adhesions. Diagnostic needle aspiration yielded simple ascites without infection. Note lack of mass effect. *B,* Loculated infected fluid in a postoperative patient. Note mass effect by rounded fluid collection and higher density of debris layering posteriorly *(arrows).*

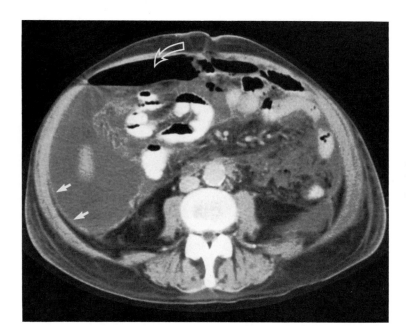

FIGURE 24–14 ■ Peritonitis with infected intraperitoneal fluid and thickening of peritoneum *(straight arrows).* Patient has large hydropneumoperitoneum from perforated jejunum. Note free air anteriorly *(curved arrow).*

is water-density intraperitoneal fluid[10] and contraction of the gallbladder in a fasting patient (Fig. 24–16). Cholescintigraphy may be useful in documenting bile leakeage, although diagnostic needle aspiration is more efficacious. Intraperitoneal rupture of the urinary bladder can be suggested on CT scans by water-density intraperitoneal fluid and large filling defects in the bladder representing clots. Chylous ascites is rare following blunt trauma. Rupture of the cysterna chyli results in a characteristic CT appearance of both intra- and extraperitoneal water-density fluid as chyle leaks along collateral pathways from the gut, as well as from retroperitoneal organs. (Fig. 24–17).[11] Often a specific diagnosis of the type of water-density fluid cannot be made by CT alone, and guided needle aspiration is required.

Intraperitoneal hemorrhage may occur following blunt abdominal trauma,[12] or excessive anticoagulation[13] or from spontaneous rupture of abdominal neoplasms, including hepatic adenomas, hepatomas, cavernous hemangioma, or angiosarcoma. Because of its high protein content, acute intraperitoneal hemorrhage has a CT attenuation value generally greater than 30 H in patients scanned within 48 hours of injury (Fig. 24–18).[12–14] Clotted blood has even higher attenuation values. On MRI scans, intraperitoneal blood demonstrates a relatively high signal intensity in both T1- and T2-weighted images (Fig. 24–19). Occasionally, exudative ascites (particularly from tuberculous peritonitis) may have attenuation values of 15 to 30 H.[15]

Pseudomyxoma peritonei is an uncommon disorder characterized by intraperitoneal accumulations of gelatinous material. It most often occurs secondary to rupture of a mucinous cystadenocarcinoma of either the ovary or appendix or to rupture of a metastatic, cystic, mucin-producing implant in the peritoneum. Rarely it occurs postoperatively from intraperitoneal seeding following a retroperitoneal lymphadenectomy (Fig. 24–20).[16] The characteristic CT features of pseudomyxoma peritonei are a scalloping of the lateral contour of the liver, produced by the gelatinous masses, and the presence of septations extending from the liver margin to the lateral peritoneal surface.[17,18] At times, pseudomyxoma peritonei produces a CT appearance indistinguishable from that of loculated ascites. Chronic pseudomyxoma peritonei may calcify (Fig. 24–21).

INTRAPERITONEAL ABSCESSES

In recent decades, the epidemiology of abdominal abscesses has changed, and now postoperative abscesses, rather than intestinal perforations, predominate. Despite improved antibiotic and supportive therapies, abdominal abscesses continue to be a major source of morbidity and mortality.[19,20] Even with surgical drainage there is a 30 per cent mortality in upper abdominal abscesses.[19] One of the major contributing factors to this continuing morbidity has been delay in diagnosis.

Plain films of the abdomen in patients with suspected abscesses are often helpful in demonstrating ectopic gas or fluid collections. However, if the abdominal film is nondiagnostic, an additional imaging procedure should be employed. In our institution, as in others, computed tomography has become one of the primary diagnostic modalities in detecting abdominal abscesses.[21–33] The advantages of CT are that it is noninvasive, has a high degree of accuracy, and is capable of imaging the entire abdomen in severely ill patients. In addition, CT can be used to guide diagnostic needle aspiration to obtain bacteriologic specimens, as well as direct placement of percutaneous abscess drainage for definitive therapy.[22–27]

The CT appearance of intraabdominal and pelvic

Text continued on page 1156

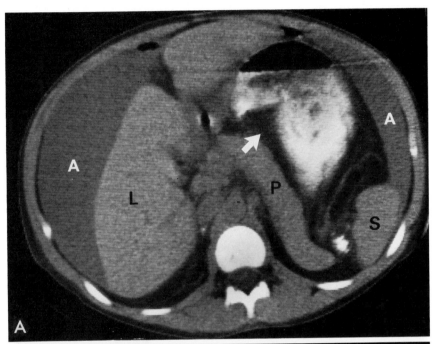

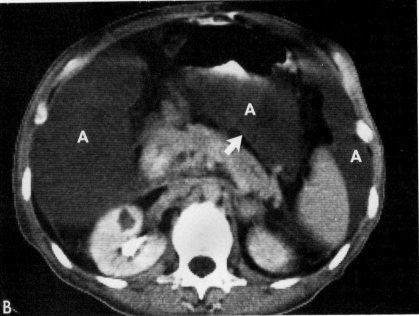

FIGURE 24–15 ■ Patterns of ascites in benign and malignant disease. *A*, Benign ascites (A) in the peritoneal cavity displaces the liver (L) and extends anteriorly to the spleen (S) but does not enter the lesser sac *(arrow)*. P = Pancreas. *B*, Malignant ascites (A) secondary to ovarian carcinoma is distributed equally in the peritoneal cavity and lesser sac *(arrow)*.

Illustration continued on following page

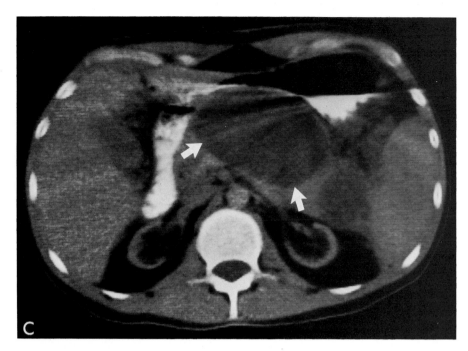

FIGURE 24–15 *Continued C, Fluid (arrows)* confined to the lesser sac in a patient with acute pancreatitis.

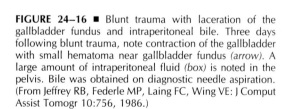

FIGURE 24–16 ■ Blunt trauma with laceration of the gallbladder fundus and intraperitoneal bile. Three days following blunt trauma, note contraction of the gallbladder with small hematoma near gallbladder fundus *(arrow)*. A large amount of intraperitoneal fluid *(box)* is noted in the pelvis. Bile was obtained on diagnostic needle aspiration. (From Jeffrey RB, Federle MP, Laing FC, Wing VE: J Comput Assist Tomogr 10:756, 1986.)

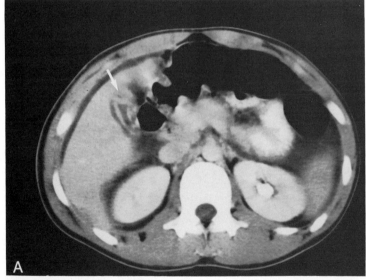

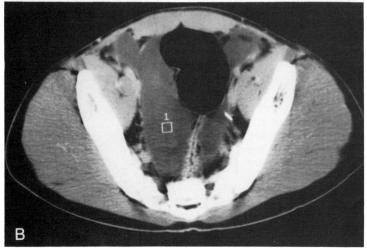

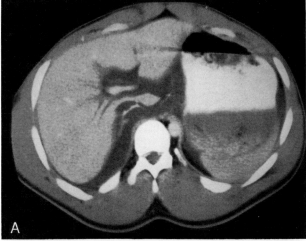
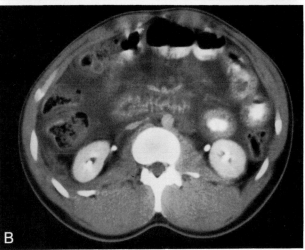

FIGURE 24–17 ■ Rupture of cisterna chyli following blunt abdominal trauma. CT performed 4 hours after trauma demonstrates diffuse intra- and extraperitoneal, water-density chylous fluid demonstrated by CT. Note extraperitoneal fluid around the inferior vena cava. (From Watanabe AT, Jeffrey RB: J Comput Assist Tomogr 11:175, 1987.)

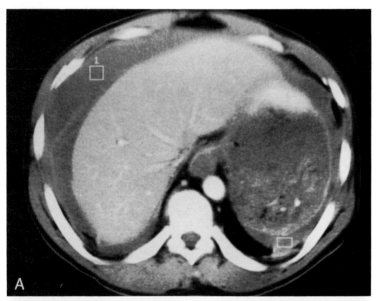

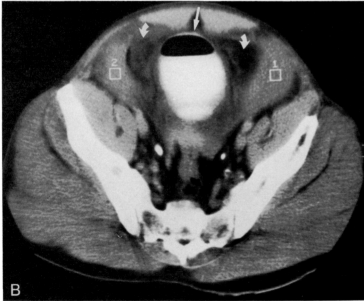

FIGURE 24–18 ■ Acute hemoperitoneum following blunt abdominal trauma secondary to mesenteric artery laceration. A diagnostic peritoneal lavage was attempted prior to CT and was thought to be negative for hemoperitoneum. *A,* CT scan reveals massive hemoperitoneum *(boxes)* and *(B)* documents that water-density lavage fluid (saline) was instilled extraperitoneally in the prevesicle space *(curved arrows).* Note adjacent high-density intraperitoneal blood in paravesicle fossae *(cursor boxes)* and air on contrast in bladder *(straight arrow).*

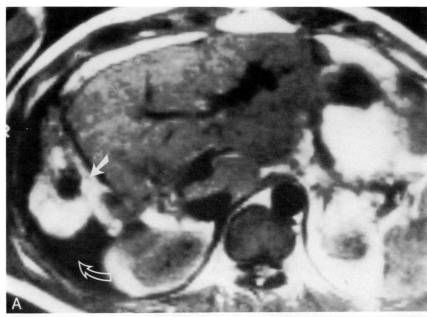

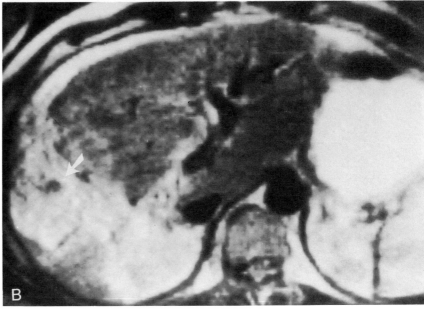

FIGURE 24–19 ■ MR scan of postoperative intraperitoneal hemorrhage. Note high signal on both *(A)* T1- and *(B)* T2-weighted images *(solid arrow)*. Adjacent serous ascites is of low signal intensity *(open arrow)* on T1-weighted image.

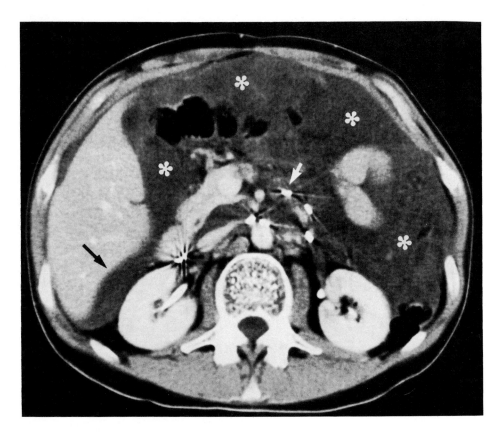

FIGURE 24–20 ■ Diffuse intraperitoneal gelatinous metastasis from mucin-producing teratocarcinoma of the testis. Peritoneal cavity was seeded during retroperitoneal lymphadenectomy. Note low-density tumor scalloping inferior contour of liver *(black arrow)* and complete filling peritoneal cavity by tumor *(asterisk)*. White arrow indicates surgical clips from lymphadenectomy. (From Barakos JA, Jeffrey RB, McAninch JW, Bottles K: J Urol 136:680, 1986.)

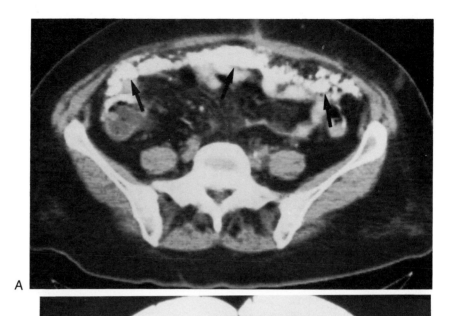

FIGURE 24–21 ■ *A,* Pseudomyxoma peritonei producing a dense band of calcification *(arrows)* in the peritoneal cavity that simulates a barium-filled colon. *B,* MR scan of pseudomyxoma peritonei in another patient with ovarian carcinoma. T1-weighted image demonstrates multiple low-density, rounded masses compressing the spleen and left lobe of the liver *(arrows)*. *C,* T2-weighted image demonstrates higher signal intensity compatible with gelatinous masses of pseudomyxoma peritonei *(straight arrows)*. Note peritoneal implant along the posterior aspect of the right lobe of the liver *(curved arrow)*.

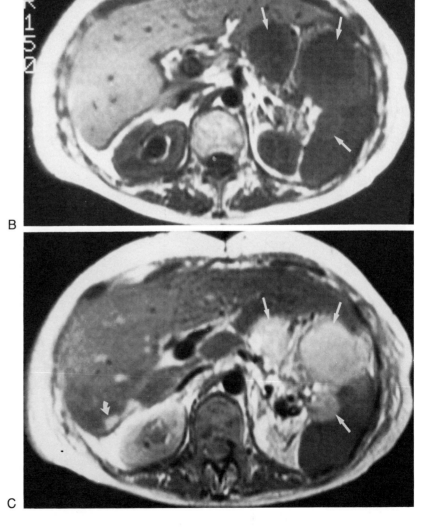

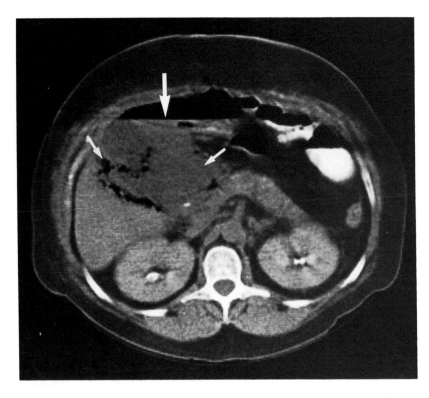

FIGURE 24–22 ■ Gas-forming subhepatic abscess *(small arrows)* and free air *(large arrow)* following anastomotic leak from a gastrojejunostomy.

abscesses is varied. Typically, abscesses are loculated fluid collections with mass effect. The most specific CT feature of an intraabdominal or pelvic abscess is the presence of extraluminal gas (Fig. 24–22).[27] Gas is found in slightly more than one third of abscesses[18] and may be present as multiple small bubbles of gas or a larger gas collection having an air-fluid interface (Figs. 24–23 and 24–24).[25] When a large air-fluid level is identified, special attenuation must be given to the possibility of a perforated viscus or an intestinal fistula (see Fig. 24–14). Often abscesses appear as rounded, oval, or biconvex, rather homogenous low-

density masses having density values between 15 and 35 H (Fig. 24–25).[25,29] A definable wall and low-density center are seen in about one third of abscesses and are signs of a mature, drainable chronic abscess. The wall or rim of an abscess is frequently more clearly identified after intravenous contrast administration because of the highly vascularized connective tissue that comprises the wall of the abscess.

Abscesses commonly produce obliteration of extraperitoneal fat and thickening of adjacent muscles, fascial planes, mesentery, or bowel wall. On occasion

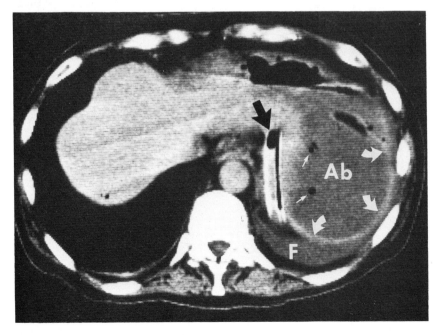

FIGURE 24–23 ■ Left subphrenic abscess (Ab) containing small gas bubbles *(small white arrows)* following splenectomy. A surgically placed drainage tube *(black arrow)* is seen medial to the abscess. A small amount of pleural fluid (F) is present. The diaphragm is well seen *(large white arrows)*.

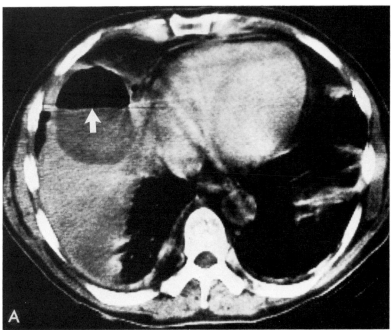

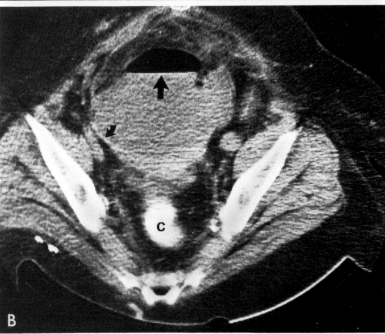

FIGURE 24–24 ■ Abscesses with air-fluid levels. *A,* Subphrenic abscess with an air-fluid level *(arrow).* Note that it is difficult to distinguish whether an abscess is intrahepatic or subphrenic on a single transverse scan. Sagittal reformations are most helpful in these cases. *B,* Large pelvic abscess with air-fluid level *(straight arrow)* following gynecologic surgery. A hypervascular rim *(curved arrow)* is seen around part of the abscess. Note also contrast in the rectosigmoid colon (C).

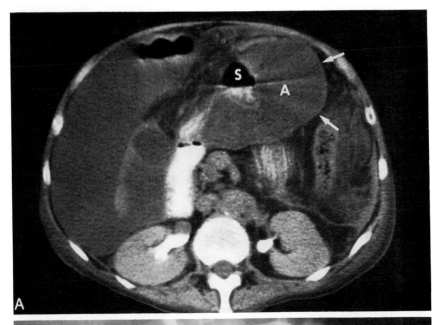

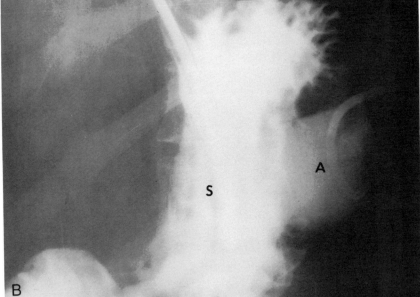

FIGURE 24–25 ■ *A* demonstrates lesser sac abscess (A) within inferior recess. Abscess appears as a homogeneous, water-density mass bulging gastrosplenic ligaments *(arrows)*. S = Stomach. There is no ascites in the right flank. *B,* Following successful percutaneous drainage, abscess sinogram reveals relationship of abscess to contrast-filled stomach. A = Abscess; S = stomach.

the CT characteristics of an abscess provide a clue to its etiology. Identification of a high-density object within a postoperative abscess suggests a sponge abscess (Fig. 24–26); a calcific density in a right lower quadrant abscess or pelvic abscess is evidence of a periappendiceal abscess (Fig. 24–27). Gas in the lesser sac in a patient with pancreatitis and fever is diagnostic of a pancreatic abscess (Fig. 24–28). Commonly encountered associated findings in patients with abdominal or pelvic abscesses are ascites, pleural effusions, and parenchymal consolidation.

Although almost all abscesses are detected on a well-performed CT examination, the CT features are often nonspecific. Low-density abdominal masses can be produced by hematomas, bile collections, peritoneal implants, pseudocysts, necrotic tumors, loculated ascites, lymphocoeles, and benign simple cysts. The CT features of abscesses overlap with these pathologic processes. The presence of gas may be found in a necrotic but noninfected tumor, and following intravenous contrast, hypervascular rims may be identified in tumors, hematomas, and pseudocysts. However, in the proper clinical setting, the findings of an intraabdominal or pelvic mass having

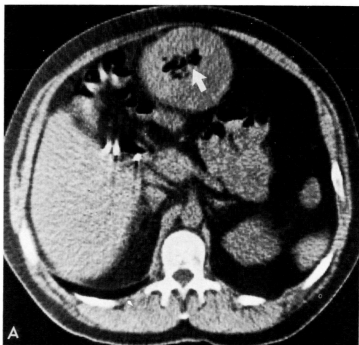

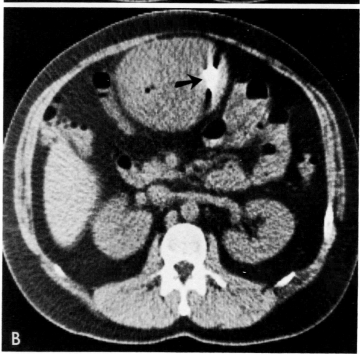

FIGURE 24–26 ■ Sponge abscess. *A,* A soft tissue mass containing gas *(arrow)* is present in the peritoneal cavity. *B,* Scan at a lower level demonstrates a high-density object *(arrow)*, proven to be a retained sponge.

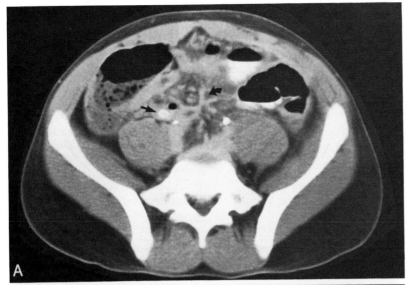

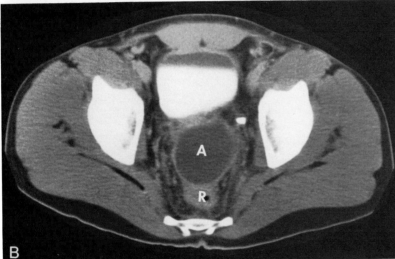

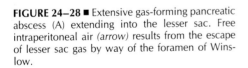

FIGURE 24–27 ■ Pelvic extension of periappendiceal abscess. *A* demonstrates calcified appendicolith *(straight arrow)* and infiltration of adjacent mesentery *(curved arrow)*. *B* demonstrates pelvic extension of abscess into retrovesicle space. A = abscess; R = rectum.

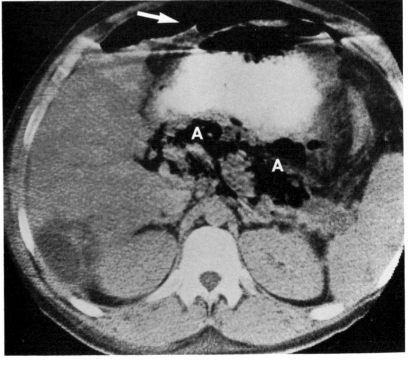

FIGURE 24–28 ■ Extensive gas-forming pancreatic abscess (A) extending into the lesser sac. Free intraperitoneal air *(arrow)* results from the escape of lesser sac gas by way of the foramen of Winslow.

the CT criteria of an abscess is most likely an abscess. Should any doubt exist, a diagnostic needle aspiration using a 22- or 20-gauge needle has proven to be a reliable, safe, and accurate method of providing a definitive diagnosis.

The question of which imaging modality should be employed to diagnose abdominal and pelvic abscesses is still being debated. In a prospective study comparing computed tomography, ultrasound, and gallium imaging, McNeil and colleagues noted that all three modalities had similar sensitivities (> 90 per cent) in the detection of abscesses.[28] The overall diagnostic yield could be increased slightly by combining two of the studies.[28] In a retrospective study of 170 patients with possible abscesses, a comparison of CT, ultrasound and indium-labeled leukocyte scans demonstrated that the diagnostic accuracy of CT was 96 per cent; that of ultrasound, 90 per cent; and that of indium-labeled leukocyte scans, 92 per cent.[28] Koehler and Moss[27] found CT to be 93 per cent accurate and to have a sensitivity of 99 per cent in 110 patients evaluated for possible abscesses. A number of other reports have documented CT accuracy rates for abscess detection to be greater than 90 per cent.[29-33]

Currently patients who are not critically ill and have no focal signs of an abscess are initially imaged by an indium-labeled leukocyte scan. However, in critically ill patients, CT and ultrasound afford a more rapid and specific diagnosis. Because intestinal ileus, surgical wounds, drainage tubes, and ostomy appliances can restrict the usefulness of ultrasound in the postoperative patient, CT is usually selected to study these patients. The relationship of an abscess to surrounding structures is best displayed by CT, and because of this, CT is becoming the imaging procedure of choice to evaluate patients with possible abscesses. If an abscess is detected, CT also permits planning of the most appropriate route for percutaneous or surgical drainage.

PERITONEAL MASSES

The majority of solid peritoneal masses occur secondary to metastatic implants from abdominal or pelvic malignancies. Peritoneal metastasis occurs in a variety of abdominal malignancies, with carcinomas of the ovary, pancreas, stomach, and colon being the most common primary lesions. The CT demonstration of peritoneal metastasis may be the only evidence of recurrent disease, and the detection of a peritoneal nodule can help distinguish benign from malignant ascites.[34,35] Comparing CT with laparoscopy, the modalities may be complementary, as CT is capable of evaluating regions of the peritoneum not amenable to laparoscopy because of obscuration by adhesions or mass.[35]

On CT scans, peritoneal implants appear as nodular plaque- or sheetlike masses of soft tissue density along the peritoneal surface, often outlined by ascites (Figs. 24–29 through 24–31). Occasionally a peritoneal implant has a cystic appearance and simulates

an intraabdominal abscess, pseudocyst, or mesenteric cyst (Fig. 24–32). One of the easiest sites to detect peritoneal implants is along the lateral peritoneal surface of the liver, where the identification of neoplastic nodules is not hampered by loops of small intestine. In patients with known malignancies that characteristically seed by way of the peritoneum, this area, as well as all peritoneal surfaces, should be carefully scrutinized for the presence of peritoneal nodules. Nonopacified loops of small bowel may mimic peritoneal implants, and therefore to avoid misdiagnosis, it is important to opacifiy the entire small bowel with dilute oral contrast. Because of the superficial location of many peritoneal nodules, CT-directed aspiration biopsies to confirm recurrent malignancy are easily and safely performed.

The overall sensitivity of CT in detecting peritoneal implants is not known. However, because of the small size of most metastatic implants and the extensive surface of the peritoneum, CT is relatively insensitive when compared with endoscopic techniques, which directly visualize the peritoneal surface. In studies comparing laparoscopy with CT, small peritoneal implants (i.e., less than 1 to 2 cm) were not detected by CT but were easily seen by laparoscopic methods.[35,36]

OMENTAL MASSES

The normal greater omentum is comprised mainly of fat and is readily identified on CT scans anterior to the stomach and transverse colon. Soft tissue infiltration of the omentum frequently occurs in carcinomatosis and in widespread peritoneal metastases.[37] Confluent omental masses are often referred to as omental *cakes* (Fig. 24–33). With early involvement, nodular infiltrates can be demonstrated by CT. This appearance is not specific for peritoneal metastases and may be seen in tuberculous peritonitis.

FREE INTRAPERITONEAL AIR

Although plain abdominal radiographs are the preferred method of diagnosing free air, on occasion the diagnosis of a perforated viscus is not suspected clinically, and a patient is referred for CT scanning to exclude an abscess or other acute abdominal disorder. Free air evidenced on CT scans can generally be distinguished from gas within a segment of dilated bowel as a result of its nondependent location and lack of haustral or small bowel folds (Figs. 24–34 and 24–35). In supine patients, free intraperitoneal air collects anteriorly beneath the abdominal musculature in the midabdomen. Small amounts of free intraperitoneal air may be noted by CT up to 7 days after surgery and should not be interpreted as anastomotic breakdown or abdominal infection. However, loculated gas within a fluid or solid mass is almost always indicative of an abdominal abscess. CT may detect even minute quantities of pneumoperitoneum and is superior to plain abdominal radiographs in this regard.[38]

Text continued on page 1167

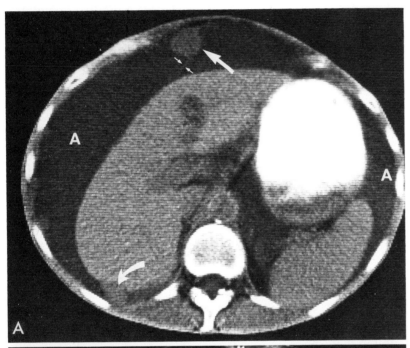

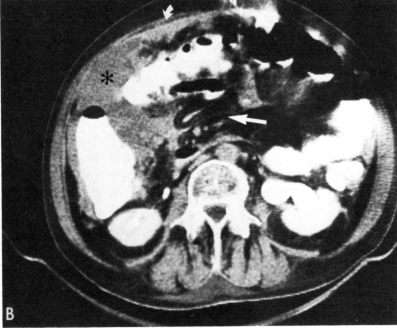

FIGURE 24-29 ■ The varied CT appearance of peritoneal implants. *A,* Nodular implant *(large straight arrow)* resulting from ovarian carcinoma, located adjacent to the falciform ligament *(small arrows)* and along the lateral peritoneal surface of the liver *(curved arrow).* Massive ascites (A) is present in the peritoneal cavity, but only a small amount is present in the lesser sac. *B,* Plaquelike peritoneal implant *(curved arrow)* in ovarian carcinoma. Adjacent ascites *(asterisk)* and marked angulation and kinking of the mesentery *(straight arrow)* by serosal adhesions are shown.

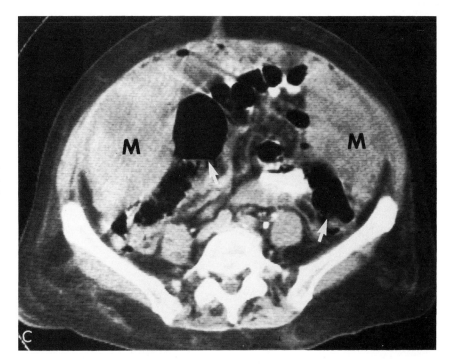

FIGURE 24–29 *Continued* C, Sheetlike peritoneal masses (m) displacing the bowel *(arrows)* centrally as a result of peritoneal metastasis from endometrial carcinoma.

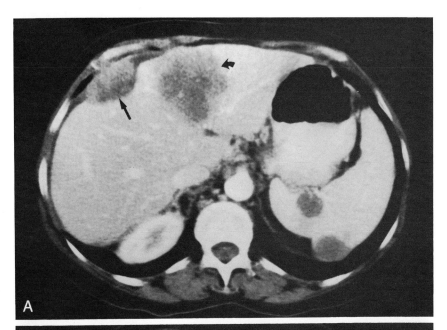

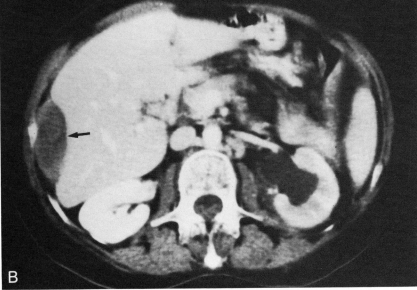

FIGURE 24–30 ■ Peritoneal metastases from colon carcinoma. *A*, Solid peritoneal metastasis *(straight arrow)* impressing on the lateral aspect of the liver. Note left lobe hepatic parenchymal metastasis *(curved arrow)*, as well as splenic metastasis. B, An additional solid peritoneal implant can be seen at a lower level *(arrow)*. Note left hydronephrosis.

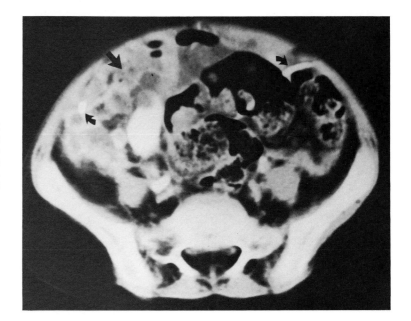

FIGURE 24–31 ■ Intraperitoneal seeding of malignant brain tumor by way of a ventriculoperitoneal shunt in a nine-year-old child with a malignant tumor of the pineal region. The tumor spread via CSF into the peritoneal cavity through a shunt catheter *(curved arrows)*. Note solid and cystic peritoneal implant *(straight arrow)* next to shunt catheter.

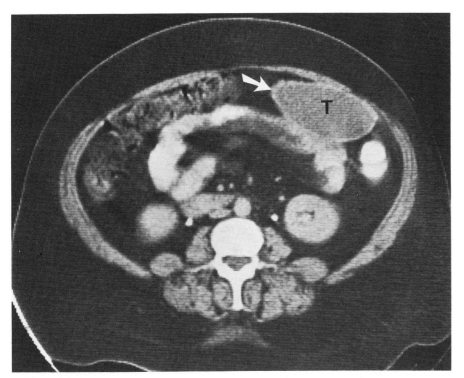

FIGURE 24–32 ■ Cystic peritoneal tumor implant (T) from carcinoma of the ovary; the implant simulates a peritoneal abscess. The center of the implant has a density that approaches that of water, and there is a well-defined rim *(arrow)* that enhances after contrast administration.

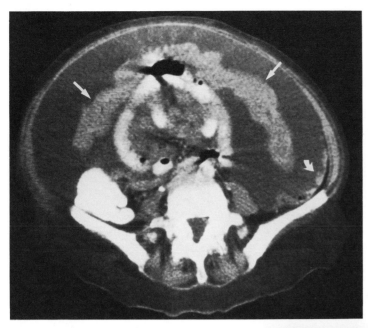

FIGURE 24–33 ■ Omental and peritoneal metastases from breast carcinoma. A large omental "cake" is seen anteriorly in the midabdomen *(straight arrows)*. Note the plaquelike peritoneal implants *(curved arrow)*. (From Jeffrey RB, Federle MP, Wall SP: J Comput Assist Tomogr 7:825, 1983.)

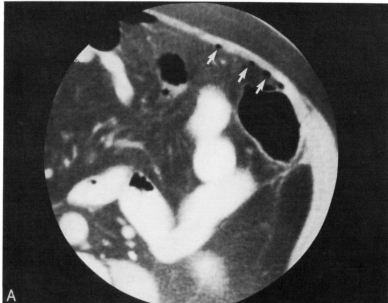

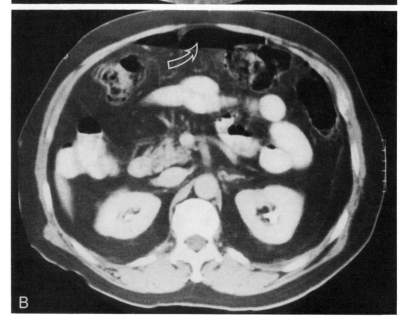

FIGURE 24–34 ■ Pneumoperitoneum from diverticulitis. *A,* Magnified view demonstrates tiny ectopic gas bubbles *(arrows)* anteriorly along the peritoneal surface. *B,* Typical pneumoperitoneum layering anteriorly in midabdomen *(arrow)*.

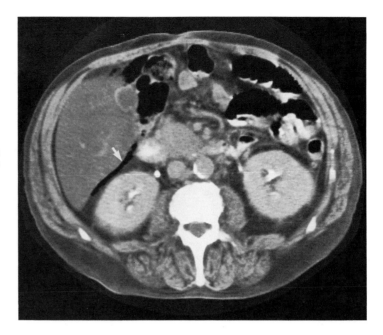

FIGURE 24–35 ■ Pneumoperitoneum following perforation of peptic ulcer. Free air in subhepatic space *(arrow)* is also shown.

LESSER SAC ABNORMALITIES

Computed tomography is an extremely useful method in evaluating suspected lesser sac abnormalities.[5,6,39,40] Conventional radiologic studies such as plain abdominal films and upper gastrointestinal examination often provide only indirect evidence of lesser sac pathologic abnormalities such as a retrogastric mass or gas collection. CT directly images the lesser sac and can generally distinguish primary lesions of the lesser sac from pancreatic, adrenal, or retroperitoneal masses.

In axial projections, fluid collections in the inferior recess of the lesser sac are usually diagnosed by their characteristic position posterior to the stomach and anterior body of the pancreas and spleen (Figs. 24–36 and 24–37; see also Figs. 24–25 and 24–28). Abnormalities in the superior recess of the lesser sac are identified immediately adjacent to the caudate lobe of the liver, extending into the fissure of the ligamentum venosum (Fig. 24–38).

In most CT series, lesser sac abnormalities are most often pancreatic pseudocysts.[5,6] However, a variety of lesser sac abnormalities may occur, including abscesses, hematomas, perforated ulcers, or, rarely, neoplastic invasion. The CT findings must be considered in conjunction with the clinical setting in differentiating between these entities. Should the diagnosis still be in doubt, a CT-guided diagnostic needle aspiration or biopsy can be performed to distinguish infected from noninfected fluid collections or to diagnose neoplastic disease. The lesser sac can be safely approached percutaneously through a variety of access sites, including transhepatic and transgastric routes.[40,41] Nunez et al.[41] have emphasized that a transgastric approach may be the optimal method of percutaneously draining lesser sac pancreatic pseudocysts, as a fistulous tract is created from the stomach to cyst by the catheter.

Mesentery

Although barium studies are the optimal methods for diagnosing mucosal abnormalities of the gut, they provide only an indirect image of the outer bowel wall and mesentery. In contrast, the outer wall of the small and large bowel mesentery can be directly imaged by computed tomography. Thus CT is capable of more accurately reflecting the true extent of extramural neoplasms and inflammatory processes that affect the mesentery than are conventional radiographic methods.

Anatomy

The mesentery of the small bowel is formed by a reflection of the posterior parietal peritoneum, which connects the jejunum and ileum to the posterior wall of the abdomen and thus acts as a suspensory ligament. The root of the mesentery extends from the right sacroiliac joint, across the origin of the superior mesenteric artery and vein, to the left upper lumbar spine. At the intestinal margin, the peritoneum divides into two layers, or leaves, which encase the small bowel and surround the superior mesenteric artery, lymph nodes, and adjacent fat. Thus the small bowel mesentery is a compartment that contains mainly fat but also vascular and lymphatic channels and numerous mesenteric lymph nodes. The transverse mesocolon appears as a similar fatty structure containing lymphatic channels and vessels along the posterior medial aspect of the colon.

In patients with abundant fat, the mesentery is seen on CT scans as a structure having a density closely approximating that of abdominal and subcutaneous adipose tissue (Figs. 24–39 and 24–40). Normal mesenteric lymph nodes measuring less than 1 cm in diameter can be identified, but usually only

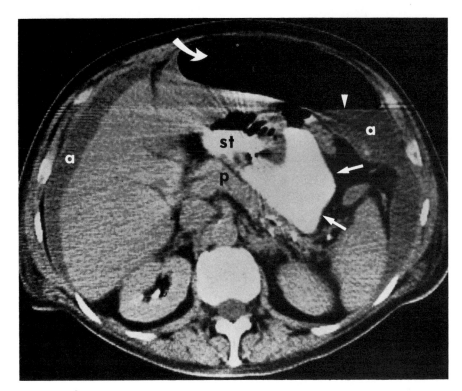

FIGURE 24–36 ■ A large amount of free air *(curved arrow)* is seen to collect anteriorly following perforation of a gastric ulcer. Note air-fluid level *(arrowhead)*. Oral contrast material has extravasated from the stomach (st) to outline the lesser sac *(straight arrows)* just anterior to the pancreas. a = Ascites. (From Jeffrey RB, Federle MP, Goodman PC: Radiology 141:117, 1981.)

FIGURE 24–37 ■ Posttraumatic lesser sac biloma following a gunshot wound to the porta hepatis that lacerated the common hepatic duct. Postoperative biliary dilatation *(solid curved arrow)* and subcapsular hematoma of the liver *(open curved arrow)*. A biloma *(straight arrow)* is present in the lesser sac and displaces the stomach anteriorly to the left. (From Jeffrey RB, Federle MP, Goodman PC: Radiology 141:117, 1981.)

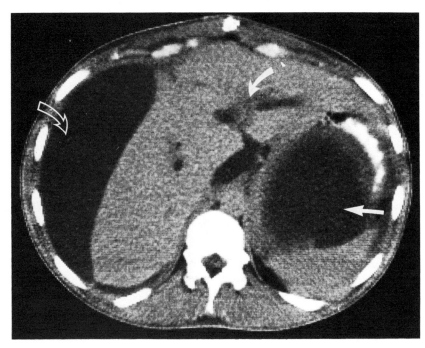

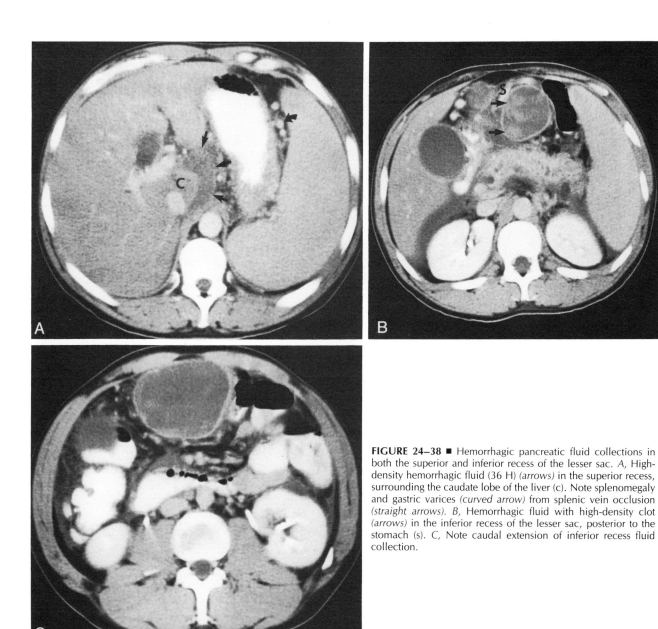

FIGURE 24–38 ■ Hemorrhagic pancreatic fluid collections in both the superior and inferior recess of the lesser sac. *A,* High-density hemorrhagic fluid (36 H) *(arrows)* in the superior recess, surrounding the caudate lobe of the liver (c). Note splenomegaly and gastric varices *(curved arrow)* from splenic vein occlusion *(straight arrows). B,* Hemorrhagic fluid with high-density clot *(arrows)* in the inferior recess of the lesser sac, posterior to the stomach (s). *C,* Note caudal extension of inferior recess fluid collection.

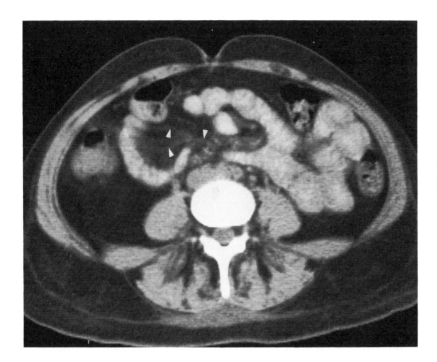

FIGURE 24–39 ■ Normal mesentery appears as a structure containing fat and vessels *(arrowheads)*. Occasionally a few normal-sized lymph nodes can be detected.

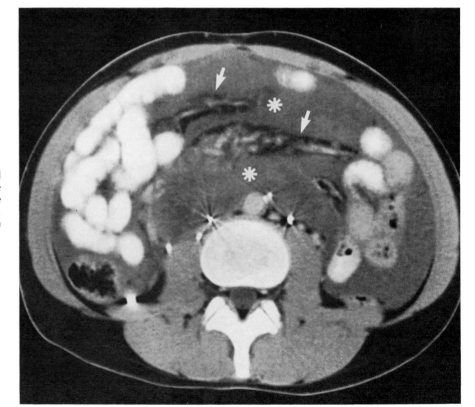

FIGURE 24–40 ■ Mesenteric fat and vasculature *(arrows)* encased by diffuse intraperitoneal tumor *(asterisk)*, from the same patient shown in Figure 24–20. (From Barakos JA, Jeffrey RB, McAninch JW, Bottles K: J Urol 136:680, 1986.)

two or three are clearly demonstrated on any one CT section.

Scanning Technique

Detection of mesenteric abnormalities is made easier by the presence of ample mesenteric fat and by complete opacification of both the large and small bowel with contrast material. At least 480 mL of oral contrast material (1 per cent diatrizoate meglumine [Gastrografin] or barium) is given 30 to 45 minutes before and another 250 to 300 mL just prior to the CT examination. To better define the sigmoid mesentery, the colon is filled with an enema of the same material. CT examinations are performed at 1-cm intervals, through the area of interest. Intravenous contrast administered with a bolus injection permits identification of the mesenteric vessels when a mesenteric mass is detected.

Pathology

LYMPHADENOPATHY: NEOPLASMS

Computed tomography can detect a variety of lesions involving the mesentery, including adenopathy, hematomas, abscesses, cysts, and inflammatory thickening.[42–48] Mesenteric lymphadenopathy is not opacified during bipedal lymphangiography but is readily detected by computed tomography (Fig. 24–41). The CT appearance of mesenteric lymphadenopathy varies from multiple small, round, soft tissue densities to large, irregular, bulky masses (see Figs. 24–40 and 24–41).[42–47] Advanced mesenteric adenopathy produces a characteristic CT appearance in which enlarged nodes between the dorsal and ventral leaves of the mesentery encase the superior mesenteric vessels, producing a "sandwichlike" appearance (Fig. 24–42).[42]

Bulky mesenteric adenopathy frequently occurs in non-Hodgkin's lymphoma, and more than 50 per cent of patients have mesenteric nodal involvement at the time of the initial diagnosis.[46] The ability of CT to diagnose mesenteric adenopathy is an important contribution of CT in the evaluation of lymphomas (see Figs. 24–41 and 24–42), as mesenteric lymphadenopathy cannot be detected by lymphangiography, and the detection of mesenteric involvement has important therapeutic and prognostic implications in all forms of lymphoma.

In addition to lymphoma, CT may demonstrate mesenteric involvement in other neoplastic disorders, including carcinoid tumors, leukemia, and metastatic disease (Figs. 24–43 and 23–44).[43,44] Carcinoid and desmoid tumors may produce mesenteric masses, as well as an intense desmoplastic infiltration resulting in tethering and kinking of the mesentery. Similar findings can be seen in other lesions that produce a dense fibroblastic infiltration of the mesentery, such as retractile mesenteritis or metastatic carcinoma of the breast or pancreas.[45]

INFLAMMATORY DISEASE

In addition to neoplastic lesions, computed tomography can also diagnose a variety of benign lesions of the mesentery. In patients with necrotizing pancreatitis, the inflammatory reaction may extend directly down the transverse mesocolon (Fig. 24–45; see also Fig. 24–11). This is the mechanism for the often-associated ileus of the transverse colon, or the "colon cutoff" sign. Pancreatic pseudocysts and abscesses may also dissect down the transverse mesocolon and may result in perforation of the colon and peritonitis.

In the later stages of Crohn's disease, there is often secondary inflammation of the mesentery adjacent

Text continued on page 1176

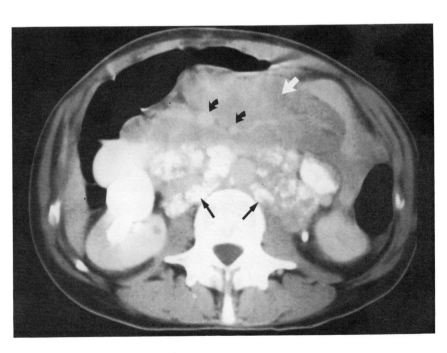

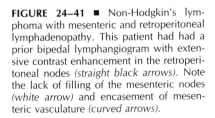

FIGURE 24–41 ■ Non-Hodgkin's lymphoma with mesenteric and retroperitoneal lymphadenopathy. This patient had had a prior bipedal lymphangiogram with extensive contrast enhancement in the retroperitoneal nodes (*straight black arrows*). Note the lack of filling of the mesenteric nodes (*white arrow*) and encasement of mesenteric vasculature (*curved arrows*).

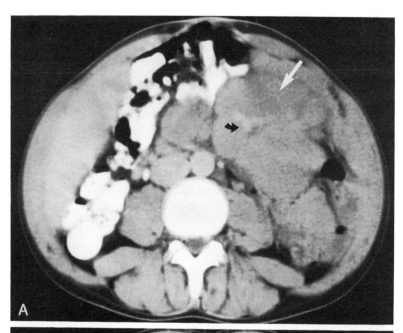

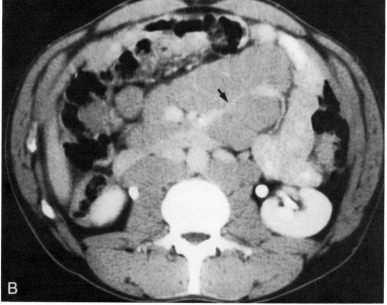

FIGURE 24–42 ■ *A*, Mesenteric adenopathy in non-Hodgkin's lymphoma *(white arrow)* encasing mesenteric vasculature *(black arrow)*, resulting in the "sandwich sign." *B*, Note flattening of the mesenteric vessel *(arrow)*.

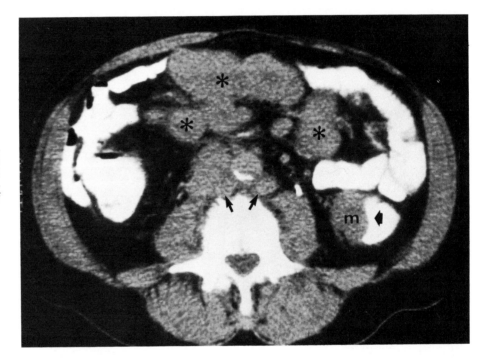

FIGURE 24–43 ■ Melanoma metastatic to paraaortic *(thin arrows)* and mesenteric nodes *(asterisks)*. A mural metastases (m) is seen along the medial margin *(thick arrow)* of a loop of small intestine.

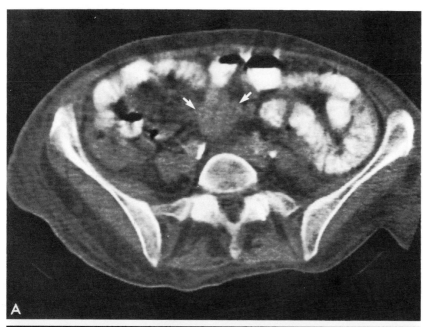

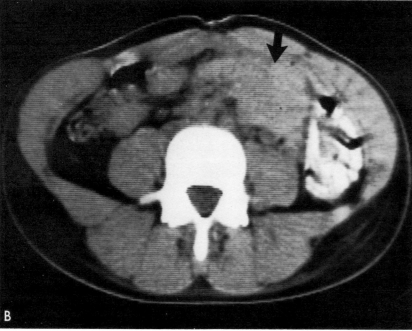

FIGURE 24–44 ■ *A,* Carcinoid tumor involving the mesentery *(arrows),* resulting in a mesenteric mass. *B,* Mesenteric desmoid tumor *(arrow)* in a patient with Gardner's syndrome, presenting as solid mesenteric mass.

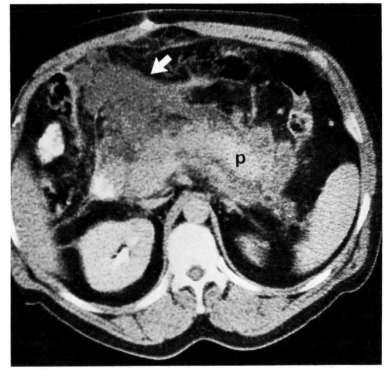

FIGURE 24–45 ■ Acute pancreatitis. *A,* An inflammatory exudate encases the pancreas (p) and extends into the transverse mesocolon *(arrow). B,* In another patient, mesenteric inflammatory exudate is seen adjacent to mesenteric vasculature *(arrows).*

to diseased loops of small bowel or colon. The mesenteric thickening may be related to sinus tracts that extend into the mesentery, forming microabscesses, or by direct extension of the transmural inflammatory process. Mesenteric lymphatic obstruction by adjacent granulomatous reaction also occurs, which contributes to thickening of the small bowel folds in Crohn's disease. The CT appearance is that of a fibrofatty mass surrounding the affected bowel and an increase in density of the adjacent mesenteric fat (Fig. 24–46).[48,49] Infectious processes such as tuberculosis may cause nodular infiltration of the mesentery (Fig. 24–47) or calcification of mesenteric nodes (Fig. 24–48). These nodes are readily identified by CT as rounded soft tissue density structures in the mesentery.

TRAUMA

Blunt trauma to the abdomen, excessive anticoagulation, or postoperative bleeding may result in mesenteric hematomas.[50,51] At times a specific diagnosis of mesenteric hematoma may be made by CT because of the relatively high attenuation coefficient of acute hematoma within the mesentery (Fig. 24–49). Although most small mesenteric hematomas following trauma do not require surgical evacuation, they are an important finding and indicate possible injury to the bowel wall that may result in delayed stenosis or perforation.[50,51]

ABSCESSES

Mesenteric abscesses can occur following pancreatitis, Crohn's disease, surgery, or penetrating inju-

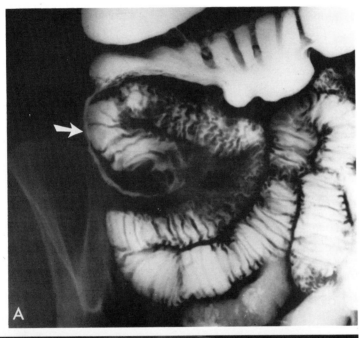

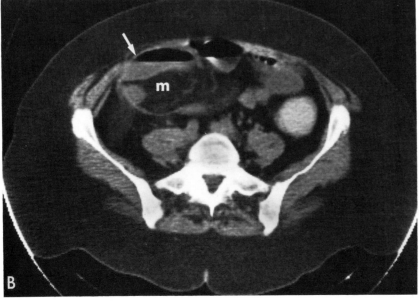

FIGURE 24–46 ■ Recurrent Crohn's disease with fibrofatty thickening of the adjacent mesentery. *A*, Barium enema demonstrates stenosis *(arrow)* of the small bowel following ileocolostomy for Crohn's disease. *B*, CT scan reveals a fibrofatty mass (m) in the right lower quadrant adjacent to the bowel *(arrow)*. The CT number of normal mesenteric fat in this patient was −80 H; the CT number of the fibrofatty mass was −40 H.

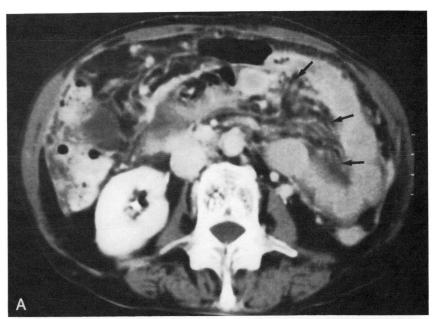

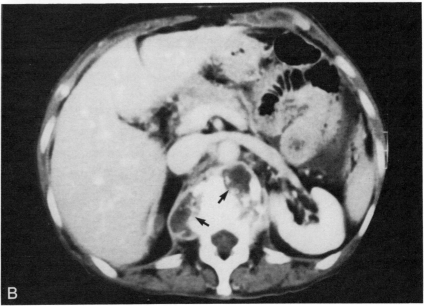

FIGURE 24–47 ■ *A,* Tuberculous peritonitis with subtle soft tissue infiltration of mesentery *(arrows). B,* Note paraspinous abscess and osteomyelitis *(arrows).*

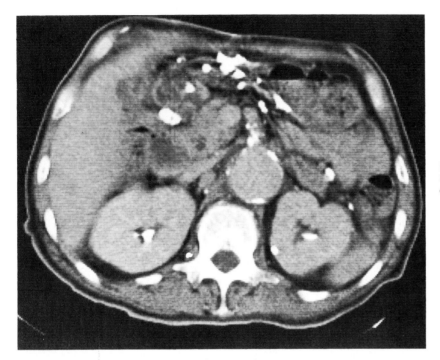

FIGURE 24–48 ■ Multiple calcified mesenteric nodes resulting from tuberculosis are readily detected by computed tomography.

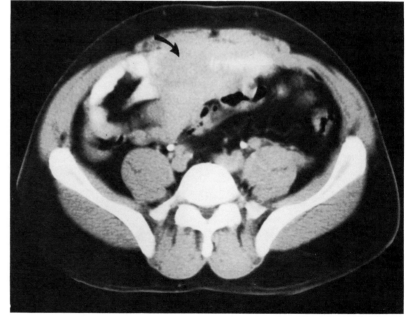

FIGURE 24–49 ■ Acute mesenteric hematoma *(arrow)* encasing the small bowel following blunt abdominal trauma.

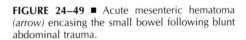

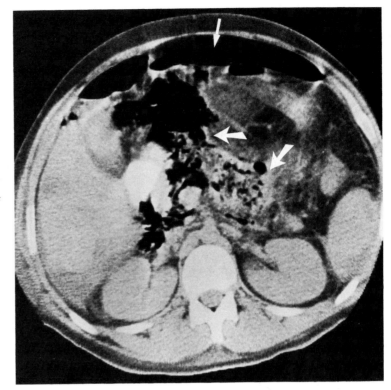

FIGURE 24–50 ■ A pancreatic gas-forming abscess has extended into the root of the mesentery *(large arrows).* Free air is noted anteriorly *(small arrow)* from passage of gas through the foramen of Winslow.

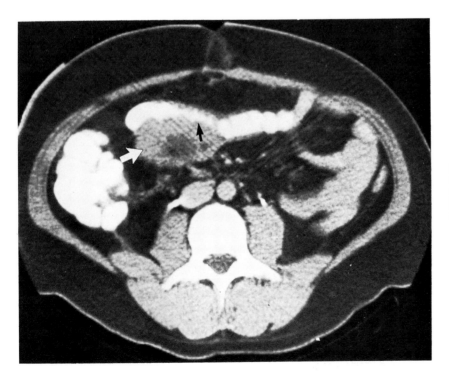

FIGURE 24–51 ■ Abscess *(white arrow)* in the mesentery of the transverse colon following pancreatitis. There is marked thickening of the folds of the transverse colon with narrowing of the lumen *(black arrow).*

ries. Mesenteric abscesses have a CT appearance similar to that of other abscesses and range from ill-defined areas of low density to well-encapsulated fluid collections with or without gas (Figs. 24–50 and 24–51). As with mesenteric pseudocysts, pancreatic abscesses may extend into the bowel wall, causing perforation.[52]

Abscesses may also point to the skin and result in an abdominal sinus being formed. CT can delineate the sinus abstract and determine its relationship to adjacent mesenteric and peritoneal structures. CT provides three-dimensional information concerning the extent of fistula or sinus tracts that is complementary to information obtained from conventional sinograms or fistulograms.

References

1. Meyers MA: Dynamic Radiology of the Abdomen. Normal and Pathologic Anatomy. New York, Spinger-Verlag, 1976.
2. Meyers MA: Peritoneography: normal and pathologic anatomy. AJR 123:67–73, 1975.
3. Meyers MA: The spread and localization of acute intraperitoneal effusions. Radiology 95:547, 1970.
4. Meyers MA: Roentgen significance of the phrenicocolic ligament. Radiology 95:539, 1970.
5. Jeffrey RB, Federle MP, Goodman PC: Computed tomography of the lesser peritoneal sac. Radiology 141:117, 1981.
6. Dodds WJ, Foley WD, Lawson TL, Stewart ET, Taylor A: Anatomy and imaging of the lesser peritoneal sac. AJR 144:567, 1985.
7. Dunnick NR, Jones RB, Poppman JL, Speyer J, Myers CE: Intraperitoneal contrast infusion for assessment of intraperitoneal fluid dynamics. AJR 133:221, 1979.
8. Jolles H, Coulam CM: CT of ascites: differential diagnosis. AJR 135:315, 1980.
9. Gore RM, Callen PW, Filly RA: The incidence and significance of lesser sac fluid in general peritoneal ascites. AJR 139:71, 1982.
10. Jeffrey RB, Federle MP, Laing FC, Wing VE: Computed tomography of blunt trauma to the gallbladder. J Comput Assist Tomogr 10:756, 1986.
11. Watanabe AT, Jeffrey RB: CT diagnosis of traumatic rupture of the cisterna chyli. J Comput Assist Tomogr 11:175, 1987.
12. Federle MP, Goldberg HI, Kaiser JA, Moss AA, Jeffrey RB, Mall JC: Evaluation of abdominal trauma by computed tomography. Radiology 138:637, 1981.
13. Lewin JR, Patterson EA: Recognition of spontaneous intraperitoneal hemorrhage complicating anticoagulant therapy. AJR 134:1271, 1980.
14. Federle MP, Jeffrey RB: Hemoperitoneum studied by computed tomography. Radiology 148:187, 1983.
15. Hanson RD, Hunter TB: Tuberculous peritonitis: CT appearance. AJR 144:931, 1985.
16. Barakos JA, Jeffrey RB, McAninch JW, Bottles K: Computerized tomography diagnosis of diffuse intraperitoneal metastases after retroperitoneal lymphadenectomy for testicular carcinoma. J Urol 136:680, 1986.
17. Seshal MB, Coulam CM: Pseudomyxoma peritonei. Computed tomography and sonography. AJR 136:803, 1981.
18. Mayes GB, Chaang VP, Fisher RB: CT of pseudomyxoma peritonei. AJR 136:807, 1981.
19. Connell TR, Stephens DH, Carlson HC, Brown ML: Upper abdominal abscess: a continuing and deadly problem. AJR 134:759, 1980.
20. Ariel IM, Kazarian KK: Diagnosis and Treatment of Abdominal Abscesses. Baltimore, Williams & Wilkins, p 174, 1971.
21. Wolverson MK, Janannadharaob SM, Joyce PF, Riaz MA, Shields JB: CT as a primary diagnostic method in evaluating intraabdominal abscess. AJR 133:1089, 1979.
22. Haaga JR, Weinstein AJ: CT guided percutaneous aspiration and drainage of abscesses. AJR 135:1187, 1980.
23. Harter LP, Moss AA, Goldberg HI: Computed tomographic guided fine needle aspirations for neoplastic and inflammatory disease. AJR 140:363, 1983.
24. Van Sonnenberg E, Mueller PR, Ferrucci JT Jr: Percutaneous drainage of 250 abdominal abscesses and fluid collections. Part I: results, failures and complications. Radiology 151:337, 1984.
25. Callen PW: Computed tomographic evaluation of abdominal and pelvic abscesses. Radiology 131:171, 1979.
26. Knochel JQ, Koehler PR, Lee TG, Welch DM: Diagnosis of abdominal abscesses with computed tomography, ultrasound and indium-111 leukocyte scans. Radiology 137:425, 1980.
27. Koehler PR, Moss AA: Diagnosis of intra-abdominal and pelvic abscesses by computerized tomography. JAMA 244:49, 1980.
28. McNeil BJ, Sanders R, Alderson PO, Hessel SJ, Fenberg H, et al: A prospective study of computed tomography, ultrasound and gallium imaging in patients with fever. Radiology 139:647, 1981.
29. Scneekloth G, Terrier F, Fuchs WA: Computed tomography of intraperitoneal abscesses. Gastrointest Radiol 7:35–42, 1982.
30. Korobkin M, Callen PW, Filly RA, Hoffer PB, Shimshak RR, Kressel HY: Comparison of computed tomography, ultrasonography, and gallium-67 scanning in the evaluation of suspected abdominal abscess. Radiology 129:89, 1978.
31. Aronberg DJ, Stanley RJ, Levitt RG, Sagel SS: The evaluation of abdominal abscesses with computed tomography. J Comput Assist Tomogr 2:384, 1978.
32. Wolverson MK, Jagennadharao B, Sundaram M, Joyce PF, Riaz MA, Shields JB: CT as a primary diagnosis method in evaluating intraabdominal abscess. AJR 133:1089, 1979.
33. Halber MD, Daffner RH, Morgan CL, Trought WS, Thompson WM, et al: Intraabdominal abscess. Current concepts in radiologic evaluation. AJR 133:9, 1979.
34. Jeffrey RB: CT demonstration of peritoneal implants. AJR 135:323, 1980.
35. Barth RA, Jeffrey RB Jr, Moss AA, Liberman MS: A comparison study of computed tomography and laparoscopy in the staging of abdominal neoplasms. Dig Dis Sci 26:253, 1981.
36. Whitley NO, Bohlman ME, Baker LP: CT patterns of metastatic disease. J Comput Assist Tomogr 6:490, 1982.
37. Cooper C, Jeffrey RB Jr, Silverman PM, Federle MP, Chun GH: Computed tomography of omental pathology. J Comput Assist Tomogr 10:62, 1986.
38. Jeffrey RB, Federle MP, Wall SP: Use of computed tomography in detecting occult gastrointestinal perforation. J Comput Assist Tomogr 7:825, 1983.
39. Siegelman SS, Copeland BE, Sabe GB, Cameron JR, Sanders RC, Zerhouni BA: CT of fluid collections associated with pancreatitis. AJR 134:1121, 1980.
40. Mueller PR, Ferrucci JT Jr, Simeons JE, Butch RJ, Willenberg J, et al: Lesser sac abscess and fluid collections: drainage by transhepatic approach. Radiology 155:615, 1985.
41. Nunez DJR, Yrizarry JM, Russell E, Sadighi A, Casilas J, et al: Transgastric drainage of pancreatic fluid collections. AJR 145:815, 1985.
42. Mueller PR, Ferrucci JT, Harbin WP, Kirkpatrick RH, Simeone JF, Wittenberg J: Appearance of lymphomatous involvement of the mesentery of ultrasonography and body computed tomography: the "sandwich sign." Radiology 134:467, 1980.
43. Bernardino ME, Jing BS, Wallace S: Computed tomography diagnosis of mesenteric masses. AJR 132:33, 1979.
44. Siegel RS, Kuhns LR, Borlaza GS, McCormick TL, Simons JR: Computed tomography and angiography in ileal carcinoid tumor and retractile mesenteritis. Radiology 134:437, 1980.
45. Ellert J, Kreel L: The role of computed tomography in the initial staging and subsequent management of the lymphomas. J Comput Assist Tomogr 4:368, 1980.
46. Harell GS, Breiman RS, Glatstein EJ, Marshall WH, Castellino RA: Computed tomography of the abdomen in the malignant lymphomas. Radiol Clin North Am 15:391, 1977.

47. Lee JKT, Stanley RJ, Sagel SS, Levitt RG: Accuracy of computed tomography in detecting intraabdominal and pelvic adenopathy in lymphoma. AJR 131:311, 1978.
48. Goldberg HI, Gore RM, Margulis AR, Moss AA, Baker EL: Computed tomography in the evaluation of Crohn disease. AJR 140:277, 1983.
49. Gore RM: Cross-sectional imaging of inflammatory bowel disease. Radiol Clin North Am 25:115, 1987.
50. Shuck JM, Lowe RG: Intestinal disruption due to blunt abdominal trauma. Am J Surg 136:668, 1978.
51. Donahue JH, Federle MP, Griffiths BG, Trunkey DD: Computed tomography in the diagnosis of blunt intestinal and mesenteric injuries. J Trauma 27:11, 1987.
52. Jeffrey RB, Federle MP: CT of mesenteric involvement in fulminant pancreatitis. Radiology 147:184, 1983.

CHAPTER 25

COMPUTED TOMOGRAPHY AND MAGNETIC RESONANCE IMAGING OF THE PELVIS

LESLIE M. SCOUTT ▪ *SHIRLEY M. McCARTHY* ▪ *ALBERT A. MOSS*

Computed tomography (CT) and, more recently, magnetic resonance imaging (MRI) have become important tools in the radiographic examination of the pelvis in patients with suspected pelvic disease. The widespread use of CT is largely related to the excellent anatomic detail this technique provides, whereas the ability of MRI to display axial, coronal, and sagittal views of the pelvis ensures optimal display of normal and abnormal anatomy. Thus CT and MRI scanning of the ovary, prostate, seminal vesicles, bladder, uterus, and cervix have become important for both diagnosis and treatment planning.

Techniques of Examination

Computed Tomography

Optimal CT scanning of the pelvis requires that all intestinal structures be well filled with contrast ma-terial at the time of the examination. To ensure that the distal small bowel and colon are opacified, each patient is asked to drink 500 to 1000 mL of two per cent diatrizoate meglumine or two per cent barium sulfate the evening before the examination. In addition, all patients are given 350 to 500 mL of two per cent diatrizoate meglumine or barium sulfate solution to drink 45 minutes before the CT study. This method of administering oral contrast material ensures good filling of the distal small bowel and proximal colon and helps eliminate the diagnostic dilemma produced by nonopacified small-bowel loops that project into the pelvis and simulate soft tissue masses. To ensure better definition of the rectum and distal colon, either 300 mL of one per cent solution of diatrizoate sodium (Hypaque) or air is administered by way of the rectum just prior to the examination. In selected instances, 1 mg of glucagon is injected to paralyze the small bowel and distend the colon. In female patients, vaginal tampons may be inserted prior to the CT examination to mark the exact position of the vagina and cervix. Intravenous contrast material is routinely administered as a bolus injection of 150 mL of 60 per cent ionic or nonionic contrast material to define the ureters and to distinguish vessels from enlarged lymph nodes.

When the bladder is being evaluated for a primary tumor or for determining whether invasion of the bladder wall is present, a single- or double-contrast examination of the bladder may be performed. For a single-contrast examination of the urinary bladder, 150 mL of contrast material is administered by rapid bolus (1 to 2 mL/sec) before scanning.[1, 2] For a double-contrast examination of the urinary bladder, a Foley catheter is inserted into the bladder, and 100 to 300 mL of air and 100 mL of dilute contrast material (30 per cent diatrizoate meglumine) are instilled for better definition of the bladder wall. The double-contrast technique has been shown to be particularly helpful for evaluation of the anterior portion of the bladder dome[3] and accurately demonstrates intraluminal and intramural tumor extension.

Following air and contrast instillation, patients are scanned in the appropriate supine, decubitus, or prone position. A scout view or digital radiograph of the pelvis permits localization of the bladder, prostate, inguinal canal, intrauterine contraceptive devices, ischial spines, and occasionally, pelvic masses prior to obtaining an axial CT scan.

The routine CT examination of the pelvis is performed using contiguous sections 10 mm thick from the iliac crest to the symphysis during shallow breathing or suspended expiration. For staging of prostate, ovarian, uterine and bladder tumors, scans 5 mm thick are employed at 5-mm intervals. When searching for undescended testes, contiguous scan sections 5 mm thick are taken from the pubic symphysis to the anterior superior iliac spine, and if the testes are not identified, scans through the lower abdomen at 10-mm intervals up to the lower pole of the kidney are obtained. In patients being evaluated for superficial rectal tumors, 300 mL of air are administered by rectal tube, 1 mg of glucagon is injected to ensure maximum colonic distention, and scanning is initiated at the level of the symphysis. For tumor staging, the initial scans of the pelvis then are followed by contiguous sections 1 cm thick through the abdomen, starting from the dome of the liver to identify metastases to the liver, adrenals, spine, and mesenteric or retroperitoneal lymph nodes.

Maximum resolution is obtained by performing scans using the smallest field of view that includes the entire pelvis. Reformation of transverse CT images into sagittal and coronal sections is not routinely performed but has proven useful in some patients in determining tumor extension into the bladder or prostate.[4] Direct coronal or sagittal computed tomography of the pelvis has been described and offers improved image quality by avoiding partial volume averaging and patient motion disturbance.[5, 6]

Measurement of the volume of an organ can be readily calculated by tracing the organ of interest with an electronic computer cursor and summating the surface area measurements obtained on the individual scans. This area is then multiplied by the slice thickness to determine the segmental volume. The total volume of the organ to be measured is computed by the addition of all segmental volumes.

Magnetic Resonance Imaging

In MRI scanning of the female pelvis, T2-weighted pulse sequences are essential, as internal organ anatomy and most disease entities are optimally demonstrated using this pulse sequence. The addition of T1-weighted images increases the ability to characterized tissues and is particularly useful when considering the presence of hemorrhage or fat. Additionally, T1-weighted scans provide high contrast between pelvis fat and viscera. For this reason, T1-weighted sequences are useful for demonstrating transserosal spread of neoplasms. Using a synthetic imaging program, Duberg et al.[7] have demonstrated that zonal anatomy is visible using a short TR and long TE pulse sequence. However, it is not known whether pelvic pathology can be adequately visualized using this technique. Gradient-echo sequences are useful for assessing vessel patency, differentiating between lymph nodes and vessels, and occasionally confirming the presence of hemorrhage. The field of view should be kept as small as possible, usually between 24 and 32 cm, depending on the patient's size, to optimize spatial resolution. A 128 × 256 matrix is usually adequate, although a 256 × 256 matrix may be helpful when delineating very small structures such as ovarian follicles. Depending on the size of the lesion, a slice thickness of 5 to 10 mm with a 1- to 5-mm gap is used.

Because respiratory motion degrades images of the pelvis, respiratory compensation techniques should be used routinely. The use of 0.5 to 1.0 mg of intravenous glucagon decreases artifact from bowel peristalsis.[8] Glucagon should be administered slowly to minimize nausea and vomiting[9] and should not be administered to patients with a history suggestive of pheochromocytoma, insulinoma, or with a known hypersensitivity to glucagon.[10] An intravenous injection of glucagon results in immediate bowel hypotonicity, which lasts for 15 to 20 minutes. Therefore glucagon should be administered immediately prior to acquisition of T2-weighted sequences.

A recent advance in MR software technology that will greatly impact imaging of the female pelvis is fast spin-echo (FSE) imaging. The FSE sequence provides T2-weighted images up to sixteen times more rapidly than conventional spin-echo sequences. The signal-to-noise ratio (SNR) of fast spin-echo sequences is inherently greater than conventional spin-echo sequences. In addition, the rapid scan time greatly reduces phase ghosts from respiratory motion, bowel peristalsis, and vascular pulsation. This obviates the need for respiratory compensation techniques as well as the use of IV glucagon.

In the body coil, FSE standard resolution T2-weighted images of the female pelvis can be obtained in 1.5 minutes per imaging plane. The quality and lesion detection capability of this sequence is actually superior to conventional spin-echo sequences[10a] (Fig. 25-1A and B). When combined with a phased-array multicoil, the FSE sequence can provide images with in-plane resolution up to four times greater than that of conventional sequences in under 5 minutes.[10b] These images provide detailed anatomy that cannot be visualized using conventional sequences (Fig. 25-1C and D).

Anatomy

At the level of the sacral promontory, the right colon is usually located anterior to the right psoas major and iliacus muscles, and the descending colon is positioned similarly on the left side. Ileal loops are located anteriorly, immediately below the rectus abdominis muscle and anterior to the sigmoid colon. The ileal loops are separated by the mesentery from the jejunal loops, which are located on the left side anterior to the psoas and iliacus (Fig. 25–2A). In the midpelvis the sigmoid colon is identified by the one or two loops it forms prior to joining the descending colon in its retroperitoneal location (Fig. 25–2B. Dis-

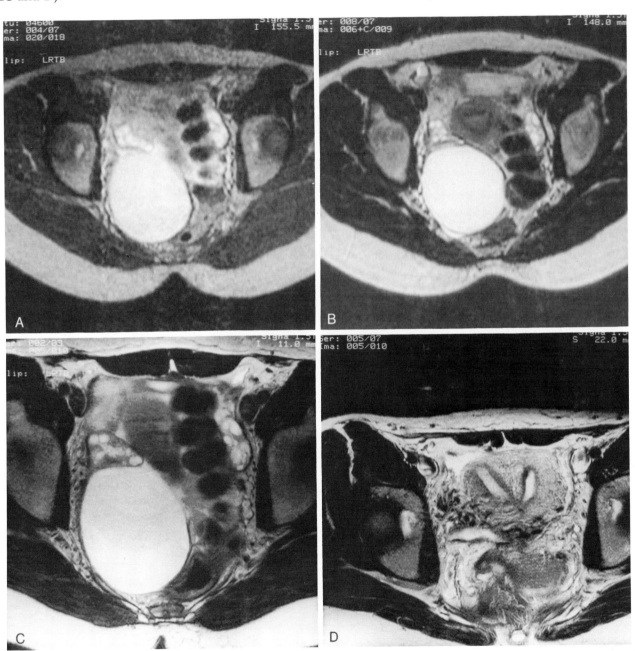

FIGURE 25–1 ■ Comparison of conventional spin-echo (CSE) and fast spin-echo (FSE) techniques. *A*, Body coil CSE sequence of patient with a paratubal cyst (scan time 9:18). *B*, Same slice location as *A*, using body coil FSE sequence (scan time 1:46). *C*, High-resolution image at same slice location, using phased array multicoil with FSE sequence (scan time 4:46). *D*, High-resolution multicoil FSE image of a patient with a septate uterus.

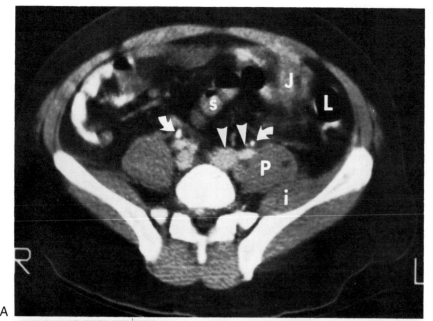

A

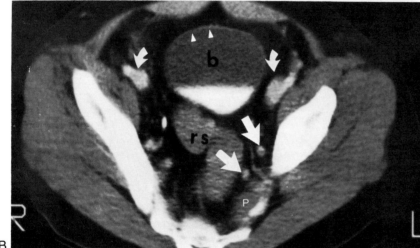

B

FIGURE 25–2 ■ *A*,CT section at the level of the sacral promontory shows the common iliac arteries and veins *(arrowheads)* anteromedial to the psoas muscle (P). The ureters *(curved arrows)* are located anterior to the vessels. i = iliacus muscle; J = jejunal loops; L = left colon; s = sigmoid colon. *B*, CT scan through the midpelvis. A bolus of contrast material shows the location of internal *(straight arrows)* and external *(curved arrows)* iliac arteries and veins. Nodes accompanying the vessels are not identified in this normal patient. The rectosigmoid (rs) and bladder (b) also are well demonstrated. The bladder wall *(arrowheads)* is thin and has a smooth outer margin. The piriformis muscle (P) is seen on the left side, but not on the right, because of a slight tilt of the pelvis in the gantry.

FIGURE 25–3 ■ CT scan through the distal pelvis. A bolus of contrast material outlines the femoral artery *(large solid arrow)* and vein *(curved arrow)*. Seminal vesicles *(open arrows)* are well delineated as oval structures between the bladder (b) and rectum (r), which is midline in position just anterior to the sacrum *(arrowhead)*. Small arrows = Coccygeal muscle; g = gluteus maximus muscle; i = internal obturator muscle; ig = inferior gemellus muscle.

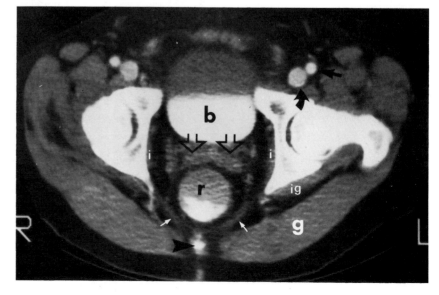

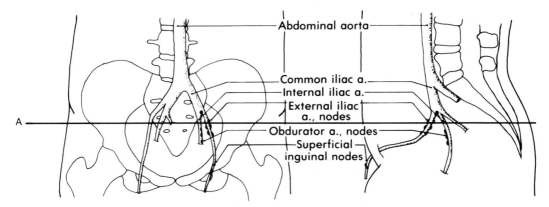

FIGURE 25–4 ■ Diagram demonstrating the relationship of pelvic lymph nodes to pelvic arterial supply. Line A = level of CT scan shown in Figure 25–2. (Modified from Walsh JW, Amendola MA, Konerding KF, Tisnado J, Dazra TA: Computed tomographic detection of pelvic and inguinal lymph node metastases from primary and recurrent pelvic malignant disease. Radiology 137:157, 1980.)

tally the rectum occupies a midline position surrounded by fat, just ventral to the sacrum (Fig. 25–3).

On CT scans the urinary bladder is a homogeneous midline structure of water density whose size and configuration varies greatly depending on the amount of urine present. The outer margin of the bladder wall is smooth and usually well delineated by perivesicle fat (see Fig. 25–2B). The bladder wall (2 to 5 mm thick) appears as a rim of soft tissue whose inner margins are better identified if the bladder contains only urine or if air, carbon dioxide, or oil has been instilled into the bladder.

The ureters are best seen after intravenous administration of iodinated contrast material. At the level of the sacral promontory, the ureters are located anteromedial to the psoas major and anterior to the common iliac artery or lateral to the external iliac artery (see Fig. 25–2A). The ureters then course medially and posteriorly to the external iliac arteries until they reach the midportion of the internal obturator muscle. At this level, they course anteromedially to reach the trigonum of the bladder.

The pelvic muscles (psoas, iliacus, obturator internus, piriformis, and levator ani) are well outlined on cross sections of the pelvis and are symmetric in the normal patient (see Fig. 25–3). Pelvic lymph nodes accompany the common iliac, external iliac, and obturator vessels (Fig. 25–4), and although normal-size pelvis lymph nodes often cannot be identified on CT scans (see Fig. 25–2), if pelvic lymph nodes are enlarged, calcified, or contain ethiodized oil (Ethiodol), they are readily identified. In the male pelvis, the seminal vesicles are seen dorsal to the bladder and anterior to the rectum (Figs. 25–3 and 25–5). They are oval to tear-shaped structures and are clearly displayed as a result of the abundance of perirectal and perivesical fat. The position of the seminal vesicles is not fixed in the pelvis, and their location and configuration change slightly depending on the patient's position. On CT scans the prostate is a homogeneous round structure of soft tissue density, 2 to 4 cm in length, located just beneath the symphysis pubis immediately anterior to the rectum (Fig. 25–6).

On MRI scans the normal zonal anatomy of the

FIGURE 25–5 ■ Normal male pelvis. The seminal vesicles are seen as oval to elliptical masses of soft tissue density (arrows) posterior to the bladder and anterior to the rectum.

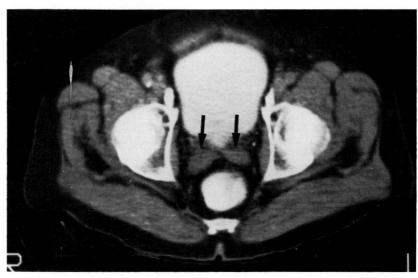

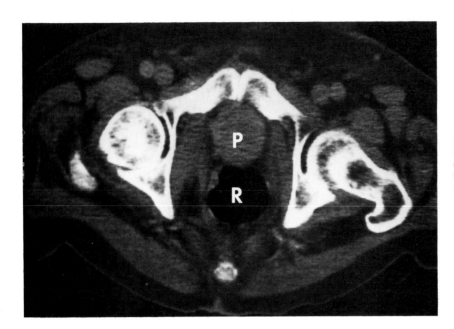

FIGURE 25–6 ■ Male pelvis. A slightly enlarged prostate (P) is seen as a round soft tissue density posterior to the symphysis and anterior to the rectum (R). At higher levels, the prostate is related to the base of the bladder.

FIGURE 25–7 ■ Normal prostate. *A*, A TR 2000/TE 20 MR scan reveals the central zone *(straight arrow)* to have a lower signal intensity than the peripheral zone *(arrowheads)* and urethra *(wavy arrow)*. *B*, A T2-weighted MR scan more clearly demonstrates the high-intensity peripheral zone surrounding the low-intensity central zone. Arrow = periprostatic venous plexus; Arrowhead = anterior fibromuscular band; b = bladder; r = rectum.

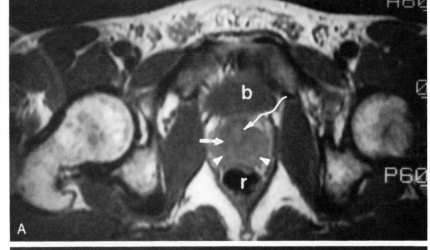

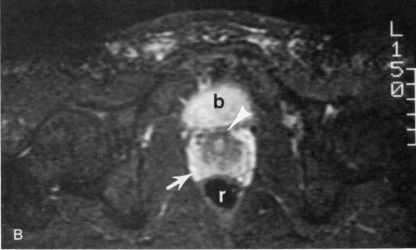

prostate is readily displayed (Fig. 25–7). The central zone is of intermediate to low signal intensity and is surrounded by the high-intensity peripheral zone. The anterior fibromuscular band, transitional zone, and seminal vesicles are also readily demonstrated.[11–15]

On CT scans the spermatic cord with the vas deferens and testicular artery and vein can be recognized on lower cross sections of the pelvis. The spermatic cord appears as a circular or oval mass of soft tissue density (Fig. 25–8*A*) or as a thin-walled, ringlike structure containing a small dot or linear streak of soft tissue density representing the vas deferens and the spermatic vessels (Fig. 25–8*B*). The normal testes appear as oval structures measuring 1 to 3 cm in anteroposterior diameter and 4 to 5 cm in length. The parenchyma of the testes is of low attenuation and is surrounded by the denser tunica albuginea.

On CT scans the uterus is seen as a homogeneous round, oval, or triangular soft tissue mass located dorsal to the bladder, which may contain a central area of low attenuation (Fig. 25–9*A–C*). CT clearly demonstrates the pouch of Douglas as a recess between the uterus and rectum (Fig. 25–9*A*). Unless they are enlarged, the ovaries are not generally identified as discrete structures, and the oviducts are seen only if markedly abnormal in size, as found in an ectopic pregnancy. The demarcations between the vagina, cervix, and uterus are poorly delineated by CT scans. Insertion of a vaginal tampon prior to CT demonstrates the close relationship between the wall of the vagina, urinary bladder, and rectum (Fig. 25–10) and permits delineation of the cervix and uterus.

On MRI scans the anatomy of the vagina, cervix, and uterus is well displayed. The upper one third of the vagina is demarcated by the lateral fornices, whereas the bladder base and urethra demarcate the lower third of the vagina. Unlike on CT images, the internal anatomy of the vagina can be visualized on MRI scans and is best detected using T2-weighted scans in the axial or sagittal planes (Fig. 25–11).[16–20] The appearance of the vagina changes during the

FIGURE 25–8 ■ Male pelvis. *A,* The normal spermatic cords are shown as oval densities *(arrows)* anterior to the pectineal muscles (P). *B,* In an individual with sufficient fat, following intravenous administration of contrast medium the spermatic vessels *(curved arrows)* can be seen as small dots of high density within the spermatic cords *(straight arrows)*.

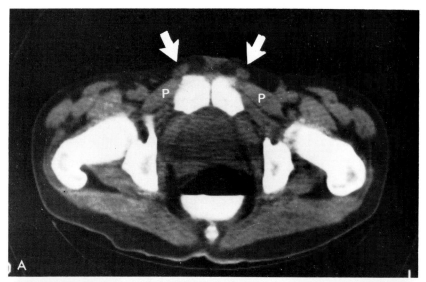

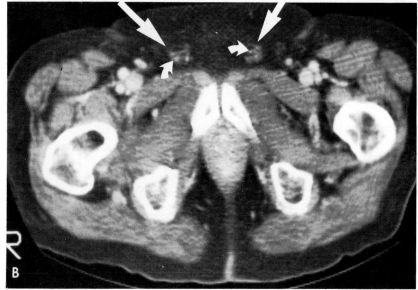

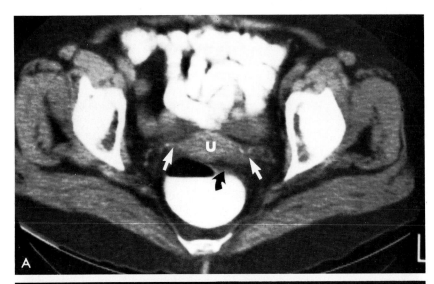

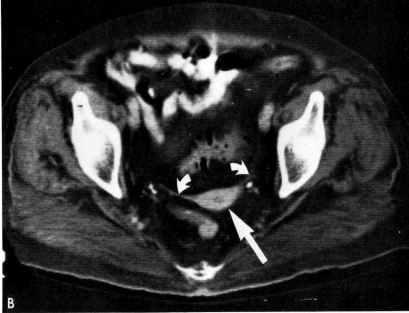

FIGURE 25–9 ■ Normal female pelvis. *A*, The normal uterus (u) is identified as an oval structure with deltoid extensions *(arrows)* on either side representing the adnexal structures. Pouch of Douglas is represented by a curved arrow. *B*, CT scan at a higher level shows the uterine cavity as an area of low attenuation *(arrow)*. Broad ligaments *(curved arrows)* extend from the body of the uterus.

FIGURE 25–10 ■ A tampon *(arrowheads)* outlines the vagina between the rectum (r) and bladder (b).

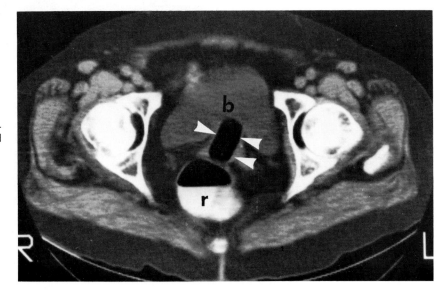

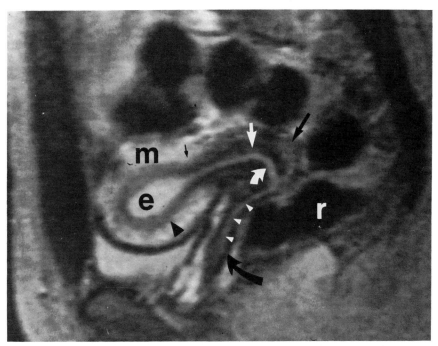

FIGURE 25–11 ■ Normal uterus and cervix. A T2-weighted sagittal image of the pelvis demonstrates the normal zonal anatomy of the cervix and uterus. Note high signal intensity of the endometrium (e), low signal intensity of the junctional zone *(black arrowhead)*, intermediate signal intensity of the myometrium (m), internal cervical os *(short straight black arrow)*, endocervical canal *(curved white arrow)*, fibrous cervical stroma *(straight white arrow)*, and outer layer of the cervix *(long straight black arrow)*. Note also the vaginal wall *(curved black arrow)*, vaginal cavity *(white arrowheads)*, and air within the rectum (r).

menstrual cycle.[19] The vaginal wall and mucus within the vaginal cavity are highest in signal intensity and thickest during the midsecretory phase. However, maximal contrast between the signal intensity of the vaginal wall and the surrounding fat occurs during the early or late secretory phase. For this reason, it is recommended that MR examination of the vagina be performed at this time. A vaginal tampon is not necessary for localization of the vagina or external os of the cervix and in fact will obscure structural detail.

In postmenopausal women, the signal intensity of the vaginal wall decreases, and the central mucus is thinned.[19] However, in postmenopausal women on exogenous estrogen replacement therapy, the vagina is similar in appearance to the vagina of a reproductive-age woman.[19] The external cervical os is readily identified on T2-weighted images, as it protrudes into the high-signal vaginal cavity. The internal os is appreciated by a well-defined constriction or decrease in width of the myometrium and an increase in the width of the low-signal-intensity band as the junctional zone merges with the thicker fibrous cervical stroma.

On T2-weighted sagittal images, the zonal anatomy of the cervix is observed (see Fig. 25–11).[16, 17, 20–22] Centrally, a stripe of high signal intensity most likely represents mucus within the endocervical lumen and epithelial glands. Surrounding the central stripe is a cylinder of low signal intensity that is continuous with the junctional zone of the uterine corpus. This cylinder most likely represents the fibrous cervical stroma. An outer zone of intermediate signal intensity, isointense to and continuous with the outer myometrium, is present in many patients.[16, 21, 22] This outer zone has been shown to contain fewer cells than the band of low signal intensity.[23] The appear-

ance of the cervix does not vary during the menstrual cycle[20, 21] or in women taking oral contraceptives (Fig. 25–12).[20] In reproductive-age women, the cervix measures 2.7 to 2.9 cm in length and 2.2 to 2.7 cm in width. The central high-signal-intensity stripe measures 3.8 to 4.5 cm, and the low-signal-intensity cylinder measures from 3.8 to 4.2 mm in width.[20]

Benign masses may involve the cervix. Nabothian cysts, frequently visualized with MRI, appear on T2-

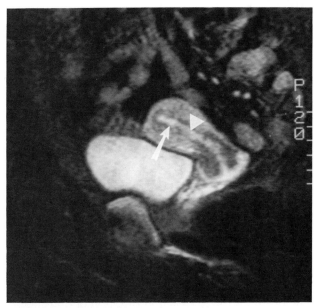

FIGURE 25–12 ■ Normal uterus in women taking oral contraceptives. A sagittal MR scan using a short TI inversion recovery (STIR) pulse sequence (TR, 2000; TE, 43; TI, 160) reveals typical anatomy of the cervix, but the junctional zone of the uterus *(arrow)* and endometrium is thin *(arrowhead)*.

weighted images as focal areas of high signal intensity located within the fibrous cervical stroma. They also occasionally have high signal intensity on T1-weighted images. Cervical fibroids appear as focal areas of low signal intensity on both T1- and T2-weighted images, either displacing the cervix or distorting the normal zonal architecture, depending on their size.

The dimensions of both the corpus and uterine zonal anatomy vary depending on the patient's hormonal status. In reproductive-age women, the uterine corpus averages 4 cm in width and 5 cm in length.[20] The total uterine volume increases slightly during the midsecretory phase.[24] A characteristic zonal anatomy of the corpus has been described on MRI scans that is not visualized with either CT or ultrasound (see Fig. 25–11).[16] The high-signal-intensity stripe represents the normal endometrium and endometrial cavity.[25–28] The endometrium is thinnest during menstruation. As estrogen levels rise during the follicular phase, the endometrium increases in width and widens further, although at a slower rate, during the secretory phase as a result of stimulation from both estrogen and progesterone.[20–22] The endometrium reaches maximum width during the midsecretory phase, averaging 5 to 7 mm on MR examination.[20, 21] A band of low signal intensity on T2-weighted images, the junctional zone (JZ), borders the high-signal-intensity central stripe. The JZ averages 5 mm in width, and its thickness or signal intensity have not been noted to vary during the menstrual cycle.[20, 21, 29] The JZ represents the innermost aspect of the myometrium,[25–28] and at the level of the internal os, it merges with the low-signal-intensity band of the fibrous cervical stroma. An increase in nuclear area, primarily reflecting an increase in cellularity, has been demonstrated by Scoutt et al.[28] within the JZ. McCarthy et al.[27] have shown that the water content of the JZ is decreased in comparison with the outer myometrium. The outer myometrium is intermediate in signal intensity on T2-weighted images. Changes in myometrial width parallel changes in endometrial width, and the myometrium reaches a maximum width, averaging 2.5 cm, during the midsecretory phase.[24] An increase in the signal intensity of the myometrium has also been described at this time.[21, 24]

In women taking oral contraceptives, the size of the uterine corpus and the width of the endometrium and JZ are diminished in comparison with those of other reproductive-age women (see Fig. 25–12). The average thickness of the endometrium is only 2 mm, and it does not vary in width.[20, 24] The myometrial signal intensity is increased in comparison with non–oral contraceptive users, most likely reflecting an increase in water content or edema within the corpus.[20, 24] Both the dosage and duration of oral contraceptive use affect the appearance of the uterus.[20, 24]

In postmenopausal women, the uterine corpus decreases in size until it approximates the length of the cervix. The endometrium is thinned and does not usually exceed 3 mm in width.[24, 30] Myometrial signal intensity is diminished in comparison with women of reproductive age, and this results in a decrease in endometrial-to-myometrial contrast.[24, 30] Although the JZ is usually visible, it is often thinner and less well defined than in premenopausal women. In postmenopausal women on exogenous estrogen replacement therapy, the appearance of the uterus on MRI scans is similar to that of a reproductive-age female.[24] Prior to menarche, the uterus appears similar to the postmenopausal uterus. The length of the corpus approximates the length of the cervix and usually does not exceed 2.5 cm. The endometrium is thinned, the JZ is less distinct, and the myometrial signal intensity is diminished in comparison with the uterus of a normal reproductive-age woman.[24] The appearance of the uterine zonal anatomy is important in the detection of pathologic abnormalities but must be interpreted in the context of the patient's hormonal status.

Urinary Bladder

Pathology

BENIGN DISEASE

Masses seen on intravenous urography impressing, compressing, or displacing the bladder are readily evaluated by CT. True masses are easily distinguished from bladder impressions produced by loops of bowel present in the pelvis, if the bowel loops are adequately filled with contrast material. Alterations in the shape of the bladder can be produced by retroperitoneal fibrosis, pelvic lipomatosis, hematoma, lymphoceles, or inferior vena caval thrombosis.[31–33] In these benign conditions, CT reveals elevation and narrowing of the bladder in such a way that the bladder appears pear-shaped. The cause of the pear-shaped bladder often can be determined by pelvic CT examinations. Large amounts of low-density fat surrounding the pelvic organs are present in pelvic lipomatosis (Fig. 25–13). Lymphoceles are cystic masses that compress the bladder and have sharp borders and a CT density close to that of water. Acute hematomas have a density greater than that of surrounding muscles, and contrast-enhancing perivesical collateral vessels together with a filling defect in the inferior vena cava confirm a diagnosis of an inferior vena caval occlusion. Schistosomiasis can result in extensive bladder wall calcification.[34] If a mass has an irregular shape, obliterates perivesical fat planes, or appears to invade adjacent pelvic organs in the presence of a pear-shaped bladder, the most likely underlying cause is a pelvic malignancy.[35]

Extravesical inflammatory processes may extend to involve the bladder. Diverticulitis and inflammatory bowel disease can produce a localized thickening of the bladder wall that can be difficult to differentiate from tumorous thickening. These inflammatory conditions can result in intravesical air as a result of enterovesical fistula formation.[36] On rare occasions,

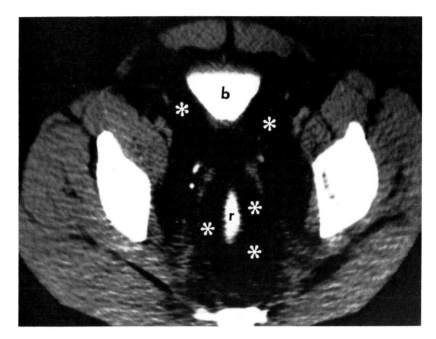

FIGURE 25–13 ■ Pelvic lipomatosis. CT scan demonstrates excessive pelvic fat *(asterisks)* compressing the rectum (r) and bladder (b).

localized irregular bladder wall thickening may be caused by endometriosis or malacoplakia of the urinary bladder.[37–39] In cases of endometriosis, ultrasound or CT—together with a history of classic cyclicity (seen in approximately 25 per cent of cases) and cystoscopy with biopsy—usually leads to the correct diagnosis.

Malacoplakia of the bladder is an unusual inflammatory granulomatous lesion characterized by mucosal plaques or firm nodules. The masses are composed of macrophages that contain basophil inclusions called *Michaelis-Gutmann bodies*.[38, 39] The CT features are those of a solid bladder mass, which may have areas of calcification, central necrosis, or cyst formation. The origin is unknown but is thought to be an altered host response to bladder infection. Malacoplakia is four times more common in females, and although it is usually self-limited, antibiotic therapy is often employed.

Care must be taken not to confuse thickening of the bladder wall related to incomplete distention, trabeculation resulting from urinary outflow obstruction, radiation edema, or fibrosis (Fig. 25–14A) with thickening of the bladder wall related to a malignancy.

Nonmalignant bladder tumors are rare, but bladder fibromas, nephrogenic adenomas,[40, 41] pheochromocytomas[42] (see Fig. 25–14B), and angiomas appear as smooth, intravesical filling defects. Distinguishing these from a noncalcified bladder calculus or intravesical blood clot is usually easy, because calculi have a high CT attenuation, and blood clots change position as the patient is scanned in the prone or decubitus position. Cystitis emphysematosa is a condition of the urinary bladder characterized by gas-filled vesicles in the bladder wall and often gas in the bladder lumen (Fig. 25–15).[43] Hemorrhagic cys-

titis can produce marked and diffuse bladder wall thickening (Fig. 25–16).

Bladder injury in pelvic trauma may cause intra- or extraperitoneal rupture or a contusion with bladder wall hematoma. CT cystography is highly accurate in classifying bladder injuries and is more accurate than plain cystography in detecting the location and extent of injury.

MALIGNANT DISEASE

Bladder Carcinoma ■ The standard methods of examining patients with suspected bladder tumors are cystoscopy, biopsy using a transurethral approach, excretory urography, cystography, lymphangiography, arteriography, and bimanual examination under anesthesia. The Jewett-Marshall system or the TNM method can be used to stage bladder tumors (Table 25–1).[44] Although there is extensive experience with the Jewett-Marshall system, Kenny and associates[45] reported an accuracy rate of only 56 per cent for preoperative staging of bladder tumors using standard methods. Superficial tumors and tumors infiltrating the wall without extension beyond the margin

TABLE 25–1 ■ Bladder Carcinoma: Methods of Staging

JEWETT-MARSHALL	TNM	PATHOLOGY
O	T1s	Carcinoma in situ
A	T1	Confined to lamina propria
B1	T2	Microinvasion of superficial muscle
	T3	Microinvasion of deep muscle
B2	T3a	Deep muscle invasion
C	T3b	Perivesical invasion
D1	T4, N1–N3	Spread to adjacent organs, positive pelvic lymph nodes
D2	M1,N4	Distant metastasis

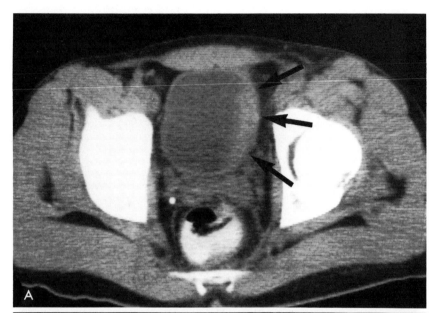

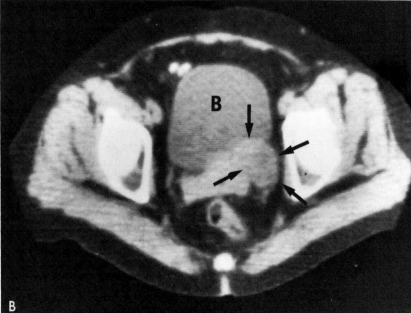

FIGURE 25–14 ■ Benign bladder abnormalities. *A,* Irregular thickening of the left lateral wall of the bladder *(arrows)* is caused by radiation cystitis but mimics a tumor. The clinical history is necessary for correct intepretation of bladder wall thickening. *B,* A soft mass *(arrows)* representing a pheochromocytoma arising in the posterior wall of the bladder (B). The histologic nature of this mass cannot be determined by CT without biopsy or without confirming clinical evidence of a pheochromocytoma.

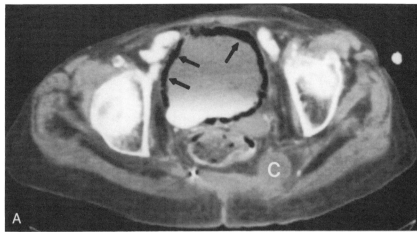

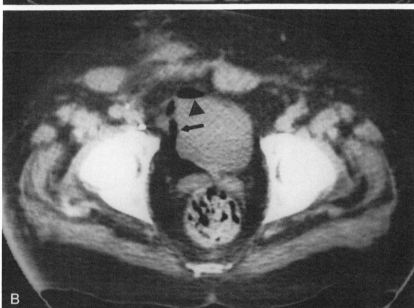

FIGURE 25–15 ■ Cystitis emphysematosa. *A,* Extensive air in the bladder wall *(arrows).* The patient has a sacral chordoma *(C). B,* Another patient with air in the bladder wall *(arrow)* and lumen *(arrowhead).*

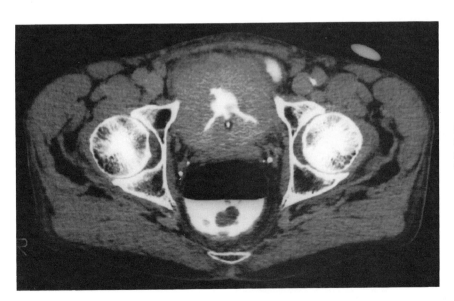

FIGURE 25–16 ■ Hemorrhagic cystitis. Contrast has been instilled via a Foley catheter and demonstrates a diffusely markedly thickened bladder wall.

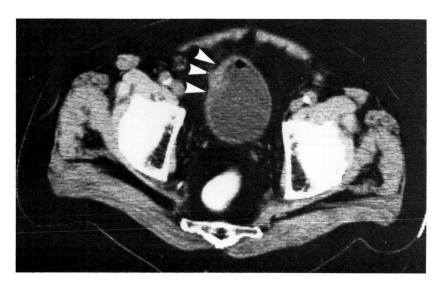

FIGURE 25–17 ■ Bladder carcinoma. Focal thickening of the wall of the urinary bladder (*arrowheads*) from a stage B2 transitional cell carcinoma. Air in the bladder was introduced during cystoscopy.

of the bladder wall generally were diagnosed accurately, but extension of tumor behond the bladder wall (stages C, D1, D2 or T3b, T4, M1) were not adequately determined using conventional modalities.

Improvement in staging of bladder carcinoma has been obtained by the use of ultrasound, computed tomography, and magnetic resonance imaging.[46, 47] Ultrasonographic examination of the bladder by means of an intravesical transducer is highly accurate,[48] but accurate depiction of infiltration into surrounding pelvic structures is difficult to determine because of the somewhat limited depth penetration of the intraluminal transducer. Transabdominal ultrasonography of the bladder is also useful, but tumors in the bladder outlet or in the anterior wall near the outlet are difficult to evaluate by transabdominal ultrasonography. Accurate ultrasonographic evaluation of the extension of tumor into seminal vesicles or the prostate is best done by transrectal ultrasonographic scanning.[49, 50]

CT of the pelvis is easy to perform, is noninvasive, and can detect mucosal or mural abnormalities. In general, CT cannot distinguish among stages A (T1) B1 (T2), and B2 (T3a) bladder carcinoma,[46, 47, 51] because CT cannot differentiate the various layers of the wall of the urinary bladder. However, CT is very useful in determining extension of tumor to neighboring structures, pelvic sidewalls, and distant sites.[46, 47, 51] Tumor confined to the bladder wall appears as thickening of the bladder wall with sharp borders. The tumor may produce localized bladder wall thickening (Fig. 25–17) or papillary projections into the lumen (Fig. 25–18) or involve a large portion of the bladder wall. Bladder wall thickening is usually caused by malignant disease, but inflammatory or radiation changes may mimic malignant wall thickening (see Figs. 25–14A and 25–16).

Poor definition of the borders of the urinary bladder with loss of distinctness of the surrounding fat suggests perivesical tumor extension of disease (Fig. 25–19). If CT examination demonstrates a loss of tissue planes and a tumor mass that clearly extends into the perivesical fat or involves neighboring structures such as seminal vesicles or obturator muscles, a diagnosis of stage D1 (T4) carcinoma can be made (Fig. 25–20). Hydronephrosis frequently is seen in advanced malignancies, but distinction by CT between a stage C (T3b) and a D1 (T4) tumor may not be possible. Stage D2 (MI) is characterized by meta-

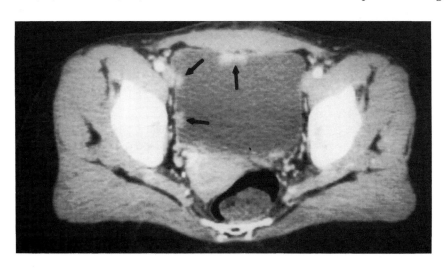

FIGURE 25–18 ■ Multifocal transitional cell carcinoma of the bladder is seen as numerous small localized nodular projections into the urine-filled bladder (*arrows*).

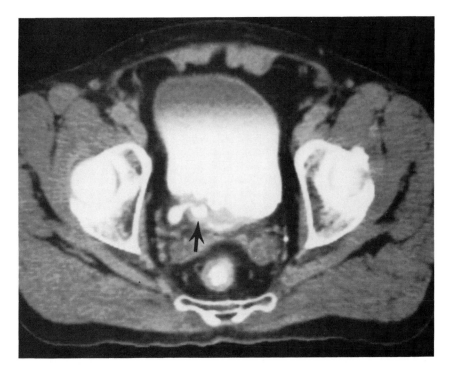

FIGURE 25–19 ■ Stage C transitional cell carcinoma. A CT scan shows irregular thickening of the bladder wall. The tumor has spread to involve the distal right ureter *(arrow)*, producing partial ureteral obstruction.

static disease, usually in the form of retroperitoneal adenopathy or metastases to the liver or lungs.

The reported accuracy rate for staging bladder tumors by CT has ranged from 40 per cent to 90 per cent.[46, 47, 51–53] CT has proven superior to cystography for detecting extension of tumor mass beyond the bladder wall and is particularly helpful in the evaluation of anterior or posterior bladder wall lesions. Axial CT scans frequently detect posterior spread of tumor into the seminal vesicles, but extension of carcinoma into the prostate is only rarely demonstrated. Sagittal and coronal image reformation can be used to evaluate craniocaudal extension of tumor, to determine the relationship of the tumor mass to the seminal vesicles and prostate gland,[5] and to identify lesions located in the dome and base of the urinary bladder.[51] Kellet and co-workers found that in untreated patients, CT tended to reveal a more advanced stage than did clinical examination.[54] This was particularly true among obese patients in whom

increased fat facilitated CT differentiation of pelvic organs.

Although CT is a useful method for staging bladder carcinoma, it cannot reliably predict microscopic invasion of muscle or perivesical fat by intrinsic bladder tumors.[46, 47, 51, 52, 54] In one study, eight per cent of bladder tumors were understaged by CT, largely because microscopic invasion of tumor to surrounding structures was not detectable. CT can also overstage bladder tumors when insufficient body fat makes delineation of tissue planes impossible.

Magnetic resonance imaging has proven to be very useful in the detection and staging of bladder cancer (Fig. 25–21).[46, 47, 52, 55–60] The normal bladder wall is visualized as a linear low-intensity structure on T2-weighted images, and disruption of the homogeneity of this line has been positively correlated with deep muscle infiltration.[46, 52, 55, 58] Heavily T2-weighted sequences are best employed for delineating tumor extension into the bladder wall, whereas T1-weighted

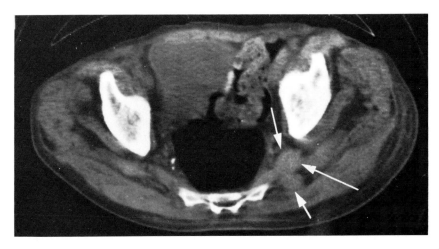

FIGURE 25–20 ■ Stage D1 transitional cell carcinoma of the bladder. Metastases from bladder carcinoma *(arrows)* are adjacent to and are invading the left piriformis muscle.

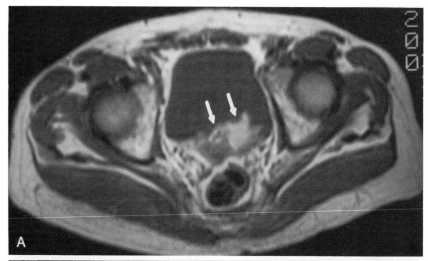

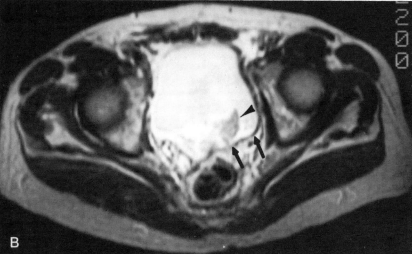

FIGURE 25–21 ■ Transitional cell carcinoma of the bladder. *A*, An intermediate-weighted MR scan reveals a large papillary neoplasm *(arrows)* of mixed high and low signal intensity arising from the base of the bladder. *B*, A T2-weighted MRI sequence reveals the bladder wall *(arrows)* to be intact, indicating that the tumor has not extended to the perivesical tissues. The area of low signal intensity *(arrowhead)* proved to be an area of fibrosis within the tumor.

sequences best demonstrate perivesical extension and lymph node enlargement (Fig. 25–21*B*).

Data to date indicate MRI to be very comparable to CT in staging bladder carcinoma.[46, 47, 52, 55, 58, 60] Staging accuracies ranging from 60 per cent to 95 per cent have been reported.[46, 47, 52, 58, 60] However, both CT and MRI have difficulty depicting microscopic tumor extension into adjacent organs,[61] detecting normal-size lymph nodes, and separating T2, T3a, and T3b lesions. Improved MRI staging may become possible with MR contrast agents[62] or as new surface coil[56] or intravesical imaging coils are developed.

Following radiotherapy, CT and MRI have been used in an attempt to distinguish recurrent tumor from radiation fibrosis.[63, 64] The recognition of fibrosis is important, because patients with recurrent tumor not extending to the pelvic walls can undergo curative cystectomy.[65] Fibrosis has a low signal intensity on T2-weighted or short T1 inversion recovery (STIR) images, whereas cancer typically has a higher signal intensity (Figs. 25–21 and 25–22).[64] However, acute radiation change, infection, or inflammation can produce regions of high signal, and microscopic tumor spread into areas of fibrosis may not be detectable.

The major methods to evaluate for lymph node metastases from bladder carcinoma are lymphangiography, CT, MRI, and lymphadenectomy. Although ultrasound is employed for screening of abdominal or pelvic adenopathy in some institutions, this method, despite reported accuracy rates of 78 per cent, remains limited in its use.[66] The reported accuracy rates of lymphangiography in detecting lymph node metastases from bladder tumors range between 90 per cent and 94 per cent,[67, 68] whereas histologically confirmed CT accuracy rates for differentiation of lymph node metastases from pelvic tumors and for evaluation of pelvic lymph nodes in patients with bladder carcinoma have ranged from 73 per cent to 77 per cent.[69, 70] Preliminary reports indicate no definite evidence that MRI is superior to CT in demonstrating cancer metastatic to pelvic lymph nodes.[47, 55] CT and MRI routinely demonstrate enlarged celiac, renal pelvic, iliac, and obturator nodes that are not usually filled during lymphangiography. Lymph nodes are considered abnormal if they are larger than 1.5 cm in diameter,[69–71] but CT and MRI cannot distinguish between benign and malignant lymphadenopathy. Lymphangiography detects smaller me-

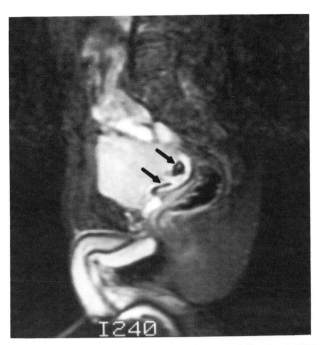

FIGURE 25-22 ■ Bladder carcinoma with areas of fibrosis. A STIR image (TR, 2000; TE, 40; TI, 120) done in the sagittal plane demonstrates the bladder carcinoma to have areas of very high signal surrounding central low-signal foci *(arrows)*, which were shown to be areas of fibrosis.

tastases and distinguishes between benign and malignant lymphadenopathy and thus is the most sensitive method of diagnosing pelvic lymph node metastases. However, lymphangiography is limited, because it cannot detect microscopic metastases and fails to distinguish certain groups of nodes in which metastases are often found.

In practice, a CT scan is initially obtained to detect abnormal lymph nodes in patients with bladder carcinoma. If abnormal lymph nodes are demonstrated by CT examination, no further evaluation is performed unless histologic confirmation is required prior to institution of therapy. CT-guided percutaneous needle biopsy can be performed to obtain tissue from the abnormal nodes. If CT results are negative, lymphangiography may be performed.

Evaluation of Therapy ■ Several reports have documented the value of CT in planning external beam radiation portals in patients with tumors of the bladder.[51, 72, 73] The use of computerized radiotherapy-planning programs, coupled with anatomic and densitometric CT data, has increased the accuracy of portal planning and permitted the use of computerized dosimetry. Often, based on CT results, treatment plans are changed, radiation ports adjusted, and dosages modified.

A major role of CT and MR imaging in bladder tumors is to determine those patients in whom radical surgery should be avoided. Both modalities also can detect early recurrence following radiation therapy or resection. More data with larger series and longer follow-up periods are necessary to establish whether the additional information provided by CT and MRI will produce an overall improved survival rate.

Carcinoma of the Urachus ■ Urachal carcinoma is a rare malignancy (less than one per cent of bladder carcinomas) that arises from the intra- or juxtavesical segment (90 per cent), the middle segment (six per cent), or the umbilical end (four per cent) of the urachus.[74] Of urachal carcinomas, 75 per cent to 80 per cent occur in males 40 to 70 years of age, and although most are adenocarcinoma (94 per cent), transitional, squamous, and anaplastic carcinomas are found. Patients most commonly present with hematuria (78 per cent), passage of mucoid material in the urine (ten per cent), and discharge of blood or mucus from the umbilicus; dysuria and abdominal pain are less frequent clinical manifestations. Plain radiography detects calcifications in less than five per cent of tumors. Urachal tumors can deform the bladder outline, cause lateral displacement of the ureters, or produce no abnormality. Urachal carcinoma is treated with radiation and partial cystectomy, but patient prognosis is poor, with the 5-year survival rates ranging from 6.5 per cent to 15 per cent.[74]

On CT scans, urachal carcinoma is seen as a midline soft tissue or cystic mass that may contain calcium (Fig. 25-23). Typically the mass is located anterior to the bladder, extending toward the umbilicus and anterior abdominal wall.[75-77] CT examination also provides information concerning extent of tumor spread, resectability, and local recurrence, which unfortunately occurs in 30 per cent of patients following partial cystectomy. MRI has demonstrated urachal carcinoma to have a signal close to that of urine on T1-weighted scans.[76]

Rare Tumors ■ Although decidedly uncommon, osteogenic sarcoma, lymphoma, and chloromas (Fig. 25-24) can arise in the bladder.

CT and MRI Following Cystectomy ■ A treatment regimen of preoperative radiation and radical cystectomy (consisting of a total cystectomy, pelvic lymphadenectomy, prostatectomy, and removal of seminal vesicles in men and total abdominal hysterectomy and bilateral salpingo-oophorectomy in women) has reduced the rate of recurrence of bladder tumors. However, postoperative complications following such extensive surgery are not uncommon. Abscesses and urinary leaks at the anastomotic site can occur immediately, and CT has proved to be a highly accurate method of detecting immediate postcystectomy complications.[78] CT scans are not hampered by drains or surgical packing and can be performed with intravenous and oral contrast media to permit distinction of bowel from abscess and urine leak from hematoma or lymphocyst. MRI has proven useful in distinguishing lymphocysts from nodal metastases (Fig. 25-25).

Continent urinary diversions are commonly performed following cystectomy. A variety of surgical procedures are being employed using either small

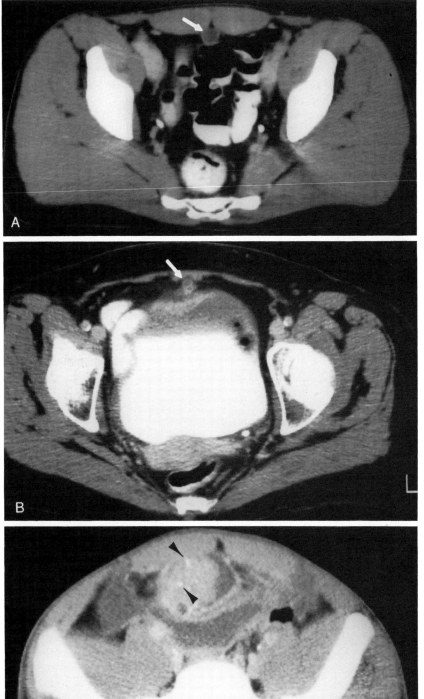

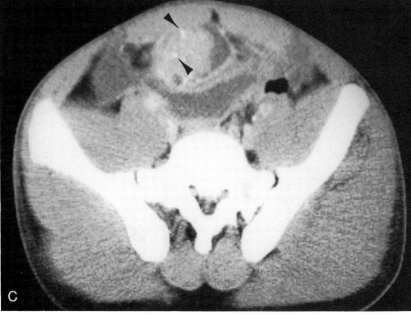

FIGURE 25–23 ■ Carcinoma of the urachus. *A*, A small midline cystic mass *(arrow)*. *B*, A small, solid midline mass *(arrow)* with associated thickening of the anterior wall of the bladder. *C*, A large mass that has both solid and cystic components. The tumor contains several areas of calcification *(arrowheads)*.

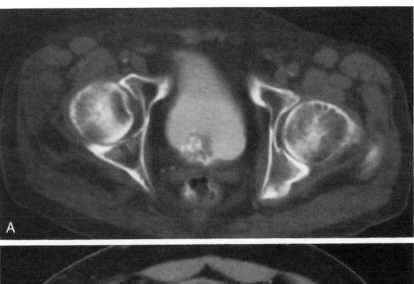

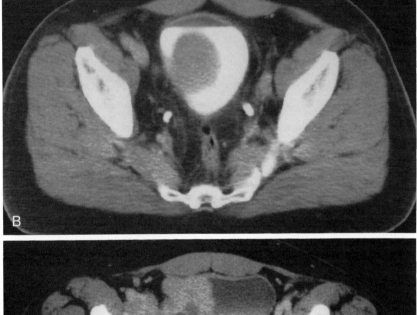

FIGURE 25–24 ■ Rare bladder malignancies. *A*, Osteogenic sarcoma arising in the base of the bladder has foci of calcification. *B*, A primary bladder lymphoma produces a rounded, sharply delineated, entirely luminal polypoid mass. *C*, A large bladder chloroma has both solid and cystic components. The right half of the bladder wall is irregular, and the tumor extends to the pelvic side wall.

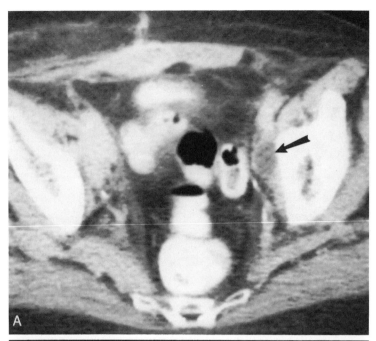

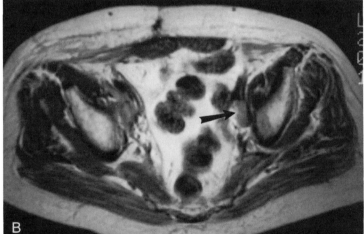

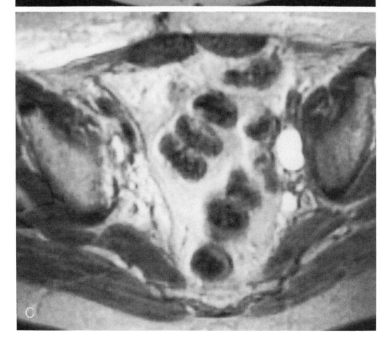

FIGURE 25–25 ■ Postcystectomy lymphocyst. *A*, CT scan reveals a low-density mass *(arrow)* along the left pelvic sidewall. *B*, T1-weighted MRI scan shows the mass *(arrow)* to have a low signal intensity. *C*, T2-weighted spin-echo image demonstrates the lymphocele to be hyperintense.

bowel alone or terminal ileum and cecum to create a reservoir pouch.[79] Typically, CT scans demonstrate the pouch as a fluid-filled right-sided mass, which may contain air. It is important not to mistake the pouch for an abscess. Contrast instilled into the pouch will readily demonstrate small leaks or fistulas. **Recurrent Bladder Tumors** ■ Recurrent tumor appears as a soft tissue mass with or without central necrosis. Any pelvic mass detected more than 3 months after cystectomy should be considered a tumor recurrence. However, a percutaneous biopsy may be necessary to differentiate a tumor from post-treatment fibrosis.

Prostate

The prostate is well visualized by CT and MRI in almost every male patient, and as a result of the clear delineation of the prostate, prostatic size and volume can be accurately measured. In men 30 years old and younger, the average craniocaudal diameter measures 3 cm; the anteroposterior diameter, 2.3 cm; and the lateral diameter, 3.1 cm. In the 60- to 70-year-old group, these average measurements increase to 5 cm for the craniocaudal diameter, 4.3 cm for the anteroposterior diameter, and 4.8 cm for the lateral diameter.[80]

Pathology

The prostate should not be considered enlarged if a scan 1 cm above the symphysis does not vizualize the prostate. Prostatic enlargement can be diagnosed if the prostate is seen 2 to 3 cm or more above the symphysis, in which instances it is usually surrounded by the bladder. The actual volume of prostatic tissue can be calculated by summating prostatic volumes on sequential CT or MRI scans.

Prostatic calcifications are detected by CT more frequently with increasing patient age, reaching 60 per cent in the 50- to 70-year-old group.[46] The calcifications usually appear as punctate, scattered, rounded densities that may not be identified on plain radiographs (Fig. 25–26). Large foci of calcification with irregular margins also are demonstrable.

BENIGN DISEASE

The margins of different prostatic lobes cannot be distinguished by CT, and prostatic gland tissue cannot be differentiated from the prostatic capsule; thus CT is a reliable indicator of prostatic disease only when the prostate either is grossly enlarged or contains gas, fluid, or calcium. In the presence of an enlarged prostate with sharp, smooth borders, it is impossible to distinguish on CT between prostatic hypertrophy and a small focal adenocarcinoma of the prostate (Fig. 25–27).

MRI is readily able to display the zonal anatomy of the prostate.[11–13, 81] The central zone (25 per cent of gland) has an intermediate to low signal intensity, in contrast to the high signal intensity of the peripheral zone (70 per cent of gland) (see Fig. 25–7). The anterior fibromuscular band has a very low signal intensity. The transitional zone (five per cent gland volume) has signal intensity characteristics close to those of the central zone in young males. As benign hypertrophy develops, this zone enlarges and signal intensity becomes more variable (Fig. 25–28).[11–13] Like CT, MRI has found it difficult to distinguish between benign hypertrophy and small adenocarcinomas (Fig. 25–29).[81–90] As the measured T1 and T2 values of these processes overlap, endorectal MRI probes may provide superior images of the prostate, but we must await more data before diagnostic accuracy is known.[14, 91, 92]

Sonographically, benign hypertrophy presents as symmetric enlargement having a homogeneous texture and sharp margination.[93] The accuracy of transrectal ultrasonography in detecting benign prostatic hypertrophy ranges from 91 per cent to 97 per cent and is 89 per cent in detecting prostatitis.[94] Although the value of ultrasound in differentiating among benign diseases of the prostate is still unclear, it appears that ultrasonography is currently more specific than CT or MRI in evaluating benign prostatic disease.

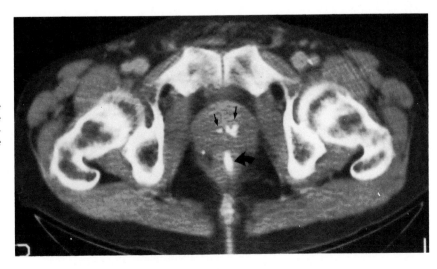

FIGURE 25–26 ■ Calcifications *(arrows)* are demonstrated within the prostate gland. The rectum *(curved arrows)* contains contrast material and cannot be clearly separated from the prostate.

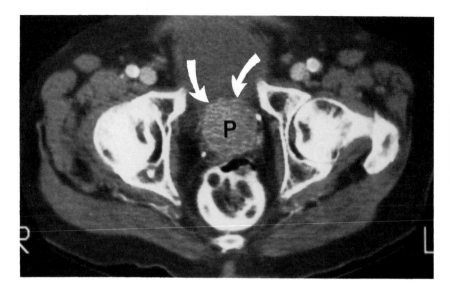

FIGURE 25–27 ■ Stage B prostatic carcinoma producing symmetric enlargement of the prostate (P). The margins *(arrows)* are smooth, and there is no evidence of extension of tumor beyond the prostate. Distinction between benign prostatic hypertrophy and carcinoma is not possible.

MALIGNANT DISEASE

Prostatic Carcinoma ■ The diagnosis of prostatic carcinoma usually is made by physical examination and biopsy.[89] Despending on the clinical and surgical findings, prostatic carcinoma is placed in one of four stages (Table 25–2):

1. Stage A carcinoma is not clinically detectable.

2. Stage B malignancy produces a palpable mass that is confined to the prostate and causes no symptoms or abnormal laboratory tests.

3. Stage C tumor extends beyond the prostatic capsule or, if confined to the prostate, is associated with symptoms of prostatism and/or elevation of serum acid phosphatase levels.

4. Patients with stage D prostatic cancer have distant metastatic disease. Elevated serum acid phos-

phatase levels are present in two thirds of patients, and lymph node metastases are present in 35 per cent to 85 per cent of such patients.[95]

The major role of CT and MRI in prostatic carcinoma is not diagnosis, but staging and evaluation of therapy. CT can neither diagnose stage A disease nor detect stage B carcinoma unless the tumor mass alters the contour of the prostate gland (see Fig. 25–27). Based on the attenuation coefficient, a carcinoma confined within the capsule cannot be distinguished from a normal prostate gland.[51] A nodular contour or focally altered margin suggests the presence of a carcinoma, and a smooth contour in an enlarged gland suggests benign prostatic hypertrophy, but the separation is imprecise. A smooth outer prostatic margin does not exclude a small, confined carcinoma, nor is an irregular margin pathognomonic of prostatic malignancy.

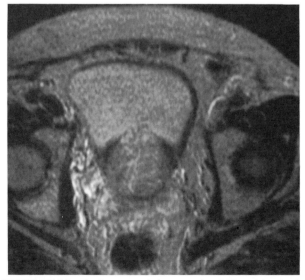

FIGURE 25–28 ■ Benign prostatic hypertrophy. A T2-weighted spin-echo MRI scan demonstrates prostatic enlargement and loss of the normal zonal anatomy. The signal intensity is intermediate. The large prostate is indenting the bladder.

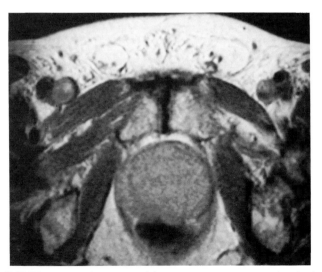

FIGURE 25–29 ■ Carcinoma of the prostate: stage B. A T2-weighted spin-echo MR image shows prostatic enlargement, loss of normal zonal anatomy, and a mixed signal intensity. This is similar to the MR features of benign prostatic hypertrophy.

TABLE 25–2 ■ Staging Prostatic Cancer

STAGE	DESCRIPTION
A (Microscopic)	Occult; incidentally found
A1	Focal; <5 per cent of tissue examined; low grade
A2	Diffuse (>5 per cent) or high grade
B (Macroscopic)	Palpable; confined to capsule
B1	Nodule less 1.5 cm
B2	Nodule greater 1.5 cm
C (Extracapsular)	Localized clinically
C1	Periprostatic, not fixed to sidewall (<70 g)
C2	Fixed to sidewall (>70 g)
D (Metastatic)	
D1	Confined to pelvis
D2	Extrapelvic spread

MRI also has limitations in detection and separation of stage A and B disease and in distinguishing benign prostatic hyperplasia from adenocarcinoma (Figs. 25–28, 25–29, and 25–30 through 25–32).[84, 85, 87–90] Extraprostatic extension of prostatic carcinoma (stage C or D) can be accurately assessed by computed tomography, MRI, or transrectal ultrasonography. Extension of prostatic carcinoma most frequently involves the seminal vesicles and bladder, producing loss of tissue fat planes (Fig. 25–33). Invasion of the seminal vesicles is found in 17 per cent of patients with newly diagnosed prostatic carcinoma,[96] whereas bladder and rectal invasion occurs less frequently.

Stage D prostatic carcinoma is diagnosed when metastatic lesions in the pelvis, spine, long bones, liver, lung, or retroperitoneal lymph nodes (Fig. 25–34) are demonstrated. Bone metastases occur most frequently in the bony pelvis, lumbar vertebrae, and proximal femur[96] and appear as osteoblastic (80 per cent), mixed osteolytic-osteoblastic (10 per cent to 15 per cent), or osteolytic (five per cent) lesions.[51]

Evaluation of pelvic and retroperitoneal lymph nodes for metastatic prostatic carcinoma can be done by lymphangiographic CT or MRI methods. Lymphangiographic accuracy ranges from 48 per cent to 80 per cent,[51, 98] with false-negative lymphangiogram results usually caused by nonfilling of internal iliac, obturator, or sacral lymph nodes that contain metastatic foci of prostatic carcinoma. Improvement in lymphangiographic accuracy is unlikely, because earliest lymphatic spread of prostatic carcinoma occurs by way of the obturator and internal iliac nodes (see Fig. 25–34),[99] and in 30 per cent of patients with lymphatic metastases, these are the only lymph nodes involved.

The reported accuracy of CT in detecting pelvic and retroperitoneal nodal metastases from prostatic carcinoma ranges from 33 per cent to 93 per cent,[51, 100] whereas that of MRI ranges from 44 per cent to 69 per cent.[87, 89] Levine and colleagues found CT to be more accurate than lymphangiography (93 per cent versus 55 per cent) in differentiating lymph node metastasis from prostate carcinoma[100] and attributed the greater accuracy of CT to its ability to demonstrate metastases to internal iliac and obturator nodes. Both CT and MRI detect nodal metastases on the basis of nodal enlargement, and thus metastatic deposits that do not produce lymphadenopathy go undetected. Therefore a negative CT or MRI examination does not exclude lymph node metastasis, and pelvic lymphadenectomy must be performed if optimal staging of prostatic carcinoma is required.[64]

Percutaneous needle biopsy can be used to document metastasis in patients with abnormal or suspicious lymph nodes seen on lymphangiography, CT, or MRI (Fig. 25–35).[101] MRI examination following biopsy can demonstrate a hyperintense region in the peripheral zone that cannot be distinguished from a carcinoma (Fig. 25–36).

The overall accuracy of CT for staging prostatic carcinoma is 67 per cent to 75 per cent.[51, 89] Most errors are a result of the inability of CT to recognize depth of tumor within the gland and to detect microscopic invasion of surrounding fatty tissues or metastatic foci in normal-sized lymph nodes.

The reported overall accuracy of MRI for staging prostatic carcinoma ranges from 61 per cent to 85 per cent.[82, 85, 87–89] Most errors result from difficulty deter-

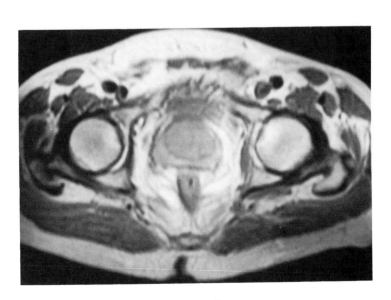

FIGURE 25–30 ■ Stage B prostatic carcinoma. T1-weighted image demonstrates prostatic enlargement with an enlarged central zone and a normal peripheral zone. No focal masses are seen.

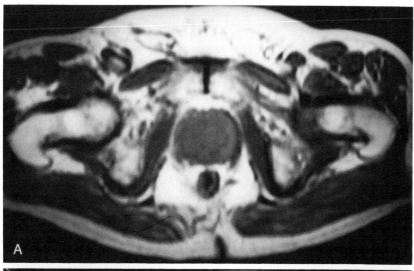

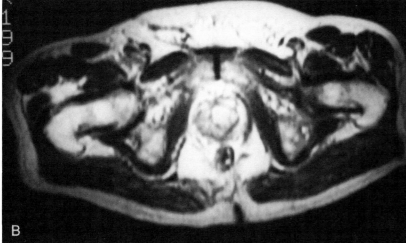

FIGURE 25–31 ■ Stage B prostatic carcinoma. *A*, Spin-density MR image shows prostatic enlargement with an increase in size of the central zone. *B*, T2-weighted spin-echo image reveals the prostate to have a heterogenous signal intensity, with areas of high signal intensity mixed with lower intensity regions.

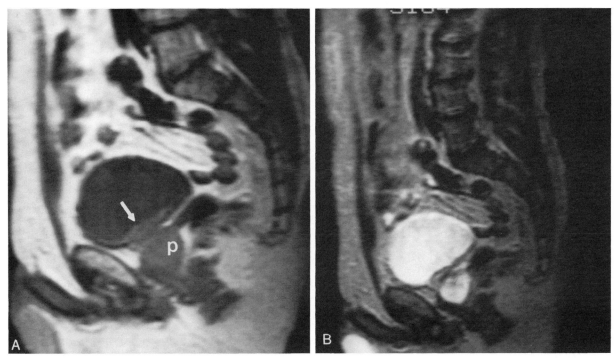

FIGURE 25–32 ■ Prostatic hyperplasia and bladder carcinoma. *A,* An intermediate-weighted spin-echo MRI scan demonstrating a focal bladder mass *(arrows)* and an enlarged prostate (p) of low signal intensity. *B,* On a T2-weighted sequence, the bladder lesion continues to have low signal intensity; biopsy revealed carcinoma with fibrosis. The prostate has a heterogeneous hyperintense signal intensity; biopsy revealed benign hyperplasia.

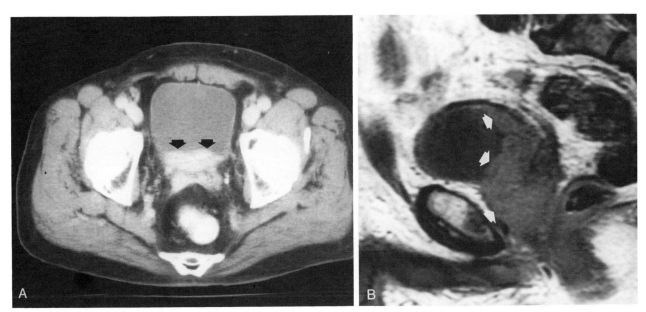

FIGURE 25–33 ■ Prostatic carcinoma invading the bladder. *A,* CT scan reveals thickening of the base of the bladder *(arrows).* *B,* A sagittal MRI scan better displays the extent of the carcinoma *(arrows),* which is invading the bladder base.

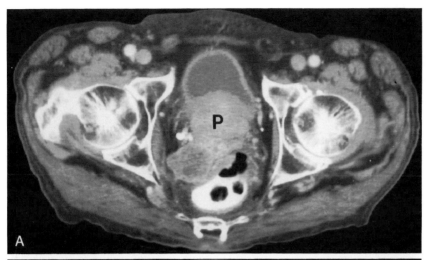

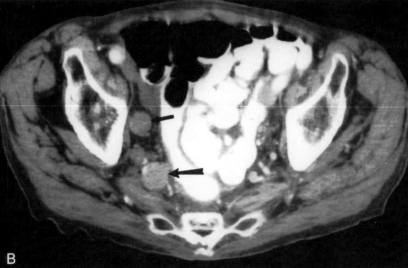

FIGURE 25–34 ■ Stage D prostatic carcinoma. *A,* A very large prostatic carcinoma (P) is seen invading the bladder and rectum and extending to the right pelvic sidewall. *B,* Enlarged obturator and internal iliac lymph nodes *(arrows)* proven to be caused by metastatic prostate carcinoma.

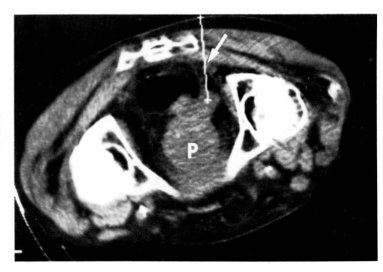

FIGURE 25–35 ■ Prone CT scan demonstrating a stage C prostatic carcinoma (P) extending beyond the capsule into surrounding tissue. A cursor line *(arrow)* indicates the proposed path for placement of a biopsy needle.

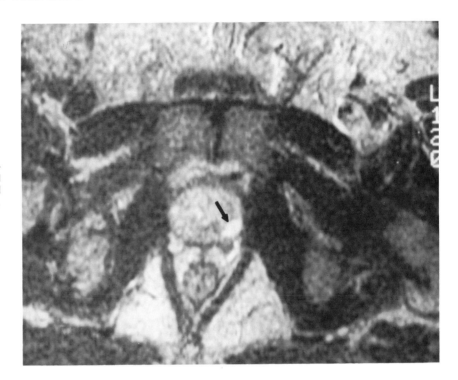

FIGURE 25–36 ■ Benign prostatic hypertrophy following biopsy. A T2-weighted MRI scan reveals a bright region in the peripheral zone on the left *(arrow)* 24 hours after biopsy. Biopsy findings were benign.

mining direct extracapsular spread, nodal involvement, and periprostatic venous plexus involvement. Distinguishing stage B from stage C or D disease appears possible in approximately 80 per cent of cases.[87–89]

Postoperative Complications ■ Following prostatic surgery, CT is useful for evaluating the pelvis for postoperative changes and a variety of complications such as pelvic lymphoceles, hematomas, and/or abscesses that may follow pelvic lymphadenectomy.[102]

Lymphoceles occur in the early postoperative period, usually within the first 10 postoperative days. They are usually located anterolateral to the bladder and within 3 cm of the anterior abdominal wall. Spring and colleagues[102] found lymphoceles in 27 per cent of 22 prospectively studied patients undergoing surgical staging of prostatic carcinoma. Lymphoceles appear as sharply delineated cystic masses having

an attenuation value close to that of water (see Fig. 25–25). Internal septations may be present. Small lymphoceles without septations tend to resolve spontaneously, whereas large (greater than 30 cm)[3] lymphoceles and lymphoceles with septations often require surgical intervention.

Evaluation of Therapy ■ CT has proven to be a useful method for assessing the adequacy of portals for external beam radiation and for calculating the volume and average dimensions of the prostate for correct dosimetry of iodohippurate sodium ^{125}I seeds (Fig. 25–37).[51, 96, 103–106] Based on CT results, error rates of 18 per cent to 25 per cent were found in clinical estimation of treatment volume, thus requiring an adjustment in field size to ensure optimum external beam radiation therapy.[51, 96, 103]

Localized carcinoma of the prostate (stages A and B) can be effectively treated by prostatic implantation

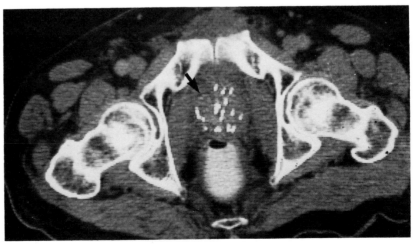

FIGURE 25–37 ■ CT scan shows the distribution of ^{125}I seeds within the prostate. The right anterior portion of the prostate *(arrow)* demonstrates a lack of ^{125}I seeds.

of iodohippurate sodium ^{125}I seeds.[104–106] This procedure reduces the incidence of impotence and other complications that frequently occur following radical prostatectomy or external beam radiation. Optimal therapy is given when there is even distribution of seeds, and CT has proven capable of precisely assessing the distribution of seeds within the prostate and of determining whether extraprostatic radioactive seeds have been placed (see Fig. 25–37). In one study, CT detected inhomogeneous seed distribution (usually involving the cephalic portion of the prostate) or extraprostatic seeds in 85 per cent of the patients examined.[103] Depending on clinical and CT findings, external radiation may be directed to areas that are not adequately treated by the ^{125}I seeds.[105, 107]

Testes

Pathology

Undescended Testes

The absence of a palpable testis may be related to agenesis, dysgenesis, acquired atrophy, or incomplete descent. It is important to identify an undescended testis (cryptorchidism), because there is a loss of fertility if the testis remains undescended and a 12- to 40-fold increased incidence of neoplasm, particularly in those testes located in the abdominal cavity.[108] In the prepubertal patient, generally an undescended testis is brought into the scrotum, whereas in the postpubertal patient, orchidectomy is usually performed because of the high incidence of malignancy in cryptic testes in older males.

Bilateral anorchidism is diagnosed readily by endocrinologic tests in patients younger than 35 years, and no exploratory surgery or radiologic examination is needed. In patients older than 35 years, endocrinologic tests are unreliable, because even if testes are present, their prolonged intraabdominal position results in severe atrophy, which prevents a response to hormonal stimulation. If only one testis is absent, endocrinologic tests will be normal and the distinction between unilateral agenesis of the testis and cryptorchidism must be made by other means.

The testes develop from embryonic gonads located ventral to the mesonephric ridge. During the descent of the gonads from their abdominal position, the vascular structures, nerve supply, and ductal connections are brought down into the inguinal canal and scrotum. The external descent, with migration of the testes through the inguinal canal into the scrotum, begins at about the thirty-sixth week of gestation.[109] This process is usually completed at birth but may continue for 4 to 6 weeks after birth in a full-term infant and for up to 12 weeks in a premature infant. The incidence of undescended testes is less than one per cent at 1 year of age.[110]

Arrest of the migration of the testes may occur anywhere along the developmental pathway from the lower pole of the kidney to the external inguinal ring. In 80 per cent of patients with undescended testes, the testis is palpable in the superficial inguinal region. When the testis is impalpable, it may be because the testis is absent or is very small and atrophic or dysplastic. Most nonpalpable undescended testes lie near the external ring located in the superficial inguinal pouch or at the neck of the scrotum. In some patients the testes lie just above the inguinal ring, deep below the muscle layer of the anterior abdominal wall and close to the iliac vessels. In rare instances, a cryptic testis is located higher on the posterior abdominal wall.[111]

The current approach to nonpalpable testes is to attempt preoperative localization using ultrasonography, CT, or MRI.[110–112] Detection of undescended testes by CT is based on recognition of an oval-shaped soft tissue mass along the course of the testicular descent (Fig. 25–38). CT scan sections must be carefully examined for the presence or absence of a cryptic testis between the inguinal ring, which lies approximately 5 to 6 cm caudal to the anterosuperior iliac spine, and the external ring, which is located just cephalic to the pubic ramus. Because the normal structures in the inguinal area and lower pelvis are symmetric, even a small extra soft tissue mass can be detected easily by CT. Detection by CT of testes located higher in the pelvis or in the abdomen is more difficult, because the testis may be confused with bowel loops, vascular structures, or lymph nodes.[110, 113] Lack of demonstration of a spermatic cord is found in both agenesis of the testes (Fig. 25–39) and in cases of undescended testes (see Fig. 25–37).

Lymph nodes in the inguinal region can be distinguished from testicular tissue by their location: inferior to the inguinal ligament or adjacent to femoral and iliac vessels, deep and lateral to the inguinal canal. In equivocal cases, a bolus injection of contrast material will permit separation of vascular structures from nonvascular soft tissue masses.

Experience using CT to detect undescended testes has demonstrated the method to be highly accurate.[113, 114] Ultrasonography has also been successfully used to detect undescended testes located in the inguinal canal.[111] The sonographic diagnosis of an undescended testis is based on recognition of an oval mass with medium-level echoes along the course of the testicular descent. However, ultrasound is less useful in detecting undescended testes located in the lower abdomen and is difficult to perform when there is an inguinal hernia present.

MRI has been used to locate undescended testes.[110, 112] Fritzche et al.[112] correctly located 15 of 16 undescended testes in 12 patients. The undescended testes were best located by using contiguous transverse scans through the inguinal region. Intracanalicular testes were seen as elliptical masses having an intermediate signal, whereas atrophic fibrotic testes were shown to have an abnormal low signal intensity on T2-weighted images.

Our approach to examining patients with an nonpalpable testis is to initially perform an ultrasono-

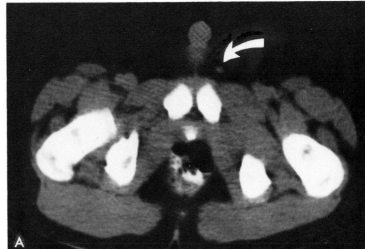

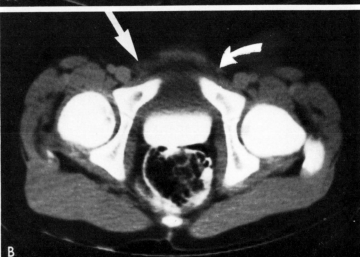

FIGURE 25–38 ■ Undescended right testis in a 10-year-old boy. *A,* CT scan at the base of the scrotum demonstrates a spermatic cord on the left side *(curved arrow)* but no spermatic cord on the right. A palpable testis was present on the left side but not on the right. *B,* CT scan at a higher level reveals an oval area of soft tissue density in the right inguinal canal *(straight arrow)* that is larger than the normal spermatic cord *(curved arrow)* identified in the left inguinal canal. A right inguinal testis was found at surgery.

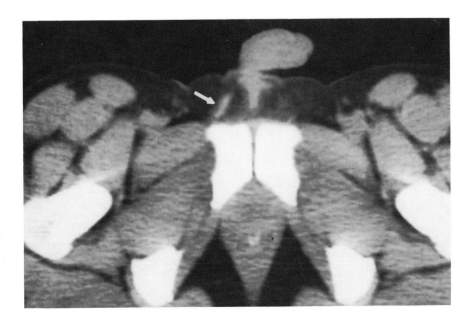

FIGURE 25–39 ■ Agenesis of the left testes. There is a normal spermatic cord on the right *(arrow),* but no spermatic cord is identified on the left.

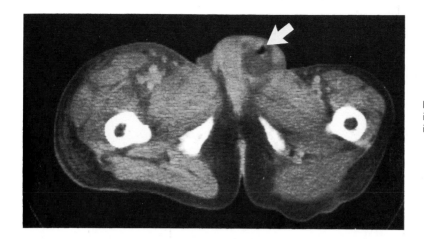

FIGURE 25–40 ■ A left inguinal hernia descending into the scrotum is seen in a low-density area containing air *(arrow)*.

graphic study. Because more than 70 per cent of undescended testes are located in the inguinal canal, ultrasonography will detect the vast majority of ectopic testes. If the ultrasound results are equivocal or negative, CT or MRI is performed. CT is usually favored because of its lower cost and greater availability. When spermatic cord structures but no testes are identified or when the testes cannot be localized unequivocally by CT or MRI, testicular venography or arteriography may be used for further evaluation.

BENIGN TESTICULAR DISEASE

CT has not been widely used to examine the scrotum and testes, because CT carries some radiation risk, whereas ultrasound is highly accurate and completely risk free.[115–118]

Extratesticular lesions such as hernias, hydroceles,[119] varicoceles, or spermatoceles can be easily demonstrated by CT (Figs. 25–40 and 25–41). Traumatic dislocation of the testes has also been demonstrated by CT (Fig. 25–42).

MRI now offers another completely safe method to examine the testes.[120–123] MRI appears to be highly accurate in differentiating intra- from extratesticular disease. The normal testis has a homogeneous inter-

mediate signal on T1 images and a high signal intensity on T2-weighted scans. The tunica albuginea is seen as a surrounding layer of low signal intensity. The MRI appearance of hydroceles, infarcts, hematomas, and testicular atrophy have been reported,[120–123] but insufficient data are available to determine the role of MRI in evaluating benign testicular disease.

MALIGNANT TESTICULAR NEOPLASMS

The yearly incidence of testicular carcinoma in the United States is 2.5 to 3.7 per 100,000 men.[124] Although accounting for only two per cent of all malignancies in men, they are the most common cause of death in men between the ages of 24 and 35 years. The most common malignant testicular tumor is seminoma, closely followed by embryonal carcinoma and teratoma.[125] The rarest primary tumor of the testes is choriocarcinoma.

Localized testicular pain is the most common presenting symptom, but many patients present with symptoms related to tumor spread at the time of diagnosis. Testicular tumors commonly metastasize via lymphatics to the iliac, paraaortic, mediastinal, and supraclavicular lymph nodes. When hematogenous spread occurs, metastases can involve any or-

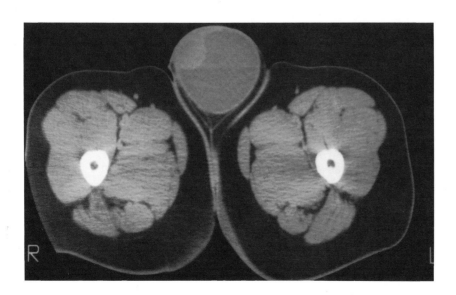

FIGURE 25–41 ■ A large oval mass of water density was proven to be a hydrocele.

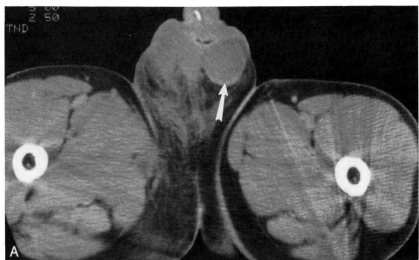

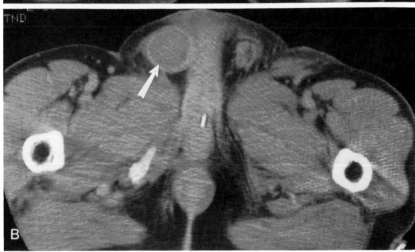

FIGURE 25–42 ■ Traumatic dislocation of the testes. *A,* CT scan through the scrotum demonstrates a normal left testes *(arrow)* and an absence of the right testes. *B,* Scan at a higher level reveals the right testes *(arrow)* to be displaced cephalad.

gan, but the lungs, liver, and kidney are the most frequent sites.

Prognosis and treatment of testicular malignancy depend on cell type and the stage of the disease when it is first diagnosed (Table 25–3). Because testicular tumors commonly metastasize by way of the lymphatic system, staging has relied heavily on lymphangiography. Lymphangiography is 62 per cent to 89 per cent accurate, 50 per cent to 90 per cent sensitive, and 67 per cent to 100 per cent specific in demonstrating lymphatic spread of testicular neoplasms.[126–128] Metastases may be missed because of the microscopic size of the metastatic focus or because involved nodes are not visualized on bipedal lymphangiography. An example of the latter is the group of lymph nodes near the renal hilum that receive lymphatic drainage directly from the testes but are often insufficiently opacified.[129] False-positive lymphangiographic interpretations can be the result of fibrosis, fatty replacement, or inflammatory disease,[128] all of which produce areas of incomplete lymph node filling.

CT, ultrasound, and MRI have all been used to stage testicular tumors.[120, 130–133a] Reported accuracies of CT in demonstrating lymph node metastases range from 74 per cent to 87 per cent; ultrasound accuracy ranges from 75 per cent to 81 per cent.[134, 135] Although the overall accuracy rates are comparable with those achieved with lymphangiography, lymphangiography is slightly more accurate, as it can detect metastases in nonenlarged nodes. However, CT is superior for detecting abnormal nodes in the upper retroperitoneum and inferior mediastinum and provides visualization of enlarged nodes in the mesentery and renal hilar areas (Fig. 25–43*A*).[125, 136–138] In addition, CT can evaluate extranodal tissue in the liver, kidney,

TABLE 25–3 ■ Staging of Testicular Tumors

STAGE	EXTENT OF CARCINOMA
I	Tumor clinically limited to the testis and spermatic cord
II	Clinical or radiographic evidence of tumor spread beyond the testis and spermatic cord but limited to the regional lymphatics below the diaphragm
IIA	Moderate-size retroperitoneal metastasis
IIB	Massive retroperitoneal metastasis
III	Metastasis beyond the diaphragm
IIIA	Extension beyond the diaphragm but still confined to the mediastinum or supraclavicular lymphatics
IIIB	Extranodal metastasis

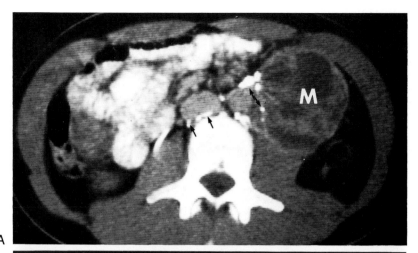

A

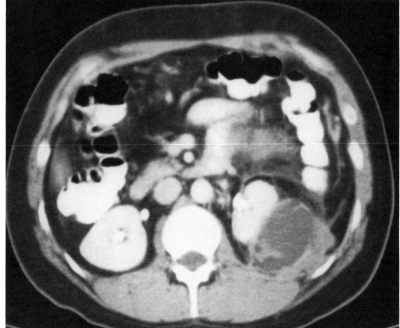

B

FIGURE 25–43 ■ *A*, Massive lymph node metastases (M) from seminoma of the left testis. Normal-sized lymph nodes filled with lymphangiographic contrast material *(arrows)* are displaced by the nonopacified low-density, septated tumor mass. *B*, Seminoma invading the left posterior pararenal space and displacing the left kidney.

bone, and lungs during a single examination (see Fig. 25–43*B*).

We perform a CT study as the initial staging procedure in patients with testicular neoplasms. Lymphangiography is performed only in patients having normal or equivocal CT examination results. Neither phlebography nor excretory urography is necessary for staging testicular tumors.[134, 137]

Evaluation of Therapy ■ CT findings in patients undergoing chemotherapy and/or orchidectomy have been correlated with clinical and surgical results and the level of serum tumor markers.[133, 138–140] CT readily demonstrates changes in the attenuation value and size of nodal metastases following chemotherapy[130, 141–144] and has been useful in detecting metastatic lung disease[141] and differentiating bleomycin-induced pulmonary fibrosis from recurrent metastatic disease.[145]

Following therapy, measurement of CT attenuation values of nodal metastases has been reported to provide useful information concerning changes in tumor composition. Conversion of a solid to a cystic mass during therapy has been reported to be evidence that viable tumor no longer remains or that a tumor such as an embryonal cell carcinoma has matured into a cystic teratoma.[142] However, other investigators have demonstrated that low-density postchemotherapy masses contained necrosis and viable tumor.[146] A decrease in CT number during or following therapy suggests that a residual mass does not contain tumor, irrespective of the final absolute CT number,[144] but an increase in CT density during treatment suggests viable malignant tissue.[144]

More than 85 per cent of recurrences following treatment of nonseminomatous germ cell tumors occur in the first year, 96 per cent within 2 years.[133, 140] The median recurrence interval is 3 months. Recurrence was most common in the initial disease site only (61 per cent), whereas in another 26 per cent it was in both a new and the initial site. Eighteen per cent of patients with recurrence had only a positive CT study, whereas eight per cent had positive serum markers only.[140] CT examinations every 6 months for the first year coupled with serum marker determinations is the current recommended method of following the effect of therapy and detecting recurrent disease. It is advocated that CT be used at 3-month intervals in the first year after therapy to demonstrate lack of growth and then at yearly intervals for the next 3 years.[139]

Serial CT studies in patients with seminoma have demonstrated tumor masses to resolve totally or partially or remain unchanged.[139] However, the presence of residual tumor in masses in patients with pure seminoma is rare, and there appears to be no correlation between CT attenuation values and the presence or absence of malignancy in posttherapy masses.

Pelvis

Pathology

PELVIC INADEQUACY

CT pelvimetry is employed whenever a vaginal delivery is being considered for a patient with a fetal breech presentation in order to avoid the high fetal morbidity that results from delivery of an aftercoming unmolded head through an inadequate maternal pelvis. In addition, predelivery identification of a hyperextended fetal head permits avoidance of damage to the umbilical cord. Gonadal radiation dose to the fetus using conventional pelvimetry is estimated to be 0.0885 mGy,[147] and technical failures necessitating additional radiographs often further increase the radiation dose to the mother and fetus.

Pelvimetry using digital radiography alone or combined with a single CT scan at the level of the fovae of the femoral heads has largely replaced conventional pelvimetry.[148–151] Digital radiographs of the abdomen and pelvis are obtained in the anteroposterior and lateral positions, and pelvic measurements are made using the CT console (Fig. 25–44). The technique is rapid, positioning problems are avoided, and radiation exposure is markedly reduced compared with standard techniques. The abdominal pelvic digital radiograph gives a maximum entrance skin dose of less than 10 mGy and fetal dose of approximately 22 mGy. Using the Federle technique, the CT scan (see Fig. 25–44) taken at the level of the ischial spines, exposed with reduced factors of 80 mA, 2.2-ms pulse width, and a 5.7-sec scan time, results in an average absorbed dose of 380 mGy.[148] Claussen et al.[149] and Adam et al.[150] employed only anteroposterior and lateral scout views and reported fetal doses ranging from 0.048 to 0.17 mGy. MRI can be also

used to perform pelvimetry (see Fig. 25–44D) and does not result in any radiation hazard.

Measurements ■ The pelvic inlet or true conjugate is measured on the lateral scout view from the sacral promontory to the upper portion of the symphysis pubis (normal, >11.0 cm) (see Fig. 25–44A). The transverse diameter of the pelvis is measured on the anteroposterior scout view as the largest transverse diameter in the pelvis (normal, >12.0 cm) (see Fig. 25–44B). The interspinous distance (midpelvic diameter) is measured between two points connecting the ischial spines on a CT section obtained at the level of the fovae of the femoral heads (normal, >10 cm) (see Fig. 25–44C). The measurements obtained with the electronic cursor do not require adjustments for magnification and are highly accurate.[148] Pelvimetry using digital radiography therefore offers the advantage of lower radiation exposure to fetus and mother and higher accuracy of measurements when compared with conventional pelvimetry. However, movement by the fetus while the scout film is being taken can result in artifacts that simulate fractures of the long bones.[152]

Ovaries

The ovaries generally are not identified on CT scans as separate structures, unless they are enlarged as a result of ovarian cysts, benign tumors, tuboovarian abscesses, or malignant neoplasms. CT readily demonstrates most ovarian masses and can usually determine whether the mass is fluid-containing or hemorrhagic but often gives little information concerning internal architecture. When very large ovarian masses are present, it may be difficult to identify the ovary as the origin of the mass because of the marked distortion of intrapelvic organ relationships.

On MRI scans the ovaries are homogeneous ovoid structures of low signal intensity on T1-weighted images. They are well marginated by the high signal intensity of the surrounding fat but may be obscured by loops of bowel. On T2-weighted images, the ovarian stroma remains of low signal intensity, but fluid within follicular cysts becomes of high signal intensity (Fig. 25–45). In premenopausal women, Zawin et al.[153] have reported that the ovaries are routinely identified on MR examination in 96 per cent of cases. However, in postmenopausal women with enlarged uteri, the ovaries are less frequently visualized because of atrophy and absence of follicular cysts.[154]

Pathology

BENIGN OVARIAN TUMORS

Teratomas account for approximately 10 per cent to 15 per cent of all ovarian neoplasms and typically occur in women during their reproductive years, being rare before puberty and not developing after menopause.[155–157] The overwhelming majority of cystic teratomas are benign, with less than three per

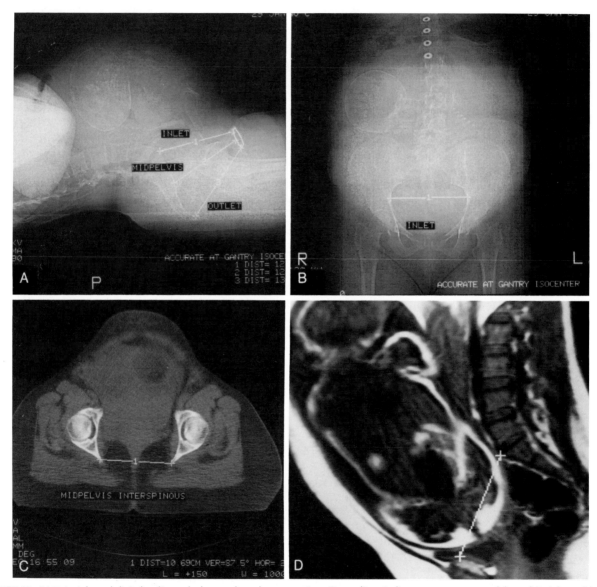

FIGURE 25–44 ■ *A,* A lateral digital radiograph shows a breech presentation. Cursor lines indicate measurements of the pelvic inlet, midpelvis, and outlet. *B,* Transverse diameter, normal pelvic inlet. A breech presentation is shown. The pelvic inlet measures 13 cm. *C,* CT scan at the level of the femoral fovea permits easy measurement of the interspinus diameter. *D,* Sagittal MRI scan with cursor measurement of pelvic inlet.

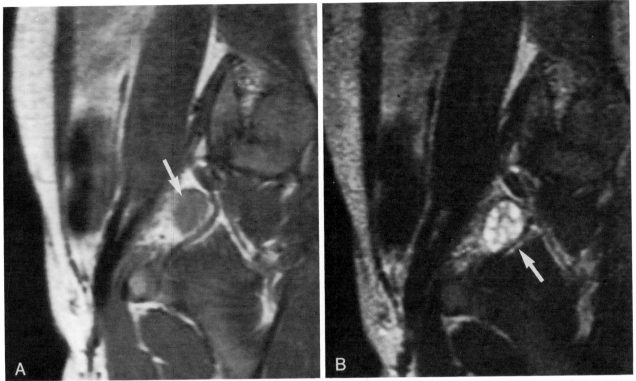

FIGURE 25–45 ■ Normal ovaries. *A,* Sagittal T1-weighted image. *B,* Sagittal T2-weighted image demonstrates a normal ovary *(arrow).* Note numerous small follicular cysts of increased signal intensity.

cent undergoing malignant degeneration.[155, 158] Teratomas are believed to arise from pluripotential embryonal cells and also may involve the mediastinum. If a cystic teratoma contains only one derivative of the germ layer, the ectoderm, it is called a *dermoid cyst.*

On plain radiographs, approximately 40 per cent of ovarian teratomas show specific diagnostic characteristics.[159] These consist of a mass containing calcific densities, often formed into patterns suggesting the presence of teeth or abortive bone, and a low-density mass with or without curvilinear calcification. The CT features of ovarian teratomas are sufficiently pathognomonic to permit a correct histologic diagnosis to be made in approximately two thirds of patients.[155]

The CT findings in ovarian teratomas vary depending on the components that are present in the mass. Most commonly CT examination reveals a low-density mass containing a mixture of fat, hair, debris, and fluid (Fig. 25–46*A*). In addition, calcifications (teeth or abortive bone) can often be seen, and a solid projection (dermoid plug) arising from the cystic wall is often present (Fig. 25–46*B*). A definitive CT diagnosis of cystic teratoma can be made when a gravity-dependent layering within a fatty mass or a fat-fluid level is present. Additional CT features are cystic masses with curvilinear calcifications and water-density masses containing solid tissue components and globular calcifications. If neither fat nor calcium is present in the cyst and if the contents of

the teratoma consist only of proteinaceous fluid, necrosis, hemorrhage, and/or hair and debris, the CT findings are nonspecific.[160, 161] Invasion of surrounding tissue by a malignant teratoma is detected by CT as loss of tissue fat planes and extension of a mass into the bladder, pelvic muscles, or bowel.

The classic sonographic features of ovarian teratomas consist of a mass in an axial location cephalic to the urinary bladder, having a solid mural component, which usually is echogenic, demonstrating acoustic shadowing and "fluid" and "hair-fluid" levels (see Fig. 25–46*B*).[160, 162–164] However, in one study,[165] one or more of these features were seen only in 17 of 40 teratomas; in another, only 33 per cent of 51 cystic teratomas had a focal area of increased echogenicity, and almost 25 per cent of the teratomas were not detected by ultrasound.[163] Difficulties in ultrasonographic diagnosis occur when teratomas appear as solid masses or complex masses with highly reflective echoes that are confused with bowel. Often hematomas, abscesses, or endometriosis cannot be distinguished ultrasonographically from teratomas. Thus although ultrasound is recommended as the initial study in patients with a suspected ovarian mass, CT or MRI can often provide more specific diagnostic information. Specifically, teeth and bone within a teratoma can be diagnosed with more certainty, and fat within a teratoma can be specifically diagnosed because of its characteristic CT density.

The key to diagnosing a dermoid cyst on MR examination is the identification of fat within an

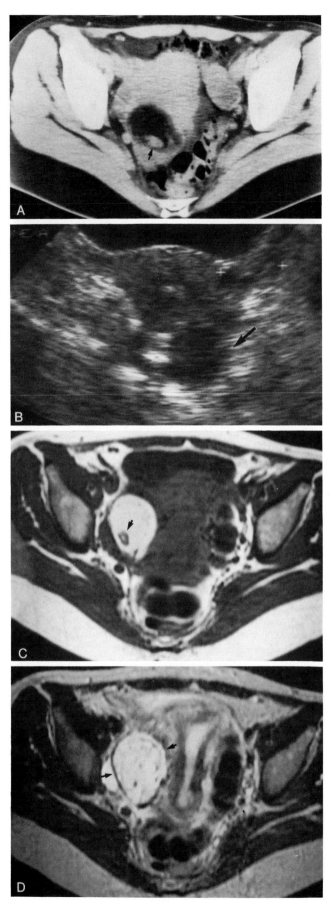

FIGURE 25–46 ■ Cystic teratoma of the ovary. *A,* CT section reveals a well-demarcated mass having areas of fat density, as well as a soft tissue nodule *(arrow)* representing a dermoid plug (Rokitansky's protuberance). *B,* Axial ultrasound image demonstrates a hypoechoic mass *(arrow)* containing low-level echoes posterior to the uterus. The left ovary *(cross marks)* is normal. *C,* Axial T1-weighted image demonstrates a right adnexal mass that is isointense to fat. A mass of low signal intensity *(arrow)* represents the Rokitansky's protuberance. *D,* Axial T2-weighted image confirms that the mass is isointense to fat and demonstrates atypical chemical shift artifact *(arrows)* and internal speckling.

adnexal mass (see Fig. 25–46C,D).[134, 166–170] On MRI scans, fat is confidently identified when the signal intensity of the mass (or part of it) is isointense to fat on all pulse sequences and internal or external chemical-shift artifact, indicating a fat-water interface, is present. Generally, fat is slightly lower in signal intensity on T2-weighted images than hemorrhage. However, hemorrhage and possibly even proteinaceous fluid may mimic the appearance of fat, as all three tissues may be bright on both T1- and T2-weighted images.[154, 168, 169] Therefore the presence of chemical shift artifact may be key in discriminating between these tissues.[170a] Specific pulse sequences that suppress signal from fat or water can be used to differentiate fat from hemorrhage. Several characteristic morphologic features favor the diagnosis of a dermoid, including layering, floating debris, palm tree–like protrusions, dermoid plugs, speckling, and calcifications.[166, 170] In addition, dermoid cysts can contain predominantly serous fluid rather than fatty liquid,[156] and such dermoids will be indistinguishable from simple cysts on either ultrasound or MR examination.[168, 170] MRI is less sensitive than CT in detecting calcifications in adnexal masses.

MRI is more sensitive and specific than ultrasound in identifying cystic teratomas of the ovaries. Togashi et al.[170] reported that MRI accurately diagnosed 20 out of 23 dermoids, whereas ultrasound diagnosed only 16 out of 23 dermoids. The relative accuracy of MRI in detecting dermoids in comparison with CT is not known. Recently, Scoutt et al.[166] reported that 19 of 19 dermoids were accurately diagnosed with MRI, whereas only 9 of 15 were confidently diagnosed with ultrasound.

OVARIAN CYSTS AND TUBO-OVARIAN ABSCESSES

The majority of ovarian cysts are asymptomatic and are detected by ultrasound[121, 123] as smooth-walled masses having no internal echoes and excellent through-transmission. On CT scans, ovarian cysts appear as smooth-walled masses having a central density close to that of water.[171] A rim of soft tissue surrounds the cyst, but internal septations are usually not identified (Fig. 25–47).

Most ovarian cysts are solitary small (less then 4 cm) masses, but large multiple or bilateral cysts are not infrequent (Figs. 25–47 and 25–48). A serous, follicular cyst cannot be distinguished from a cyst of the corpus luteum by CT, but acute hemorrhagic cysts may be diagnosed because of the high density of blood within the cyst (Fig. 25–49).

Tubo-ovarian abscesses are seen on CT scans as thick-walled, complex adnexal masses with centers of low-attenuation septations and shaggy margins (Fig. 25–50).[172] If air is present within the mass, a diagnosis of an abscess can be made with confidence, but when no gas is present, differentiation of abscess from neoplasm is usually not possible without a percutaneous fine-needle aspiration.[173] A hydrosalpinx can be diagnosed on CT when a tubular cystic mass in the adnexal region is identified that does not fill with oral contrast material.[174] Following surgical transplantation of the ovary, the ovary can be shown on CT scans as a rounded mass in the iliac fossa (Fig. 25–51).

On MR examination, serous ovarian cysts are homogeneous, with a thin wall and signal intensity isointense to urine on all pulse sequences.[154, 166–169] Occasionally cystadenomas (Fig. 25–52) and cystic teratomas may mimic the ultrasound and MR appearance of simple cysts.[166, 167, 169, 170, 175–178] Rarely, a serous cyst has high signal intensity on T1-weighted images; the reason for this is not certain.[166–168]

A paratubal cyst may be recognized on MR examination in some cases by its characteristic tubular configuration often encircling the adjacent ovary.[166] Tubo-ovarian abscesses (TOAs) have a serpiginous, tubular configuration and tend to be heterogeneous and ill defined on T2-weighted images (Fig. 25–53).[166, 168] Solid areas or septations may be present, and hemorrhage has been described in 40 per cent of patients in one series.[168] A pelvic abscess appears

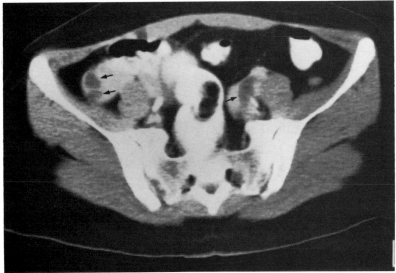

FIGURE 25–47 ■ Bilateral corpus luteal cysts (arrows) are identified as water-density ovarian masses.

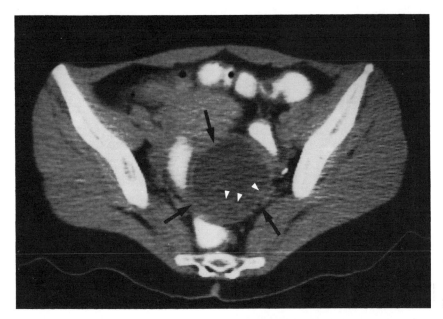

FIGURE 25–48 ■ A serous ovarian cyst measuring 8 cm in diameter is seen as a water-density mass having a smooth rim *(arrows)*. Several internal septations *(arrowheads)* are also identified.

FIGURE 25–49 ■ Acute hemorrhage into an ovarian cyst. CT scan reveals a cystic mass *(arrows)* containing areas of mixed low and high attenuation. The rim of the cyst is slightly enhanced. Ultrasound confirmed an ovarian cyst containing interal echoes characteristic of acute hemorrhage into the cyst.

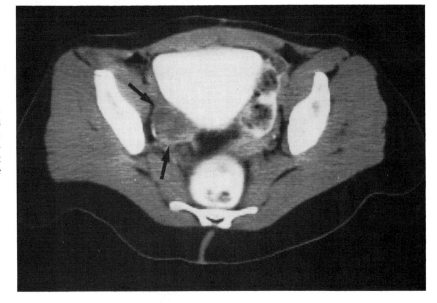

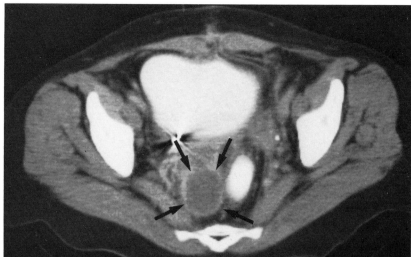

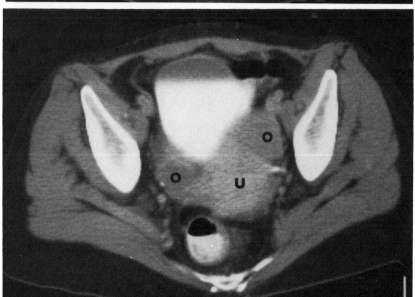

FIGURE 25–50 ■ *A*, Tubo-ovarian abscess producing a well-defined oval mass having a low attenuation center surrounded by a thin rim *(arrows)*. On CT scanning, differentiation of a tubo-ovarian abscess from a simple ovarian cyst or cystadenoma cannot be made unless septations or gas are present. *B*, Bilateral tubo-ovarian abscesses (o) are identified as ill-defined areas of low density on each side of the uterus (u).

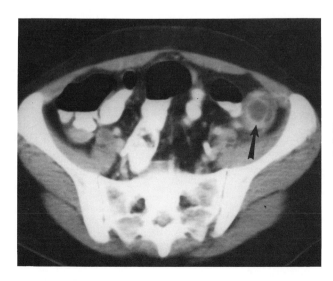

FIGURE 25–51 ■ Transplanted ovary. CT scan reveals the transplanted ovary as a rounded mass having a low-density center surrounded by a rim of soft tissue.

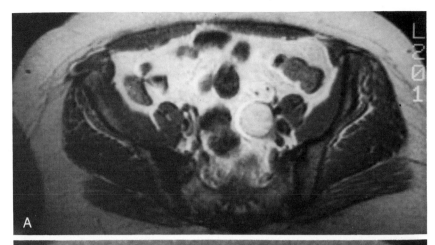

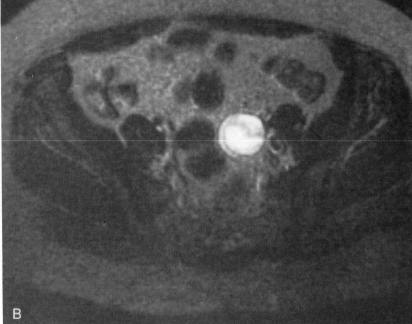

FIGURE 25–52 ■ Cystadenoma of left ovary. *A*, T1-weighted MR scan reveals a 3-cm, round left pelvic mass with a well-defined low-intensity rim. *B*, T2-weighted scan demonstrates marked signal enhancement of the cystadenoma. Internal septations are clearly shown.

FIGURE 25–53 ■ Tubo-ovarian abscess. Sagittal T2-weighted image demonstrates a serpiginous heterogeneous structure of predominantly high signal intensity *(arrows)* superior to the bladder and uterus (u).

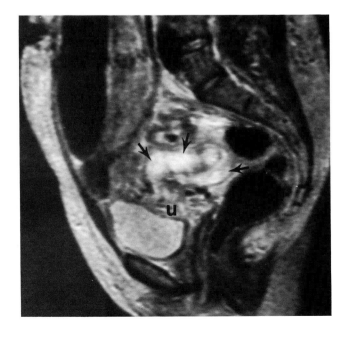

as a predominately low-signal-intensity mass on T1-weighted images, with a variable increase in signal intensity on T2-weighted images. Adjacent organs and blood vessels may be displaced or compressed by the mass, and surrounding inflammation may be manifested as ill-defined areas of increased signal intensity within the muscles on T2-weighted images.[179] In comparison with CT, MR examination better delineates the extent of inflammatory changes in the surrounding tissues and does not require intravenous contrast. Additionally, images are not degraded by artifact from surgical clips.[179] However, MRI is less sensitive than CT in differentiating bowel from pelvic abscesses or in identifying bony destruction or calcifications, and these may be significant limitations.[179]

On MR examination, hemorrhagic cysts are bright on both T1- and T2-weighted images. Layering and/or an hematocrit effect may be observed.[154, 166, 168, 169] However, when hemorrhage occurs in other lesions, these may be indistinguishable from hemorrhagic cysts on MRI.

On ultrasound examination, hemorrhagic cysts demonstrate increased through-transmission and often contain diffuse low-level echoes. Hemorrhagic cysts can also demonstrate diffuse increased echogenicity or contain echogenic masses representing blood clots and thereby mimic the ultrasonic appearance of endometriomas, dermoid cysts, or ovarian neoplasms.[180]

There is wide variability in the clinical manifestations of polycystic ovarian disease (PCOD), with only a fraction of patients presenting with the classic triad of hirsutism, menstrual irregularity, and reduced fertility. PCOD is diagnosed by hormonal assay. Pathologic findings include subcapsular cyst formation with multiple cysts <8 mm in diameter and subcapsular fibrosis. On ultrasound examination, approximately 71 per cent of patients have enlarged ovaries, but cysts will be visualized in only 39 per cent to 58 per cent of patients.[181, 182] Subcapsular cysts are more often visualized on transvaginal ultrasound (TVUS).[183] On MR examination, small cysts of high signal intensity are visualized in a ringlike configuration in the periphery of the ovary on T2-weighted images. Although subcapsular cysts have been documented on MR examination even when transabdominal ultrasonic examination is negative, the sensitivity and specificity of this appearance is not known.[184]

MALIGNANT OVARIAN TUMORS

Ovarian cancer ranks sixth among cancers in women, with one in seven newborn females expected to develop cancer of the ovary.[185] The patient prognosis is poor, with the overall 5-year survival rate for all stages and grades of ovarian cancer being less than 25 per cent, largely because two thirds of patients with ovarian cancer present initially with stage III or IV disease. The delay in detection of ovarian cancer is primarily because of the absence of early symptoms and the nonspecific nature of many of the symptoms.[186]

The most common primary malignant ovarian tumors are adenocarcinoma (papillary or undifferentiated) (Fig. 25–54), serous or mucinous cystadenocarcinoma (Fig. 25–55), and endometrioid carcinoma.[187] Less frequently encountered are malignant teratoma, endodermal sinus tumor, mixed müllerian tumor (Fig. 25–56), malignant thecoma, and dysgerminoma. A frequent ovarian tumor, the Krukenberg tumor (Fig. 25–57), is actually a metastatic tumor to the ovary from the gastrointestinal tract.[188]

The most generally accepted classification of ovarian carinoma is the one proposed by the International Federation of Gynecologists and Obstetricians (FIGO).[189] However, the FIGO staging has been simplified for use in classifying ovarian tumors using CT

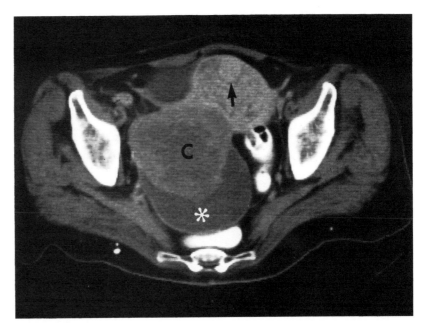

FIGURE 25–54 ■ Adenocarcinoma of the ovary. CT scan demonstrates a poorly differentiated adenocarcinoma of the ovary (C) producing an inhomogeneous pelvic mass containing cystic (asterisk), solid (arrow), and mixed solid and cystic components.

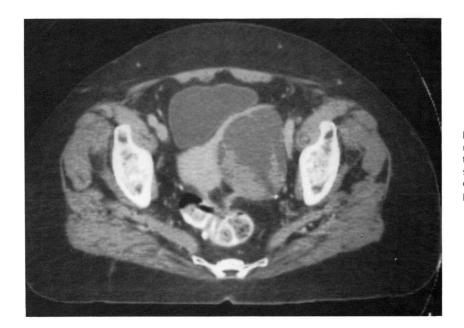

FIGURE 25–55 ■ Papillary serous cystadenocarcinoma of the ovary. CT reveals the tumor as a predominantly cystic mass having slightly irregular margins and a soft tissue component projecting into the low-density portion of the tumor.

scanning (Table 25–4). The main difference between the two classifications is the elimination of subgroups in stage I and II disease.

On CT sections, primary and metastatic ovarian tumors can appear as abdominal or pelvic masses (see Figs. 25–54 and 25–55), as cul-de-sac lesions (Fig. 25–58), or as uni- or bilateral adnexal masses (see Figs. 25–55 and 25–57).[187, 190] Cystadenocarcinomas usually appear on CT as large, predominantly cystic tumors having CT attenuation values ranging from 10 to 20 Hounsfield units (H). The margins of the tumor are irregular, and often there are soft tissue components within the cystic central portion

of the tumor (Figs. 25–55 and 25–59). These features usually permit differentiation between simple cysts and cystadenocarcinomas. Thickened walls, papillary projections, and solid portions were seen in 94 per cent of malignant tumors, but in only 4.8 per cent of benign tumors. Amorphous calcifications and internal septations commonly found in benign cystadenomas are less frequently present in cystadenocarcinomas.

Other ovarian tumors present as mixed solid-cystic (see Fig. 25–57) or predominantly solid masses (see Fig. 25–58) with density readings of 40 to 50 H.[191] CT distinction between histologic types of solid or mixed

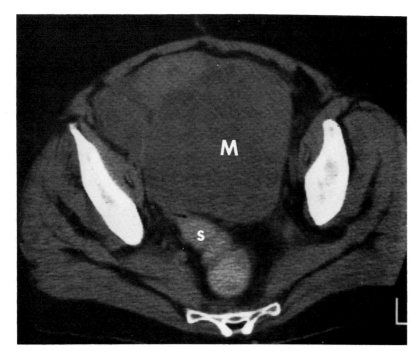

FIGURE 25–56 ■ A malignant, mixed müllerian tumor of the ovary (M) producing a large, inhomogeneous pelvic mass that displaces the sigmoid colon (s) and extends to, but does not invade, the pelvic side walls.

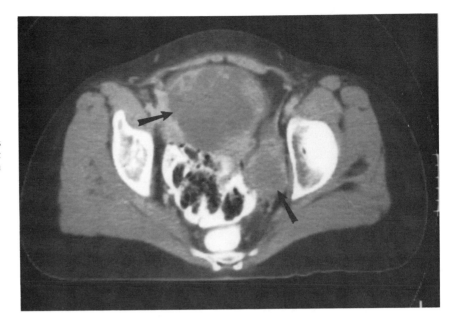

FIGURE 25–57 ■ Bilateral Krukenberg tumors *(arrows)* caused by metastasis from a colonic carcinoma. The ovarian metastases have a mixed cystic and solid appearance.

solid-cystic ovarian tumors is usually not possible, and at times even determining whether a tumor originates from the ovary is impossible (see Figs. 25–56 and 25–58).[192] Invasion of the bladder (see Fig. 25–58), small bowel, or colon can be suggested when there is a loss of adjacent soft tissue planes, but caution must be taken to avoid false-positive diagnoses in thin patients and in situations when a tumor is touching but not invading an adjacent organ. The presence of even small amounts of ascites can be diagnosed accurately by CT, and peritoneal implants and retroperitoneal adenopathy are frequently detected by CT when larger than 2 cm (Fig. 25–60).[191] When recurrent ovarian tumor is present, CT identifies abdominal masses, retroperitoneal or inguinal adenopathy, ascites (see Fig. 25–60), and/or soft tissue masses in the pelvis or cul-de-sac.[193–195]

On MR examination, no morphologic or tissue characteristics of adnexal masses have been reported that are specific for ovarian malignancy, and hence MRI is no more accurate than ultrasound or CT in differentiating benign from malignant ovarian neoplasms.[154, 166–169, 196, 197] However, it has been demonstrated that MRI may be more accurate than either CT or ultrasound in localizing small ovarian tumors.[198]

Although the imaging literature reports that certain morphologic characteristics (e.g., the presence of solid tissue, septations, indistinct margins, mural nodules, or ascites) make an ovarian mass more likely

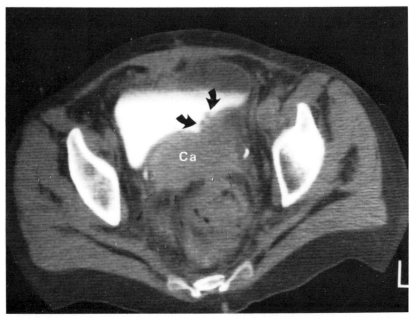

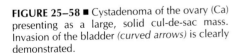

FIGURE 25–58 ■ Cystadenoma of the ovary (Ca) presenting as a large, solid cul-de-sac mass. Invasion of the bladder *(curved arrows)* is clearly demonstrated.

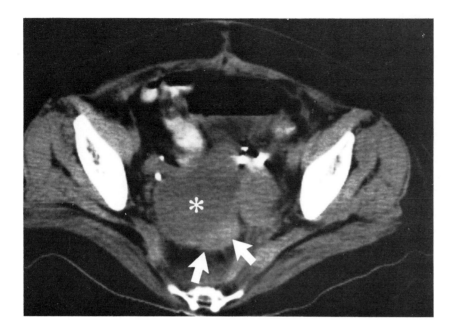

FIGURE 25–59 ■ Papillary cystadenocarcinoma of the ovary. CT scan reveals a large cystic mass *(asterisk)* with slightly irregular margins and a solid component *(arrows)* projecting into the cystic portion of the tumor.

to be malignant, there are many exceptions to these rules.[154, 175, 178, 199] For example, large, solid ovarian masses may be benign, (e.g., fibromas) (Fig. 25–61).[166] Similarly, the MR appearance of cystadenomas, as well as cystadenocarcinomas, has been reported to range from that of a simple cyst to a complex mass containing septations, mural nodules, and both solid and cystic components (Figs. 25–62 and 25–63).[166–168] MR examination has not been shown to differentiate accurately between serous and mucinous epithelial tumors.[166] Hemorrhage has been reported more frequently in serous tumors,[166, 168, 169] whereas mucinous tumors tend to be larger and more septated.[167] In pseudomyxoma peritonei, a complication of mucinous cystadenoma or cystadenocarcinoma of the ovary, MR examination has been reported to demonstrate numerous intraperitoneal masses of high signal intensity on T2-weighted images.[200]

TABLE 25–4 ■ Staging of Ovarian Carcinoma

STAGE		DESCRIPTION
I		Tumor confined to ovaries
	IA	Limited to ovary, no ascites
		1. No tumor on surface
		2. Tumor on external surface; capsule rupture
	IB	Limited to both ovaries
		1. No tumor on surface
		2. Tumor on surface; capsule rupture
	IC	Stage IA or IB with ascites
II		Tumor in one or both ovaries with pelvic extension
	IIA	Uterus or Fallopian tubes involved
	IIB	Other pelvic structures involved
	IIC	Stage IIA or IIB with ascites
III		Tumor involving one or both ovaries; intraperitoneal spread or retroperitoneal nodes; tumor limited to the pelvis but involving bowel or omentum
IV		Tumor involving one or both ovaries with distant metastasis

Although MRI is more accurate in identifying fat, fibrous tissue, and hemorrhage within adnexal masses than are ultrasound and CT (with the possible exception of CT's ability to identify fat),[166, 168] this knowledge is still frequently inadequate to formulate a specific histologic diagnosis. For example, although MRI can readily identify fat in an adnexal mass, MRI has not been reported to be able to differentiate between benign and malignant ovarian teratomas.[166] Because simple fluid, hemorrhage, soft tissue, and fibrous tissue may occur in a wide spectrum of pelvic abnormalities, the lack of specificity of even the most accurate tissue characterization should be not surprising.[200]

Staging ■ Because ultrasonography is safe and inexpensive, it is widely employed as the initial study in evaluating suspected ovarian tumors.[191, 201] However, in one report, accurate sonographic staging was achieved in only 48 per cent of patients with malignant ovarian tumors,[202] as small amounts of ascites were undetected, lymph node metastases were often missed, and small omental and peritoneal implants were not detectable in 55 per cent of patients with ovarian tumors.[202]

Lymphangiography is less helpful in staging ovarian tumors than in staging other pelvic tumors, because a preferential site of nodal involvement cannot be predicted,[201, 203] and microscopic nodal spread is common.

CT has been widely used in staging, in following the effects of therapy, and as an aid to radiation therapy. The principal limitation of CT when compared with second-look surgery has been its low sensitivity in detecting peritoneal, omental, or hepatic implants less than 2 cm in diameter.[194, 195, 204–206] Various authors have reported sensitivity rates ranging from 32 per cent to 52 per cent.[207–209] However, using newer CT techniques, Megibow et al.[195] were

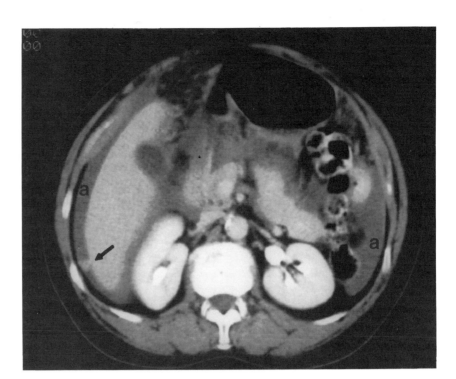

FIGURE 25–60 ■ Ovarian carcinoma. CT scan demonstrates ascites (a) and a small metastatic peritoneal implant *(arrow).*

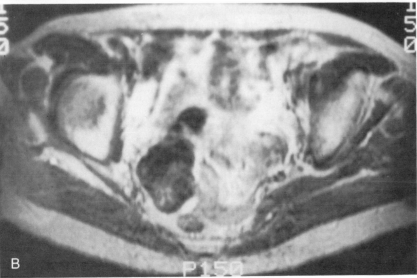

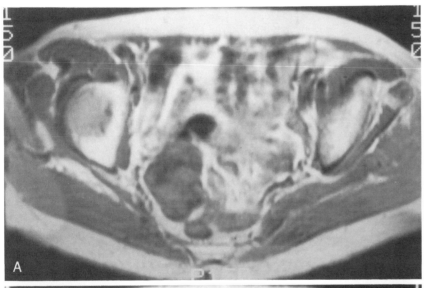

FIGURE 25–61 ■ Ovarian fibroma. *A,* T1-weighted MR scan demonstrates a large, right lobulated ovarian mass of mixed signal intensity. *B,* On a T2-weighted image, the tumor remains predominantly hypointense. Surgery revealed an ovarian fibroma with extensive fibrotic tissue.

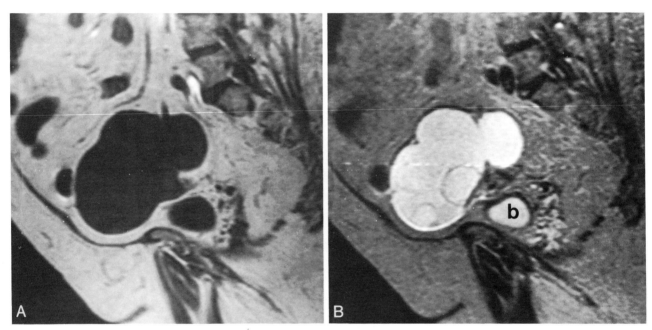

FIGURE 25–62 ■ Mucinous cystadenoma. *A,* Sagittal T1-weighted image demonstrates a lobular mass of homogeneous low signal intensity in the right adnexa. *B,* On T2-weighted images the mass is of high signal intensity, isointense to bladder (b), and internal septations are seen.

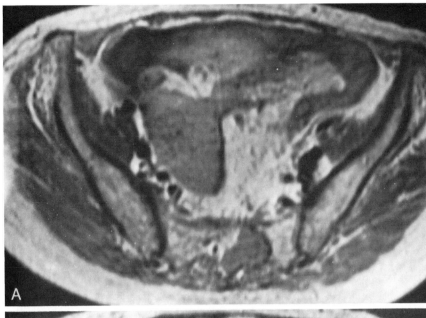

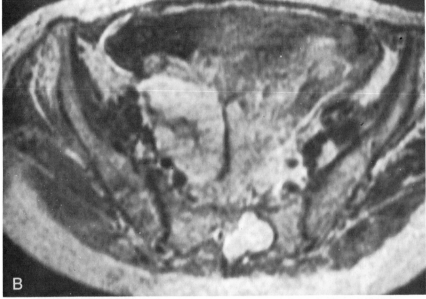

FIGURE 25–63 ■ Serous papillary cystadenocarcinoma. *A*, Intermediate-weighted axial image demonstrates a mass of intermediate signal intensity in the right adnexa. *B*, On T2-weighted images the mass is high signal intensity, and a central low-signal soft tissue area is seen. *C*, Corresponding axial CT scan demonstrates ascites, but no definite mass is seen. Note cystic lesion with a sclerotic margin in the sacrum. The appearance is most consistent with a CSF diverticulum or Tarlov's cyst.

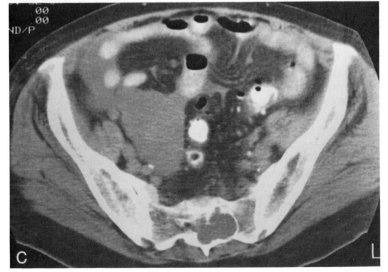

able to increase sensitivity to 78 per cent, and Buy et al. reported a 71 per cent detection rate of metastatic disease in a carefully performed prospective study.[194] It appears that the usefulness of CT in detecting metastatic leasions depends on the location of the implants and the presence of adjacent ascites, rather than on lesion size (see Fig. 25–60).[194]

In the staging of ovarian carcinoma, CT is probably superior to MRI, particularly outside the pelvis, because of a lack of obscuration of peritoneal surfaces by peristalsis during the shorter scan times of CT.[197, 207, 208] Following debulking surgery and chemotherapy, MRI has been reported to be equivalent to CT in the demonstration of persistent or recurrent disease, such as lymph node metastases and peritoneal masses.[209] However, because both imaging modalities may miss small (less than 2 cm) serosal implants, some investigators feel that neither CT nor MRI can replace second-look surgery.[198, 200, 207–210] However, a positive CT or MR examination may help the clinician by either making second-look surgery unnecessary or directing the surgeon to the location of recurrent disease.[210]

Uterus

Pathology

BENIGN ABNORMALITIES

Most benign uterine conditions can be effectively evaluated with a combination of bimanual pelvic examination and ultrasonography. Ultrasound is the primary method of locating intrauterine contraceptive devices (IUDs);[211] examining suspected molar pregnancy;[212] detecting endometrial fluid collections unassociated with pregnancy[213] and hydrocolpos and hydrometrocolpos;[214] viewing the persistently retroverted gravid uterus; examining the gravid uterus for gestational age; and checking for suspected abnormal pregnancy, ectopic pregnancy, endouterine abnormalities, endometriosis, myomas, and fetal anomalies.[215–217] In many of these abnormalities CT has proven to be a valuable complementary method for examining the uterus. More recently, MRI has been demonstrated to be able to provide valuable and unique information in a variety of uterine abnormalities.

Intrauterine Devices ■ Although ultrasonography has been the method of choice for locating intrauterine devices (IUDs), the sonographic differentiation among various types of IUDs is accurate only for the Lippes loop (78 per cent to 94 per cent) and the Copper-7 device (81 per cent), and precise sonographic localization of extrauterine devices can be difficult.[211] If the ultrasonographic findings are equivocal, CT can be used to determine the type of device and identify an intra- or extrauterine location of the IUD (Fig. 25–64).[218]

When performing a CT examination, radiation exposure should be kept to an absolute minimum. A preliminary digital scout radiograph can locate the position of the IUD and thus reduce the number of CT scans necessary to locate and characterize the IUD. Additional radiation reduction is achieved by performing CT scans for IUD localization at the lowest possible exposure factors.

Endometriosis ■ Endometriosis is defined as the presence of functioning endometrium located outside the uterus. The ectopic endometrium is responsive to ovarian hormonal stimulation and, like the normotopic endometrium, undergoes repeated cycles of hemorrhage. The end result is the development of endometriomas, or chocolate cysts. The cysts are often multiple and coalesce. Adhesions, fibrosis, and scarring frequently occur. Endometriosis most frequently involves the ovary (50 per cent bilateral), uterosacral ligaments, cul-de-sac, posterior wall of the lower uterus, and fallopian tubes, but implantation can occur on any intraperitoneal serosal surface, and distant spread to lymph nodes, lung, muscle, and bone have been reported.[219, 220]

Endometriosis has an incidence ranging from 8 to 30 per cent in women undergoing gynecologic surgery.[221] Patients most commonly present with pelvic pain, dysmenorrhea, infertility, or dyspareunia. The severity of the symptoms is not necssarily related to the pathologic extent of disease. Patients are treated either surgically or with hormonal therapy, depending on the severity of symptoms and the extent of disease.[219, 220]

Endometriosis usually produces sharply delineated spherical lesions, most frequently located in the cul-de-sac, that sonographically appear as cystic or predominantly cystic adnexal masses, with echoes confined to the periphery or dependent portion of the mass.[156] However, a specific diagnosis of endometriosis can be suggested by ultrasound only if it is strongly supported by the clinical history, as similar sonographic features are seen in a variety of gynecologic abnormalities.[222]

The CT findings in endometriosis are varied.[223, 224] There may be a thickening of the tissues adjacent to the ovaries or uterus or involvement of the bladder, rectum (Fig. 25–65), small bowel, or abdominal wall by single or multiple solid masses or fluid-filled cysts. The cul-de-sac of the pelvis is the most common site for endometriosis (see Fig. 25–65); however, even when endometriosis is present, a definitive CT diagnosis cannot be made without a typical history. If extensive chronic disease is present, a correct CT diagnosis is very difficult, as the loss of tissue planes mimics a primary or metastatic pelvic malignancy.

On MRI examination, endometriosis typically appears as multiple cystic lesions with signal behavior consistent with the presence of varying stages of hemorrhage (Figs. 25–66 and 25–67).[225–228] Most commonly, endometriotic cysts have high signal intensity on both T1- and T2-weighted sequences and are higher in signal intensity than either fat or fluid (urine) (see Fig. 25–67).[228] However, lesions may be hypointense on both T1- and T2-weighted sequences or even hyperintense on T1-weighted images and

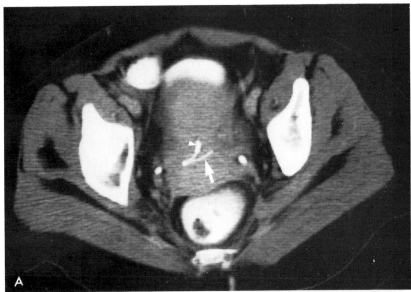

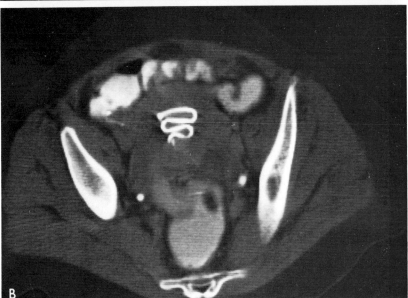

FIGURE 25–64 ■ CT documentation of intrauterine position of two intrauterine devices (IUDs). *A,* CT cross section reveals a Copper-7 *(arrow)* and Lippes loop *(arrowhead)* IUD within the intrauterine lumen. The uterus contains multiple leiomyomas. *B,* The Lippes loop is better demonstrated on a CT scan obtained at a higher level.

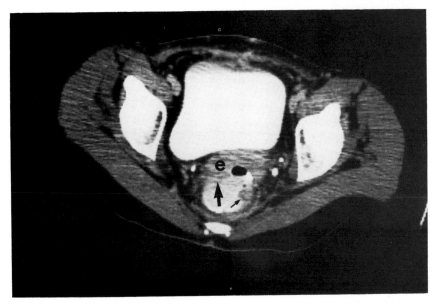

FIGURE 25–65 ■ Endometriosis (e) located in the cul-de-sac, producing irregularities in the anterior rectal wall *(large arrow)*. A small focus of endometriosis *(small arrow)* involves the left lateral wall of the rectum.

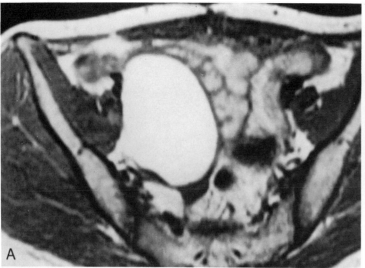

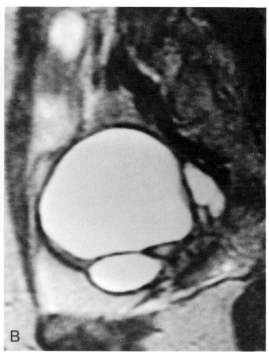

FIGURE 25–66 ■ Endometriosis. *A*, Axial T1-weighted image *B*, Sagittal T2-weighted image demonstrates numerous cysts with angular margins in the right adnexa. Note that at least two of these cysts are hyperintense on both T1- and T2-weighted images, which is consistent with the presence of subacute hemorrhage.

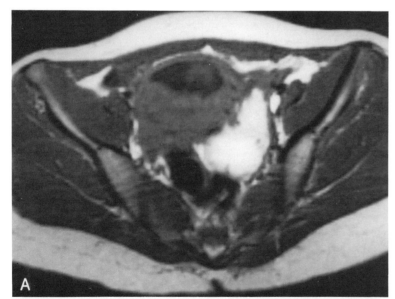

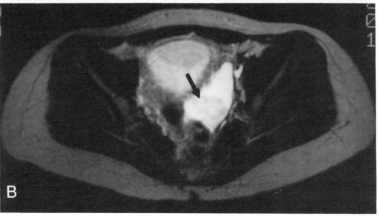

FIGURE 25–67 ■ Endometriosis. *A*, T1-weighted MR scan reveals a left pelvic mass of very high signal intensity. *B*, On a T2-weighted pulse sequence, the endometrioma has portions that are much brighter than fat. There are also nodular and papillary excrescences seen as regions of lower signal intensity within the endometrioma *(arrow)*.

becoming hypointense on T2-weighted scans. Hazy, ill-defined areas of low signal intensity within endometriotic cysts, described as shading, may be observed on the T2-weighted images (see Fig. 25–67).[225, 226] Signal void areas, reflecting chronic hemorrhage with the accumulation of hemosiderin-laden macrophages, may also be present.[227] Similarly, a hypointense or signal void rim can be seen and is believed to represent either fibrosis or the presence of peripheral hemosiderin-laden macrophages. The edges of the cyst are often hazy or angular because of the presence of adhesions.[225, 226] Rectal tethering is highly suggestive of endometriosis, and the classic appearance on MRI is of a tear-shaped rectum with the point directed toward the ovary or uterus.[226]

MRI is superior to both CT and ultrasound in accurately diagnosing endometriosis.[229, 230] The sensitivity of MRI in diagnosing endometriosis has ranged from 64 per cent to 71 per cent and the specificity from 60 per cent to 83 per cent.[225–227] Although hemorrhagic cysts and even mesenteric fat may have a MR appearance similar to that of endometriosis,[225–227] when multiple cystic lesions with acutely angulated margins and signal behavior consistent with the presence of hemorrhage are visualized on MR examination, endometriosis should be considered first in the differential diagnosis.[228] Although MRI should not replace laparoscopy for either the staging or diagnosis of endometriosis, it is useful as a screening test for establishing the presence of endometriosis in a patient with questionable clinical or ultrasound presentation or in a patient with an adnexal mass of uncertain cause.[166] Additionally, MRI has been shown to be helpful in monitoring response to therapy or in evaluating patients with pelvic adhesions that hamper adequate surgical evaluation.[227]

Adenomyosis ■ Adenomyosis is defined as the presence of endometrium inside the myometrium. The heterotopic endometrium is usually resistant to hormonal stimulation, and hemorrhage is infrequently observed.[231] Foci of adenomyosis are surrounded by hypertrophied smooth muscle, which interdigitates with the smooth muscle of the normal myometrium without forming a sharp border. Adenomyosis may be microscopic, focal, or diffuse. Although the exact incidence is unknown, adenomyosis has been found in 8 per cent to 20 per cent of hysterectomy specimens.[231]

Adenomyosis is most commonly diagnosed in multiparous, premenopausal women during the fifth decade. Hypermenorrhea, dysmenorrhea, and an enlarged uterus are the most common presenting symptoms, but these are nonspecific complaints and may be seen in patients with dysfunctional uterine bleeding or leiomyomas. Although the definitive treatment of adenomyosis is hysterectomy, dysfunctional uterine bleeding may be controlled with dilatation and curettage (D and C) and symptomatic leiomyomas may be removed via myomectomy. Hence the differentiation between these entities is important for patient management.

Although CT and ultrasonography have little to offer, several recent studies have reported that MRI is highly accurate in the diagnosis of adenomyosis.[232–234] Togashi et al.[234] were able to distinguish adenomyosis from leiomyoma in 92 of 93 women who presented with the uterine enlargement. They and other authors describe focal adenomyosis on T2-weighted images as ill-defined areas of low signal intensity located within the myometrium, but contiguous with the junctional zone.[232–234] Diffuse adenomyosis is characterized by generalized thickening, either even or uneven (>5 mm), of the junctional zone (Fig. 25–68).[232] Occasionally small foci of increased signal intensity on both T1- and T2-weighted images are seen in adenomyosis that pathologically correspond to small foci of hemorrhagic endometrium.[233] Focal adenomyosis often has an ill-defined border, whereas the border around leiomyomas is sharp. However, small leiomyomas (<2 to 3 cm) may also occasionally have ill-defined borders and may therefore not be distinguishable from focal adenomyosis on MR examination.

Uterine Leiomyoma ■ Leiomyomas are smooth muscle cell tumors containing varying amounts of fibrous tissue. The smooth muscle cells have a swirling configuration and are sharply demarcated from surrounding myometrium. The uterine leiomyoma or fibroid is a common benign tumor in adult women, affecting approximately 20 per cent of women older than 30 years of age. Although many patients are asymptomatic, others may present with menorrhagia, dysmenorrhea, infertility, habitual second trimester abortion, or pelvic pain or pressure.[231] In general, the lobulated masses projecting from the outer surfaces of the uterus are subserosal, the intracavitary masses are submucosal, and the masses obliterating the uterine cavity are intramural in location. Habitual abortion or infertility may be caused by any leiomyoma that distorts the endometrial cav-

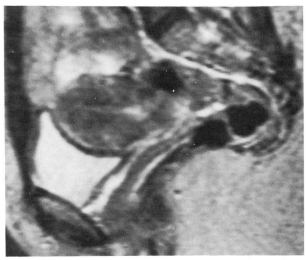

FIGURE 25–68 ■ Adenomyosis. Sagittal T2-weighted image through the uterus demonstrates diffuse irregular thickening of the junctional zone.

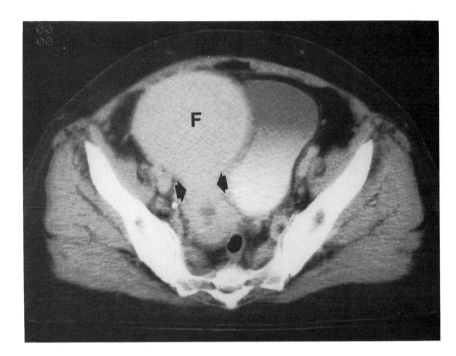

FIGURE 25–69 ■ Pedunculated uterine fibroid. CT scan reveals a large, solid, enhancing mass (F) arising from the uterus on a narrow stalk *(arrows)*.

ity or blocks the oviducts. Menorrhagia is most commonly associated with submucosal leiomyomas.

Major CT features suggesting a diagnosis of a uterine leiomyoma include (1) a focal solid mass causing a lobulation and/or protrusion from the outer margin of the uterus (Fig. 25–69), (2) soft tissue masses that distort or obliterate the uterine cavity (Fig. 25–70), (3) areas of calcification within uterine masses (Fig. 25–71), and (4) irregular, low-density areas within uterine masses representing degeneration of a leiomyoma (Figs. 25–70 and 25–72).[235]

Occasionally myomas produce diffuse enlargement of the uterus. Solid noncalcified uterine myomas usually cannot be distinguished from other solid uterine masses, but occasionally a diagnosis of a

uterine lipoleiomyoma can be made when CT demonstrates a well-encapsulated uterine mass that is predominantly the density of fat (-70 to -100 H).[236]

Other investigations have demonstrated MRI to be the most accurate imaging modality for the detection and localization of leiomyomas.[153, 234, 237–240] Leiomyomas are low signal intensity on T2-weighted images in comparison with the intermediate signal intensity of the surrounding myometrium. They are sharply marginated and usually homogeneous in signal intensity unless degenerated, in which case they contain central areas of increased signal intensity on T2-weighted images (Fig. 25–73). Lesions as small as 0.3 cm are easily classified on MR examination as submucosal, intramural, subserosal, or cervical in loca-

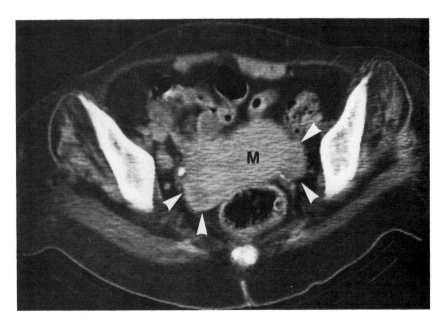

FIGURE 25–70 ■ Uterine myoma (M) producing a lobulated uterine mass. The mass obliterates the uterine cavity and has two rounded protrusions *(arrowheads)* with low-density centers.

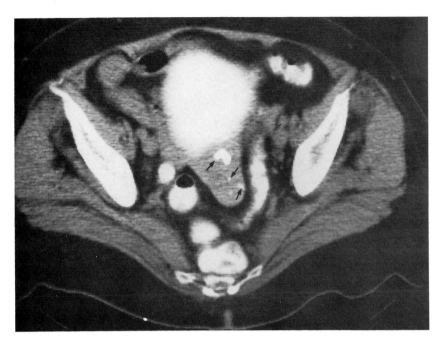

FIGURE 25–71 ■ Typical calcifications (arrows) in a smoothly lobulated myoma of the uterus.

tion. In a recently reported series, Hricak et al.[237] accurately identified nine of nine subserosal, 37 of 37 intramural, and 10 of 11 subserosal leiomyomas. It is generally not possible to differentiate malignant degeneration from hyaline, myxomatous, fatty, or mucinous degeneration on MR examination.[237] Malignant degeneration, however, occurs only infrequently (0.1 to 0.6 per cent of cases).[231] However, when a sharply marginated border is not definable on MR examination or when a leiomyoma enlarges suddenly following menopause, malignant degeneration should be considered.

In the evaluation of a woman presenting with an adnexal mass, MRI is more specific than ultrasound or CT.[166, 168, 209] A recent prospective study of 127 pelvic masses demonstrated that MRI had a sensitivity of 100 per cent with a specificity of 99 per cent in diagnosing cystic teratomas of the ovary, a sensitivity of 90 per cent with a specificity of 100 per cent in diagnosing uterine leiomyomas, and a sensitivity of 93 per cent with a specificity of 91 per cent in diagnosing endometriosis.[166] In addition, MRI is extremely useful in clarifying whether a mass is ovarian or uterine in origin in the face of an equivocal ultrasound, CT, or physical examination (Fig. 25–74).[153, 166, 168, 240]

Endometrial Polyps ■ Endometrial polyps are focal areas of hyperplasia of both the glands and stroma of the basal endometrium found in approximately ten per cent of hysterectomy specimens.[231] Polyps are usually located in the uterine fundus and are solitary and either sessile or pedunculated masses 2 to 4 cm in diameter. Invasive carcinoma is extremely rare.[231]

FIGURE 25–72 ■ Degenerating fibroids. CT scan demonstrates very large mass lesions having a predominantly cystic appearance. A more solid-appearing leiomyoma (M) has not yet undergone cystic degeneration.

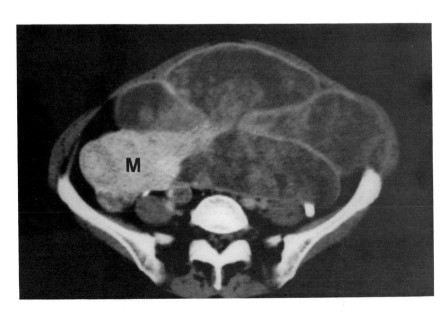

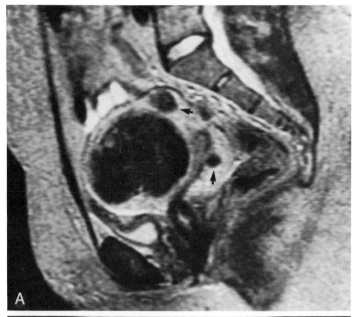

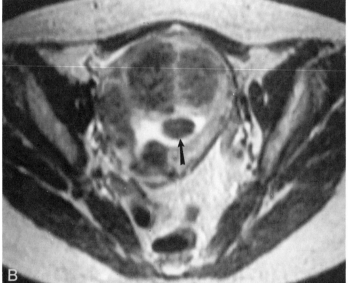

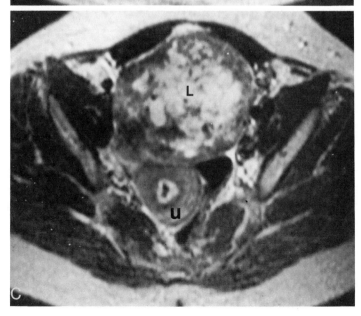

FIGURE 25–73 ■ Leiomyoma. *A,* Sagittal T2-weighted image through the uterus demonstrates two small, well-circumscribed areas of low signal intensity within the myometrium *(arrows).* These represent small intramural leiomyomas. A large intramural leiomyoma is also seen. *B,* Axial T2-weighted image of a submucosal leiomyoma. Note the mass of low signal intensity within the endometrial cavity *(arrow).* Several intramural leiomyomas are also present. *C,* Axial T2-weighted image demonstrates a large subserosal leiomyoma (L). Ill-defined areas of central increased signal intensity within this mass are indicative of degeneration. Signal void area within the endometrial cavity most likely represents clot. u = Uterus.

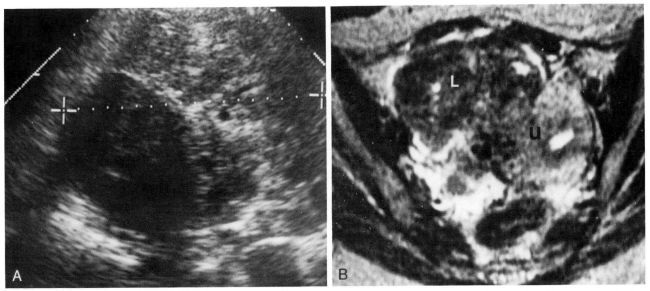

FIGURE 25–74 ■ *A,* Oblique ultrasound image demonstrates a hypoechoic mass adjacent to the uterus. Ultrasound could not clarify whether the mass was adnexal or a subserosal leiomyoma. *B,* Axial T2-weighted MRI scan demonstrates a predunculated low-signal-intensity lobular mass in the right adnexa consistent with a subserosal leiomyoma (L). u = Uterus.

On MR examination, an endometrial polyp may be suspected when a mass of intermediate signal intensity is noted within the endometrial cavity (Fig. 25–75). A peripheral linear area of low signal intensity may be noted, possibly representing fibrous tissue within the stalk of the polyp. The normal uterine zonal architecture is preserved. However, if the polyp is small or sessile, the uterus may appear entirely normal or demonstrate nonspecific widening of the endometrial cavity. It is not known whether an endometrial polyp can be accurately differentiated from noninvasive or superficial endometrial cancer.

MISCELLANEOUS UTERINE ABNORMALITIES

Congenital Anomalies ■ In women presenting with infertility or repeated spontaneous abortions, the incidence of congenital anomalies of the female reproductive tract has been reported to be as high as nine per cent.[241] A spectrum of anomalies can occur (Table 25–5). Renal anomalies, most frequently renal agenesis or ectopia, are often associated with congenital anomalies of the female reproductive tract.[242]

Clinical manifestations vary widely. Patients with uterus didelphys may be asymptomatic and lead a normal reproductive life. However, uterine anoma-

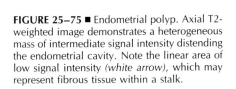

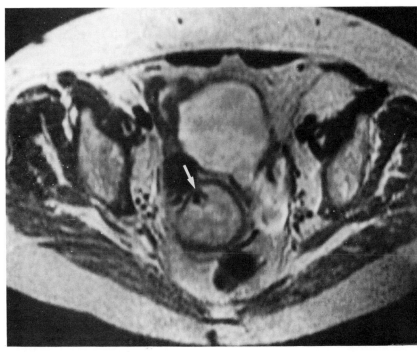

FIGURE 25–75 ■ Endometrial polyp. Axial T2-weighted image demonstrates a heterogeneous mass of intermediate signal intensity distending the endometrial cavity. Note the linear area of low signal intensity *(white arrow),* which may represent fibrous tissue within a stalk.

TABLE 25–5 ■ Classification of Congenital Uterine Anomalies

TYPE	ANOMALY
I	Segmental müllerian agenesis or hypoplasia Vaginal, cervical, fundal, tubal, or combined
II	Unicornuate uterus A. Rudimentary horn present that may or may not communicate with main uterine cavity B. No rudimentary horn
III	Uterus didelphys
IV	Bicornuate uterus A. Septation complete to internal os B. Partial C. Arcuate uterus
V	Septate uterus A. Septation complete to internal/external os B. Partial
VI	Uterus with internal luminal changes

Source: Adapted from Buttram VC, Gibbons WE: Mullerian anomalies: a proposed classification (an analysis of 144 cases). Fertil Steril 32:40–46, 1979. Reproduced with permission of the publisher, The American Fertility Society.

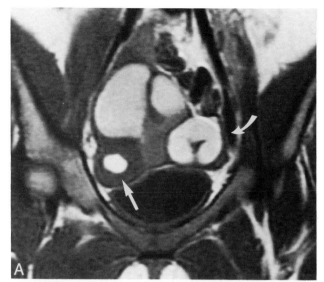

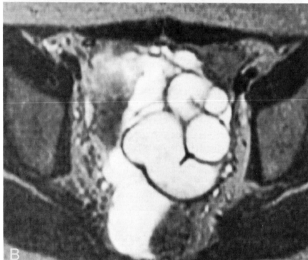

FIGURE 25–76 ■ Vaginal septum. *A,* Coronal T1-weighted image demonstrates hematometra *(straight arrow)* and hematosalpinx *(curved arrow)*. *B,* Axial T2-weighted image demonstrating hematosalpinx.

lies, particularly the septate uterus, may be associated with infertility or fetal loss as a result of repeated spontaneous abortion, premature labor, and/or fetal malpresentation.[243, 244] Because the clinical management of the different uterine anomalies varies considerably, precise preoperative diagnosis is critical.

Except for demonstrating abnormalities in position, CT has had little impact on the diagnosis of congenital anomalies of the reproductive tract. Hysterosalpingography (HSG) and ultrasound have been the primary imaging modalities, but each has its own limitations.

Several recent studies have demonstrated that MRI can accurately distinguish between the bicornuate and septate uterus.[245, 246] On MRI examination, it is important to obtain scans coronally through the corpus. Hence oblique scans through the pelvis may be required depending on the degree of uterine flexion. The demonstration of a fundal notch or indentation is diagnostic of a bicornuate uterus. An outwardly convex fundal contour documents a septate uterus.[245–248]

Other uterine anomalies are also readily identified with MRI. The unicornuate uterus has an elongated, banana-like shape that is quite unlike the triangular shape of a normal uterus.[246, 248] The arcuate uterus is diagnosed by its heart-shaped endometrial cavity and flat fundal contour.[246] In uterus didelphys, two separate uteri and cervices are visualized. Differentiating a double cervix from a cervical septation can be difficult,[248] as transverse septations or segmental hypoplasia may be difficult to resolve. However, the obstruction created by a vaginal septum can produce a hematosalpinx, hematometra, or hematocolpos that can be readily diagnosed on MR examination (Fig. 25–76). MRI can be used to document the uterine hypoplasia, hydrosalpinx, and/or T-shaped, constricted uterine cavity that occur in patients exposed in utero to diethylstilbestrol.

Abscess ■ Uterine abscesses following surgery and pyometrium (Fig. 25–77) from a variety of origins are

readily demonstrated by CT. Gas within the wall of the uterus may be indicative of an intrauterine abscess, especially if the inner margins of the uterus are irregular. Differentiating a pyometrium from other causes of uterine fluid collections is possible if gas is noted within the area of low density.

Intrauterine gas also can result from malignant uterine tumors (Fig. 25–78) or can be iatrogenically introduced or follow surgery. Bacterial metabolism of necrotic neoplastic tissue is thought to be the major mechanism responsible for the production of intrauterine gas in patients with uterine malignancy.

Gravid Uterus ■ CT is not usually used to study the gravid uterus, but occasionally a pelvic scan will be performed in a patient who does not know she is pregnant. In early pregnancies, CT demonstrates an enlarged, thick-walled uterus containing a fluid-filled gestational sac. CT scans performed later in preg-

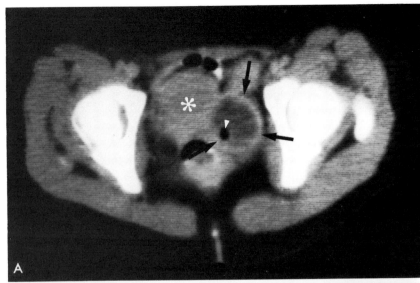

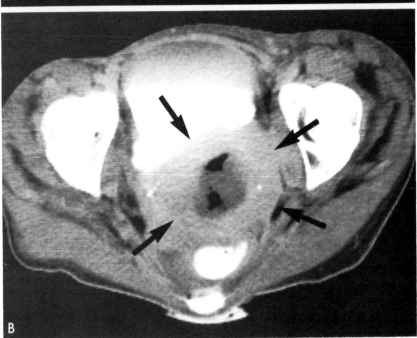

FIGURE 25–77 ■ Pyometrium of the uterus. *A,* An oval low-density mass *(arrows)* containing air *(arrowhead)* represents a pyometrium in a patient with a bicornuate uterus and an obstructed left horn. The unobstructed right horn *(asterisk)* has a normal soft tissue density. *B,* An enlarged thick-walled uterus *(arrows)* containing a central collection of fluid and air represents a hydrocolpos and pyometrium in a patient with cervical carcinoma obstructing the uterus.

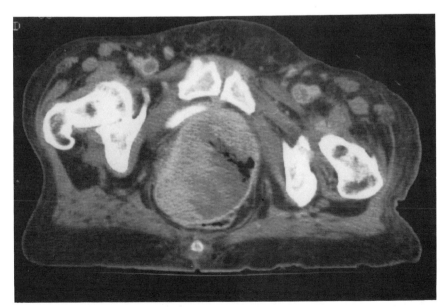

FIGURE 25–78 ■ CT scan of a uterine sarcoma demonstrates that the tumor contains small foci of gas.

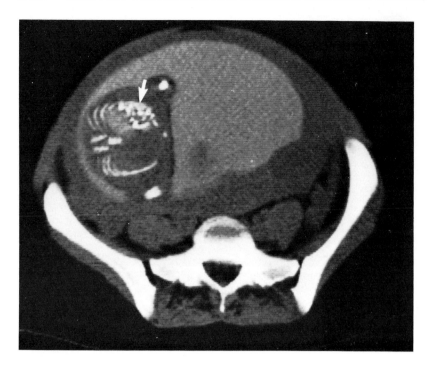

FIGURE 25–79 ■ A CT scan following instillation of contrast material into the amniotic sac reveals a single intrauterine pregnancy and contrast-filled bowel *(arrow)* present within the left chest, resulting from the presence of a fetal diaphragmatic hernia.

nancy demonstrate the fetal skeleton and, rarely, detect fetal anomalies (Fig. 25–79). CT scans obtained shortly after delivery reveal an enlarged uterus with a diffusely thickened wall and a central cavity (Fig. 25–80).

MALIGNANT UTERINE DISEASE

Endometrial Carcinoma ■ Endometrial carcinoma is the most frequent invasive gynecologic malignancy, most commonly presenting with postmenopausal bleeding in women older than 50 years.[250] Choice of treatment is dependent on depth of myometrial invasion, histologic grade, and tumor stage (Table 25–6).[251] Simple curettage, hysterectomy, surgery followed by radiotherapy, radiation with subsequent hysterectomy or chemotherapy, and external irradia-

tion are used, depending on extent and histologic features of the tumor.[252–254]

Clinical assessment of tumor extent has historically been unreliable, but CT, ultrasonography and (more recently) MRI have been utilized in an attempt to decrease the number of treatment failures by more accurately staging endometrial carcinoma.

Transabdominal ultrasonography has been evaluated as a method to detect and stage endometrial carcinoma.[164, 255, 256] Results to date have not shown ultrasonography to have a major role in detecting stage I or II endometrial carcinoma. Transabdominal ultrasonography cannot be used to exclude a tumor and is insensitive for detecting depth of tumor invasion and extrauterine extension and thus has a limited role in staging endometrial carcinoma.

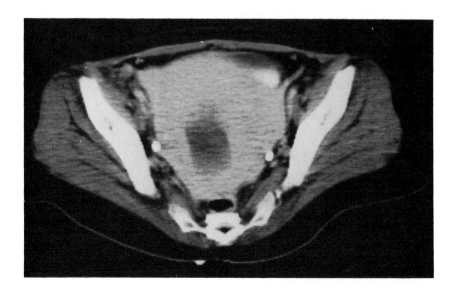

FIGURE 25–80 ■ A CT scan shortly following delivery demonstrates a normally enlarged uterus with thick walls and a central fluid cavity.

TABLE 25–6 ■ FIGO Staging System for Endometrial Cancer

STAGE	DESCRIPTION
I	Carcinoma confined to uterine corpus
A G123	Tumor limited to endometrium
B G123	Tumor invasion through < 50% myometrial wall thickness
C G123	Tumor invasion through > 50% myometrium
II	Carcinoma has invaded cervix
A G123	Endocervical glandular involvement only
B G123	Cervical stromal invasion
III	Carcinoma has invaded true pelvis without bladder or rectal invasion but including pelvic and para-aortic lymph nodes
IV	Carcinoma has extended outside true pelvis, including bladder or rectal invasion

Source: Creasman WT: New gynecologic cancer staging. Obstet Gynecol 75:287–288, 1990.

CT has been widely employed to detect, stage, and follow the effects of therapy in patients with endometrial carcinoma.[257–263] Endometrial carcinoma is demonstrated on contrast-enhanced CT scans as a hypodense lesion surrounded by densely opacified normal endometrium (Fig. 25–81).[260, 261] The hypodense area represents necrotic tumor of varying degree. On CT sections, submucosal leiomyomas, particularly if they undergo cystic changes, cannot be differentiated from endometrial carcinoma (see Fig. 25–72). However, only five per cent of leiomyomas occur in a submucosal location, and these tend to regress after menopause, reducing the likelihood of confusion with endometrial carcinoma.

Carcinoma of the endometrium usually produces focal or global enlargement of the uterine body (Figs. 25–81 and 25–82). The attenuation values of endo-

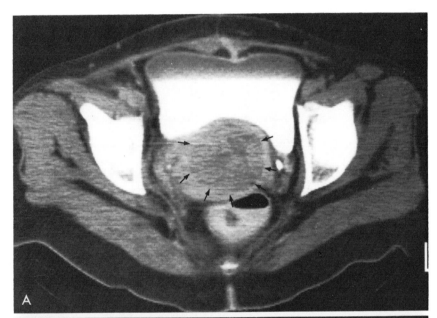

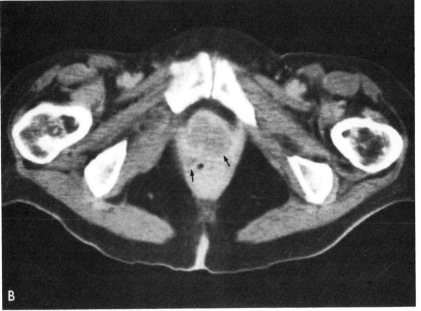

FIGURE 25–81 ■ Endometrial carcinoma. *A,* CT scan following intravenous infusion of contrast material demonstrates a hypodense lesion *(arrows)*, representing necrotic tumor, sharply demarcated from normal endometrium. *B,* Postcontrast CT study demonstrates that uterine tissue enhances more than foci of endometrial carcinoma *(arrows)*.

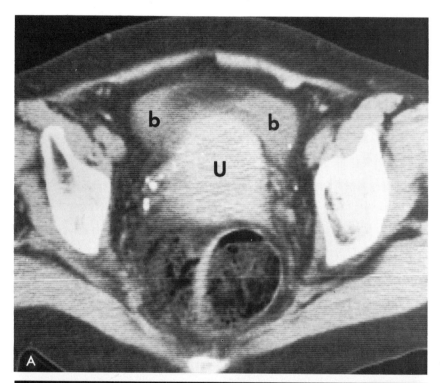

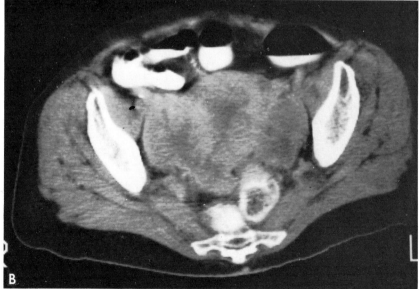

FIGURE 25–82 ■ Endometrial carcinoma producing focal enlargement of the uterus (U). In this patient, the carcinoma has a uniform solid appearance. There is preservation of the fat planes between the uterus and rectum and uterus and bladder (b), indicating lack of direct tumor spread. *B*, Global enlargement of the uterus. There are multiple areas of tumor necrosis, and the tumor fills the entire pelvis.

MR examination, or the endometrial stripe may be widened but have a normal, homogeneous high signal intensity on T2-weighted images. Occasionally a mass of intermediate to high signal intensity on T2-weighted images distends the endometrial cavity without disrupting the junctional zone.[30, 268–274] Experience to date indicates MRI to be 74 per cent to 85 per cent accurate in differentiating noninvasive superficial endometrial cancer from invasive disease.[30, 271–274] However, endometrial polyps, adenomatous hyperplasia, and hemorrhage have all been reported to have similar appearances on MRI examinations,[30, 272] and Ascher et al.[276] have reported that blood clot within the endometrial cavity can appear as a linear area of signal void 1 week after D and C.

MRI also can accurately depict cervical invasion by endometrial carcinoma, as positive results have been reported even when fractional endocervical curettage (ECC) is negative or inconclusive.[271, 274] However, the number of reported cases with pathologic proof is far too small to generate accuracy values. Stage IIA carcinoma, invasion of the endocervical glands, may be suspected on T2-weighted images by distention of the endocervical canal with or without visualization of a mass isointense to the primary tumor.[269] Deep cervical spread to the fibrous cervical stroma, stage IIB, is diagnosed on T2-weighted images when a mass isointense to the primary tumor invades and disrupts the low signal intensity of the fibrous cervical stoma.[30, 270–274]

Extrauterine spread of endometrial carcinoma is most commonly found in patients with deep myometrial invasion, papillary serous carcinomas, or histologic grade III tumors.[30, 277, 278] Direct extension of the tumor mass through the serosal surface of the uterus disrupting the signal intensity of the parametrial fat is indicative of parametrial spread.[30, 268] Ovarian metastases most commonly appear as masses of intermediate signal intensity replacing the normal signal intensity of the ovarian stroma.[30, 271, 273] The criterion for diagnosing lymph node metastases by tumor is length greater than 1.5 cm in the pelvic or periaortic regions.[30, 268, 271] Peritoneal or omental tumor implants usually have an intermediate signal intensity on T1-weighted images and higher signal intensity on T2-weighted images. Because of the small number of patients with pathologic correlation, the sensitivity and specificity of documenting extrauterine spread of endometrial cancer on MR examination is not known, although MRI has been reported to compare favorably with CT.[30] However, microscopic spread of disease to lymph nodes, ovaries, parametria, or cervix, as well as small (<2 cm) peritoneal or omental implants, will not be routinely identified on MR examination.[30, 268, 271, 273, 274]

CT is useful in planning intracavitary irradiation by providing measurements of the uterus and cervix, as well as three-dimensional anatomic information that enables selection of the appropriate applicator for proper implantation of radioactive sources.[278] CT accurately determines the relationship of the applicator to adjacent structures, and based on CT, radiation treatment can be individualized in regard to total radiation dose and the number and spatial distribution of radioactive sources.[257]

Recurrent Endometrial Carcinoma ■ Recurrent disease most frequently is confined to the pelvis, producing symptoms of low back or sciatic pain, leg edema, or obstructive uropathy. CT can be employed to assess the pelvis for recurrent endometrial carcinoma. Data obtained by CT regarding the presence or absence of a tumor mass (Fig. 25–87A) and extension of tumor (Fig. 25–87B, C) complement the physical examination and facilitate appropriate therapeutic decisions.

CT can detect recurrent uterine carcinoma with greater than 80 per cent accuracy. Most false-positive results are related to radiation changes that simulate recurrent tumor. MRI shows promise of aiding in this differentiation. False-negative results on MRI are related to small superficial tumor deposits in the perineum or vagina.

Sarcoma ■ Although sarcomas are rare uterine tumors, accounting for only three per cent of malignant uterine neoplasms, they are the most lethal of all uterine malignancies.[250] Leiomyosarcoma is the most common uterine sarcoma and is believed to arise in preexisting leiomyomas,[250] although malignant degeneration must be extremely rare, considering the prevalence of benign myomas. CT demonstrates uterine enlargement with inhomogeneity and zones of low attenuation. Although foci of calcification may be present, the CT features are usually identical to those of endometrial carcinoma and do not permit a preoperative diagnosis of uterine sarcoma to be made.

Gestational Trophoblastic Neoplasia ■ Gestational trophoblastic neoplasia (GTN) is a spectrum of proliferative abnormalities of trophoblasts ranging from partial and complete hydatiform mole to persistent (invasive) GTN and choriocarcinoma.[212, 279] The biologic behavior varies from the rarely invasive hydatidiform mole to the highly aggressive choriocarcinoma. A complete mole is characterized by swelling of chorionic villi, which are enveloped by atypical, hyperplastic trophoblasts. Partial moles exhibit only focal swelling of chorionic villi.[279] Persistent GTN refers to both locally invasive disease and distant metastases. Metastases occur most frequently to the lungs (80 per cent), vagina (30 per cent), pelvis (20 per cent), liver, and brain.[279, 280] Persistent GTN most commonly follows a complete hydatidiform mole but may occur subsequent to any gestational event, including abortion, ectopic pregnancy, or term pregnancy. Treatment varies according to degree of invasion and presence of metastases. Evacuation of a molar pregnancy is curative in most patients. Patients are usually followed by measuring serum β-human chorionic gonadotropin (β-hCG) levels, which are sensitive indicators of the presence of disease. A rise or plateau in the serum β-hCG level following evac-

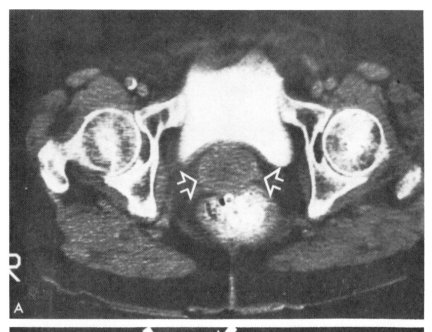

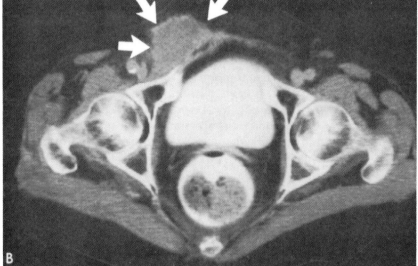

FIGURE 25–87 ■ Patterns of recurrent endometrial carcinoma. *A,* A solid pelvic mass *(arrows)* following total hysterectomy. *B,* Invasion of the abdominal wall *(arrows)* by a large necrotic tumor mass. *C,* Endometrial carcinoma encasing the left ureter *(arrow).*

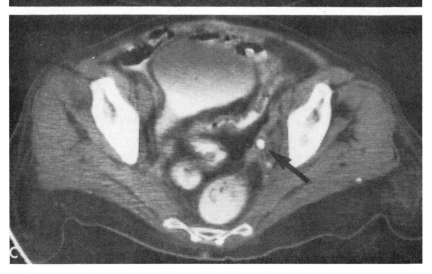

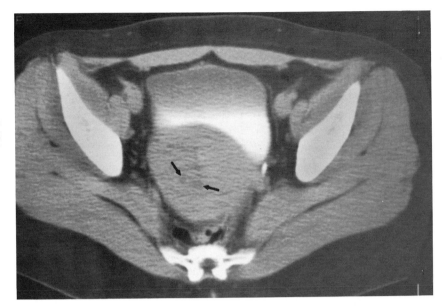

FIGURE 25–88 ■ Gestational trophoblastic neoplasia producing a uterine mass having sharp margins and several central foci of low attenuation value *(arrows)*.

uation is diagnostic of invasive or persistent GTN. Peristent GTN is extremely sensitive to chemotherapy, and even patients with distant metastases have a cure rate approaching 100 per cent.

Although the diagnosis of hydatidiform mole and persistent GTN is made clinically using serum β-hCG levels, diagnostic imaging can play a useful role in certain clinical settings. Ultrasound excludes the presence of a normal intrauterine gestation and may demonstrate distention of the uterine cavity by a soft tissue mass containing numerous small cystic spaces. However, hydropic degeneration of the placenta, missed abortions, and degenerating fibroids may have a similar appearance. In patients with persistently elevated serum β-hCG levels following molar evacuation, ultrasound is useful to exclude intrauterine pregnancy and may demonstrate focal areas of increased echogenicity within the uterus.[279] CT scanning of the chest, abdomen, and pelvis is used to detect both local extension of disease and distant metastases in patients with gestational trophoblastic disease. The CT scan usually demonstrates a normal-size uterus with areas of hypodensity, an enlarged inhomogeneous uterus with a central area of low attenuation (Fig. 25–88), or hypodense foci surrounded by highly enhanced areas in the myometrium.[280, 281] An associated CT finding is the presence of bilaterally enlarged ovaries containing multiple corpus luteum cysts (Fig. 25–89).

On T2-weighted images, a hydatidiform mole appears as a heterogeneous mass of high signal intensity that distends the endometrial cavity. Numerous cystic spaces may be present in the mass.[282, 282a, 283] In persistent GTN, heterogeneous masses distorting the uterine zonal architecture are demonstrated (Figs. 25–90 and 25–91).[283, 284]

Following chemotherapy, CT can be employed to document response of the enlarged uterus and areas of tumor extension or metastases. MRI will reveal a reappearance of normal uterine zonal anatomy, a decrease in uterine volume, and disappearance of the theca luteal cysts.[284] Research is ongoing to de-

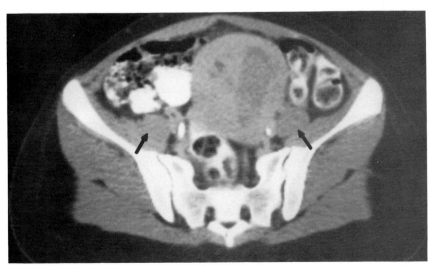

FIGURE 25–89 ■ Gestational trophoblastic neoplasia. CT scan demonstrating a uterine mass having cystic and solid components and enlarged ovaries *(arrows)* containing multiple corpus luteum cysts.

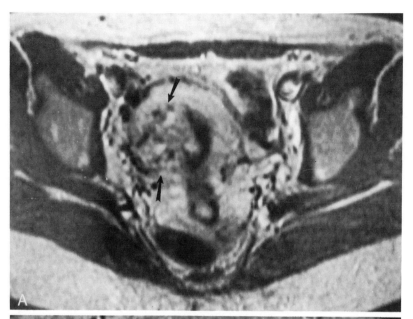

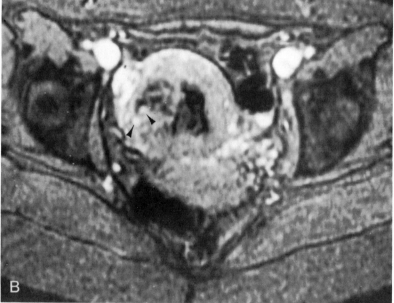

FIGURE 25–90 ■ Gestational trophoblastic neoplasia. *A,* Axial T2-weighted image demonstrates a heterogeneous vascular mass *(arrows)* distending the endometrial cavity and invading the myometrium on the right in this patient with persistent gestational trophoblastic neoplasia. *B,* Gradient-recalled acquisition in the steady state (GRASS) image confirms the vascular nature of this mass as several low-intensity structures become hyperintense *(arrowheads).*

termine whether a MRI examination can be used to predict patients who will develop persistent GTN or who will respond to chemotherapy.[285]

Metastasis ■ Uterine metastasis most commonly arise from tumors originating in the ovary, whereas extrapelvic neoplasms that metastasize to the uterus most frequently arise in the breast and gastrointestinal tract. Metastatic tumors produce lobular, homogeneous soft tissue masses that are nonspecific in appearance and indistinguishable from benign or malignant primary uterine neoplasms.

Cervical Carcinoma ■ Cervical carcinoma is the most frequent gynecologic malignancy, with 13,500 new cases and 6000 deaths occurring yearly in the United States, according to Silverberg et al.[283a] Approximately 75 per cent of new cases will be detected as carcinoma in situ by a cervical smear cytologic examination. Peak incidence of invasive cervical carci-

noma occurs in women younger than 50 years of age; 95 per cent are squamous cell carcinomas arising in the external surface of the cervix and vagina, and 4.5 per cent are adenocarcinomas arising from endocervical epithelium (Table 25–7).[159]

Accurate staging of cervical carcinoma is vital in selecting optimal therapy. Hysterectomy is usually performed only in patients with cancer limited to the cervix (stage I) or with slight extension to the proximal vagina (stage IIA).[286] Radiation therapy is utilized for tumors beyond stage IIB. Although bimanual pelvic examination, cystoscopy, excretory urography, sigmoidoscopy, and lymphangiography are used to evaluate extent of disease in patients with invasive cervical carcinoma, when compared with surgical findings, these methods have been found to have error rates ranging from 35 per cent to 39 per cent.[287]

The overall accuracy of CT in staging patients with

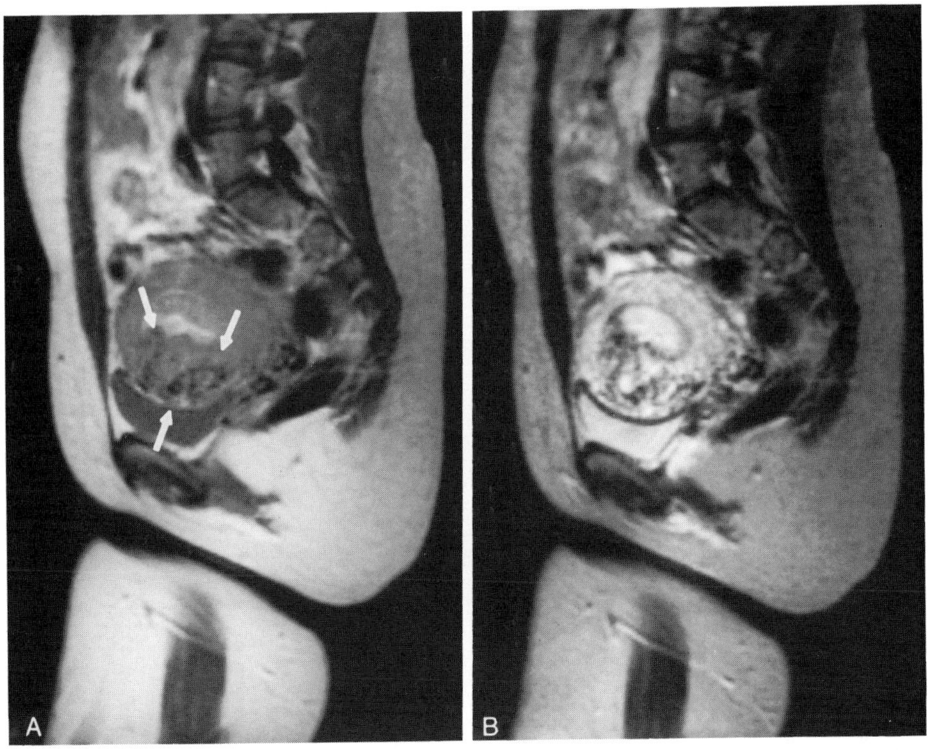

FIGURE 25–91 ■ Persistent gestational trophoblastic neoplasia. *A,* An intermediate-weighted sagittal MR scan demonstrates a focal uterine mass *(arrows)* that has areas of low signal intensity. *B,* A T2-weighted scan shows the mass to be heterogeneous and predominantly of high signal intensity.

cervical carcinoma has been reported to range between 66 per cent and 80 per cent.[265, 288] However, CT has had a disappointing accuracy of only 30 per cent to 58 per cent in evaluating parametrial extension of cervical cancer[286] and has not been able to differentiate stage IB lesions from IIB lesions. Thus it has not played a major role in decisions regarding surgical versus nonsurgical therapy.[286, 289] CT staging is more accurate than clinical staging but is less accurate than staging using a combination of clinical and cystoscopic techniques.[286] The normal cervix on CT scans has smooth outer cervical margins sharply delineated by paravaginal fat. The overall size of the cervix is usually less than 3 cm in diameter. Invasive carcinoma of the cervix typically produces a mass of

soft tissue density that may be confined to the cervix or extend into the uterus and parametrium (Fig. 25–92). Areas of tumor necrosis are seen as foci of decreased attenuation within the tumor (see Fig. 25–92). Extension of the tumor to the parametrium produces irregularity or poor delineation of the cervical margins; an irregular, lobulated, or triangular eccentric parametrial mass; parametrial soft tissue strands; and/or obliteration of the perirectal fat planes, (Figs. 25–93, 25–94, and 25–95).[286]

The overall accuracy of MRI in staging carcinoma of the cervix has been reported to range from 76 per cent to 83 per cent.[18, 289, 290] In most series, MRI is reported to be comparable to clinical staging and superior to CT.[268, 269, 289] In addition, MRI is more accurate than CT in estimating primary tumor volume.[268, 269, 289, 291] T2-weighted images provide maximal contrast between tumor and the normal cervical stroma, and T1-weighted images provide maximal contrast between invasive tumor and the parametrial fat. Axial images are recommended for evaluating the extent of cervical, vaginal, and parametrial disease, as well as tumor extension to the pelvic sidewall. Sagittal images are useful for depicting invasion of the lower uterine segment, bladder, or rectum. Coronal images are useful for evaluation of the parametria, pelvic sidewall, and lower uterine segment.[18]

Localized cervical carcinoma, stage I, appears on T2-weighted images as a mass of moderate signal intensity either expanding the endocervical canal or disrupting the low signal intensity of the fibrous cervical stoma (Fig. 25–96).[18, 268, 269, 289–293] The lateral margin of the cervix should appear smooth, without

TABLE 25–7. ■ **FIGO Staging System for Carcinoma of the Cervix**

STAGE	DESCRIPTION
0	Carcinoma in situ
I	Carcinoma is confined to the cervix
Ia	Microscopic invasion
Ib	Lesions extending deeper than 5 mm from the base of the epithelium and wider than 7 mm
II	Carcinoma extends beyond the cervix, but not to the pelvic side wall or the lower third of the vagina
IIa	No obvious parametrial involvement
IIb	Obvious parametrial involvement
III	Carcinoma extends to the lower third of the vagina or to the pelvic side wall, including all cases with hydronephrosis
IV	Carcinoma extends beyond the true pelvis or involves bladder or rectal mucosa

Source: Pettersson F., ed: Annual Report on the Results of Treatment in Gynecological Cancer, Vol 20. Stockholm, Panorama Press AB, 1988, p 30.

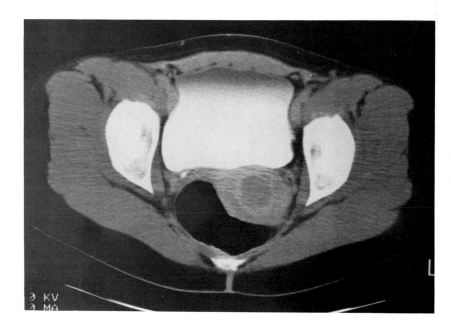

FIGURE 25–92 ■ Cervical carcinoma. An axial CT scan demonstrates an enlarged cervix containing a central hypodense region that represents tumor necrosis.

FIGURE 25–93 ■ Carcinoma of the cervix. CT demonstrates a mixed-density cervical mass extending to encase the left ureter *(arrowhead)*. The gas in the right parametrium is caused by a vaginal tampon.

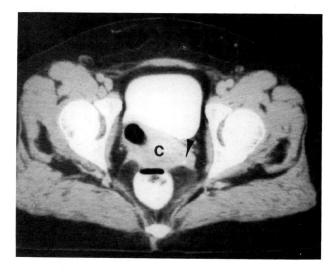

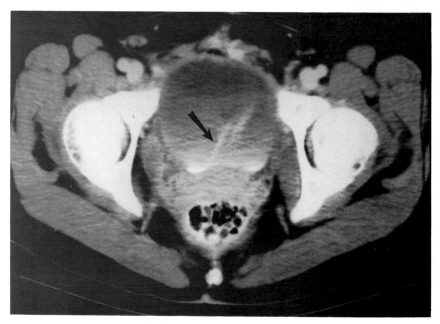

FIGURE 25–94 ■ Cervical carcinoma has invaded the base of the bladder and extends to obliterate the fat plane between the cervix and rectum. Extension to the right parametrial region is also present. A nice example of a jet of contrast coming into the bladder is shown *(arrow)*.

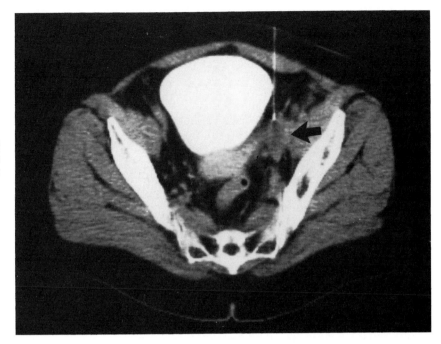

FIGURE 25–95 ■ Needle biopsy of cervical carcinoma. Extension of cervical carcinoma into the left parametrium *(arrow)*, proven by CT-guided biopsy.

soft tissue masses or stranding in the surrounding fat on T1-weighted images. Hricak et al.[18] reported that MRI was 70 per cent accurate in determining tumor size to within 0.5 cm of the surgical specimen. Togashi et al.[290] reported that MRI was 100 per cent specific and 92 per cent sensitive in detecting invasive stage I cervical carcinoma. Patients should be examined with MRI before biopsy, as postbiopsy changes are indistinguishable from primary tumors on MR examination.[18] MRI surpasses visual examination in demonstrating stromal invasion by cervical carcinoma below a normal-appearing epithelium and in evaluating exophytic tumors.[18, 289–291] However, carcinomas in situ or superficial tumors are not usually detectable on MR examination, although they are readily visualized at culposcopy.

MRI is less accurate in evaluating more advanced stages of cervical carcinoma,[18, 290] and the small number of reported patients with advanced disease in whom surgical correlation has been obtained has

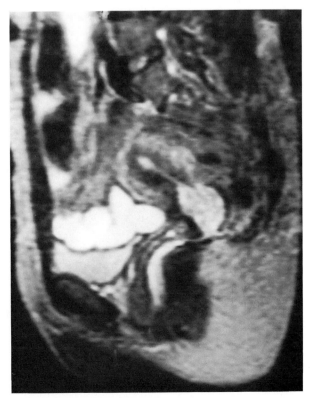

FIGURE 25–96 ■ Cervical carcinoma. Sagittal T2-weighted image demonstrates a heterogeneous mass of predominately high signal intensity attenuating the normal low signal intensity of the fibrous cervical stroma. A peripheral rim of low signal intensity indicates that there is no parametrial invasion.

prohibited statistical analysis. The criteria for documenting advanced disease on MRI are similar to those for CT. In patients with vaginal invasion (stage IIA disease), tumor invades the upper two thirds of the low-signal-intensity vaginal wall.[18, 290, 293] However, false-positive examination results occur, because tumors may prolapse into the vagina without frankly invading the vaginal wall. Parametrial invasion (stage IIB) is suggested when full-thickness loss of the normal signal intensity of the cervical stroma is accompanied by an irregular lateral cervical margin or areas of abnormal signal intensity within the parametrial fat. T1-weighted images are particularly useful for evaluation of the lateral cervical margin and parametrial fat. MRI has been reported to be between 88 per cent and 92 per cent accurate in the detection of parametrial extension of tumor.[18, 289, 290] However, microscopic disease is not identified by MR examination, and exophytic stage I tumors or inflammatory changes may cause false-positive results.[18, 290] In patients with stage IIIA disease, the normal low signal intensity of the lower one third of the vaginal wall is disrupted by the tumor mass. Stage IIIB disease is diagnosed when soft tissue masses or stranding extend to the pelvic sidewall or when hydronephrosis is present (Fig. 25–97). Focal disruption of the normal low signal intensity of the bladder or rectal wall, loss of perivesical/perirectal fat planes, asymmetric nodular wall thickening, or intraluminal masses are seen with bladder or rectal involvement (stage IV disease).[18, 268, 289, 291]

Although lymph node metastases are not part of the FIGO staging system, their presence adversely affects patient prognosis and eliminates the possibility of surgical cure.[280] Both CT and MRI rely on measurements of size to distinguish between normal and abnormal lymph nodes. Lymph nodes larger than 1.5 cm are considered to be abnormal, and lymph nodes between 1.0 and 1.5 cm are considered suspicious.[18, 294] Neither the signal intensity nor calculated T1 or T2 values have been helpful in discriminating normal from pathologically abnormal lymph nodes.[295, 296] The sensitivity of CT in detecting lymph node metastases has approximated 70 per cent, with up to 30 per cent false-negative and 22 per cent false-positive interpretations.[259, 265, 267, 288] MRI has been reported to be equivalent to CT in detecting lymph node metastases.[297] Neither modality can demonstrate microscopic disease, and lymph nodes enlarged by inflammatory disease may result in a false-positive diagnosis.[18, 289, 290, 298, 299] The only way to document metastatic disease in lymph nodes of normal size is via lymphangiography (LAG).[296, 298] However, very small deposits of microscopic disease (<3 mm) may not be visualized on LAG, and failure of opacification of involved lymph nodes or total replacement of a lymph node by tumor may also result in false-negative examination results on LAG. The diagnostic accuracies of MRI, CT, and LAG for the diagnosis of lymph node metastases from cervical carcinoma are essentially equivalent, ranging from 75 per cent to 85 per cent.[267, 289, 290, 294, 300, 301] CT has applications in the planning of radiotherapy for cervical carcinoma. Calculation of tumor volume and determination of extent is useful for the planning of radiation portals, and CT examination after insertion of a radiation applicator permits accurate dosimetric calculations.[257, 278]

Recurrent Cervical Carcinoma ■ Carcinoma of the cervix most frequently recurs within 2 years after treatment, with approximately 50 per cent of patients having pelvic recurrences and 50 per cent having distant metastases.[302]

On CT, recurrent tumor typically produces an irregular pelvic mass that can be either uniformly solid or have an area of central necrosis. Pelvic sidewall extension is commonly present and produces either irregular linear soft tissue strands extending to the internal obturator muscle or a solid tumor mass that invades muscle and obliterates the pelvic fat planes. Recurrent tumor can also be detected by demonstrating lymphadenopathy, rectal or bladder invasion, or liver or bone metastasis.[302]

Patients with pelvic recurrence may be treated with pelvic exenteration if the disease remains confined to the true pelvis and does not invade the pelvic sidewall.[303] In a patient with a recurrent mass following radiation therapy, the key differentiation is between radiation fibrosis and tumor, and CT cannot reliably make this distinction. On MRI scans, recurrent tumor usually has a high signal intensity on T2-weighted images, and radiation fibrosis imaged at least 12 months after therapy usually is of low signal intensity.[303–305] However, MRI does not reliably differentiate local recurrence from early postradiation changes.[305]

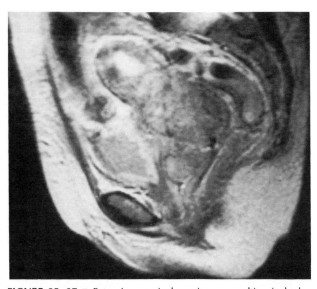

FIGURE 25–97 ■ Extensive cervical carcinoma resulting in hydrometra of the uterus. Very large bulky mass of mixed signal intensity is seen to invade the lower portion of the uterus and destroy normal cervical anatomy.

Vagina

Pathology

SQUAMOUS CELL CARCINOMA

Squamous cell carcinoma accounts for more than 90 per cent of the relatively rare primary vaginal neoplasms. Although the tumor is readily diagnosed by clinical examination, CT gives additional information regarding local extension, nodal metastasis, and bladder or rectal invasion. On CT scans, carcinoma of the vagina typically produces a mass caudal to the uterus that contains areas of low attenuation representing necrotic tumor (Fig. 25–98).[98]

Carcinoma of the vagina appears on T2-weighted images as either a diffuse or a focal area of increased signal intensity interrupting the normal low signal intensity of the vaginal wall.[304] Advanced disease (e.g., invasion of the ischiorectal fat, pelvic sidewall, or bones) is readily identified (Fig. 25–99). The MRI criteria for diagnosing advanced disease are similar to those for CT—namely, soft tissue masses or linear densities within the pelvic fat—and are best seen on T1-weighted images.

Patients with carcinoma of the vagina are most commonly treated with radiation therapy.[280] Therefore in a patient with a recurrent vaginal mass, differentiation between tumor recurrence and radiation fibrosis is important but is not possible with CT (Fig. 25–100). On MRI scans, a mass resulting from radiation fibrosis typically has low signal intensity on both T1- and T2-weighted images. A recurrent vaginal mass of increased signal intensity on T2-weighted images most often represents recurrent tumor, but Chang et al.[304] reported two patients with masses of high signal intensity on T2-weighted images in whom only nonspecific inflammation was found at biopsy.

Uterine or cervical carcinomas may also invade the vagina. On MR examination, a mass of signal intensity similar to that of the primary tumor can be noted disrupting the low signal intensity of the vaginal wall. However, it should be recognized that false-positive diagnoses of tumor invasion of the anterior fornix are commonly made, as vascular congestion and inflammation may produce focal areas of increased signal intensity in this region.[304]

Radiation may damage the vagina, rectum, sigmoid colon, distal small bowel, and bladder.[306] The most common changes demonstrated by CT after pelvic irradiation are widening of the presacral space, an increase in perirectal fat, thickening of the perirectal fibrous tissue and bladder wall, and fibrotic connection between the sacrum and rectum (Fig. 25–101).[63]

In contrast to changes found with recurrent tumor, postradiation changes usually are symmetric. Increased pelvic fat secondary to irradiation can be distinguished from pelvic lipomatosis by demonstration of presence of fibrosis in the fatty tissue.

RHABDOMYOSARCOMA (SARCOMA BOTRYOIDES)

Rhabdomyosarcoma is a rare vaginal tumor usually occurring in children younger than 5 years. It is highly malignant, despite a relatively innocuous microscopic appearance. CT reveals a large solid pelvic mass having multiple zones of decreased attenuation. The mass is often so large and local invasion so extensive that it can be difficult to identify the organ of origin.

Soft Tissue

In addition to displaying pathologic changes in the pelvic organs, CT is valuable in detecting a variety of primary tumors of pelvic soft tissue and osseous structures (Figs. 25–102 and 25–103). Among the more common pelvic soft tissue masses are anterior meningoceles, lumbosacral lipomas, and hemophilic pseudotumors.

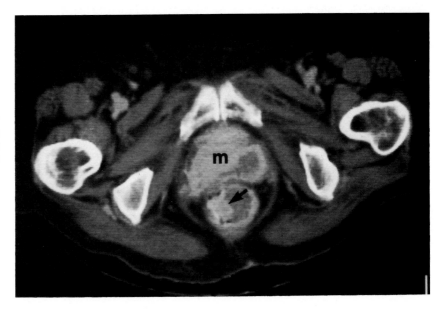

FIGURE 25–98 ■ Carcinoma of the vagina. CT scan in a patient with squamous cell carcinoma of the vagina demonstrates a soft tissue mass (m) with areas of decreased density. The rectum is partially filled with tumor (*arrow*).

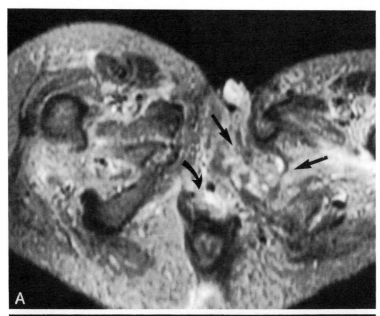

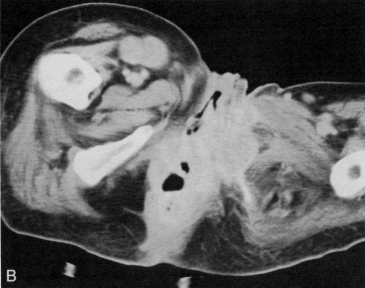

FIGURE 25–99 ■ Vulvar carcinoma. A, Axial T2-weighted image demonstrates a heterogeneous mass disrupting the normally low signal intensity of the vaginal wall *(curved arrow)*. The mass also invades the left adductor muscles and left inferior pubic ramus *(straight arrows)*. B, Axial CT scan also demonstrates a mixed-attenuation mass invading adjacent musculature on the left.

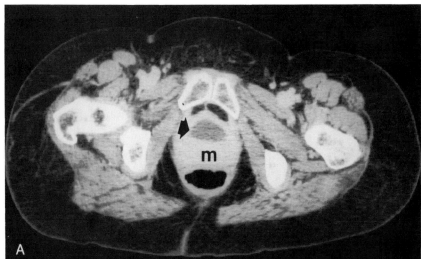

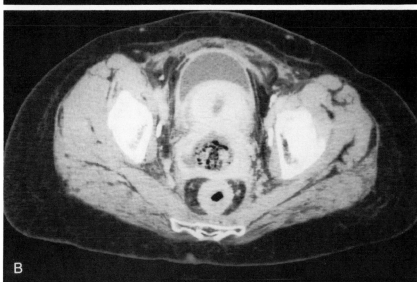

FIGURE 25–100 ■ Vaginal stenosis secondary to radiation therapy. *A,* A soft tissue mass (M) is demonstrated in the vagina. Fluid above the stenosis is seen as a water-density mass *(arrow). B,* CT scan at a higher level reveals the vagina to be distended and filled with fluid and gas.

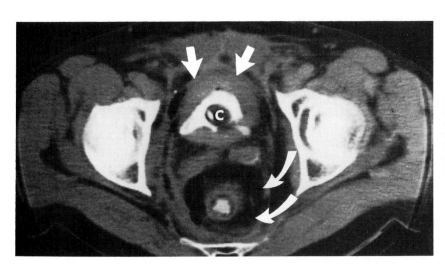

FIGURE 25–101 ■ Postradiation changes. The bladder wall *(straight arrows)* is markedly thickened because of radiation cystitis. Increased fat surrounds the rectum *(curved arrows).* There is thickening of the perirectal tissue and narrowing of the rectum as a result of pelvic irradiation. A catheter (c) is present in the bladder.

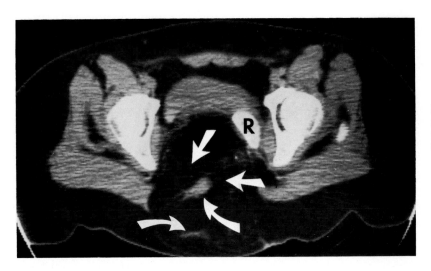

FIGURE 25–102 ■ Pelvic liposarcoma. A pelvic mass is shown to have fatty *(straight arrows)* and solid *(curved arrows)* components in a patient with a large liposarcoma, displacing the rectum (R).

Pathology

ANTERIOR MENINGOCELE

The anterior sacral meningocele usually herniates through a ventral defect in the sacrum or through an enlarged intervertebral or sciatic foramen.[307] It can present as a soft tissue mass either anterior to the sacrum or in the gluteal region. An anterior sacral bony defect, which is smooth and well demarcated, is commonly identified. The tip of the sacrum and coccyx is seen to hook under the meningocele, producing a scimitar appearance.

The diagnosis of an anterior sacral meningocele is made from plain radiography of the sacrum, excretory urography, and/or myelography. CT is usually not necessary for diagnosis but can determine the relationship of the meningocele to the intrapelvic organs and, in equivocal cases, exclude other tumors. On CT scans, a sacral meningocele appears as a smooth, well-defined mass of low attenuation lying anterior to the sacrum. The differential diagnosis includes chordoma, dermoid cyst, teratoma, lipoma, chondroma, and neurogenic tumor.

LUMBOSACRAL LIPOMA

Lumbosacral lipomas are rare benign tumors that are often associated with neural defects. The CT examination demonstrates the lipomatous nature of the tumor, defines the superior and inferior extent of the lesion, gives detailed information about extension into the neighboring tissue, outlines the origin of the tumor, and identifies bony abnormalities in the sacrum and cartilaginous tissue within the lipoma.

HEMOPHILIC PSEUDOTUMOR

Hemophilic pseudotumors are old hematomas surrounded by thick fibrous capsules and filled with coagulum. Hemophilic pseudotumors of the pelvis occur as rare complications of bleeding in one per cent to two per cent of patients with severe hemophilia. They may be contained exclusively within soft tissue or may originate in subperiosteal or intraosseous sites (Fig. 25–104). In patients with bony involvement, CT examination of the pelvis demonstrates a soft tissue mass destroying bone and

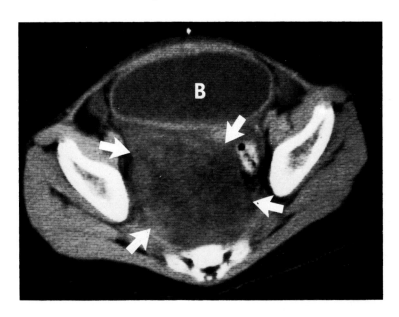

FIGURE 25–103 ■ Rhabdomyosarcoma producing a large soft tissue mass containing areas of low attenuation. The appearance of the rhabdomyosarcoma is similar to that of a large endometrial carcinoma. B = Bladder.

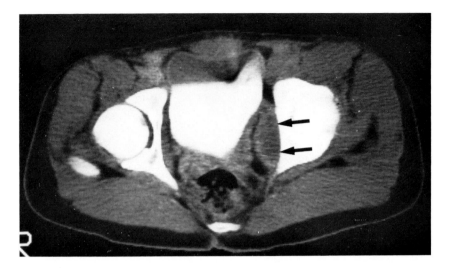

FIGURE 25–104 ■ Hemophilic pseudotumor. A pelvic CT scan reveals enlargement of the left internal obturator muscle (*arrows*) in a hemophiliac boy. The low-density component of the mass represents a partially organized hematoma. Without the clinical history, a malignant mass could not be excluded based on the CT appearance.

extending into the external oblique, iliopsoas, or gluteus muscles.[308] If only a soft tissue pseudotumor is present, CT examination reveals a noncalcified pelvic mass containing regions of low or high density, suggesting fresh and old hemorrhage.

ILIOPSOAS BURSITIS

The iliopsoas bursa overlies the hip capsule, lies behind the iliopsoas muscle, and is lateral to the femoral vessels. A communication between the hip joint and bursa exists in 15 per cent of autopsies. Bursal enlargement may occur if the bursa is inflamed, and if significant enlargement is present, CT scans will reveal a mass of low attenuation, lateral to the femoral vessels, that displaces the iliopsoas muscle.[309] If bursal enlargement extends beneath the inguinal ligament, CT examination may reveal compression of the sigmoid colon, cecum, ureter, or bladder by the water-density mass.

MUSCULOAPONEUROTIC FIBROMATOSIS (DESMOID TUMOR)

These tumors derive from the musculoaponeurotic supporting tissues. The majority arise in the anterior abdominal wall (Fig. 25–105). Desmoid tumors occur most commonly in women, frequently following pregnancy, and may manifest as a painful mass requiring differentiation from a sarcoma. The etiology of these tumors is uncertain but may relate either to trauma (e.g., severe muscle contractions during labor) or to endocrinologic disturbances.

Fluid Collections

Abnormal fluid collections within the pelvis may be caused by ascites, free blood, pelvic hematomas, abscesses, necrotic tumors, or lymphoceles. Although it is not always possible to differentiate among various pelvic fluid collections, certain CT findings give clues as to the true nature of pelvic fluid.

Pathology

ASCITES

The most frequently observed pelvic fluid collection is ascites. Usually ascitic fluid has a CT density close to that of water but can have an attenuation value of 10 to 30 H, depending on the protein content of the fluid. Initially ascites collects in the rectovesical or rectouterine (pouch of Douglas) recesses. Larger amounts fill the lateral paravesical recesses and extend up along the paracolic gutters to be contiguous with fluid in the perihepatic and perisplenic spaces. The accuracy of CT in detecting ascites approaches 100 per cent,[310] with CT readily demonstrating even small amounts of intraabdominal and pelvic fluid. Ascitic fluid conforms to surrounding structures, insinuating around and between organs. Bowel loops tend to float out of the pelvis, except when a tense ascites develops and they are displaced to one side. Distinction between benign and malignant ascites is not usually possible on the basis of the attenuation value of the fluid. However, demonstration of peritoneal implants, matted bowel loops, and lymphadenopathy are factors indicating that the ascitic fluid is malignant. Differentiation between blood and ascitic fluid is possible only in the acute circumstance, when fresh blood has a CT attenuation value significantly greater than water.

HEMATOMA

Pelvic hematomas are usually caused by trauma, excessive anticoagulation, hemophilia, surgical error, or neoplasia. The CT features of an acute hematoma consist of a soft tissue mass of relatively high density (20 to 60 H) with sharp margins. As in hematomas elsewhere in the body, the attenuation value of the hematoma decreases with time as the hemoglobin content decreases and the water content increases. Hematomas 2 to 4 weeks old can be confused with other pelvic fluid collections, because they appear on CT as a cystic structure of low density. A necrotic- or cystic-appearing tumor or an abscess can mimic

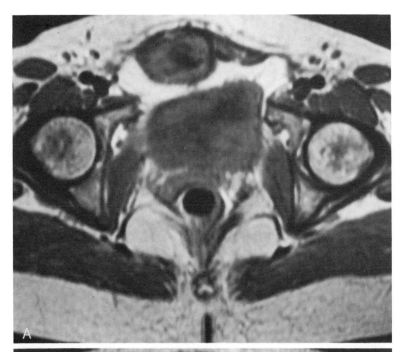

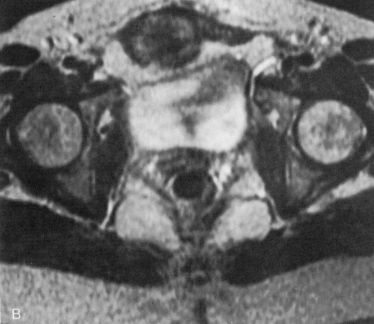

FIGURE 25–105 ■ Desmoid tumor. *A*, Proton density, and *B*, T2-weighted, axial images, obtained in a woman 3 months following a vaginal delivery, reveal an inhomogeneous, predominantly low signal intensity mass arising from the right rectus abdominus muscle anterior to the bladder.

FIGURE 25–106 ■ Acute pelvic abscess. A large oval area of low density *(box)* posterior to the small bowel and anterior to the rectum (R) is seen in a patient with a large abscess in the cul-de-sac resulting from perforation of the sigmoid colon. The abscess does not have well-defined walls.

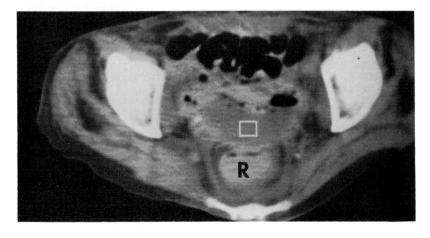

an old hematoma and require percutaneous needle aspiration to make the correct diagnosis.

ABSCESS

Pelvic abscesses most often are related to inflammatory adnexal disease, appendicitis, or diverticulitis, but they are also found to be secondary to Crohn's disease, pelvic surgery, carcinoma, trauma, or colonic perforation. Gluteal abscesses may be caused by infection of degenerated hematomas or seromas following trauma or surgery (particularly hip surgery), a necrotic neoplasm,[311] or extension of an abscess along the iliacus,[311] or they may be the result of a pelvic abscess spreading to the buttocks and hip through the greater and lesser sciatic foramen.

As in other areas of the body, CT has proved to be an accurate method for detecting and documenting the extent and size of pelvic abscesses.[312] On CT scans, an acute pelvic abscess usually appears as a low-density mass having either a sharp or an irregular outer margin (Fig. 25–106). The wall or rim of the abscess is often irregular and is best demonstrated following intravenous administration of contrast material. Chronic abscesses have a better defined rim, and the internal contents are generally of lower density. When an abscess obscures adjacent fat planes, CT can exclude a cyst or seroma, both of which leave the tissue planes intact. If an abscess is caused by a gas-forming organism, air bubbles may be identified within the fluid collection. Without the presence of intraluminal gas (seen in 38 per cent in one series),[313] hematomas, noninfected inflammatory masses, or cystic or necrotic tumors cannot be excluded. Not all gas collections within a mass are caused by infection, as gas within a mass also may be secondary to ischemia and subsequent necrosis, be iatrogenically administered, or result from fistula formation.

CT has proven to be superior to ultrasonography in the postoperative patient, as postoperative ileus, abdominal surgical dressings, and drains often prevent an adequate ultrasonographic examination.[312] In addition, CT is of greater help in demonstrating fistulous tracts and in guiding placement of percutaneous drainage catheters into pelvic abscesses. Currently, CT is used as the initial imaging procedure in high-risk postoperative patients and in patients undergoing percutaneous drainage procedures.

References

1. Hamlin DJ, Cockett AT: Modification for computerized tomographic staging of infiltrative bladder carcinoma. J Urol 123:489, 1980.
2. Hamlin DJ, Burgener FA: Positive and negative contrast agents in CT evaluation of the abdomen and pelvis. J Comput Tomogr 5:82, 1981.
3. Seidelmann FE, Cohen WN, Bryan PJ, Temes SP, Kraus D, Schoenrock G: Accuracy of CT staging of bladder neoplasms using the gas-filled method: report of 21 patients with surgical confirmation. AJR: 130:735, 1978.
4. Hamlin DJ, Cockett AK, Burgener FA: Computed tomography of the pelvis: sagittal and coronal image reconstruction in the evaluation of infiltrative bladder carcinoma. Comput Assist Tomogr 5:27, 1981.
5. van Waes PF, Zonnveld FW: Patient positioning for direct coronal computer tomography of the entire body. Radiology 142:531, 1982.
6. Osborn AG, Koehler PR, Gibbs FA, Leavitt DD, Anderson RE, et al: Direct sagittal computed tomographic scans in the radiographic evaluation of the pelvis. Radiology 134:255, 1980.
7. Lange RC, Duberg AD, McCarthy SM: Determination of optimal contrast within the normal and pathologic uterus via synthetic MRI. Magn Reson Med 17:279–284, 1991.
8. Weinreb JC, Maranilla KR, Redman HC, Nunally R: Improved MR imaging of the upper abdomen with glucagon and gas. J Comput Assist Tomogr 8:835–838, 1984.
9. Chernish SM, Maglinte DT: Glucagon: common untoward reactions—review and recommendations. Radiology 177:145, 1990.
10. Chernish SM, Maglinte DT, Brunelle RL: The laboratory response to glucagon dosages used in gastrointestinal examinations. Invest Radiol 23:847, 1988.
10a. Smith RC, Reinhold C, Lange RC, McCauley TR, Kier R, et al: Comparison of conventional and fast spin-echo body coil MR imaging of the female pelvis. (In press.)
10b. Reinhold C, Smith RC, McCauley TR, Lange RC, McCarthy S: High-resolution fast spin-echo MR imaging of the female pelvis using a phased array multicoli. (In press.)
11. Bryan PJ, Butler HE, Nelson AD, LiPuma JP, Kopiwoda SY, et al: Magnetic resonance imaging of the prostate. Am J Roentgenol 146:543–548, 1986.
12. Hricak H, Dooms GC, McNeal JE, Mark AS, Marotti M, et al: Imaging of the prostate gland: normal anatomy. Am J Roentgenol 148:51–58, January 1987.
13. Sommer FG, McNeal JE, Carrol CL: MR depiction of zonal anatomy of the prostate at 1.5 T. J Comput Assist Tomogr 10(6):983–989, 1986.
14. Schnall MD, Lenkinski RE, Pollack HM, Imai Y, Kressel HY: Prostate: MR imaging with an endorectal surface coil. Radiology 172:570–574, 1989.
15. Koslin DB, Kenneyh PJ, Koehler RE, Van Dyke JA: Magnetic resonance imaging of the internal anatomy of the prostate gland. Invest Radiol 22:947–953, 1987.
16. Hricak H, Alpers C, Crooks LE, Sheldon PE: Magnetic resonance imaging of the female pelvis: initial experience. AJR 141:1119, 1983.
17. Hricak H: MRI of the female pelvis: a review. AJR 146:1115, 1986.
18. Hricak H, Lacey CG, Sandles LG, Chang YCF, Winkler ML, Stern JL: Invasive cervical carcinoma: comparison of MR imaging and surgical findings. Radiology 166:623, 1988.
19. Hricak H, Chang YCF, Thurnher S: Vagina: evaluation with MR imaging. Part 1. Normal anatomy and congenital anomalies. Radiology 169:109, 1988.
20. McCarthy S, Tauber C, Gore J: Female pelvic anatomy: MR assessment of variations during the menstrual cycle and with use of oral contraceptives. Radiology 160:119, 1986.
21. Haynor DR, Mack LA, Soules MR, Shuman WP, Montana MA, Moss AA: Changing appearance of the normal uterus during the menstrual cycle: MR studies. Radiology 161:459, 1986.
22. McCarthy S: Magnetic resonance imaging of gynecological anatomy. Magn Reson Imaging 5:171, 1986.
23. McCauley TR, Scoutt LM, Flynn SB, Luthringer D, McCarthy SM: Zonal anatomy of the cervix: MR pathological correlation in hysterectomy specimens. J Magn Reson Imaging 1:197, 1991.
24. Demas BE, Hricak H, Jaffe RB: Uterine MR imaging: effects of hormonal stimulation. Radiology 159:123, 1986.
25. Lee JKT, Gersell DJ, Balfe DM, Worthington JL, Picus D, Gapp G: The uterus: in vitro MR-anatomic correlation of normal and abnormal specimens. Radiology 157:175, 1985.
26. Worthington BS, Powell M, Womack C, Buckley J, Symonds EM: The low-intensity band on spin-echo images of the

uterus: an anatomic and clinicopathologic study. Radiology 157(P):310, 1985.

27. McCarthy S, Scott G, Majumdar S, Shapiro B, Thompson S, et al: Uterine junctional zone: MR study of water content and relaxation properties. Radiology 171:241, 1989.

28. Scoutt LM, Flynn SD, Luthringer D, McCauley T, McCarthy SM: The junctional zone of the uterus: MRI-histologic correlation in hysterectomy specimens. Radiology 179:403–407, 1991.

29. Zawin M, McCarthy S, Scoutt L, Lange R, Lavy G, Vulte J: Monitoring therapy with a gonadotropin-releasing hormone analog: utility of MR imaging. Radiology 175:503, 1990.

30. Hricak H, Stern JL, Fisher MR, Shapeero LG, Winkler ML, Lacey CG: Endometrial carcinoma staging by MR imaging. Radiology 162:297, 1987.

31. Church PA, Kazam E: Computed tomography and ultrasound in diagnosis of pelvic lipomatosis. Urology 14:631, 1979.

32. Harris RD, Bendon JA, Robinson CH, Seat SG, Herwig KR: Computed tomographic evaluation of pear-shaped bladder. Urology 14:528, 1979.

33. Hueber F, De Faveri D, Franceschi L, Canciani L: Su di un caso di lipomatosi pelvica constrittiva: rilievi con la TAC. Radiol Med (Torino) 66:277, 1980.

34. Jorulf H, Lindstedt E: Urogenital schistosomiasis: CT evaluation. Radiology 157:745–749, 1985.

35. Brun B, Kristensen JK: Computed tomography in the evaluation of a pelvic tumor. J Comput Assist Tomogr 3:547, 1979.

36. Merine D, Fishman E, Kuhlman J, Bronwyn J, Bayless TK, Siegelman S: Bladder involvement in Crohn disease: role of CT in detection and evaluation. J Comput Assist Tomogr 13(1):90–93, 1989.

37. Goodman JD, Macchia RJ, Macasaet MA, Schneider M: Endometriosis of the urinary bladder: sonographic findings. AJR 135:625, 1980.

38. Epstein BM, Patel V, Porteous PH: Case report: CT appearance of bladder malakoplakia. J Comput Assist Tomogr 7(23):541–543, 1983.

39. Bidwell JK, Dunne MG: Computed tomography of bladder malakoplakia. J Comput Assist Tomogr 11(5):909–910, 1987.

40. Zingas AP, Kling GA, Crotte E, Shumaker E, Vazquez PM: Computed tomography of nephrogenic adenoma of the urinary bladder. J Comput Assist Tomogr 10(6):979–982, 1986.

41. Patel PS, Wilbur AC: Nephrogenic adenoma presenting as a calcified mass. AJR 150:1071–1072, 1988.

42. Warshawsky R, Bow SN, Waldbaum RS, Cintron J: Bladder pheochromocytoma with MR correlation. J Comput Assist Tomogr 13(4):714–716, 1989.

43. Ney C, Kumar M, Billah K, Doerr J: Clinical image. J Comput Assist Tomogr 11(3):552–553, 1987.

44. Marshall VF: The relation of the preoperative estimate to the pathologic demonstration of the extent of vesical neoplasms. J Urol 68:714, 1952.

45. Kenny GM, Hartoner GJ, Moore RM, Murphy GP: Current results from treatment of stage C & D bladder tumors at Roswell Park Memorial Institute. Urology 107:56, 1972.

46. Bryan PJ, Butler HE, LiPuma JP, Resnick MI, Kursh ED: CT and MR imaging in staging bladder neoplasms. J Comput Assist Tomogr 11(1):96–101, 1987.

47. Husband JES, Olliff JFC, Williams MP, Heron CS, Cherryman GR: Bladder cancer: staging with CT and MRI imaging. Radiology 173:435–440, 1989.

48. Nakamura S, Nijima T: Staging of bladder cancer by ultrasonography: a new technique by transurethral intravesical scanning. J Urol 124:341, 1980.

49. Harada K, Igari D, Tanahashi Y, Watanabe H, Saiton M, Mishina T: Staging of bladder tumors by means of transrectal ultrasonography. J Clin Ultrasound 5:388, 1977.

50. Gammelgaard J, Hom HH: Transurethral and transrectal ultrasonic scanning in urology. J Urol 124:863, 1980.

51. Morgan CL, Calkins RF, Cavalcanti EJ: Computed tomography in the evaluation, staging, and therapy of carcinoma of the bladder and prostate. Radiology 140:751, 1981.

52. Amendola MA, Glazer GM, Grossman HB, Aisen AM, Francis IR: Staging of bladder carcinoma: MRI-CT-surgical correlation. Am J Roentgenol 146:1179–1183, 1986.

53. Froedin L, Hemmingsson A, Johannson A, Wicklund HL: Computed tomography in staging of bladder carcinoma. Acta Radiol (Diagn) 21:763, 1980.

54. Kellett MJ, Oliver RT, Husband JE, Fry IK: Computed tomography as an adjunct to bimanual examination for staging bladder tumors. Br J Urol 52:101, 1980.

55. Buy J-N, Moss AA, Guinet C, Ghossain MA, Malbec L, et al: MR staging of bladder carcinoma: correlation with pathologic findings. Radiology 169:695–700, 1988.

56. Barentsz JO, Lemmens JAM, Ruijs SHJ, Boskamp EB, Hendrikx AJM, et al: Carcinoma of the urinary bladder: MR imaging with a double surface coil. Am J Roentgenol 151:107–112, 1988.

57. Koelbel G, Schmiedl U, Griebel J, Friedrich H, Kueper K: MR imaging of urinary bladder neoplasms. J Comput Assist Tomogr 12(1):98–103, 1988.

58. Rholl KS, Lee JKT, Heiken JP, Ling D, Glazer HS: Primary bladder carcinoma: evaluation with MR imaging. Radiology 163:117–121, 1987.

59. Fisher MR, Hricak H, Crooks LE: Urinary bladder MR imaging. Radiology 157:467–470, 1985.

60. Fisher MR, Hricak H, Tanagho EA: Urinary bladder MR imaging. Radiology 157:471–477, 1985.

61. Jeffrey RB, Palubinskas AJ, Federle MP: CT evaluation of invasive lesions of the bladder. J Comput Assist Tomogr 5:22, 1981.

62. Neuerburg JM, Bohndorf K, Sohn M, Feufl F, Guenther RW, Daus HJ: Urinary bladder neoplasms: evaluation with contrast-enhanced MR imaging. Radiology 172:739–743, 1989.

63. Doubleday LC, Bernardino ME: CT findings in the perirectal area following radiation therapy. J Comput Assist Tomogr 4:634, 1980.

64. Glazer HS, Lee JKT, Levitt RG, Heiken JP, Ling D, et al: Radiation fibrosis: differentiation from recurrent tumor by MR imaging. Radiology 156:721–726, 1985.

65. Wallace DM, Bloom HJG: The management of deeply infiltrating (T3) bladder cancer: controlled trial of radical radiotherapy versus preoperative radiotherapy and radical cystectomy. Br J Urol 48:587, 1976.

66. Beyer D, Peters PE: Real-time ultrasonography—an efficient screening method for abdominal and pelvic lymphadenopathy. Lymphology 13:142, 1980.

67. Wajsman Z, Baumgartner G, Murphy GP, Merrin C: Evaluation of lymphangiography for clinical staging of bladder tumors. J Urol 114:712, 1975.

68. Johnson DE, Kaesler KE, Kaminsky S, Jing BS, Wallace S: Lymphangiography as an aid in staging bladder carcinoma. South Med J 69:28, 1976.

69. Walsh JW, Amendola MA, Konerding KF, Tisnado J, Dazra TA: Computed tomographic detection of pelvic and inguinal lymph node metastases from primary and recurrent pelvic malignant disease. Radiology 137:157, 1980.

70. Lee JK, Stanley RJ, Sagel SS, McClennan BL: Accuracy of CT in detecting intraabdominal and pelvic lymph node metastases from pelvic cancers. AJR 131:675, 1978.

71. Castellino RA, Marglin SI, Carroll BA, Young SW, Narell GS, Blank N: The radiographic evaluation of abdominal and pelvic lymph nodes in oncologic practice. Cancer Treat Rev 7:153, 1980.

72. Schlager B, Asbell SO, Baker AS, Aklaroff DM, Seydel MG, Ostrum BJ: The use of computerized tomography scanning in treatment planning for bladder carcinoma. Int J Radiol Oncol Biol Phys 5:99, 1979.

73. Brizel HE, Livingston PA, Grayson EV: Radiotherpeutic applications of pelvic computed tomography. J Comput Assist Tomogr 3:453, 1979.

74. Kwok-Liu JP, Zikman JM, Cockshott WP: Carcinoma of the urachus: the role of computed tomography. Radiology 137:731, 1980.

75. Korobkin M, Cambier L, Drake J: Computed tomography of urachal carcinoma. J Comput Assist Tomogr 19(6):981–987, 1988.

76. Brick SH, Friedman AC, Pollack HM, Fishman EK, Radecki PD, et al: Urachal carcinoma: CT findings. Radiology 169:377–381, 1988.

77. Narumi Y, Sato T, Kuriyama K, Fujita M, Saiki S, et al:

Vesical dome tumors: significance of extravesical extension on CT. Radiology 169:383–385, 1988.

78. Lee JK, McClennan BL, Stanley RJ, Levitt RG, Sagel SS: Use of CT in evaluation of postcystectomy patients. AJR 136:483, 1981.

79. Amis ES, Newhouse JH, Olsson CA: Continent urinary diversions: review of current surgical procedures and radiologic imaging. Radiology 168:395–401, 1988.

80. Van Engelshoven JM, Kreel L: Computed tomography of the prostate. J Comput Assist Tomogr 3:45, 1979.

81. Carrol CL, Sommer FG, McNeal JE, Stamey TA: The abnormal prostate: MR imaging at 1.5 T with histopathologic correlation. Radiology 163:521–525, 1987.

82. Ling D, Lee JKT, Heiken JP, Balfe DM, Glazer HS, McClennan BL: Prostatic carcinoma and benign prostatic hyperplasia: inability of MR imaging to distinguish between the two diseases. Radiology 158:103–107, 1986.

83. Griebel JH, Hess CF, Schmiedl U, Koelbel G: MR characteristics of prostatic carcinoma and benign prostatic hyperplasia at 1.5 T. J Comput Assist Tomogr 12(6):988–994, 1988.

84. Kahn T, Burrig K, Schmitz-Drager B, Lewin JS, Furst G, Modder U: Prostatic carcinoma and benign prostatic hyperplasia: MR imaging with histopathologic correlation. Radiology 173:847–851, 1989.

85. Schiebler JL, Tomaszewski JE, Bezzi M, Pollack HM, Kressel HY, et al: Prostatic carcinoma and benign prostatic hyperplasia: correlation of high-resolution MR and histopathologic findings. Radiology 172:131–137, 1989.

86. Hruban RH, Zerhouni EA, Dagher AP, Pessar ML, Hutchins GM: Morphologic basis of MR imaging of benign prostatic hyperplasia. J Comput Assist Tomogr 11(6):1035–1041, 1987.

87. Bezzi M, Kressel HY, Allen KS, Schiebler ML, Altman HG, et al: Prostatic carcinoma: staging with MR imaging at 1.5 T. Radiology 169:339–346, 1988.

88. Biondetti PR, Lee JKT, Ling D, Catalona WJ: Clinical stage B prostate carcinoma: staging with MR imaging. Radiology 162:325–329, 1987.

89. Hricak H, Dooms GC, Jeffreey RB, Avallone A, Jacobs D, et al: Prostatic carcinoma: staging by clinical assessment, CT, and MR imaging. Radiology 162:331–336, 1987.

90. Platt JF, Bree RL, Schwab RE: The accuracy of CT in the staging of carcinoma of the prostate. AJR 149:315–318, 1987.

91. Narayan P, Vigneron DB, Jajodia P, Anderson CM, Hedgcock MW, et al: Transrectal probe for ^{1}H MRI and ^{31}P MR spectroscopy of the prostate gland. Magn Reson Med 11:209–220, 1989.

92. Martin JF, Hajek P, Baker L, Gylys-Morin V, Fitzmorris-Glass R, Mattrey RR: Inflatable surface coil for MR imaging of the prostate. Radiology 167:268–270, 1988.

93. Resnick MI: Ultrasound evaluation of the prostate and bladder. Semin Ultrasound 1:69, 1980.

94. Harada K, Tanahashi Y, Igari D, Numata I, Orikasa S: Clinical evaluation of inside echo patterns in gray scale prostatic echography. J Urol 124:216, 1980.

95. Whitehead ED, Leiter E: Prostatic carcinoma: clinical and surgical staging. NY state J Med 81:184, 1981.

96. Pilepich MV, Perez CA, Prasas S: Computed tomography in definitive radiotherapy of prostatic carcinoma. Int J Radiat Oncol Biol Phys 6:923, 1980.

97. Hovsepian JA, Byar DP: Quantitative radiology for staging and prognosis of patients with advanced prostatic cancer. Urology 14:145, 1979.

98. Prando A, Wallace S, Von Eschenbach AC, Jing BS, Rosengren JE, Hussey DM: Lymphangiography in staging of carcinoma of the prostate. Radiology 131:641, 1979.

99. McLaughlin AP, Saltzstein SL, McCullough DL, Gittes RF: Prostatic carcinoma: incidence and location of unsuspected lymphatic metastases. J Urol 115:89, 1976.

100. Levine MS, Arger PH, Coleman BG, Mulhern CB Jr, Pollack HM, Wein AJ: Detecting lymphatic metastases from prostatic carcinoma: superiority of CT. AJR 137:207, 1981.

101. Goethlin JH, Hoiem L: Percutaneous fine-needle biopsy of radiographically normal lymph nodes in the staging of prostatic carcinoma. Radiology 141:351, 1981.

102. Spring DB, Schroeder D, Babu S, Agee R, Gooding GAW: Ultrasonic evaluation of lymphocele formation after staging lymphadenectomy for prostatic carcinoma. Radiology 141:479, 1981.

103. Gore RM, Moss AA: Value of computed tomography in interstitial I-125 brachytherapy of prostatic cancer. Radiology 146:453–458, 1983.

104. Lytton B, Schiff M, Shonk CR: Treatment of early stage prostate cancer by implantation of Iodine-125. Surg Clin North Am 60:1215, 1980.

105. Goffinet DR, Alvaro M, Freiha F, Toolers DM, Pistenma DA, et al: ^{125}Iodine prostate implants for recurrent carcinomas. Cancer 45:2717, 1980.

106. Ambrose SS: Transcoccygeal ^{125}Iodine prostatic implantation for adenocarcinoma. J Urol 125:365, 1981.

107. Elkon D, Kim JA, Constable WC: Anatomic localization of radioactive gold seeds of the prostate by computer-aided tomography. Comput Tomogr 5:89, 1980.

108. Pinch L, Aceto T JR, Meyer-Bahlburg HFL: Cryptorchidism: a pediatric review. Urol Clin North Am 1:573, 1974.

109. Scorer CG: The descent of the testis. Arch Dis Child 39:605, 1964.

110. Friedland GW, Chang P: The role of imaging in the management of the impalpable undescended testis. AJR 151:1107–1111, 1988.

111. Madrazo BL, Klugo RC, Parks JA, Diloretto R: Ultrasonographic demonstration of undescended testes. Radiology 113:181, 1979.

112. Fritzsche PJ, Hricak H, Kogan BA, Winkler ML, Tanagho EA: Undescended testis: value of MR imaging. Radiology 164:169–173, 1987.

113. Lee JK, McClennan BL, Stanley RJ, Sagel SS: Utility of computed tomography in the localization of the undescended testis. Radiology 135:121, 1980.

114. Wolverson MK, Jagannadharao B, Sundaram M, Riaz MA, Nalesnik WJ, Houttuin E: CT in localization of impalpable cryptorchid testes. AJR 134:725, 1980.

115. Hricak H, Filly RA: Ultrasonography of the scrotum. Invest Radiol 18:112, 1983.

116. Leopold GR, Woo VL, Scheible W, Nachtsheim D, Gosink BB: High-resolution ultrasonography of scrotal pathology. Radiology 131:719, 1979.

117. Phillips GN, Schneider M, Goodman JD, Macchia RJ: Ultrasonic evaluation of the scrotum. Urol Radiol 1:157, 1979.

118. Rodriguez DD, Rodriguez WC, Rivera JJ, Rodriguez S, Otero AA: Doppler ultrasound versus testicular scanning in the evaluation of the acute scrotum. J Urol 125:343, 1981.

119. Bernardy MO, Umer MA, Flanigan RC: Computed tomography of hydrocele of the tunica vaginalis. J Comput Assist Tomogr 9(1):203–204, 1985.

120. Thurnher S, Hricak H, Carroll PR, Pobiel RS, Filly RA: Imaging the testis: comparison between MR imaging and US. Radiology 167:631–636, 1988.

121. Baker LL, Hajek PC, Burkhard TK, Dicapua L, Leopold GR, et al: MR imaging of the scrotum: normal anatomy. Radiology 163:89–92, 1987.

122. Seidenwurm D, Smathers RL, Lo RK, Carrol CL, Bassett J, Hoffman AR: Testes and scrotum: MR imaging at 1.5 T. Radiology 164:393–398, 1987.

123. Rholl KS, Lee JKT, Ling D, Heiken JP, Glazer HS: MR imaging of the scrotum with a high-resolution surface coil. Radiology 163:99–103, 1987.

124. Holder LE, Martire JR, Holmes ER, Wagner HN: Testicular radionuclide angiography and static imaging: anatomy, scintigraphic interpretation, and clinical indications. Radiology 125:739, 1977.

125. Beard CM, Benson RC Jr, Kelalis PP, Elveback LR: Incidence of malignant testicular tumors in the population of Rochester, Minnesota, 1935 through 1974. Mayo Clin Proc 52:8, 1977.

126. Lackner K, Weissbach L, Boldt I, Scherholz K, Brecht G: Computed tomographic demonstration of lymph node metastases in malignant tumors of the testicles: comparison of results of lymphography and computed tomography. ROFO 130:636, 1979.

127. Storm PB, Kern A, Leoning SA, Brown RC, Culp DA: Evaluation of pedal lymphangiography in staging non-seminomatous testicular carcinoma. J Urol 118:1000, 1977.

128. Kademian M, Wirtanen G: Accuracy of bipedal lymphangiography in testicular tumors. Urology 9:218, 1977.

129. Zaubauer W, Kunz R, Lauppi R: Diagnostic reliability of lymphography in patients with malignant testicular tumors. Fortschr Roentgenstr 126:335, 1977.

130. Husband JE, Peckham MJ, MacDonald JS, Hendry WF: The role of computed tomography in the management of testicular teratoma. Clin Radiol 30:243, 1979.

131. Glazer HS, Lee JKT, Melson GL, McClennan BL: Sonographic detection of occult testicular neoplasms. AJR 138:673, 1982.

132. Poskitt KJ, Cooperberg P, Sullivan LD: Sonography and CT in staging nonseminomatous testicular tumors. AJR 144:939–944, 1985.

133. Stomper PC, Fung CY, Socinski MA, Jochelson MS, Garnick MB, Richie JP: Detection of retroperitoneal metastases in early-stage nonseminomatous testicular cancer: analysis of different CT criteria. AJR 149:1187–1190, 1987.

133a. Williams MP, Husband JE, Heron CW: Stage I nonseminomatous germ cell tumors of the testis: radiologic follow-up after orchidectomy. Radiology 164:671–674, 1987.

134. Burney BT, Klatte EC: Ultrasound and computed tomography of the abdomen in the staging and management of testicular carcinoma. Radiology 132:415, 1979.

135. Williams RD, Reinberg SB, Knight LC, Fraley EE: Abdominal staging of testicular tumors using ultrasonography and computed tomography. J Urol 123:872, 1980.

136. Lee JK, McClennan BL, Stanley RJ, Sagel SS: Computed tomography in the staging of testicular neoplasms. Radiology 130:387, 1978.

137. Lien HH, Kolbenstvedt A, Kolmannskog F, Liverud K, Aakhus T: Computer tomography, lymphography and phlebography in metastases from testicular tumors. Acta Radiol (Diagn) 21:505, 1980.

138. Javadpour N, Doppman JL, Bergmann SM, Anderson T: Correlation of computed tomography and serum tumor markers in metastatic retroperitoneal testicular tumor. J Comput Assist Tomogr 2:176, 1978.

139. Stomper PC, Jochelson MS, Friedman EL, Garnick MC, Richie JP: CT evaluation of advanced seminoma treated with chemotherapy. AJR 146:745–748, 1986.

140. Stomper PC, Socinski MA, Kaplan WD, Garnick MB: Failure patterns of nonseminomatous testicular germ cell tumors: radiographic analysis of 51 cases. Radiology 167:641–646, 1988.

141. Husband JE, Barrett A, Peckham MJ: Evaluation of computed tomography in the management of testicular teratoma. Br J Urol 53:179, 1981.

142. Javadpour N, Anderson T, Doppman JL: Computed tomography in evaluation of testicular cancer during intensive chemotherapy. J Urol 122:565, 1979.

143. Soo CH, Bernardino ME, Chuang VP, Ordonez N: Pitfalls of CT findings in post-therapy testicular carcinoma. J Comput Assist Tomogr 5:39, 1981.

144. Husband JE, Hawkes DJ, Peckham MJ: CT estimations of mean attenuation values and volume in testicular tumors: a comparison with surgical and histologic findings. Radiology 144:553, 1982.

145. Nachman JB, Baum ES, White H, Chuang VP, Ordonez N: Bleomycin-induced pulmonary fibrosis mimicking recurrent metastatic disease in a patient with testicular carcinoma. Cancer 47:236, 1981.

146. Scatarige JC, Fishman EK, Kuhajda FP, Taylor GA, Siegelman SS: Low attenuation nodal metastasis in testicular carcinoma. J Comput Assist Tomogr 7:682–687, 1983.

147. Osborn SB: The implications of the reports of the Committee on Radiological Hazards to Patients (Adrian Committee). A symposium given at the Annual Congress of the British Institute of Radiology, April 27, 1962. I. Variations in the radiation dose received by the patient in diagnostic radiology. Br J Radiol 36:230, 1963.

148. Federle MP, Cohen HA, Rosenwein MF, Brant-Zawadzki MN, Cann CE: Pelvimetry by digital radiography, a low dose examination. Radiology 143:733, 1982.

149. Claussen C, Koehler D, Christ F, Golde G, Lochner B: Pelvimetry by digital radiography and its dosimetry. J Perinatal Med 13:287–292, 1985.

150. Adam Y, Alberge S, Castellano M, Kassab M, Escude B: Pelvimetry by digital radiography. Clin Radiol 36:327–330, 1985.

151. Moore MM, Shearer DR: Fetal dose estimates for CT pelvimetry. Radiology 171:265–267, 1989.

152. Brody AS, Saks BJ, Field DR, Skinner ST, Capra RE: Artifacts seen during CT pelvimetry: implications for digital systems with scanning beams. Radiology 160:269–271, 1986.

153. Zawin M, McCarthy S, Scoutt LM, Comite F: High-field MRI and US evaluation of the pelvis in women with leiomyomas. Magn Reson Imaging 8:371, 1990.

154. Dooms GC, Hricak H, Tscholakoff D: Adnexal structures: MR imaging. Radiology 158:639, 1986.

155. Friedman AC, Pyatt RS, Hartman DS, Downey EF, Olson WB: CT of benign cystic masses. AJR 138:659, 1982.

156. Griffiths CT, Berkowitz RS: The ovary. In Kistner RW (ed): Gynecology: Principles and Practice. Chicago, Year Book Medical Publishers, 1986.

157. Scully RE: Tumors of the ovary and mal-developed gonads. In Hartmass WH (ed): Atlas of Tumor Pathology, 3d ed. Washington, DC, Armed Forces Institute of Pathology, 1979.

158. Skaane P, Huebenerm KH: Computed tomography of cystic ovarian teratomas with gravity-dependent layering. J Comput Assist Tomogr 7(5):837–841, 1983.

159. Sloan RD: Cystic teratoma (dermoid) of the ovary. Radiology 81:847, 1963.

160. Sheth S, Fishman EK, Buck JL, Hamper UM, Sanders RC: The variable sonographic appearances of ovarian teratomas: correlation with CT. AJR 151:331–334, 1988.

161. Cawley KM, Mahoney PD, Wilmot MD, Longacre TL: Ovarian dermoid: unusual CT presentation. J Comput Assist Tomogr 7(6):1116–1117, 1983.

162. Quinn SF, Erickson S, Black WC: Cystic ovarian teratomas: the sonographic appearance of the dermoid plug. Radiology 155:477–478, 1985.

163. Laing FC, Van Dalsem VF, Marks WM, Burton JL, Martinez DA: Dermoid cysts of the ovary: their ultrasonographic appearances. Obstet Gynecol 57:99, 1981.

164. Walsh JW, Taylor KJ, Wasson JF, Schwartz PE, Rosenfeld AT: Gray-scale ultrasound in 204 proved gynecologic masses: accuracy and specific diagnostic criteria. Radiology 130:391, 1979.

165. Sandler MA, Silver TM, Karo JJ: Gray-scale ultrasonic features of ovarian teratomas. Radiology 131:705, 1979.

166. Scoutt LM, McCarthy SM, Lange R, Bourque A, Schwartz PE: Evaluation of ovarian masses on MRI with ultrasound correlation. (In press).

167. Mawhinney RR, Powell MC, Worthington BS, Symonds EM: Magnetic resonance imaging of benign ovarian masses. Br J Radiol 61:179, 1988.

168. Mitchell DG, Mintz MC, Spritzer CE, Gussman D, Arger PH, et al: Adnexal masses: MR imaging observations at 1.5 T, with US and CT correlation. Radiology 162:319, 1987.

169. Nyberg DA, Porter BA, Olds MO, Olson DO, Andersen R, Wesby GE: MR imaging of hemorrhagic adnexal masses. J Comput Assist Tomogr 11:664, 1987.

170. Togashi K, Nishimura K, Itoh K, Fujisawa I, Sago T, et al: Ovarian cystic teratomas: MR imaging. Radiology 162:669, 1987.

170a. Smith RC, Lange RC, McCarthy SM: Chemical shift artifact. Dependence on shape and orientation of the lipid-water interface. (In press).

171. Sawyer RW, Vick CW, Walsh JW, McClure PH: Computed tomography of benign ovarian masses. J Comput Assist Tomogr 9(4):784–789, 1985.

172. Wilbur A: Computed tomography of tuboovarian abscesses. J Comput Assist Tomogr 14(4):625–628, 1990.

173. Shamam OM, Bennet WF, Teteris NJ, Finer RM: Primary Fallopian tube adenocarcinoma presenting as a hydrosalpinx: CT appearance. J Comput Assist Tomogr 12(4):674–675, 1988.

174. Togashi K, Nishimura K, Itoh K, Nakano Y, Torizuka K, et al: Computed tomography of hydrosalpinx following tubal ligation. J Comput Assist Tomogr 10(1):78–80, 1986.
175. Moyle JW, Rochester D, Sider L, Shrock K, Krause P: Sonography of ovarian tumors: predictability of tumor type. AJR 141:985, 1983.
176. Sandler MA, Silver TM, Karo JJ: Gray-scale ultrasonic features of ovarian teratomas. Radiology 131:705, 1979.
177. Sheth S, Fishman EK, Buck JL, Hamper UM, Sanders RC: The variable sonographic appearances of ovarian teratomas: correlation with CT. AJR 151:331, 1988.
178. Walsh JW, Taylor KJW, Rosenfield AT: Gray scale ultrasonography in the diagnosis of endometriosis and adenomyosis. AJR 132:87, 1979.
179. Wall SD, Fisher MR, Amparo EG, Hricak H, Higgins CB: Magnetic resonance imaging in the evaluation of abscesses. AJR 144:1217, 1985.
180. Baltarowich OH, Kurtz AB, Pasto ME, Rifkin MD, Needleman L, Goldberg BB: The spectrum of sonographic findings in hemorrhagic ovarian cysts. AJR 148:901, 1987.
181. Hann LE, Hall DA, McArdle CR, Seibel M: Polycystic ovarian disease: sonographic spectrum. Radiology 150:531, 1984.
182. Yeh H, Futterweit W, Thornton JC: Polycystic ovarian disease: US features in 104 patients. Radiology 163:111, 1987.
183. Mendelson EB, Bohn-Velez M, Neiman HL, Russo J: Transvaginal sonography in gynecologic imaging. Semin Ultrasound Comput Tomogr Magn Reson 9:102, 1988.
184. Mitchell D, Gefter W, Spritzer C, Blasco L, Nulson J, et al: Polycystic ovaries: MR imaging. Radiology 160:425, 1986.
185. Silverberg BS: Gynecologic Cancer: Statistical and Epidemiological Information. American Cancer Society Professional Education Publication 6–8, 1975.
186. Watring WG, Edinger DD, Anderson B: Screening and diagnosis in ovarian cancer. Clin Obstet Gynecol 22:745, 1979.
187. Brammer HM, Buck JL, Hayes W, Sheth S, Tavassoli FA: Malignant germ cell tumors of the ovary: radiologic-pathologic correlation. RadioGraphics 10:715–724, 1990.
188. Cho KC, Gold BM: Computed tomography of Krukenberg tumors. AJR 145:285–288, 1985.
189. Rutledge F, Boronow RC, Wharton JT: Gynecologic Oncology. New York, John Wiley & Sons, 1976, p 160.
190. Fukuda T, Ikeuchi M, Hashimoto H, Shakudo M, Oonishi M, et al: Computed tomography of ovarian masses. J Comput Assist Tomogr 10(6):990–996, 1986.
191. Amendola MA, Walsh JW, Amendola BE, Tisnado J, Hall DJ, Goplerud DR: Computed tomography in the evaluation of carcinoma of the ovary. J Comput Assist Tomogr 5:179, 1981.
192. Megibow AJ, Hulnick DH, Bosniak MA, Balthazar EJ: Ovarian metastases: computed tomographic appearances. Radiology 156:161–164, 1985.
193. Photopulos GJ, McCartney WH, Walton LA, Staab EV: Computerized tomography applied to gynecologic oncology. Am J Obstet Gynecol 135:381, 1979.
194. Buy JN, Moss AA, Ghossain MA, Sciot C, Malbec L, et al: Peritoneal implants from ovarian tumors: CT findings. Radiology 169:691–694, 1988.
195. Megibow AJ, Bosniak MA, Ho AG, Beller U, Hulnick DH, Beckman EM: Accuracy of CT in detection of persistent or recurrent ovarian carcinoma: correlation with second-look laparotomy. Radiology 166:341–345, 1988.
196. Smith FW, Cherryman GR, Bayliss AP, Fullerton WT, Law ANR, et al: A comparative study of the accuracy of ultrasound imaging, x-ray computerized tomography and low field MRI diagnosis of ovarian malignancy. Magn Reson Imaging 6:225, 1988.
197. Fishman-Javitt M, Lovecchio JL, Stein HL: MR imaging of ovarian neoplasms. Radiology 165:123, 1987.
198. Ayalon D, Graid M, Hetman-Peri M, et al: Diagnosis of a small ovarian tumor (androgen secreting) by magnetic resonance: a new noninvasive procedure. Am J Obstet Gynecol 159:903, 1988.
199. Fukuda T, Ikeuchi M, Hashimoto H, Shakudo M, Oonishi M, et al: Computed tomography of ovarian masses. J Comput Assist Tomogr 10:990, 1986.
200. Weigert F, Linder P, Rohde U: Computed tomography and magnetic resonance of pseudomyxoma peritonei. J Comput Assist Tomogr 9:1120, 1985.
201. Requard CK, Mettler FA, Wicks JD: Preoperative sonography of malignant ovarian neoplasms. AJR 137:79, 1981.
202. Musumeci R, De Palo G, Kenda R, Tesoro-Tess JD, Di Re F, et al: Retroperitoneal metastases from ovarian carcinoma: Reassessment of 365 patients studied with lymphography. AJR 134:449, 1980.
203. Dunnick NR, Fisher RI, Chu EW, Young RC: Percutaneous aspiration of retroperitoneal lymph nodes in ovarian cancer. AJR 135:109, 1980.
204. Silverman PM, Osborne M, Dunnick NR, Bandy LC: CT prior to second-look operation in ovarian cancer. AJR 150:829–832, 1988.
205. Warde P, Rideout DF, Herman S, Majesky IF, Sturgeon JFG, et al: Computed tomography in advanced ovarian cancer, inter- and intraobserved reliability. Invest Radiol 21:31–33, 1986.
206. Johnson RJ, Blackledge G, Eddleston B, Crowther D: Abdominopelvic computed tomography in the management of ovarian carcinoma. Radiology 146:447–452, 1983.
207. Clarke-Pearson DL, Bandy LC, Dudzinski M, Heaston D, Creasman WT: Computed tomography in evaluation of patients with ovarian carcinoma in complete clinical remission. JAMA 255(5):627–630, 1986.
208. Brenner DE, Shaff MI, Jones HW, Grosh WW, Greco A, Burnett LS: Abdominopelvic computed tomography: evaluation in patients undergoing second-look laparotomy for ovarian carcinoma. Obstet Gynecol 645:715–719, 1985.
209. Goldhirsch A, Triller JK, Greiner R, Dreher E, Daves BW: Computed tomography prior to second-look operation in advanced ovarian cancer. Obstet Gynecol 62:630–633, 1983.
210. Silverman PM, Osborne M, Dunnick NR, Bandy LC: CT prior to second-look operation in ovarian cancer. AJR 150:829, 1988.
211. Callen PW, Filly RA, Munyer TP: Intrauterine contraceptive devices: evaluation by sonography. AJR 135:797, 1980.
212. Wittmann BK, Fulton L, Cooperberg PL, Lyons EA, Miller C, Shaw D: Molar pregnancy: early diagnosis by ultrasound. J Clin Ultrasound 9:153, 1981.
213. Laing FC, Filly RA, Marks WM, Brown TW: Ultrasonic demonstration of endometrial fluid collections unassociated with pregnancy. Radiology 137:471, 1980.
214. Wilson DA, Stacy TM, Smith EI: Ultrasound diagnosis of hydrocolpos and hydrometrocolpos. Radiology 128:451, 1978.
215. Laing FC: Sonography of a persistently retroverted gravid uterus. AJR 136:413, 1981.
216. Chinn DH, Filly RA, Callen PW: Prediction of intrauterine growth retardation by sonographic estimation of total intrauterine volume. J Clin Ultrasound 8:125, 1981.
217. Brown TW, Filly RA, Laing FC, Barton J: Analysis of ultrasonographic criteria in the evaluation for ectopic pregnancy. AJR 131:967, 1978.
218. Richardson ML, Kinard RE, Watters DH: Location of intrauterine devices: evaluation by computed tomography. Radiology 142:690, 1982.
219. Barbieri R, Kistner RW: Endometriosis. In Kistner RW (ed): Gynecology: Principles and Practice. Chicago, Year Book Medical Publishers, 1986.
220. Clarke-Pearson DL, Dawood MY: Endometriosis. In Clarke-Pearson DL, Dawood MY (eds): Green's Gynecology. Boston, Little, Brown, 1990.
221. William TJ, Pratt JH: Endometriosis in 1,000 consecutive celiotomies: incidence and management. Am J Obstet Gynecol 129:245, 1977.
222. Coleman BG, Arger PH, Mulhern CH: Endometriosis: clinical and ultrasonic correlation. AJR 132:747, 1979.
223. Fishman EK, Scatarige JC, Saksouk FA, Rosenshein NB, Siegelman SS: Computed tomography of endometriosis. J Comput Assist Tomogr 7(2):257–264, 1983.
224. Amato M, Levitt R: Abdominal wall endometrioma: CT Findings. J Comput Assist Tomogr 8(6):1213–1214, 1984.
225. Arrivé L, Hricak H, Martin MC: Pelvic endometriosis: MR imaging. Radiology 171:687, 1989.
226. Nishimura K, Togashi K, Itoh K, Fujisawa I, Noma S, et al:

Endometrial cysts of the ovary: MR imaging. Radiology 162:315, 1987.

227. Zawin M, McCarthy S, Scoutt L, Comite F: Endometriosis: appearance and detection at MR imaging. Radiology 171:693, 1989.

228. Togashi K, Kimura I, Nakano Y, Konishi J, Mori T: Endometrial cysts: diagnosis with MR imaging. Radiology 177(P):242, 1990.

229. Friedman H, Vogelzang RL, Mendelson EB, Neiman HL, Cohen M: Endometriosis detection by US with laparoscopic correlation. Radiology 157:217, 1985.

230. Fishman EK, Scatarige JC, Saksouk FA, Rosenhein NB, Siegelman SS: Computed tomography of endometriosis. J Comput Assist Tomogr 7:257, 1983.

231. Kistner RW: The uterine corpus. In Kistner RW (ed): Gynecology: Principles and Practice. Chicago, Year Book Medical Publishers, 1986.

232. Mark AS, Hricak H, Heinrichs LW, Hendrickson MR, Winkler ML, et al: Adenomyosis and leiomyoma: differential diagnosis with MR imaging. Radiology 163:527, 1987.

233. Togashi K, Nishimura K, Itoh K, Fujisawa I, Noma S, et al: Adenomyosis: diagnosis with MR imaging. Radiology 166:111, 1988.

234. Togashi K, Ozasa H, Konishi I, Itoh H, Nishimura K, et al: Enlarged uterus: differentiation between adenomyosis and leiomyomas with MR imaging. Radiology 171:531, 1989.

235. Tada S, Tsukioka M, Ishii C, Tanaka H, Mizunuma K: Computed tomographic features of uterine myoma. J Comput Assist Tomogr 5:866–869, 1981.

236. Oppenheimer DA, Carroll BA, Young SW: Lipoleiomyoma of the uterus. J Comput Assist Tomogr 6:640, 1982.

237. Hricak H, Tscholakoff D, Heinrichs L, Fisher M, Dooms G, et al: Uterine leiomyomas: correlation of MR, histopathologic findings, and symptoms. Radiology 158:385, 1986.

238. Dudiak CM, Turner DA, Patel SK, Archie JT, Silver B, Norusis M: Uterine leiomyomas in the infertile patient: preoperative localization with MR imaging versus US and hysterosalpingography. Radiology 167:627, 1988.

239. Hamlin DJ, Pettersson H, Fitzsimmons J, Morgan LS: MR imaging of uterine leiomyomas and their complications. J Comput Assist Tomogr 9:902, 1985.

240. Weinreb JC, Barkoff ND, Megibow A, Demopoulos R: The value of MR imaging in distinguishing leiomyomas from other solid pelvic masses when sonography is indeterminate. AJR 154:295, 1990.

241. Zanetti E, Ferrari LR, Rossi G: Classification and radiographic features of uterine malformations: hysterosalpingogram study. Br J Radiol 51:161, 1978.

242. Woolf RB, Allen WM: Concomitant malformations: the frequent simultaneous occurrence of congenital malformations of the reproductive and urinary tracts. Obstet Gynecol 2:236, 1953.

243. Buttram VC: Mullerian anomalies and their management. Fertil Steril 40:159, 1983.

244. Golan A, Langer R, Bukovsky I, Caspi E: Congenital anomalies of the mullerian system. Fertil Steril 51:747, 1989.

245. Pellerito J, McCarthy S, Doyle M, Meyer W, De Cherney A: Relative accuracy of MRI, transvaginal ultrasound, and hysterosalpingography in the diagnosis of uterine anomalies. Radiology 177(P):105, 1990.

246. Carrington BM, Hricak H, Nuruddin RN, Secaf E, Laros RK, Hill EC: Mullerian duct anomalies: MR imaging evaluation. Radiology 176:715, 1990.

247. Fedele L, Dorta M, Brioschi D, Massari C, Candiani GB: Magnetic resonance evaluation of double uteri. Obstet Gynecol 74:844, 1989.

248. Mintz MC, Thickman DI, Gussman D, Kressel HY: MR evaluation of uterine anomalies. AJR 148:287, 1987.

249. Gross BH, Jafri SZH, Glazer GM: Significance of intrauterine gas demonstrated by computed tomography. J Comput Assist Tomogr 7(5):842–845, 1983.

250. Kistner RW: Gynecology Principles and Practice, 3d ed. Chicago, Year Book Medical Publishers, 1979, pp 255–276.

251. Staging as recommended by the Cancer Committee of the International Federation of Gynecology and Obstetrics. Gynecol Oncol 4:13, 1976.

252. De Saia PJ, Creasman WT: Clinical Gynecologic Oncology. St Louis, CV Mosby, 1981, pp 128–152.

253. Jobson VW, Girtanner RE, Averette HE: Therapy and survival of early invasive carcinoma of the cervix uteri with metastases to the pelvic nodes. Surg Obstet Gynecol 151:27, 1980.

254. Baker HW, Makk L, Morrissey RW, Ockstein H: Stage I adenocarcinoma of the endometrium: a clinical and histopathological study of 65 cases treated with preoperative radium. Obstet Gynecol 54:146, 1979.

255. Requard CK, Wicks JD, Mettler FA: Ultrasonography in the staging of endometrial adenocarcinoma. Radiology 140:781, 1981.

256. Schlensker KH, Beckers H: The use of ultrasound in the diagnosis of pelvic pathology. Arch Gynecol 229:91, 1980.

257. Lee KR, Mansfield CM, Dwyer SJ, Cox HL, Levine E, Templeton AW: CT for intracavitary radiotherapy planning. AJR 135:809, 1980.

258. Chen SS, Kumari S, Lee L: Contribution of abdominal computed tomography (CT) in the management of gynecologic cancer: correlated study of CT image and gross surgical pathology. Gynecol Oncol 10:162, 1980.

259. Walsh JW, Amendola MA, Karsten FK, Tisnado J, Hazra TA: Computed tomographic detection of pelvic and inguinal lymph-node metastases from primary and recurrent pelvic malignant disease. Radiology 137:157, 1980.

260. Hamlin DJ, Burgener FA, Beecham JB: CT of intramural endometrial carcinoma: contrast enhancement is essential. AJR 137:551, 1981.

261. Dore R, Moro G, D'Andrea F, Fianza A, Franchi M, Bolis PF: CT evaluation of myometrium invasion in endometrial carcinoma. J Comput Assist Tomogr 11(2):282–289, 1987.

262. Walsh JW, Goplerud DR: Computed tomography of primary, persistent and recurrent endometrial malignancy. AJR 139:1149–1154, 1982.

263. Balfe DM, Dyke JV, Lee JKT, Weyman PJ, McClennan BL: Computed tomography in malignant endometrial neoplasms. J Comput Assist Tomogr 7(4):677–681, 1983.

264. Scott WW, Rosenheim NB, Seigelman SS, Sander RC: The obstructed uterus. Radiology 141:767, 1981.

265. Whitley NO, Brenner DE, Francis A, Villa Santa U, Aisner J, et al: Computed tomographic evaluation of carcinoma of the cervix. Radiology 142:439, 1982.

266. Musumeci R, de Palo G, Conti U, Kenda R, Mangioni C, et al: Are retroperitoneal lymph node metastases a major problem in endometrial adenocarcinoma? Cancer 46:1887, 1980.

267. Ginaldi S, Wallace S, Jing BS, Bernardino ME: Carcinoma of the cervix: lymphangiography and computed tomography. AJR 136:1087, 1981.

268. Javitt MCF, Stein HL, Lovecchio JL: MRI in staging of endometrial and cervical carcinoma. Magn Reson Imaging 5:83, 1987.

269. Worthington JL, Balfe DM, Lee JKT, Gersell DJ, Heiken JP, et al: Uterine neoplasms: MR imaging. Radiology 159:725, 1986.

270. Belloni C, Vigano R, del Maschio A, Sironi S, Taccagni GL, Vignali M: Magnetic resonance imaging in endometrial carcinoma staging. Gynecol Oncol 37:172, 1990.

271. Chen SS, Rumancik WM, Spiegel G: Magnetic resonance imaging in stage I endometrial carcinoma. Obstet Gynecol 75:274, 1990.

272. Long F, Scoutt L, McCarthy S, Lange R, Zawin M, et al: MRI & synthetic imaging of endometrial carcinoma. Abstract. In Book of Abstracts: SMRI 1988. Sixth Annual Meeting Program and Abstracts, 62, 1988.

273. Posniak HV, Olson MC, Dudiak CM, Castelli MJ, Dolan J, et al: MR imaging of uterine carcinoma: correlation with clinical and pathologic findings. RadioGraphics 10:15, 1990.

274. Yazigi R, Cohen J, Munoz AK, Sandstad J: Magnetic resonance imaging determination of myometrial invasion in endometrial carcinoma. Gynecol Oncol 34:94, 1989.

275. DiSaia PJ, Creasman WT, Boronow RC, Blessing JA: Risk factors and recurrent patterns in Stage I endometrial cancer. Am J Obstet Gynecol 151:1009, 1985.

276. Ascher SM, Scoutt LM, McCarthy SM, Lange RC, DeCherney AH: Uterine changes after dilatation and curettage. MR imaging findings. Radiology 180:433–435, 1991.

277. Boronow RC, Morrow CP, Creasman WT, DiSaia PJ, Silverberg SG, et al: Surgical staging in endometrial cancer: clinical-pathology findings of a prospective study. Obstet Gynecol 63:825, 1984.

278. Yu WS, Sagerman RH, Chung CT, King GA, Dalal PS, et al: Anatomical relationships in intracavitary irradiation demonstrated by computed tomography. Radiology 143:537, 1982.

279. Callen PW: Ultrasound evaluation of gestational trophoblastic disease. In Callen PW (ed): Ultrasonography in Obstetrics and Gynecology. Philadelphia, WB Saunders Company, 1988.

280. Schwartz P: Gynecologic cancer in clinical medicine. In Spittell JA (ed): Clinical Medicine. Philadelphia, Harper & Row, 1985.

281. Miyasaka Y, Hachiya J, Furuya Y, Seki T, Watanabe H: CT evaluation of invasive trophoblastic disease. J Comput Assist Tomogr 9(3):459–462, 1985.

282. Sanders C, Rubin E: Malignant gestational trophoblastic disease: CT findings. AJR 148:165–168, 1987.

282a. Powell MC, Buckley J, Worthington BS, Symonds EM: Magnetic resonance imaging and hydatidiform mole. Br J Radiol 59:561, 1986.

283. Barton JW, McCarthy S, Scoutt LM, Lange R, Kohorn EI: Gestational trophoblastic neoplasia: a role for MR imaging? Radiology 173:372, 1989.

283a. Silverberg E, Boring CC, Squires TS: Cancer statistics, 1990. CA 40:18–19, 1990.

284. Hricak H, Demas BE, Braga CA, Fisher MR, Winkler ML: Gestational trophoblastic neoplasm of the uterus: MR assessment. Radiology 161:11, 1986.

285. Kohorn EI, Barton JW, McCarthy SM, Scoutt LM: Magnetic resonance imaging as an aid in the diagnosis of gestational trophoblastic neoplasia. Abstract. In Book of Abstracts: International Society for the Study of Trophoblast. London, Fifth World Congress on Gestational Trophoblastic Diseases, 1990.

286. Vick CW, Walsh JW, Wheelock JB, Brewer WH: CT of the normal and abnormal parametria in cervical cancer. AJR 143:597–603, 1984.

287. Walsh JW, Rosenfield AT, Jaffe CC, Schwartz PE, Simeone J, et al: Prospective comparison of ultrasound and computed tomography in the evaluation of gynecologic pelvic masses. AJR 131:955, 1978.

288. Kilcheski, Arger PH, Mulhern CB, Coleman BG, Kressel HY, Mikuta JI: Role of computed tomography in the presurgical evaluation of carcinoma of the cervix. J Comput Assist Tomogr 5:378, 1981.

289. Kim S, Choi B, Lee H, Kang S, Choi Y, et al: Uterine cervical carcinoma: comparison of CT and MR findings. Radiology 175:45, 1990.

290. Togashi K, Nishimura K, Sagoh T, Minami S, Noma S, et al: Carcinoma of the cervix: staging with MR imaging. Radiology 171:245, 1989.

291. Rubens D, Thornbury JR, Angel C, Stoler M, Weiss S, et al: Stage 1B cervical carcinoma: comparison of clinical, MR and pathologic staging. AJR 150:135, 1988.

292. Togashi K, Nishimura K, Itoh K, Fujisawa I, Asato R, et al: Uterine cervical cancer: assessment with high-field MR imaging. Radiology 160:431, 1986.

293. Waggenspack GA, Amparo EG, Hannigan EV: MR imaging of uterine cervical carcinoma. J Comput Assist Tomogr 12:409, 1988.

294. Bandy LC, Clarke-Pearson DL, Silverman PM, Creasman WT: Computed tomography in evaluation of extra pelvic lymphadenopathy in carcinoma of the cervix. Obstet Gynecol 65:73, 1985.

295. Dooms GC, Hricak H, Moseley ME, Bottles K, Fisher M, Higgins CB: Characterization of lymphadenopathy by magnetic resonance relaxation times: preliminary results. Radiology 155:691, 1985.

296. Lee JKT, Heiken JP, Ling D, Glazer HS, Balfe DM, et al: Magnetic resonance imaging of abdominal and pelvic lymphadenopathy. Radiology 153:181, 1984.

297. Dooms GC, Hricak H, Crooks LE, Higgins CB: Magnetic resonance imaging of the lymph nodes: comparison with CT. Radiology 153:719, 1984.

298. Ginaldi S, Wallace S, Jing BS, Bernardino ME: Carcinoma of the cervix: lymphangiography and computed tomography. AJR 136:1087, 1981.

299. Whitley NO, Brenner DE, Francis A, Villa Santa U, Aisner J, et al: Computed tomographic evaluation of carcinoma of the cervix. Radiology 142:439, 1982.

300. Piver MS, Wallace S, Castro JR: The accuracy of lymphangiography in carcinoma of the uterine cervix. AJR, Rad Ther Nucl Med 111:278, 1971.

301. Brown RC, Buchsbaum HJ, Tewfik HH, Platz CE: Accuracy of lymphangiography in the diagnosis of paraaortic lymph node metastases from carcinoma of the cervix. Obstet Gynecol 54:571, 1979.

302. Walsh JW, Amendola MA, Hall DJ, Tisnado J, Goplerud DR: Recurrent carcinoma of the cervix: CT diagnosis. AJR 136:117, 1981.

303. Waggenspack GA, Amparo EG, Hannigan EV, O'Neal MF: MRI of cervical carcinoma. Semin Ultrasound CT MR 9:158, 1988.

304. Chang YCF, Hricak H, Thurnher S, Lacey CG: Vagina: evaluation with MR imaging Part II. Neoplasms. Radiology 169:175–179, 1988.

305. Ebner F, Kressel HY, Mintz MC, Carlson J, Cohen E, et al: Tumor recurrence versus fibrosis in the female pelvis: differentiation with MR imaging at 1.5 T. Radiology 166:333, 1988.

306. Mayer JE: Review: radiography of the distal colon and rectum after irradiation of carcinoma of the cervix. AJR 136:691, 1981.

307. De Klerk DJJ, McCusker I, Loubser JS: Anterior sacral meningoceles. S Afr Med J 54:361, 1978.

308. Sundaram M, Wolverson MK, Joist JH, Riaz MA, Rao BJ: Case report 133. Skeletal Radiol 6:54, 1981.

309. Penkava RR: Iliopsoas bursitis demonstrated by computed tomography. AJR 135:175, 1980.

310. Jolles H, Coulam CM: CT of ascites: differential diagnosis. AJR 135:315, 1980.

311. Wolverson MK, Jagannadharoa B, Sundaram M, Heiberg E, Grider R: Computed tomography in the diagnosis of gluteal abscesses and other peripelvic fluid collections. J Comput Assist Tomogr 5:34, 1981.

312. Koehler PR, Moss AA: Diagnosis of intraabdominal and pelvic abscesses by computerized tomography. JAMA 244:49, 1980.

313. Callen PW: Computed tomographic evaluation of abdominal and pelvic abscesses. Radiology 131:171, 1979.

CHAPTER 26

PEDIATRIC BODY IMAGING

EDWARD WEINBERGER ▪ *DAVID K. BREWER*

In this chapter we offer the radiologist an introduction to pediatric body computed tomography (CT), including (1) technical guidelines for performing pediatric CT exams, (2) suggestions for selection among imaging methods, and (3) descriptions of pediatric diseases most often studied with CT. In some areas of pediatric body imaging, magnetic resonance (MR) clearly provides more information than CT (e.g., in tumors of the musculoskeletal system). Appropriate applications of MR are discussed.

Amplification of such a brief chapter will no doubt be necessary. Among the references, we especially recommend the books by Daneman,[1] Siegel,[2] and Cohen and Edwards.[3]

Techniques

Radiographic Techniques

Radiographic factors are adjusted to achieve a balance between good spatial resolution and low radiation exposure. Slice thickness depends on the body part of interest but is usually thinner in children than in adults. For example, a 5-mm slice is often used in examination of infants and small children. Spacing of slices varies with the clinical problem. A field of view is selected so that the area of interest fills the imaging screen. Short exposure time is important. We use a 2-sec exposure for children who cannot hold their breath and a 3.5-sec exposure for those who can. The milliamperes and peak kilovolts vary with body size, slice thickness, and capabilities of individual machines.

Radiation dose during CT examinations is expressed as computed tomography dose index (CTDI) or multiple scan average dose (MSAD). Manufacturers provide CTDI values for their machines, and several reports have assessed these values in children.[4–6]

For a given milliampere setting a child usually receives a higher dose than an adult.[5] Thus the CTDI, which is based on adult phantoms, may underestimate the pediatric dose. Radiation dose varies with milliamperes but is less dependent on slice thickness.[6] By lowering the milliamperes for pediatric patients and carefully monitoring the number of slices, the radiologist can control the radiation dose.

Sedation

Experienced personnel and modern, fast CT scanners reduce the need for sedation. Approximately 30 per cent of our patients are sedated, and most of these are between the ages of 6 months and 3 years.

Standard principles of care for sedated patients should be observed regardless of the sedative agent. The American Academy of Pediatrics (AAP) has published guidelines for the elective use of sedation, and radiologists supervising pediatric sedation should be familiar with them.[7–9] A pulse oximeter and an automatic sphygmomanometer simplify the monitoring of a sedated child. A radiology department nurse provides valuable assistance in caring for these patients.

Selection among the numerous sedative agents is best left to the radiologist's preference and experience.[8] We prefer chloral hydrate because of its ease of oral administration and its relative lack of respiratory depression. We administer 50 to 75 mg/kg body weight, with a maximum dose of 1000 mg for children less than 3 years old and a maximum dose of 2000 mg for children 3 years and older. The intestinal absorption of the drug is improved by not allowing the child anything by mouth before sedation, as described by AAP guidelines, and by adding metoclopramide (0.4 mg/kg; maximum dose, 5 mg), which assists in gastric emptying. The onset of sedation then becomes more rapid and predictable.

Chloral hydrate sedation is unsuccessful in about five per cent of uncooperative patients, particularly older, retarded children. We generally resort to intravenous sedation given by an anesthesiologist in these cases. A person other than an anesthesiologist may, of course, be qualified to administer intravenous sedation.[10, 11] This practice may become more widespread as the increasing use of MR examinations increases the need for efficient sedation. We have tried to avoid intramuscular agents (e.g., mixtures of meperidine hydrochloride, promethazine hydrochloride, and chlorpromazine) because of a prolonged sedative effect and an increased risk of respiratory complications.[9, 12]

Gastrointestinal Contrast

Gastrointestinal contrast is necessary in almost every abdominal examination.[13] Most of our patients are willing to drink a 2.5 per cent diatrizoate meglumine (Hypaque) solution made by mixing diatrizoate meglumine powder with decarbonated soda pop such as cola. The contrast solution is put back in the soda pop can to make it psychologically more pleasing. Flavored barium products are less well accepted. Infants younger than 8 months receive up to 150 mL of oral contrast. Children between the ages of 8 months and 2 years receive 250 mL. Those older than 2 years receive 400 mL, and teenagers drink about 800 mL. The child drinks the contrast over a 30-minute period, and the exam starts shortly after he or she finishes. If a child needs sedation, it is given first, and the oral contrast is given about 15 minutes later while the child is still awake. In children 2 years old and younger, we often use a nasogastric tube to give oral sedation and contrast expeditiously. The colon is identified by gas and stool contents. Contrast enemas are used only when the colon is of particular concern, as in complex pelvic abscess.

Intravenous Contrast

Intravenous contrast is almost always used in abdominal examinations and is often helpful in thoracic and musculoskeletal examinations.[14] We use nonionic contrast agents (300 mg I/mL) because of the low incidence of vomiting during bolus injection. We limit total contrast dose to 2 mL/kg body weight (maximum dose, 100 mL). Contrast is injected by hand as a bolus, and scanning starts after about half the contrast has been injected.

Thorax

Technical Considerations

Modern CT machines with scan times of 1 to 2 seconds cannot completely eliminate respiratory and cardiac motion artifact in the small child. Because cine-CT is not widely available, most radiologists will continue to face this limitation.[15] The small central lesion in the small patient may remain elusive.

Large mediastinal masses can severely compress the trachea, and sedation may compound the risk of airway obstruction.[16] The radiologist must be particularly cautious in sedating these patients.

Bolus injection of intravenous contrast is important in studying mediastinal problems. Contrast is of less benefit in other thoracic abnormalities and is not routinely used.

TABLE 26–1 ■ Mediastinal Masses

ANTERIOR	MIDDLE	POSTERIOR
Thymus, normal	Foregut duplication cysts	Neurogenic tumors
Thymus, enlarged (thymoma, cyst)	(bronchogenic, enteric)	Neurenteric cyst
Lymphoma/leukemia	Adenopathy (inflammatory, neoplastic)	
Germ cell tumors		
Lymphangioma (cystic hygroma)		

Mediastinum

The mediastinum is the most frequent location of childhood chest masses, and nearly all these masses are discovered on plain chest films.[17] Dividing the mediastinum into anterior, middle, and posterior compartments remains a useful method to categorize masses (Table 26–1).[18] Since these divisions are not true anatomic spaces, masses may not be neatly restricted to one compartment.

ANTERIOR MEDIASTINUM

Computed tomography demonstrates the thymus in all normal children. Because of its variable size, shape, and location, the normal thymus eventually "tricks" every radiologist into a misdiagnosis of pathologic mass. Familiarity with the numerous descriptions of normal thymic appearance will reduce this error.[19–23] In general, the thymus occupies the upper anterior mediastinum. Either lobe may lie adjacent to the lateral border of the heart, and thymic tissue may extend posteriorly to reach the spine. The normally large thymus of young children often has convex lateral borders and seems to envelop the great vessels anteriorly (Fig. 26–1). In older children the thymus is smaller and less likely to extend away from the upper anterior mediastinum. It usually has a triangular shape with straight or concave lateral borders (Fig. 26–2). The borders of a normal thymus are smooth rather than nodular. The normal thymus never displaces other mediastinal structures such as

trachea and great vessels. Normal thymic tissue in young children is homogeneous before and after intravenous contrast. Fat in the thymus of older children produces a more heterogeneous appearance. The abnormal thymus is identified by increased size, nodular contours, displacement of normal mediastinal structures, and excessively heterogeneous tissue density. In cases of questionable enlargement of the thymus, quantitative measurements may be helpful.[19–21, 24] Magnetic resonance provides information similar to that given by CT. Although heterogeneous MR signal suggests an abnormal thymus, the signal intensity alone does not reliably distinguish normal from abnormal thymus.[25, 26]

Lymphoma is the most frequent mass in the anterior mediastinum.[27, 28] Lymphomas are often lobulated, may have irregular enhancement, and may cause severe tracheal compression.[16, 29] When compared with chest films, CT more accurately defines the extent of thoracic lymphoma. The additional information provided by CT modifies therapy often enough to warrant routine use of CT in most, and perhaps all, children with lymphoma.[30–33] Computed tomography aids radiation therapy planning and allows more accurate evaluation of small masses during treatment. Early detection of recurrence is probably best accomplished with CT. The normal thymus may regrow after treatment and can be confused with tumor recurrence.[34, 35]

Other anterior mediastinal masses may have CT

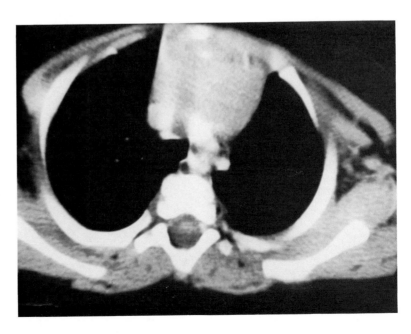

FIGURE 26–1 ■ Normal thymus in a 9-month-old girl. At this age, the thymus is homogeneous in appearance and usually has convex or straight lateral margins. This pattern may persist into the early teenage years, when the thymus assumes a configuration more like an arrowhead or a triangle (see Figure 26–2).

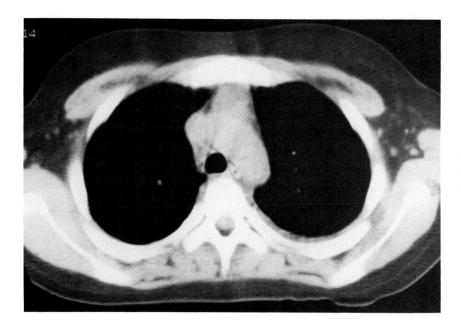

FIGURE 26–2 ■ Normal thymus in an 11-year-old girl. By this age the thymus has assumed a configuration more like an arrowhead or a triangle. Slightly heterogeneous parenchyma is normal at this age. The presence of an anterior junction line may not be seen until the third decade of life. Small left pleural effusion is unrelated.

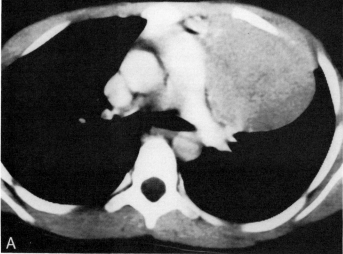

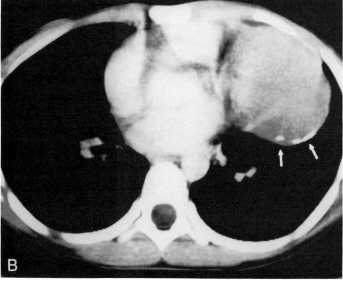

FIGURE 26–3 ■ Thymoma in an 11-year-old girl with myasthenia gravis. CT scans show a large, left-sided anterior mediastinal mass of soft tissue density. Calcification *(arrows)* would be distinctly unusual in lymphoma but may also be present in teratoma.

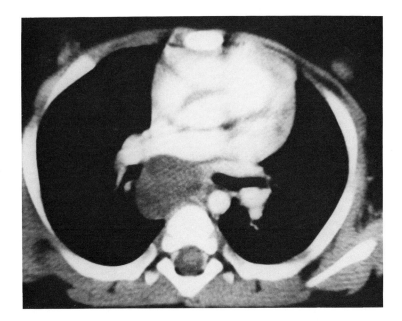

FIGURE 26–4 ■ Bronchogenic cyst in a 9-month-old girl. There is a nonenhancing, well-circumscribed, round subcarinal mass of fluid density that compresses and displaces the right pulmonary artery anteriorly and the right bronchus superiorly (not shown in this section). These findings are typical for bronchogenic cyst.

features that distinguish them from lymphoma.[28] Teratomas, for example, often contain fat and calcifications. Thymomas may contain calcification (Fig. 26–3). Lymphangioma, or cystic hygroma, is a benign congenital malformation of lymphatic tissue that may form a network of small lymphatic channels or a collection of large cystic spaces. Most lymphangiomas occur in the neck and axilla. The cervical tumors may extend into the anterior mediastinum. Occasionally lymphangiomas are found in other mediastinal compartments. CT shows a hypodense mass without calcification or enhancement; thin septations may be visible. Lymphangiomas may displace normal structures.

MIDDLE MEDIASTINUM

Hilar adenopathy and benign cysts account for most of the masses in the middle mediastinum. Computed tomography has limited use in evaluation of inflammatory adenopathy. Lymphoma in hilar nodes usually is studied with CT for the reasons mentioned in the preceding section.

The benign cysts include bronchogenic cysts and enteric duplication cysts. These are usually recognized as cysts because of their low CT attenuation numbers (Fig. 26–4). Occasionally the fluid in the cyst has a high CT number, and the cyst appears to be solid tissue.[36] These cysts may also be shown by MR (Fig. 26–5).

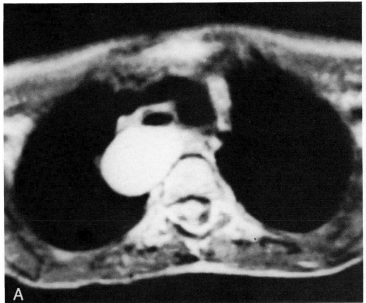
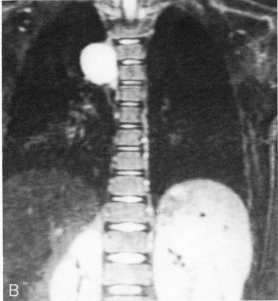

FIGURE 26–5 ■ Bronchogenic cyst in a 10-year-old boy. *A*, Axial (SE, 2000/25) and *B*, coronal (SE, 2000/80) MR images show a well-circumscribed, right paravertebral mass of high signal intensity, consistent with proteinaceous fluid. The mass displaces the trachea anteriorly and has its center anterior to the paravertebral sympathetic chain. Findings are suggestive of bronchogenic or enteric cyst.

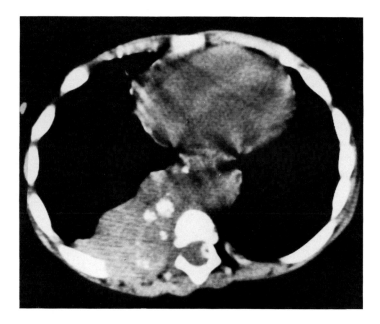

FIGURE 26–6 ■ Intraspinal extension of thoracic neuroblastoma in an 8-month-old boy. CT scan performed after a myelogram demonstrates a large, partially calcified, predominantly right-sided paravertebral mass that extends into the spinal canal and displaces the thecal sac to the left. The ring of density within the spinal canal represents contrast within the subarachnoid space. About 15% of neuroblastomas extend into the spinal canal, but subarachnoid extension is extremely unusual.

POSTERIOR MEDIASTINUM

About 40 per cent of mediastinal masses arise in the posterior mediastinum. Nearly all of these masses are neuroblastomas, ganglioneuromas, or other neurogenic tumors. Characteristic plain film features, including distortion of adjacent ribs and tumor calcification, usually allow confident diagnosis, but CT is critically important in evaluating intraspinal extension.[37] Such extension may be asymptomatic and should be demonstrated before surgery. The CT examination after subarachnoid contrast injection accurately defines the intraspinal extradural tumor (Fig. 26–6). However, a high-resolution CT examination without subarachnoid contrast can often clearly show extradural fat and may thus indicate whether tumor

is in the canal (see Fig. 26–19).[38] MR offers excellent demonstration of paraspinal masses and intraspinal extension of tumor (Fig. 26–7; see also Fig. 26–21). Because subarachnoid contrast is not needed in MR exams, MR will likely replace CT as the most important imaging method to detect posterior mediastinal masses.[39]

Lung Parenchyma and Bronchi

Computed tomography is the most effective method to search for metastatic tumor nodules in children's lungs.[40, 41] The examination occupies an important position in the "protocol" workup of patients with tumors such as Wilms' tumor, osteogenic

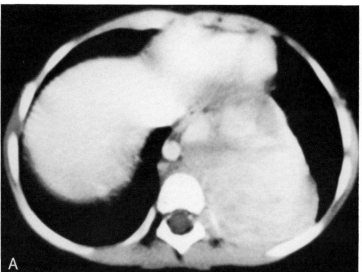

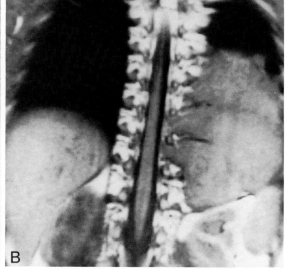

FIGURE 26–7 ■ Thoracic neuroblastoma in an 8-month-old girl. About one third of neuroblastomas have their origin outside the abdomen. A, CT scan demonstrates large left paravertebral mass consistent with tumor originating from the paravertebral sympathetic chain. The mass extends into the neural foramen but does not displace the contents of the thecal sac. B, Coronal MR T1-weighted image (SE, 600/20) more dramatically illustrates the mass, which extends into multiple neural foramina without displacing the thecal sac. These findings are typical of neuroblastoma. A large neurofibroma could give similar appearance.

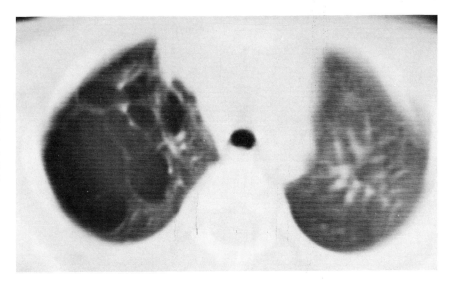

FIGURE 26–8 ■ Cystic adenomatoid malformation in an 11-month-old girl with recurrent upper respiratory tract infections. A multilocular cystic mass is present in the right upper lobe. Chest films suggested that this abnormality had been present since birth. Cystic adenomatoid malformation may have both solid and cystic components.

sarcoma, and rhabdomyosarcoma. The nodules are often in a subpleural or peripheral location. Benign nodules, although less common in children than in adults, slightly reduce the specificity of the CT examination.[42] In addition, nodules may still be visible after chemotherapy has transformed malignant cells into "benign" scar tissue.[43]

Nonmetastatic masses in lung tissue are rare in children and are generally adequately displayed with chest films. Computed tomography may be helpful in distinguishing solid neoplasms from masslike inflammatory processes.

Most congenital malformations of the lung are adequately demonstrated by plain films. CT has limited use in evaluating such lesions as congenital cystic adenomatoid malformation and sequestration, but it may help in confirming the diagnosis and planning surgery (Fig. 26–8).[44–46]

Bronchial abnormalities have been evaluated with CT. Thin-section, or high-resolution, CT can demonstrate bronchiectasis, for example.[47] Aspirated foreign bodies are usually recognized with plain film techniques, but CT can be helpful in confusing cases.[48]

Other pulmonary parenchymal diseases are being studied by high-resolution CT, but the utility of this application of CT in children is not clear.[49, 50]

Chest Wall and Pleura

Computed tomography offers clear delineation of chest wall masses and may give some clues about their histology (Table 26–2). This information is helpful mainly in preparing for surgery. Because many

TABLE 26–2 ■ Chest Wall Masses

BENIGN	MALIGNANT
Lipoma	Rhabdomyosarcoma
Lymphangioma/hemangioma	Neuroblastoma
Neurofibroma	Small round cell tumors (Ewing's, Askin's)

chest wall tumors are cosmetically deforming or malignant,[51] surgery is at least contemplated in most cases.

Useful therapeutic information may be obtained from CT examination of complicated pleural effusions. Loculated inflammatory effusions may be localized and distinguished from adjacent pulmonary abnormalities.[52] CT will define the mass associated with a malignant effusion (Fig. 26–9).

Cardiovascular System

Standard CT techniques have limited value in imaging congenital anomalies of the heart and thoracic vessels. Ultrafast CT, gated MR, and dynamic MR have the potential to become important diagnostic methods in congenital heart disease.[53–57]

Abdomen and Pelvis

In children, as in adults, an integrated imaging approach is used to evaluate the abdomen and pelvis. It is unusual for CT to be the initial modality employed. If a mass is suspected, plain films should be obtained first. If the problem clearly relates to the gastrointestinal tract (such as bowel obstruction or atresia), the appropriate gastrointestinal study is performed. Otherwise, ultrasound is usually performed after plain films, as it is easier to perform than CT and can often localize the abnormality. Relative lack of fat makes ultrasound ideally suited for the evaluation of the young infant. Ultrasound also has the benefit of being able to "move" with the patient; even with 1- and 2-sec scan times, considerable degradation of information may occur on CT if the child is small and breathing rapidly. In general, if a solid mass is discovered, CT or MR should be performed to more accurately characterize the lesion, evaluate its relationship to adjacent structures, and determine coexistent abnormalities. Cystic abnormalities are usually benign and most often are ade-

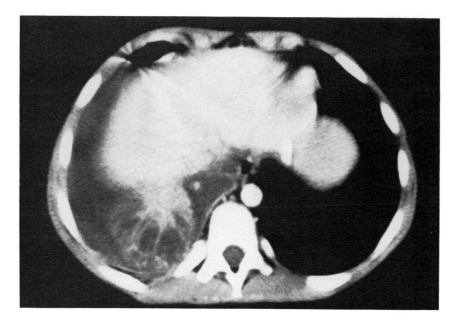

FIGURE 26–9 ■ Pleural metastasis in a 9-year-old boy, who presented with shortness of breath 1 year after surgery and chemotherapy for testicular germ cell tumor. Chest film showed homogeneous opacity of the right lower hemithorax, thought to represent pleural effusion. CT scan shows the effusion, as well as a diaphragmatic-based mass "hidden" by the effusion on chest film.

quately characterized by ultrasound. With renal cystic abnormalities, radionuclide scintigraphy and contrast urographic studies are often employed as ancillary studies.

CT is often the first modality employed in abdominal trauma or in abnormalities known to be difficult to evaluate by ultrasound (e.g., interloop abscess). CT and MR are the best imaging choices to evaluate the pelvic bones and adjacent soft tissues, as well as intraspinal extension of mass. MR appears to be as good or better than CT in evaluating hepatic neoplasms and neuroblastoma.[39, 58, 59]

Liver

CT of the liver is most often performed in children for the evaluation of primary masses[60, 61] and metastases, abdominal trauma, and (less commonly) diffuse parenchymal disease. Sonography usually precedes CT evaluation and in many cases obviates the need for CT. For example, virtually all major diseases of the pediatric biliary tract (e.g., biliary atresia and choledochal cyst) are best evaluated with ultrasound and hepatobiliary scintigraphy.[62] Ultrasound may also be definitive in the evaluation of cysts and abscesses if the appearance is characteristic. The ability of MR to delineate intrahepatic venous anatomy better than CT suggests that it may become the imaging modality of choice for liver tumors, as vascular landmarks are crucial in determining location and resectability of a mass.[63] One study suggests that the accuracy of MR imaging is comparable to that of CT in the diagnosis of primary liver tumors in children, with neither modality always accurate in discriminating malignant from benign disease.[59]

BENIGN MASSES

Cysts ■ Liver cysts are rare. If multiple, the diagnoses of tuberous sclerosis and autosomal dominant polycystic kidney disease should be considered.[64]

Choledochal cyst is usually adequately characterized with ultrasound and scintigraphy, but its CT appearance has been described.[65]

Abscesses ■ Hepatic abscesses most often occur in immunologically deficient children.[66] We usually rely on ultrasound and the clinical context for the diagnosis, but CT can be performed[67, 68] and may sometimes show lesions not seen by sonography.[69] Hepatic abscesses usually appear as well-defined areas of low attenuation that may have rim enhancement.

Mesenchymal Hamartoma ■ Mesenchymal hamartoma usually presents in the first 2 years of life. It is thought to be a developmental anomaly consisting of bile ducts and mesenchymal tissue. Both ultrasound and CT demonstrate a multilocular cystic mass, with variation in the size of the septae and cystic spaces.[70, 71]

Infantile Hemangioendothelioma. ■ Infantile hemangioendothelioma is the most common vascular liver tumor of infancy,[72] with over 85 per cent of patients presenting before 6 months of age.[73] Accurate diagnosis is important and may obviate surgery because most of these benign tumors regress spontaneously within 2 years. There are potential complications, including congestive heart failure, consumptive coagulopathy, and thrombocytopenia.[72, 74] Noncontrast CT demonstrates one or several low-attenuation masses. Bolus contrast enhancement produces striking early edge enhancement and variable delayed central enhancement, which causes the tumor to become nearly isointense with surrounding liver (Fig. 26–10).[73, 75] Although this tumor may present with congestive heart failure, hepatomegaly or mass is more often noted. Up to 45 per cent may have associated cutaneous hemangiomata. Both sonography and CT may demonstrate large draining veins and a dilated proximal aorta.[72, 73] Differential diagnostic possibilities include hepatoblastoma and metastatic neuroblastoma (discussed later).

Miscellaneous Lesions ■ Hepatic adenoma and focal

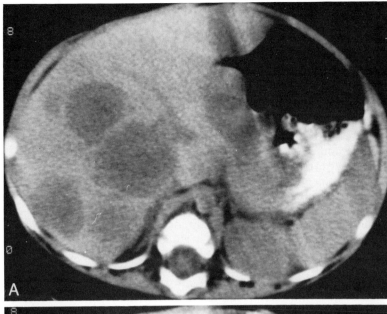

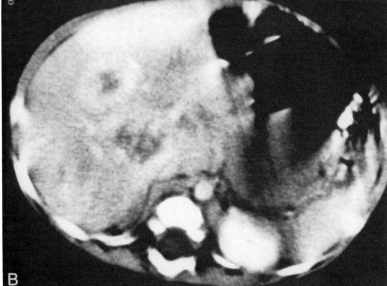

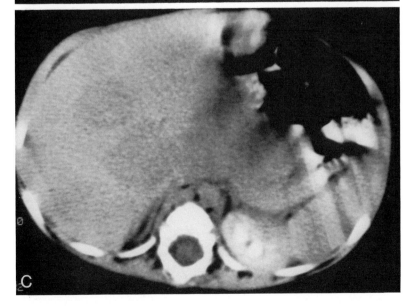

FIGURE 26–10 ■ Multiple hemangioendotheliomas of the liver in a 4-month-old boy. *A,* Precontrast CT scan. There are multiple masses of lower density than the surrounding liver. *B,* Immediate postbolus CT scan. There is early, predominantly peripheral enhancement of the lesions. *C,* Delayed (15-minute) postcontrast scan. The masses are nearly isodense with liver. This pattern is most consistent with multiple hemangioendotheliomas.

nodular hyperplasia are uncommon in children.[61, 76] Hepatic adenoma is usually associated with glycogen storage disease.[61]

MALIGNANT MASSES

Hepatoblastoma ■ Hepatoblastoma, a poorly differentiated tumor, usually occurs in children under the age of 3 years.[77, 78] It is most often solitary[60] but may be multinodular or even diffuse.[77] Definition of tumor margin and presence of calcification are variable.[66, 77] The tumor is usually hypodense with minimal enhancement (Fig. 26–11).[77] Rarely, rim enhancement[77] and central enhancement that increases with time mimic the appearance of hemangioendothelioma;[66] in these cases, a persistently and markedly elevated alpha-fetoprotein level helps support the diagnosis of hepatoblastoma. Metastases to lung occur.

Hepatocellular Carcinoma ■ Hepatocellular carcinoma is histologically more mature than hepatoblastoma and tends to occur in children older than 5 years.[66] It is most often multicentric in origin, with multiple confluent masses,[60] but it may also be solitary. The tumor is usually of lower attenuation than surrounding liver parenchyma and exhibits variable enhancement. Calcification and ring enhancement may occur (Fig. 26–12).[66] Age of presentation and multicentricity help differentiate this lesion from hepatoblastoma. The chest is the most common site for metastases.[66]

Metastases ■ Many malignancies metastasize to liver, but the most common ones include neuroblastoma, Wilms', lymphoma, leukemia, and rhabdomyosarcoma. In general, metastases are of lower attenuation and enhance less than normal liver.

Neuroblastoma is the most frequent tumor to metastasize to liver at time of diagnosis. In the young infant, neuroblastoma may cause extensive replacement of hepatic parenchyma,[66] and an erroneous diagnosis of primary liver tumor may be made if the primary tumor is not identified (Fig. 26–13). In these cases, elevation of urinary catecholamine levels helps support the diagnosis of neuroblastoma. Ring enhancement may occur.[61]

Leukemic infiltration may only demonstrate nonspecific hepatomegaly.

TRAUMA

The role of CT in the evaluation of the child with blunt abdominal trauma has been well established.[79–87] Pediatric injuries most commonly involve the liver and spleen, with the kidneys, pancreas, and gastrointestinal tract less commonly involved.[83, 88] Nonoperative management in the hemodynamically stable patient is becoming more common. This is especially true with splenic injury because of the known increased risk of sepsis following splenectomy.[89] Brick et al.[79] found no correlation between the presence of hemoperitoneum and extent of hepatic and splenic parenchymal damage and the need for emergent laparotomy. They concluded that the decision for emergent surgery should be based on the clinical condition of the child rather than on the extent of injury as shown on CT. An adult study of hepatic injuries[90] made a similar conclusion. Nonetheless, CT is important to help establish patient management and ascertain resolution of the injuries.

Most hepatic injuries involve the right lobe, especially the posterior segment.[82, 90] Lesions of the left lobe are less common but are likely to be more extensive.[82]

DIFFUSE PARENCHYMAL DISEASE

Fatty infiltration (sometimes seen in patients with cystic fibrosis) results in areas of diffuse or focal lower attenuation. Similar findings may be seen in patients receiving steroids and in association with chemotherapy for malignant disease. Iron deposition in the liver (seen in patients with multiple transfu-

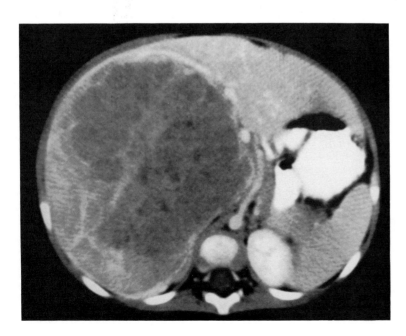

FIGURE 26–11 ■ Hepatoblastoma in a 19-month-old boy. Contrast-enhanced CT scan demonstrates a large hypodense mass within the right lobe of the liver.

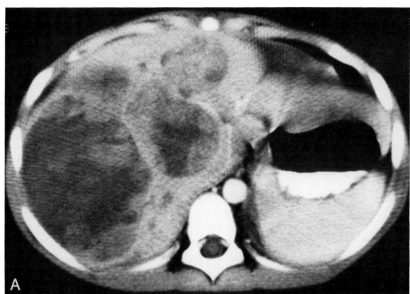
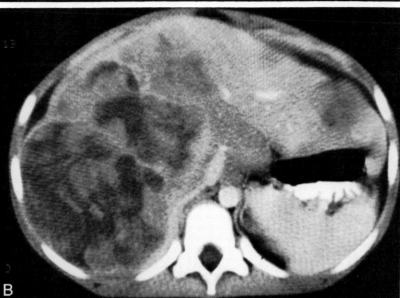

FIGURE 26–12 ■ Hepatocellular carcinoma in a 6-year-old boy. Two images from contrast-enhanced CT scan show multiple, partially confluent, hypodense masses, suggesting multicentric origin. Age of patient and multicentricity help to differentiate this lesion from hepatoblastoma, which tends to be solitary and usually occurs in younger patients.

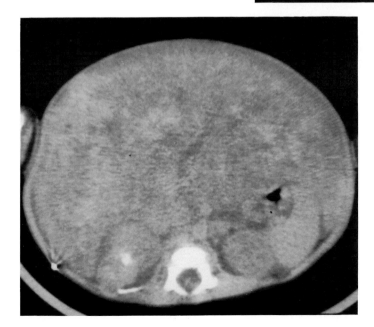

FIGURE 26–13 ■ Disseminated neuroblastoma in a 2-month-old boy. Non–contrast-enhanced CT scan shows a small, partially calcified, right adrenal mass and a markedly enlarged, heterogeneous liver, suggesting diffuse metastatic involvement. The adrenal mass displaced the right kidney inferiorly.

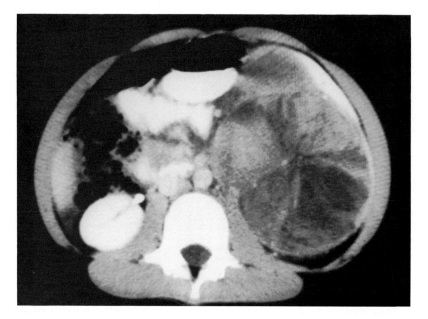

FIGURE 26–14 ■ Large left Wilms' tumor in a 9-year-old boy. Contrast-enhanced CT scan shows a large soft tissue mass containing hypodense areas posteriorly that represent regions of cyst formation, hemorrhage, and necrosis. An enhancing rim of compressed renal parenchyma is noted anterolaterally. Although the tumor extends to the midline, the aorta is not encased. Vascular encasement is more common in neuroblastoma (see Figs. 26–20 and 26–21).

sions) results in diffuse increased attenuation. Changes caused by cirrhosis in children are similar to those seen in the adult.[66]

Kidneys

Most pediatric renal problems are first evaluated with ultrasound. Hydronephrosis (the most common neonatal abdominal mass), renal cystic disease, congenital renal anomalies, and urinary tract infection are usually adequately studied by a combination of ultrasound, radionuclide scintigraphy, and excretory urography.[91–95] Although CT may offer information on these conditions,[96–102] it is most useful in the evaluation of tumor and trauma. The role of pediatric renal MR is being defined[103, 104] and appears most useful in delineating renal origin of a tumor.

WILMS' TUMOR

Wilms' tumor and neuroblastoma are the two most common primary abdominal neoplasms of childhood.[105] Most children with Wilms' tumor present between 1 and 5 years of age, with a peak incidence between 3 and 4 years.[100] Patients are usually asymptomatic and present with an abdominal mass. Associated congenital anomalies include aniridia and hemihypertrophy.[100] Hypertension may occur.[105] Ultrasound is usually performed first and in the uncomplicated case demonstrates a predominantly solid intrarenal mass that displaces and distorts the collecting system. CT complements ultrasound in defining the extent of the mass and its relationship to adjacent structures and in evaluating possible metastases to lung, contralateral kidney, liver, and lymph nodes.

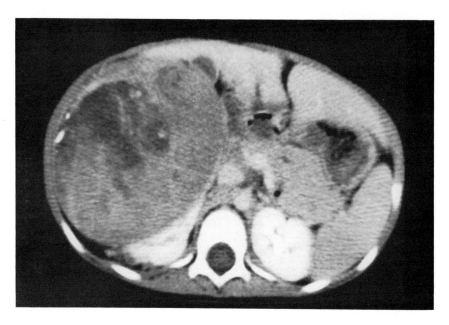

FIGURE 26–15 ■ Large right Wilms' tumor in a 14-month-old girl. Contrast-enhanced CT scan shows a large right tumor mass. A rim of functioning renal tissue posteromedially indicates intrarenal origin of the mass. Although the tumor is large and extends to the midline, it does not encase the great vessels. Punctate calcification along the right lateral margin of the tumor is unusual for a Wilms' tumor.

CT shows a large, spherical, intrarenal solid mass, often with central hypodense areas representing cysts, necrosis, and hemorrhage.[106, 107] Calcification is unusual. An enhancing rim of compressed renal parenchyma (pseudocapsule) is frequently seen (Figs. 26–14 and 26–15)[108] and is helpful in establishing intrarenal origin of the mass.

The tumor may have a large exophytic component that compresses adjacent liver. In these cases it may be difficult to establish renal origin of the mass, and on axial CT, liver metastasis may be simulated. Sagittal sonography or MR is often helpful in these cases.[58, 104] Extension of tumor into the renal vein and inferior vena cava is not uncommon, and both sonography and MR may help in differentiating vascular invasion from extrinsic compression.[58]

OTHER RENAL TUMORS

Renal cell carcinoma is rare in the first two decades of life.[100, 102] This tumor may be smaller than Wilms' tumor at presentation, but CT appearance is nonspecific and may simulate Wilms' tumor.[109]

Mesoblastic nephroma is a benign renal tumor. It usually presents in the neonatal period and is the most common renal neoplasm to present in the first 3 months of life.[100, 110] Complete surgical resection is curative. CT findings are nonspecific and do not directly permit differentiation from malignant lesions,[100] although age at presentation helps to differentiate it from Wilms' tumor.

Multilocular cystic nephroma is an uncommon, usually benign neoplasm characterized by a well-circumscribed encapsulated mass containing multiple fluid-filled locules. It affects predominantly male children and female adults. CT usually shows a well-defined multilocular mass with septa.[111]

Children with tuberous sclerosis may have renal angiomyolipomas and/or cysts. Small lipomas may be better shown on CT than on ultrasound.[112, 113]

Nephroblastomatosis represents persistence and proliferation of the metanephric blastema.[114] Although spontaneous regression may occur, malignant degeneration has been described,[114] and coexistence with Wilms' tumor is known.[115] Contrast-enhanced CT is probably more sensitive than ultrasound in demonstrating deposits of nephroblastomatosis.[115]

Renal involvement with lymphoma may present as solitary or multiple intrarenal masses, as well as diffuse infiltration with nephromegaly.[100, 116] Lymphomatous tissue tends to enhance less than normal renal tissue.[100] CT may show renal lymphoma masses better than ultrasound (Fig. 26–16).[117]

RENAL INFECTION

Although CT does not play a primary role in the evaluation of pediatric urinary tract infection,[92] it may be helpful in the evaluation of renal parenchymal infections (e.g., pyelonephritis and abscess),[101, 118] some of which may be missed or underestimated by sonography (Fig. 26–17).[99, 101]

RENAL TRAUMA

In children presenting with blunt abdominal trauma, contrast-enhanced CT can provide both anatomic and functional information about the kidneys. CT can accurately distinguish minor from major trauma by defining the extent of parenchymal injury, perirenal hemorrhage, and urinoma (Fig. 26–18)[119–123] and by suggesting renal artery injury.[124] Most renal injuries can be treated conservatively, but if renal pedicle injury is identified, angiography and surgery are usually necessary.[100] CT may be used to define the extent of healing after injury.[125]

The significance of hematuria in children following blunt abdominal trauma is still in question. Karp et al.[126] found no correlation between the severity of renal injury and the amount of hematuria. On the

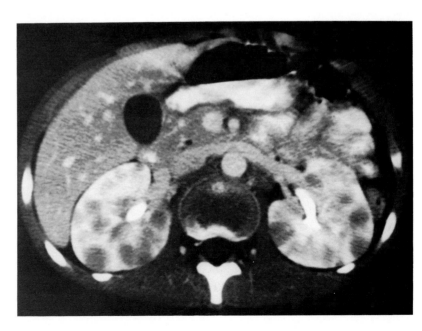

FIGURE 26–16 ■ Renal lymphoma in a 13-year-old girl with disseminated non-Hodgkin's lymphoma. Contrast-enhanced CT scan shows circumferential enlargement of the kidneys with multiple well-defined, low-density nodules. Nodules of lymphoma may be difficult to delineate on a noncontrast study.

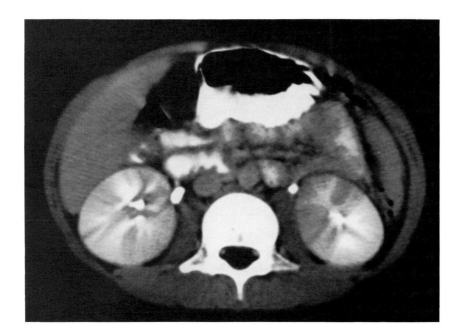

FIGURE 26–17 ■ Pyelonephritis in an 8-year-old boy. Contrast-enhanced CT scan shows striated and wedge-shaped zones of decreased enhancement. No focal well-defined areas of low attenuation were seen to suggest abscess. Concurrent ultrasound suggested questionable renal enlargement and showed a slight prominence of the renal pelves. Cystogram demonstrated bilateral grade III reflux (reflux into dilated, blunted calyces) and intrarenal reflux.

other hand, Stalker et al.[127] found a direct correlation between the amount of hematuria and the severity of injury. In both studies the presence of radiographic renal injury correlated closely with abdominal symptoms and physical findings. Thus a child with a normal physical examination and hematuria is unlikely to have significant renal injury, especially if there are fewer than 50 red blood cells per high power field.[127]

Adrenals

Neonatal adrenals are large and easy to visualize on ultrasound. Subsequently the cortex involutes, making visualization difficult. The child suspected of having an adrenal lesion often has sonography performed first, but if the suspicion of disease is high,

CT is usually performed. The most common use for pediatric adrenal CT is in the evaluation of neuroblastoma, but MR is being increasingly used, as it can show intraspinal extent of tumor[39, 128] and vascular encasement.[39, 129]

NEUROBLASTOMA

Neuroblastoma and the more differentiated neural tumors, ganglioneuroblastoma and ganglioneuroma, arise from primitive sympathetic neuroblasts of the embryonic neural crest.[130] Neuroblastoma and Wilms' tumor are the most common extracranial malignant tumors in children.[105, 131, 132] Most neuroblastomas occur before 5 years of age, with a peak incidence at 2 years.[132] Sixty-five per cent are located in the abdomen, and approximately two thirds of these arise in the adrenal gland. However, they may arise

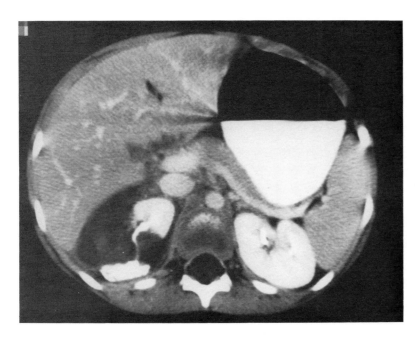

FIGURE 26–18 ■ Renal injury in a 7-year-old boy involved in a motor vehicle accident. Contrast-enhanced CT scan demonstrates a complete renal laceration that extends into the collecting system and results in extravasation of urine.

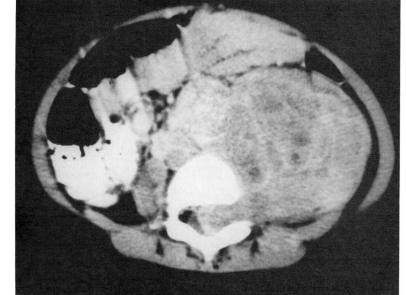

FIGURE 26–19 ■ Extraadrenal neuroblastoma extending into the spinal canal in a 3-year-old girl. This CT scan was performed without intrathecal contrast. Slice at the L4 level shows a large left-sided heterogeneous mass that is difficult to separate from partially opacified gut medially. The mass extends through the left neural foramen into the spinal canal, where it displaces the thecal sac and obliterates the left extradural fat. This case demonstrates that intraspinal extension of tumor can be identified without intrathecal contrast.[38]

anywhere along the paravertebral sympathetic chain extending from the neck to the sacrum. Ten per cent are disseminated, without known site of origin.[130]

Neuroblastoma often presents as a mass. There is a high frequency of increased catecholamine secretion. Disseminated disease is common at time of diagnosis, with metastatic sites including skeleton, liver (see Fig. 26–13), lymph nodes, bone marrow, and skin.[130] Imaging workup usually includes plain films, ultrasound, bone scintigraphy, and CT or MR. Both CT and MR are used to depict the extent of the primary lesion and its relationship to surrounding structures and to evaluate for the presence of metastases. These modalities thus play a critical role in staging.[37, 39, 129, 131, 133–135] Intraspinal extension of tumor occurs in approximately 15 per cent of patients, and

in these patients, CT with subarachnoid contrast or MR is important for surgical planning.[39, 128] The use of CT in demonstrating occult neuroblastoma in children presenting with opsomyoclonus has been well demonstrated.[136–138]

CT demonstrates an inhomogeneous mass usually of lower attenuation than surrounding tissue. Margins of the tumor are often irregular. Extension of tumor across the midline and liver metastases are common. CT features helpful in distinguishing neuroblastoma from Wilms' tumor include (1) clear extrarenal location, (2) presence of calcification (see Fig. 26–6), (3) retroperitoneal lymphadenopathy, (4) extension of tumor into the spinal canal (Figs. 26–6 and 26–19), and (5) encasement of mesenteric and great vessels (Fig. 26–20).[139] The last two features are well shown by MR (Figs. 26–7 and 26–21).

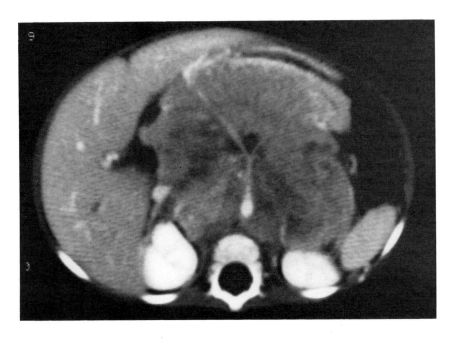

FIGURE 26–20 ■ Unresectable neuroblastoma in a 13-month-old girl. A large soft tissue mass with low-density regions is present in the upper abdomen. The mass encases the aorta and superior mesenteric artery. This encasement of vessels is often seen in advanced neuroblastoma but is distinctly unusual for Wilms' tumor.

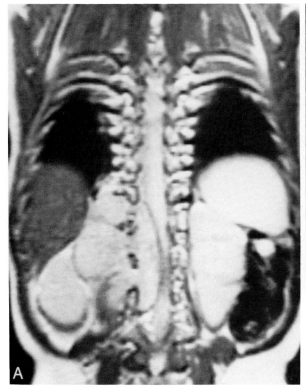

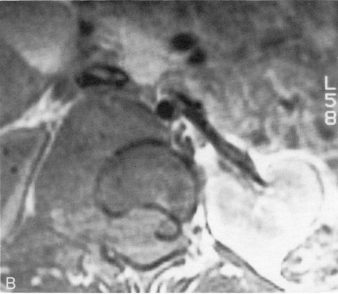

FIGURE 26–21 ■ MR images of a large right paraspinal neuroblastoma with intraspinal extension in a 15-month-old girl. *A*, Coronal image (SE, 1800/50) shows the large, multilobulated right paraspinal mass, which extends into the spinal canal through multiple neural foramina and displaces the thecal sac to the left. *B*, Axial image (SE, 700/20) at the level of the left renal vein shows the large intraspinal component of the mass. In addition, the mass barely extends across the midline, displacing the inferior vena cava and aorta anteriorly. These findings are typical of neuroblastoma.

PHEOCHROMOCYTOMA

Five per cent of pheochromocytomas arise in children.[132] They are extremely unusual in the child younger than 5 years.[140] In children, sustained, rather than intermittent, hypertension is often a presenting finding.[132] Up to 30 per cent may be extraadrenal in location and, like neuroblastoma, may arise anywhere along the sympathetic chain. The upper abdomen is the most common extraadrenal site.[140] Pheochromocytomas may be multiple, especially if associated with multiple endocrine adenomatosis. In evaluating patients with suspected pheochromocytoma, CT of the abdomen and pelvis is usually performed first; if negative, chest CT can be performed. Imaging with ^{131}I-metaiodobenzylguanidine (MIBG) is a complementary technique that may help localize extraadrenal or metastatic tumor.[141] Finding a pheochromocytoma is important, as it is potentially curable if completely resected.[142] Most are greater than 2 cm at time of presentation and, if adrenal in location, may have a homogeneous appearance. Enhancement with contrast is not characteristic but may occur.[140] The role of CT in the detection of pheochromocytoma has been well established.[140, 143–145] CT without contrast has been advocated as the initial screening test to avoid the small risk of hypertensive crisis associated with intravenous injection of urographic contrast medium.[142] MR also appears to be useful in the evaluation of pheochromocytoma.[146–149]

ADRENOCORTICAL TUMORS

Adrenocortical tumors (e.g., carcinomas and adenomas) are rare in children, and unlike those in adults, they are usually hormonally active.[150, 151] Differentiating benign from malignant lesions is difficult, as the CT appearance is variable (Fig. 26–22).[151, 152]

ADRENAL HEMORRHAGE

Adrenal hemorrhage is most commonly seen in neonates. Although it can be demonstrated by CT and MR,[153–155] ultrasound is preferable for evaluation and follow-up. Any cystic mass in a neonate should be followed to ensure complete resolution, as both adrenal hemorrhage and neuroblastoma may be cystic (Fig. 26–23).[156–157]

Pancreas

Imaging of the pancreas in children is usually performed to evaluate pancreatitis and its complications, abdominal trauma, and pancreatic tumor. Except in the setting of generalized trauma, sonography

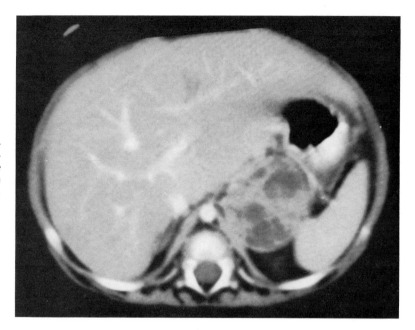

FIGURE 26–22 ■ Functioning adrenocortical adenoma in a 4-month-old girl. A predominantly hypodense mass originates from the left adrenal gland. The patient was cushingoid and hirsute. The differentiation of adenoma from carcinoma was made histologically.

is the initial modality of choice for evaluating pancreatic abnormality in children. Both CT and ultrasound may be useful in demonstrating fatty replacement of the pancreas in patients with cystic fibrosis and Shwachman-Diamond syndrome.[158]

PANCREATITIS

The etiology of pancreatitis in children differs from that in adults, in whom alcoholism and biliary tract disease are the most common causes. In children, trauma, infection, drugs, and congenital anomalies of the biliary tract are major considerations.[62] Pancreatitis may also occur as a familial trait. We use sonography to initially diagnose pancreatitis and to follow its sequelae, especially pseudocyst. In some cases (e.g., fulminant pancreatitis or complex pseudocyst), CT may better demonstrate the extent of disease.[159–161]

TRAUMA

Although injury to the pancreas is unusual (liver, spleen, and renal injuries being much more common), it is the most common cause of pancreatitis and pseudocyst formation in early childhood.[162] Traumatic pancreatitis may be a presenting feature in child abuse. Pancreatic fractures, contusions, and posttraumatic pseudocysts have been demonstrated by CT.[163]

TUMORS

Tumors of the pancreas are extremely rare in children and include functioning lesions (e.g., islet cell adenomas and carcinomas[164] and neisidioblastosis) and nonfunctioning tumors such as pancreaticoblastoma and adenocarcinoma.[165] Adjacent neuroblastoma or lymphadenopathy may be inseparable from the pancreas.[62]

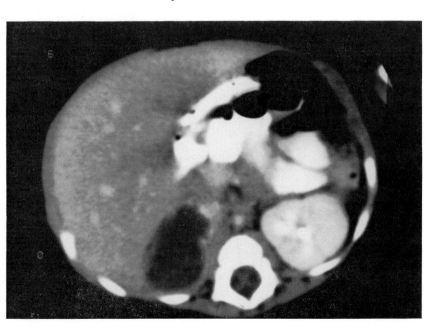

FIGURE 26–23 ■ Right adrenal hemorrhage in a 3-week-old boy. Both ultrasound and CT studies demonstrated a cystic mass in the right adrenal fossa that displaced the kidney inferiorly. Urinary catecholamine levels were normal, and there were no liver metastases. These findings strongly argue against a cystic neuroblastoma. A follow-up ultrasound confirmed the diagnosis of hemorrhage by showing complete resolution of the cystic mass.

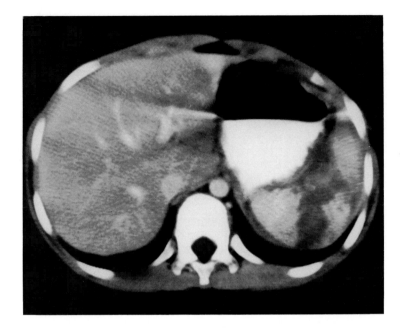

FIGURE 26–24 ■ Splenic trauma in an 11-year-old girl who fell off a horse. Irregular areas of low density within the spleen suggest laceration and hematoma.

FIGURE 26–25 ■ Splenic trauma in a 13-year-old girl. A, Two hypodense areas within the spleen suggest hematoma. B, A large amount of blood in the pelvis outlines the uterus and cystic ovaries (best seen on the left side). Hemoperitoneum frequently accompanies splenic trauma. The patient was managed medically and did well.

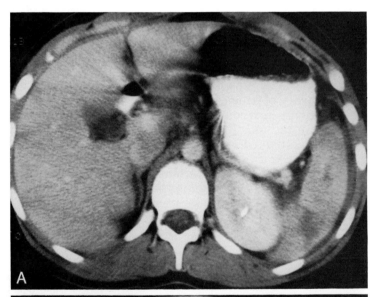

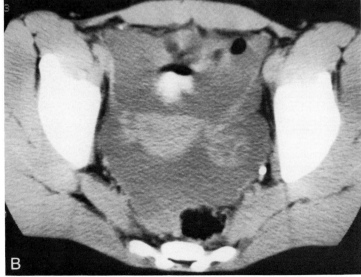

Spleen

The spleen is frequently involved in pediatric blunt abdominal trauma,[83] with injuries including splenic laceration, focal intraparenchymal injury, subcapsular hematomas, and hemoperitoneum (Figs. 26–24 and 26–25).[81] If the patient is hemodynamically stable, splenectomy is usually not performed so that the complications of splenectomy (e.g., severe infection) can be avoided.[89] Streak artifacts originating from ribs or bowel gas may create confusion by giving the spleen an inhomogeneous appearance.

Lymphomatous involvement of the spleen may manifest as diffuse homogeneous enlargement and, less commonly, ill-defined areas of lower attenuation.[166]

Incidental findings include punctate calcifications relating to granulomatous disease, simple epithelial cysts, and accessory spleens.[166]

Gastrointestinal Tract

It is rare for CT to be the primary imaging modality of the pediatric gastrointestinal tract: Gastrointestinal studies and ultrasound (such as for pyloric stenosis) are the modalities of choice.[62] However, certain entities deserve mention.

BOWEL WALL THICKENING

The normal appearance of the bowel wall has been described in the adult.[167, 168] Both in children and in adults, a thickened wall often suggests edema (Fig. 26–26), inflammatory disease, or neoplasm,[167, 169] especially lymphoma (Figs. 26–27 and 26–28).[169–171] Eo-sinophilic gastroenteritis, pediatric hypertrophic gastropathy, and *Helicobacter pylori* (formerly *Campylobacter pylori*) infection may cause thickening of the gastric wall and simulate malignancy (Fig. 26–29).[172–174]

ABSCESS, APPENDICITIS, AND TYPHLITIS

Initial evaluation for abscess is usually done by ultrasound. CT is useful in delineating the full extent of an abscess when it is large, involves musculoskeletal structures, or is intimately associated with bowel (interloop abscess). Complications of inflammatory bowel disease (e.g., abscess and fistula) are often best shown by CT.[175] In general, abscesses appear as areas of low attenuation that may have some rim enhancement on contrast study. A right lower quadrant abscess associated with calcification is highly suggestive of a ruptured appendix. Immunocompromised children (especially those with leukemia) with right lower quadrant pain may have typhlitis, a necrotizing inflammation of the cecum. In these cases CT may show marked cecal wall thickening with associated pericolic inflammatory changes (Fig. 26–30).[176–178]

INTUSSUSCEPTION

The diagnosis of intussusception is usually not made by CT, but this entity should not be overlooked in the patient who has a CT examination for the evaluation of abdominal pain or intestinal obstruction.[179–181] Ileoileal intussusception is distinctly unusual in children and usually has a pathologic lead point (e.g., intramural hematoma in Henoch-Schönlein purpura [Fig. 26–31]).[182]

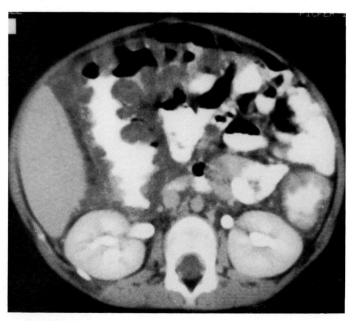

FIGURE 26–26 ■ Colitis in a 3-year-old immunosuppressed girl. The colitis was caused by *Clostridium difficile*. CT scan shows severe mucosal edema in the right and left sides of the colon.

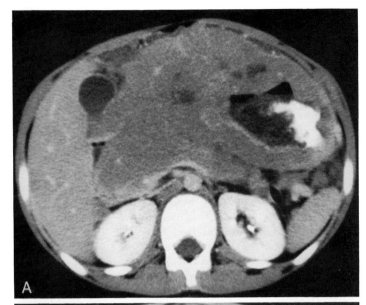

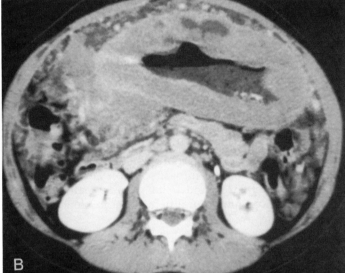

FIGURE 26–27 ■ Gastric lymphoma in an 11-year-old boy. Lymphomatous infiltration markedly thickens the gastric wall and adjacent mesentery.

FIGURE 26–28 ■ Burkitt's lymphoma in a 6-year-old boy. Multiple mesenteric and bowel wall masses were seen on CT scans. This image shows marked thickening of the bowel wall with centrally located lumen filled with gas and contrast.

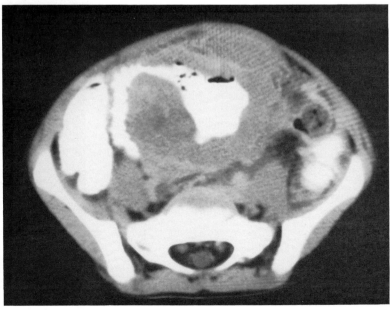

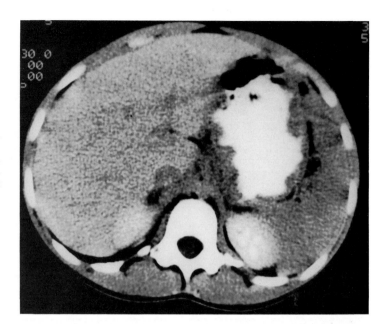

FIGURE 26–29 ■ *Helicobacter pylori* infection in a 12-year-old girl who presented with abdominal pain. The stomach wall is irregularly thickened. *H. pylori* is one of many causes of a thick stomach wall. In this patient the diagnosis was made by endoscopic biopsy and histology, and the patient responded to medical therapy.

TRAUMA

Blunt abdominal trauma in the child rarely results in gastrointestinal tract injury (e.g., hematoma or intestinal perforation).[86] Pneumoperitoneum suggests viscus rupture. However, other causes for peritoneal gas may be present (e.g., pneumomediastinum dissecting into peritoneal cavity), and not all viscus rupture leads to radiographically detectable free air.[87]

Retroperitoneum

LYMPH NODES

Lymph nodes are evaluated in all patients suspected of having malignant disease, especially those with Hodgkin's disease and testicular tumors.[183] Because there are no strict criteria for what constitutes an abnormally large lymph node in the young child, anything larger than several millimeters should be viewed with suspicion in the appropriate clinical setting.[183]

SOFT TISSUES

Retroperitoneal inflammation may be assessed by CT and MR. Inflammation and infection of bones or bowel (e.g., appendicitis) may involve the contiguous retroperitoneal soft tissues. Soft tissue tumors are rare and include neurofibroma, teratoma, and rhabdomyosarcoma.[183]

VESSELS

In a CT examination, a dynamic bolus contrast study is necessary for good visualization of vessels. The following abnormalities may be seen:

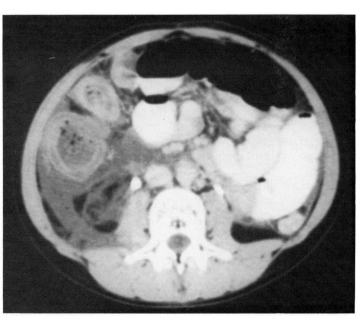

FIGURE 26–30 ■ Typhlitis in a 12-year-old girl with acute myelogenous leukemia. The wall of the cecum is thickened and has a hypodense central layer of inflammation and edema. Pericecal inflammatory changes are also seen posteromedial to the cecum. These findings, especially in the appropriate clinical setting, are typical of typhlitis.

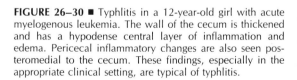

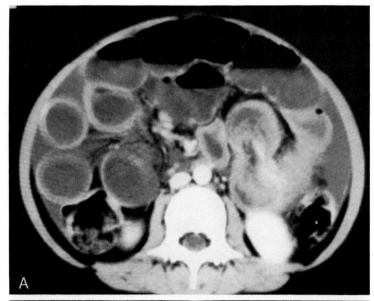

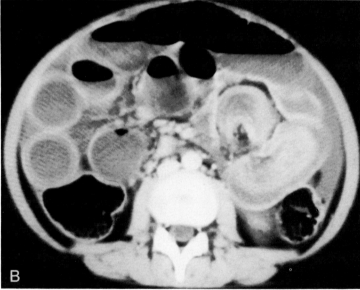

FIGURE 26–31 ■ Small bowel obstruction resulting from intussusception in a 3-year-old boy with Henoch-Schön-lein purpura. Hemorrhage into the bowel wall may act as a lead point of intussusception. Multiple loops of small bowel are dilated and have thick walls. The sausage-shaped mass in the left side of the abdomen represents proximal bowel intussuscepted into the more distal segment. The small areas of lower density within the center of the mass represent invaginated mesenteric fat and/or admixtures of intestinal gas and fluid.

1. Intravenous extension of tumor. Ultrasound and MR often help to differentiate tumor extension from flow artifact.

2. Vascular anomalies, such as azygous continuation of the inferior vena cava and superior mesenteric vein rotation. With the latter, the superior mesenteric vein at or just below the level of the uncinate process lies on the left rather than the right ventral aspect of the superior mesenteric artery. This abnormal position of the vein is highly suggestive of midgut malrotation.[184]

3. Abnormalities of the portal venous system, such as cavernous transformation of the portal vein.

MR is an excellent alternative for the evaluation of vascular abnormalities.

Pelvis

Ultrasound usually adequately evaluates pelvic cystic masses and genitourinary abnormalities. Pelvic MR or CT is useful in the delineation of soft tissue mass (tumor and inflammation),[185] the evaluation of the musculoskeletal system, the search for undescended testes, and (rarely) the evaluation of anomaly.[186, 187] MR of the pelvis can provide more information than CT[188] and is likely to become the modality of choice.

MASSES

The etiology of a pelvic mass can often be deduced on the basis of location and appearance. Adjacent bony destruction and extension into the spinal canal are well delineated with CT and MR.

Presacral lesions include extragonadal germ cell tumors (especially endodermal sinus tumor and sacrococcygeal teratoma), neuroblastoma, anterior meningomyeloceles, and (rarely) duplication cysts.[189] The demonstration of both fat and calcification helps in making the diagnosis of teratoma.[190, 191] CT nicely demonstrates associated sacral anomalies of anterior meningomyelocele.

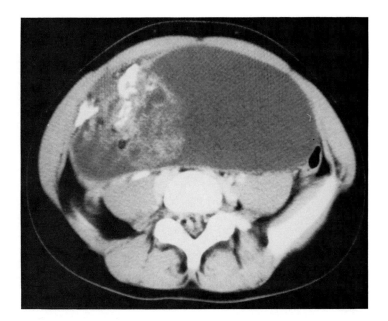

FIGURE 26–32 ■ Cystic ovarian teratoma in a 12-year-old girl. Image through the upper pelvis shows a large fluid-density mass that also contains focal areas of calcification and fat. These findings are typical of cystic teratoma.

Most bladder and genital lesions are evaluated with sonography and cystography. Pelvic rhabdomyosarcoma and the rare ovarian neoplasm may require further evaluation with CT or MR (Fig. 26–32).[191, 192] Rhabdomyosarcoma accounts for the majority of soft tissue sarcomas in childhood.[189] In the pelvis, the prostate, bladder, uterus, and vagina are the most frequently involved sites (Fig. 26–33).[193]

Lateral pelvic masses usually represent lymphadenopathy from lymphoma and sarcoma.

Lesions of the pelvic bones include primary tumors (e.g., Ewing's sarcoma) and osteomyelitis. CT helps in defining the extent of disease. MR is particularly useful in defining the extent of soft tissue and marrow involvement.[194, 195]

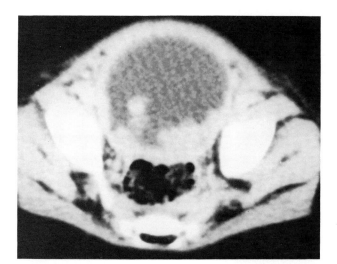

FIGURE 26–33 ■ Bladder rhabdomyosarcoma in a 10-month-old boy. Image through the lower pelvis demonstrates irregular thickening of the posterior wall of the bladder and a lobulated soft tissue mass extending into the bladder lumen. The remainder of the bladder wall is thick, presumably because of bladder outlet obstruction.

UNDESCENDED TESTES

Undescended testes are usually located within the inguinal canal or superficial inguinal pouch; rarely, they may be intraabdominal in location. Ultrasound, CT, and MR have all been used with varying success to locate the undescended testis,[196–199] with the undescended intraabdominal testicle being the most difficult to detect. We prefer ultrasound as our initial screening exam and concur that there is no good modality to find the intraabdominal testicle.

Musculoskeletal System

Tumors

Computed tomography has been successfully used to evaluate soft tissue tumors and bone tumors. The major advantage of CT is its ability to demonstrate the extent of tumor.[200, 201] In primary soft tissue tumors such as rhabdomyosarcoma, CT identifies involvement of muscle groups, neurovascular bundles, and adjacent bones.[202] In primary bone tumors such as osteogenic sarcoma and Ewing's sarcoma, CT can display bone marrow involvement, skip metastases, the size of an associated soft tissue mass and its effect on neurovascular bundles, and joint involvement. Such an evaluation is particularly important in planning limb salvage surgery.[203]

Despite its proven usefulness in this area, CT will probably be replaced by MR. Comparative studies show that MR is superior to CT in almost every aspect of tumor definition (Fig. 26–34).[195, 204–209] Magnetic resonance may have some limitation in showing tumor calcification and fine detail of cortical bone abnormalities.

Infection

Computed tomography has been used to assess acute and chronic osteomyelitis.[200, 201, 210] We have

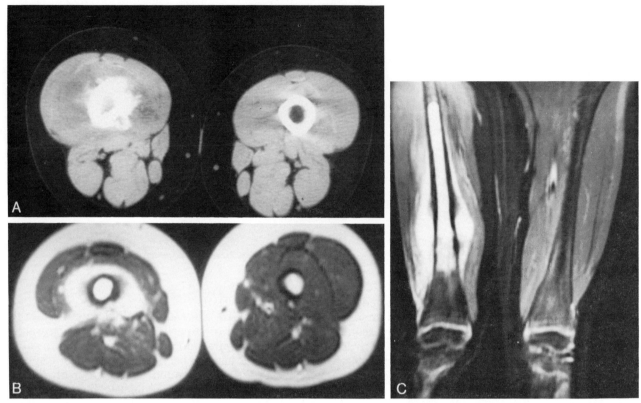

FIGURE 26–34 ■ Right femoral osteosarcoma in a 10-year-old girl. *A,* CT scan shows marked thickening and spiculation of bone, increased density of marrow, and the suggestion of a circumferential soft tissue mass. *B,* T2-weighted MR image (SE, 2000/80) more clearly demonstrates the circumferential mass. The relatively sharp boundary suggests that the mass is tumor, not simply edema. On this pulse sequence, it is difficult to separate tumor from normal marrow, as both have relatively high signal intensity. *C,* Coronal MR image using inversion recovery fat suppression technique causes fat to appear dark. Marrow and soft tissue abnormalities are dramatically shown.

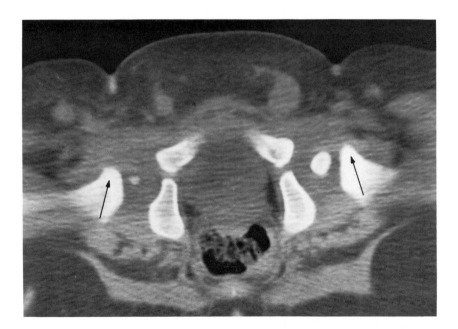

FIGURE 26–35 ■ Normal femoral head position in a 7-month-old girl. Prior dislocation of the right hip resulted in delayed ossification of the right femoral head. Both femoral heads, which are mostly cartilaginous, are directed in joint. The upturn of femoral metaphyses *(arrows)* indicates that the proper section through the femoral head has been obtained.[200]

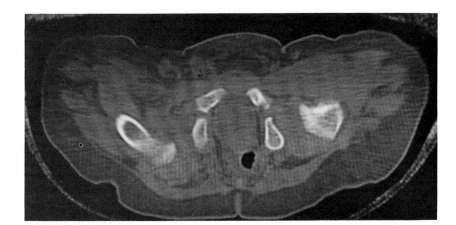

FIGURE 26–36 ■ Right hip dislocation in a 4-month-old girl. CT scan of the hips with the child in a cast shows normal location of the left, unossified femoral head and posterior dislocation of the right femoral head.

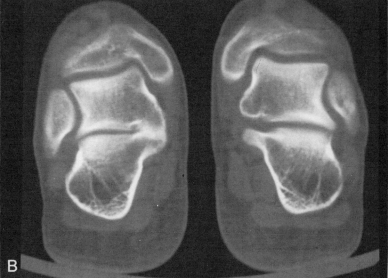

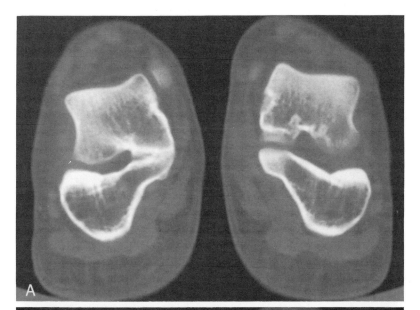

FIGURE 26–37 ■ Tarsal coalition in an 11-year-old girl. Coronal images show broad-based right talo-calcaneal coalition. The appearance of coalition may range from narrowed irregular joint space to bony fusion.[200]

found CT particularly helpful in osteomyelitis of the pelvis, as symptoms may be confusing, and plain films are difficult to interpret. Magnetic resonance will undoubtedly displace CT in evaluation of osteomyelitis.[211-213] One report suggests that MR may become a worthwhile complement to bone scintigraphy, because it can help differentiate between soft tissue inflammation and bone infection.[212]

Trauma

CT is most useful in demonstrating complex fractures of the pelvis, calcaneus, and distal tibia ("triplane fracture").[214-217]

Congenital Dislocation of the Hip

Computed tomography has little value in the initial or routine evaluation of congenital dislocation of the hip, but it may add information during treatment of more difficult cases. Computed tomography can show the position of the femoral head while the patient is in a cast (Figs. 26–35 and 26–36), and CT may reveal reasons for incomplete reduction.[200, 218, 219] MR can display cartilage and bone in axial and coronal projections and will become important in imaging congenital hip problems.[220]

Tarsal Coalition

Fibrous or bony tarsal coalition may be suspected but is often difficult to diagnose on plain films. CT performed perpendicular to the plane of the joint in question can easily evaluate for possible coalition (Fig. 26–37).[221, 222]

Femoral Anteversion

Derotational osteotomy may be necessary in patients with excessive femoral torsion or anteversion. CT offers a simple way to measure the degree of anteversion.[223]

References

1. Daneman A: Pediatric Body CT. London, Springer-Verlag, 1987.
2. Siegel MJ (ed): Pediatric Body CT. New York, Churchill Livingstone, 1988.
3. Cohen MD, Edwards MK (eds): Magnetic Resonance Imaging of Children. Philadelphia, BC Decker, 1990.
4. Fearon T, Vucich J: Normalized pediatric organ-absorbed doses from CT examinations. AJR 148:171–174, 1987.
5. Lassen MN: Dedicated CT technique for scanning neonates. Radiology 161:363–366, 1986.
6. Fearon T, Vucich J: Pediatric patient exposures from CT examinations: GE CT/T 9800 scanner. AJR 144:805–809, 1985.
7. Pruitt AW, Striker TW, et al: Guidelines for the elective use of conscious sedation, deep sedation, and general anesthesia in pediatric patients. Pediatrics 76:317–321, 1985.
8. Keeter S, Benator RM, Weinberg SM, Hartenberg MA: Sedation in pediatric CT: national survey of current practice. Radiology 175:745–752, 1990.
9. Fisher DM: Sedation of pediatric patients: an anesthesiologist's perspective. Radiology 175:613–615, 1990.
10. Strain JD, Campbell JB, Harvey LA, Foley LC: IV Nembutal: safe sedation for children undergoing CT. AJNR 9:955–959, 1988.
11. Diament MJ, Stanley P: The use of Midazolam for sedation of infants and children. AJR 150:377–378, 1988.
12. Mitchell AA, Louik C, Lacouture P, Slone D, Goldman P, Shapiro S: Risks to children from computed tomographic scan premedication. JAMA 247:2385–2388, 1982.
13. Kaufman RA: Technical aspects of abdominal CT in infants and children. AJR 153:549–554, 1989.
14. Siegel MJ: Practical CT techniques. In Siegel MJ, (ed): Pediatric Body CT. New York, Churchill Livingstone, 1988, pp 1–28.
15. Frey EE, Sato Y, Smith WL, Franken EA: Cine CT of the mediastinum in pediatric patients. Radiology 165:19–23, 1987.
16. Kirks DR, Fram EK, Vock P, Effmann EL: Tracheal compression by mediastinal masses in children: CT evaluation. AJR 141:647–651, 1983.
17. Hope JW, Borns PF, Koop CE: Radiological diagnosis of mediastinal masses in infants and children. Radiol Clin North Am 1:17–50, 1963.
18. Kirks DR, Korobkin M: Computed tomography of the chest in infants and children: Techniques and mediastinal evaluation. Radiol Clin North Am 19:409–419, 1981.
19. St Amour TE, Siegel MJ, Glazer HS, Nadel SN: CT appearances of the normal and abnormal thymus in childhood. J Comput Assist Tomogr 11:645–650, 1987.
20. Salonen OLM, Kivisaari ML, Somer JK: Computed tomography of the thymus of children under 10 years. Pediatr Radiol 14:373–375, 1984.
21. Francis IR, Glazer GM, Bookstein FL, Gross BH: The thymus: Reexamination of age-related changes in size and shape. AJR 145:249–254, 1985.
22. Heiberg E, Wolverson MK, Sundaram M, Nouri S: Normal thymus: CT characteristics in subjects under age 20. AJR 138:491–494, 1982.
23. Baron RL, Lee JKT, Sagel SS, Peterson RR: Computed tomography of the normal thymus. Radiology 142:121–125, 1982.
24. Baron RL, Lee JKT, Sagel SS, Levitt RG: Computed tomography of the abnormal thymus. Radiology 142:127–134, 1982.
25. Siegel MJ, Glazer HS, Wiener JI, Molina PL: Normal and abnormal thymus in childhood: MR imaging. Radiology 172:367–371, 1989.
26. de Geer G, Webb WR, Gamsu G: Normal thymus: Assessment with MR and CT. Radiology 158:313–317, 1986.
27. Daneman A: Mediastinum. In Daneman A (ed): Pediatric Body CT. London, Springer-Verlag, 1987, pp 27–53.
28. Donaldson JS: Mediastinum. In Siegel MJ (ed): Pediatric Body CT. New York, Churchill Livingstone, 1988, pp 29–79.
29. Mandell GA, Lantieri R, Goodman LR: Tracheobronchial compression in Hodgkin lymphoma in children. AJR 139:1167–1170, 1982.
30. Hopper KD, Diehl LF, Lesar M, Barnes M, Granger E, Baumann J: Hodgkin disease: clinical utility of CT in initial staging and treatment. Radiology 169:17–22, 1988.
31. Cohen MD, Siddiqui A, Weetman R, Provisor A, Coates T: Hodgkin disease and non-Hodgkin lymphomas in children: utilization of radiological modalities. Radiology 158:499–505, 1986.
32. Castellino RA, Blank N, Hoppe RT, Cho C: Hodgkin disease: contributions of chest CT in the initial staging evaluation. Radiology 160:603–605, 1986.
33. Khoury MB, Godwin JD, Halvorsen R, Hanun Y, Putnam CE: Role of chest CT in non-Hodgkin lymphoma. Radiology 158:659–662, 1986.
34. Cohen M, Hill CA, Cangir A, Sullivan MP: Thymic rebound after treatment of childhood tumors. AJR 135:151–156, 1980.
35. Heron CW, Husband JE, Williams MP: Hodgkin disease: CT of the thymus. Radiology 167:647–651, 1988.
36. Mendelson DS, Rose JS, Efremidis SC, Kirschner PA, Cohen BA: Bronchogenic cysts with high CT numbers. AJR 140:463–465, 1983.
37. Armstrong EA, Harwood-Nash DCF, Ritz CR, Chuang SH, Pettersson H, Martin DJ: CT of neuroblastomas and ganglioneuromas in children. AJR 139:571–576, 1982.

38. Fredericks BJ, Boldt DW, Tress BM, Cattapan E: Diseases of the spinal canal in children: diagnosis with noncontrast CT scans. AJNR 10:1233–1238, 1989.

39. Dietrich RB, Kangarloo H, Lenarsky C, Feig SA: Neuroblastoma: the role of MR imaging. AJR 148:937–942, 1987.

40. Vanel D, Henry-Amar M, Lumbroso J, et al: Pulmonary evaluation of patients with osteosarcoma: roles of standard radiography, tomography, CT, scintigraphy, and tomoscintigraphy. AJR 143:519–523, 1984.

41. Cohen M, Grosfeld J, Baehner R, Weetman R: Lung CT for detection of metastases: solid tissue neoplasms in children. AJR 139:895–898, 1982.

42. Cohen M, Smith WL, Weetman R, Provisor A: Pulmonary pseudometastases in children with malignant tumors. Radiology 141:371–374, 1981.

43. Hidalgo H, Korobkin M, Kinney TR, Falletta J, Heaston DH, Kirks DR: The problem of benign pulmonary nodules in children receiving cytotoxic chemotherapy. AJR 140:21–24, 1983.

44. Ikezoe J, Murayama S, Godwin JD, Done SL, Verschakelen JA: Bronchopulmonary sequestration: CT assessment. Radiology 176:375–379, 1990.

45. Mata JM, Caceres J, Lucaya J, Garcia-Conesa JA: CT of congenital malformations of the lung. RadioGraphics 10:651–674, 1990.

46. Donaldson JS, Siegel MJ: Lungs, pleura, and chest wall. In Siegel MJ (ed): Pediatric Body CT. New York, Churchill Livingstone, 1988, pp 81–102.

47. Grenier P, Maurice F, Musset D, Menu Y, Nahum H: Bronchiectasis: assessment by thin-section CT. Radiology 161:95–99, 1986.

48. Berger PE, Kuhn JP, Kuhns LR: Computed tomography and the occult tracheobronchial foreign body. Radiology 134:133–135, 1980.

49. Webb WR: High-resolution CT of the lung parenchyma. Radiol Clin North Am 27:1085–1097, 1989.

50. Klein J, Gamsu G: High resolution computed tomography of diffuse lung disease. Invest Radiol 24:805–812, 1989.

51. Shamberger RC, Holcombe EG, Weinstein HJ, Perez-Atayde AR, Tarbell NJ: Chest wall tumors in infancy and childhood. Cancer 63:774–785, 1989.

52. Cleveland RH, Foglia RP: CT in the evaluation of pleural versus pulmonary disease in children. Pediatr Radiol 18:14–19, 1988.

53. Mirowitz SA, Lee JKT, Gutierrez FR, Brown JJ: Magnetic resonance imaging of congenital heart disease. Top Magn Reson Imaging 2:49–60, 1990.

54. Gomes AS: MR imaging of congenital anomalies of the thoracic aorta and pulmonary arteries. Radiol Clin North Am 27:1171–1181, 1989.

55. Bank ER, Hernandez RJ: CT and MR of congenital heart disease. Radiol Clin North Am 26:241–262, 1988.

56. Higgins CB: MR of the heart: anatomy, physiology, and metabolism. AJR 151:239–248, 1988.

57. Didier D, Higgins CB, Fisher MR, Osaki L, Silverman NH, Cheitlin MD: Congenital heart disease: gated MR imaging in 72 patients. Radiology 158:227–235, 1986.

58. Boechat MI, Kangarloo H: MR imaging of the abdomen in children. AJR 152:1245–1250, 1989.

59. Boechat MI, Kangarloo H, Ortega J, et al: Primary liver tumors in children: comparison of CT and MR imaging. Radiology 169:727–732, 1988.

60. Miller JH, Greenspan BS: Integrated imaging of hepatic tumors in childhood. Part I: malignant lesions. Radiology 154:83–90, 1985.

61. Miller JH, Greenspan BS: Integrated imaging of hepatic tumors in childhood. Part II: benign lesions. Radiology 154:91–100, 1985.

62. Blumhagen JD, Weinberger E: Pediatric gastrointestinal ultrasonography. In Sanders RC, Hill MC (eds): Ultrasound Annual. New York, Raven, 1986, pp 99–140.

63. Weinreb JC, Cohen JM, Armstrong E, Smith T: Imaging the pediatric liver: MRI and CT. AJR 147:785–790, 1986.

64. Levine E, Cook LT, Grantham JJ: Liver cysts in autosomal-dominant polycystic kidney disease: clinical and computed tomographic study. AJR 145:229–233, 1985.

65. Araki T, Itai Y, Tasaka A: CT of choledochal cyst. AJR 135:729–734, 1980.

66. Daneman A: Liver. In Daneman A (ed): Pediatric Body CT. London, Springer-Verlag, 1987, pp 173–196.

67. Merten DF, Kirks DR: Amebic liver abscess in children: the role of diagnostic imaging. AJR 143:1325–1329, 1984.

68. Miller JH, Greenfield LD, Wald BR: Candidiasis of the liver and spleen in childhood. Radiology 142:375–380, 1982.

69. Pastakia B, Shawker TH, Thaler M, O'Leary T, Pizzo PA: Hepatosplenic candidiasis: wheels within wheels. Radiology 166:417–421, 1988.

70. Stanley P, Hall TR, Woolley MM, Diament MJ, Gilsanz V, Miller JH: Mesenchymal hamartomas of the liver in childhood: sonographic and CT findings. AJR 147:1035–1039, 1986.

71. Ros PR, Goodman ZD, Ishak KG, et al: Mesenchymal hamartoma of the liver: radiologic-pathologic correlation. Radiology 158:619–624, 1986.

72. Lucaya J, Enriquez G, Amat L, Gonzalez-Rivero MA: Computed tomography of infantile hepatic hemangioendothelioma. AJR 144:821–826, 1985.

73. Dachman AH, Lichtenstein JE, Friedman AC, Hartman DS: Infantile hemangioendothelioma of the liver: a radiologic-pathologic-clinical correlation. AJR 140:1091–1096, 1983.

74. Stanley P, Gates GF, Eto RT, Miller SW: Hepatic cavernous hemangiomas and hemangioendotheliomas in infancy. AJR 129:317–321, 1977.

75. Siegel MJ: Liver and biliary tract. In Siegel MJ (ed): Pediatric Body CT. New York, Churchill Livingstone, 1988, pp 103–134.

76. Atkinson GO Jr, Kodroff M, Sones PJ, Gay BB Jr: Focal nodular hyperplasia of the liver in children: a report of three new cases. Radiology 137:171–174, 1980.

77. Dachman AH, Pakter RL, Ros PR, Fishman EK, Goodman ZD, Lichtenstein JE: Hepatoblastoma: radiologic-pathologic correlation in 50 cases. Radiology 164:15–19, 1987.

78. Amendola MA, Blane CE, Amendola BE, Glazer GM: CT findings in hepatoblastoma. J Comput Assist Tomogr 8:1105–1109, 1984.

79. Brick SH, Taylor GA, Potter BM, Eichelberger MR: Hepatic and splenic injury in children: role of CT in the decision for laparotomy. Radiology 165:643–646, 1987.

80. Taylor GA, Fallat ME, Eichelberger MR: Hypovolemic shock in children: abdominal CT manifestations. Radiology 164:479–481, 1987.

81. Federle MP, Griffiths B, Minagi H, Jeffrey RB Jr: Splenic trauma: evaluation with CT. Radiology 162:69–71, 1987.

82. Stalker HP, Kaufman RA, Towbin R: Patterns of liver injury in childhood: CT analysis. AJR 147:1199–1205, 1986.

83. Kaufman RA, Towbin R, Babcock DS, et al: Upper abdominal trauma in children: imaging evaluation. AJR 142:449–460, 1984.

84. Berger PE, Kuhn JP: CT of blunt abdominal trauma in childhood. AJR 136:105–110, 1981.

85. Brody AS, Seidel FG, Kuhn JP: CT Evaluation of blunt abdominal trauma in children: comparison of ultrafast and conventional CT. AJR 153:803–806, 1989.

86. Kaufman RA: CT of blunt abdominal trauma in children: a five-year experience. In Siegel MJ (ed): Pediatric Body CT. New York, Churchill Livingstone, 1988, pp 313–347.

87. Bulas DI, Taylor GA, Eichelberger MR: The value of CT in detecting bowel perforation in children after blunt abdominal trauma. AJR 153:561–564, 1989.

88. Taylor GA, Guion CJ, Potter BM, Eichelberger MR: CT of blunt abdominal trauma in children. AJR 153:555–559, 1989.

89. Oakes DD, Charters AC: Changing concepts in the management of splenic trauma. Surg Gynecol Obstet 153:181–185, 1981.

90. Foley WD, Cates JD, Kellman GM, et al: Treatment of blunt hepatic injuries: role of CT. Radiology 164:635–638, 1987.

91. Kirks DR, Rosenberg ER, Johnson DG, King LR: Integrated imaging of neonatal renal masses. Pediatr Radiol 15:147–156, 1985.

92. Lebowitz RL, Mandell J: Urinary tract infection in children: putting radiology in its place. Radiology 165:1–9, 1987.
93. Kangarloo H, Gold RH, Fine RN, Diament MJ, Boechat MI: Urinary tract infection in infants and children evaluated by ultrasound. Radiology 154:367–373, 1985.
94. Fong KW, Rahmani MR, Rose TH, Skidmore MB, Connor TP: Fetal renal cystic disease: sonographic-pathologic correlation. AJR 146:767–773, 1986.
95. Grossman H, Rosenberg ER, Bowie JD, Ram P, Merten DF: Sonographic diagnosis of renal cystic diseases. AJR 140:81–85, 1983.
96. Bosniak MA: The current radiological approach to renal cysts. Radiology 158:1–10, 1986.
97. Morehouse HT, Weiner SN, Hoffman JC: Imaging in inflammatory disease of the kidney. AJR 143:135–141, 1984.
98. Gold RP, McClennan BL, Rottenberg RR: CT appearance of acute inflammatory disease of the renal interstitium. AJR 141:343–349, 1983.
99. Hoddick W, Jeffrey RB, Goldberg HI, Federle MP, Laing FC: CT and sonography of severe renal and perirenal infections. AJR 140:517–520, 1983.
100. Daneman A: Kidneys. In Daneman A (ed): Pediatric Body CT. London, Springer-Verlag, 1987, pp 145–171.
101. Soulen MC, Fishman EK, Goldman SM, Gatewood OMB: Bacterial renal infection: role of CT. Radiology 171:703–707, 1989.
102. Cohen MD: Kidneys. In Siegel MJ (ed): Pediatric Body CT. New York, Churchill Livingstone, 1988, pp 135–175.
103. Dietrich RB, Kangarloo H: Kidneys in infants and children: evaluation with MR. Radiology 159:215–221, 1986.
104. Belt TG, Cohen MD, Smith JA, Cory DA, McKenna S, Weetman R: MRI of Wilms' tumor: promise as the primary imaging method. AJR 146:955–961, 1986.
105. Kirks DR, Merten DF, Grossman H, Bowie JD: Diagnostic imaging of pediatric abdominal masses: an overview. Radiol Clin North Am 19(3):527–545, 1981.
106. Siegel MJ: Pediatric applications. In Lee JKT, Sagel SS, Stanley RJ (eds): Computed body tomography. New York, Raven, 1983, pp 517–534.
107. Cohen MD. Kidneys. In Siegel MJ (ed): Pediatric Body CT. New York, Churchill Livingstone, 1988, pp 135–175.
108. Reiman TAH, Siegel MJ, Shackelford GD: Wilms tumor in children: abdominal CT and US evaluation. Radiology 160:501–505, 1986.
109. Chan HSL, Daneman A, Gribbin M, Martin DJ: Renal cell carcinoma in the first two decades of life. Pediatr Radiol 13:324–328, 1983.
110. Hartman DS, Lesar MSL, Madewell JE, Lichtenstein JE, Davis CJ Jr: Mesoblastic nephroma: radiologic-pathologic correlation of 20 cases. AJR 136:69–74, 1981.
111. Madewell JE, Goldman SM, Davis CJ Jr, Hartman DS, Feigin DS, Lichtenstein JE: Multilocular cystic nephroma: a radiographic-pathologic correlation of 58 patients. Radiology 146:309–321, 1983.
112. Mitnick JS, Bosniak MA, Hilton S, Raghavendra BN, Subramanyam BR, Genieser NB: Cystic renal disease in tuberous sclerosis. Radiology 147:85–87, 1983.
113. Kuhn JP, Berger PE: Computed tomography of the kidney in infancy and childhood. Radiol Clin North Am 19(3):445–461, 1981.
114. Montgomery P, Kuhn JP, Berger PE, Fisher J: Multifocal nephroblastomatosis: clinical significance and imaging. Pediatr Radiol 14:392–395, 1984.
115. Fernbach SK, Feinstein KA, Donaldson JS, Baum ES: Nephroblastomatosis: comparison of CT with US and urography. Radiology 166:153–156, 1988.
116. Jafri SZH, Bree RL, Amendola MA, et al: CT of renal and perirenal non-Hodgkin lymphoma. AJR 138:1101–1105, 1982.
117. Weinberger E, Rosenbaum DM, Pendergrass TW: Renal involvement in children with lymphoma: comparison of CT with sonography. AJR 155:347–349, 1990.
118. Sty JR, Wells RG, Starshak RJ, Schroeder BA: Imaging in acute renal infection in children. AJR 148:471–477, 1987.
119. Lang EK, Sullivan J, Frentz G: Renal trauma: radiological studies. Radiology 154:1–6, 1985.
120. Rhyner P, Federle MP, Jeffrey RB: CT of trauma to the abnormal kidney. AJR 142:747–750, 1984.
121. Pollack HM, Wein AJ: Imaging of renal trauma. Radiology 172:297–308, 1989.
122. Fanney DR, Casillas J, Murphy BJ: CT in the diagnosis of renal trauma. RadioGraphics 10:29–40, 1990.
123. Siegel MJ, Balfe DM: Blunt renal and ureteral trauma in childhood: CT patterns of fluid collections. AJR 152:1043–1047, 1989.
124. Lupetin AR, Mainwaring BL, Daffner RH: CT diagnosis of renal artery injury caused by blunt abdominal trauma. AJR 153:1065–1068, 1989.
125. Yale-Loehr AJ, Kramer SS, Quinlan DM, La France ND, Mitchell SE, Gearhart JP: CT of severe renal trauma in children: evaluation and course of healing with conservative therapy. AJR 152:109–113, 1989.
126. Karp MP, Jewett TC Jr, Kuhn JP, Allen JE, Dokler ML, Cooney DR: The impact of computed tomography scanning on the child with renal trauma. J Pediatr Surg 21:617–623, 1986.
127. Stalker HP, Kaufman RA, Stedje K: The significance of hematuria in children after blunt abdominal trauma. AJR 154:569–571, 1990.
128. Siegel MJ, Jamroz GA, Glazer HS, Abramson CL: MR imaging of intraspinal extension of neuroblastoma. J Comput Assist Tomogr 10:593–595, 1986.
129. Fletcher BD, Kopiwoda SY, Strandjord SE, Nelson AD, Pickering SP: Abdominal neuroblastoma: magnetic resonance imaging and tissue characterization. Radiology 155:699–703, 1985.
130. Bousvaros A, Kirks DR, Grossman H: Imaging of neuroblastoma: an overview. Pediatr Radiol 16:89–106, 1986.
131. Stark DD, Moss AA, Brasch RC, et al: Neuroblastoma: diagnostic imaging and staging. Radiology 148:101–105, 1983.
132. Daneman A: Adrenals. In Daneman A (ed): Pediatric Body CT. London, Springer-Verlag, 1987, pp 121–143.
133. Stark DD, Brasch RC, Moss AA, et al: Recurrent neuroblastoma: the role of CT and alternative imaging tests. Radiology 148:107–112, 1983.
134. Boechat MI, Ortega J, Hoffman AD, Cleveland RH, Kangarloo H, Gilsanz V: Computed tomography in stage III neuroblastoma. AJR 145:1283–1287, 1985.
135. Cohen MD, Weetman R, Provisor A, et al: Magnetic resonance imaging of neuroblastoma with a 0.15-T magnet. AJR 143:1241–1248, 1984.
136. Donaldson JS, Gilsanz V, Miller JH: CT scanning in patients with opsomyoclonus: importance of nonenhanced scan. AJR 146:781–783, 1986.
137. Farrelly C, Daneman A, Chan HSL, Martin DJ: Occult neuroblastoma presenting with opsomyoclonus: utility of computed tomography. AJR 142:807–810, 1984.
138. Baker ME, Kirks DR, Korobkin M, Bowie JD, Filston HC: The association of neuroblastoma and myoclonic encephalopathy: an imaging approach. Pediatr Radiol 15:184–190, 1985.
139. Lowe RE, Cohen MD: Computed tomographic evaluation of Wilms tumor and neuroblastoma. RadioGraphics 4:915–928, 1984.
140. Farrelly CA, Daneman A, Martin DJ, Chan HSL: Pheochromocytoma in childhood: the important role of computed tomography in tumour localization. Pediatr Radiol 14:210–214, 1984.
141. Francis IR, Glazer GM, Shapiro B, Sisson JC, Gross BH: Complementary roles of CT and ^{131}I-MIBG scintigraphy in diagnosing pheochromocytoma. AJR 141:719–725, 1983.
142. Radin DR, Ralls PW, Boswell WD Jr, Colletti PM, Lapin SA, Halls JM: Pheochromocytoma: detection by unenhanced CT. AJR 146:741–744, 1986.
143. Thomas JL, Bernardino ME, Samaan NA, Hickey RC: CT of pheochromocytoma. AJR 135:477–482, 1980.
144. Laursen K, Damgaard-Pedersen K: CT for pheochromocytoma diagnosis. AJR 134:277–280, 1980.
145. Welch TJ, Sheedy PF II, van Heerden JA, Sheps SG, Hattery RR, Stephens DH: Pheochromocytoma: value of computed tomography. Radiology 148:501–503, 1983.
146. Reinig JW, Doppman JL, Dwyer AJ, Johnson AR, Knop RH:

Adrenal masses differentiated by MR. Radiology 158:81–84, 1986.

147. Fink IJ, Reinig JW, Dwyer AJ, Doppman JL, Linehan WM, Keiser HR: MR imaging of pheochromocytomas. J Comput Assist Tomogr 9:454–458, 1985.

148. Dunnick NR: Adrenal imaging: current status. AJR 154:927–936, 1990.

149. Quint LE, Glazer GM, Francis IR, Shapiro B, Chenevert TL: Pheochromocytoma and paraganglioma: comparison of MR imaging with CT and I-131 MIBG scintigraphy. Radiology 165:89–93, 1987.

150. Hamper UM, Fishman EK, Hartman DS, Roberts JL, Sanders RC: Primary adrenocortical carcinoma: sonographic evaluation with clinical and pathologic correlation in 26 patients. AJR 148:915–919, 1987.

151. Fishman EK, Deutch BM, Hartman DS, Goldman SM, Zerhouni EA, Siegelman SS: Primary adrenocortical carcinoma: CT evaluation with clinical correlation. AJR 148:531–535, 1987.

152. Daneman A, Chan HSL, Martin J: Adrenal carcinoma and adenoma in children: a review of 17 patients. Pediatr Radiol 13:11–18, 1983.

153. Ling D, Korobkin M, Silverman PM, Dunnick NR: CT demonstration of bilateral adrenal hemorrhage. AJR 141:307–308, 1983.

154. Brill PW, Jagannath A, Winchester P, Markisz JA, Zirinsky K: Adrenal hemorrhage and renal vein thrombosis in the newborn: MR imaging. Radiology 170:95–98, 1989.

155. Boechat MI: Adrenal glands, pancreas, and retroperitoneal structures. In Siegel MJ (ed): Pediatric Body CT. New York, Churchill Livingstone, 1988, pp 177–217.

156. Atkinson GO Jr, Zaatari GS, Lorenzo RL, Gay BB Jr, Garvin AJ: Cystic neuroblastoma in infants: radiographic and pathologic features. AJR 146:113–117, 1986.

157. Forman HP, Leonidas JC, Berdon WE, Slovis TL, Wood BP, Samudrala R: Congenital neuroblastoma: evaluation with multimodality imaging. Radiology 175:365–368, 1990.

158. Robberecht E, Nachtegaele P, Van Rattinghe R, Afschrift M, Kunnen M, Verhaaren R: Pancreatic lipomatosis in the Shwachman-Diamond syndrome. Pediatr Radiol 15:348–349, 1985.

159. Silverstein W, Isikoff MB, Hill MC, Barkin J: Diagnostic imaging of acute pancreatitis: prospective study using CT and sonography. AJR 137:497–502, 1981.

160. Balthazar EJ, Ranson JHC, Naidich DP, Megibow AJ, Caccavale R, Cooper MM: Acute pancreatitis: prognostic value of CT. Radiology 156:767–772, 1985.

161. Williford ME, Foster WL Jr, Halvorsen RA, Thompson WM: Pancreatic pseudocyst: comparative evaluation by sonography and computed tomography. AJR 140:53–57, 1983.

162. Daneman A: Pancreas. In Daneman A (ed): Pediatric Body CT. London, Springer-Verlag, 1987, pp 107–120.

163. Jeffrey RB Jr, Federle MP, Crass RA: Computed tomography of pancreatic trauma. Radiology 147:491–494, 1983.

164. Rossi P, Baert A, Passariello R, Simonetti G, Pavone P, Tempesta P: CT of functioning tumors of the pancreas. AJR 144:57–60, 1985.

165. Robey G, Daneman A, Martin DJ: Pancreatic carcinoma in a neonate. Pediatr Radiol 13:284–286, 1983.

166. Daneman A: Spleen. In Daneman A (ed): Pediatric Body CT. London, Springer-Verlag, 1987, pp 209–220.

167. James S, Balfe DM, Lee JKT, Picus D: Small-bowel disease: categorization by CT examination. AJR 148:863–868, 1987.

168. Fisher JK: Normal colon wall thickness on CT. Radiology 145:415–418, 1982.

169. Siegel MJ, Evans SJ, Balfe DM: Small bowel disease in children: diagnosis with CT. Radiology 169:127–130, 1988.

170. Megibow AJ, Balthazar EJ, Naidich DP, Bosniak MA: Computed tomography of gastrointestinal lymphoma. AJR 141:541–547, 1983.

171. Vade A, Blane CE: Imaging of Burkitt lymphoma in pediatric patients. Pediatr Radiol 15:123–126, 1985.

172. Teele RL, Katz AJ, Goldman H, Kettell RM: Radiographic features of eosinophilic gastroenteritis (allergic gastroenteropathy) of childhood. AJR 132:575–580, 1979.

173. Marks MP, Lanza MV, Kahlstrom EJ, Mikity V, Marks SC, Kvalstad RP: Pediatric hypertrophic gastropathy. AJR 147:1031–1034, 1986.

174. Morrison S, Dahms BB, Hoffenberg E, Czinn SJ: Enlarged gastric folds in association with Campylobacter pylori gastritis. Radiology 171:819–821, 1989.

175. Riddlesberger MM Jr: CT of complicated inflammatory bowel disease in children. Pediatr Radiol 15:384–387, 1985.

176. Abramson SJ, Berdon WE, Baker DH: Childhood typhlitis: its increasing association with acute myelogenous leukemia. Radiology 146:61–64, 1983.

177. Merine DS, Fishman EK, Jones B, Nussbaum AR, Simmons T: Right lower quadrant pain in the immunocompromised patient: CT findings in 10 cases. AJR 149:1177–1179, 1987.

178. Balthazar EJ, Megibow AJ, Hulnick D, Gordon RB, Naidich DP, Beranbaum ER: CT of appendicitis. AJR 147:705–710, 1986.

179. Parienty RA, Lepreux JF, Gruson B: Sonographic and CT features of ileocolic intussusception. AJR 136:608–610, 1981.

180. Iko BO, Teal JS, Siram SM, Chinwuba CE, Roux VJ, Scott VF: Computed tomography of adult colonic intussusception: clinical and experimental studies. AJR 143:769–772, 1984.

181. Merine D, Fishman EK, Jones B, Siegelman SS: Enteroenteric intussusception: CT findings in nine patients. AJR 148:1129–1132, 1987.

182. Glasier CM, Siegel MJ, McAlister WH, Shackelford GD: Henoch-Schonlein syndrome in children: gastrointestinal manifestations. AJR 136:1081–1085, 1981.

183. Daneman A: Retroperitoneum. In Daneman A (ed): Pediatric Body CT. London, Springer-Verlag, 1987, pp 89–105.

184. Nichols DM, Li DK: Superior mesenteric vein rotation: a CT sign of midgut malrotation. AJR 141:707–708, 1983.

185. Siegel MJ, Glasier CM, Sagel SS: CT of pelvic disorders in children. AJR 137:1139–1143, 1981.

186. Kohda E, Fujioka M, Ikawa H, Yokoyama J: Congenital anorectal anomaly: CT evaluation. Radiology 157:349–352, 1985.

187. Sato Y, Pringle KC, Bergman RA, et al: Congenital anorectal anomalies: MR imaging. Radiology 168:157–162, 1988.

188. Dietrich RB, Kangarloo H: Pelvic abnormalities in children: assessment with MR imaging. Radiology 163:367–372, 1987.

189. Daneman A: Pelvic viscera and soft tissues. In Daneman A (ed): Pediatric Body CT. London, Springer-Verlag, 1987, pp 221–244.

190. Friedman AC, Pyatt RS, Hartman DS, Downey EF Jr, Olson WB: CT of benign cystic teratomas. AJR 138:659–665, 1982.

191. Buy J-N, Ghossain MA, Moss AA, et al: Cystic teratoma of the ovary: CT detection. Radiology 171:697–701, 1989.

192. Togashi K, Nishimura K, Itoh K, et al: Ovarian cystic teratomas: MR imaging. Radiology 162:669–673, 1987.

193. Siegel MJ: Pelvic organs and soft tissues. In Siegel MJ (ed): Pediatric Body CT. New York, Churchill Livingstone, 1988, pp 219–251.

194. Vogler JB III, Murphy WA: Bone marrow imaging. Radiology 168:679–693, 1988.

195. Aisen AM, Martel W, Braunstein EM, McMillin KI, Phillips WA, Kling TF: MRI and CT evaluation of primary bone and soft-tissue tumors. AJR 146:749–756, 1986.

196. Fritzsche PJ, Hricak H, Kogan BA, Winkler ML, Tanagho EA: Undescended testis: value of MR imaging. Radiology 164:169–173, 1987.

197. Wolverson MK, Houttuin E, Heiberg E, Sundaram M, Shields JB: Comparison of computed tomography with high-resolution real-time ultrasound in the localization of the impalpable undescended testis. Radiology 146:133–136, 1983.

198. Wolverson MK, Jagannadharao B, Sundaram M, Riaz MA, Nalesnik WJ, Houttuin E: CT in localization of impalpable cryptorchid testes. AJR 134:725–729, 1980.

199. Kier R, McCarthy S, Rosenfield AT, Rosenfield NS, Rapoport S, Weiss RM: Nonpalpable testes in young boys: evaluation with MR imaging. Radiology 169:429–433, 1988.

200. Hernandez RJ: Musculoskeletal system. In Siegel MJ (ed): Pediatric Body CT. New York, Churchill Livingstone, 1988, pp 253–291.

201. Daneman A: Bones. In Daneman A (ed): Pediatric Body CT. London, Springer-Verlag, 1987, pp 329–347.
202. Weekes RG, McLeod RA, Reiman HM, Pritchard DJ: CT of soft-tissue neoplasms. AJR 144:355–360, 1985.
203. Schreiman JS, Crass JR, Wick MR, Maile CW, Thompson RC Jr: Osteosarcoma: role of CT in limb-sparing treatment. Radiology 161:485–488, 1986.
204. Bloem JL, Taminiau AHM, Eulderink F, Hermans J, Pauwels EKJ: Radiologic staging of primary bone sarcoma: MR imaging, scintigraphy, angiography, and CT correlated with pathologic examination. Radiology 169:805–810, 1988.
205. Demas BE, Heelan RT, Lane J, Marcove R, Hajdu S, Brennan MF: Soft-tissue sarcomas of the extremities: comparison of MR and CT in determining the extent of disease. AJR 150:615–620, 1988.
206. Boyko OB, Cory DA, Cohen MD, Provisor A, Mirkin D, DeRosa GP: MR imaging of osteogenic and Ewing's sarcoma. AJR 148:317–322, 1987.
207. Petasnick JP, Turner DA, Charters JR, Gitelis S, Zacharias CE: Soft-tissue masses of the locomotor system: comparison of MR imaging with CT. Radiology 160:125–133, 1986.
208. Totty WG, Murphy WA, Lee JKT: Soft-tissue tumors: MR imaging. Radiology 160:135–141, 1986.
209. Zimmer WD, Berquist TH, McLeod RA, et al: Bone tumors: magnetic resonance imaging versus computed tomography. Radiology 155:709–718, 1985.
210. Wing VW, Jeffrey RB Jr, Federle MP, Helms CA, Trafton P: Chronic osteomyelitis examined by CT. Radiology 154:171–174, 1985.
211. Tang JSH, Gold RH, Bassett LW, Seeger LL: Musculoskeletal infection of the extremities: evaluation with MR imaging. Radiology 166:205–209, 1988.
212. Unger E, Moldofsky P, Gatenby R, Hartz W, Broder G: Diagnosis of osteomyelitis by MR imaging. AJR 150:605–610, 1988.
213. Fletcher BD, Scoles PV, Nelson AD: Osteomyelitis in children: detection by magnetic resonance. Radiology 150:57–60, 1984.
214. Scuderi G, Bronson MJ: Triradiate cartilage injury. Clin Orthop 217:179–189, 1987.
215. Heger L, Wulff K, Seddiqi MSA: Computed tomography of calcaneal fractures. AJR 145:131–137, 1985.
216. Feldman F, Singson RD, Rosenberg ZS, Berdon WE, Amodio J, Abramson SJ: Distal tibial triplane fractures: diagnosis with CT. Radiology 164:429–435, 1987.
217. Cone RO, Nguyen V, Flournoy JG, Guerra J Jr: Triplane fracture of the distal tibial epiphysis: radiographic and CT studies. Radiology 153:763–767, 1984.
218. Toby EB, Koman LA, Bechtold RE, Nicastro JN: Postoperative computed tomographic evaluation of congenital hip dislocation. J Pediatr Orthop 7:667–670, 1987.
219. Hernandez RJ, Tachdjian MO, Dias LS: Hip CT in congenital dislocation: appearance of tight iliopsoas tendon and pulvinar hypertrophy. AJR 139:335–337, 1982.
220. Johnson ND, Wood BP, Jackman KV: Complex infantile and congenital hip dislocation: assessment with MR imaging. Radiology 168:151–156, 1988.
221. Lee MS, Harcke HT, Kumar SJ, Bassett GS: Subtalar joint coalition in children: new observations. Radiology 172:635–639, 1989.
222. Deutsch AL, Resnick D, Campbell G: Computed tomography and bone scintigraphy in the evaluation of tarsal coalition. Radiology 144:137–140, 1982.
223. Hernandez RJ, Tachdjian MO, Poznanski AK, Dias LS: CT determination of femoral torsion. AJR 137:97–101, 1981.

CHAPTER 27

INTERVENTIONAL COMPUTED TOMOGRAPHY

ALBERT A. MOSS

Many imaging techniques—including fluoroscopy,[1–4] angiography,[5] endoscopic retrograde cholangiopancreatography (ERCP),[6] ultrasonography,[7–12] nuclear imaging,[13] computed tomography (CT),[14–25] and magnetic resonance imaging (MRI)[26–28]—have been used to guide interventional procedures. Each technique has advantages and limitations in guiding specific interventional procedures, and selection of the most appropriate technique demands the consideration of a variety of factors.

Since its introduction, CT has been used to guide percutaneous interventional procedures.[29] CT precisely defines the relationship of a needle to the surrounding tissues. Thus if the needle tip is demonstrated by CT, its precise position is ensured, limited only by the thickness of the CT section. In a CT section 5 mm thick, the needle tip can be located within a 2.5-mm range on the z-axis, and thus the actual location of the needle is known within very narrow limits. Because CT can identify and localize lesions less than 1 cm in diameter, the size of the smallest lesion that can undergo biopsy depends more on the technical skill of the radiologist in placing the needle into a small mass than on detecting the lesion.

A major advantage of CT over other imaging techniques is its capacity to image materials ranging in density from air to metal. The capability of CT to image materials with high attenuation values permits the use of oral, rectal, and intravenous contrast material as aids in locating lesions on CT and in distinguishing an abnormality from surrounding normal structures or tissue. An abscess can be readily distinguished from bowel when the bowel is filled with contrast medium, and a lymph node can be readily differentiated from an adjacent vessel. Intravenous contrast medium permits better definition of the relationship of a mass to nearby vascular structures, improves the detectability of certain mass lesions, and provides an assessment of tumor vascularity before biopsy. Injection of iodinated urographic contrast medium into cysts, abscesses, or fistulas delineates the true extent of the abnormal cavity, reveals any communicating tracts, and permits assessment of the inner margin of the cystic space. In addition, CT images are not significantly degraded by external dressings, open wounds, ostomy devices, or drainage catheters, and low-density lesions can be imaged even if they are adjacent to high-density material.

The indications for percutaneous interventional procedures are rapidly evolving as new equipment is developed, experience is accumulated, and the risks and benefits are defined. Lesions readily demonstrated by conventional radiographic techniques are sampled under fluoroscopic guidance, and ultrasonography is employed whenever ultrasound clearly images a lesion and a safe approach can be ensured.

CT is most frequently used to guide the following interventional procedures:

1. Biopsy of lesions not easily demonstrated by other imaging techniques
2. Masses less than 3 cm in diameter
3. Lesions positioned close to bone, blood vessels, or bowel
4. Deep lesions
5. Mediastinal masses
6. Pulmonary parenchymal lesions that cannot be sampled fluoroscopically
7. Intraabdominal or pelvic abscesses requiring catheter drainage
8. Neurolysis
9. Repeated biopsies when a biopsy has been unsuccessful by other methods
10. Implantation of radiotherapy seeds

CT-guided interventional procedures require expensive, often heavily used scanning instruments, and therefore such procedures are more costly than those guided by fluoroscopy or ultrasound.

CT-Guided Percutaneous Biopsies

Whenever possible, a full diagnostic CT scan is performed before a CT-guided biopsy. The biopsy is scheduled after review of the diagnostic CT scan, history, physical findings, and laboratory results with the referring physician. Selection of the type of needle and technique to be used is based on the depth and location of the abnormality and its relationship to bone, vascular structures, bowel, or pleura.

Patient Preparation

Patients are placed on a clear liquid diet on the day of the biopsy to minimize the chance of aspiration if emesis occurs. Biopsies are performed on an outpatient basis, unless the patient is hospitalized for another reason. Informed consent is obtained, and the procedure, including possible complications, is fully explained to the patient. Premedication is not routinely given except to pediatric patients. As a precaution, a prothrombin time and platelet count

are obtained before performing a biopsy with a needle larger than 20 gauge. A low platelet count or a prothrombin time more than 50 per cent above normal are relative contraindications to a percutaneous biopsy; in these situations, we attempt to correct the abnormality before proceeding with the biopsy. If a bleeding tendency still persists after attempted correction, the indications for the biopsy should be carefully reassessed in view of the increased hazards of the procedure. If a biopsy is still clinically indicated, the smallest needle possible should be used, and typed and cross-matched whole blood should be readily available. Following a biopsy, patients are kept in the outpatient department for an observation period of 1 to 2 hours. Biopsies can be performed to obtain cytologic material, histologic material, or both.

Materials

NEEDLES FOR CYTOLOGIC ASPIRATION

Material for cytologic evaluation can be aspirated using a variety of fine-gauge needles (Figs. 27–1 and 27–2). Because each needle for cytologic aspiration has advantages and limitations, a complete selection should be kept available in the CT scanning suite. The original Chiba 22-gauge needle had an outer diameter of 0.028 inch and an inner diameter of 0.015 inch[30]; a more flexible needle with the same outer diameter and a larger inner diameter (0.020 inch) is also available (Cook, Inc., Bloomington, IN).[30]

The thinner-walled needle permits slightly more material to be obtained but is somewhat more difficult to direct, as the extreme flexibility of the needle often causes it to bend or deflect when passing through materials of different consistencies. Both needles are made of flexible steel and have an inner stylet. The original Chiba needle had a noncutting bevel of 30°, which was modified to 24° to facilitate introduction of the needle and dislodgement of bits of tissue as the needle was rotated (Fig. 27–3A).[30] Needles of the same design are available in 18- to 23-gauge sizes. Usually 21- to 22-gauge needles are employed for cytologic aspiration, because larger needles permit aspiration of more blood, but little additional cytologic material. Biopsies of deep-seated lesions or masses in obese patients are more easily performed using larger gauge needles, which provide improved direction control as they are passed through the abdomen, retroperitoneum, and subcutaneous tissue.

Cytologic aspiration can also be done with spinal needles of various lengths and gauges (see Figs. 27–1A,B). Spinal needles are less flexible and easier to control than thinner-walled needles; their short length makes them ideal for biopsies of superficial lesions.

NEEDLES FOR HISTOLOGIC SAMPLING

Many cutting needles are available for obtaining tissue for histologic analysis. Some needles are designed for biopsy of a particular organ, such as liver when the needle is rotated. The Madayag needle (Cook, Inc.) has a 90° bevel and a conical stylet (see Fig. 27–3E). The Green needle (Cook, Inc., Bloomington, IN) is identical to the Madayag needle, except for its multifaceted, diamond-shaped stylet (see Fig. 27–3F).

Larger gauge needles permit larger pieces of tissue to be obtained, and the tissue specimens can be fixed and stained in a conventional manner. The TruCut needle (Travenol Laboratories, Inc., Deerfield, IL) (see Fig. 27–3G) has been widely used for biopsies of pleural, chest wall, liver, renal, retroperitoneal, and soft tissue lesions.[4, 21, 31, 32] The needle has an outer cutting cannula through which an inner component containing a 2-mm specimen slot is passed. After insertion of the needle, the cutting cannula is slid over the inner component, slicing the specimen and holding it for retrieval. The Lee and Westcott needles (Becton-Dickinson, Inc., Franklin Lakes, NJ) are similar to the TruCut but have a smaller gauge.

The Rotex biopsy instrument (Travenol Laboratories, Inc.) is designed to collect tissue without significant dilution of the specimen by blood (Figs. 27–2 and 27–4). The instrument consists of two parts: a stainless steel needle, whose distal end consists of a tapered screw, and an outer cannula. The needle is passed through the cannula and rotated into the mass by the small handle on the needle. The outer cannula slides over the screw, and the needle and

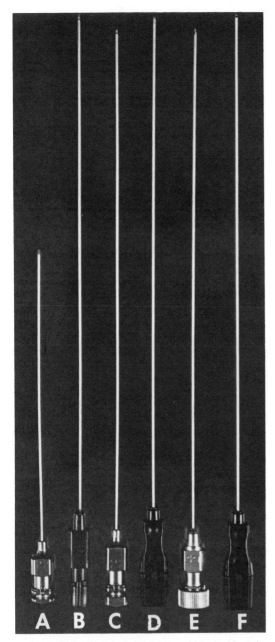

FIGURE 27–1 ■ Various 22-gauge needles used for cytologic biopsies. A = Spinal needle; B = Green needle; C = Madayag needle; D = Turner needle; E = Franseen needle; F = Chiba needle.

or bone, whereas others are general-purpose biopsy needles. Histologic needles are of two general types: thin-walled, small-gauge needles and larger gauge, stiffer needles.

Thin-walled needles, designed to obtain tissue for histologic analysis, are available in 22-, 20-, and 18-gauge sizes (see Fig. 27–3). The Franseen needle (Cook, Inc.) has three cutting teeth that detach pieces of tissue when the needle is rotated (see Fig. 27–3C). The Turner needle (Cook, Inc.) consists of a cutting cannula with a flat, 45° beveled cutting tip and a fitted obturator (see Fig. 27–3D). The tip of the Turner needle occasionally makes entry difficult, but it cuts a core of tissue that remains in the needle

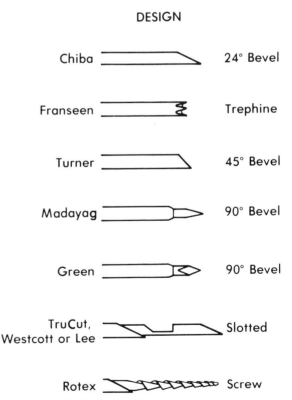

FIGURE 27–2 ■ Needles frequently employed in CT-directed biopsies. (Modified from Lieberman RP, Hafez CR, Crummy AB: AJR 138:561, 1982. © 1982 American Roentgen Ray Society. Used with permission.)

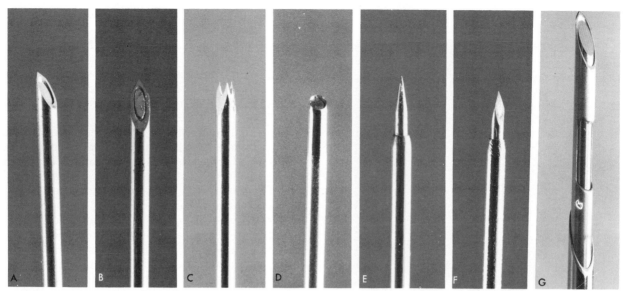

FIGURE 27–3 ■ Close-up photographs of tips of various biopsy needles. *A*, Chiba needle; tip has short (24°) noncutting bevel. *B*, Spinal needle; tip has slightly longer, cutting bevel. *C*, Franseen needle; trephine tip with three cutting teeth. *D*, Turner needle; beveled tip (45°) with inner cutting edge. *E*, Madayag needle; beveled tip (90°) with a conical stylet. *F*, Green needle; beveled tip (90°) with a diamond-shaped stylet. *G*, TruCut, Lee, or Westcott needle; slotted, three pieces.

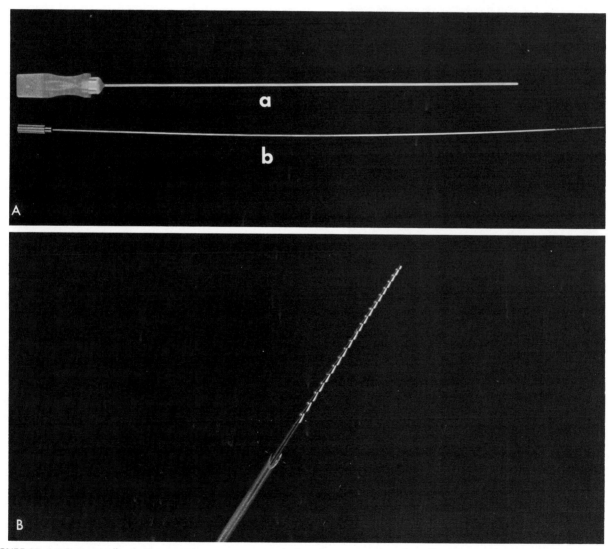

FIGURE 27–4 ■ Rotex needle. *A*, Components: a = outer cannula; b = inner screw-shaped needle. *B*, Tapered screw passing through outer cannula (magnified view).

1300

cannula are removed together. A small-gauge version has been introduced for cytologic sampling.[32]

The Menghini needle is a cutting instrument used primarily for biopsy of the liver and solid avascular abdominal or pelvic masses. The needle is available in 15- to 20-gauge sizes and various lengths[32] and comes with calibrations on the shaft (Fig. 27–5B). A stop on the shaft of the needle can be adjusted to the depth of the lesion. The needle is inserted to the premeasured depth and withdrawn in a single motion.

The Vim-Silverman (Becton-Dickinson, Inc.) (Fig. 27–6) is a 14- or 18-gauge cutting needle that provides a larger core of tissue and is used primarily for liver biopsies.

Several automated biopsy devices have been introduced for obtaining histologic samples.[34] Some of these instruments create a set amount of suction by employing a locking syringe (Fig. 27–7) or Vacutainer.[35] Other approaches have employed automatic biopsy guns (Fig. 27–8).[35] These devices usually come in 14- or 18-gauge sizes and in short (0.9 cm) or long throw (1.7 cm) models. A notch needle of the TruCut type is generally employed.

The Bard biopsy gun (C. R. Bard, Covington, GA) uses an 18-gauge cutting needle.[36] The handle can be attached after the needle is placed and is activated by pushing a button.

The Cook biopsy gun (Cook, Inc.) has a reusable handle through which the needle is inserted; an 18-gauge needle is used. The gun is activated by first cocking the gun manually, which retracts the outer cannula and exposes the side notch of the needle. Pushing a button rapidly advances the cannula.

The Klear Kut biopsy gun (The Percy Group, St. Louis, MO) has both 14- and 18-gauge needles. The handle and needle are attached. After needle placement, the plunger is manually advanced. The stylet is then driven forward by pulling the gun's trigger.

Needles for biopsy of bone are pointed instruments consisting of an outer cannula, a pointed obturator, and a cutting inner cannula. The Turkel needle is a 10-gauge triephine instrument that has a slightly blunt obturator beveled to wedge into the bone. The inner cannula has three sharp teeth that are rotated by two hexagonal metal pieces that attach to the hub of the inner cannula and act as a handle. The Craig needle has a serrated inner cannula and a very large bore (3.5-mm inner diameter). Blunt stylets are provided for all triephine needles to expel the biopsy material.

The Jamshide needle (Baxter Healthcare, Valencia,

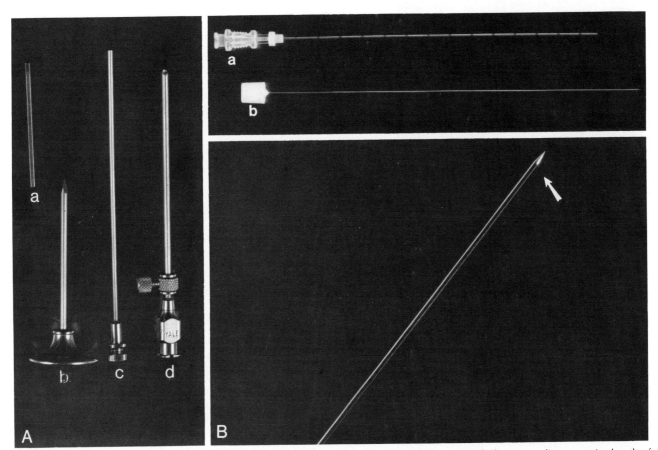

FIGURE 27–5 ■ *A*, Menghini needle (classic type). a = Biopsy-retaining pin to prevent biopsy sample from extending up entire length of cannula or extruding into syringe; b = trocar for initial skin puncture; c = stylet to push biopsy specimen out of needle; d = thin-wall needle with a bevel of 45° to 50° and sharpened edge (side stop can be adjusted to ensure biopsy at premeasured depth). *B*, New model components. a = Outer calibrated cannula; b = inner needle. Magnified view of inner needle with a conical tip *(arrow).*

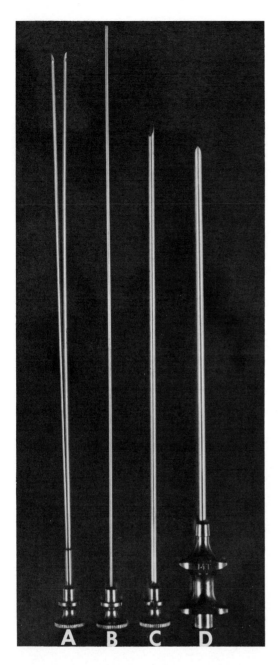

FIGURE 27–6 ■ Vim-Silverman needle. A = 17-gauge inner split cutting cannula; B = blunt stylet for removing tissue from split cannula; C and D = 14-gauge outer beveled cannula with fitted stylet.

CA) combines the features of cutting and triephine needles. It is available in 11- to 17-gauge sizes and consists of a cannula with a sharp beveled tip and a flat obturator.

A short (5-cm) 17-gauge bone biopsy needle (E-Z-EM, Inc., Westbury, NY) has a sharp inner stylet and an outer cannula with screwlike threads scored into its outer surface (Fig. 27–9).

A number of specialized needles are available to perform certain tasks. The Onik needle[37, 38] (Medical Instrument Development Laboratories, San Leandro, CA) is a needle specifically designed for percutaneous diskectomy, coaxial needles[37, 38, 39] permit repeated biopsy sampling, and the Mick applicator (Mick Radionuclear Instruments, Bronx, NY) is designed for implantation of ^{125}I seeds.[40, 41] The Trough

needle[42] is particularly useful for biopsy of lung cancer, and Pais et al.[43] designed a triephine bone biopsy system.

Methods

The diagnostic CT study should be carefully reviewed to select the biopsy site and determine the position in which the patient will be placed for biopsy. An anterior transabdominal or transthoracic approach with the patient in the supine position is used, except for biopsy of paravertebral and deep retroperitoneal masses. Generally the supine position is easier for the patient to maintain than the prone or decubitus position.

The abnormality undergoing biopsy is relocated on

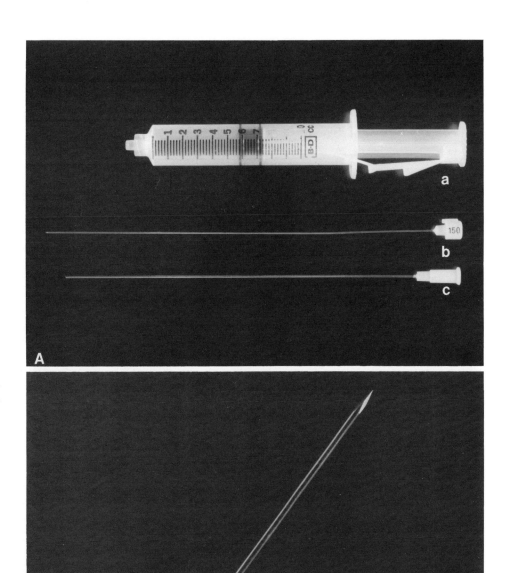

FIGURE 27–7 ■ Cutting biopsy needle with vacuum syringe and positioning clips (E-Z-EM, Inc.). *A*, Components: a = locking syringe; b = inner 19.5-gauge needle; c = outer stylet. *B*, Magnified view of inner needle showing diamond-shaped tip.

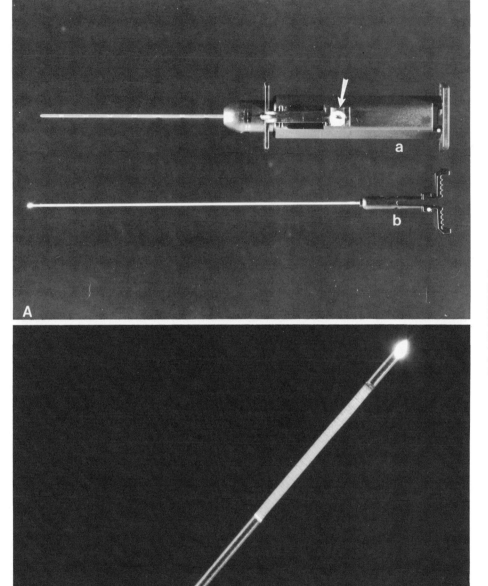

FIGURE 27-8 ■ Hand-held biopsy gun with TruCut needle. *A*, Components: a = integrated handle and outer cannula. The outer cannula has markings every 1 cm. The triggering button is indicated by the arrow; b = inner cutting needle. *B*, Magnified view of inner notched needle.

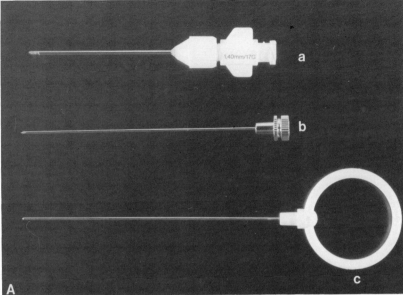

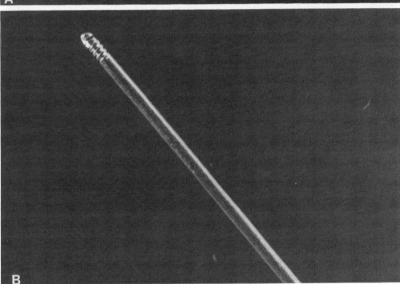

FIGURE 27–9 ■ Bone biopsy needle (E-Z-EM, Inc.). *A*, Components: a = outer cannula (17-gauge); b = inner needle; c = blunt stylet for pushing biopsy material from cannula. *B*, Magnified view of outer cannula with screw-like threads.

a series of scans at levels preselected from the diagnostic study. The distance from the midabdominal or midthoracic line to the entry site, the depth from the skin to the anterior and posterior margins of the lesion, and the angle of insertion of the needle are measured on the CT monitor console (Fig. 27–10). Currently I most frequently use a hand-held guidance device (GE Medical Systems, Milwaukee, WI) to perform biopsy and drainage procedures.[44] This device is designed to permit placement of a needle at any angle to the horizontal. It incorporates a bubble level to indicate when the base is horizontal, and vertical to the base is a protractor with an attached movable arm that serves as the needle guide. A ruler on the protractor arm permits accurate measurement of the depth of the needle (Fig. 27–11).

The entry site is marked with a radiopaque marker, and a repeat CT scan is performed to confirm that the entry site is appropriate. The entry site is marked with indelible ink, the marker is removed, the skin is cleansed with povidone iodine (Betadine), and the area is sterilely draped. A small cut in the skin is made, the angle to the horizontal is set by the guidance device, and the needle is inserted to the premeasured depth following leveling of the base by using the bubble level (Fig. 27–12).

Once the needle is placed, the guidance device is removed from the needle, and a scan is obtained to verify position. Needles of any size and trocars up to no. 9 French can be guided with this device.

A great variety of other methods are employed to guide biopsy needles. These include the tandem-needle technique first described by Ferrucci and Wittenberg (Fig. 27–13),[15] the single-needle free-hand technique (Fig. 27–14), coaxial needle systems,[45-47] guidance of biopsy pathways using light guidance systems, gantry tilt or triangulation methods (Fig. 27–15), guidance by simple geometric calculations, and even guidance using elaborate, expensive stereotaxic instruments (Fig. 27–16).[48] Each method has

Text continued on page 1310

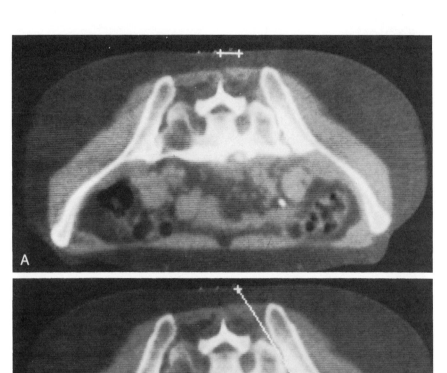

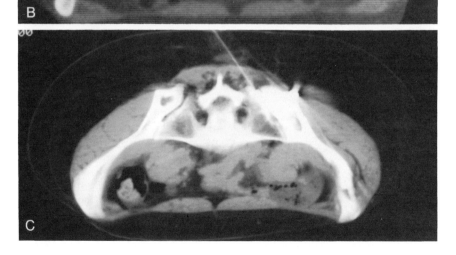

FIGURE 27–10 ■ Method of CT-guided biopsy. *A*, CT scan in the prone position. There is sclerosis of the right sacroiliac joint with slight widening of the joint space. A distance of 1.6 cm was measured from the midline and selected as the site of needle entry. *B*, Simulated placement of needle into the joint space. CT console–measured depth was 8.3 cm at an angle of −55°. *C*, CT confirmation of satisfactory needle placement in sacroiliac joint. Diagnosis: nonpyogenic sacroiliitis.

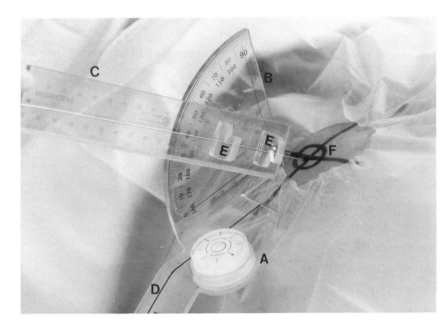

FIGURE 27–11 ■ Hand-held biopsy device. A = Bubble level mounted to base of device; B = protractor fixed to base at 90° angle; C = hinged arm with ruler; D = baseline, E = needle guides; F = marked entry point.

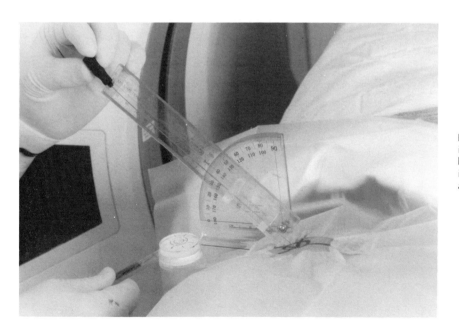

FIGURE 27–12 ■ Use of hand-held biopsy instrument. The radiologist is leveling the base using the bubble level and is ready to insert the needle to the premeasured depth at the angle measured from the CT console.

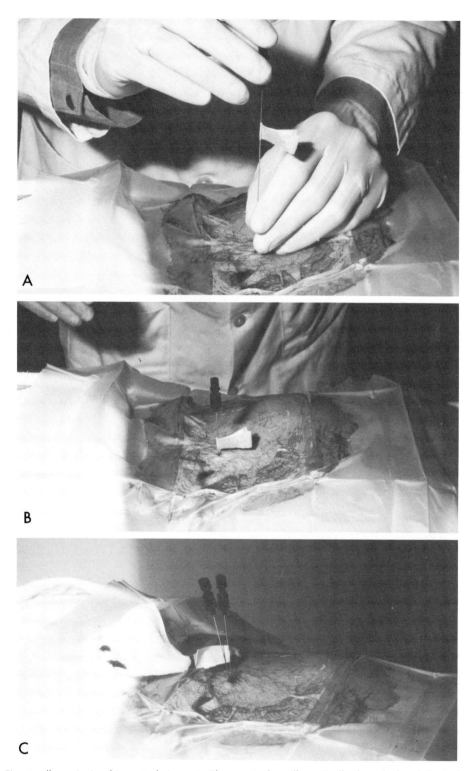

FIGURE 27–13 ■ Fine-needle aspiration biopsy technique. *A,* Placement of needle vertically through the abdominal wall. The needle is flexible, and holding it near the entry point helps stabilize it. Tape is placed around needle at the desired depth. *B,* Needle positioned vertically up to tape. *C,* Second needle is placed using the first needle as a guide.

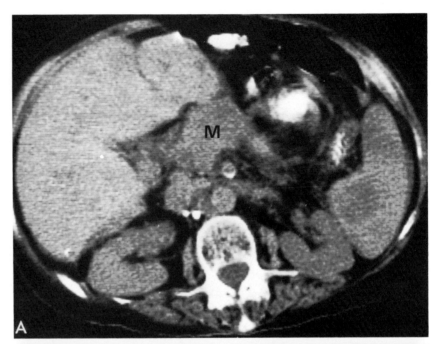

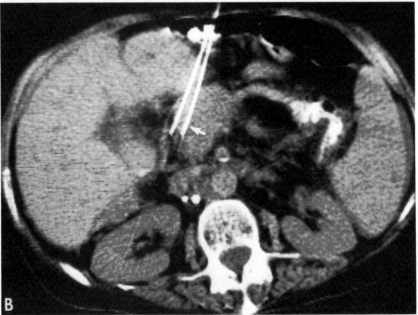

FIGURE 27–14 ■ CT-guided pancreatic biopsy using the tandem technique. *A,* A small mass (M) is identified in the head of the pancreas. *B,* Two needles are placed into the pancreatic mass. The tip of one needle (*arrow*) appears to be just in the pancreas.

Illustration continued on following page

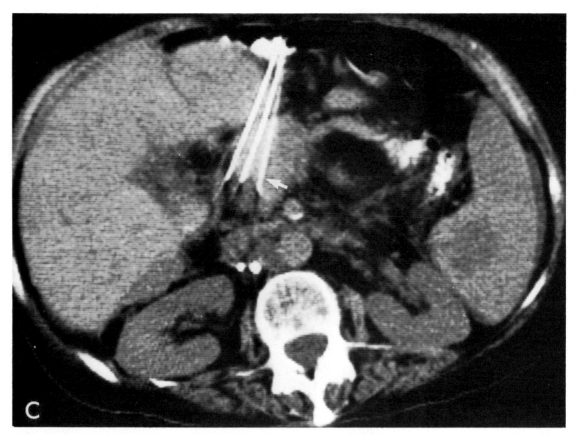

FIGURE 27–14 *Continued C,* Placement of another needle (*arrow*) into the pancreatic mass. Diagnosis: carcinoma of the pancreas.

advantages and disadvantages, and various investigators each have their favorite. What is important is not what method is employed to place a needle, but that the needle is precisely placed and the biopsy proceeds safely and has success rates comparable to those reported in the literature.

CYTOLOGIC BIOPSY TECHNIQUES

Following insertion of a thin-walled 22-gauge needle, CT scans are obtained until the needle tip is shown to be in the lesion. When included within the scan slice, the needle tip will appear square,[14] and the needle will have a uniform density throughout its length. To minimize radiation exposure, CT scans for needle verification should be performed at the lowest possible exposure factors.

I have found it easier to place the biopsy needle accurately if the needle is inserted perpendicular to the lesion through the abdominal wall or chest. This usually can be accomplished in the abdomen, as a 22-gauge needle can be passed through bowel without complication.[49] Whether the needle is being guided by a mechanical device or by hand injection, it is important when the needle is being passed to maintain it on a straight path, because a slight deviation at skin level will produce a larger deviation within the body. If the needle is directed incorrectly, its course cannot be corrected by altering the position of the needle hub; the entire needle must be removed

and reintroduced. Coaxial methods employ a thin-walled needle that serves as a cannula through which a smaller needle can be passed.[28, 39]

If the physician is using the tandem method,[15] once the needle tip is verified to be within the lesion, a second needle is passed parallel to the first needle into the mass (see Fig. 27–13). This method permits multiple cytologic aspirations to be obtained without repeat CT scans to verify the position of subsequent needle placements.

Increased resistance to passage of the needle may be felt as the mass is reached. When resistance is met, the needle should be advanced slightly into the lesion and rotated several times to dislodge cellular material from around the needle tip. However, there is debate as to what to do next. Although Fagelman and Chess[50] employ a nonaspiration technique to obtain fine-needle cytologic samples, other investigators have stressed the need to apply suction to obtain adequate samples when using fine-needle techniques.[51, 52] Hueftle and Haaga[51] found suction necessary to obtain adequate specimens but did not find any significant increase in sample size as suction pressure was increased from 5 to 30 mL. Sample size was 20 per cent larger if suction was maintained during needle removal.[51]

Kreula et al.[52] also found suction necessary to obtain adequate samples. They reported that needle movement without suction, suction without needle

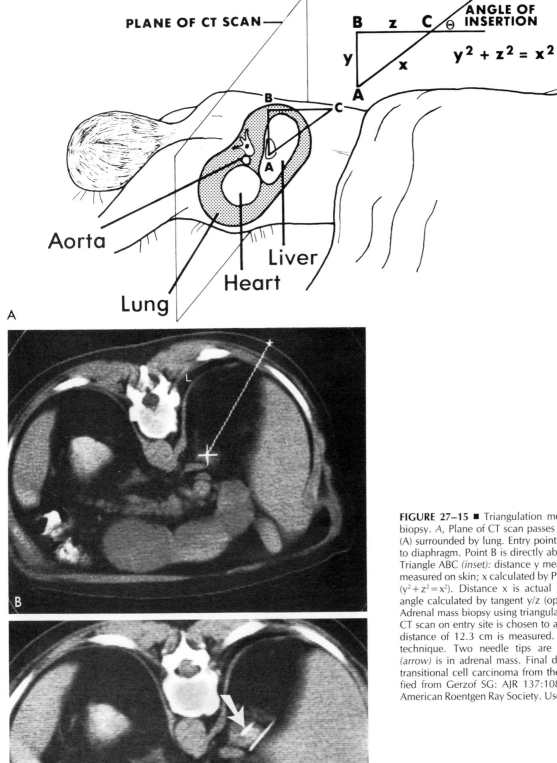

PLANE OF CT SCAN

ANGLE OF INSERTION

$$y^2 + z^2 = x^2$$

Aorta

Lung

Heart

Liver

A

B

C

FIGURE 27–15 ■ Triangulation method of CT-guided biopsy. *A,* Plane of CT scan passes through liver lesion (A) surrounded by lung. Entry point (C) selected caudal to diaphragm. Point B is directly above liver lesion (A). Triangle ABC *(inset):* distance y measured from scan; z measured on skin; x calculated by Pythagorean theorem $(y^2 + z^2 = x^2)$. Distance x is actual needle path. Entry/angle calculated by tangent y/z (opposite/adjacent). *B,* Adrenal mass biopsy using triangulation method. Prone CT scan on entry site is chosen to avoid the lung (L). A distance of 12.3 cm is measured. *C,* Tandem needle technique. Two needle tips are demonstrated; one *(arrow)* is in adrenal mass. Final diagnosis: metastatic transitional cell carcinoma from the bladder. (*A* modified from Gerzof SG: AJR 137:1080, 1981. © 1981, American Roentgen Ray Society. Used with permission.)

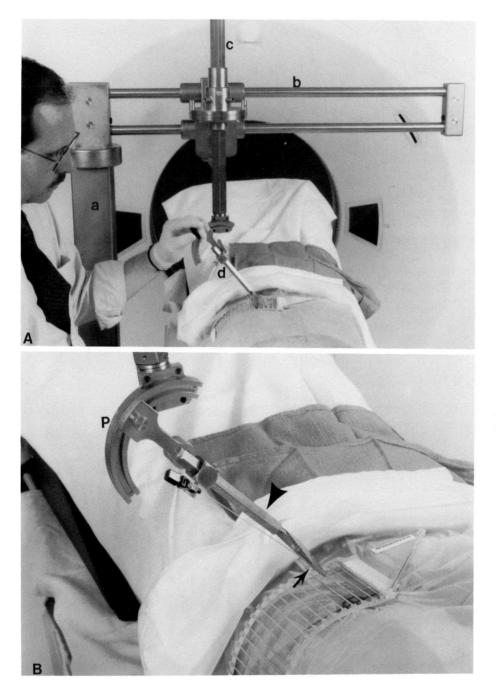

FIGURE 27–16 ■ Use of stereotaxic CT biopsy instrument. *A*, Overview of system showing the instrument's base stand (a), horizontal arm (b), vertical arm (c), and needle holder and guidance system (d). *B*, Close-up view of needle holder *(arrow)* and guidance arm with ruler *(arrowhead)* and integrated protractor (P), which permits needle to be inserted at a premeasured angle. Tubes of various sizes are placed on the patient's skin to facilitate measurement of entry point.

movement, rate of application of suction, and duration of suction had no effect on sampling.[52]

Kreula[53] also studied the effect of sampling technique on specimen size and found technique to be extremely important. Specimen size increased linearly with the number of passes, provided the needle sampled in different directions. The amplitude of the needle pass also is important, as specimen weight increases linearly above an excursion of 3 to 4 mm. Specimens were larger when fewer and longer excursions were made, compared with a large number of passes with small needle movements.[53] Small-bore needles with acute bevels appear superior to flat-bevel needles of similar gauge.[54]

It appears that optimal aspiration techniques using thin-walled needles will entail use of an acute-beveled needle; excursion of the needle of at least 4 mm, the longer the better; 10 to 20 mL of suction applied during needle movement and maintained as the needle is withdrawn; samples obtained from different portions of the mass, if multiple needles are to be inserted or multiple passes performed; and discontinuance of suction if blood is aspirated. When the pleura, lung, or a critical vascular structure intervenes between the lesion and the site of entry for a biopsy performed in the same plane, the needle can be angulated into the mass by simple triangulation (see Fig. 27–15).[44, 47, 55, 56]

PREPARATION OF CYTOLOGIC SPECIMENS

The accuracy of diagnosis depends to a great degree on the skill of the cytopathologist and the quality of the biopsy material. The cytopathologist is notified at the beginning of the biopsy and, if possible, is present during the biopsy to prepare the specimens. Specimens are immediately smeared on glass slides and fixed with 95 per cent ethanol or, if the aspirate is bloody, a modified Carnoy's solution (ethyl alcohol and 5 per cent glacial acetic acid). Although specimens can first be placed in a preservative solution and then centrifuged, smeared on ground-glass slides, and postfixed in 95 per cent ethanol, rapid wet fixation better preserves the entire cell and prevents distortion, shrinkage, and swelling. Immediately after fixation, the specimen is stained, and the cytopathologist views the specimen to determine whether the sample is adequate (Fig. 27–17). A final diagnosis is made after the aspirated material is permanently stained.

The value of immediate microscopic evaluation of aspiration specimens is debatable. Inadequate specimens can be detected and repeat aspirations performed, but Miller et al.[57] were unable to demonstrate that immediate assessment improved accuracy rates or lowered complications. Obviously the presence of a cytopathologist at the time of aspiration does not reduce accuracy rates, provides greater educational benefits, and improves overall communication.

Knowledge of the expected diagnosis can influence the diagnostic approach. Because epithelial tumors such as adenocarcinomas and squamous cell carcinomas usually provide adequate cellular material,

fine-needle cytologic aspiration biopsy specimens are usually satisfactory.[58, 59] However, solid mesodermal tumors tend to have great cellular cohesiveness and may not yield adequate specimens unless histologic samples are obtained. Therefore the radiologist and pathologist must be prepared to obtain and preserve histologic as well as cytologic material. Fortunately, supplementary tissue core material can often be obtained from fine-needle aspiration biopsies.[60]

HISTOLOGIC BIOPSY TECHNIQUES

Tissue core biopsies can be obtained with flexible 20- or 22-gauge needles, as well as with large-bore needles.[33, 54, 60–64] The technique for obtaining histologic material depends largely on the organ undergoing biopsy and the needle used to obtain the material. Obtaining core biopsies with thin needles requires only a slight modification of the technique used for cytologic aspiration biopsies. Patient preparation is identical, and no additional laboratory studies are obtained. Following placement of the thin needle by any technique, a syringe containing 1 mL of normal nonbacteriostatic saline is attached to the needle, and continuous suction is applied as the needle is advanced and rotated. Suction should be maintained continually during withdrawal of the aspirating needle.[60] When blood or bits of tissue are aspirated into the syringe, the needle and syringe should be removed together and the contents of the syringe injected into a sterile test tube. The tissue fragments are individually removed in the pathology laboratory and processed using the usual histologic techniques. The remaining portion of the supernatant may be filtered and processed for cytologic analysis.

Larger tissue samples can be obtained with various larger and more rigid needles (Fig. 27–18).[22, 34, 36, 42, 43, 54, 61] To avoid complications, vascular structures, bowel, and solid parenchymal organs should not be traversed. The use of various "angled" techniques,[15, 45–47] decubitus positioning,[65] and even injection of CO_2 intraperitoneally to move critical structures out of a needle's path have been advocated.[66] Solid superficial masses without intervening lung or bowel can be safely sampled. Prior to obtaining a biopsy, the vascularity of the lesion may be determined by injecting a bolus of contrast material and performing a dynamic CT scan sequence. If a lesion is hypervascular, the decision to perform a large-bore biopsy should be reconsidered.

Large-bore biopsies are performed only on patients who do not have any coagulopathy. Patients are screened by measuring prothrombin time and partial thromboplastin time and performing platelet counts.[67]

Most studies have demonstrated that better histologic specimens can be obtained using large cutting needles.[22, 54, 68–70] If a single-needle technique is employed, the entry site, depth of biopsy, and needle angulation are determined and anesthesia accomplished in a manner identical to that used in a cytologic aspiration biopsy.

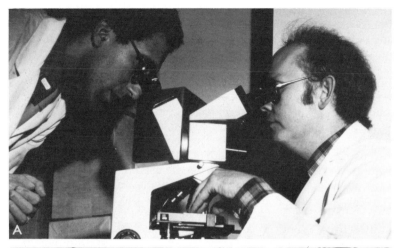

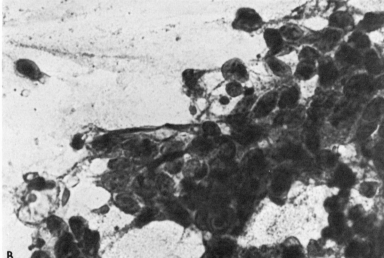

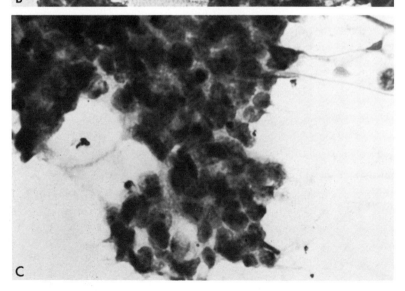

FIGURE 27–17 ■ *A,* Immediate viewing of cytologic specimen to determine whether sample is adequate for diagnosis. *B,* Cytologic material from hepatic aspirate of metastatic carcinoma is stained with toluidine blue. Excellent preservation of cytologic characteristics permits a preliminary diagnosis and termination of the aspiration procedure. *C,* The same aspirate stained with the final Papanicolaou stain. Cytologic detail is excellent and is not affected by prior toluidine blue stain.

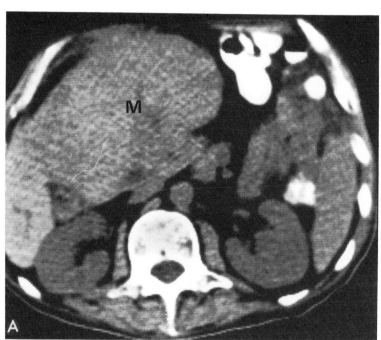

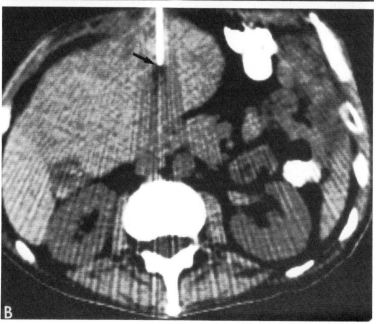

FIGURE 27–18 ■ Large-bone biopsy of hepatic tumor. *A,* A large hepatic mass (M) is demonstrated in the left lobe of the liver. The mass was not highly vascular on a dynamic CT scan series performed following a bolus injection of contrast. *B,* Histologic biopsy using an 18-gauge needle. The tip of the needle appears square *(arrow).* Streak artifacts are caused by the hub of the needle. Diagnosis: metastatic adenocarcinoma.

The double-needle technique involves placing a thin needle into the lesion and using it as a guide for inserting the cutting needle into the mass. A verifying CT scan is not performed, and the tissue sample is obtained immediately.

Complications

Although fine-needle biopsy has become a routine diagnostic procedure and is considered safe, it is not completely free of complications that may be severe and sometimes fatal. Smith[71] reviewed the world literature and found 33 deaths and 23 instances of malignant seeding of needle tracts. The frequency of deaths ranged from 0.006 per cent to 0.1 per cent, whereas needle tract seeding ranged from 0.003 per cent to 0.009 per cent. Twenty of the deaths involved biopsy of liver lesions, only two of which were hemangiomas. Most hepatic deaths occurred in patients with hepatomas or metastases. Six deaths involved pancreatic biopsies. Seventeen of the deaths following liver biopsy were a result of bleeding, and five of six deaths occurring after pancreatic biopsies were secondary to pancreatitis. Pancreatic carcinoma was the most common malignancy to seed along needle tracts.[71]

Hemorrhage may occur immediately after biopsy or be delayed.[72, 73] Yankaskas et al.[72] found a 3 per cent or more drop in hematocrit in 12.7 per cent of patients undergoing fine-needle abdominal biopsies, although only 1 to 2.9 per cent of patients require transfusion following renal biopsy.[73] Use of a hemostatic protein polymer sheath[74] and embolization of biopsy tracts with Gelfoam, clotted blood, or metallic coils have been advocated to reduce hemorrhagic complications.[75] However, no technique has proven totally effective in preventing complications, and all patients should be monitored closely for 1 to 2 hours after biopsy; if treated on an outpatient basis, patients should be instructed to return to the emergency department immediately if they have persistent or increasing pain, fever, or signs of bleeding.

Biopsy of Specific Organs

PANCREAS

The most frequent indication for a thin-needle pancreatic biopsy is to differentiate pancreatic carcinoma from chronic pancreatitis in a patient with abdominal pain, weight loss, and a pancreatic mass. This distinction remains difficult despite advances in ultrasonography, CT, endoscopic pancreatography, and angiography. Intraoperative diagnosis is also frequently difficult.[76] Percutaneous pancreatic aspiration biopsy is an accurate, nonoperative method of providing cytologic or histologic proof of pancreatic malignancy.[1, 3, 5, 6, 14, 18, 62, 64, 77–80]

After CT localization of the pancreatic mass to be biopsied, various techniques can be employed to obtain cytologic or histologic material. If cytologic material is to be obtained, most frequently a 21- or 22-gauge thin-walled needle is directed vertically through the abdominal wall, stomach, and intervening bowel directly into the pancreatic mass (Figs. 27–14 and 27–19).[15, 78, 79] Additional needles often can be placed into the pancreatic mass using the tandem-needle technique (see Fig. 27–14),[15, 78] or a coaxial needle biopsy can be performed through the initial needle. Histologic samples may be obtained using a biopsy gun[80] fitted with an 18-gauge needle.

Pancreatic aspiration biopsies provide cytologic material of excellent quality. The high yield of cytologic specimens probably stems from the fact that the cells are obtained directly from pancreatic glands and not from surrounding scar, fibrotic, or necrotic tissue.

The reported accuracy of CT-directed pancreatic biopsies has varied from 70 per cent to 95 per cent.[18, 62, 77–79] An overall accuracy of 96 per cent in CT-directed pancreatic biopsies and a 95 per cent accuracy in diagnosis of pancreatic adenocarcinoma was reported by Harter et al.[81] Using current techniques, an accuracy rate of about 90 per cent should be achievable in most CT laboratories.

Complications after a fine-needle pancreatic biopsy are uncommon but are not rare. Although most investigators report no significant complications,[3, 18, 58, 78, 79, 81] there have been reports of sepsis,[58, 71] hematomas,[58] spread of pancreatic carcinoma along the needle tract,[78, 81, 82] pancreatitis,[71] and death.[71]

LIVER

Percutaneous liver biopsy is commonly used to obtain tissue for diagnosis of hepatic abnormalities.[83] Blind, undirected biopsies using the Vim-Silverman or Menghini needle provide a large core of hepatic tissue sufficient for a diagnosis of most diffuse hepatic diseases. However, the diagnostic yield of blind hepatic biopsies in patients with malignant disease ranges from 50 per cent to 71 per cent,[84, 85] with only a 20 per cent accuracy in patients with focal hepatic metastasis.[85] Significant complications occur in 10 per cent to 17 per cent of patients after a large-bore hepatic biopsy.[86]

Overall accuracy rates of 65 per cent to 100 per cent have been obtained using CT-guided biopsy techniques.[21, 50, 58, 63, 64, 67, 70, 81, 87] Several factors account for this increased accuracy. The biopsy needle is directed toward a focal lesion, and the needle's position within the mass is verified before the sample is obtained. In addition, thin-gauge needles are longer than the traditional large-bore needles used for blind biopsies and thus can reach deeper lesions and be safely used for biopsy of lesions in the left hepatic lobe.[87]

Fine-needle hepatic cytologic biopsy is similar to other fine-needle biopsy procedures, and accuracy rates of more than 90 per cent have been reported.[50, 81] Necrotic lesions should be sampled at the periphery as well as the center (Fig. 27–20). Cystic hepatic lesions can be punctured and the fluid aspirated for analysis.

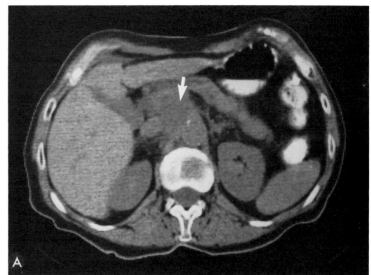

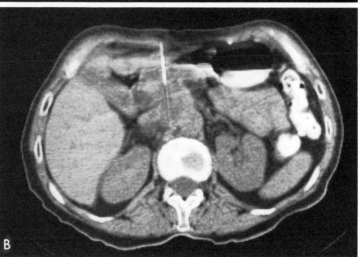

FIGURE 27–19 ■ CT-guided biopsy of a small pancreatic mass. *A*, Prebiopsy CT scan demonstrates a solid mass *(arrow)* in the head of the pancreas. The mass obliterates fat planes around the aorta and vena cava. *B*, CT scan documents placement of a 22-gauge needle into the anterior portion of the pancreatic mass. Diagnosis: pancreatic adenocarcinoma.

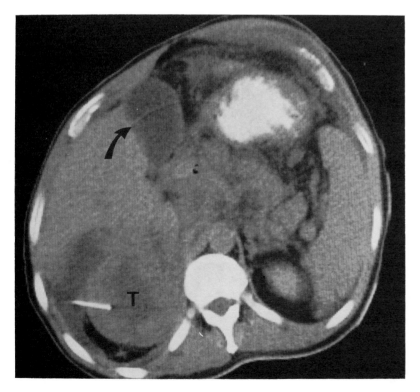

FIGURE 27–20 ■ Necrotic tumor (T) presenting as a mass off the edge of the right lobe of the liver. CT-guided biopsy of the periphery of the lesion yielded cytologic material positive for hepatoma. Material from the center of the lesion was nondiagnostic necrotic debris. Curved arrow points to the gallbladder.

Histologic biopsies of the liver are coming to be preferred by many investigators.[21, 33, 62, 67, 70] Histologic samples can be obtained using single-needle techniques or by employing one of a variety of biopsy guns or devices. Although the overall complication rate following directed hepatic biopsy has been reported to range from 0.83 per cent to 1.67 per cent,[70] a number of severe and even fatal complications have been reported.[21, 64, 70–72] Hemorrhage, sepsis, fistula formation, carcinoid crisis, needle tract seeding, and death have been documented using both cutting and noncutting needles.[71] Of 21 fatal liver biopsies reported, seven occurred in patients with hepatoma, two in patients with hemangiomas, two in patients with angiosarcomas, and ten in patients with metastatic foci.[71]

RETROPERITONEUM, PELVIS, KIDNEYS, AND ABDOMEN

Percutaneous biopsy of lesions involving the pelvis, retroperitoneum, kidneys, adrenals, and abdomen have been successfully performed.[15, 17, 18, 19, 21, 29, 57, 58, 62, 64, 65, 67, 69, 88–91] The usual indications for a CT-guided needle biopsy are as follows:

1. To demonstrate metastatic disease to stage a known neoplasm
2. To diagnose the cell type of a lesion in order to better plan a therapeutic regimen
3. To make or exclude a diagnosis of lymphoma
4. To determine the presence of viable or recurrent tumor after therapy

Both aspiration and cutting biopsies can be performed. The techniques are similar to those used in pancreatic and liver biopsies, although small posterior masses are often best approached with the patient in the prone position (Fig. 27–21).

Biopsy of renal and perirenal lesions has seldom been guided by CT,[15, 17, 18] as biopsies guided by fluoroscopy or ultrasonography are simple and provide a high diagnostic yield.[69, 91] However, CT has been valuable for guiding biopsy of renal lesions that are small, located near major vascular structures, or poorly seen on ultrasonography (Fig. 27–22). The accuracy of CT-guided biopsies of renal masses and cysts has been found to be greater than 90 per cent.[31]

Accuracy rates of 66 per cent to 100 per cent have been reported for CT-directed pelvic and retroperitoneal biopsies.[15–18, 31, 58, 62] The reported accuracy rates are higher for epithelial than for lymphomatous masses.[17, 31, 62] The greater success rate for biopsy of nonlymphomatous masses is probably a result of a combination of the greater retrieval rate of adequate tissue and the easier cytologic diagnosis of epithelial malignancy. If it is suspected that metastatic disease is present in normal-size lymph nodes, a fluoroscopically guided thin-needle biopsy of the node that appears most abnormal by lymphangiography is preferred to a CT-guided approach.[88,89] CT is used to direct biopsies of diffuse lymphatic abnormalities, critically positioned lymphatic masses, and necrotic lymphatic lesions. Histologic sampling is preferred, because histologic architecture is helpful in arriving at a definitive diagnosis.

Major complications of transabdominal pelvic or retroperitoneal biopsy guided by CT are unusual, with most investigators reporting no significant complications.[18, 62, 87] However, Yankaskas et al.[72] found a hematocrit drop of 3 per cent or more in 12.7 per cent of patients, and death and needle tract seeding have been reported following pelvic and retroperitoneal biopsy.[71]

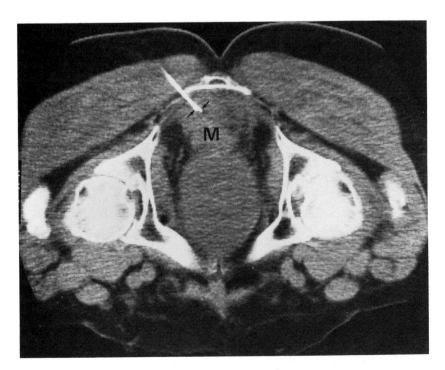

FIGURE 27–21 ■ Presacral mass (M) in a patient 1 year after an abdominoperineal resection for rectal carcinoma. CT scan in the prone position shows two needles *(arrows)* in mass. Final diagnosis: recurrent adenocarcinoma.

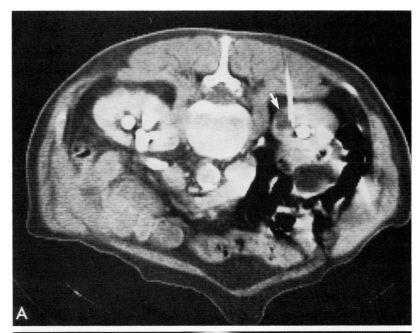

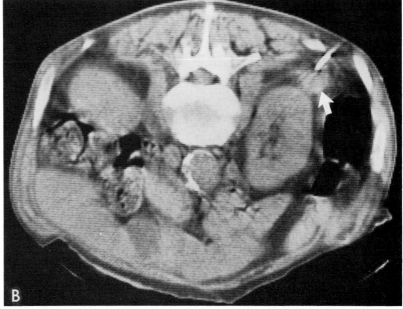

FIGURE 27–22 ■ Use of CT to guide biopsy of renal and perirenal masses with patient in the prone position. *A,* A small intrarenal mass *(arrow)* of indeterminate density undergoes biopsy using the tandem needle technique. Final diagnosis: hemorrhagic cyst. *B,* A small perirenal mass *(arrow)* having a soft tissue density undergoes biopsy using an angulated approach from the lateral flank. Final diagnosis: perirenal abscess.

LUNG AND MEDIASTINUM

Fluoroscopically guided needle biopsy of pulmonary, pleural, and mediastinal abnormalities is an easily performed procedure with an overall accuracy rate of 79 per cent to 96.5 per cent.[4, 24, 92, 93] As a rule, therefore, fluoroscopic guidance is preferred for biopsy of such masses. However, CT has been useful in guiding the biopsies of small pulmonary or mediastinal lesions that cannot be clearly delineated by fluoroscopy or of masses that are deep or near major vascular structures (Figs. 27–23 and 27–24).[20, 21, 24, 93–96]

The mass to be sampled is located by CT while the patient suspends respiration at end-expiratory volume. Distances and angles required for accurate needle placement are measured, and either a single- or double-needle (Fig. 27–25) biopsy technique is used. The double-needle method requires placing a guidance cannula at the margin of the lesion; a 22- to 23-gauge biopsy needle is then passed through the cannula into the mass (Figs. 27–23 and 27–26). Another approach is to initially place a 22- or 23-gauge needle with a removable hub into the mass; the hub is removed, and a 19-gauge needle is coaxially passed over the inner thin needle.[24]

Pneumothorax is the principal complication of CT-guided transthoracic biopsies. Rates ranging from 14 per cent to 61 per cent have been reported.[20, 24, 60, 92, 97] This is somewhat higher than the rate of pneumothorax reported for fluoroscopically guided transthoracic needle aspiration biopsies.[4, 93, 98, 99] Most patients with pneumothorax require no therapy, but 3 per cent to 10 per cent may require placement of a

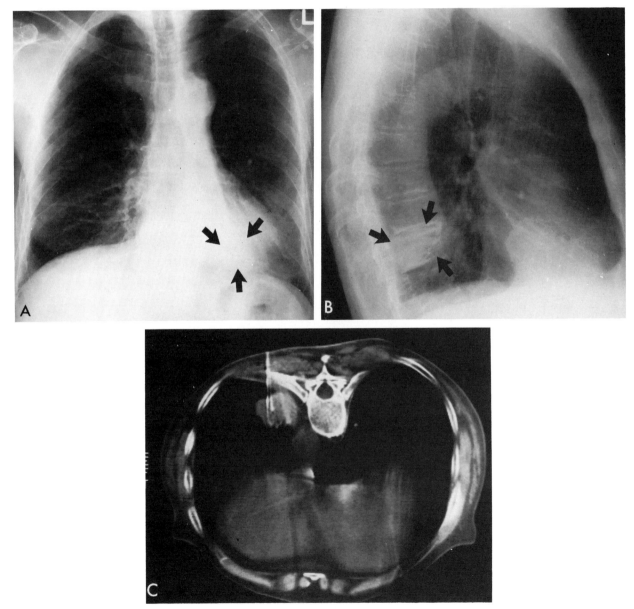

FIGURE 27–23 ■ CT-guided biopsy of pleural-based, paraaortic left lung mass. *A* and *B*, Posteroanterior and lateral chest radiographs demonstrate a vague retrocardiac, paraaortic mass *(arrows)*. *C*, Tandem needle biopsy of mass performed in the prone position. Final diagnosis: chronic inflammatory mass.

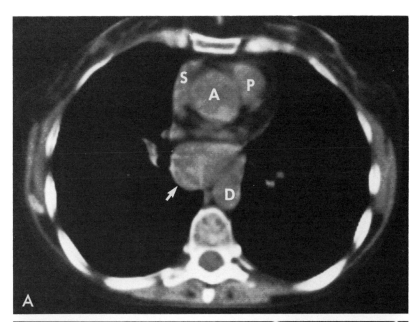

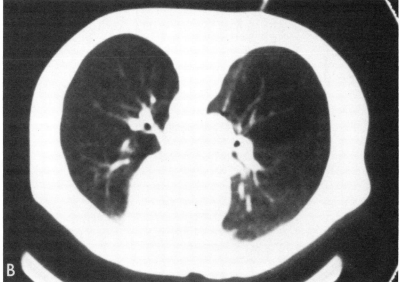

FIGURE 27–24 ■ CT-directed biopsy of mediastinal mass. *A,* CT scan demonstrating a rounded, predominantly right-sided mediastinal mass *(arrow).* A = Root of aorta; D = descending aorta; P = main pulmonary artery; S = superior vena cava. *B,* Biopsy of mass performed in the prone position using a single-needle technique. Final diagnosis: oat cell carcinoma.

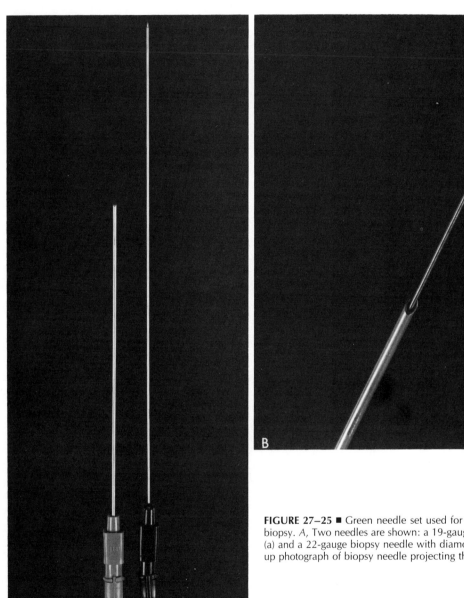

FIGURE 27–25 ■ Green needle set used for double-needle method of lung biopsy. *A*, Two needles are shown: a 19-gauge guidance cannula with stylet (a) and a 22-gauge biopsy needle with diamond-shaped stylet (b). *B*, Close-up photograph of biopsy needle projecting through guidance cannula.

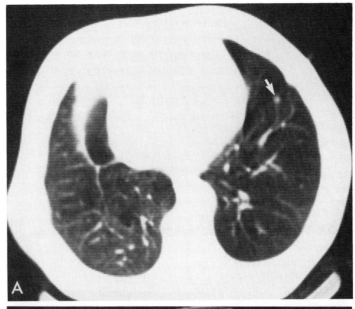

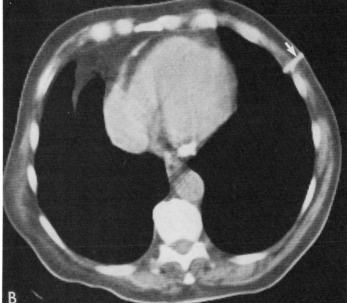

FIGURE 27–26 ■ Double-needle technique for CT-guided biopsy of pulmonary nodule. *A*, CT scan demonstrates a small nodule *(arrow)* in the left lung. *B*, The short guidance cannula *(arrow)* is directed toward the lung nodule. *C*, CT scan after placement of the thin biopsy needle *(small arrow)* through the guidance cannula *(large arrow)* into the pulmonary nodule. Final diagnosis: metastatic adenocarcinoma.

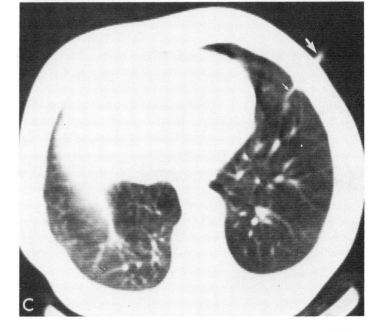

no. 7 or 8 French chest catheter.[4, 99] Thus the means to treat a pneumothorax rapidly and effectively should be available whenever transthoracic biopsy is performed.

If a pneumothorax occurs during a CT-directed lung biopsy, the biopsy is usually stopped, because additional needle punctures increase the hazard to the patient and the changing position of the mass relative to the entry point makes the initial localizing measurements no longer accurate. This problem is not as severe if a mediastinal or paraspinous mass is being sampled. If the needle misses the lesion on the initial placement, the needle and stylet may be left in position and a second attempt made using the first needle as a guide. After the biopsy, injection of 5 to 10 mL of clotted blood through the guidance needle has been employed in an attempt to seal the needle track, but this technique has not significantly reduced the incidence of pneumothorax. After biopsy, an expiratory chest radiograph is obtained, and if a small pneumothorax is present, the patient is closely monitored for at least 4 hours. If after 4 hours a major pneumothorax has not developed, the patient is permitted to go home.

SKELETAL SYSTEM

Percutaneous bone biopsies are utilized to diagnose primary bone tumors, metastasis, or infection. Most investigators prefer to perform bone biopsies using fluoroscopic guidance, because the technique is safe, convenient, and familiar and has an accuracy rate of greater than 90 per cent.[100]

Despite the ease and accuracy of fluoroscopically guided skeletal biopsy, CT can provide information that permits more accurate prebiopsy planning. Hardy and colleagues[101] reported that in patients referred for percutaneous bone biopsy, CT influenced the choice of needle, biopsy site, or needle path in 37 per cent and demonstrated that no biopsy should be performed in 21 per cent. When a vertebral biopsy is indicated, CT guidance can make a percutaneous

large-bore biopsy of the spine (Fig. 27–27) safer, and in other instances, CT may permit smaller, less invasive needles to be used.[43] The use of CT for planning and guiding percutaneous bone biopsies has increased as more experience has been obtained.

CT-Guided Therapeutic Procedures

Abscess Aspiration and Drainage

Computed tomography has contributed much to the diagnosis of intraabdominal and pelvic abscesses. More than 90 per cent of abscesses are detected by CT, and in many centers, CT is the preferred procedure for detecting abscess.[102, 103] CT precisely localizes an abscess and defines its relationship to adjacent organs and peritoneal spaces. This information is vital in planning surgical procedures, aspirating abscesses for culture, and determining suitability for percutaneous drainage.

PATIENT SELECTION

CT-guided needle aspiration of a suspected abscess is indicated to confirm the diagnosis and to provide material or culture to aid in selecting antibiotics. Fine-needle aspiration for culture can be performed in virtually any patient. Percutaneous drainage of a documented abscess is indicated when there is a well-defined abscess cavity and a safe drainage route and the surgeon and radiologist agree the procedure is warranted. Percutaneous drainage was initially used in patients who were poor surgical risks[104, 105] or who had simple unilocular abscesses, but it has become the preferred initial therapy in virtually all patients.[106–112]

TECHNIQUES

The site of entry for diagnostic and drainage procedures is determined by the size, location, and relationship of the abscess to surrounding organs.

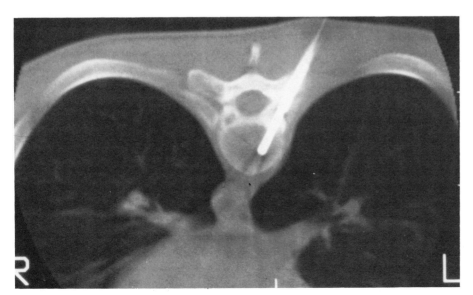

FIGURE 27–27 ■ Large-bore needle biopsy of vertebral body. CT scan demonstrates the tip of a Craig needle in the center of the body of a thoracic vertebra. Despite the large-bore needle, the use of the extended scale (−1000 to +3000 H) permits CT scans of nonmoving high-density objects to be obtained that are relatively free of artifacts. Final diagnosis: compression fracture; no tumor or infection.

FIGURE 27–28 ■ Ring catheter–stylet combination (Cook, Inc.). An inner trocar stylet and outer no. 5 French polyethylene catheter is used for diagnostic aspiration of intraabdominal or pelvic abscesses. If necessary, a guide wire can be passed through the sheath and a larger gauge catheter placed into the abscess to aspirate pus that is too thick to be aspirated through the smaller Teflon sheath.

Following a diagnostic CT scan, the shortest straight line from the skin to the abscess that does not traverse bowel or other organs is measured. The skin is marked, cleansed, and anesthetized as for a percutaneous needle biopsy. Whenever possible, an extraperitoneal approach is employed.

Diagnostic Aspiration ■ If the lesion has an accessible, safe aspiration route, a diagnostic aspiration can be performed using either a Teflon-sheathed (Fig. 27–28) or a nonsheathed 18- to 20-gauge needle. If a sheathed needle is employed, a small incision is made in the skin to facilitate entry. The needle is inserted into the abscess to the premeasured depth, the stylet is removed, and a small amount of abscess is aspirated for culture and Gram stain.

Aspiration of small, deep, or critically positioned abscesses requiring needle passage through bowel or solid parenchymal organs is performed with a 22-gauge needle. The location of the needle should be verified by CT before aspiration (Fig. 27–29). Often only thin, nonviscous material can be aspirated through a 22-gauge needle, but usually enough material is obtained for culture and smear. Thin-needle aspiration is useful for diagnostic purposes only, as the contents of an abscess can seldom be completely aspirated through a small-gauge needle.

Therapeutic Drainage ■ Successful drainage requires placement of a drainage catheter (or catheters) of sufficient size to drain the viscous material present within most abscesses. Most frequently percutaneous

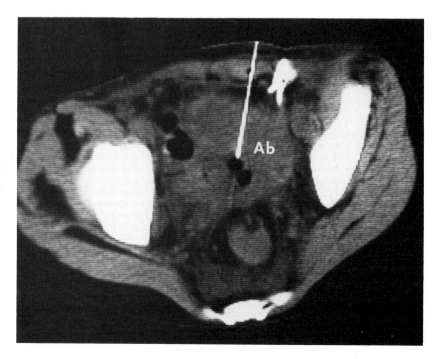

FIGURE 27–29 ■ Diagnostic aspiration of pelvic abscess (Ab), resulting from Crohn's disease, with a 22-gauge needle. The thin needle was used because the abscess could not be clearly separated from bowel, and because it provided an extra margin of safety.

abscess drainage is a multiple-step procedure. Initial abscess drainage is done under CT or ultrasonographic guidance following placement of a sheathed needle into an abscess located with a thin-walled 20- to 22-gauge needle. Subsequent guidance of needle placement, tract dilatations, and placement of additional or larger bore catheters is then done under fluoroscopy.[109]

The placement of a drainage catheter entails a series of steps. After the abscess is located and the needle path planned, a diagnostic aspiration of the abscess is performed using a sheathed catheter. A guide wire is passed through the sheath and into the abscess, and the sheath is removed. The track is dilated with an angiographic dilator, and the appropriate-size catheter is passed over the guide wire into the abscess. The position of the catheter can be documented by CT or fluoroscopy. A variety of catheter sizes and shapes can be employed. Drainage of very thin, nonviscous fluid has been done using no. 8 to no. 10 French pigtail catheters (Fig. 27–30). The pigtail shape prevents perforation of the catheter through the wall of the abscess and protects against dislodgement. Continuous drainage is promoted, because the drainage holes are on the inner curve of the pigtail, where they will not be occluded if the catheter lodges against the wall of the abscess.

Following successful catheter placement, the abscess is aspirated to dryness by manual suction. Water-soluble contrast material injected into the abscess cavity permits detection of undrained loculated portions of the abscess, outlines fistulous tracts, and documents catheter position (Fig. 27–31).

Abscesses can also be drained using a variety of large-bore (no. 12 to no. 16 French) trocar catheters (Fig. 27–32). After diagnostic aspiration of the abscess, the large trocar catheter is passed into the abscess along the same path and to the same depth as the needle used for the diagnostic aspiration. During the passage of the trocar catheter, solid parenchymal organs, bowel, and the pleural space must be avoided. The recent introduction of a blunt needle for abscess drainage may lower the potential hazard of sharp-tipped needles lacerating bowel, vessels, or parenchymal organs.[113] Once the catheter is advanced into the abscess, the stylet is removed, and the contents of the abscess are totally drained. Placement of large-bore catheters is usually best done using Seldinger or trocar techniques monitored fluoroscopically.

After evacuation of the abscess, the catheter is securely fastened to the skin using a molnar disk to prevent inadvertent dislodgement. A drainage bag is attached to the catheter, and the system is left to drain by gravity or is attached to continuous low-pressure suction. If the abscess contents are viscous, the drainage catheter is irrigated frequently with sterile saline.

Following 4 to 6 days of drainage or when there is cessation of drainage, a follow-up CT scan or abscessogram of the cavity is performed. Clinical response is frequently immediate and almost always occurs by 96 hours,[104–108] but it can take 15 to 30 days of drainage before all of the conditions for catheter removal are met.[105, 108] Patients who have an enteric communication usually require a longer period of drainage. Catheter drainage has been maintained for up to 120 days without complications.[105, 108]

RESULTS AND COMPLICATIONS

Properly performed percutaneous catheter drainage is a safe and effective method of treating abdominal abscesses. Gerzof and colleagues[105] successfully drained 86 per cent of 71 abscesses and Haaga and Weinstein[106] successfully treated 28 of 33 abscesses (85 per cent) by CT-guided percutaneous catheter drainage. Other investigators report similar success rates.[81, 107, 108, 114] Failure occurs most frequently in patients with multiple very large or multiloculated abscesses, infected tumors, pancreatic phlegmons, or enteric fistulas, intrarenal abscesses, and abscesses containing material too thick to be drained by large-bore catheters.[105, 106, 108–110, 115–118]

Complications occur in approximately 10 per cent to 15 per cent of patients undergoing drainage procedures.[105] Sepsis is the most common, but empyema, hemorrhage, and fistula formation are also encountered.[105, 106, 108, 119] Although vanSonnenberg et al.[108] had only one death (0.004 per cent) in 250 percutaneous drainage procedures, Sones[107] reported a 4 per cent mortality rate. These rates are significantly lower than the 11 per cent to 43 per cent mortality and 14 per cent to 49 per cent recurrence rates after surgery.[120, 121] These results indicate that percutaneous drainage should be performed before surgical drainage in most patients.[108, 110, 118] Virtually

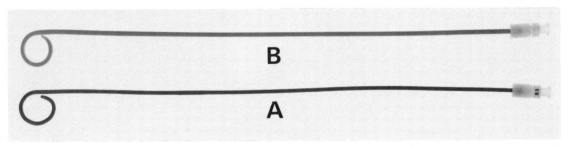

FIGURE 27–30 ■ Pigtail catheters (Cook, Inc.) used for percutaneous drainage of abscesses. A = Black no. 8.3 French catheter; B = white no. 10 French catheter.

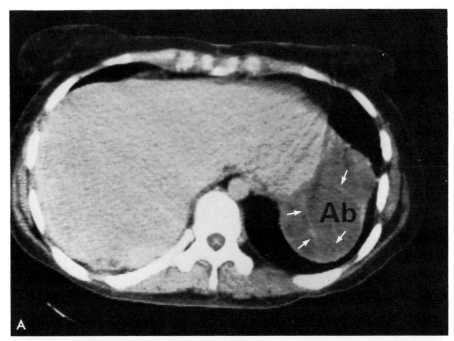

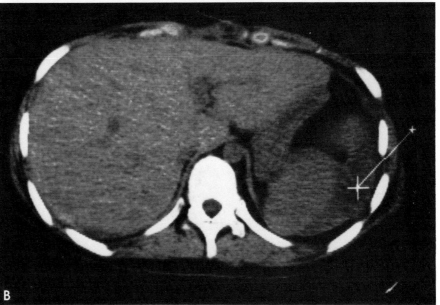

FIGURE 27–31 ■ Percutaneous drainage of left subphrenic abscess using pigtail catheter. *A*, A well-defined multiseptated *(arrows)* abscess (Ab) in the left subphrenic space. *B*, CT scan at a slightly lower level demonstrating the projected path of the drainage catheter chosen to avoid the pleural space. The distance from skin to abscess center is approximately 5.7 cm.

Illustration continued on following page

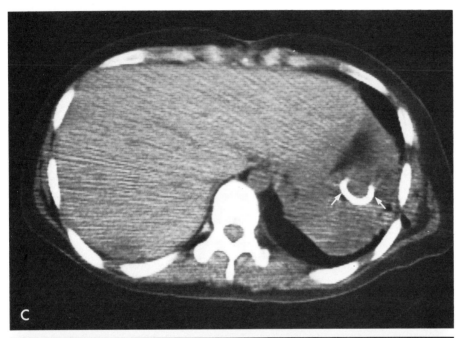

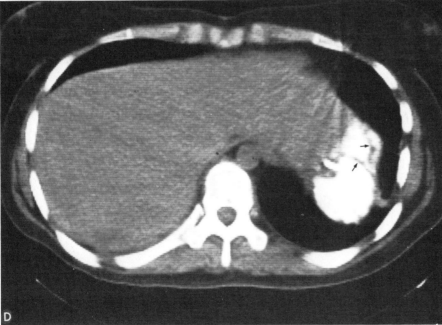

FIGURE 27–31 *Continued C*, CT scan through the curved tip of the pigtail catheter *(arrows)* documents the catheter in the abscess. *D*, Contrast medium injection into abscess cavity confirms catheter communication with abscess. Contrast material fills the entire abscess despite the presence of septations *(arrows)*. No extravasation of contrast into the pleural space is noted.

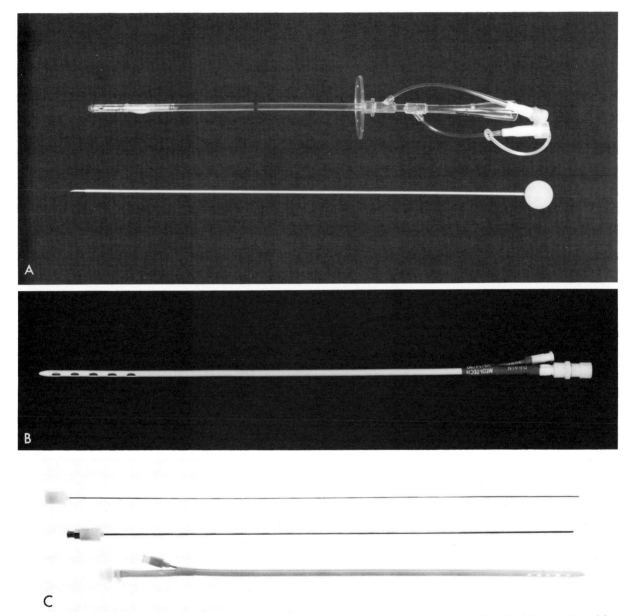

FIGURE 27–32 ■ Large-bore catheters used for drainage of abscesses. *A,* Ingram trocar catheter (Sherwood Medical Group). Special features include a very stiff metal stylet for introduction, a balloon tip to contain the catheter in the abscess, a flange for anchoring the catheter to the skin, and a separate injection port. *B,* vanSonnenberg catheter (Medi-Tech, Inc.). Special features include a stiff metal stylet for introduction when used as a trocar catheter, a distal hole permitting passage over a guide wire, multiple large side holes, a separate injection port, long length, and extreme flexibility. *C,* Ring-McLean abscess drainage catheter (Cook, Inc.). Special features include true sump design, a pointed stylet that fits through a metal stiffening cannula for introduction when used as a trocar catheter, catheter and metal cannula with end hole for easy passage over a guide wire, multiple large side holes, separate injection port, long length, and extreme flexibility.

no immediate catastrophic complications have occurred, and whenever percutaneous drainage proves inadequate, surgical intervention can be performed. In some cases, percutaneous catheter drainage can be used as an intermediate step; a patient who is a poor operative candidate can be made fit to undergo surgical drainage.[110]

Pancreatic Pseudocyst Aspiration and Drainage

PATIENT SELECTION

Conventional surgical management of pancreatic pseudocysts is internal drainage of a mature pseudocyst into an adjacent viscus.[122] Surgical internal drainage carries a 21 per cent to 53 per cent morbidity and a 2 per cent to 10 per cent mortality and requires a 6- to 8-week waiting period while the cyst wall matures sufficiently to permit a satisfactory enteric anastomosis.[122–124] Although more than 10 per cent of pseudocysts resolve during the wait for cyst wall maturation,[122,125] others can become infected, expand rapidly, and cause severe unrelenting pain, duodenal or biliary obstruction, or hemorrhage. Surgical intervention before the cyst wall is mature is difficult and is associated with high morbidity and mortality.[126]

Although experience is still limited, results indicate that percutaneous aspiration and drainage of pancreatic pseudocysts via catheters or internalized double-J catheter (MediTech, Inc., Watertown, MA) percutaneous transgastric cystogastrostomy can safely and effectively relieve symptoms and nonsurgically treat pancreatic pseudocysts.[105, 125, 127, 128]

TECHNIQUES

The technique employed is similar to that used for diagnostic aspiration of abscesses (Fig. 27–33). A thin-walled needle is inserted into the cyst and appropriately sized drainage catheters are placed using CT or fluoroscopic guidance. If a percutaneous transgastric cystogastrostomy is to be performed, a slightly different procedure is followed.[125] Puncture is made with the 21-gauge needle of a Cope introducer set (Cook, Inc.). The needle is passed through the abdominal wall and both walls of the stomach and into the pseudocyst.[125] After aspiration of fluid for culture and chemistry, fluoroscopy guidance is used. Guide wire placement, dilatation of the track to permit a no. 8 to no. 10 French catheter, and placement of a ureteral double-J stent are accomplished so that one end of the catheter is in the stomach and the other in the pseudocyst. Communication of a pseudocyst with the main pancreatic duct has been shown by injecting contrast material into a pseudocyst.[128]

RESULTS AND COMPLICATIONS

Pain is usually relieved immediately after drainage, and serious complications have not been reported.[125, 128] The incidence of recurrence after percutaneous drainage is unknown; MacErlean's group[129] reported that effectively drained pseudocysts did not recur for up to a year, and Gerzof and associates[105]

successfully treated patients without recurrence or complications.

In patients who develop sepsis and who are not surgical candidates, pseudocysts should be aspirated. If the fluid is purulent or gram positive, antibiotics and catheter drainage therapy can be instituted immediately.

CT-guided aspiration and drainage of uncomplicated pancreatic pseudocysts has become a valuable therapeutic procedure, but the success rate of treating nontumorous, semisolid, phlegmonous pancreatic masses by percutaneous drainage has been reported to be only 40 per cent.[125]

Percutaneous diagnostic needle aspiration of noncystic pancreatic masses is a useful, accurate method of determining whether a pancreatic abscess is present. In patients with pancreatitis and a suspected pancreatic abscess, fluid aspirated with an 18- or 20-gauge needle is immediately stained and examined for bacteria. If the aspirate contains a large number of bacteria, the patient is considered to have a pancreatic abscess, and appropriate therapy is instituted.

Miscellaneous Aspiration and Drainage Procedures

PERCUTANEOUS NEPHROSTOMY

Percutaneous nephrostomy is a well-established procedure that is usually performed under fluoroscopic or ultrasonic guidance. Although rarely used to place the drainage catheter, CT can be used to guide percutaneous nephrostomies in patients in whom placement of catheters by fluoroscopy or ultrasound has failed. In patients with absent renal function, CT visualization of the renal collecting system without injection of contrast medium permits accurate placement of the drainage catheter. The use of CT also permits the nephrostomy catheter to be placed laterally, allowing the patient to lie more comfortably during drainage.

The technique of percutaneous nephrostomy is similar to that used in abscess puncture and drainage.[117, 118] A sheathed needle is inserted into the collecting system. A J-shaped guide wire is then passed through the sheath, and the sheath is removed, leaving the wire in place. The needle tract is dilated, and the appropriate-size catheter is inserted for drainage. A follow-up CT scan confirms the catheter's position. Haaga and co-workers[130] reported successful placement in 93 per cent of CT-guided percutaneous nephrostomies without serious complications.

BILIARY DECOMPRESSION

CT can be used to guide the puncture of a dilated biliary radicle and to place a drainage catheter to effect biliary decompression. However, because biliary decompression can almost always be performed under fluoroscopic guidance, CT is not often recommended to guide this procedure. CT can be used to guide drainage of a locally obstructed biliary sys-

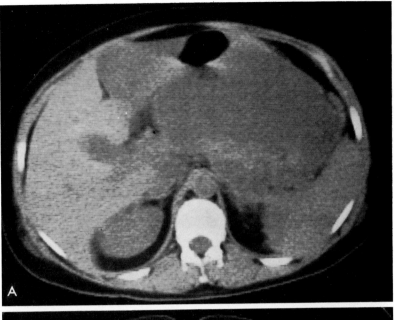

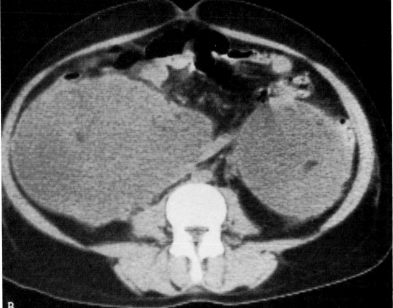

FIGURE 27–33 ■ Percutaneous drainage of multiple extrapancreatic pseudocysts in a patient with congenital excess of serum triglycerides. *A,* CT scan at level of pancreas demonstrates large extrapancreatic pseudocysts. *B,* Pseudocysts extend down into the flanks. *C,* Drainage catheters placed into cyst located in the right flank.

Illustration continued on following page

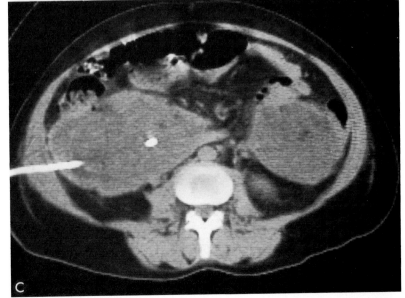

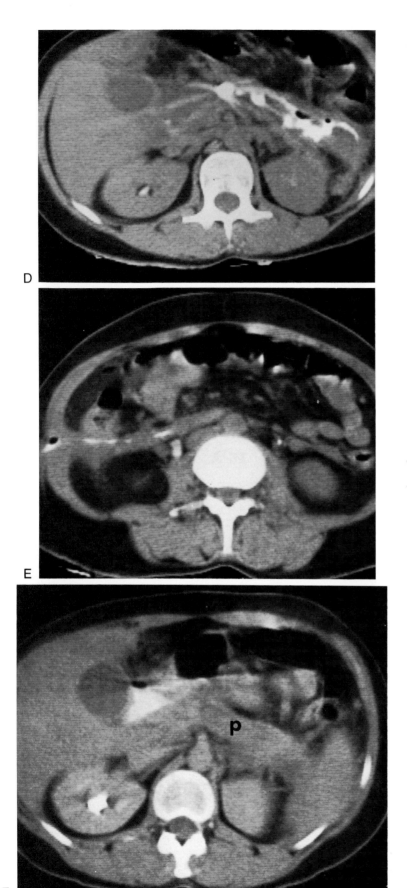

D

E

F

FIGURE 27–33 *Continued D* and *E,* Five weeks after drainage was initiated, pseudocysts have almost resolved. *F,* Three months after initiation of drainage, the abdomen is almost normal. p = Pancreas.

tem when drainage guided by fluoroscopy or ultrasound has failed.

HEMATOMA EVACUATION

Chronic subcapsular and intrahepatic hematomas that have undergone liquefaction can be aspirated and evacuated using CT to guide catheter placement.[131] CT usually reveals a low-density mass lesion that can be completely evacuated. Even if the hematoma is not infected, evacuation decreases the mass effect on the liver and promotes hepatic healing.[131]

EMPYEMA AND LUNG ABSCESSES

Standard treatment for empyema includes thoracentesis, drainage via a thoracostomy catheter, and administration of antibiotics. Open thoracostomy, excision of a rib or ribs, and thoracostomy are performed when simpler measures fail.[23] Inadequate drainage resulting from a malpositioned thoracostomy tube and complications of pain, subcutaneous emphysema, leakage, chylothorax, and hypotension from pleural tubes have led to only a 10 per cent cure rate for empyema by thoracic tube drainage alone.[132]

vanSonnenberg et al.[23] used CT, ultrasound, or both to position catheters to drain empyemas in patients who had failed to improve on chest tube drainage; they reported an 88 per cent success rate. Following aspiration of the fluid for culture, a drainage catheter was inserted using trocar and Seldinger techniques. Larger catheters were thought to be more effective. CT scans are useful to determine whether the empyema has been completely drained or whether undrained loculations persist that require further procedures.[23]

Lung abscesses such as empyema that have not responded to conventional antibiotic and drainage therapy often require surgery for cure, despite a reported 9 per cent to 28 per cent mortality rate for lung abscesses, even those treated with surgery.[25] Lung abscesses drained by catheters placed under CT guidance were cured in 100 per cent of instances, and surgery was avoided in 84 per cent.[25] Catheter placement is best accomplished through an abscess-pleura syndesis. Complications reported have been minor (e.g., hemothorax and clogged catheters). CT-directed catheter drainage of lung abscesses appears to be a viable alternative to surgery in some patients who do not respond to conventional measures.

GASTROINTESTINAL INTERVENTIONS

CT has been used as an aid in performing percutaneous gastrostomy,[125] cecostomy,[133, 134] drainage of an obstructed afferent loop,[135] or decompression of the colon.[136] Although fluoroscopy is usually the method employed to guide these procedures, CT offers the ability to plan a safe path for catheter placement, employ a retroperitoneal route, and confirm satisfactory catheter position.

Neurolysis

Splanchnic nerve neurolysis in the management of upper abdominal pain was first described in 1919 by Kappis[137] and during the past decade has become an accepted form of therapy for treating intractable back or upper abdominal pain.[138, 139]

Using fluoroscopy and bony landmarks to direct the placement of needles prior to the alcohol injection, the overall complication rate is low (less than 5 per cent), although there is a 1 per cent incidence of serious complications such as paralysis and peritonitis.[139, 140] The relationship of the needle tips to surrounding structures and the spread of the neurolytic agent in the retroperitoneum cannot be accurately determined by conventional radiologic techniques; this has led to the use of CT to guide some neurolytic procedures.

TECHNIQUES

The celiac artery reliably indicates the position of the celiac ganglia.[141] Because the celiac artery has a variable position relative to the spine, reliance on bony landmarks is an imprecise way to ensure proper needle position. CT, by displaying the aortic, celiac, and superior mesenteric arteries, can provide reliable guidance for celiac ganglion neurolysis in almost every patient.[142, 143] The splanchnic nerves are in a retrocrural location on either side of the aorta (Fig. 27–34). If a splanchnic block is to be performed, CT demonstration of the diaphragmatic crura permits accurate retrocrural needle placement.

CT-guided splanchnic nerve and celiac ganglion neurolysis has been described by several investigators.[130, 142, 143] A computed radiograph of the upper abdomen is obtained with the patient prone. The T12 level is identified, and CT scans at 0.5- to 1-cm intervals are obtained from the bottom of T11 until the celiac axis is clearly demonstrated.

Visceral sympathetic neurolysis may be accomplished by celiac plexus or splanchnic nerve ablation. Both techniques require accurate insertion of two 20- to 22-gauge needles. The needle tips are positioned either retrocrurally (classic splanchnic nerve neurolysis) or transcrurally, with the needle tips located anterior and lateral to the aorta at the level of the celiac artery (see (Fig. 27–34). The distances from the midline to the puncture site, the angle of the needle entry, and the depth of the site of injection are measured directly from the CT scan with the scan cursor (Fig. 27–35). To avoid the kidneys and lungs, the needles are angled in a cephalocaudal direction. The location of the needle tips are verified by CT before the injection of the neurolytic agent (see Fig. 27–35B).

Neurolysis is accomplished by injecting 18 to 22 mL of absolute alcohol mixed with 2 to 3 mL of contrast through each needle, following which CT scans are obtained to assess the spread of alcohol around the celiac ganglia or splanchnic nerves (see Fig. 27–35C).

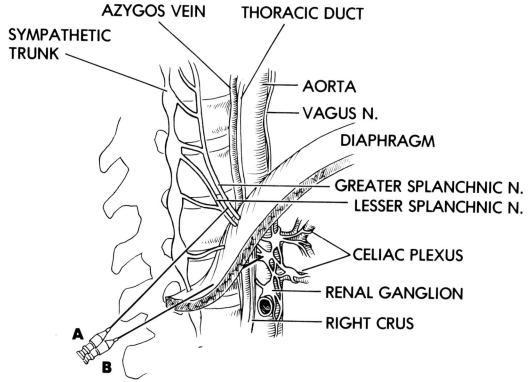

FIGURE 27–34 ■ Diagram showing location of needle tips for retrocrural splanchnic nerve neurolysis (A) and transcrural celiac plexus neurolysis (B). (From Buy J-N, Moss AA, Singler RC: J Comput Assist Tomogr 6:315, 1982.)

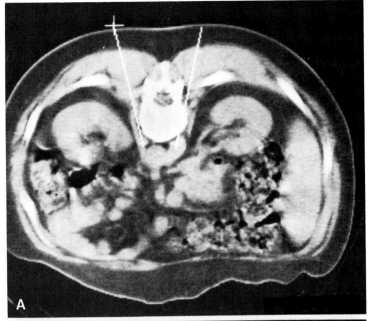

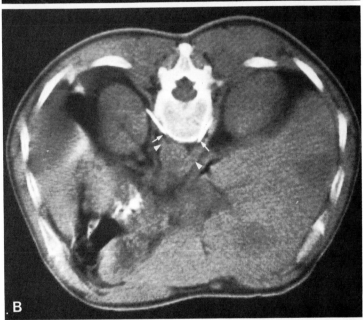

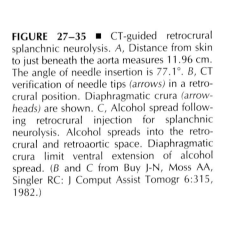

FIGURE 27–35 ■ CT-guided retrocrural splanchnic neurolysis. *A,* Distance from skin to just beneath the aorta measures 11.96 cm. The angle of needle insertion is 77.1°. *B,* CT verification of needle tips *(arrows)* in a retrocrural position. Diaphragmatic crura *(arrowheads)* are shown. *C,* Alcohol spread following retrocrural injection for splanchnic neurolysis. Alcohol spreads into the retrocrural and retroaortic space. Diaphragmatic crura limit ventral extension of alcohol spread. (*B* and *C* from Buy J-N, Moss AA, Singler RC: J Comput Assist Tomogr 6:315, 1982.)

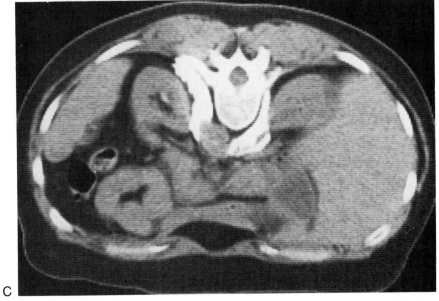

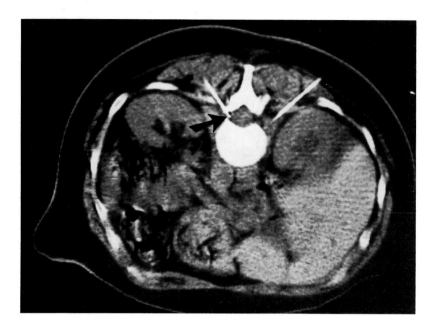

FIGURE 27–36 ■ CT documentation of needle malposition during a neurolytic procedure. Left needle tip *(arrow)* was placed into spinal canal. Injection of alcohol in this position could have produced paralysis. (From Buy J-N, Moss AA, Singler RC: J Comput Assist Tomogr 6:315, 1982.)

In addition to ablation procedures, CT has been used to guide peripheral nerve root blocks at a variety of locations.[143] Guided nerve blocks can be performed to determine the clinical significance of disk herniation, foraminal stenosis, or as a preablation test in patients with pain caused by malignancy. CT is used to guide a 22-gauge needle into or within 1 to 2 mm of the nerve to be blocked. A mixture of 3 mL of 1 per cent lidocaine and 1 mL of 60 per cent contrast media is injected to temporarily block the nerve. CT scans are used to confirm needle position and spread of the lidocaine.[143]

RESULTS AND COMPLICATIONS

Success in relieving pain with percutaneous sympathetic nerve blocks has been reported to vary from 33 per cent[144] to 98 per cent.[143] In our experience, 86 per cent of ablation procedures relieve pain at least partially,[142] whereas Quinn et al.[143] reported only a 63 per cent success rate. Because pain relief is subjective, it is difficult to quantitate the degree of success in relieving abdominal and back pain with neurolytic techniques.[141–143] Pain relief has varied from total for up to 9 months to partial for 1 to 2 weeks; it is unclear why some patients have excellent results and others experience poor results.

Serious complications of splanchnic blocks occur in less than 1 per cent of patients.[139] When the needle tip is inadvertently placed into the peritoneal cavity, chemical peritonitis may follow the injection of alcohol, and paralysis occurs after a direct subarachnoid injection or spread of alcohol along nerve roots into the subarachnoid space.[139] Back pain and moderate hypotension are common minor complications that are usually transient.[141, 142] No serious complications have been reported after CT-guided neurolytic procedures.[130, 142, 143] CT guidance and verification of needle position should detect needle malpositions (Fig. 27–36) and avoid inadvertent subarachnoid in-

jections. Transcrural needle placement virtually eliminates the chance of alcohol flowing back along nerve roots into the spinal canal.

References

1. Goldstein H, Zornoza J, Wallace S: Percutaneous fine needle aspiration biopsy of pancreatic and other abdominal masses. Radiology 123:319,1977.
2. Göthlin JH: Post-lymphographic percutaneous fine needle biopsy of lymph nodes guided by fluoroscopy. Radiology 120:205, 1976.
3. Pereiras RV, Meiers W, Kunhardt B, Troner M, Hutson D, et al: Fluoroscopically guided thin needle aspiration biopsy of the abdomen and retroperitoneum. AJR 131:197, 1978.
4. Westcott JL: Direct percutaneous needle aspiration of localized pulmonary lesions: results in 422 patients. Radiology 137:31, 1980.
5. Tylen U, Arnesjo B, Lindberg LG, Lunderquist A, Akerman M: Percutaneous biopsy of carcinoma of the pancreas guided by angiography. Surg Gynecol Obstet 142:737, 1976.
6. Ho C-S, McLoughlin MJ, McHattie JD, Tao L-C: Percutaneous fine needle aspiration biopsy of the pancreas following endoscopic retrograde cholangiopancreatography. Radiology 125:351, 1977.
7. Holm HH, Pedersen JF, Kristensen JK, Rasmussen SN, Hancke S, Jensen E: Ultrasonically guided percutaneous puncture. Radiol Clin North Am 13:493, 1975.
8. Juul N, Torp-Pedersen S, Gronvall S, et al: Ultrasonically guided fine needle aspiration biopsy of renal masses. J Urol 133:579–581, 1985.
9. Spamer C, Brambs H-J, Kich HK, et al: Benign circumscribed lesions of the liver diagnosed by ultrasonically guided fine-needle biopsy. J Clin Ultrasound 14:83–88, 1986.
10. Bret M, Sente J-M, Bretagnolle M, et al: Ultrasonically guided fine-needle biopsy in focal intrahepatic lesions: six years experience. J Can Assoc Radiol 37:5–8, 1986.
11. Reading CC, Charboneau JW, Felmlee JP, et al: US-guided percutaneous biopsy: use of a screw biopsy stylet to aid needle detection. Radiology 163:280–281, 1987.
12. Solbiati L, Livraghi T, DePra L, et al: Fine-needle biopsy of hepatic hemangioma with sonographic guidance. AJR 144:471–474, 1985.
13. Johansen P, Svendsen KN: Scan-guided needle aspiration biopsy in malignant hepatic disease. Acta Cytol 22:292, 1978.

14. Haaga JR, Alfidi RJ: Precise biopsy localization by computed tomography. Radiology 118:603, 1976.

15. Ferrucci JT Jr, Wittenberg J: CT biopsy of abdominal tumors: aids for lesion localization. Radiology 129:739, 1978.

16. Jaques PF, Staab E, Richey W, et al: CT-assisted pelvic and abdominal aspiration biopsies in gynecological malignancy. Radiology 128:651, 1978.

17. Haaga JR: New techniques for CT-guided biopsies. AJR 133:633, 1979.

18. Ferrucci JT Jr, Wittenberg J, Mueller PR, et al: Diagnosis of abdominal malignancy by radiologic fine-needle aspiration biopsy. AJR 143:323–330, 1980.

19. Sundaram M, Wolverson MK, Heiberg E, et al: Utility of CT-guided abdominal aspiration procedures. AJR 139:1111–1115, 1982.

20. Gobien RP, Stanley JH, Vujic I, et al: Thoracic biopsy: CT guidance of thin-needle aspiration. AJR 142:827–830, 1984.

21. Welch TJ, Sheedy PF, Johnson CD, et al: CT-guided biopsy: prospective analysis of 1,000 procedures. Radiology 171:493–496, 1989.

22. Charboneau JW, Reading CC, Welch TJ: CT and sonographically guided needle biopsy: current techniques and new innovations. AJR 154:1–10, 1990.

23. vanSonnenberg E, Nakamoto SK, Mueller PR, et al: CT and ultrasound guided catheter drainage of empyemas after chest-tube failure. Radiology 151:349–353, 1984.

24. vanSonnenberg E, Casola G, Ho M, et al: Difficult thoracic lesions: CT-guided biopsy experience in 150 cases. Radiology 167:457–461, 1988.

25. vanSonnenberg E, D'Agostino HB, Casola G, et al: Lung abscess: CT-guided drainage. Radiology 178:347–351, 1991.

26. Mueller PR, Stark DD, Semeone JF: MR-guided aspiration biopsy: needle design and clinical trial. Radiology 161:608–609, 1986.

27. Lufkin R, Teresi L, Chiu L, et al: A technique for MR-guided needle placement. AJR 151:193–196, 1988.

28. Lufkin R, Layfield L: Coaxial needle system of MR- and CT-guided aspiration cytology. J Comput Assist Tomogr 13:1105–1107, 1989.

29. Alfidi RJ, Haaga JR, Meany TF, et al: Computed tomography of the thorax and abdomen: A preliminary report. Radiology 117:257, 1975.

30. Okuda K, Tanikawa K, Emura T, et al: Nonsurgical percutaneous transhepatic cholangiography—diagnostic significance in medical problems of the liver. Am J Digest Dis 19:21, 1974.

31. Zornoza J: Abdomen. In Zornoza J (ed): Percutaneous Needle Biopsy. Baltimore, Williams & Wilkins, 1981, pp 102–140.

32. Murphy FB, Barefield KP, Steinberg HV, et al: CT- or sonography-guided biopsy of the liver in the presence of ascites: frequency of complications. AJR 151:485–486, 1988.

33. Haaga JR, Vanek J: Computed tomographic guided liver biopsy using the Menghini needle. Radiology 133:405, 1979.

34. Hopper KD, Baird DE, Reddy VV, et al: Efficacy of automated biopsy guns versus conventional biopsy needles in the pygmy pig. Radiology 176:671–676, 1990.

35. Fornage BD: Fine-needle aspiration biopsy with a vacuum test tube. Radiology 169:553–554, 1988.

36. Parker SH, Hopper KD, Yhakes W, et al: Image-directed percutaneous biopsies with a biopsy gun. Radiology 171:663–669, 1989.

37. Onik G, Helms CA, Ginsberg L, et al: Percutaneous lumbar diskectomy using a new aspiration probe: porcine and cadaver model. Radiology 155:251–252, 1985.

38. Onik G, Helms CA, Ginsburg L, et al: Percutaneous lumbar diskectomy using a new aspiration probe. AJR 144:1137–1140, 1985.

39. Frederick PR, Miller MH, Bahr AL, et al: Coaxial needles for repeated biopsy sampling. Radiology 170:273–274, 1989.

40. Heelan RT, Hilaris BS, Anderson LL, et al: Percutaneous implantation of 1-125 sources with CT treatment planning. Radiology 164:735–740, 1987.

41. Sider L, Mittal BB, Nemcek AA, et al: CT-guided placement of iodine-125 seeds for unresectable carcinoma of the lung. J Comput Assist Tomogr 12:515–517, 1988.

42. Qin D: Technical note: a new needle for puncture biopsy. AJR 147:543, 1986.

43. Pais MJ, Lightfoote JB, Burnett K, et al: Trephine bone biopsy system: a refined needle for radiologists. Radiology 153:253–254, 1984.

44. Palestrant AM: Comprehensive approach to CT-guided procedures with a hand-held guidance device. Radiology 174:270–272, 1990.

45. Frederick PR, Brown TH, Miller MH, et al: A light-guidance system to be used for CT-guided biopsy. Radiology 154:535–536, 1985.

46. Yueh N, Halvorsen RA, Letourneau JG, et al: Gantry tilt technique for CT-guided biopsy and drainage. J Comput Assist Tomogr 13:182–184, 1989.

47. Axel L: Simple method for performing oblique CT-guided needle biopsies. AJR 143:341–342, 1984.

48. Onik G, Cosman ER, Wells T, et al: CT body stereotaxic instrument for percutaneous biopsy and other interventive procedures. Invest Radiol 20:525–530, 1989.

49. Coel MN, Niwayama G: Safety of percutaneous fine-needle pancreatic biopsy: a porcine model. Invest Radiol 13:547, 1978.

50. Fagelman D, Chess Q: Nonaspiration fine-needle cytology of the liver. A new technique for obtaining diagnostic samples. AJR 155:1217–1219, 1990.

51. Hueftle MF, Haaga JR: Effect of suction on biopsy sample size. AJR 147:1014–1016, 1986.

52. Kreula J, Virkkunen P, Bondestam S: Effect of suction on specimen size in fine-needle aspiration biopsy. Invest Radiol 25:1175–1181, 1990.

53. Kreula J: Effect of sampling technique on specimen size in fine needle aspiration biopsy. Invest Radiol 25:1294–1298, 1990.

54. Andriole JG, Haaga JR, Adams RB, et al: Biopsy needle characteristics assessed in the laboratory. Radiology 148:659–662, 1983.

55. Gerzof SG: Triangulation: indirect CT guidance for abscess drainage. AJR 137:1080, 1981.

56. vanSonnenberg E, Wittenberg J, Ferrucci JT Jr, et al: Triangulation method for percutaneous needle guidance: the angled approach to upper abdominal masses. AJR 137:757, 1981.

57. Miller DA, Carrasco CJ, Katz RI, et al: Fine needle aspiration biopsy: the role of immediate cytologic assessment. AJR 147:155–158, 1986.

58. Mueller PR, Wittenberg J, Ferrucci JT Jr: Fine-needle aspiration biopsy of abdominal masses. Semin Roentgenol 16:52, 1981.

59. Boyd DP: Computer tomography. In Margulis AR, Burhenne HJ (eds): Alimentary Tract Radiology: Abdominal Imaging. St Louis, CV Mosby, 1979, pp 3–11.

60. Greene R, Szyfelbein WM, Isler RJ, et al: Supplementary tissue-core histology from fine-needle transthoracic aspiration biopsy. AJR 144:787–792, 1985.

61. Lukeman JM: Cytological diagnosis and techniques. In Zornoza J (ed): Percutaneous Needle Biopsy. Baltimore, Williams & Wilkins, 1981, pp 1–12.

62. Isler RJ, Ferrucci JT Jr, Wittenberg J, et al: Tissue core biopsy of abdominal tumors with a 22 gauge cutting needle. AJR 136:725, 1991.

63. Kasugai H, Yamamoto R, Tatsuta M, et al: Value of heparinized fine needle aspiration biopsy in liver malignancy. AJR 144:243–244, 1985.

64. Bernardino ME: Percutaneous biopsy. AJR 142:41–45, 1985.

65. Heiberg E, Wolverson MK: Ipsilateral decubitus position for percutaneous CT-guided adrenal biopsy. J Comput Assist Tomogr 9:217–218, 1985.

66. Haaga JR, Beale SM: Use of CO_2 to move structures as an aid to percutaneous procedures. Radiology 161:829–830, 1986.

67. Gazelle GS, Haaga JR: Guided percutaneous biopsy of intraabdominal lesions. AJR 153:929–935, 1989.

68. Haaga JR, LiPuma JP, Bryan PJ, et al: Clinical comparison of small and large-caliber cutting needles for biopsy. Radiology 146:665–667, 1983.

69. Mostbeck GH, Wittich GR, Derfler K, et al: Optimal needle size for renal biopsy: in vitro and in vivo evaluation. Radiology 173:819–822, 1989.
70. Martino CR, Haaga JR, Bryan PJ, et al: CT-guided liver biopsies: eight years' experience. Radiology 152:755–757, 1984.
71. Smith EH: Complications of percutaneous abdominal fine-needle biopsy. Radiology 178:253–258, 1991.
72. Yankaskas BC, Staab EV, Craven MB, et al: Delayed complications from fine-needle biopsies and solid masses of the abdomen. Invest Radiol 21:325–328, 1986.
73. Low RN, Jeffrey RB: Intraperitoneal hemorrhage after renal biopsy: a grave prognostic sign. AJR 151:113–114, 1988.
74. Gazelle GS, Haaga JR, Neuhauser D: Hemostatic protein-polymer sheath: new method to enhance hemostasis at percutaneous biopsy. Radiology 175:671–674, 1990.
75. Crummy AB, McDermott JC, Wojtwoycz M: A technique for embolization biopsy tracts. AJR 153:67–68, 1989.
76. Arnesjo B, Stormby N, Akerman M: Cytodiagnosis of pancreatic lesions by means of fine-needle biopsy during operation. Acta Chir Scand 138:363, 1972.
77. Goldstein HM, Zornoza J: Percutaneous transperitoneal aspiration biopsy of pancreatic masses. Digest Dis Sci 23:840, 1978.
78. Hall-Craggs MA, Lees WR: Fine-needle aspiration biopsy: pancreatic and biliary tumors. AJR 147:399–403, 1986.
79. Cohan RHJ, Illescas FF, Braun SD, et al: Fine needle aspiration biopsy in malignant obstructive jaundice. Gastrointest Radiol 11:145–150, 1986.
80. Elvin A, Andersson T, Scheibenpflug L, et al: Biopsy of the pancreas with a biopsy gun. Radiology 176:677–679, 1990.
81. Harter LP, Moss AA, Goldberg HI: Computed tomographic guided fine needle aspirations for neoplastic and inflammatory diseases. AJR 140:363, 1983.
82. Ferrucci JT Jr, Wittenberg J, Margolies MN, et al: Malignant seeding of the tract after thin-needle aspiration biopsy. Radiology 130:345, 1979.
83. Menghini G: One-second biopsy of the liver—problems of its clinical application. N Engl J Med 283:582, 1970.
84. Ovlisen B, Baden H: Liver biopsy by the method of Menghini. Nord Med 83:297, 1970.
85. Conn HO, Yesner RA: A re-evaluation of needle biopsy in the diagnosis of metastatic cancer of the liver. Ann Intern Med 59:53, 1963.
86. Madden RE: Complications of needle biopsy of the liver. Arch Surg 83:778, 1961.
87. Zornoza J, Wallace S, Ordonez N, et al: Fine-needle aspiration biopsy of the liver. AJR 134:331, 1980.
88. Zornoza J, Cabanillas FF, Altoff TM, et al: Percutaneous needle biopsy in abdominal lymphoma. AJR 136:97, 1981.
89. Dunnick NR, Fisher RI, Chu EW, et al: Percutaneous aspiration of retroperitoneal lymph nodes in ovarian cancer. AJR 135:109, 1980.
90. Bret PM, Fond A, Casola G, et al: A prospective study of clinical efficacy of percutaneous fine-needle biopsy. Radiology 159:345–346, 1986.
91. Bogan MR, Kopecky KK, Kraft JL, et al: Needle biopsy of renal allografts: comparison of two techniques. Radiology 174:273–274, 1990.
92. Stevens GM, Jackman RJ: Outpatient needle biopsy of the lung: its safety and utility. Radiology 151:301–304, 1984.
93. Cohan RH, Newman GE, Braun SD, et al: CT assistance for fluoroscopically guided transthoracic needle aspiration biopsy. J Comput Assist Tomogr 8:1093–1098, 1984.
94. Williams RA, Haaga JR, Karagiannis E: CT guided paravertebral biopsy of the mediastinum. J Comput Assist Tomogr 8:575–578, 1984.
95. Morettin LB, Allen TE: Thoracic duct cyst: diagnosis with needle aspiration. Radiology 161:437–438, 1986.
96. Doppman JL, Loughlin T, Miller DL, et al: Identification of ACTH-producing intrathoracic tumors by measuring ACTH levels in aspirated specimens. Radiology 163:501–503, 1987.
97. Fink I, Gamsu G, Harter LP: CT-guided aspiration biopsy of the thorax. J Comput Assist Tomogr 6:958–962, 1982.
98. Lalli AF, McCormack LJ, Zelch M, et al: Aspiration biopsies of chest lesions. Radiology 127:35, 1978.
99. Stevens GM, Jackman RJ: Outpatient needle biopsy of the lung: its safety and utility. Radiology 151:301–304, 1984.
100. DeSantos LA, Zornoza J: Bone and soft tissue. In Zornoza J (ed): Percutaneous Needle Biopsy. Baltimore, Williams & Wilkins, 1981, pp 141–178.
101. Hardy DC, Murphy WA, Gilula LA: Computed tomography in planning percutaneous bone biopsy. Radiology 134:447, 1980.
102. Koehler PR, Moss AA: Diagnosis of intraabdominal and pelvic abscesses by computed tomography. JAMA 144:49, 1980.
103. Haaga JR, Alfidi RJ, Havrilla TR, et al: CT detection and aspiration of abdominal abscesses. AJR 128:465, 1977.
104. Gerzof SG, Robbins AH, Birkett DH, et al: Percutaneous catheter drainage of abdominal abscesses guided by ultrasound and computed tomography. AJR 133:1, 1979.
105. Gerzof SG, Robbins AH, Johnson WC, et al: Percutaneous catheter drainage of abdominal abscesses: a five year experience. N Engl J Med 305:653, 1981.
106. Haaga JR, Weinstein AJ: CT-guided percutaneous aspiration and drainage of abscesses. AJR 135:1187, 1980.
107. Sones PJ: Percutaneous drainage of abdominal abscesses. AJR 142:35–39, 1984.
108. vanSonnenberg E, Mueller PR, Ferrucci JT: Percutaneous drainage of 250 abdominal abscesses and fluid collections. Intervent Radiol 151:337–341, 1984.
109. Lambiase RE, Cronan JJ, Dorfman GS, et al: Percutaneous drainage of abscesses in patients with Crohn disease. AJR 150:1043–1045, 1988.
110. vanSonnenberg E, Wing VW, Gasola G, et al: Temporizing effect of percutaneous drainage of complicated abscesses in critically ill patients. AJR 142:821–826, 1984.
111. Stanley P, Atkinson JB, Reid BS, et al: Percutaneous drainage of abdominal fluid collections in children. AJR 142:813–816, 1984.
112. Mueller PR, Ferrucci JT, Wittenberg J, et al: Iliopsoas abscess: treatment by CT-guided percutaneous catheter drainage. AJR 142:359–362, 1984.
113. Akins EW, Hawkins IR, Mladinich C, et al: The blunt needle: a new percutaneous access device. AJR 152:181–182, 1989.
114. Martin EC, Karlson FB, Fankuchen E, et al: Percutaneous drainage in the management of hepatic abscesses. Surg Clin North Am 61:157, 1981.
115. Mueller PR, White EM, Glass-Royal M, et al: Infected abdominal tumors: percutaneous catheter drainage. Radiology 173:627–629, 1989.
116. Abbitt PL, Armstrong P: Percutaneous catheter drainage of necrotic tumors: CT demonstration. J Comput Assist Tomogr 13:437–439, 1989.
117. Cronan JJ, Amis ES, Dorfman GS: Percutaneous drainage of renal abscesses. AJR 142:351–354, 1984.
118. Lang EK: Renal, perirenal and pararenal abscesses: percutaneous drainage. Radiology 174:109–113, 1990.
119. Mueller PR, Ferrucci JT, Butch RJ, et al: Inadvertent percutaneous catheter gastroenterostomy during abscess drainage: significance and management. AJR 145:387–391, 1985.
120. vanSonnenberg J, Simeone JF: Percutaneous drainage of abscesses and fluid collections: technique, results and applications. Radiology 142:1–10, 1982.
121. Deck KB, Berne TV: Selective management of subphrenic abscesses. Arch Surg 114:1165, 1979.
122. Anderson MC: Management of pancreatic pseudocysts. Am J Surg 123:209, 1972.
123. Wade JW: Twenty-five year experience with pancreatic pseudocysts. Are we making progress? Ann Surg 149:705–708, 1985.
124. O'Malley VP, Cannon JP, Posteir RG: Pancreatic pseudocysts: cause, therapy and results. Am J Surg 150:680–682, 1985.
125. Sacks BA, Greenberg JJ, Porter DH, et al: An internalized double-J catheter for percutaneous transgastric cystogastrostomy. AJR 152:523–526, 1989.
126. Polk HC, Zeppa R, Warren WD: Surgical significance of

differentiation between acute and chronic pancreatic collections. Ann Surg 169:444, 1969.

127. Bernardino ME, Amerson JR: Percutaneous gastroaptostomy: a new approach to pancreatic pseudocyst drainage. AJR 143:1096–1097, 1984.

128. Haaga JR, Highman LM, Cooperman AV, et al: Percutaneous CT-guided pancreatography and pseudocystography. AJR 132:829, 1979.

129. MacErlean DP, Bryan DJ, Murphy JL: Pancreatic pseudocyst: management by ultrasonically guided aspiration. Gastrointest Radiol 5:255, 1980.

130. Haaga JR, Reich NE, Havrilla TR, et al: Interventional CT scanning. Radiol Clin North Am 15:449, 1977.

131. Bhatt G, Jason RS, Delany HM, et al: Hepatic hematoma: percutaneous drainage. AJR 135:1287, 1980.

132. Davis WC, Johnson LF: Adult thoracic empyema revisited. Am Surg 44:362–368, 1978.

133. Morrison MC, Lee MJ, Stafford SA, et al: Percutaneous cecostomy: controlled transperitoneal approach. Radiology 176:574–576, 1990.

134. Haaga JR, Bick RJ, Zollinger RM: CT-guided percutaneous catheter cecostomy. Gastrointest Radiol 12:166–168, 1987.

135. Maile CW, Hanna PD: Direct percutaneous drainage of an obstructed afferent loop. AJR 152:521–522, 1989.

136. Crass JR, Simmons RL, Frick MD, et al: Percutaneous decompression of the colon using CT guidance in Ogilvie syndrome. AJR 144:475–476, 1985.

137. Kappis M: Sensibilitat und lokale Anästhesie und chirurgischen Gebiet der Bauchhole mit besonderer Berücksichtigung der Splanchnicus Anästhesis. Beitr zur Klin Chir 115:161, 1919.

138. Bell SN, Cole R, Robert-Thomson IC: Celiac plexus block for control of pain in chronic pancreatitis. Br Med J 281:1064, 1980.

139. Thompson GE, Moore DC, Bridenbaugh LD, et al: Abdominal pain and alcohol celiac plexus nerve block. Anesth Analg Curr Res 56:1, 1977.

140. Boas RA: Sympathetic blocks in clinical practice. Int Anesthesiol Clin 16:149, 1978.

141. Ward EM, Rorie DK, Nauss LA, et al: The celiac ganglia in man: normal anatomic variations. Anesth Analg 58:461, 1979.

142. Buy J-N, Moss AA, Singler RC: CT-guided celiac plexus and splanchnic nerve neurolysis. J Comput Assist Tomogr 6:315, 1982.

143. Quinn SF, Murtagh FR, Chatfield R, et al: CT-guided nerve root block and ablation. AJR 151:1213–1216, 1988.

144. Elmgilie RC, Slavotinek AH: Surgical objectives in unresected cancer of the head of the pancreas. Br J Surg 59:508, 1972.

CHAPTER 28

PRINCIPLES OF MAGNETIC RESONANCE IMAGING

PETER L. DAVIS

Basic Principles

Nuclear Magnetic Resonance

The basis of nuclear magnetic resonance (NMR) is that the nuclei of many atoms have magnetic fields.[1-4] These nuclear magnetic fields exist because the protons and neutrons in the nuclei spin. For the remainder of this chapter the hydrogen atom will be used as the principal example.

The hydrogen atom's nucleus consists of a single proton. The proton has a positive charge that is distributed throughout the proton. The proton spins. The positive charge that is revolving in the nucleus is a moving charge and hence produces a magnetic field along the axis of the proton's spin. Like any other magnet, this "proton" magnet can be attracted or repelled by another magnetic field.

If a group of protons is placed in a static magnetic field, they will tend to align their spins with the static magnetic field. If another magnetic field is added, the proton will be attracted or repulsed by this field. However, because of the proton's spin, the proton will actually tilt not toward the new field, but perpendicular to it. This will cause the proton to tip from its alignment with the static magnetic field. Once the additional magnetic field is turned off, the

protons, which are tipped with respect to the static magnetic field, will be pulled by the static magnetic field back into realignment. Again, because of the spin of the proton, the proton will wobble or precess around the axis of the static magnetic field, analogous to a spinning top wobbling in the earth's gravitational field.

As the proton precesses, its magnetic field precesses also. If a coil of wire is placed near the precessing proton, this coil of wire will experience a changing magnetic field as the proton precesses. According to Faraday's Law of Electromagnetic Induction, a changing magnetic field induces an electrical current in a conductor. This is exactly what happens with the proton's precessing magnetic field near a coil: a changing electrical current is induced in the coil of wire. This is the received NMR signal.

To summarize, because the proton has both charge and spin, it has a magnetic field along its axis of spin. When placed in an external static magnetic field, the proton tends to align with the external field. If the proton is exposed to another magnetic field, it will be tipped from its alignment with the static field. Once tipped, the proton precesses. As the proton precesses, so does its magnetic field. This precessing magnetic field is a changing magnetic field with respect to a stationary coil. Therefore the changing magnetic field induces electrical current within the coil. This electrical signal is the received NMR signal.

Spatial Localization

To create an image, the magnetic resonance imaging (MRI) equipment must determine where in the body a specific NMR signal originates.[5] The basis of this is the Larmor relationship. This relationship states that the frequency that the proton precesses at, and hence the frequency of the received NMR signal, is proportional to the strength of the magnetic field the proton finds itself in when it is precessing.

Hence if the strength of the magnetic field can be varied through space, protons at different locations will precess at different frequencies. All of these different frequencies will be received together by the receiving antenna, also known as the *radiofrequency (RF) coil*, and brought into the MR computers. Using a mathematic tool known as the *Fourier transform*, the computers can determine how much signal is present for each frequency. Because frequency corresponds to magnetic field strength and magnetic field strength corresponds to a position in the body, it would be possible to plot a three-dimensional map of signal strength versus three-dimensional location.

Unfortunately it is not possible to vary the mag-netic field strength in all three dimensions uniquely at the same time. Instead, most MR equipment superimposes a small, linearly changing magnetic field known as a *magnetic gradient* on top of the static magnetic field. This superposition is effectively done one dimension at a time.[6] By applying gradients in all three dimensions in a particular sequence, it is possible to uniquely identify the MR signal in any location in the body and then generate the image.

Imaging Pulse Sequences

General Principles

MRI involves large numbers of protons simultaneously. Eighteen milliliters of water contain more than 10^{23} protons. Although thermodynamics allows just a small fraction of these protons to participate in the NMR phenomenon, this is still an extremely large number of protons. Hence the NMR experiment is a group phenomenon.

For example, when a tissue is placed in a perfectly homogeneous static magnetic field and exposed to a small radiofrequency magnetic field to tip the protons, then once the small magnetic field is turned off, an extremely large number of protons will be precessing. All of these precessing magnetic fields induce an electrical current in the RF coil. If we

$$(I_0\,e^{-a/T2})$$

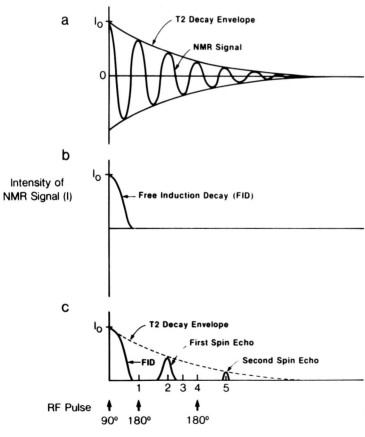

FIGURE 28–1 ■ Relationship of T2 decay and NMR signal intensity in spin-echo imaging. *a,* Exponential decay of free induction decay signal following 90° RF pulse in an ideal uniform magnetic field. *b,* Free induction decay in an actual nonuniform magnetic field occurs more rapidly than in the ideal uniform field and is associated with time constant T2*. *c,* NMR signal intensity at various intervals following 180° RF pulse (time 1). At time 2, a radio signal, first spin echo, is received with an intensity strongly dependent on the tissue's T2 relaxation time. The intensity of the signal rapidly decays (time 3). If another 180° RF pulse is performed at time 4, a second weaker radio signal (second spin echo) is received at time 5. A tissue's T2 relaxation time can be calculated by placing the two different intensities from the two spin-echo signals into equation 28–5 (see text).

observe this current with an oscilloscope, the wave form demonstrated in Figure 28–1A is observed. The received signal decays approximately exponentially with time.

This decay occurs because the protons in the object are subject to local magnetic field inhomogeneities. Because of Larmor's relationship, these inhomogeneities cause neighboring protons to precess at slightly different frequencies. As they precess at slightly different frequencies, they are no longer precessing synchronously, but instead are out of phase with each other. As they become out of phase, their magnetic fields begin to cancel each other, and the induced electrical current decays.

These local magnetic field inhomogeneities are caused by two factors: the very small magnetic fields of neighboring molecules within the object itself, and the inhomogeneities of the external static and gradient magnetic fields. The time constant associated with dephasing caused by just the effects of the molecular magnetic field interactions is called T2. The time constant associated with dephasing caused by both of these effects together is called T2*. T2* is always shorter than T2. The rapidly decaying signal associated with T2* is known as the free induction decay (FID) (Fig. 28–1B).

As discussed previously, additional magnetic gradients must be turned on and off to determine where the NMR signal is coming from within the body. A sequence of such gradient pulses is shown in Figure 28–2. After the RF pulse, which tips the protons and starts them precessing, a small NMR FID occurs. However, it is extremely short because of the presence of the slice-selective magnetic gradient, which causes T2* to be extremely short. A phase-encoding gradient and a readout gradient are sequentially superimposed to vary the magnetic field in the other two dimensions. The dephasing effects of the slice-selective gradient can be counteracted by reversing its direction. Similarly, the readout gradient causes dephasing effects, but if it is preceded by a reversed lobe of appropriate length at the center of the readout gradient, its dephasing effects are also canceled. When the dephasing effects of both the readout and the slice-selective gradient are canceled by the gradient reversals, the FID signal recurs. This is known as a *gradient echo*. Observe that the effects of the phase-encoding gradient are not canceled. This dephasing effect is actually used to determine spatial localization information.

This gradient-echo pulse sequence is quite simple and with modern MRI equipment can be quite short in duration. The limiting factor is how rapidly the gradient magnetic fields can be turned on and off. Initially such rapid changes could not be performed, and other sequences such as the spin-echo sequence and the inversion recovery pulse sequences were (and still are) utilized. The spin-echo sequence has the advantage that the dephasing effects of external magnetic fields can be canceled, and a much larger NMR signal can be received based on T2 decay,

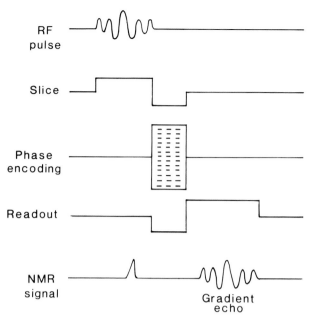

FIGURE 28–2 ■ Gradient refocused–echo pulse sequence. After the RF pulse, the FID signal is cut short by the dephasing caused by the slice-selective magnetic gradient. This dephasing effect is cancelled by reversing the direction of the gradient later. Similarly, the readout gradient begins with a reversed lobe, and halfway through the main lobe, after all gradient dephasing effects are cancelled, the gradient echo occurs. The phase-encoding gradient is not cancelled, as its dephasing effect is used to determine spatial localization information.

compared with the gradient-echo approach, which is dependent on the shorter T2* decay. We will illustrate the spin-echo and inversion recovery sequences in the following discussion of how image contrast among different tissues is formed in MR images.

NMR Tissue Properties

For there to be contrast between different tissues, tissues must have differences in their NMR properties. There are three basic NMR properties: hydrogen density and the T1 and T2 relaxation times.[1–3] In general, the more hydrogen that is present, the more NMR signal generated. Most hydrogen is located in either water or lipids.

T1, also called the *thermal*, *longitudinal*, or *spin-lattice relaxation time*, is related to the time it takes a group of protons to align with a static magnetic field. This is not an instantaneous process. Liquids are held by weaker forces than solids, take a shorter time to align, and thus have a shorter T1 time than solids. Because this process is dependent on the motion and vibration of other molecules in the lattice, T1 has been referred to as the *spin-lattice relaxation time*. Liquid molecules move more rapidly than solids, and T1 is thus shorter for liquids than solids.

The T2 relaxation time was introduced previously. It is related to the time it takes a group of signal-emitting precessing hydrogen protons to lose synchronization after being synchronized by the tipping magnetic field. T2 is termed the *spin-spin* or *transverse relaxation time* and is a measure of how long the substance holds the temporary transverse magnetism induced by the RF pulse, which is perpendicular to the external magnetic field. Synchronization is lost as a result of small variations of the local magnetic field within the tissue itself. Liquids have weaker internal fields and thus maintain synchronization longer (in seconds). Solids with strong internal fields have short T2 values (in microseconds). As synchronization decays at the rate of T2, the longitudinal component grows at a rate of T1. The T1 and T2 relaxation times are affected by many properties of the physical state of a tissue, including its temperature, viscosity, composition, and molecular structure.

The T1 and T2 relaxation times play an important role in providing contrast between different soft tissues.[7, 8] This is because although the hydrogen content of most soft tissues varies over a range of approximately 20 per cent, T1 and T2 can vary over a range of 500 per cent. In actual practice, the received NMR signal intensity is usually a synthesis of the hydrogen concentration and the T1 and T2 relaxation times of the hydrogen. How these three components are combined depends on the imaging methods employed.

Basic to an understanding of nuclear magnetic resonance is a knowledge of the mechanism by which different T1 and T2 relaxation times translate into image contrast. There are many imaging techniques, each one combining the hydrogen concentration and the T1 and T2 effects differently. Three basic techniques will be elucidated in detail: saturation recovery, inversion recovery, and spin echo.

SATURATION RECOVERY

In the saturation recovery imaging technique (proton imaging), the protons in the magnetic field are tipped by an RF pulse at 90° to the static magnetic field. Image contrast is dependent on a variety of factors in saturation recovery imaging but depends most strongly on proton density and the T1 relaxation time of the tissues.

When protons are placed in a magnetic field, they do not align in the direction of the field instantaneously but instead align in an exponential manner. Initially alignment occurs rapidly, but the rate of alignment gradually decreases with the length of time the protons are in the magnetic field. The process of proton alignment in a magnetic field can be described by the equation:

$$A = (1 - e^{-b/T1}) \qquad (28-1)$$

where A is the fraction of the protons aligned after being placed in a magnetic field for a specific period of time, T1 is the T1 relaxation time of the protons in the tissue, and b is the amount of time the protons have had to align with the magnetic field. Therefore the protons in tissues with short T1 times align faster than those with long T1 times (Fig. 28–3).

Each time the protons are tipped by the 90° RF pulse, they lose all their alignment with the magnetic field and thus b and A become 0 (Fig. 28–4). As time passes and b increases, A also increases as more protons realign with the magnetic field. As a rule, at any particular time b, tissues with different T1 relaxation times will have different fractions (A) of their protons in alignment with the magnetic field. However, there are two exceptions to this rule. As shown in Figure 28–3, immediately after the protons are flipped, they are totally out of alignment, and b = 0, A = 0; also, when b = ∞, then A = 1, indicating that all protons are in alignment. For practical purposes, A = 1 when b is greater than four to five times the T1 time of a tissue.

The intensity (I) of the induced signal received after the protons are tipped is proportional to the total number of protons aligned with the magnetic field just before the 90° pulse. The total number of protons aligned with the field is the fraction of protons in alignment (A) multiplied by the hydrogen density (H) of the tissue. This relationship can be described by the equation:

$$I = k \cdot H \cdot A \qquad (28-2)$$

where I is the signal intensity and k is a proportionality constant. As shown by equation (28–2), the more protons that are aligned, the more intense the NMR signal will be when the protons are tipped. From the relationship of equation (28–2) to equation (28–1), it is apparent that

$$I = k \cdot H \cdot A = k \cdot H \cdot (1 - e^{-b/T1}) \qquad (28-3)$$

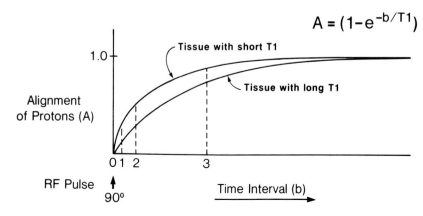

$$A = (1-e^{-b/T1})$$

FIGURE 28–3 ■ Saturation recovery imaging technique: alignment of protons in the magnetic field following 90° pulse. Alignment is 0 immediately after the RF pulse. A = 1 when b is four to five times the T1 value of the tissue. Tissue with a short T1 time aligns more quickly than tissue with a long T1 time. Contrast between the two tissues varies with time.

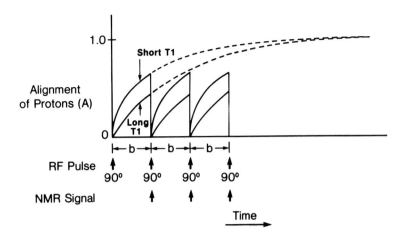

FIGURE 28–4 ■ Saturation recovery imaging sequence. Alignment of protons following RF pulse drops to 0 just after 90° RF pulse. Alignment of protons increases with time but is different for tissues having unequal T1 times. The repeated time interval b between each RF pulse is called the *TR time.*

and that, as shown in Figure 28–4, a tissue with a short T1 time will produce a more intense NMR signal than a tissue with a long T1 time.

The contrast between two tissues is equal to the ratio of the signal intensities, assuming that the hydrogen densities of the two tissues are similar. This assumption is reasonably true for most soft tissues in the body; thus tissue contrast is dependent largely on the ratio of the fraction (A) of protons in each tissue that have aligned prior to being tipped by the RF pulse.

Tissue contrast can be displayed graphically as a ratio of the heights of the exponential curves. In Figure 28–3, for example, the contrast between the two tissues will be different at times 1, 2, and 3.

Thus it is clear that NMR imaging employing only a single time, b, will probably not be sufficient to obtain optimum contrast between normal and abnormal tissue in every instance. Using the saturation recovery technique, if b is varied from time 2 to time 3 (see Fig. 28–3), the signal intensity received for each tissue will be different, and thus the contrast between tissues is changed.

Presently most MRI equipment requires that many, usually 128 or 256, repetitions of the pulse sequence be performed to obtain adequate information to generate an image. During each of these repetitions, the phase-encoding gradient is changed slightly. The repeated time interval between each RF pulse is called the *TR time.*

INVERSION RECOVERY

In the saturation recovery technique, the protons are tipped 90° and lose their alignment with the magnetic field. In the inversion recovery technique, the protons are tipped 180°. The maximum number of protons is aligned against the field immediately after the 180° tip. Once the protons are tipped, they begin to realign with the magnetic field according to their T1 times (Fig. 28–5) and as follows:

$$A = (1 - 2e^{-b/T1}) \qquad (28-4)$$

To obtain an NMR signal, the protons must undergo a 90° tip in addition to the 180° tip. Thus a complete inversion recovery sequence (Fig. 28–6) consists of a 180° tip, followed by a period of realignment (t_r, also called *TI*), then a 90° tip, at which time the NMR signal is received. The protons are then allowed to realign with the external magnetic field before the 180° pulse is repeated. This latter realignment follows equation (28–1) and may be complete or partial, depending on the amount of time ($b - t_r$) allowed and the T1 of the tissue.

Contrast between tissues in the inversion recovery images is highly dependent on the time at which the 90° tip is performed. This is a result of the fact that the net negative alignment (Fig. 28–7A) that occurs after the 180° tip generates a positive image intensity (see Fig. 28–7B). If the 90° tip is performed at time 1, tissue with a long T1 has a higher intensity than tissue with a short T1 time. If the 90° tip is performed at time 2, the tissue having a short T1 has no intensity and appears black on the NMR image, thus ensuring high contrast between the two tissues. At time 3, the long T1 tissue appears more intense than the short T1 tissue, but the contrast between the two tissues is less than that present at time 2. At time 4, both tissues have the same intensity and are indistinguish-

FIGURE 28–5 ■ Inversion recovery imaging technique: alignment of protons in the magnetic field following 180° RF pulse. Immediately after 180° RF pulse, the maximum number of protons are aligned against the magnetic field, but once flipped, they realign with the magnetic field according to their T1 times. Tissues with short T1 values align more rapidly than tissues with long T1 times.

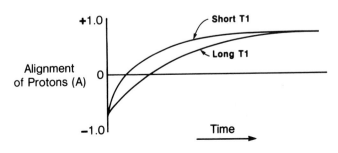

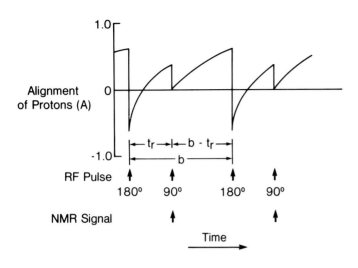

FIGURE 28–6 ■ Inversion recovery imaging sequence. The complete sequence consists of a 180° RF pulse, followed by a period of realignment (t, also called TI), and then a 90° RF pulse, at which time the NMR signal is received. Protons are then allowed to realign before the 180° RF pulse is repeated. b = Time between 180° RF pulses, also called TR.

able. If tipped at time 5, however, the tissue with the short T1 appears more intense than the tissue with a long T2 time. Images generated at time 6 reveal tissue with a long T1 time to have no intensity, thus ensuring high contrast between the two tissues. Images obtained at time 7 still demonstrate the tissue having a short T1 as more intense than tissue with a longer T1 value; however, the image contrast is less than at time 6.

Thus it is evident that image contrast in the inversion recovery technique is strongly dependent on hydrogen density, a tissue's T1 value, and the time at which the 90° tip occurs. The chief advantage of the inversion recovery technique is that it provides relatively high-contrast images over a narrow range of T1 relaxation times. For example, if liver tumors are being searched for, the t_r (TI) can be set so that the 90° tip occurs when normal liver tissue is at the baseline or "bounce point" and therefore produces no signal. However, the liver tumor, which usually has a longer T1 than normal liver, will produce signal and be readily seen in the dark background. This corresponds to time 2 and is the basis of the short TI inversion recovery (STIR) imaging technique.

SPIN ECHO

Magnetic resonance images can also be obtained using a spin-echo technique. This method involves an initial 90° tip followed at a later time by a 180° tip.[1–3, 8] The images obtained by the spin-echo method are dependent on both the T1 and T2 relaxation times of the tissue.

In a perfectly homogeneous magnetic field, the NMR radio signal decays exponentially following a 90° tip (see Fig. 28–1A):

$$D = I_0 e^{-a/T2} \qquad (28\text{–}5)$$

In this equation, a is the time since the 90° tip has occurred, D is the amplitude of the NMR signal at time a (also called the *TE time*), I_0 is the signal's initial

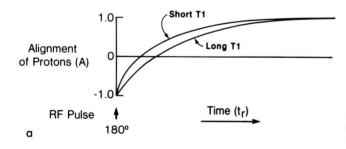

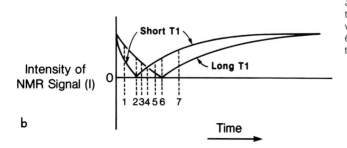

FIGURE 28–7 ■ Variation in contrast between tissues using an inversion recovery imaging technique. *a,* A net negative alignment of protons occurs immediately after the 180° RF pulse. Tissues with different T1 times then realign at unequal rates. *b,* Intensity of NMR signal. Just after the 180° RF pulse (time 0), the intensity of the NMR signal is positive. If the 90° RF pulse is performed at time 1, the signal intensity of tissue with long T1 is greater than that of tissue with short T1 time. At time 2, tissue with a short T1 will have no signal intensity and appear black on the image, ensuring high contrast between tissues. Tissue contrast is less at time 3, whereas at time 4 the tissues will have equal intensities and will be indistinguishable. At times 5, 6, and 7, tissue with a short T1 time will appear more intense than tissue with a long T1 time.

value at time a = 0, and T2 is the T2 relaxation time of the tissue.

The exponential decay of FID signal is shown graphically in Figure 28–1A. As discussed previously, after a 90° tip, the protons are synchronized and emit their signals in a synchronized fashion. According to Larmor's relationship, the frequency of the signals generated by each proton at any moment is dependent on the strength of the magnetic field enveloping the proton. Within each tissue are small variations of the local magnetic field caused by tissue structure; those protons in areas having stronger fields will emit signals of higher frequencies than those protons in regions of weaker fields. As a result of the inhomogeneity of tissue magnetic fields, the signals generated from the two areas will gradually lose synchronization, finally canceling each other so that no signal is received. The loss of synchronization is independent of the realignment of the protons, which is occurring simultaneously.

Loss of synchronization occurs rapidly and, except for pure fluid, is usually more rapid than proton realignment. Because the nonuniformity of the static magnetic field is usually stronger than the internal tissue field variations, FID signal decays more rapidly than it would in a perfectly homogeneous static magnetic field (see Fig. 28–1B).

The spin-echo technique temporarily corrects for inhomogeneities of the external magnetic field by performing a 180° proton tip at an interval following the initial 90° tip (see Fig. 28–1C, time 1). With this approach, the relative differences in synchronization losses among protons can be reversed, so that after a delay equal to the interval between the 90° and 180° tip, the individual signals are again synchronized, and a radio signal—the spin echo—is received (see Fig. 28–1C, time 2). Because this technique corrects only the external field variations, the maximum intensity of the signal received will be strongly dependent on the tissue's T2 relaxation time. After the signals have become resynchronized, synchronization immediately begins to be lost, and the intensity of the signal decays (see Fig. 28–1C, time 3). If another 180° tip is performed (see Fig. 28–1C, time 4), the protons can be resynchronized and an equal time later (see Fig. 28–1C, time 5) a second spin echo received. In practice, the timing and number of 180° tips are under operator control.

The contrast between two tissues having different T2 relaxation times is dependent on the time interval between the 90° tip and occurrence of the spin-echo signal. In Figure 28–8 the contrast between tissues having long and short T2 relaxation times is greater at time 2 than at time 1. Although the contrast between tissues using the spin-echo technique is strongly dependent on differences in T2 relaxation times, the T1 tissue relaxation time also influences final tissue contrast.

In the example shown in Figure 28–8, it was assumed that both tissue signals had the same initial intensity after the 90° tip. Actually this assumption is not necessarily true, because the intensity of the initial signal is dependent on the percentage of protons aligned with the external magnetic field, which is dependent on the T1 relaxation times of the tissues. Thus the interrelationship of T1 and T2 times to signal intensity is complex (Fig. 28–9). After the initial 90° tip, the FID signal occurs; then 180° tips cause spin echoes to be generated at the same time the protons are realigning.

The relationship of T1 and T2 relaxation times to tissue contrast using spin-echo imaging techniques is demonstrated in Figure 28–10. Following the 90° tip, the intensity from tissue A is greater than the intensity from tissue B (see Fig. 28–10A). If tissue A has a longer T2 time than tissue B (see Fig. 28–10B), the contrast between tissues will be greater at time 2 than at time 1. If tissue A has a shorter T2 time than tissue B (see Fig. 28–10C), the contrast can vary drastically, depending on the time the signal is obtained. For example, at time 3, tissue A is more intense than tissue B; at time 4, tissue A has the same intensity as tissue B; and at time 5, tissue A is less intense than tissue B. Thus contrast between tissues using spin-echo techniques is variable, depending on the timing parameters employed, as well as inherent T1 and T2 relaxation times.

The intensity equation for the spin-echo technique is simply the product of equations (28–3) and (28–5):

$$I = kH\, e^{-a/T2}\, (1 - e^{-b/T1}) \qquad (28-6)$$

Although the effects of hydrogen density have largely been ignored in this discussion, as shown in equation (28–6), hydrogen density does affect the intensity and tissue contrast obtained by the spin-echo technique.

FIGURE 28–8 ■ Effect of tissue T2 differences on spin-echo signal intensity. Contrast between tissues is dependent on the time interval between the 90° pulse and the time at which spin echo occurs. Contrast is greater at time 2 than at time 1, even though signal intensity for both tissues is greater at time 1.

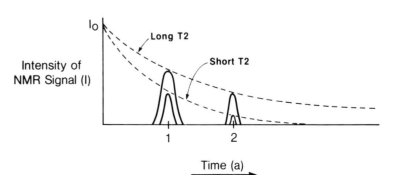

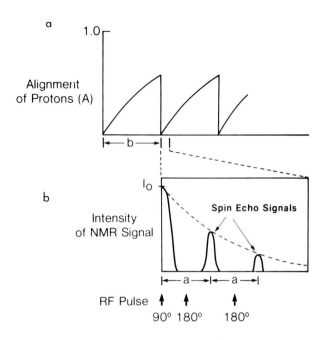

FIGURE 28–9 ■ Interrelationships of T1 and T2 times to signal intensity in spin-echo sequence. *a*, Alignment of protons (A) is dependent on T1 time of tissue. *b*, Detailed diagram of events occurring shortly after the initial 90° RF pulse. An FID signal occurs after the 90° RF pulse, and then 180° RF pulses cause spin-echo signals to be generated at the same time protons are realigning. The intensity of signal is strongly dependent on the tissue's T1 and T2 times. Time interval a is also known as the *TE time.*

Fast Scanning

There are two primary goals in decreasing scan time: to increase patient through-put and decrease motion artifacts.[9, 10] The latter is particularly relevant to body imaging, because historically chest and abdominal CT scan quality improved substantially once scans could be readily obtained in the time period that an ill person could hold his or her breath. In addition, cine-CT scanning has demonstrated the utility of cardiac imaging when image times are fast enough to stop cardiac motion.

Scan time T for the routinely used two-dimensional Fourier transform (2DFT) imaging technique is given by the following equation:

$$T = N_p \cdot TR \cdot NEX \qquad (28\text{–}7)$$

where N_p is the number of phase encodings, TR is the pulse repetition time, and NEX is the number of signal excitations averaged. This latter term is also called the *number of averages or acquisitions.* The greater the NEX, the greater the signal-to-noise ratio is. To decrease scan time, one or several of these variables

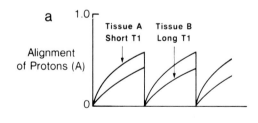

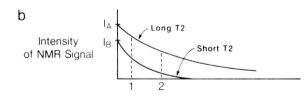

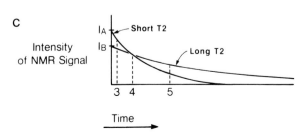

Time

FIGURE 28–10 ■ Relationship of T1 and T2 times to tissue contrast using spin-echo imaging techniques. *a*, Following the 90° RF pulse, alignment of protons (and signal intensity) will be greater for tissue A with a short T1 time than for tissue B with a long T1 time. *b*, If tissue A has a longer T2 time, contrast will be greater at time 2 than at time 1. *c*, If tissue A has a shorter T2 time, contrast can vary depending on the time the signal is obtained. At time 3, tissue A is more intense than B. At time 4, the intensities are equal. At time 5, tissue A is less intense than B.

must be decreased. With the overall improvement of the signal-to-noise ratio, it has been possible to decrease NEX to one. N_p is typically 128 or 256.[6] Decreasing this while maintaining the same field of view reduces the spatial resolution in the phase-encoding direction. Therefore N_p can only be decreased with a corresponding decrease in spatial resolution. However, an examination of the mathematics involved in the Fourier transformation of the phase-encoding information reveals that half of the phase-encoding data can in theory be calculated from the other half.[11] Therefore only half of the phase-encoding steps are required. In actuality, imperfections in the imaging equipment, particularly of the static and radiofrequency magnetic fields, prevent the ideal case from being fully realized.[12] Somewhat more than half of the phase encodings must therefore be performed. This technique has been labeled *NEX = 1/2*, although it is actually a partial or half-Fourier imaging technique.

It is also possible to increase the number of phase-encoding intervals collected per TR interval. For example, when a multi–spin-echo technique is being implemented, the phase encoding can be stepped between every echo. Therefore instead of obtaining several different images, one image can be obtained in a proportional fraction of the N_p. These images will be heavily T2 weighted, as T2 signal decay occurs across the echoes. This method has been termed *rapid acquisition with relaxation enhancement* (*RARE*).[13]

Decreasing the TR time will decrease the scan time. Gradually this has become more possible because of the continuing improvements in MR equipment signal-to-noise ratio, magnetic field homogeneity, and faster and stronger magnetic gradients. As TR shortens, several limitations in the technique become apparent. First, the 180° RF pulse becomes the time-limiting factor. It can be eliminated, but only at the price of using a T2* decay factor rather than a T2 decay factor. If the 180° pulse is removed, then the pulse sequence becomes a gradient-echo sequence. To further decrease the TR requires that the TE time be decreased. This is accomplished by decreasing the amount of time the gradients can be switched on. To compensate for this, the gradients must turn on faster and be stronger. However, an advantage of decreasing the TE time is that more signal is obtained, as less T2* decay has occurred.

The next limiting factor as TR shortens is that with a standard 90° tip, there will be very few protons in alignment after the TR interval to provide signal for the next pulse sequence. To get around this problem, instead of using a 90° tip, a smaller tip is performed. What this effectively does is leave the protons in partial alignment, which enables more signal to be generated at the next partial tip.

In summary, TR can be shortened considerably by removing the 180° RF pulse needed to generate a spin echo and instead generating a gradient echo, by using faster and stronger gradients that allow the TE to be shortened, and by using tip angles less than 90°, which increases the number of protons aligned with the external magnetic field when the next RF pulse is delivered. The prototype of this pulse sequence was developed by Hasse et al. in 1986 and termed *fast low-angle shot* (*FLASH*).[14] Images can now be generated with this technique in slightly less than 1 second.[15]

There are several implications to this technique. First, how does the tip angle, more commonly called the *flip angle*, affect the tissue contrast? Essentially, at small flip angles, the signal intensity is independent of T1 and primarily dependent on proton density.[16] TE still affects the T2* contribution. As the flip angle increases toward 90°, the T1-dependent effects contribute more. However, there is a side effect of going to very short TR times, which can be either an advantage or a disadvantage, depending on the application, and has resulted in a plethora of variations on the FLASH technique.

This side effect occurs when TR becomes substantially less than the T2* relaxation time of a tissue. When this situation happens, a substantial number of protons are still in phase when the next RF pulse is given. These in-phase protons can add or subtract to the various tissue intensities depending on their T2. Tissues with longer T2 times (e.g., cerebrospinal fluid) will have more protons in phase when the next RF pulse is administered.[17] Because this situation is a dynamic equilibrium, it is called a *steady state*.[18] By adjusting the RF pulses and the gradients, it is possible to either reinforce this steady-state situation or to destroy it. Several examples will be illustrated.

Gradient-recalled acquisition in the steady state (GRASS), also known as *fast imaging with steady-state precession* (FISP) is an example of adjusting the phase-encoding gradients in such a way that the steady state is partially reinforced.[9] At small flip angles, tissue contrast remains primarily dependent on hydrogen density. However, at larger flip angles, tissue intensity is dependent on the ratio of T2 to T1. Because this ratio is quite similar for most tissues, including pathologically abnormal tissues, tissue contrast is relatively low. The exception to this is fluids such as cerebrospinal fluid that have a much larger T2:T1 ratio and therefore are usually quite bright.

The steady-state free precession (SSFP) or contrast-enhanced fast acquisition in the steady state (CE-FAST) technique balance the gradients even further to reinforce the steady-state effect.[19] As a result, these pulse sequences can generate considerable T2 weighting even at very short TR times.

Spoiled grass (SPGR) uses a variety of techniques to destroy the steady-state effect.[20] The result is T1-weighted images at all but the lowest flip angles.

To further increase the T1 weighting of the fast scan techniques, Hasse has used a conditioning RF pulse before the fast imaging sequence.[16] For example, if a 180° tip is performed sometime before the fast scan, the T1 weighting of the inversion recovery is superimposed on the fast scan. This technique is known as magnetization-prepared rapid gradient-echo imaging (MP RAGE).[21] It is based on the fact that if the entire image acquisition can be performed in a time period that is small compared with the T1 of the tissue, the entire image data acquisition will be weighted by the preconditioning pulse. The preconditioning pulse, in addition to being an inversion recovery technique, could also be a spin-echo technique. Hence T2 weighting could be obtained with fast scanning techniques.

Echo Planar Imaging

The previously described fast scanning techniques can decrease scan times down to less than a second. The echo planar technique can decrease the scanning time to the order of 50 ms, short enough to freeze the motion of the heart.[22, 23] The echo planar technique applies the gradient-echo techniques to the RARE pulse sequence.

To review, the RARE sequences performed multiple spin echoes, each of which had a different phase encoding, so that several phase encodings could be obtained per TR interval to decrease the scan time. In the echo planar technique, instead of doing spin echoes, multiple gradient echoes are performed. Using very fast and strong gradients, 64 or 128 gradient echoes can be generated in a TE interval of 30 to 40 ms. Each of the gradient echoes have a slightly different phase encoding. Hence all the data needed to generate an image is performed in one pulse sequence. Such rapidly changing gradients require specially designed gradient coils that must operate in a resonant mode.

Flow

General Principles

In addition to hydrogen density and the T1 and T2 relaxation times, movement also affects the NMR intensity.[24–26] For the spin-echo pulse sequence at least two RF pulses must be performed. If the protons move out of the volume element being imaged before they can experience both pulses, their contribution to the NMR signal is lost. This effect will increase as the velocity of the blood flow increases. Hence rapidly flowing blood usually images with little or no intensity. Slower flowing blood may demonstrate more intensity. This effect is known as a *washout effect*.

While the washout effect is occurring, a wash-in effect is also occurring. This wash-in effect can increase signal intensity. This is caused by the fully aligned protons that flow into the plane between RF excitations. These protons emit considerable signal when flipped as compared with the stationary protons in the plane. These stationary protons, having experienced repeated RF exposure, are not fully aligned with the external magnetic field and therefore emit less signal at the subsequent RF pulse.

This wash-in effect is more effective in single-slice gradient-echo images. There are several reasons for this. First, because only one RF pulse is necessary to generate the gradient echo, as compared with the two required for the spin-echo technique, the washout effect will not occur. Hence even rapidly flowing venous and arterial structures will demonstrate increased signal. Second, because shorter TR times are usually used in gradient-echo techniques when compared with spin-echo techniques, the realignment of the stationary protons will be much less compared with the fully aligned protons entering in the flowing blood. Hence, when appropriately designed, a single-slice gradient-refocused echo pulse sequence can produce a signal where the flowing structures are quite high in intensity and the stationary structures are quite low in intensity.[27]

MR Angiography

If many such gradient-echo images were obtained of contiguous planes and if the images were superimposed and displayed in proper spatial location, an angiographic effect would be obtained. Such manipulations can now be readily performed with modern computer work stations. This is the basis of time-of-flight MR angiography (MRA).[28, 29] Once the data is entered into the computer work station, using appropriate software it can be rotated to any desired view.

The second technique to obtain the MRA effect is phase-contrast angiography (PCA).[30] This technique is based on the observation that moving protons in a magnetic gradient change their phase at a different rate than stationary protons in the gradient. By performing certain gradient manipulations, it is possible to subtract out the signal from stationary objects involved while the signal from flowing objects remains.

A present limitation of MR angiography is the signal loss resulting from turbulence. Turbulence causes random dephasing of the proton. This dephasing causes signal loss. This effect can be seen in stenoses and even sharply curved vessels.

MR Contrast Agents

A variety of agents can be placed into the body that can increase the image contrast between normal and abnormal tissues and help identify normal structures such as bowel. These agents are analogous to those provided by the iodinated or barium-based compounds used in x-ray studies. MR contrast agents work by affecting the basic three NMR properties of tissue, namely T1, T2, and hydrogen density.[31]

Paramagnetic Agents

Some atoms or molecules have unpaired electrons.[32] When these atoms or molecules are placed in a magnetic field, they generate their own small magnetic fields that add and/or subtract from the main magnetic field in the local volume. The effect of these compounds is to shorten both T1 and T2 relaxation times. On a T1-weighted imaging sequence, these compounds will initially cause increased intensity of the agent-containing tissue, but as the concentration of the compounds increases, intensity loss will occur.[33]

There are three main types of paramagnetic compounds. The first type is metal ions of the first transition series and the lanthanide series. The former includes copper, iron, and manganese ions, and the latter includes gadolinium. The second type is nitroxide-free radicals, and the third is molecular oxygen.

Gadolinium (Gd) is one of the strongest paramagnetic ions because of its seven unpaired electrons. Because gadolinium is quite toxic in its free form, it is chelated with diethylenetriaminepentaacetate (DTPA) to make it safe for human use. Gd-DTPA has an extracellular distribution similar to that of the iodinated contrast agents used in radiography.[34] Gadolinium and other paramagnetic ions have been chelated to other molecules such as DOTA, EDTA, and TETA, with varying results.[35] The chelates have been attached to larger molecules such as proteins and monoclonal antibodies.[36] Unfortunately the amount of paramagnetically labeled antibody that reaches the target site is inadequate to change the NMR signal sufficiently to enable detection.

Other complexes can be targeted at the hepatobiliary system. Iron (III) ethylene-bis-(2-hydroxyphenylglycine) (Fe-EHPG) is taken up by the liver cell.[37] Early reports have shown that this compound can improve the contrast between normal liver and liver metastases.

Superparamagnetic Agents

To understand superparamagnetism, ferromagnetism must first be explained. Ferromagnetism is the basis of permanent magnets.[32] Unlike paramagnetism, which is based on an individual atom or molecule, ferromagnetism is based on the interaction of a closely packed group of atoms or molecules, usually in a crystalline form. Ferromagnetic materials include iron, nickel, and cobalt. When these paramagnetic compounds are closely packed, their individual magnetic fields are coupled and will tend to align parallel to each other. Hence their magnetic effects are additive. Small foci of the magnetically aligned regions are called *domains*. In large samples that contain multiple domains, the net magnetization is zero because of random ordering. However, once the sample is placed in an external magnetic field, the individual domains will align with the external magnetic field. This alignment will remain even after the external magnetic field is removed. In addition, the parallel alignment of all of these paramagnetic moments creates a relatively large magnetic field compared with the individual paramagnetic ions.

When a ferromagnetic crystal is made smaller and

smaller, finally a single-domain particle is produced. When a large number of these single-domain particles are subjected to an external magnetic field, they will exhibit the properties of ferromagnetism and generate a strong magnetic field. However, because of their small size, thermal agitation will randomly reorient the particles once the external field is removed. Therefore superparamagnetic materials demonstrate the strong magnetic field characteristics of a ferromagnetic material, but similar to a paramagnetic compound, it is only present in the presence of an external magnetic field.[38]

The end result is that the strong magnetic fields produced by superparamagnetic material cause large inhomogeneities in local magnetic fields. This increases proton dephasing. This dephasing shortens T2. Hence superparamagnetic materials primarily cause T2 relaxation time shortening. T2 shortening will cause signal intensity decrease on both T1- and T2-weighted pulse sequences.

Ferrite magnetite (Fe_3O_4) is a superparamagnetic iron oxide (SPIO) crystal.[38, 39] These crystals can be made 5 to 50 nm in size. However, larger composite particles can be formed up to 1000 nm in size. These particles can be made biocompatible by coating them with materials such as dextran, lipid, protein, or glycoproteins. The size of the particle and its coating will determine its biodistribution.

AMI-25 (Advanced Magnetics, Inc.; Cambridge, MA) is a SPIO coated with dextran that has a mean diameter of approximately 72 nm.[38, 39] After injection it has a blood clearance half-life of approximately 10 minutes. It is primarily cleared by the reticuloendothelial system (RES) in the liver and spleen. Because of the strong dephasing effects of these particles, even in very small doses, they shorten the T2 relaxation time of the liver and spleen so much that there is complete signal loss from these organs. However, because neoplasms do not contain RES cells, tumors in these organs will not decrease in intensity but instead will remain at normal intensity. Hence there will be large signal differences between the normal RES-containing tissue and the tumor. In initial clinical trials, SPIO substantially improved the detection of hepatic neoplasms.[40]

If SPIOs are made approximately 12 nm in diameter and coated with arabinogalactin, a galactose-containing polysaccharide, they are not scavenged by the RES cells.[41, 42] Instead they are selectively taken up by receptors on hepatocytes. This uptake also causes the T2 relaxation times to be shortened and the corresponding MR intensity to decrease. Because these receptors are lost during malignant transformation and are not present in metastatic tumors, these tumors will not take up this SPIO. Again, normal liver will appear dark, and tumor will appear with higher intensity. This has been demonstrated in animal models.

Hydrogen Density Agents

Agents that either increase or decrease the hydrogen density present have primarily been targeted at the gastrointestinal tract. Because pure water has long T1 and T2 relaxation times, on T1-weighted images it will appear dark. If a paramagnetic compound such as Gd-DTPA is added, the bowel content can be made hyperintense.[43] Mineral oil will also increase the hydrogen content of the bowel and the image intensity.[44] However, patient acceptance of mineral oil was very poor.

The hydrogen content of the bowel has been decreased by two techniques. First, air can be placed into the bowel using effervescent agents.[45] Second, clinical investigations have also been performed with perfluorohexylbromide (PFHB),[46] a liquid that does not contain any hydrogen and therefore appears as a void in the bowel loops. None of these agents work as well as the iodinated or barium-based compounds used in x-ray studies.

Presently, extensive development of MR contrast agents is occurring. Tissue targeting is a primary aim of many of these new agents.

Radiofrequency Coils

The radiofrequency coil is the only piece of MRI hardware discussed in detail in this chapter, because it is the only piece of hardware that can be changed between examinations and must in fact be properly selected to optimize the examination. To review, the tasks of the radiofrequency coil are (1) to produce the changing magnetic field that tips the proton and (2) to be the coil in which the changing magnetic fields of the precessing proton induce the current that generates the NMR signal. Although a coil can be both a receiver and a transmitting coil, these functions have different demands and will be discussed separately.

There are basically two types of receiving coils: volume coils and surface coils.[47, 48] Volume coils are coils that typically completely wrap around the volume being studied. Typical examples are head coils, body coils, and extremity coils. Surface coils are usually smaller and just receive signal from a small volume near the coil. Two conflicting effects must be balanced to decide what type of coil to use. First, every coil has associated with it a volume in space where it optimally sees the changing magnetic fields of the precessing protons. Therefore the coil must be chosen so that the desired volume is seen. However, a larger volume is not helpful, as it will also pick up electrical noise produced by thermal motion of ions in tissues that are not relevant to the examination. When the receiving coil's sensitive volume matches the desired imaging volume, the coil is defined as having a high filling factor. As a general rule, to choose between a surface coil or a volume coil or between types of surface coils, if the volume to be studied is within approximately one radius of the surface coil, the surface coil will be a better choice than the volume coil. If the volume to be imaged is quite large or quite deep, the volume coil is usually the better choice. The volume coil is also the better choice when uniformity of signal is desired throughout the image, especially if T1 or T2 relaxation measurements will be made.

The transmitting RF coil is usually designed to produce a uniform field to ensure that the protons are uniformly tipped throughout the tissue. As a result, most transmitting coils are volume type coils. Usually a volume coil can be used for both transmission and reception. When a surface coil is used for reception, a volume coil is simultaneously used for transmission.

Safety of MR Imaging

Although MR uses no ionizing radiation, three different types of magnetic fields are used: the static magnetic field, the changing magnetic gradients, and the radiofrequency magnetic fields. Each of these fields has potential safety concerns.[49–51] In addition, other environmental effects associated with MR imaging must be considered.

The biologic effects of the static magnetic fields used in MR imaging are uncertain. Although no definite deleterious effects have been observed, complete safety cannot be proven. A large number of investigations have not demonstrated any biologic effect of strong static magnetic fields in a large number of experimental systems.[52–55] However, other studies did show some effect of a static magnetic field on a variety of animal systems.[56, 57] Research in this area is continuing.

A definite safety concern of static magnetic fields is the force or torque exerted on ferromagnetic objects by the magnetic field. These ferromagnetic objects can be in, on, or even remote from the subject and the equipment operators. The ferromagnetic objects entering the field can become missiles, causing severe injury to the patient or the operator. Ferromagnetic material within the body can similarly be pulled or twisted into alignment with the magnetic field. Of particular concern are a few types of aneurysmal vascular clips and shrapnel that is located in or near the central nervous system or the eyes.[58] The magnetic force or torque on implanted metallic devices or prostheses may also make these contraindications to MRI.[59, 60] Lists of such objects are given in the literature.[61]

Cardiac pacemakers should be considered a contraindication for MR examination.[62] Frequently they contain ferromagnetic material, and most contain a magnetically activated relay switch that can close in fields as low as 5 to 20 gauss. The pacemaker leads may act as an antenna, and the changing magnetic fields may possibly induce electrical current that would pace the heart directly.

Changing magnetic fields are created by both the magnetic gradients and the RF magnetic fields. By Faraday's Law, changing magnetic fields can induce electrical currents.[63] Presently the currents induced by the magnetic gradients are lower than the threshold currents necessary to cause the stimulation of nerve or muscle cells, including those of the heart. However, the rapid changes of the magnetic field gradients of echo planar imaging may approach the threshold of peripheral muscle stimulation.[64]

Induced current may also cause heating effects.[63] The currents caused by the magnetic gradients are insufficient to cause any significant heating. However, the RF magnetic field can induce substantial currents within the patient that can generate heat.[65–67]

This RF power deposition is specified by the specific absorption rate (SAR). The SAR cannot be readily measured and is usually estimated. The Food and Drug Administration (FDA) limits the SAR to which the body can be exposed.[68] This in turn may cause limitations on the pulse sequences being applied in MRI.[66]

The complexity of the MR equipment is such that it may create adverse effects in the environment, affecting not only the subject, but also the operating personnel. In addition to the ferromagnetic effects mentioned previously, electrical currents induced in wire such as for ECG monitoring may cause burns.[69] The rapid changes of the gradient magnetic fields can induce considerable noise for which ear plugs are suggested.[70] The cryogens used in superconductive systems can cause asphyxiation and frost bite or other tissue damage if they are not properly ventilated and handled.[50]

A thorough review of this subject has been published by Kanal and co-workers.[50] In addition the Safety Committee of the Society of Magnetic Resonance Imaging (SMRI) has released a report of policies, guidelines, and recommendations for MR imaging safety and patient management.[71]

References

1. Gore JC, Emery EW, Orr JS, Doyle FH: Medical nuclear magnetic resonance imaging: I. Physical principles. Invest Radiol 16:269, 1981.
2. Bradley WG, Tosteson H: Basic principles of NMR. In Kaufman L, Crooks LE, Margulis AR (eds): Nuclear Magnetic Resonance in Medicine. Tokyo, Kgaku-Shoin, 1981, pp 11–29.
3. Pykett IL, Newhouse JH, Buonanno FS, Brady TJ, Goldman MR, et al: Principles of nuclear magnetic resonance imaging. Radiology 143:157, 1982.
4. Pykett IL: NMR imaging in medicine. Sci Am 246:78, 1982.
5. Lauterbur PC: Image formation by induced local interactions: examples employing NMR. Nature 242:190, 1973.
6. Edelstein WA, Hutchison JMS, Johnson G, Redpath T: Spin warp imaging and applications to human whole-body imaging. Phys Med Biol 25:756–759, 1980.
7. Herfkins RJ, Davis PL, Crooks LE, Kaufman L, Price DC, et al: Nuclear magnetic resonance imaging of atherosclerotic disease. Radiology 141:211, 1981.
8. Crooks L, Arakawa M, Hoenninger J, Watts J, McRee R, et al: Nuclear magnetic resonance whole-body imager operating at 3.5 KGauss. Radiology 143:169, 1982.
9. Haacke EM, Tkach J: A review of fast imaging techniques and applications. AJR 155:951, 1990.
10. Wehrli FW: Fast-Scan Magnetic Resonance: Principles and Applications. New York, Raven Press, 1991.
11. Feinberg DA, Hale JD, Watts JC, Kaufman L, Mark A: Halving MR imaging time by conjugation: demonstration at 3.5 kG. Radiology 161:527–531, 1986.
12. MacFall JR, Pelc N, Vavrek RM: Correction of spatially dependent phase shifts in partial Fourier imaging. Magn Reson Imaging 6:143–155, 1988.
13. Hennig J, Nauerth A, Friedburg H: RARE imaging: fast imaging method for clinical MR. Magn Reson Med 3:823–833, 1986.
14. Haase A, Frahm J, Matthaei D, Itänicke W, Merboldt KD: FLASH imaging: rapid NMR imaging using low flip angle pulses. J Magn Reson 67:258–266, 1986.
15. Frahm J, Merboldt KD, Bruhn H, Coyngell ML, Itänicke W, et al: 0.3-second FLASH MRI of the human heart. Magn Reson Med 13:150–157, 1990.
16. Haase A: Snapshot FLASH MRI. Applications to T1, T2 and chemical-shift imaging. Magn Reson Med 13:77–89, 1990.
17. Perkins TG, Wehrli FW: CSF signal enhancement in short TR gradient echo images. Magn Reson Imaging 4:465–467, 1986.
18. Hawkes RC, Patz S: Rapid Fourier imaging using steady-state free precession. Magn Reson Med 4:9–23, 1987.
19. Gyngell ML: The application of steady-state free precession in rapid 2DFT NMR imaging: fast and CE-FAST sequences. Magn Reson Imaging 6:415–419, 1988.
20. Crawley AP, Wood ML, Henkelman RM: Elimination of transverse coherences in FLASH MRI. Magn Reson Med 8:248–260, 1988.
21. Mugler JP III, Brookeman JR: Three-dimensional magnetization-prepared rapid gradient-echo imaging (3D MP RAGE). Magn Reson Med 15:152–157, 1990.
22. Rzedzian RR, Pykett IL: Instant images of the human heart using a new, whole-body MR imaging system. AJR 149:245–250, 1987.
23. Pykett IL, Rzedzian RR: Instant images of the body by magnetic resonance. Magn Reson Med 5:563–571, 1987.
24. Bradley WG Jr, Waluch V: Blood flow: magnetic resonance imaging. Radiology 154:443–450, 1985.
25. Axel L: Blood flow effects in magnetic resonance imaging. AJR 143:1157–1166, 1984.
26. Wehrli FW, Shimakawa A, Gullberg GT, MacFall JR: Time-of-flight MR flow imaging: selective saturation recovery with gradient refocusing. Radiology 160:781–785, 1986.
27. Atlas SW, Mark AS, Fram EK, Grossman RI: Vascular intracranial lesions: applications of gradient-echo imaging. Radiology 169:455–461, 1988.
28. Keller PJ, Drayer BP, Fram EK, Williams KD, Dumoulin CL, Souza SP: MR angiography with two-dimensional acquisition and three-dimensional display: work in progress. Radiology 173:527–532, 1989.
29. Masaryk TJ, Modic MT, Ross JS, Ruggieri PM, Laub GA, et al: Intracranial circulation: preliminary clinical results with three-dimensional (volume) MR angiography. Radiology 171:793–799, 1989.
30. Dumoulin CL, Souza SP, Walker MF, Wagle W: Three-dimensional phase contrast angiography. Magn Reson Med 9:139–149, 1989.
31. Saini S, Modic MT, Hamm B, Hahn PF: Advances in contrast-enhanced MR imaging. AJR 156:235–254, 1991.
32. Saini S, Frankel RB, Stark DD, Ferrucci JT: Magnetism: a primer and review. AJR 150:735–743, 1988.
33. Davis PL, Parker DL, Nelson JA, Gillen JS, Runge VM: Interactions of paramagnetic contrast agents and the spin echo pulse sequence. Invest Radiol 23:381–388, 1988.
34. Weinmann HJ, Brasch RC, Press WR, Wesby GE: Characteristics of gadolinium-DTPA complex: a potential NMR contrast agent. AJR 142:619–624, 1984.
35. Allard M, Doucet D, Kien P, Bonnemain B, Caille JM: Experimental study of DOTA-gadolinium: pharmacokinetics and pharmacologic properties. Invest Radiol 23(suppl 1):S271–S274, 1988.
36. Schmeidl U, Ogan M, Paajanen H, Marotti M, Crooks LE, et al: Albumin labeled with Gd-DTPA as an intravascular, blood-pool enhancing agent for MR imaging: biodistribution and imaging studies. Radiology 162:205–210, 1987.
37. Lauffer RB, Grief WL, Stark DD, Vincent AC, Saini S, et al: Iron-EHPG as an hepatobiliary MR contrast agent: initial

imaging and biodistribution studies. J Comput Assist Tomogr 9:431–438, 1985.

38. Saini S, Stark DD, Hahn PF, Wittenberg J, Brady TJ, Ferrucci JT: Ferrite particles: a superparamagnetic MR contrast agent for the reticuloendothelial system. Radiology 162:211–216, 1987.

39. Stark DD, Weissleder R, Elizondo G, Hahn PF, Saini S, et al: Superparamagnetic iron oxide: clinical application as a contrast agent for MR imaging of the liver. Radiology 168:297–301, 1988.

40. Ferrucci JT, Stark DD: Iron oxide-enhanced MR imaging of the liver and spleen: review of the first 5 years. AJR 155:943–950, 1990.

41. Weissleder R, Reimer P, Lee AS, Wittenberg J, Brady TJ: MR receptor imaging: ultrasmall iron oxide particles targeted to asialoglycoprotein receptors. AJR 155:1161–1167, 1990.

42. Reimer P, Weissleder R, Lee AS, Wittenberg J, Brady TJ: Receptor imaging: application to MR imaging of liver cancer. Radiology 177:729–734, 1990.

43. Laniado M, Kornmesser W, Hamm B, Clauss W, Weinmann H-J, Felix R: MR imaging of the gastrointestinal tract: value of Gd-DTPA. AJR 150:817–821, 1988.

44. Ang PGP, Li KCP, Tart RP, Storm B, Rolfes R: Geritol oil emulsion: ideal positive oral contrast agent for MR imaging. Radiology 173(P):522, 1989.

45. Weinreb JC, Maravilla KR, Redman HC, Nunnally R: Improved MR imaging of the upper abdomen with glucagon and gas. J Comput Assist Tomogr 8:835–838, 1984.

46. Mattrey RF: Perfluorooctylbromide: a new contrast agent for CT, sonography, and MR imaging. AJR 152:247–252, 1989.

47. Axel L: Surface coil magnetic resonance imaging. J Comput Assist Tomogr 8(3):381–384, 1984.

48. Surface/specialty coil devices and gating techniques in magnetic resonance imaging. Health Technology Assessment Report, 1990, no 3. Rockville, MD: US Dept of Health and Human Services, Public Health Service, Agency for Health Care Policy and Research.

49. Budinger TF: Nuclear magnetic resonance (NMR): in vivo studies. Known thresholds for health effects. J Comput Assist Tomogr 5:800–811, 1981.

50. Kanal E, Shellock FG, Talagala L: Safety considerations in MR imaging. Radiology 176:593–606, 1990.

51. Persson BRR, Stahlberg F: Health and safety of clinical NMR examinations. Boca Raton, FL: CRC Press, 1989.

52. Schwartz JL, Crooks LE: NMR imaging produces no observable mutations or cytotoxicity in mammalian cells. AJR 139:583, 1982.

53. Wolff S, Crooks LE, Brown P, Howard R, Painter RB: Tests for DNA and chromosomal damage induced by nuclear magnetic resonance imaging. Radiology 136:707, 1980.

54. Wolff S, James TL, Young GB, Margulis AR, Bodycote J, Afzal V: Magnetic resonance imaging: absence of in vitro cytogenetic damage. Radiology 155:163–165, 1985.

55. Geard CR, Osmak RS, Hall EJ, Simon HE, Maudsley AA, Hilal SK: Magnetic resonance and ionizing radiation: a comparative evaluation in vitro of oncogenic and genotoxic potential. Radiology 152:199–202, 1984.

56. Doherty JU, Whitman GJR, Robinson MD, Harken AH, Simson MB, et al: Changes in cardiac excitability and vulnerability in NMR fields. Invest Radiol 20:129–135, 1985.

57. Marsh JL, Armstrong TJ, Jacobson AP, Smith RG: Health effect of occupational exposure to steady magnetic fields. Am Ind Hyg Assoc J 43:387–394, 1982.

58. Dujovny M, Kossovsky N, Kossovsky R, Valdivia R, Suk JS, et al: Aneurysm clip motion during magnetic resonance imaging: in vivo experimental study with metallurgical factor analysis. Neurosurgery 17:543–548, 1985.

59. New PFJ, Rosen BR, Brady TJ, Buonanno FS, Kistler JP, et al: Potential hazards and artifacts of ferromagnetic and nonferromagnetic surgical and dental materials and devices in nuclear magnetic resonance imaging. Radiology 147:139–148, 1983.

60. Teitelbaum GP, Bradley WG Jr, Klein BD: MR imaging artifacts, ferromagnetism, and magnetic torque of intravascular filters, stents, and coils. Radiology 166:657–664, 1988.

61. Shellock FG: MR imaging of metallic implants and materials: a compilation of the literature. AJR 151:811–814, 1988.

62. Pavlicek W, Geisinger M, Castle L, Borkowski GP, Meaney TF, et al: The effects of nuclear magnetic resonance on patients with cardiac pacemakers. Radiology 147:149–153, 1983.

63. Bottomley PA, Edelstein WA: Power deposition in whole body NMR imaging. Med Phys 8:510–512, 1981.

64. Fischer H: Physiological effects by fast oscillating magnetic field gradients. Radiology 173(P):382, 1989.

65. Shellock FG, Crues JV III: Temperature, heart rate, and blood pressure changes associated with clinical MR imaging at 1.5 T. Radiology 163:259–262, 1987.

66. Shellock FG, Schaefer DJ, Crues JV: Alterations in body and skin temperatures caused by MR imaging: is the recommended exposure for radiofrequency radiation too conservative? Br J Radiol 62:904–909, 1989.

67. Bottomley PA, Reddington RW, Edelstein WA, Schenck JF: Estimating radiofrequency power deposition in body NMR imaging. Magn Reson Med 2:336–349, 1985.

68. Guidance for content and review of a magnetic resonance diagnostic device 510(k) application. Federal Register, August 2, 1988.

69. Kanal E, Shellock FG: Burns associated with clinical MR examinations. Letter. Radiology 175:585, 1990.

70. Brummett RE, Talbot JM, Charuhas P: Potential hearing loss resulting from MR imaging. Radiology 169:539–540, 1988.

71. Shellock FG, Kanal E, and the SMRI Safety Committee: Policies, guidelines, and recommendations for MR imaging safety and patient management. J Magn Reson Imaging 1:97–101, 1991.

CHAPTER 29

PRINCIPLES OF COMPUTED TOMOGRAPHY

DOUGLAS P. BOYD · DENNIS L. PARKER · MITCHELL M. GOODSITT

Principles of Reconstructive Imaging

The primary purpose of CT is to produce a two-dimensional representation of the linear x-ray attenuation coefficient distribution through a narrow planar cross section of the human body (or any general object). Because tissues of different structures within the body are of different elemental compositions, they also tend to exhibit different x-ray attenuation qualities. Thus in generating cross-sectional images of the x-ray attenuation coefficients, an image is formed that delineates various structures within the body, showing the relative anatomic relationships. The mathematic and physical processes used to generate the image are discussed next.

Basic Principles of Computed Tomography

When a beam of monochromatic x-rays passes through a homogeneous medium, it diminishes in intensity because of interactions with the medium. In the diagnostic energy range, these interactions are primarily molecular ionizations resulting from Compton scattering and photoelectric absorption. In traversing a very small thickness of the medium, the decrease in the beam (i.e., the number of x-ray photons removed from the beam) is proportional to the initial number of photons and the thickness traversed. This can be expressed as

$$\Delta I = -\mu I \Delta s,$$

where I is the incident intensity, Δs is the thickness, and μ is the proportionality constant; μ is also known as the linear attenuation coefficient. When the medium is thick, this relationship can be solved by giving an exponential relationship for the attenuation:

$$I = I_o e^{-\mu s}$$

or

$$\ln[I_o/I] = \mu s.$$

The logarithm of the ratio of the incident x-ray intensity to the transmitted intensity is just the product of the x-ray linear attenuation coefficient of the medium and the thickness along the line of transmission. A typical line of transmission might be from point (C) to point (D) as shown in Figure 29–1A. The line from (C) to (D) is completely specified by the angle θ and the distance r along a perpendicular line through the origin. In the case of objects such as the human body that are not homogeneous, the linear attenuation coefficient may be different at various positions. Because the change is generally gradual in adjacent positions, it can be assumed that the linear attenuation coefficient is constant over very small distances. The logarithm of the ratios of the intensities is directly related to the sum of each small

distance multiplied by the corresponding linear attenuation coefficient. This can be expressed as

$$\ln[I_o/I] = \int \mu(E,s) \, ds.$$

The E indicates that μ changes as a function of the x-ray energy. This weighted summation of the linear attenuation coefficients is referred to as a *projection of the attenuation distribution along a line.*

In 1917, Radon[1] became the first to derive equations describing the reconstruction of the two-dimensional distribution in a plane of an object from its projections. His equations require the projections along all possible lines through the plane of the object. The set of projections along all possible lines is thus referred to as the *radon transformation.* The operations that generate the reconstructed image from the radon transformation are sometimes referred to as the *inverse radon transformation.*

The most simple visualization of the geometry of making the projection measurements along lines can be seen in Figure 29–2. In the original EMI scanner, a single pencil x-ray beam traverses the slice to be examined at multiple view angles. An x-ray detector records the transmitted x-ray intensity during each crossing, as shown in the figure. This set of measurements is referred to as a *parallel ray projection of*

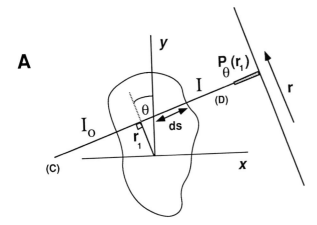

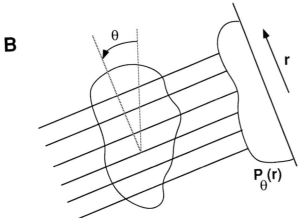

FIGURE 29–1 ■ Geometry of projection imaging (radon transformation) for computed tomography. *A,* Ray sum along line from (C) to (D). This line may be specified by two numbers: r, the distance of the line from the origin; and θ, the angle of inclination of the line. The ray sum for this particular line is indicated as Pθ(r$_1$). *B,* The projection at angle θ. This projection is the set of ray sums or line integrals at angle θ and is represented as Pθ(r).

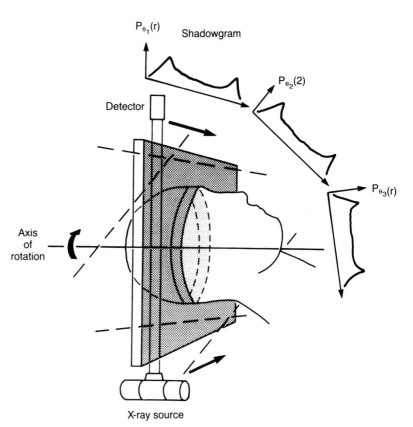

FIGURE 29–2 ■ CT scanning pencil beam. Translate-rotate two-motion scanning of head with a single x-ray beam. $P_\theta(r) = \ln[Io/I]_\theta(r)$.

the section being examined (see Fig. 29–1B). It is also often referred to as a *profile* or *parallel ray view.* Each point in the profile represents the transmitted intensity at each point along the traverse; a separate profile is obtained for each angle.

Examples of a radon transformation are shown in Figure 29–3. In Figure 29–3A a simple diagram composed of ellipses of different "densities" is shown. Two high-density "calcified" points are at the lower right. If the set of all projections is computed, it can be displayed as shown in Figure 29–3B, with θ as the y-axis and r and θ as polar coordinates, as in Figure 29–3C. Displays of the radon transformation in the format of Figure 29–3B are generally referred to as *sinograms,* because a point in the object traces out a sine curve in the display, as seen for the pair of points (also see Fig. 29–7). In the polar coordinate display, a point in the object becomes a circle.

The objective of the computer reconstruction program is to convert or transform a series of profiles into a CT image. This procedure is illustrated in Figure 29–4. In Figure 29–4A the profiles of a point object in the scanned slice of four view angles separated by 45° steps are shown. One approach to reconstruction would be to simply project the profiles back across the CT image, as shown in Figure 29–4B, similar to the principle of axial tomography. This procedure produces a starlike reconstruction. If a large number of views are used, the radial streaks merge together and the point reconstruction becomes a smooth image with a peak at the center and falling off as l/r, where r is the distance from the center of

the point. Such streaks may occasionally appear in scanners when the number of views are only marginally adequate; they are referred to as *angular aliasing streaks* or the *angular undersampling artifact.*

One method of accurate reconstruction is to mathematically remove the l/r blurring from the back-projected image. Such a technique is referred to as *unfolding* or *deconvolution.* If the profiles are accumulated at equal angular intervals from 0° to 180°, this process of deconvolution may be accomplished by first modifying the profiles prior to their back-projection. The modification is produced by applying a mathematic "filter" or "convolution" function to the profile so that the resulting reconstructed image more closely resembles the original object from which the original, unmodified profiles were obtained. The modified profiles and resulting modified back-projected image are indicated in Figure 29–4C. This technique of modified or filtered back-projection is essentially the image reconstruction process used by all modern CT scanners.[2] Thus the principle of CT rests on the premise that it is possible to accurately reconstruct a two-dimensional object from many angles of view. Similarly, a three-dimensional image may be reconstructed from a series of two-dimensional projections.

Practical Implementation of Computed Tomography

As might be inferred, the ideal implementation of computed tomography would reconstruct a contin-

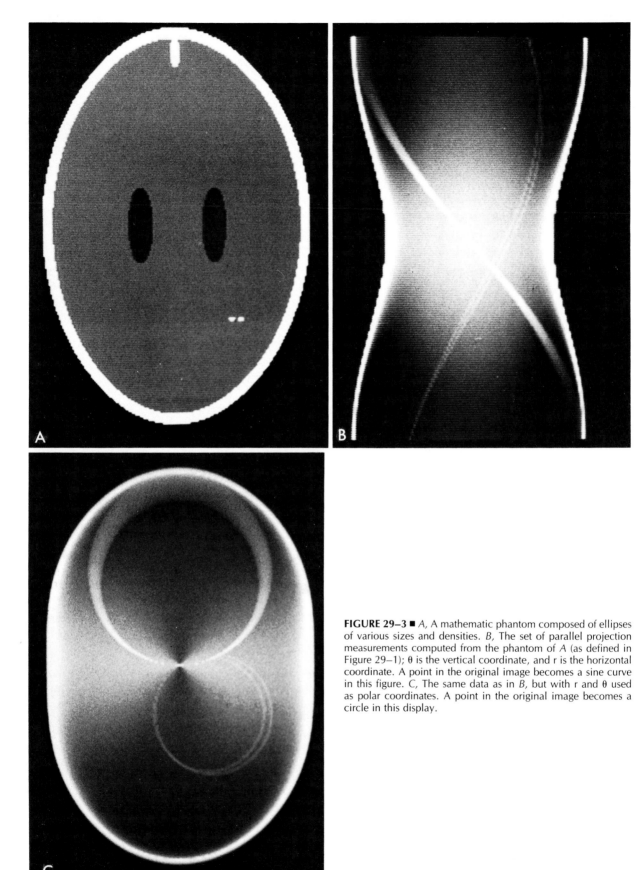

FIGURE 29–3 ■ *A,* A mathematic phantom composed of ellipses of various sizes and densities. *B,* The set of parallel projection measurements computed from the phantom of *A* (as defined in Figure 29–1); θ is the vertical coordinate, and r is the horizontal coordinate. A point in the original image becomes a sine curve in this figure. *C,* The same data as in *B,* but with r and θ used as polar coordinates. A point in the original image becomes a circle in this display.

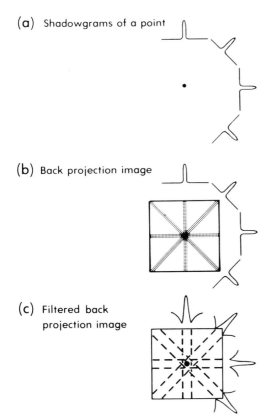

(a) Shadowgrams of a point

(b) Back projection image

(c) Filtered back projection image

FIGURE 29–4 ■ Principle of filtered back-projection reconstruction.

uous distribution of attenuation coefficient measurements within a plane or slice through the object of interest. The distribution would be known accurately and precisely at all points within the two-dimensional object plane. The reconstruction of a continuous distribution requires that measurements be made of all possible projections, along lines of negligible width, through the object within the imaging plane. Because the lines are of negligible width, this requires a very large (infinite) number of projection measurements. The negligible width requirement also means that the x-ray source and detector elements must all have negligible width. Thus, the reconstruction of a continuous distribution (at very high resolution) is impractical because of the large amount of measurements required, as well as the constraints on smallness of the x-ray source and detectors.

The reconstructed CT image is represented by a two-dimensional matrix of CT numbers. Because of the practical limitations of finite beam width and the finite number of projection measurements, the spatial resolution possible in the reconstructed image is compromised. Intuitively, this is seen to happen because of the blurring effect of scanning very fine details by a rather coarse beam. Typically the effective width of the beam created by the geometry of the source, detector, and associated collimators varies from about 3 mm down to less than 0.5 mm among various commercially available CT scanners. The

number of individual projection measurements varies between about 65,000 and 1 million.

It is generally true that the number of elements in the final display matrix should not be greater than the number of individual projection measurements, which gives the number of resolution elements that can be determined. This would mean that the final reconstruction matrix should be between 256 × 256 and 1000 × 1000. The matrix size of commercial CT scanners is found to vary between 256 × 256 and 1024 × 1024 picture elements (pixels). The maximum matrix size is typically restricted to 512 pixels × 512 pixels. This restriction is partially a result of the fact that a substantial increase in x-ray dose is required in CT if it is desired to increase spatial resolution while maintaining contrast resolution for the smaller pixels. Indeed, it is found that the pixel variance varies inversely with the cube of the linear dimension of the in-plane resolution element.[3] Because of the long-range negative correlation of noise in CT images, the dose required for the more common task of perceiving contrast differences in large (many pixel) areas is relatively unaffected by decreasing pixel dimensions. This conclusion is substantiated by the experimental observation of Cohen and DiBianca that the minimum perceptible area contrast was the same for the GE 7800 and 8800 CT scanners, where the only difference was spatial resolution.[4] It should also be noted that higher resolution reconstructions of local regions (target reconstructions) within the full image can generally be obtained to utilize the full resolution capabilities of the scanner without increasing the dose when the number of display elements is significantly less than the number of measurements.

Another geometric limitation in CT scanners is the fact that the beam does not have negligible width in the direction perpendicular to the scan plane. To obtain sufficient x-ray signals, this width is generally between 2 and 20 mm and can often be varied under operator control. Thus the CT number corresponds to the mean value of density or, more accurately, the linear attenuation coefficient within the volume of tissue denoted by a particular pixel. This volume element has a depth, L, which is the CT section thickness or slice thickness as indicated in Figure 29–5.

Limitations Inherent in Computed Tomography of the Body

In addition to geometric considerations, there are other limitations that are directly related to the number and energy distribution of the photons within the beam. These affect the accuracy and precision of the measurements and lead to artifacts, which are discussed later.

The number of photons that are detected directly affects the precision with which the attenuation coefficient can be measured. For example, the total attenuation of an x-ray beam that passes through the

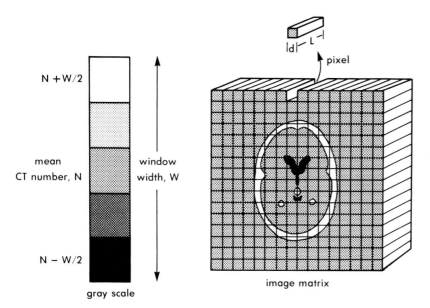

FIGURE 29-5 ■ Gray scale CT image matrix.

thicker parts of the body is considerably greater than that of beams used in head scanning. The practical implementation of whole-body CT is thus much more difficult than that of head CT because of this greatly increased constraint on the dynamic range that is observed by the detection system. Also, because the body is larger, either more detectors or longer scan times (or both) are required to produce images of contrast and spatial resolution comparable to those of head CT. Finally, internal motion of organs (lung, heart, digestive tract) is much more problematic in body CT than in head CT.

Definition of Numbers in Computed Tomography

As mentioned, the linear attenuation coefficient of any medium is a strong function of x-ray energy. To determine a tissue characteristic (such as density) using the values of the reconstructed linear attenuation coefficient, it is necessary that the energy spectrum of the x-ray beam be known. Because the spectrum varies from scanner to scanner, as well as for various points along the penetrating beam path of each measurement of a given scanner, an approximation based on the use of CT numbers is commonly used. In this method the measured linear attenuation coefficient for water for a specific scanner is used to transform the measured attenuation coefficient of the object into a standard relative unit called the *CT number*. The CT number is generally defined by the relationship

$$CT\ number = K\ \frac{\mu_{object} - \mu_{water}}{\mu_{water}}$$

where K is a constant. This equation assigns water the CT number of 0. Because μ_{air} is negligible relative to μ_{water}, the CT number of air is essentially equal to

−K. At the present time, nearly all manufacturers have adopted the convention that assigns K the value 1000. The resulting CT numbers are given in terms of Hounsfield units (H). For this case, air has the value −1000 H; dense (cortical) bone is between 1000 H and 2000 H, and soft tissue is in the range of +40 H to +60 H. Thus CT numbers have a range of about −1000 to +2000 on the Hounsfield scale. It is evident that a change of one Hounsfield unit corresponds to a change of 0.1 per cent in linear attenuation coefficient relative to water.

It is interesting to note that for the x-ray energies employed in CT (typically those corresponding to a highly filtered 120 kV(p) x-ray beam), the dominant x-ray attenuation mechanism is the Compton effect for which μ is proportional to mass density (p). Introducing this relationship into the previous equation and setting K equal to 1000, we have the expression

$$CT\ number \approx 1000 \frac{\rho_{object} - \rho_{water}}{\rho_{water}} = 1000(\rho_{object} - 1).$$

Thus the CT number is approximately linearly related to the mass density of the attenuating tissue. CT numbers calculated using this approximation for a variety of tissues are listed in Table 29-1. The CT values in the table are in fairly good agreement with those that are actually measured. However, the linear attenuation coefficient of a tissue, and hence its CT number, is dependent on the x-ray energy, which is not reflected in this table. Thus the CT numbers of fat, muscle, and bone that are measured using an 80 kV(p) x-ray beam are different than those that are measured using a 120 kV(p) beam. The approximation also tends to be less accurate for high-atomic-number materials such as bone and iodine for which there is substantial attenuation as a result of the photoelectric effect.

TABLE 29–1 ■ Mass Densities and Approximate CT Numbers of a Variety of Tissues

TISSUE	MASS DENSITY (g/cm³)	APPROXIMATE CT NUMBER (H)
Air	1.18×10^{-3}	−999
Fat	0.91	−90
Water	1.0	0
Muscle	1.05	+50
Bone	1.92	+920

Numeric Illustration of the Partial Volume Effect

As has been mentioned earlier, the fact that the CT scanner slice thickness is finite in dimension can lead to an error in the measured CT numbers. This error is referred to as the *partial volume effect* and occurs whenever more than one tissue is present within a volume element or voxel. Indeed, the CT number within a voxel is equal to the sum of the CT numbers of the constituents within the voxel weighted by their volume fractions. For example, if a voxel within a bone marrow cavity contains bone and fat with volume fractions of 0.15 and 0.85, respectively, the CT number within that voxel would be

$$CT\ Number_{bone} \times v_{bone} + CT\ Number_{fat} \times v_{fat} =$$
$$1000 \times 0.15 + -90 \times 0.85 = 65,$$

which is approximately equal to the CT number of muscle.

A number of excellent articles have been published that summarize the important principles and physical concepts in computed tomography.[5-9]

History of Computed Tomography

The almost sudden success of computed tomography has been a result of the fact that highly developed technologies from various branches of the sciences were simultaneously acquired. Thus although the commercial development of CT began in the early 1970s, a complete history of CT must include many developments in various technologies during the many decades preceding the first implementation. These include the mathematic achievements of Radon and others, the development of x-ray technology—specifically medical x-ray technology—as well as general radiology, and the introduction of inexpensive mini- and microcomputers and array processors. Developments in each of these areas occurred in such a way that by the late 1960s, all the necessary technical elements required for the invention of CT scanning were in place.

From the early discovery of x-rays, it was soon apparent that transmission images of the human body could yield an immense amount of interesting and often diagnostically useful information. However, because a three-dimensional structure was being "projected" onto a two-dimensional display, much information about a specific internal structure was masked by the shadows of overlying and underlying structures. To eliminate the unwanted structural detail in the final image, various "tomographic" techniques were developed. In conventional linear tomography, a tomographic section or plane of interest is held in focus while overlying and underlying layers are blurred, owing to relative motion of the source and film receptor. Thus noise (i.e., unwanted structure information) caused by superimposed layers is converted to a background noise similar to that caused by scattered radiation.

The radiation dose can be quite high for a complete examination, as the planes above and below the focal plane are exposed to the full x-ray beam for each exposure. This problem is avoided by the technique of axial tomography as introduced by Takahashi.[10] In axial tomographic systems a fan x-ray beam rotates around the body, exposing only a single transverse axial cross section of the body. A radiographic film cassette on the opposite side of the body rotates together with the source. The film is nearly parallel to the x-ray fan but is tilted slightly so that the transmitted fan beam exposes the entire film at each angle of rotation. This causes the fan beam projection to be smeared or "back-projected" across the film during the scan. The final image is an approximate representation of the density distributions of the scanned section but contains considerable blurring, which limits the utility of this method. The blurring results from the fact that an axial tomographic or back-projection image is only a first-order approximation to the true density cross section. The solution to this problem of blurring requires a computer program specifically designed to accomplish the required deblurring. Such a technique is referred to as *computed axial tomography*.

Since Radon's contribution,[1] a variety of mathematic techniques for reconstruction have been developed by many authors. These methods are sometimes jointly referred to as the *inverse radon transformation*. During the 1950s and 1960s, these techniques were applied to scientific problems in many fields, including radio astronomy and electron microscopy.[11, 12]

Cormack first applied the techniques of image reconstruction from projections to radiography and carried out demonstration experiments using "phantoms."[13] Kuhl and Edwards[14] applied these principles to nuclear medicine and developed computed emission tomography. Hounsfield developed the first clinically viable CT scanner, the EMI neuroscanner, which became an immediate success during the early 1970s. Cormack and Hounsfield[15] later shared the Nobel prize for medicine in 1980.

Shortly after the tremendous diagnostic capabilities of CT were recognized, a dozen or more x-ray equipment manufacturers joined EMI in the production of CT scanners. The performance and technical sophistication of CT equipment evolved rapidly in this

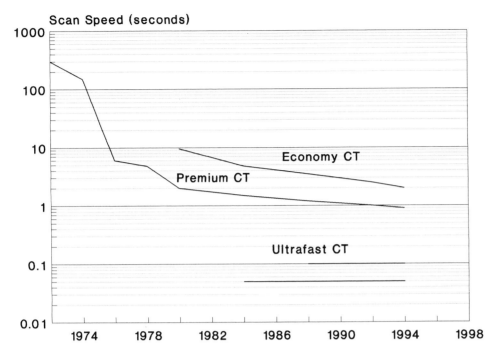

FIGURE 29-6 ■ This chart illustrates the history of speed improvements in CT. Premium scanners are the most widely used scanners in the United States and currently have a fast scan speed of about one second. Economy scanners are generally slower, with maximum speeds in the three to five second range. The Ultrafast CT scanner was introduced in 1984 with a low-resolution 50-millisecond speed for cardiac studies. In 1988, the Ultrafast CT was upgraded with a 100-millisecond, high-resolution mode designed for general head and body applications.

competitive atmosphere. For example, the introduction of fan beam-scanning techniques led to reductions in scan time from 300 sec to 2 sec in just 4 years (Fig. 29-6).

Design of CT Scanners

General Considerations

A modern CT facility consists of a scanning gantry that includes the collimated x-ray source and detectors, the computer data acquisition and reconstruction system, a motorized patient-handling table, and a CT viewing console. The major technical difference between various commercial scanners lies in the gantry design and involves the number and type of x-ray detectors used, as well as their scanning motion. These differences are discussed later.

Data acquisition and reconstruction systems consist of one or more minicomputers and related peripheral equipment, such as a magnetic tape unit for archival storage, a line printer for printing CT numbers in regions of interest, an operator's control keyboard and display, data acquisition electronics, and special processors to speed the reconstruction computations. The complexity of this system is related to the size of the detector array, scanning speed, and the required speed of image reconstruction. In early CT scanners with slow scan times (1 to 5 min), image reconstruction was performed during scanning, and the CT image became available for viewing after the end of the scan. In faster scanners (2 to 5 sec), image reconstruction cannot (at least at present) be performed during scanning, and the additional computation time can become a limiting factor in patient throughput. Therefore fast scanners often

employ fairly complex special hardware and array processors that produce reconstruction in as little as 4 sec.

The patient-handling table is usually motorized, with horizontal and vertical drives. The couch may be automatically indexed in the horizontal direction under computer control to position a series of adjacent tomographic sections. Laser-produced light beams are used initially to localize the patient with respect to markers recorded on a projection radiograph. Either the gantry or the couch may be designed for tilting to about ±25°

CT display systems offer a great range of options for quantifying regions of interest, image processing, radiation therapy treatment planning, and production of hard copies. Regions of interest are selected by electronically outlining the selected region on the television display monitor using a manually controlled cursor such as a brightened dot or cross. The cursor is moved by manipulating a velocity-sensitive joystick, a position-sensitive trackball, or an electronic tablet. A computer program displays the outlined region's area and calculates the mean CT number and various statistical parameters. With the image in digital format, various image manipulation routines can be applied digitally to increase visibility of desired information.

One image processing feature that is standard on all scanners is user-selectable window level and width settings for the enhancement of image contrast. A maximum of 256 gray levels are normally depicted on the image displays. This is much less than the full dynamic range of the CT scanner (−1000 H to +3000 H). The window level and width settings permit the user to display a subset of that range at full contrast. For example, to enhance muscle detail, the user might select a window level (corresponding with the center of the displayed range) of 50 H (approximately the CT number of muscle) and use a window width of 200H. Tissues having CT numbers between -50 and $+150$ will then be displayed with gray levels in the image, and those having CT numbers less than -50 will be displayed as black, while those having CT numbers greater than 150 will be displayed as white. For the same image data, the user could adjust the window level up (e.g., to $+500$) to enhance bony detail or down (e.g., to -500) to enhance lung detail. In general, the employment of narrow window widths results in images that have a great deal of contrast and noise (small fluctuations in CT number are readily apparent), whereas the employment of wide widths results in images that have less contrast and are more smooth. Scanners often incorporate push buttons for selecting default window level and width values for particular image types. Some of the default settings on the GE 9800 CT scanner are listed in Table 29–2.

One very useful image-processing option appears to be spatial smoothing to enhance the low-contrast detectability of larger lesions having a CT number very similar to surrounding tissue. Alternatively, some benefits of spatial smoothing can be accomplished by viewing the CT image with a minifying lens, by stepping back a fair distance from the image, or by using a smaller auxiliary television monitor. Many manufacturers offer software and hardware options for computing radiotherapy treatment planning using the CT image. Hard copies of CT images and related analyses are produced with multiformat cameras (most recently laser imagers) that record several CT images on a single sheet of large-format x-ray film.

Types of Scanning Gantries

There are currently three types of scanning gantries in common use. All employ a fan of x-ray beams used in combination with a position-sensitive detector array. X-ray fan angles range from 3° to greater than 90°, with the wider angles providing greater utilization of the total flux of x-radiation produced at the x-ray tube anode. Detector arrays contain from three to more than 1000 discrete detector elements. The more detectors that are simultaneously recording transmitted x-ray intensities, the faster the scanning sequence may be completed. In addition, larger detector arrays typically permit the size of an individual

TABLE 29–2 ■ Default Settings on the GE 9800 Ct Scanner

REGION	WINDOW LEVEL	WINDOW WIDTH
Abdomen	50	150
Brain	20	250
Lungs	-700	2000
Mediastinum	0	450
Spinal cord	30	350
Vertebra	300	4000

detector element to be minimized, leading to significant improvements in spatial resolution. The use of large detector arrays can be costly. Such systems are typically several times more expensive than their simpler counterparts.

For detector arrays of up to about 90 elements, the *translate-rotate* scanning sequence, similar to that of the original EMI brain scanner, is used. Scintillation crystal detectors coupled to photomultiplier tubes or xenon ionization chambers are used to detect and record the x-ray beam intensities. During each traverse, each detector records a parallel ray profile at successive angles within the x-ray fan. Following the traversing motion, the system rotates by an amount equal to the width of the fan; for example, a system with 30 detectors at $\frac{1}{3}°$ intervals requires 18 translations at 10° steps to obtain 180° of projection data, for a total of 540 profiles. In such systems, mechanical considerations limit the ultimate scanning speed obtainable to about 10 sec.

If 300 to 600 detectors can be used, it is possible to eliminate the need for a linear traverse by measuring all the sample points in a given profile simultaneously. In such systems, only pure rotary motion is required, and scanning speeds of 2 sec or faster can be achieved. Because both the detector array and x-ray source rotate, this geometry is often referred to as a *rotate-rotate* geometry.

A third type of scanning system (*rotate-stationary*) uses a stationary ring detector array with 600 or more detectors arranged in a circle about the patient. A rotating fan of x-radiation produces the scan.

These three configurations lead to important differences in performance characteristics. Figures 29–7 through 29–9 illustrate the basic differences. Transmission data recorded by the detectors may be plotted as a profile in which the x-axis represents the position of a particular measurement, and the y-axis represents the logarithm of the detected intensity divided by the incident intensity. In the following sections we compare the sequence of data collection and some inherent properties of the three scanning geometries.

TRANSLATE-ROTATE

Figure 29–7 illustrates the projection data recorded by two particular detectors of a translate-rotate fan system. The detectors and source traverse linearly from left to right at a particular gantry rotation angle or view angle θ. Peaks caused by the skull and a radiographically dense lesion are illustrated. Each detector in the fan measures a profile at a slightly different angle, providing multiple views within the fan angle. The gantry rotates, using angular steps equal to the fan angle, until a complete set of profiles covering 0° to 180° is obtained.

The completed scan data represented may be plotted as a series of profiles in a two-dimensional θ-x' graph or in matrix form similar to the format of Figure 29–3*B*. In the former, θ is the view angle of a particular measuring ray, and x' is the distance of

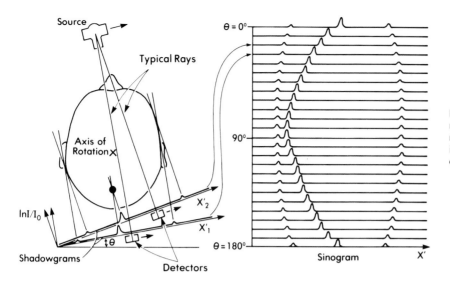

FIGURE 29–7 ■ Basic principles of translate-rotate fan scanning. Profiles produced by two representative detectors of detector array are indicated. A typical sinogram indicating peaks caused by skull and dense lesion is illustrated.

each ray from the axis of rotation. This graph is a sinogram, because the locus of points described by an object point (e.g., the dense lesion illustrated) describes a sine curve whose amplitude and phase are related to the polar coordinates of the object point. The computer reconstruction program can be considered a two-dimensional transformation of the sinogram into the CT image. The data organization of Figure 29–7 is ideally suited to the requirements of fast-modified back-projection reconstruction methods.

For a translate-rotate fan system with n detectors, every n^{th} line or profile of the sinogram represents data gathered by a particular detector. If that detector malfunctions, only the corresponding profiles are disturbed, and image degradation may be minimal, because back-projection smoothly distributes the error over the entire image. The detectors may be easily calibrated at the left- and right-hand edges of the profile, where the rays bypass the outer contours of the body. Thus long-term detector stability is not required, and inexpensive photomultiplier tube-based detectors are suitable.

ROTATE-ROTATE

Pure rotary fan systems are illustrated in Figure 29–8. In this case, a profile at a particular angle θ is recorded simultaneously by a large number of individual detector elements. Only pure rotation of the source and detector is required to form a complete set of profiles. The sinogram consists of slanted lines, because adjacent measurements within the diverging fan beam are at slightly differing angles. Reconstruction may be accomplished by reorganizing the set of fan rays into equivalent sets of equally spaced parallel rays and using standard methods. This process is

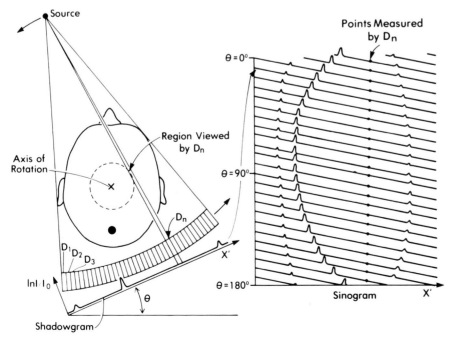

FIGURE 29–8 ■ Principle of rotary fan–rotary detector fan scanning. The profile is generated by simultaneous outputs of all detectors in the curved detector array. A typical rotary scanner is illustrated, along with location of points measured by a single detector element, D_n. Measurements of each detector describe vertical lines in sinogram that should be compared with horizontal lines measured by individual detectors in translate-rotate systems. The dashed circle illustrates the location of the ring artifact that would be produced by an error in detector D_n.

FIGURE 29–9 ■ Basic principle of data acquisition for stationary detector ring systems. Each profile is produced by recording serial outputs from each detector during scan; such measurements are referred to as *detector-fan profiles*. Measurements recorded by individual detector elements describe nearly horizontal lines in the sinogram, similar to the example of translate-rotate systems (Fig. 29–7).

often referred to as *reordering and rebinning*.[16] Alternatively, direct divergent beam reconstruction algorithms may be employed.[17]

The locus of points corresponding to a particular detector is now along a vertical line in the sinogram, as illustrated by the dots in Figure 29–8. An error along this line transforms to a circle in the reconstructed image, as illustrated by the dashed curve in the CT image. Thus small detector errors tend to produce circular or "ring" artifacts in pure rotary fan systems. In addition, the detectors cannot be continuously calibrated during the scan as in translate-rotate systems. Calibration is accomplished at infrequent intervals using a known absorber such as a cylindric water phantom. Thus the requirements for detector accuracy and stability are very high in a rotary fan system. Fortunately, xenon ionization chambers and solid-state detector arrays can be built to perform within these requirements.

ROTATE-STATIONARY

The stationary ring detector–rotary fan (Fig. 29–9) produces a sinogram similar to that of Figure 29–8. Here the divergent ray profiles are obtained by recording the output of a particular detector as the source moves on its circular path on the opposite side of the body. Such profiles are sometimes referred to as *detector fans*. The number and angular spacing of detector profiles depend on the number and spacing of detectors. The locus of points is a slanted, nearly horizontal line. Thus detector errors in stationary ring designs propagate as in translate-rotate systems, and the same advantages of insensitivity to small errors of a few detectors and the ability to perform continuous detector calibrations are inherent in the design. A disadvantage is that many more detectors are required by this system, because only a fraction are recording data at any one time.

The ability to obtain good spatial resolution and high quantum detection efficiency simultaneously can be difficult in stationary designs. Spatial resolution is strongly dependent on the width of detector

elements, but if detector element width is minimized, it is sometimes necessary to leave gaps between the detectors in the ring. Because the source x-ray fan is continuous, x-ray photons falling in the gaps between detectors contribute to patient dose but are not utilized by the scanner. Increasing the number of detectors is helpful, but the number of profiles to be reconstructed also increases thereby, and this can necessitate expensive additional computer hardware. One approach to this problem is to minimize the diameter of the detector array. This approach has been developed in one commercial scanner in which the source rotates outside of the detector ring. In this system, the detector ring wobbles, or "nutates," so that the near portion of the ring does not block the source fan.

The technical trade-offs among the various scanner types are difficult to evaluate. In general, rotary scanners have a faster scan speed and fewer motion streak artifacts. The stationary detector array version requires more, but less accurate, detectors than do the rotary detector designs. Faster rotary scanners (2 to 5 sec) are less apt to be affected by streaks caused by peristaltic motion of the bowel.

Important commercial competitive factors currently include image quality and dose, scan speed, processing speed, and economic considerations. Other features that appear to be of value are variable slice thickness, variable field size (by direct magnification or through software), high- and low-sensitivity scan selection, advanced reconstruction algorithms that correct the beam-hardening effect, cursors for outlining regions of interest, sagittal and coronal reconstructions, and dual-energy scans. All of these features are already available on many commercial scanners.

The assessment of comparative image quality and dose is often a complex task. Some manufacturers can provide contrast detail graphs at various dose levels that provide a rather complete description of the detection capability of the scanner as a function of object size. Many phantoms are available that can be scanned in a given machine to produce similar information in semiquantitative form. Any study of image quality must include consideration of the occurrence of image-degrading artifacts, particularly streak artifacts. Perhaps the best "phantom" for evaluating the frequency and intensity of streaks is the body of an actual patient that contains the necessary high-contrast, streak-producing edges and moving structures. When evaluating patient CT images, it is important to know whether the images selected are the "best" or are representative of a typical series of clinical images.

Cost is an important aspect that must take into consideration the patient load and expected throughput, as well as the initial installation and maintenance charges. Patient throughput depends on a number of factors that vary considerably among the various scanners. These include the following:

1. Image processing time.
2. Scanning time (including the tube-cooling cycle).
3. Image display, analysis, storage, and retrieval.
4. Facilities for patient preparation and staging.

Image Noise, Artifacts, and Image Quality

The evaluation of image quality in computed tomography can proceed at various levels. In the ideal (but impractical) situation, each number in the CT image is directly related to the average linear attenuation coefficient within the corresponding volume element in the original object. Furthermore, the relationship is identical for each picture element. For a variety of reasons and in various ways, the picture elements of the final image are not consistently related to the original distribution throughout the object. Generally, such variations in the final image are referred to as *artifacts* and are often given names that relate to their appearance in the image or their cause. In this section we describe several of the more common sources of artifacts and the manner in which they may be manifested in the final image.

In the 20 years since the first CT images, CT scanners have become sufficiently sophisticated to minimize most artifacts. Because of these efforts, many of the artifacts mentioned are only significantly visible when there is a major instrumental failure. Other artifacts remain and are related to limitations in instrument quality and to fundamental limitations resulting from the physical properties of the imaging process itself. The fact that some artifacts appear differently in rotate-rotate and rotate-stationary geometry scanners is a direct result of the method and relative timing of sample acquisition.

The causes of image artifacts may be divided into the following classes:

1. Measurement errors, including
   a. random noise caused by quantum statistics and electronic noise;
   b. periodic noise caused by such things as x-ray intensity oscillation; and
   c. other instrument failures, nonlinearities, and miscalibrations.
2. Fundamental geometric errors, including
   a. finite numbers of detector elements (finite numbers of views and samples per view);
   b. finite size of detector elements and x-ray source; and
   c. geometric misalignments, including detector placement and center of rotation location.
3. Uncorrected system nonlinearities, including
   a. x-ray beam-hardening and polychromatic effects;
   b. x-ray scatter; and
   c. nonlinear partial volume averaging.
4. Object-caused artifacts, including
   a. patient motions; and
   b. density fluctuation, such as that caused by contrast passage.

Artifacts Caused by Measurement Errors

Measurement error refers to errors that are system dependent and that would not exist if the specific hardware functioned properly. We include random measurement error, because this can be caused by electronic noise (resulting from thermal fluctuations in nonideal electronic components), as well as by fundamental x-ray–counting statistics.

RANDOM NOISE

Because the dose to the patient is directly related to the number of photons incident on the patient, it is desirable to obtain the best image quality for the fewest number of photons. It is therefore best that the major source of artifact (from all sources) in the CT image be caused by the number of x-ray photons detected and that all other sources of image artifact and degradation be kept below this level. When counting photons, the standard deviation in the measurement is about equal to the square root of the number of photons counted. The measured intensity can thus be considered as the expected number of photons (the value consistent with the "true" attenuation experienced) plus some random error. In addition to the randomness in the measured values caused by photon-counting statistics, there is also randomness in the electronics of the detection, amplification, and digitizing stages. All of these sources of "noise" combine to generate random errors in the measurements.

Because of the reconstruction process in which each measurement is back-projected across the image, a single spike of random noise becomes a streak across the image. Furthermore, because of the negative wings on the convolution kernel, each spike of noise causes a large parallel adjacent region of negative values to be back-projected across the image. The net effect is characteristic CT noise[18] in which the random fluctuations appear as tiny streaks in the image, and these fluctuations have a long-range negative correlation.

X-RAY INTENSITY FLUCTUATIONS

Fluctuations in x-ray intensity have very little effect on images in rotate-rotate CT geometries but appear to be a problem in rotate-stationary geometries. As shown in Figure 29–1A, these fluctuations result in a circular moire pattern that is negligible within some radius.[19] The most common cause of such fluctuations in x-ray intensity appears to be variations in the smoothness of the rotating x-ray tube anode surface, which becomes progressively pitted over time. For scanner fan angles less than about 39°, this artifact can be completely eliminated by adjusting the scan speed or anode rotation speed.

The quality of x-ray sources is such that transient spikes tend not to occur. If a transient spike in the x-ray intensity did occur in a rotate-stationary CT scanner, it would result in a set of fine streaks in the reconstructed image that converge directly to the source position at the time of the transient spike. There would be little, if any, effect in a rotate-rotate CT scanner.

INSTRUMENTAL FAILURES

Many severe problems can occur when the CT machinery is not functioning properly, and there are many ways in which a CT scanner can fail. Because of the complexity of the electronics, which results from the need for extreme accuracy and precision in measuring the low-level x-ray intensity signals, most such failures seem to relate to individual detector channels. When a detector channel does not function or when the detector does not respond uniformly, the resulting inconsistency appears as an artifact in the image. In translate-rotate or rotate-stationary designs, the artifact is generally minimal, appearing only as a low-level shift in CT numbers, similar to beam hardening. In rotate-rotate geometries, the detector channel remains at the same radius during the scan and results in a ring artifact in the final image. The amplitude (brightness) of the ring in the final image is directly proportional to the magnitude of the error caused by the detector channel. The amplitude is also inversely related to the radius of the ring. Thus to keep ring artifacts below some specified maximum brightness, it is necessary to maintain detector measurement accuracy within a tolerance that becomes very small for the most central detectors.

Artifacts Caused by Geometric Errors and Limitations

FINITE NUMBERS OF VIEWS AND SAMPLES PER VIEW

As suggested earlier, ideal image quality requires an infinite number of views and samples (rays) per view in such a manner that measurements are made along every possible line through the plane of the object. If some compromises are made in the size of

object that can be resolved and in the amount of fine structure that can exist in the object, it is possible to achieve reasonable image quality with a finite number of views and a finite number of rays (sample measurements) per view. Generally, with a finite number of ray samples per view, streaks occur in the final image and are found to emanate from sharp (high-contrast) edges and small structures of high density. These artifacts are often referred to as *aliasing artifacts* and relate directly to the ability of the scanner to resolve fine detail with a finite sample spacing.

The number of views necessary relates directly to the desired spatial resolution, the number of rays per view, and the size and angular symmetry of the object. When a finite number of views is used, each point in the reconstruction results in a starlike pattern of radial streaks. These streaks are not noticeable within a circular region around the image point. The radius of this artifact-free region is directly proportional to the number of views. Thus if a sufficient number of views are used, every point in the reconstructed image will occur within the artifact-free radius from every other point, and these view streak artifacts will not appear within the image. If insufficient numbers of views are used, streaks will be found to occur at large distances from very dense points.

FINITE SIZE OF DETECTOR ELEMENTS AND X-RAY SOURCE

For practical reasons the x-ray source and detector elements are of finite cross-sectional areas. For example, the number of x-rays collected for any given sample measurement is directly related to the size (cross-sectional area) of the detector. This finite size results in an averaging or blurring of each projection measurement over the dimensions of the x-ray source and detector elements. This blurring of the measurements in turn causes a blurring of the reconstructed image. Thus sharp density transitions in the object appear to be less sharp in the reconstructed image.

GEOMETRIC MISALIGNMENTS

Many other sources of geometric error can exist. If the center of rotation is not the same as that used by the reconstruction program, the image in a full 360° scan will be blurred. In 180° scans, this error causes an artifact that resembles a tuning fork around dense points. Imprecise or inaccurate detector positioning can result in streaks. The positioning of individual detector elements must be very accurate in rotate-rotate geometries, or rings will result. Streaks can also result if the x-ray fan beam profile is not uniformly thick, thus causing some dense, out-of-plane structures to be included in only part of the scan.

Artifacts Caused by System Nonlinearities

Several sources of image degradation occur because the physical implementation of CT deviates from the assumed simple mathematics. With the exception of detector nonlinearities, which were discussed earlier, these artifacts are independent of scanner geometry.

X-ray Beam-Hardening and Polychromatic Effects

The reconstruction mathematics assumes that the attenuation coefficient at each point is constant for all radiation beams that sample that point. This is not the case for broad diagnostic x-ray spectra used in CT x-ray tubes. Because the linear attenuation coefficient, or fraction of x-rays attenuated per centimeter, decreases as the x-ray energy increases, it is found that more of the lower energy x-ray photons are removed from the beam during the traverse of an object. In this manner, the farther a beam passes through an object, the more penetrating or "hardened" it becomes. Because those rays that pass through the edges of the object are hardened less than those passing through the center, the apparent attenuation coefficient is less at the center than at the edges. Thus a cupping or decrease in CT numbers is found to occur near the center of the reconstructed image. This result is sometimes referred to as the *beam-hardening artifact*. In the case of soft tissues that are all similar in attenuation coefficient energy dependence, it is possible to correct this artifact using a simple table lookup procedure.[20]

Polychromatic artifacts are caused by the fact that bone attenuation differs considerably in energy dependence from soft tissue. Streaks tend to occur between dense, high-atomic-number structures such as bones. This artifact can often be superimposed on partial volume streaks (see later) originating from the same bones.

X-ray Scatter

Scattered radiation that originates from photons removed from the primary beam in the object results in an artifact that is similar to beam hardening and can lead to cupping or streaks.[21] Scattered radiation can contribute several per cent of the signal recorded by detectors that are exposed to the more highly attenuated beams. Rotate-rotate scanners have much more efficient scatter collimation than rotate-stationary scanners and hence less artifact.

Edge Gradient and Partial Volume Artifacts

The reconstruction mathematics assumes that measurements are made along lines of negligible thickness. If strips are used, the mathematics still applies if the projected density (i.e., the logarithm of the x-ray intensity) is averaged over the strip width. Unfortunately, it is the x-ray intensity itself that is averaged over the strip width. Taking the logarithm of the averaged intensity ratio does not yield the average projected density. The difference is largest in the presence of dense edges or small points that are only partially included within the strip width. This inconsistency results in streaks from edges and small, dense points.[22] The appearance of these streaks is very similar to that of streaks arising from too-few samples per view, as discussed earlier.

Object-Caused Artifacts

If any part of the object moves or changes density during the course of the scan, "tuning fork"–like streaks can occur, depending on how the motion occurred relative to the scan sequence. The intensity of this streak is dependent on the speed of the scanner relative to the speed of motion.[23] The accumulated motion between the start and end of the scan causes an inconsistency between 0° and 180° profiles, leading to the most common motion streak. A small number of additional projections (i.e., overscan to 230° or so) provides measurement data that can be used to blend or "feather" the inconsistencies over a range of angles and thus reduce the intensity of this artifact.[24]

Image Quality

When the artifacts from all sources are properly addressed, the final image quality will be a function of the scanner geometry (ideally x-ray source and detector dimensions) and x-ray dose to the patient. In this case the quality of the CT image can be described in terms of spatial resolution and contrast resolution. *Spatial resolution*, or "sharpness," describes the amount of blurring of a point, line, or edge in the object. The detailed character of the blurring of a point or line is indicated by the point-spread function (PSF) or line-spread function (LSF). For most CT scanners, these functions are approximately Gaussian shaped and have a full width at half maximum of 0.5 to 2 mm. Spatial resolution as defined in this way is independent of x-ray intensity and dose.

Spatial resolution is sometimes confused with the term *resolving power*. Resolving power is a measure of the minimum separation distance between two objects, such as line pairs, for which the separation can be resolved. Resolving power depends not only on spatial resolution, but also on object contrast and noise or contrast resolution. Scanner manufacturers typically report the resolving power obtainable in the limit of very high contrast. These reported values are in the range of 5 to 20 line pairs per centimeter.

Contrast Resolution

Contrast resolution (sometimes referred to as *density resolution*) depends on the amount of variability or scatter in the CT numbers of a uniform object and is strongly dependent on x-ray intensity and dose. This variability arises from random photon and electronic statistical noise, which appears as graininess in the image, and from artifactual structured noise, such as streaks. Contrast resolution in all imaging systems depends on the object size, as the magnitude of noise fluctuations can be reduced in large areas by spatial averaging.

Contrast resolution is inversely related to the magnitude of the random fluctuations or noise in the background averaged over areas comparable in size to the object of interest. This noise may be estimated by computing the standard deviation of the mean for square-area elements of width, w, using a CT image of a uniform phantom such as a cylinder of water. When w is equal to the pixel size, $\sigma_m(w)$ is the standard deviation of the pixel values or the pixel noise, an often-quoted number. However, the pixel noise is not a good indicator of the noise or contrast resolution for large areas. The function $\sigma_m(w)$ for a typical scanner is plotted in Figure 29–10 as the dashed curve. Theoretical treatments[3] indicate that $\sigma_m(w)$ varies as $w^{-3/2}$ as a result of a unique short-range noise correlation in CT scanning.

To take advantage of the improved contrast resolution for larger objects, we must depend on the observer's eye to perform the necessary averaging. For example, an observer whose eyes have an LSF equivalent to 1 mrad will view a CT image optimally if the viewing distance is 1000 times greater than the size of the object to be detected. A typical CT image recorded as a Polaroid picture is reduced by about a factor of 6 from the original. If we wish to detect a 1-cm lesion in the liver, for instance, the optimal viewing distance would be 1000/6 = 170 cm. Alternatively, a minifying lens can be used to stimulate the effect of an increase in viewing distance.

A convenient way to express the contrast resolution or detectability of CT as a function of object contrast and size is in terms of the contrast detail diagram. This diagram is a graph of the diameter of a minimum detectable object as a function of object contrast. A typical body scanner detectability curve is illustrated in Figure 29–10. The meaning of contrast in this case is as follows:

$$\text{Contrast} = \frac{\mu_L(\text{object}) - \mu_L(\text{background})}{\mu_L(\text{object})}$$

where the μ_L is the linear attenuation coefficient of the object and background. The detectability curve is approximately five times higher than the $\sigma_m(w)$ curve for the same scanner, indicating a signal-to-noise ratio of 5:1 at optimal detectability. This implies that a signal-to-noise ratio of greater than 5:1 is necessary for object detection in this scanner. A similar detectability curve for a conventional radiographic system would be several times higher than this CT example for thick body parts in the region of w greater than 2 mm. However, for very small details (w less than 1 mm), conventional radiographic systems are generally superior, reflecting the high spatial resolution of such systems compared with CT.

A convenient rule for remembering the contrast detail characteristics of a given scanner is to recognize that the product of $\sigma_m(w)$ times w is nearly a constant in the region of a few millimeters to a few centimeters.[4, 25] In the example of Figure 29–10, $\sigma_m(w) \times w$ = 1.0 per cent per millimeter. Thus $\sigma_m(10 \text{ mm})$ = 0.1 per cent, and we may expect to detect 10-mm

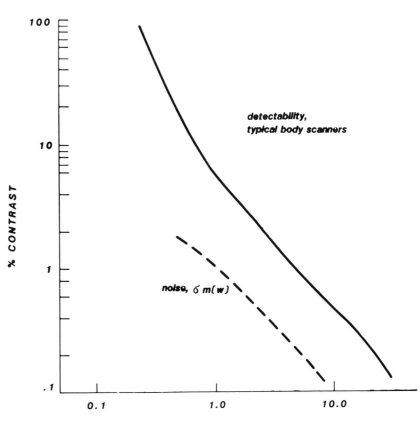

FIGURE 29–10 ■ Contrast-detail diagram illustrating the detectability relationship of a typical CT body scanner. For comparison, noise (standard deviation of mean) for corresponding variable-sized area elements is also included. Signal-to-noise ratio for minimum detectability is in the range of 5:1 to 10:1.

lesions with a contrast of 5 × 0.1 or 0.5 per cent. Similarly, detectability would be 0.25 per cent at 20 mm. The function $\sigma_m(w) \times w$ is referred to as the *noise granularity* and ranges from about 0.5 to 2 per cent per millimeter for many commercial scanners.[26]

If the scanned projection data contain no inconsistencies or errors that produce artifacts, the noise levels in the CT image depend on the total number of detected photons, *n*, and vary according to the square root of *n* law of Poisson statistics. For example, contrast resolution can be improved by a factor of 2 by increasing the number of photons, and hence the absorbed dose, by a factor of 4. In one body scanner, an optional slow scan—some four times slower than normal—is available for this purpose. In most CT scanners, the amount of the dose can be varied by adjusting tube current to produce the minimum acceptable level of contrast resolution required for a particular examination. Typical CT examination doses are in the range of 0.5 to 5 rads. Because contrast resolution depends on the number of detected photons, ideally all the radiation would be detected after exiting the body, with no additional loss because of postpatient collimators, attenuators, or poor detector efficiency. Such a scanner would make maximal use of the photon beam and could be thought of as having a dose efficiency of 100 per cent. Current scanners appear to operate below 50 per cent dose efficiency, but a definite trend toward higher efficiencies exists.

Because spatial resolution and contrast resolution are independent imaging characteristics, we do not need to seek an optimum trade-off between the two, as in collimators used in nuclear medicine gamma cameras or in the selection of various film-screen combinations in ordinary radiography.

SPATIAL RESOLUTION

In CT, spatial resolution is determined by (1) the size of the x-ray tube focal spot, (2) the width of the individual detectors (the detector aperture), (3) the separation between the detectors or the detector sampling frequency, and (4) the reconstruction field of view and matrix size. The limiting resolutions resulting from each of these parameters can be calculated using some simple equations. These equations and examples of the calculated values for a General Electric 9800 Quick CT scanner with Hi-Light detectors are given later. Values for other scanners can be determined by introducing the appropriate scanner specifications into the equations. Much of what follows is based on the work presented in Davison,[27] and the reader is referred to this reference for more detailed coverage of this topic.

To determine the limiting resolution caused by the focal spot size alone, we assume we have a perfect detector (e.g., one that can detect all spatial frequencies) and that we are imaging a line pair pattern positioned at the center of rotation of the scanner. We then find the frequency of the line pair pattern that is completely blurred out by the penumbra of the focal spot when imaged at the detector. This limiting frequency is given by the equation

$$R_{\text{focal spot}} = \frac{M}{M-1} \times \frac{1}{\text{focal spot size}}$$

where M is the geometric magnification factor, which is equal to the quotient of the focal spot–to-detector distance divided by the focal spot–to–center of rotation distance. For the GE 9800, M is equal to 1.74 (1099 mm divided by 630 mm), and the focal spot size is equal to 0.9 mm. The calculated limiting resolution caused by the focal spot is therefore 2.61 line pairs per millimeter, or 26.1 lp/cm.

To compute the limiting resolution caused by the detector aperture alone, we assume we have a perfect focal spot (e.g., a point source). The limiting resolution caused by the aperture then occurs when the projection of one line pair in the object completely fills the detector. In this limiting situation, the detector response decreases to 0. If we consider the object to be located at the center of rotation of the scanner, then the limiting resolution is given by

$$R_{\text{aperture size}} = \frac{1}{\text{aperture size}} \times M.$$

For the GE 9800, the aperture size is equal to 0.8 mm, and the associated limiting resolution is equal to 2.18 lp/mm, or 21.8 lp/cm.

According to the sampling theorem, the maximum frequency that can be reproduced is equal to half the sampling frequency. For third-generation (rotate-rotate) scanners like the GE 9800, the sampling frequency is determined by the physical distance between the centers of adjacent detectors. For fourth-generation (rotate-stationary) scanners, however, it is determined by the rate of rotation of the x-ray tube and the time between samples. For both situations, the equation that applies is

$$R_{\text{sampling frequency}} = \frac{1}{2} \times \frac{1}{\text{distance between samples at center of rotation}}$$

where 1/(distance between samples at center of rotation) is equal to the sampling frequency. For half (180°) scans on the GE 9800, the distance between samples is equal to the distance between the detectors divided by M, which is equal to 1.0166 mm divided by 1.74, or 0.58 mm. The corresponding resolution limit is 0.858 lp/mm or 8.58 lp/cm. In full (360°) scans, the GE 9800 and many other third-generation CT scanners use a technique called *quarter-offset* to effectively halve the distance between samples.[29] In this technique, the scan lines for the projections are offset or shifted relative to the center of rotation of the scanner by one quarter of the distance between the detectors. This results in the scan lines for the second half of the scan (181° to 360°) being interlaced between the corresponding lines of the first half of the scan, thus doubling the effective number of scan lines. Therefore full scans on the 9800 have a sampling frequency resolution limit of 2 × 8.58 lp/mm, or 17.16 lp/cm.

A minimum of two picture elements is required per line pair displayed in the image, one for each bar and one for each space between the bars. With this in mind, the limiting resolution caused by the reconstruction circle size and display matrix size is given by

$$R_{matrix} = \frac{1}{2} \times \frac{matrix\ size}{reconstruction\ field\ of\ view}.$$

For the GE 9800, the matrix size is 512 pixels, and the reconstruction fields of view include 25, 34.5, and 48 cm. The corresponding limiting resolutions are 10.24 lp/cm, 7.42 lp/cm, and 5.33 lp/cm.

The overall resolution of a CT scanner is equal to that of the weakest link in the reconstruction/imaging chain. In the previous example, the limiting factors are the sampling frequency and the display matrix size. The effect of the latter can be reduced by targeting the reconstruction to a smaller effective reconstruction circle size (e.g., for the GE 9800, the smallest targeted field of view is 9.6 cm).

Some examples of CT images of a resolving power phantom are given in Figure 29–11. As previously mentioned, the resolving power depends on both spatial and contrast resolution. In the four examples given, object contrast and noise were varied, and the effect on resolving power is evident. The phantom in Figure 29–11 consists of fluid-filled holes in polymerized methylmethacrylate (Lucite) ranging from 8 to 1 mm in diameter. A 13 per cent contrast fluid (water) was used on the left, and a 3 per cent contrast fluid was used on the right. The lower two images were low noise in the high-contrast, low-noise examples.

Similarly, resolving power is a strong function of spatial resolution or sharpness. Figure 29–12 schematically illustrates the effect of varying spatial sharpness and noise amplitude on resolving power. The two systems represented in the lower left and upper right have comparable resolving power. Examples of images obtained from two such systems (two actual commercial scanners) are included in Figure 29–12. Here a phantom consisting of water-filled holes in acrylic (13 per cent contrast) ranging from 1 to 3 mm in diameter was used. The system on the lower left has low noise but poor sharpness. The system at the upper right has good sharpness but a high noise level.

Precision and Accuracy

An additional aspect of CT image quality is reflected in the numeric precision and accuracy of the measured CT numbers. These values are important in tissue characterization studies and bone mineral quantitation. *Precision* describes the ability of a CT scanner to reproduce the same mean CT number in the same region of the same patient at a later scan. *Accuracy* refers to the ability to relate a given mean CT number to the true linear attenuation coefficient at a mean photon energy. The use of the "air" scan, which replaced the water bag of the original head scanners, has often been accompanied by a serious loss of both precision and accuracy. Precision is important when a particular patient needs to be followed during therapy, such as for bone mineral loss. Accuracy is important for identifying specific tissues, as in the distinction between a cyst and a solid mass—often a difference of less than ten CT numbers. Factors affecting the accuracy of CT scan-

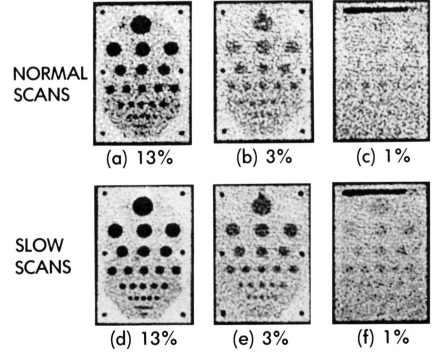

FIGURE 29–11 ■ EMI 5000 phantom scans. CT images of rods of 13 per cent or three per cent contrast (lowered density relative to background). Rod diameters are 15, 12, 9, 6, 4, 2, 1, and 0.5 mm. These comparisons indicate the dependence of detectability and resolving power on size, contrast, and noise.

NORMAL SCANS

(a) 13%   (b) 3%   (c) 1%

SLOW SCANS

(d) 13%   (e) 3%   (f) 1%

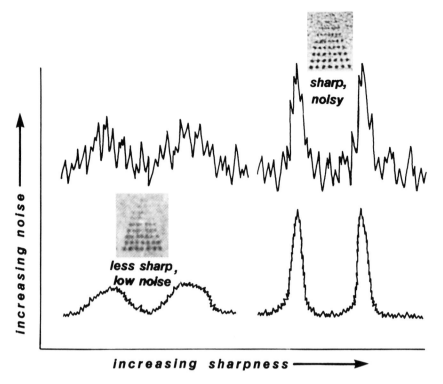

FIGURE 29–12 ■ Schematic illustration of the effect of noise and sharpness on resolving power. Curves represent CT numbers of pixels along a path passing through two nearby holes in a CT image of a resolving power phantom. As noise increases, fluctuations in CT number increase, tending to decrease the ability to resolve nearby peaks. However, the width of peaks decreases as spatial sharpness increases, and peaks may be readily resolved even in the presence of rather substantial noise fluctuations. Computed tomographic images of a resolving power phantom using a sharp, high-noise CT scanner and a less sharp, low-noise scanner are included as examples. The resolving powers of these two scanners are comparable, as is indicated in corresponding schematic illustrations.

ners include the beam-hardening artifact, detector inaccuracy (nonlinearity), motion artifacts, partial volume effects, calibration errors, and scattered radiation.

Quantitative CT (QCT)

Researchers have long been interested in using CT numbers to characterize tissues. The impetus for this is that tissues differ in their mass densities and atomic numbers, both of which affect their imaged CT numbers. The term *quantitative CT* (QCT) has been coined to describe this research specialty.

The primary purpose of most QCT applications is to quantify the amount of a specific type of tissue or chemical within a region of interest. Applications include measuring (1) the bone mineral content within the spine, hip, or radius for the assessment of osteoporosis; (2) the fat content within the spine for earlier diagnosis of osteoporosis; (3) the iron content within the liver for the evaluation of certain liver diseases; (4) the iodine content of the thyroid for the investigation of thyroid disease; (5) the fat content within the trunk of the body for the assessment of body composition; (6) the calcium content of lung nodules for the determination of disease state; and (7) the electron density within tissues for better radiotherapy treatment planning.

Unfortunately, the quantitative information provided by CT scanners is not as accurate or precise as desired. This is primarily because of deviations from the ideal monoenergetic x-ray beam, scatter-free detection situation. Specifically, the polyenergetic x-ray beams employed in all commercial CT scanners have

an associated beam-hardening artifact that results in underestimates of the true CT numbers. The magnitude of these underestimates is directly related to the amount and densities of the tissues surrounding the region of interest. Likewise, the acceptance of x-ray scatter at the detectors causes the measured attenuation values and CT numbers to be smaller than their true values, with greater errors occurring where more tissue is present. Furthermore, many CT scanners employ shaped (e.g., bow-tie) x-ray beam filters to limit the dynamic range of the x-ray intensities striking the elements of the detector array. In general, these filters cannot compensate perfectly for the shapes of all patients and introduce their own beam-hardening and scatter errors, which result in variations in the CT number of an object with its position in the scan field. The overall field nonuniformity that results from these three effects can, for example, produce a 20-H difference between the CT numbers of a bonelike substance at two locations within the CT scanner gantry.[29] Finally, the CT numbers that are measured using single-kV(p) techniques may also be in error because of volume averaging. The slice thickness is finite, and therefore the CT numbers, rather than being representative of a single tissue, are representative of the mixture of tissues that are present within the volume of interest.

QCT for Bone Mineral Analysis

QCT has been used most widely to assess the bone mineral content of lumbar vertebrae. An excellent review of this topic has been published by Cann.[30]

For most CT bone mineral studies of vertebrae, the patient is imaged in the prone position with his or her legs raised and resting on a bolster. Frequently the patient lies on a calibration phantom during the imaging procedure. Anteroposterior (AP) and lateral scout views (single scan projections) are obtained, and the technician then selects axial slices passing through four vertebrae (typically T12 to L3). These slices are usually 10-mm thick and are positioned, with the aid of the lateral scout view, to pass through the center of each vertebra along lines that are parallel to the end plates. The bone mineral content within each vertebra is computed from the axial images or scan data using one of the techniques described later. There are two basic categories of QCT bone mineral analysis techniques: preprocessing and postprocessing.

PREPROCESSING TECHNIQUE

The preprocessing technique is based on the work of Alvarez and Macovski.[31] The fundamental assumption is that the linear x-ray attenuation coefficient, and hence the CT number, may be represented as a linear combination of two independent basis functions. The original set of basis functions that were chosen represented the attenuation caused by the photoelectric effect and the attenuation caused by Compton scattering. From ray sum or line integral data measured at two separate energies (dual-energy CT), a set of two equations is obtained that can be solved for two unknowns, the coefficients of the basis functions. Thus for the original basis set, two new images could be created, one representing the amount of photoelectric absorption in each pixel and the other representing the amount of Compton scatter in each pixel. The preprocessing technique has been applied to bone mineral analysis by Kalender and colleagues.[32, 33] For this application, the x-ray attenuation of two basis materials are used as the basis functions. [It can be shown that the attenuation coefficient of any material can be expressed as a linear combination of the attenuation coefficients of two different (basis) materials.[32, 34]] The basis materials that are employed are calcium and soft tissue. The implementation of this technique involves the use of a table lookup procedure to determine the amounts of calcium and soft tissue along each ray of each CT projection, and then two new images are created, a calcium image and a soft tissue image. The bone mineral content is determined from the mean value within a region of interest that is positioned within the vertebral body in the calcium image. A key advantage of the preprocessing technique is that it is insensitive to beam-hardening errors.

POSTPROCESSING TECHNIQUES

Postprocessing techniques are applied to the final reconstructed images rather than the raw projection data. They are available in two types: single-energy and dual-energy.

Postprocessing Single-Energy QCT (SEQCT) ■ The postprocessing QCT method that is employed most frequently is the so-called "Cann-Genant" technique.[35] This is a single-energy (SE) technique in which the bone mineral content of a patient's vertebra is determined from the mean CT number (N) of the patient's vertebra and the mean CT numbers of a set of calibration standards. The latter are employed to derive a calibration line, and the mineral content of the vertebra is calculated using the equation

$$\overline{BMD}_{vertebra} = \frac{N_{vertebra} - b}{m}$$

where $\overline{BMD}_{vertebra}$ is the average bone mineral density (BMD) within a user-selected region of interest that is positioned within the trabecular region of the vertebra, $\overline{CT\ Number}_{vertebra}$ is the mean CT number in that region of interest, and m and b are the slope and intercept, respectively, of the calibration line. The m and b parameters are determined by applying a linear regression routine to the mean CT number and concentration data for the calibration standards. The BMD calculation is illustrated graphically in Figure 29–13.

The standards that are employed conventionally are five cylinders filled with solutions of 0, 50, 100, and 200 mg/mL K_2HPO_4 in water. K_2HPO_4 was selected as the calibration mineral because it attenuates x-rays, similar to actual bone mineral (calcium hydroxyapatite), and unlike that mineral, it is soluble in water and can readily be made into solutions having known concentrations.

To determine the status of a patient, the average density of the patient's four analyzed vertebrae (in mg/mL K_2HPO_4) is computed and compared with age-matched normal data. A plot depicting the QCT-determined bone mineral density in mg/mL of K_2HPO_4 as a function of age for normal women is shown in Figure 29–14.[36]

An advantage of the postprocessing SEQCT technique is that it is fairly precise (one to three per cent). However, the accuracy of SEQCT is degraded when fat is present in the marrow cavity. The CT

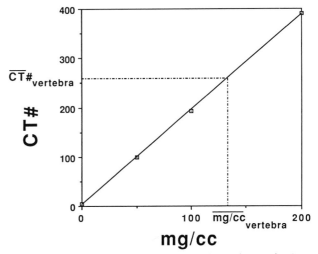

FIGURE 29–13 ■ A typical calibration line obtained using the Cann-Genant technique. The line is used to convert the measured mean CT number of the vertebra to an equivalent concentration of bone mineral in units of mg/mL.

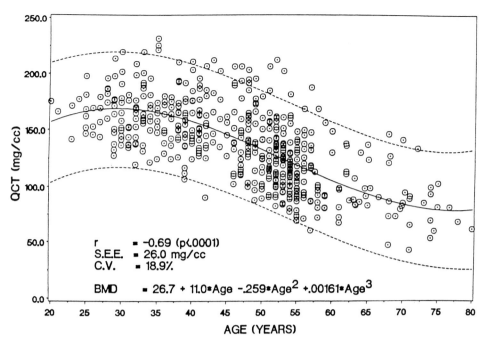

FIGURE 29–14 ■ QCT bone mineral densities (mg/mL K_2HPO_4) of normal women as a function of age. (From Block JE, Smith R, Glüer CC, Steiger P, Ettinger B, et al. J Bone Min Res 4:249–257, 1989.)

number within the selected region of interest is the volume average of the CT numbers of the trabecular bone, red marrow, and fat within that region. Fat is characterized by a relatively large negative CT number (e.g., about −100). Thus when fat is present, the CT number within the region is decreased, resulting in an underestimate of the true bone mineral content. This underestimate can be as large as −12 mg/mL K_2HPO_4 for each ten per cent fat by volume. Age-related fat corrections for SEQCT have been proposed and utilized with some success. However, when maximum accuracy is desired, researchers turn to dual-energy QCT, which is much less influenced by fat.

Postprocessing Dual-Energy QCT (DEQCT) ■ All postprocessing dual-energy QCT (DEQCT) techniques are applied to two CT scans through each vertebra, one at a high energy and one at a low energy. Although ideally the techniques should be implemented using two monoenergetic x-ray beams, in practice, two conventional polyenergetic x-ray beams are employed, one produced using a high kV(p) [e.g., 140 kV(p)] and another produced using a low kV(p) [e.g., 80 kV(p)].

Five postprocessing DEQCT techniques have been proposed, and each will be discussed briefly. The simplest and most frequently employed method[37] computes the BMD from the mean CT numbers of the vertebrae at each energy and the slopes and intercepts of the bone standard calibration lines at each energy. The equation employed is

$$\overline{BMD}_{vertebra} = \frac{[N_{vertebra}(E_1) - N_{vertebra}(E_2)] - [b(E_1) - b(E_2)]}{m(E_1) - m(E_2)}$$

where b and m represent the intercepts and slopes of the calibration lines, and E_1 and E_2 signify the high- and low-energy x-ray beams, respectively. This technique has been found to reduce the fat error to three to six per cent. However, as with other DEQCT techniques, it does so at the expense of increased x-ray exposure (the exposures for SEQCT and DEQCT are about 200 mrem and 800 mrem, respectively) and reduced precision (three to five per cent for DEQCT versus one to three per cent for SEQCT).

The other four techniques yield estimates of fat content in addition to mineral content. One proposed by Laval-Jeantet et al.[38] estimates the fat and mineral contents from the mean CT numbers of the vertebrae at the two energies and the slopes and intercepts of mineral standard and fat standard calibration lines, again at the two energies. Two techniques proposed by Goodsitt and colleagues[39, 40] make bone and fat composition estimates assuming a three-component model of bone. The techniques utilize calibration materials that simulate the x-ray attenuation properties of the three components. Presently, the materials that are simulated are bone (calcium hydroxyapatite plus collagen), fat, and fat-free red marrow.[41] The fundamental relationship that is used in both techniques is that the CT number of a mixture is equal to the sum of the CT numbers of the pure components weighted by their respective volume fractions. For example, the "three-equation" method utilizes the equations:

$$N_{vertebra}(E_1) = N_{bone}(E_1) \times B + N_{fat}(E_1) \times F + N_{marrow}(E_1) \times M$$

$$N_{vertebra}(E_2) = N_{bone}(E_2) \times B + N_{fat}(E_2) \times F + N_{marrow}(E_2) \times M$$

$$1 = B + F + M$$

where B, F, and M represent the volume fractions of bone, fat, and fat-free red marrow, respectively, and N_{bone}, N_{fat}, and N_{marrow} are the CT numbers of the pure substances. To avoid problems arising from inaccuracies in the CT number of pure bone (e.g., as a result of beam-hardening effects), a so-called "four-equation" technique was developed. This technique uses a set of lower concentration (e.g., 0, 100, 200, and 300 mg/mL) bone calibration samples.

The final technique was developed by Nickoloff et al.[42] It assumes five principal constituents of bone (bone mineral, collagen matrix, water, red marrow, and adipose tissue) and utilizes known compositional relationships rather than calibration materials to estimate fat and mineral content. The method reduces to two equations with two unknowns. Experimental values that are introduced into the equations include the mean CT numbers of the vertebra at the two energies, the effective energies of the x-ray beams as determined from the CT numbers of calibration standards, and an empiric water offset number. Because the calibration standards are only used to estimate x-ray beam energies, this method is less prone to errors caused by possible differences between the x-ray attenuation properties of the calibration materials and those of the actual bone constituents.

TYPES OF CALIBRATION PHANTOMS

Calibration phantoms are used in QCT for two general purposes: to improve the precision of the techniques and to provide a means for expressing the measurements in desired units such as mg/mL bone mineral. The phantoms can be classified according to their location in the scanning field. The phantoms that have been employed most frequently are termed *peripheral* or *external*. The patient usually lies on top of this type of phantom during a procedure, and the phantom and patient are scanned simultaneously. The primary advantage of the peripheral phantoms is that the simultaneous imaging helps correct for any short-term scan-to-scan instability in the measured CT numbers [e.g., caused by changes in kV(p)]. This was a significant problem in early QCT studies; however, with modern scanners, short-term instabilities are typically one per cent or less. One problem with peripheral phantoms that can be significant is field nonuniformity. The combined effects of beam hardening, scatter, and use of a shaped filter can result in the CT number of a bone-mimicking material at the phantom location being quite different from the CT number of the same material at the vertebral position. This adversely affects the accuracy of the measurement but should have minimal effect on reproducibility as long as the positions of the phantom, patient, and tabletop are duplicated each time the patient is imaged.

The other type of calibration phantom is termed *central* or *anthropomorphic*. The shapes and compositions of such phantoms simulate those of the patient, and the calibration standards are scanned within the phantoms at a central or vertebral location. Figure 29–15 shows a CT image of a typical anthropomorphic phantom lying on top of a typical peripheral phantom. Theoretically, central calibration phantoms should produce better corrections for the effects of x-ray beam hardening and scatter and therefore yield more accurate results. However, because the phantoms cannot match the patient size, shape and composition exactly, the corrections are imperfect. Also, anthropomorphic phantoms are more time consuming to employ, as they must be scanned separately from the patient. One group has proposed a central calibration technique that may be immune to these

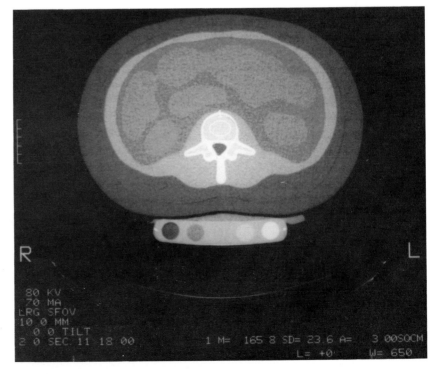

FIGURE 29–15 ■ CT image of a central calibration phantom manufactured by Computerized Imaging Reference Systems, Inc. (Norfolk, VA) lying on top of a peripheral calibration phantom manufactured by Image Analysis (Irvine, CA). The CIRS phantom includes fat rings that can be added to the periphery of the basic phantom to permit simulation of small-, medium-, and large-sized patients. The phantom that simulates a medium-sized patient is shown in this figure. Calibration and test sample inserts are placed within the vertebral cortex region of the CIRS phantom. For this image, a test insert containing 200 mg/mL bone (116 mg/mL calcium hydroxyapatite plus collagen) and 50 per cent fat was scanned. As shown, the mean CT number of this insert at 80 kVp is 165.8 H. The Image Analysis phantom contains calibration solutions consisting of 0 mg/mL, 50 mg/mL, 100 mg/mL, and 200 mg/mL of K_2HPO_4 in water.

deficiencies. The idea is to use the patient as his or her own calibration phantom. Paraspinal muscle and fat tissues are employed as internal reference standards, and initial experience with the technique has been promising.[43]

CALIBRATION PHANTOM COMPOSITION

The original Cann-Genant peripheral phantom consisting of known solutions of K_2HPO_4 in water continues to be the calibration phantom of choice in most studies. The primary advantage of K_2HPO_4 in water is the large data base that exists for normal and osteoporotic men and women. The primary disadvantage is the fact that the solutions change with time as a result of precipitation and the formation of air bubbles.

Manufacturers are now marketing solid plastic–based calibration standards. These most frequently consist of calcium hydroxyapatite in a water-equivalent epoxy resin–based material. The idea of adding fillers to epoxy resins to produce materials that simulate the x-ray attenuation properties of tissues was developed by White et al.[44] Custom resins can also be made to simulate the fat, fat-free red marrow, and bone standards that are employed in some DEQCT techniques. The materials have been found to be stable.

The only disadvantage in employing calcium hydroxyapatite in a water-equivalent plastic instead of aqueous solutions of K_2HPO_4 is that conversion relations are required to use the large K_2HPO_4 data base. The reason such relations are required is that there is a difference between the slopes of the calibration lines obtained with the two standards. In general, the calcium hydroxyapatite concentration of a vertebra has been found to be about ten per cent greater than the K_2HPO_4 concentration (C_{Ca} mg/mL $\cong 1.1 \times$ mg/mL $C_{K_2HPO_4}$ mg/mL). However, it should be noted that the conversion relation depends on the effective x-ray beam energy, which depends on the kV(p), beam filtration, and size and composition of the patient. Hence separate conversion relations may be required for each CT scanner, technique, and perhaps patient size.

Future Improvements in QCT

Although QCT techniques have great potential for characterizing tissues, they have not received as wide an application as might be expected, probably because of inaccuracies associated with the techniques. These arise in part because the scanners have been developed to produce aesthetically pleasing images using processes (e.g., spatial filtering) that often degrade the quantitative information. We conclude this section on QCT with a list of needed improvements. Although many of these have been implemented in research labs, few are employed in commercial scanners. It is our hope that this situation will change. For more successful application of QCT, the following improvements are needed:

1. Better beam-hardening and scatter corrections

should be employed to make the CT numbers more accurate. These corrections should, for example, account for estimated amounts of bone, soft tissue, and fat along each ray.

2. Special x-ray beam filters should be developed for QCT applications. These should optimize the energies of the x-ray beams for tissue analysis. An additional filter that effectively flattens a shaped (e.g., bow-tie) beam filter may be useful for reducing field nonuniformities.

3. The physical designs and desired compositions of calibration phantoms for specific applications should be decided on by noted experts in the field. There is a great need to standardize QCT techniques, and common calibration standards are required for data from one institution or scanner to be compared with that from another.

4. Automated region-of-interest (ROI) selection and positioning should be implemented to improve the reproducibility of QCT in special applications.[33, 45] Experience in bone mineral measurements, for example, has shown that manual selection and positioning of an ROI can result in errors of several per cent.[33, 45]

5. Automated slice selection should also be implemented to improve reproducibility.[46]

6. CT scanner x-ray generation and detection equipment should be designed for maximum stability and reproducibility. These factors have a direct bearing on the accuracy and reproducibility of CT numbers.

7. Shorter scan times should be implemented for DEQCT applications. Presently, with some scanners, the time interval between the high- and low-energy scans can be as long as 22 sec. Patient motion can therefore be a problem.

Ultrafast CT

Conventional CT scan times of 2.0 to 5 sec have been found to be adequate for brain imaging and most body applications. However, in imaging the body, such relatively long scan times can result in deleterious motion artifacts. Furthermore, they place severe limitations on image acquisition rates for contrast and multilevel studies. Ultrafast CT scanning refers to CT scan times less than 0.5 sec. The electron beam CT scanner was developed to address the technological constraints of conventional CT.[47] This scanner has certain advantages over real-time ultrasound and MR imaging of the body. Specifically, compared with ultrasound, ultrafast CT has superior spatial resolution and superior versatility in choice of imaging slice location (ultrasound cannot image through the ribs). Compared with MR, ultrafast CT is less susceptible to motion artifacts.

Principles of Electron Beam Scanning

A diagram of an electron beam CT scanner is shown in Figure 29–16. To achieve scan times of 50

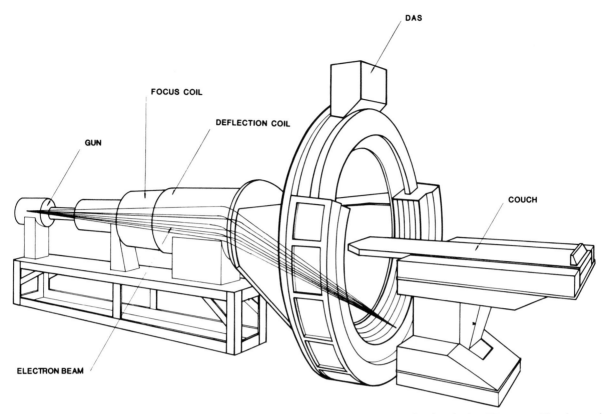

FIGURE 29–16 ■ Schematic diagram illustrating the principle of electron beam scanning as used in the ultrafast CT scanner. The electron beam is produced in the gun and steered and focused by the coils shown. X rays are produced on the target rings, sensed in a detector ring, and digitized by the data acquisition system.

ms, the electron beam CT scanner replaces the conventional mechanically rotating x-ray tube and gantry with a rotating x-ray source produced by magnetic steering of a high-powered electron beam that strikes a series of four tungsten target rings. The electron steering technique is similar to that used in television cameras and monitors. However, the electron beam is of much greater power (i.e., 130 kV and 800 mA). As shown in Figure 29–16, the design essentially surrounds the patient with an enormous x-ray tube target. Because the target rings have a large thermal mass and are directly cooled, there is not the heat-loading limitation of conventional rotating anode x-ray tubes. This CT system is capable of millisecond scanning speeds that can be repeated at a high rate to produce high-speed dynamic or cine-tomographic images.

The transmitted x-ray photons are measured in integrated scintillation crystal–photodiode array detectors and digitized by a data acquisition system at the rate of approximately 7 million 16-bit samples per second. The digitized signals are then averaged by the fast raw averager (FRA) board and temporarily stored in a scan cache memory that has a capacity of up to 160 images. The scan cache memory is transferred to disk storage at a rate of up to 0.4 sec per image.

The stored scan data are reconstructed automatically as new scan data are acquired. Asynchronous

reconstruction proceeds in parallel with scanning, patient setup, image analysis, and archival storage. Typically several images are ready for viewing prior to completion of a scanning sequence. The fastest reconstruction speed is currently 5 sec per image. The images may be viewed and analyzed on either of two independent display consoles. In addition, the system may be connected to up to 15 additional workstations to provide low-cost, remotely located, user-programmable systems.[48, 49]

The electron beam CT scanner has two modes of operation, a multislice mode (256^2 matrix) and a single-slice high-resolution mode (512^2 matrix). All images have a 12-bit gray scale. In the multislice mode of operation, there is a scan speed of 50 ms and eight 1-cm slices are acquired without moving the table. This series is produced by sequential scanning of the four tungsten target rings and using contiguous stationary detector rings having 432 channels each in 210°. Two slices are scanned at a rate of 17 scans per second with an 8-ms interscan delay time. A total of eight levels is obtained in 224 ms using all four target rings.

In the high-resolution, single-slice mode of scanning, the detectors of one ring are reconfigured into a single ring of 864 channels. A single target ring is scanned in 100 ms, giving a total of 864 views. In this mode, a special radiology collimator is used to provide improved slice collimation and to reduce scatter radiation. This collimator provides for a 6-mm and a 3-mm slice thickness. A 10-mm slice thickness is formed by incrementing the couch during scanning. Also, the FRA board makes it possible to average data to acquire scans at speeds ranging from 0.1 to 1.2 seconds at 0.1 second intervals. This allows for the option of higher dose single-slice scans while preserving the resistance to motion artifacts of the single 100-ms scan. These longer scan times are typically used in applications outside the chest in the head and body. The single-slice mode increases the spatial resolution by a factor of two when compared with the multislice mode.

CT Methods and Applications

Designed originally as a cardiac research tool, the electron beam CT system has evolved into a general purpose scanner with a wide range of applications.[50] The high-speed capabilities combined with the high-resolution capabilities give fine detail in all areas of the body, including the heart. Installation of an electron beam CT system resembles conventional CT except for the larger gantry aperture (Fig. 29–17).

The flow mode allows for sampling of a given series of slices at defined time intervals during the transit of a bolus of contrast medium through a vessel, chamber, or soft tissue. Flow studies may be acquired at up to eight levels in one study. Flow data is analyzed by determining the time-density curve in a cursor-defined region of interest and performing a numeric fit on the resulting flow curve.

The cine mode offers real-time CT scanning capabilities, which have applications primarily in the heart and include detection of wall motion abnormalities, precise quantitation of left and right ventricular volumes, and determination of function of native and prosthetic valves.[51] Applications elsewhere in the body include joint motion studies and airway function studies.

To perform high-quality images for anatomic diagnosis, the volume mode of scanning should be used. High-resolution images are best acquired in the single-slice mode with serial table incrementation. In the chest, 0.1- to 0.4-sec images are acquired and in the body a scan time of 0.4 to 1.2 sec is used. Applications include all conventional CT studies with the ability to acquire excellent examinations on pediatric, geriatric, traumatized, and very ill patients who have a difficult time lying still. Vascular imaging in general radiology of the body has been described by Lane.[52] Electron beam CT can increase contrast differentiation of soft tissues in the chest and abdomen by capturing the transient peak enhancement effects of bolus contrast injections.

An exciting application in volume imaging is coronary artery screening for atherosclerosis.[53] Because few patients with flow-limiting stenoses are free of coronary calcification, this study may evolve into a cost-effective screening test for asymptomatic patients or those with atypical symptoms.[54] With rapid image acquisition, a series of slices of the coronary arteries with electrocardiographic registration can be obtained in a single breath-holding interval. No contrast injection is required for this noninvasive screening procedure. An example of three-dimensional reformation of a coronary artery study is shown in Figure 29–18.

Ultrafast CT Performance

Image quality is the most important performance specification of a CT system. Image quality fundamentally determines the capability of the system to

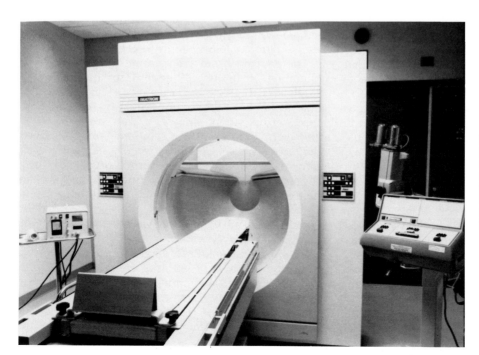

FIGURE 29–17 ■ A typical hospital installation of an electron beam CT scanner. For cardiac studies, an electrocardiogram-triggering device is placed to the left of the patient couch. A power injector used for intravenous contrast medium injection is seen to the right of the gantry.

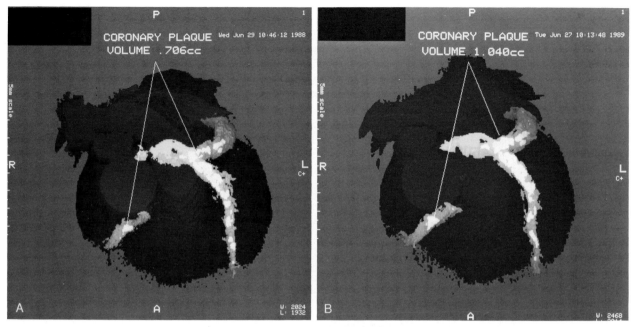

FIGURE 29–18 ■ Clinical images from a CT screening study of the coronary arteries that was reformatted into a three-dimensional image. The images were acquired in 0.1 sec, with no injection of contrast medium. The radiation dose for this study has an average quadrant skin dose of 0.4 rads covering an axial region of 6 cm. *A,* 1988 study showing severe calcification in the coronary arteries. *B,* 1989 study in the same patient shows an increased amount of calcium and additional plaques. (Images courtesy of Mt. Sinai Medical Center, Miami, FL.)

resolve details and sets the limits of precision for all quantitative applications. Image quality can be quantitatively described by the spatial resolution and the image noise. The many design factors that determine the spatial resolution have been described previously.[55] The present resolution of ultrafast CT is shown in Figure 29–19. The modulation transfer function (MTF) describes the image contrast as a function of spatial frequency. This figure shows the improvement of the CT system resulting from improved interpolation during reconstruction and compares these MTF curves to current conventional CT systems. These data were obtained using a method developed by Assimakopoulos and demonstrate the soft tissue scanning modes.[56] Because image quality is affected by any slight motion in the body, it is important to determine system resolution, which is dependent on scan acquisition times. Figure 29–20 demonstrates a comparison of the resolution of an ultrafast CT system with that of conventional systems at representative areas in the body. The MTF for a longer scan time is greatly decreased in conventional

FIGURE 29–19 ■ Comparison of MTF for the current electron beam CT scanner (FASTRAC/C-100XL), a conventional CT scanner, and the original C-100 in the soft tissue scanning modes. Optional high-resolution bone modes are available on both scanners. The improvements for the electron beam scanner primarily result from improved interpolation during reconstruction.

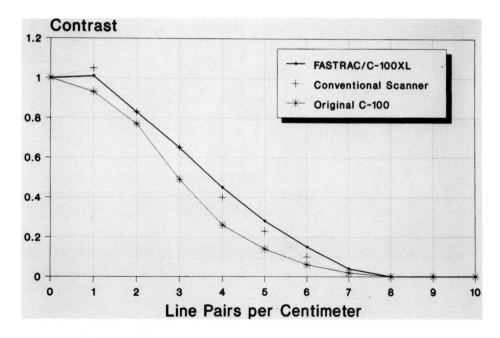

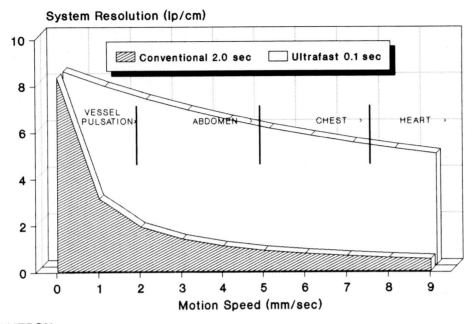

FIGURE 29–20 ■ Benefits of subsecond CT scan acquisition times. The consequences of motion in the body are shown by two MTF curves. The MTF curve for conventional CT (2-sec scan time) decreases dramatically as a result of motion in the body.

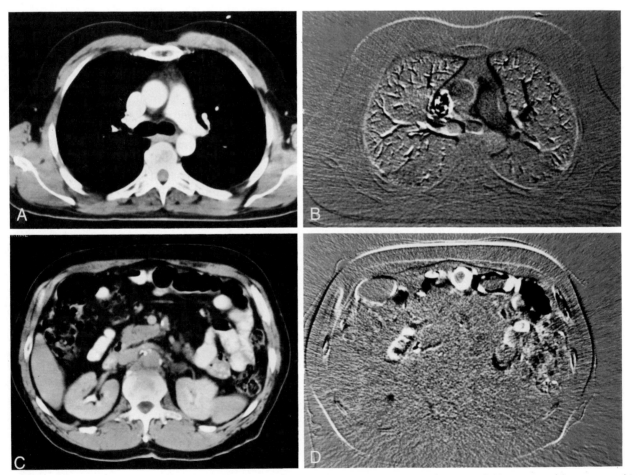

FIGURE 29–21 ■ CT images in the chest and abdomen acquired in the 100 millisecond cine mode (*A, C*). The images were then processed in the subtraction program to demonstrate the amount of motion in 2.3 seconds of scanning (*B, D*).

CT systems because of motion. Shown in Figure 29–21 are clinical studies of the chest and abdomen acquired in the cine mode and then analyzed with the subtraction program to demonstrate the amount of motion in the body.

The scanning speed of electron beam CT scanning is almost completely determined by computer restrictions. Advances in multiplexers, analog-to-digital converters, high-speed digital buses, and fast memory systems will be required to take advantage of even faster scan speeds. One goal of this increase in scan rate and scan capacity is to reduce the amount of contrast medium required to reach an accurate diagnosis. In addition, applications for CT will increase in pediatric and trauma cases with a faster scan speed.

HELICAL SCANNING

The next phase in development of faster CT scanning will be the implementation of a new scanning mode sometimes referred to as *spiral scanning* or, possibly more appropriately, *helical scanning*.[57, 58] Both terms refer to continuous gantry rotation with simultaneous continuous couch incrementation, as illustrated in Figure 29–22. In this mode a sequence of adjacent scans that may overlap are continuously obtained. A reconstruction algorithm interpolates the angular data from adjacent scans into a single parallel cross-sectional slice. The advantage of such continuous scanning over the usual scan–increment couch–scan sequence is greater speed and reduction of motion registration problems. Normal scanning is limited in speed as a result of the fact that rapid table acceleration is uncomfortable and jars the patient. The maximum acceptable speed is approximately 2 seconds for 1-cm steps in incremental scanning. In helical scanning, sequential scan speed is limited only by the speed of the CT scanner itself. Electron beam scanners and slip ring scanners (discussed later) are capable of helical scanning.

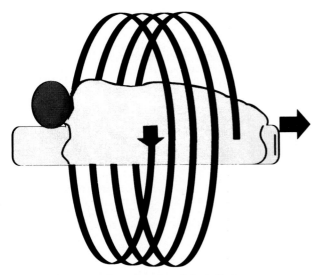

FIGURE 29–22 ■ Demonstration of the helical scan concept.

HIGH-RESOLUTION IMAGING

One of the next major advances in subsecond CT will be to improve spatial resolution by a factor of two or more. The technology for implementing such a step is currently available. This will require increasing the number of detector channels and will also require the data acquisition system to process four times as many measurements.

Based on the twofold increase in resolution described previously, all of the current imaging applications—flow, function, and anatomic studies—can be greatly enhanced. In addition, certain new applications become feasible. With a spatial resolution of 8 to 16 lp/cm, CT coronary artery imaging may begin to rival the capability of angiography. With the advent of high-resolution CT, it may be possible to measure intraluminal narrowing.

VERY FAST RECONSTRUCTION FOR REAL-TIME IMAGING

A second opportunity for greatly improved performance exists in the reconstruction processor. If processing times can be reduced to 1 second or less, then real-time fluoroscopic imaging will be feasible. Immediate access to images will provide many major benefits. It will be possible to monitor the examination and to terminate it if a problem is seen to develop. The timing of the scans to capture the peak contrast opacification will be simplified. With real-time reconstruction, it will be possible to monitor the arrival of contrast medium in the region of interest and manually trigger the study at the optimum point. Improvements will be driven by developments in the semiconductor industry, leading to faster array processors and low-cost very large scale integration (VLSI) chips that may be used in back-projectors.

IMPROVED AUTO ANALYSIS AND REPORT SOFTWARE USING ADVANCED, LOW-COST WORKSTATIONS

An important part of a diagnostic examination is the quantitative analysis of the images and extraction of a wide range of parameters. Because CT images are already in digital format, it is natural to consider automation of the analysis function. A dedicated computer workstation is the ideal method of implementing a computerized analysis and reporting system for CT studies. Fast scanners can be equipped with a network facility referred to as the *user programmable off-line workstation* (UPOW) network. The system allows export of images from the scanner to a remote workstation for off-line analysis. Nearly all commonly available workstations can be connected to this network.

Future Development of Computed Tomography

The acceptance of CT scanning as a primary tool in x-ray diagnosis is based primarily on its ability to image soft tissue abnormalities without the need for invasive interventions such as catheterization. At each stage of CT development, new applications have been introduced as speed and resolution have been improved.

Developments in CT tend to evolve around speed (i.e., scan acquisition speed, interscan delay time, and complete study time). The most obvious benefit of improved scan times is the lack of motion artifacts, particularly in the body, where there are many types of involuntary motion—cardiac, respiratory, peristalsis, and pulsatile motion in the blood vessels—in addition to general patient motion. Electron beam CT has addressed this problem with scan times in the 50- to 100-ms range and an interscan delay time of 8 ms. Another benefit of scan speed is improved diagnosis with the ability to scan a region of interest at peak contrast opacification. Using electron beam scanning, a complete 40-level, 0.4-sec abdominal study with ultrafast CT can be acquired in 60 sec.

A third benefit of scan speed is improved patient throughput. Scan time, reconstruction time, and image analysis time all must be considered when analyzing throughput of a CT system. These three factors are all dependent on the scanner and its computer system. As a result of improvements in the computer components, new computer architectures are becoming part of the modern CT systems available.

Slip Rings

Slip rings, originally developed as a means for supplying power to the x-ray tube on a rotating gantry are also used to transmit the detected signals from the gantry to the computer system. Wide-scale use of slip rings requires a large-diameter slip ring that carries a high voltage of ±70 kV and must include a provision for high-voltage insulation. It is greatly preferred to use low-voltage slip rings that do not require this insulation. The advantages are lower cost, compact size, and enhanced reliability. However, the use of low-voltage slip rings requires that the high voltage generator be placed on the gantry to rotate with the x-ray source. Then the slip rings only need to supply the 208-V three-phase power. The CT high-voltage generator must be dramatically reduced in size for this application. Current slip ring scanners have scan times of approximately 0.5 s for partial scan acquisition.

One common advantage to high-voltage and low-voltage slip ring scanners is continuous scanning capability, as the gantry may rotate continually. Issues such as computer storage capacity and x-ray tube heat capacity must then be addressed.

Solid-State Detectors

Solid-state detectors consisting of a scintillation material in contact with a photodiode array have had a major impact on CT scanners. Solid-state detector arrays have the advantages of modularity, low cost, and compact size. They have been most successful in rotate-stationary systems, where array sizes of up to 2400 elements have been used. With further cost reduction of detector electronics, array sizes should increase, with a resulting improvement in spatial resolution.

Computer Components

Phenomenal advances in microcomputers, random access memories, and disks translate directly into an improved price-to-performance ratio of CT scanners. Approximately 50 per cent of the cost of a CT scanner is in the microcomputer equipment and peripherals. As newer computer architectures are introduced into CT systems, the improvements will be in cost saving or enhanced capabilities.

References

1. Radon J: Über die Bestimmung von Funktionen durch ihre Integralwerte längs gewisser Mannigfaltigkeiten. Saechsische Akademie der Wissenschaften, Leipzig, Berichte über die Verhandlungen 69:262–277, 1917.
2. Shepp LA, Logan BF: Reconstruction in interior head tissue from x-ray transmissions. IEEE Trans Nucl Sci NS-21:228, 1974.
3. Chesler DA, Riederer SJ, Pelc NJ: Noise due to photon counting statistics in computed x-ray tomography. J Comput Assist Tomogr 1:64, 1977.
4. Cohen G, DiBianca FA: The use of contrast-detail-dose evaluation of image quality in a computed tomographic scanner. J Comput Assist Tomogr 3:189–195, 1979.
5. Brooks RA, DiChiro RA: Theory of image reconstruction in computed tomography. Radiology 117:561, 1975.
6. Brooks RA, DiChiro G: Principles of reconstructive tomography. Phys Med Biol 21:5, 1976.
7. Herman GT: Image Reconstruction from Projections: The Fundamentals of Computerized Tomography. New York, Academic Press, 1980.
8. Newton TH, Potts DG (eds): Radiology of the Skull and Brain, Vol V: Technical Aspects of Computerized Tomography. St Louis, CV Mosby, 1981.
9. Ter-Pogossian MM, Phelps ME, Brownell GL, Cox JR Jr, Davis DO, et al (eds): Reconstruction Tomography in Diagnostic Radiology and Nuclear Medicine. Baltimore, University Park Press, 1977.
10. Takahashi S: Rotational Radiography. Tokyo, Tokyo Japan Society for the Promotion of Science, 1957.
11. Bracewell RN: Strip integration in radio astronomy. Aust J Phys 9:198, 1956.
12. DeRosier DJ, Klug A: Reconstruction of three-dimensional structures from electron micrographs. Nature 217:130, 1968.
13. Cormack AM: Representation of a function by its line integrals with some radiological applications. J Appl Phys 34:2722, 1963; 35:2908, 1964.
14. Kuhl DE, Edwards RQ: Cylindrical and section radioisotope scanning of the liver and brain. Radiology 83:926, 1964.
15. Hounsfield GN: A method of an apparatus for examination of the body by radiation such as X or gamma radiation. British patent no. 1283915, 1972.
16. Dreike R, Boyd DP: Convolution reconstruction of fan beam projections. Comput Graphics Image Process 5:459, 1976.
17. Lakshminavayanan AV: Reconstruction from divergent ray data. Technical report 92. Buffalo, Department of Computer Science, State University of New York at Buffalo, 1975.
18. Hansen KM, Boyd DP: The characteristics of computed tomographic reconstruction noise and their effect on detectability. IEEE Trans Nucl Sci NS-25:160, 1978.
19. Parker DL, Couch JL, Peschmann KR, Smith V: Structured

noise in computed tomography: effects of periodic error sources. Med Phys 9:722, 1982.

20. McCullough EC: Photon attenuation in computed tomography. Med Phys 2:307, 1975.

21. Joseph PM, Spital RD: The effects of scatter in x-ray computed tomography. Med Phys 9(4):464, 1982.

22. Joseph P: Artifacts in CT. In Newton TH, Potts DG (eds): Radiology of the Skull and Brain, Vol V. St Louis, CV Mosby, 1981.

23. Boyd DP, Korobkin MT, Moss A: Engineering status of computerized-tomographic scanning. Optical Engineering 16:37–44, 1977.

24. Parker DL, Smith V, Stanley JH: Dose minimization in computed tomography overscanning. Med Phys 8:706, 1981.

25. Boyd D, Margulis AR, Korobkin M: Comparison of translate-rotate and pure rotary body scanners. SPIE Appl Opt Instrument Med VI 127:280, 1977.

26. Cohen G: Contrast-detail-dose analysis of six different computed tomographic scanners. J Comput Assist Tomogr 3:197, 1979.

27. Davison M: X-ray computed tomography. In Wells PNT (ed): Scientific Basis of Medical Imaging. New York, Churchill Livingstone, 1982.

28. Peters TM, Lewitt RM: Computed tomography with fan beam geometry. J Comput Assist Tomogr 1:429–436, 1977.

29. Cann CE: Quantitative CT applications: a comparison of current scanners. Radiology 162:257–261, 1987.

30. Cann CE: Quantitative CT for determination of bone mineral density: a review. Radiology 166:509–522, 1988.

31. Alvarez RF, Macovski A: Energy-selective reconstructions in x-ray computerized tomography. Phys Med Biol 21:733–799, 1976.

32. Kalender WA, Perman WH, Vetter JR, Klotz E: Evaluation of a prototype dual-energy computed tomographic apparatus. I. Phantom studies. Med Phys 13(3):334–339, 1986.

33. Kalender WA, Klotz E, Suess C: Vertebral bone mineral analysis: an integrated approach with CT. Radiology 164:419–423, 1987.

34. Lehmann LA, Alvarez RE, Macovski A, Brody WR, Pelc NJ, et al: Generalized image combinations in dual kVp digital radiography. Med Phys 5:659–667, 1981.

35. Cann CE, Genant HK: Precise measurement of vertebral content using computed tomography. J Comput Assist Tomogr 4:493, 1980.

36. Block JE, Smith R, Glüer CC, Steiger P, Ettinger B, Genant H: Models of spinal trabecular bone loss as determined by quantitative computed tomography. J Bone Min Res 4:249–257, 1989.

37. Cann CE, Gamsu G, Birnberg FA, Webb RW: Quantification of calcium in solitary pulmonary nodules using single and dual energy CT. Radiology 145:493–496, 1982.

38. Laval-Jeantet AM, Cann CE, Roger B, Dallant P: A post processing dual energy technique for vertebral CT density. J Comput Assist Tomogr 8:1164–1167, 1984.

39. Goodsitt MM, Rosenthal DI, Reinus WR, Coumas J: Two post processing CT techniques for determining the composition of trabecular bone. Invest Radiol 22:209–215, 1987.

40. Goodsitt MM, Rosenthal DI: Quantitative computed tomography scanning for measurement of bone and bone marrow fat content: a comparison of single- and dual-energy tech-

niques using a solid synthetic phantom. Invest Radiol 22:799–810, 1987.

41. Goodsitt MM, Johnson RH: New quantitative CT calibration phantom for estimating the fat and mineral content of vertebrae. Abstract. Radiology 173(P):415, 1989.

42. Nickoloff EL, Feldman F, Atherton JV: Bone mineral assessment: new dual-energy CT approach. Radiology 168:223–228, 1988.

43. Boden SD, Goodenough DJ, Stockham CD, Jacobs E, Dina T, Allman RM: Precise measurement of vertebral bone density using computed tomography without the use of an external reference phantom. J Digital Imaging 2:31–38, 1989.

44. White DR, Martin RJ, Darelson R: Epoxy resin based tissue substitutes. Br J Radiol 50:814–821, 1977.

45. Steiger PW, Steiger S, Block JE, Genant HK: Automated image evaluation for operator-independent vertebral bone mineral determination in longitudinal studies. Abstract. Radiology 157(P):183, 1987.

46. Kalender WA, Brestowsky H, Felsenberg D: Automated determination of the midvertebral CT slice for bone mineral measurements. Radiology 168:219–221, 1988.

47. Boyd DP: Computerized-transmission tomography of the heart using scanning electron beams. In Higgins C (ed): CT of the Heart: Experimental Evaluation and Clinical Application. Mt Kisco, NY, Futura, 1983, pp 45–59.

48. Peschmann DR, Napel S, Couch JL, Rand RE, Alei K, et al: High speed computed tomography, systems and performance, Appl Optics 24:4052–4060, 1985.

49. Ackelsberg SM, Napel S, Gould RG, Boyd DP: Efficient data archive and rapid image analysis for high speed CT. SPIE J 626:451–457, 1986.

50. Brody AS: Ultrafast CT scanning: advantages and new developments. Radiol Outlook 2:9, 1989.

51. Boyd DP: Cardiac computed tomography: technical aspects. In Brundage B (ed): Comparative Cardiac Imaging. Rockville, MD, Aspen Publishers, Inc, 1990, pp. 29–39.

52. Lane SD: Power-injected CT contrast opacifies vascular spaces. Diagn Imaging 11:308–312, 1988.

53. Janowitz WJ, Agatston AS, King D, Smoak KM, Samet P, Viamonte M: High-resolution ultrafast CT of the coronary arteries: new technique for visualizing coronary artery anatomy. Abstract number 1048. Scientific Program of the Radiological Society of North America, Chicago, November 1988, p 345.

54. Bateman TM: Commenting editorial: magnetic resonance imaging in coronary heart disease. A major breakthrough for precise noninvasive cardiac evaluation? Am J Cardiac Imaging 3(2):88–90, 1989.

55. Boyd DP, Couch JL, Napel SA, Peschmann DR, Rand RE: Ultrafast cine-CT for cardiac imaging: where have we been? What lies ahead? Am J Card Imaging 1:175–185, 1987.

56. Assimakopoulos PA, Boyd DO, Jaschke W, Lipton MJ: Spatial resolution analysis of computed tomographic images. Invest Radiol 21:260–271, 1976.

57. Kalender WA, Scissler W, Klotz E, Vock P: Spiral volumetric CT with single-breath-hold technique, continuous transport, and continuous scanner rotation. Radiology 176:181–183, 1990.

58. Rigauts H, Marchal G, Baert AL, Hupke R: Initial experience with volume CT scanning. J Comput Assist Tomogr 14(4):675–682, 1990.

INDEX

Note: Page numbers in *italics* indicate figures; those followed by *t* indicate tables.